The Truth About Cancer

A GLOBAL QUEST

A GLOBAL QUEST

COMPLETE TRANSCRIPTS OF ALL 90+ EXPERT INTERVIEWS

The TRUTH About CANCER™

educate • expose • eradicate

THE TRUTH ABOUT CANCER
"A GLOBAL QUEST"
Complete Expert Transcripts

Printed and bound in the USA

NOTICE OF RIGHTS:

DISCLAIMER:

The information and statements conteained herein have not been evaluated by the FDA and are not intended to diagnose, treat, cure, or prevent any illness. The contents of this book are for informational purposes only and are not intended to be a substitute for medical advice, diagnosis, or treatment. Never disregard professional medical advice or delay seeking treatment due to information contained herein.

Although the publisher has made every effort to ensure the accuracy and completeness of the information contained in this book, we assume no responsibilities for errors, omissions, inaccuracies, or any inconsistency herein.

DEDICATION

*This book was created for and is dedicated to **YOU** the courageous person who is seeking to reverse cancer or prevent cancer while seeking a natural approach to healing.*

Many blessings to you and your family.

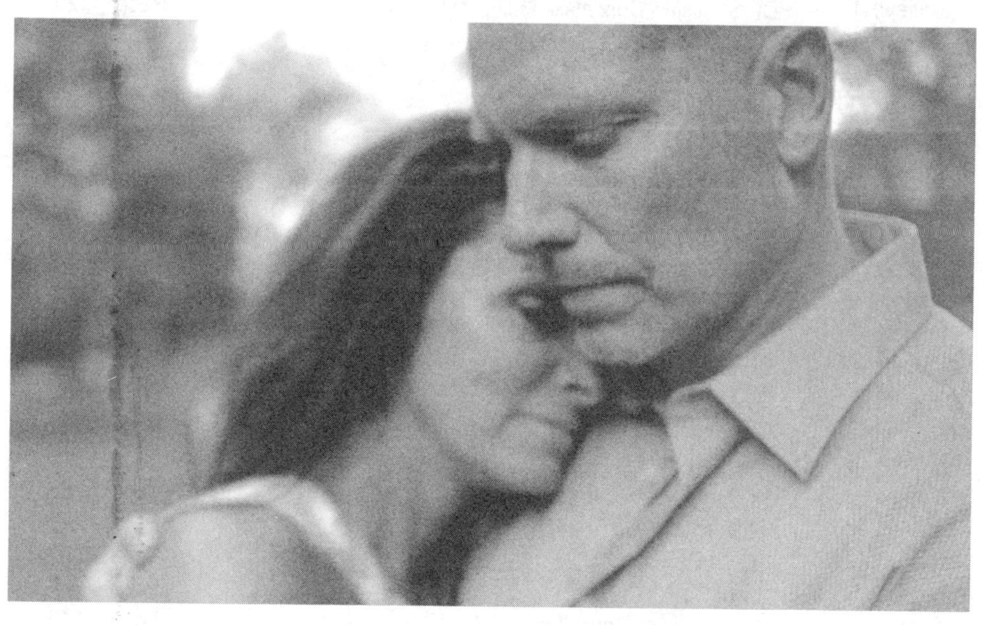

~ Ty & Charlene

TABLE OF CONTENTS

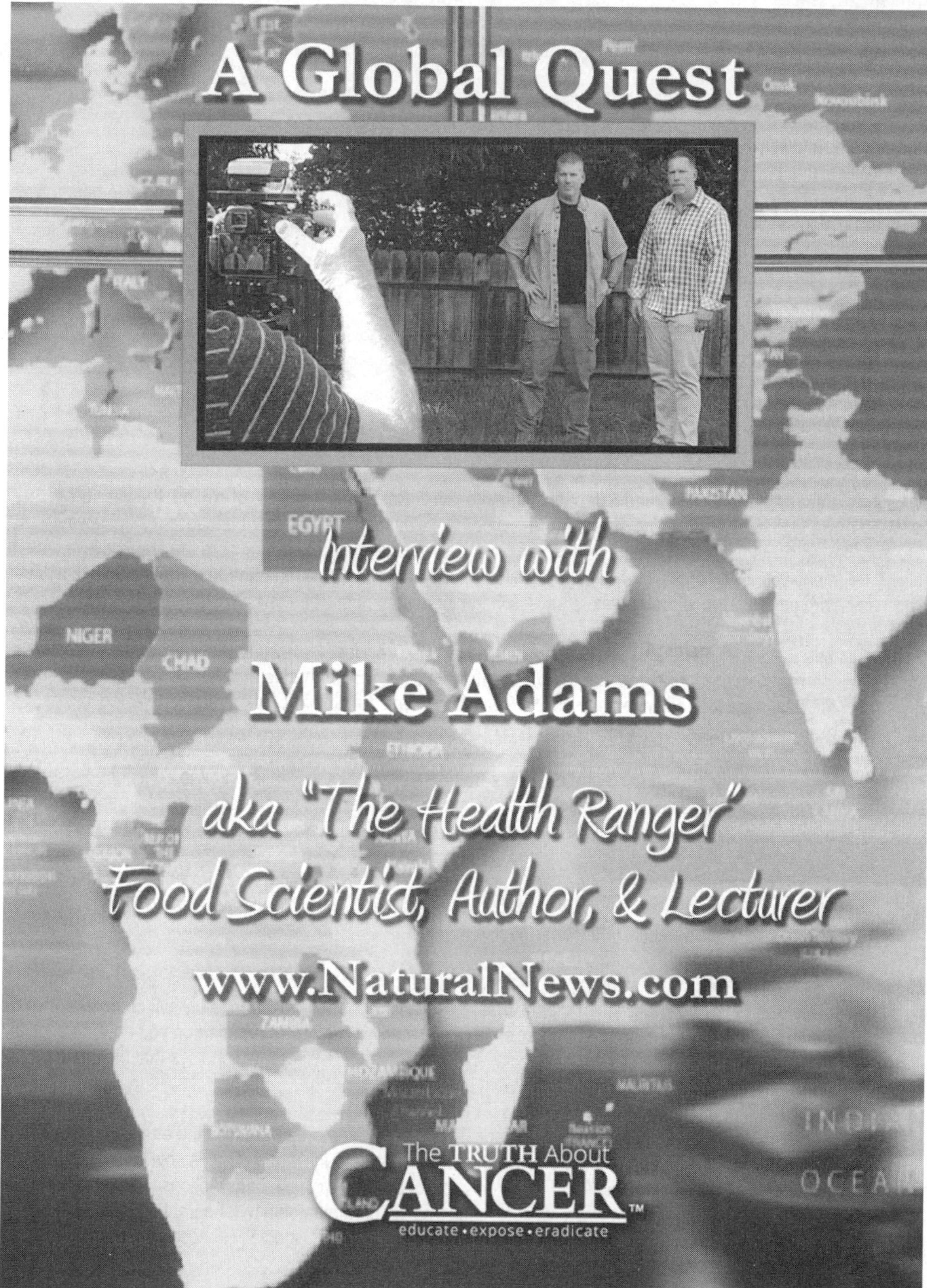
A Global Quest
Interview with
Mike Adams
aka "The Health Ranger"
Food Scientist, Author, & Lecturer
www.NaturalNews.com
The TRUTH About
CANCER™
educate • expose • eradicate

Ty: All right, I'm back in parts undisclosed here in Texas with my good buddy, Mike Adams, the Health Ranger.

Mike: Good to see you.

Ty: Or as I call you the Snake Wrangler.

Mike: Yeah, I have been relocating a lot of snakes.

Ty: Yeah. So it's good to see you again my friend. It's been a while. Last time I saw you here in person was about what, a year and a half ago.

Mike: I think so.

Ty: Fifteen months or so. 5

Mike: Time flies.

Ty: When we first did the initial interview for the *Quest for the Cures*, and since that time a lot has happened hasn't it.

Mike: Yes, a lot. Well, we've had SB 277 signed into law in California, which is, of course, the vaccine mandate for children who attend public school. It's a dangerous precedent because it strips away medical choice from parents and citizens, and it establishes a precedent where the state believes that it owns your body or the bodies of your children, and that it can then mandate that you must be injected with any substance that the state says is in the interest of public health.

Yet, that same state never talks about what is in those vaccines. They never talk about the ingredients: the mercury, the formaldehyde, the MSG, the antibiotics, the aborted fetal cells that are using them. In the past, the hidden cancer viruses like SV40, which was found in the polio vaccine injected into as many as 98 million Americans. They never talk about that.

So, if you really start digging and get to the truth, the vaccine mandate is linked to cancer because of the ingredients and it is something where the state is now denying you personal freedom and the power of your own choice to decide what interventions you want to undergo.

Ty: So, very similar with the vaccines, we're seeing these forced chemotherapy incidents. They're linked aren't they? It's an overarching tyrannical government that comes in and says, "You don't have any choice. We're going to tell you what's best."

Mike: It was best called by Jon Rappaport, "scientific totalitarianism." I think that's a great term for it. Some people call it medical fascism. It means that the so-called science, which is really just corporate driven fraudulent science, but the so-called science driven medicine is being forced upon you now in absolute violation of the American Medical Association's code of medical ethics, which says that the patient must be given the choice. The patient must be informed.

You know, they talk about informed consent. This is supposed to be a pillar of the ethical practice of medicine in the United States of America and really all around the world. That is now being stripped away. Parents are being told, "You must submit your children to these interventions whether you like it or not." That's a violation at every level of human rights, of human dignity, of parental rights, of children's health, of even the genetics of some children who are especially susceptible to these vaccine ingredients. It's a kind of genocide if you really get down to it.

Ty: It is. We interviewed Dr. Matthias Rath in Netherlands.

Mike: Great.

Ty: And he mentioned the fact that it really violates the Nuremberg Code.

Mike: Yes, it does.

Ty: The rules that were put in place after the Nuremberg trials because it's basically forced medical experimentation without any consent.

Mike: That's exactly what it is and if you read the vaccine inserts, many of them will say this vaccine has not been proven to reduce the incidence of influenza or whatever it's claiming to treat. Many vaccines, if you just read the inserts will say things—like the HPV vaccine for example, says that upon receiving this injection, you may lose consciousness and pass out or fall down and hurt yourself. This is just considered normal. Or you may have seizures, you may have fever, you may have to go to the emergency room. These are all listed on the vaccine inserts.

Somehow, the American public has been brainwashed into thinking that this is normal, healthy medicine. It isn't. If someone gives you a shot of something and you pass out, how is that not causing a neurological side effect that could damage your brain?

Ty: Sure.

Mike: I mean, think about it, if you still can. Some people can't because they've been injected with these things.

Ty: So that—the quote that you just said. They can't because they've been injected with these things. Are the vaccines affecting our mental cognition?

Mike: Yeah, the vaccines are brain damaging the population. Think about it. The vaccines still contain mercury like in flu shots. They still contain aluminum and other known neurotoxins. They still contain formaldehyde and MSG. Almost every one of these preservatives or adjuvants is a neurological poison. How can they not cause brain damage?

You know, the medical establishment today says you shouldn't smoke cigarettes because the chemicals in the cigarettes go into your body and cause damage, right. They probably say you shouldn't sniff glue, right, or you shouldn't snort crack or whatever. Why? Because those chemicals go in and cause damage. Then they're injecting you with a vaccine that contains chemicals that they know causes damage. How is that allowable? Why can't—by the way, I'm not against the theory of vaccination. Let's be clear here.

Why can't they manufacture clean vaccines without the chemicals that are single-dose vaccines that could be given with a margin of safety that doesn't exist today? And lastly on that point, if the vaccines are so safe, why does the vaccine industry have to be granted absolute legal immunity. You can't sue them. If they make a defective product that harms your child, you cannot take them to court and seek damages for that even though they messed up, and they had a faulty product.

You know, there was a town in Mexico recently where 75 percent of the children who were vaccinated wound up either in the hospital or dead. Seventy-five percent. There have been vaccines that are recalled. There was a case on the East Coast recently where dozens of children were injected with the wrong vaccines. Who knows what kinds of effects those are going to have on them over the following, subsequent years. Across Europe, $90 million in damages was just paid out by the UK government to cover children who were probably brain damaged by the swine flu vaccine. You think they would pay $90 million if it wasn't conclusively proven that that caused it? Of course not.

Ty: Of course not.

Mike: They know it caused it. That's why they're paying the money, yet the vaccine industry has complete immunity even though it's causing all of this damage. And cancer as well.

Ty: Yeah, it's interesting that you mentioned that, that you're not opposed if they excluded all of these adjuvants, these excipients, these ingredients that are toxic. On the ride over here, we were just talking about that. Alan asked, "Why include this or why include that?" Went through some different ingredients. Because they have alternate choices that they could include that are not toxic.

Mike: Yes.

Ty: But they continue to include these toxic ingredients and you'd almost think that there's some kind of an insidious purpose behind it.

Mike: There's such a scientific dictatorship out there that you're not allowed to ask any reasonable question at all. So someone who says, "Well, what if we spaced out the timing of the vaccine, so that a child could recover more before they get hit with another insult to their immune system?" Space them out. It's a reasonable thing, right. Well, you can't ask that question in the vaccine industry. Suddenly you're anti-science, you're condemned, you're a heretic.

What if you ask the question, "Well, what if we took the mercury out of the vaccines?" They've done it in Europe. They have mercury-free medicine is a pillar of the United Nations, the future of medicine. Get the mercury out of everything because it's toxic. Why do we still have mercury in flu shots that we're injecting into pregnant women, and children? But if you ask that question, you are attacked, and you are condemned.

You know, it's really a kind of insanity in the vaccine industry, just like in the cancer industry. Many people who are pushing these poisons are, themselves, clinically insane. Or they're tied to the profits in such a way that they're unable to discover the personal ethics required to tell the truth. It's sad because children are being harmed and killed every single day because of these greed-driven people or these insane people who parade as scientists, but they're not. They're the kind of scientists maybe that the Nazi regime would have loved to hire, willing to carry out experiments on Jewish prisoners. That's their ethics, but they're not the kind of scientists that we should have practicing medicine in America today.

Ty: Looks like we're in a different setting here. What happened? We got attacked by yellow jackets outside.

Mike: Oh, yeah, we were outside. It's the middle of summer in Texas insects.

Ty: Yeah, I think the yellow jackets work for the FDA, actually.

Mike: They probably do.

Ty: Yeah, they attacked us. So one of the things…

Mike: They have their little venom vaccines, you know, that they try to inject us.

Ty: Yeah, they do, they do. Maybe they're trying to get us because we won't vaccinate with regular vaccines. Maybe they're trying to get us with the yellow jackets.

Mike: Apitherapy, it's called there.

Ty: Yeah. So question for you. We were talking out there a little bit about this vaccine issue. We were also talking a little bit about this chemotherapy issue. We're talking about this insane issue. You mentioned that some of these doctors are clinically insane. So I'm thinking about this all together and I'm thinking this Dr. Farid Fata in Detroit that has been convicted recently of prescribing chemotherapy and diagnosing patients with cancer that never had cancer. Can you talk about that?

Mike: Well, importantly, he knew they didn't have cancer, so he was deliberately giving a false-positive diagnosis in order to sell the chemotherapy drugs and profit from them. So he was profiting while he was creating a toxicity and killing people. You know, chemotherapy damages the heart, damages the liver, damages the kidney, damages the brain. You know, chemo brain, right, it's a common thing.

So he subjected these people to really a torturous, chemical intervention that was medically unjustified. Now, he's been sentenced, I believe, to 45 years in prison. But the most disturbing thing about this is not that he was caught and that he has been sentenced to prison. The disturbing thing is that there are hundreds of other cancer doctors out there doing the same thing and they haven't been caught. And they get away with so much deception, violating medical ethics, lying to patients.

Most patients never question their doctor because they think the doctor is the sole authority. Most patients don't even get a second opinion. Most patients believe the explanations, the diagnoses that the cancer doctor gives them. "Oh, this shadow on this x-ray, that means you have cancer. We have to start now or you're going to die." The fear tactics that these oncologists use are highly unethical and really should be criminal.

It is completely unacceptable that oncologists profit from the treatments that are justified by their own diagnosis. It's kind of like taking your car to a greasy mechanic somewhere that's not very honest and he says, "Oh, yeah, your carburetor needs to be replaced or your car is going to blow up down the road." But he's just making that up because he wants the business. If you believe him, then you're going to have to pay all this money for a procedure that your car didn't need. Same thing happens in the cancer industry every day in America.

Ty: Not only are we getting that scenario where oncologists are prescribing chemotherapy for patients that may not even have cancer and they're making money on it, right, they make—I interviewed Dr. Sunil Pai. And he calls it a reimbursement, but it's really a kickback. Doctors, oncologists get kickbacks on chemo. That's unique among the drug world. That's, to my knowledge, the only class of drugs that they get kickbacks on is chemo.

Mike: Yeah. It's almost designed for corruption. It is a corrupt system. In almost any other industry, that activity would be illegal. Like in the Olympics. When the decision makers for the Olympics committee, if they accept bribes, which they've been caught doing, well, that's considered criminal. They might be arrested or kicked out of the committee. When doctors get kickbacks in the cancer industry, that's just considered business.

The problem is it's business that is not in the interest of the consumer. As we've seen, as in this case, consumers are being deliberately harmed and milked for money—milked for insurance money, Medicaid money, Medicare money. You see, in many cases, the patients themselves aren't making the payments, the payments come from government.

So it's a racket that involves at least four parties: the cancer doctor, the chemotherapy manufacturer/drug company, which lobbies the government, and the government makes the payments, and the patient, their body is the vessel through which all of this nefarious activity takes place, all these violations. But you got to have a patient's body in order for this racket to work, for everybody to make their money.

Truth is they don't need the patient's body. It'd be better if they left the patient out of it and just threw the chemotherapy in the trash, and billed the government, and the government paid the drug company and left the patient alone, that would be better believe it or not.

Ty: Yeah, I saw an interview with a widow of a man that had been treated by this doctor. And she said, I know that he died from the chemotherapy, which leads us to this bizarre conundrum here in the United States or worldwide, not just the United States, anybody that uses chemo, is that we have people that we know are dying from the treatments because the treatments are toxic. Yet, we still keep prescribing the treatments.

Mike: Very good point. In fact, when you look at people who die from cancer treatments, the cause of death is always listed as cancer. It is almost never recorded that they were killed by the cancer treatment. In fact, just recently there was a CEO of a large tech company that just died, I think, a couple of days ago after chemotherapy treatments. But the press reported that he died of cancer.

So chemotherapy is a medical intervention that's designed to kill cells. That's what it does, admittedly. That's what the industry says it does. That is immune from any statistical accuracy in its effects. So you know how science likes to say that it's based on cause and effect and the gold standard of evidence, well when all the evidence comes to the surface of chemotherapy damaging and killing patients, they throw that evidence away. They pretend it doesn't exist.

So we have this huge blind spot in the cancer industry where they are delusional, irrational thinkers who believe that chemotherapy can never be recorded as harming anyone, even though its sole purpose is to cause harm to cells. Now, you have to be delusional to believe the cancer industry's line of thinking along those lines. It's just insane.

Ty: It is insane. And especially in light of the fact that many of the first chemotherapy agents, as Dr. Rath shared with us, were based upon the mustard gas derivatives from world wars.

Mike: Absolutely.

Ty: They kill people. They were used to kill.

Mike: Well, yes. Again, the chemotherapy is a chemical agent whose sole purpose is to kill, to kill cells, and the thinking, the medical justification is, "Well, we're only going to kill the cancer cells." Well, even that doesn't work. If you shrink some of the cells of a tumor, you still have the cancer tumor stem cells that just regrow that same tumor. And then at the same time you poison healthy cells in the body.

So you've now reduced the ability of the body to fight future cancers and fight future insults and challenges to the immune system, which might include influenza or bird flu or Ebola someday. Who knows what's sweeping across the country that we haven't even heard of yet. All of these things you need a healthy immune system to fight them. Chemotherapy destroys the immune system. Vaccines weaken the immune system. And if you combine them, that's how you get a lot of fatalities.

You get people who are just being injected and poisoned from multiple angles, all of it under the auspices of public health. But it's really profiteering on the part of the drug companies using human bodies as the vessels of profit generation. It's like *The Matrix*. You're like the Neo character in *The Matrix*. You're in this vessel and the tubes are plugged in to you and they're generating profits off of you, and that's your only role in society according to these corporations. They just want you lined up, stacked up, towers of human bodies that they can make money off of. It's a medical matrix.

Ty: It is. It is. Talk about fear, you mentioned fear. Oncologists play on fear.

Mike: They do. Fear is their most powerful marketing tool, and they are trained to use it against patients, to lie to patients. But first, let me explain the flip side of fear, which could be called love or self-healing. The placebo effect, which is a very real effect, it's an artifact of mind-body medicine. It explains why a person who believes in their own self-healing capabilities is able to activate that healing potential inside themselves.

So a good doctor should be a good healer. A good healer is someone who should invoke the mind-body connection to unleash love, if you want to call it that, self-healing love, self-repair. The body wants to be whole. The mind wants to exist in a body that is whole, that is healthy. That's love. That's what good doctors would use.

Cancer industry uses the opposite. Fear, hatred, and self-loathing, these are the tools of oncology. They use fear, they tell you that if you don't start chemotherapy right now, you're going to be dead in six months. Self-loathing, they tell you your body is attacking you, your body is the enemy. We must kill parts of your body using this toxic chemical or you will die. So it's forcing you to go to war psychologically with part of your body that they say is cancerous.

Then there's this hatred that comes out of that because as you undergo chemotherapy, what's happening to your body. Your hair if falling out, you're losing muscle mass, you're losing appetite. You're losing your mind because of the chemo brain side effects. You're losing liver function, kidney function. You're just destroying yourself. It's a kind of self-hatred or a self-abuse, tormenting yourself in the name of chemotherapy. These are the tools of the cancer industry. So, it is the exact polar opposite of what health and healing should be or even good medicine. Good medicine should be rooted in love. The cancer industry's rooted in hatred and destruction.

Ty: Wow, Mike, that's really a great analogy the way that you contrasted the cancer industry with the way that we should be healing. It reminds me of our mutual friend, Robert Scott Bell, right. He ends his show every day, "The power to heal is yours." And it really is. He also talks a lot about this placebo effect. That's poo-pooed by the cancer industry. "Aw, we shouldn't…" He says we should harness that. It's working. Whatever it is that heals, we should embrace it.

Mike: Well, yes. There's a reason why integrative medicine is called integrative because it's about reintegrating all the parts of the body, the mind, the soul that results in healing. And what Western medicine wants to do is tear you apart piece by piece through reductionism and physiological compartmentalization. They want you to go to war with your own body really.

Everything is described as something's wrong with you, even depression. "Oh, it's a brain chemistry problem. Your brain is attacking you with its chemicals." Come on. It's absurd, but that's the way they describe it, and that's the way they sell antidepressant drugs. The truth is healing is an integrative process. It's why integrative medicine is a great word for it. Might even be better to call it holistic medicine. It's about restoring the whole. And holism is the understanding of the holistic nature of everything around us. That even a plant—you cannot take and isolate every chemical out of a plant and expect that plant to have the same healing powers.

This is why chemical cancer medicine fails 97 percent of the time, whereas plant medicine, being holistic is safer, it's more efficacious, in other words, it works better. It's more affordable, readily available and you don't have to pay patent fees to Mother Nature. So everywhere in our world—for us to heal as a civilization, to heal as a planet, we need to be moving, uplifting our ideas into a holism or holistic kind of level. We cannot stay stuck in the compartmentalization of chemicals that is based in the 1940s and 1950s understanding of science, and nutrition, and medicine. But that's what we're stuck in today with the cancer industry. We got to move past that if we hope to actually heal.

Ty: Yeah, we do. I agree. We have to move past that and I think one of the biggest atrocities that we're seeing today based upon that 1940s and 1950s still the same treatments that we had back then are being used today. Some of the same drugs.

Mike: Yes.

Ty: We have to get into this issue of forced chemotherapy and this is a really—as a father, this is an area that just makes my blood boil that we're seeing children being taken from their parents and they're being forced chemo, being forced—we did an interview with a man named Jay Matthews. You're familiar with his daughter Selena—I don't know if you're familiar with this story.

Mike: No.

Ty: We interviewed him in Detroit and he's a pharmacist, so he knows what he's talking about, and they said, "We're going to take your daughter from you if you don't give her to us." They did chemo and radiation. She recently had her arm amputated because of the radiation. He knew this, he told them all along it's going to happen, and it happened. So there's nothing that makes me angrier than this. We, just today, did another interview with a young lady named Cassandra. You're familiar with her story?

Mike: Yes.

Ty: From Connecticut. The story that she told us was just horrific. They literally strapped her to a gurney and with her screaming, saying, "I don't consent to this. I don't consent to this." And they sedated her and they put a port in her chest and they gave her five months of chemotherapy against her wishes. And she said every day she told them, "I do not consent to this." I mean, this is medical tyranny at its finest.

Mike: It's medical torture. You know the word I have for it is "chemo boarding" like water boarding. You know, we as a nation, the United States of America—I don't mean we, the people, but I mean the corrupt few in charge, they continue to condone water boarding as a form of torture in illegal prisons like Guantanamo Bay, Gitmo.

When we see a nation embody those kinds of ethics, they trickle down into the medical system, and into the economy, the business system, and many other areas. But we're seeing water boarding, torture techniques trickling down and be accepted by mainstream medicine now. What you just described is medical torture. It's a violation of the Nuremberg Code. It's an act of medical terrorism against an innocent American. There is no justification for it.

This kind of violation of medical ethics, and human rights, and human dignity, should never be tolerated in a free society. Can you imagine the outcry if any other currently politically correct group was targeted with such treatment? For example, what if doctors said that all gays and transgender people have to be strapped to the table and treated with hormones? There would be a crime against gay people, a crime against sexual orientation. There'd be a massive outcry, but it's okay if it's a kid with cancer.

Why is it not okay to treat a transgender person like that, but it's perfectly okay to treat someone who has cancer who's going to be victimized twice, once by the disease and a second time by the medical establishment. This is unacceptable. This is incompatible with a free society. And frankly, the doctors that engage in that kind of activity, the hospital staff that strap people down and force chemotherapy into these children, they should be arrested. They should go to jail just like this other oncology doctor who's serving 45 years in prison now, finally. It's time to start arresting these criminals and locking them up because they are a real danger to society.

Ty: I agree. I agree. And one of the things that Cassandra shared with us is she said that they said that we're just doing what we have to. Well, that was the most popular excuse…

Mike: On the Berlin wall.

Ty: At the Nuremberg trial.

Mike: Right. True. True. That's always the excuse of people who obey mindlessly and carry out heinous crimes against humanity.

Ty: So Mike, you've got the Natural News Food Lab that you have recently opened up.

Mike: Well, it's actually renamed the Consumer Wellness Center Laboratory, and it is a vastly expanded lab, 1,700 square feet of state-of-the-art analytical instrumentation, better than most universities by far. We've got organic chemistry, we've got the inorganic chemistry, elemental analysis instruments. We've got protein analysis, other instruments as well.

We are aiming to help consumers make informed decisions about what's in their food. Since I've been doing this testing for several years now, we've discovered some rather alarming things about toxic elements that are in certain imported foods like brown rice protein from China, for example, containing high levels of lead and sometimes tungsten and sometimes cadmium in other foods as well.

These heavy metals, by the way, are linked to cancer and they're linked to lowered IQs, and kidney problems, and skin problems, and heart disease, and cadmium is linked to cardiovascular issues as well. So most people don't know the truth about where foods are grown, and what elements they can absorb that have been deposited by pollution: factory pollution, industrial pollution, especially in China.

Most people don't know, Ty that you can grow certified organic crops on polluted soil and it can still be certified organic as long as you don't spray it with pesticide. So you can grow foods that are very high lead, high cadmium, high mercury even, and they can be certified organic and sold as organic.

So what we're trying to do—we're not trying to attack the organic industry. You know, we're pro-organic, obviously, but we want to help reward those companies that grow clean, pure foods in cleaner soils by highlighting that good news and contrasting it with the bad news of foods mostly from China that are very heavily polluted. There is huge demand now for organic produce, organic cereals, organic grains across the board. Companies like Natures Path have purchased farmland just to meet the demand for all the organic grains that they're putting into their cereal products.

Well, guess what? We tested their products. They're incredibly clean. We tested their rice in California. It's incredibly clean. The rice in Texas is also clean. It's these foods that come from China, usually, and sometimes Thailand, and Asian countries that tend to be heavily polluted. So anyway, this lab is about just giving people the answers that they need to make informed decisions to protect their health.

Ty: So you mentioned Natures Path, that's pretty clean.

Mike: Yes. Nature's Path, the entire product line is all organic.

Ty: Yeah. No, I'm glad to hear that because that's the brand that we get for our kids.

Mike: Oh, good.

Ty: So I'm just glad—okay, good. Pat myself on the back, I did something right there at least.

Mike: Yes, yes, they're great company, and they're led by an owner with passion for all of this. You can tell the difference between a company that believes in what they're doing versus a company that just wants to make shareholder profits.

Ty: Mike, earlier, you mentioned glyphosate and we were talking about the different uses for glyphosate. Many people know that are watching that it's recently been declared a probable carcinogen. But there's some unknown uses for glyphosate too that you were mentioning.

Mike: Well, most people associate glyphosate and the most popular brand name for that is Roundup or Monsanto's herbicide. But as a generic chemical, it's called glyphosate and it's sold in many, many other products for agricultural use. Glyphosate is usually associated with genetically modified crops because crops are Roundup resistant, right. You can spray the whole field with glyphosate, but the GMO crops survive.

So most people think that if they buy wheat or wheat flakes or wheat bread that it's not going to have glyphosate in it. They're wrong. Wheat farmers are spraying glyphosate on the crops right before harvest to dry them out more quickly and prepare them for harvest, and it's not just wheat, it's alfalfa and other crops. Glyphosate is being used as a chemical desiccant to reduce the waiting time after cutting and before harvesting the grains, thereby reducing the risk of the farmer to catastrophic rains that would ruin that crop.

So glyphosate is now being found in wheat products, even though wheat is not a GMO commercialized product yet. Glyphosate is toxic at low parts per billion concentrations, and some scientists even think parts per trillion concentrations may have negative hormonal effects on the body. So, obviously, there's a lot of research still being done in this area, a lot to learn about glyphosate toxicity and where it's found in the food supply, but I think this is going to be a huge issue for the next few years of people realizing just how much glyphosate they're eating and how much it's poisoning our soils, our water supply, and our food supply. It's a huge issue.

Ty: What are solutions for people? How are people going to be able to deal with this, this overabundance of glyphosate?

Mike: Really one of the best solutions is to grow as much of your own food as you can. Now, I know that's not practical for people who live in cities, for example, but you'd be surprised at what you can do. You know, I invented the Food Rising Mini-farm Grow system. You'd be surprised, you can grow tomatoes, and strawberries and lettuce—abundant lettuce, more than you can even eat—without using soil, without using electricity, and no pumps or anything. Simple system. You'd be amazed.

So you really can grow more than you think if you just try it and it doesn't take much attention. But the other thing is, you know, buy organic, certified organic, but also ask about the country of origin, so you're getting things that are grown more locally wherever possible. In the United States, most foods are not contaminated with heavy metals. Very important to know. The US is actually a clean, agricultural environment in terms of heavy metals for the most part. And Europe is also very, very clean.

Europe has even more stringent standards than the FDA by far. In fact, a lot of global companies that produce contaminated raw materials like rice protein, they can't sell it to Europe because it would be illegal. So they dump it on the US where it's packaged as organic, raw, sprouted protein and sold at health food stores.

Ty: Wow!

Mike: Yes. We are the dumping ground for a lot of these things that are grown in China where Europe would not accept them, they violate European laws. So you've got to become informed. Definitely check out our laboratory at labs.naturalnews.com where we post results for free. So people have called us kind of like the Consumer Reports of the natural products industry. We're not associated with Consumer Reports, but that's a general description that people have given. But I'm inspired by Consumer Reports because they've done a lot of good work in laboratory analysis.

Ty: You mentioned people don't think that they can grow their own food, but actually, it's not that difficult to grow some food.

Mike: That's right.

Ty: I mean, just think if the average person that's in the residential neighborhood spent as much time, and money, and effort growing a garden as they do growing their lawn and their bushes and all that. People spend a lot of money, they work really hard taking care of their yard. Robert Scott Bell, again, we'll mention our good friend. He says, "Grow gardens. Quit growing grass, grow gardens."

Mike: Exactly. You make a really excellent point. Not only are people growing grass and spending a lot of time and money on that, they're poisoning their lawns by putting all the normally, the toxic weed killers on their lawns to make it look nice and homogenized. They like homogenized milk and homogenized lawns. But both of those are bad for you.

A healthy lawn shouldn't look like there's only one species growing there. If you go out into the fields of nature, they're not mono-cropped fields. They have hundreds of species of plants, different heights, different sizes, different colors. They bloom at different times of the year. They're pollinated by different insects. They produce different kinds of food sources. They support a web of life. That's what a healthy yard should look like.

So even across America and around the world, this whole idea of what is an upscale neighborhood look like, to me it looks like death. When I drive around a neighborhood, I see a lawn, that's death. That's not life. You can't live off of that. It's not sustainable. I go out into nature like a food forest or a permaculture environment, that's life, that's food. That's probiotics in the soil. That's nutrients recycling through nature. A composting happening naturally right on the ground. That's life. We should be aiming for biodiversity in our food.

You know, culturally, it's fascinating that there's such a powerful call right now by the politically correct opinion leaders for diversity in races, diversity in gender, and diversity in sexual orientation and even marriage, right. All this call for diversity, and yet these same people, they hate diversity in the food supply. They want the same 20 things over and over again. They hate diversity on their lawn. They want a clean, green lawn that's like the eugenics of lawn care if you think about it.

So how come we can't have diversity in medicine? How come we can't have diversity in food sources, diversity in our seed supply, diversity in the foods that we grow and eat ourselves. We should have an abundance of different foods that we're consuming and that's how you prevent cancer. That's how you prevent diabetes, that's how you become healthy. Again, it's this idea of holistic living. It's always fascinating to me, the contradictions that exist out there in the culture.

Ty: It is. Yeah. It's inconsistent, a lot of inconsistent logic. It's illogical, I guess. It's not logic at all, it's illogical.

Mike: Even intellectually, in terms of science, what is demanded by California lawmakers recently with SB 277 is the complete destruction of diverse scientific opinions. Instead, everyone must obey with this one opinion that happens to coincide with the pharmaceutical industry. And that is the only one opinion that's tolerated.

So we talk about tolerance in this country. Well, there's no group that is more intolerant than the pharmaceutical industry, and the cancer doctors, and the vaccine pushers. They're completely intolerant of any other opinion. They do not welcome freedom of thought. They do not even believe in the scientific method, which involves questioning and seeking answers to those questions by letting the evidence tell you what is true.

They hate that process. They want to dictate science to you and that's a contradiction. Scientific dictatorship is like military intelligence. It doesn't exist. It shouldn't exist. Real science cannot be dictated. Real science is a process of discovery, and that process is no longer really represented in our culture today.

Ty: Yeah, I have to agree. I have to agree. That's a good oxymoron. I remember that one from when I was a kid, military intelligence.

Mike: Yeah. Jumbo shrimp.

Ty: Jumbo shrimp. That's another good one. One of the things you mentioned last year, Mike, in *The Quest for the Cures* was a quote that really resonated with a lot of people. I asked you something about plants, and herbs, and things that had anti-cancer effects and you said, "The funny thing is that when you park your car and you go walk to your oncologist's office, you probably walk through a field or a forest that had more anti-cancer effects than anything you're going to get in that office."

Mike: That's right. You can't even walk through nature without encountering medicine everywhere. There's an ancient fable in traditional Chinese medicine where a Chinese teacher challenges his students to go out into nature, walk into the forest, and try to find anything that isn't medicine. And the students point to the rocks and they say, "Well, those rocks, those aren't medicine." The teacher says, "But of course they are, they're made of minerals. The right minerals with the right treatment can be very medicinal, can be very healing. So yeah, those can be medicine too."

And the students point to, "Well, the tree bark. That's not medicine." "Well, of course tree bark is medicine." Where does cinnamon come from? Cinnamon helps regulate blood sugar. It's part of traditional Chinese medicine. Many of the medicinal substances come from bark. Even aspirin is derived from the white willow bark that was originally used by the American Indians. So, yeah, of course the tree bark is medicine."

The students point to the dirt, "Well, the dirt can't be medicine." "Ah, but the dirt is full of pro-biotics, living organisms. The right organisms can actually—if you ingest them, enhance your health, protect your health. So those can be medicine too." Everything around you—what about the sunlight? That's medicine. What about the tree leaves? That's medicine. What about the air that you're breathing? Well, you can breathe therapeutically, you can reduce stress. You can change your physiology by breathing in the right manner. The water in the stream, not just the water in the stream, but the sound of the water in the stream, vibrational medicine is all around us. And all we have to do is tap into it.

So much of Western medicine and chemical medicine is about dissociation, it's about isolating you from these real cures that really exist all around you. That's why I really appreciate your work, Ty, because you're helping people just reestablish the connection with what is real.

Ty: Thanks Mike, appreciate it. One of the things you just mentioned, it just took me to another place, sound and water. We interviewed a man, a scientist down in California that was on the Russian team after Chernobyl. They were sent to investigate why certain areas were recovering better from the radiation than others. And what he found is that there were certain areas that were drinking water that had been exposed to the natural sound vibrations that the earth makes more than other areas, and it has changed the structure of the water and it was causing them to heal. Really fascinating, so this is not quack science. This is a man that was on the team for Russia after Chernobyl and these were his findings. He's got stacks and stacks of research on this.

Mike: That's amazing. There's a lot of mystery about water structure, and that's an area that fascinates me. And it's not—I think water structure has to do with the energetics of it. You can't necessarily see it in chemistry, and certainly not physically under a microscope, but energetically, there's a lot of interesting…

Ty: There is—one of the things with animals and with plants is there's no placebo effect. Right? There is with people, but there's no placebo effect with animals and plants.

Mike: Right. I suppose so, yeah.

Ty: Well, he's been watering his lemon tree with this water and the lemons are this big. So it's like something's different about this water. There's no placebo effect with these. But anyway, just interesting story.

So let's talk real quickly Mike. I know that your time is precious and we got to roll to get out of here as well, but I want to talk real quickly about diagnostic techniques. I mean, we know the mammograms are causing cancer and we know that there's these diagnostic techniques that are not really even early detection. They're late detection before we start hitting you up with these poisons.

Mike: Well, my main message on diagnosis of cancer to everyone out there watching, number one, don't trust anyone opinion of one oncologist. Because what this guy went to jail for giving people false positives on purpose, right. So these hucksters and con artists are out there in the cancer industry and they're called oncologists. So make sure that you get at least a second opinion from a reputable person.

And make sure you talk to a naturopath. Get all your options. You don't have to—look, if you're diagnosed with a tumor and they say, "Well, you're going to die in six months unless you start today."

That's a lie. You've been growing that tumor for a decade or more probably. You're not going to die tomorrow. You'd be best served to use that extra day and that extra time to learn your options so that you can make the best informed decision with a diversity of opinions among qualified naturopaths, and alternative cancer doctors, complementary medicine, and so on. Only when you have the right information, which is why people are watching this, can you then make an informed decision that's in your own best interest.

If you think about it Ty, the cancer industry is very, very good at convincing people to make decisions that are contradicting their self-interest. The cancer industry does not want you to make a decision that protects you and your finances. The cancer industry wants you to make a decision that protects you and your finances. The cancer industry wants you to make a decision that enriches them.

Well, that is a conflict with your own self-interest. You may not want to live a life with a damaged brain, and a damaged heart, and a damaged kidney, and have all your hair fall out, all these other side effects of chemotherapy. You may not even have cancer at all. So shouldn't you do your homework up front so that you can make a decision about you? You have to be a little bit selfish as a patient here. You have to be a little bit assertive as a patient. You have to realize that that doctor has no authority over you other than what you give that doctor.

Just because that doctor has a diploma on the wall and is wearing a doctor's costume, and whatever, doesn't mean that they can command you to do something unless you're under 18 years old, in which case they call the cops and actually force you at gunpoint and strap you to a bed. But you as an adult, you have to surrender power to the doctor. You have to consent, or they can't give you that treatment.

So the key is don't let them use fear tactics, which is what terrorists use, by the way, to manipulate your decision-making process. Oncologists and ISIS use many of the same tactics of fear to manipulate your behavior. Yes, I'm comparing oncologists to a known terrorist organization because they use the same tactics to try to control people. In fact, terrorism is the use of fear—the definition is the use of widespread fear or the threat of fear, the threat of violence in order to achieve a desired behavior or decision-making outcome among people.

So by definition, what many oncologists do today is a cousin of terrorism. That's why it's unacceptable. That's why some of them are going to jail. That's why they're criminals. And that's why more of them should be arrested, and that's why you as a patient should be extremely, extremely skeptical of anything that an oncologist tells you because it is in their interest that you say yes to what they are pushing.

Ty: And if you don't have the disease, which we know that now that many of the people, that almost all the people of this doctor in Detroit treated, you may soon have it because of the treatment.

Mike: Well, exactly. It becomes a self-fulfilling prophecy. Chemotherapy treatments cause cancer. So if you didn't have cancer to begin with, you may have it in six months after undergoing chemotherapy. If you think about it—you know, people really have to understand the origins of cancer. We don't have time to go into it here, but it's not some outside invading pathogen. It's not like malaria.

Cancer is a failure of the body's own cells to communicate with each other properly—genetics, plus intercellular communication. Cancer is the mal-expression, or the inappropriate expression of your DNA. It is not something that has invaded you from the outside so you cannot look at cancer with the paradigm of carpet-bombing your body, declaring war on an invader. It's not an invader. It's something internally that is not communicating correctly at a cellular level.

So you need to become whole. You need to heal, not destroy in order to overcome cancer. Now there may be extreme cases where there's a tumor that's so large that it's pressing on an artery, or a nerve or something like that, where it has to be physically removed. I understand that. I'm not saying surgery doesn't have any place at all. It can have its place, but even then the surgery is only a temporary solution. You still have to address what has led to that tumor in the first place. And that's where it comes back to integrative healing and holistic self-love and self-healing. And that's not accomplished by chemotherapy.

Ty: It's not. As a matter of fact, the exact opposite is accomplished by chemotherapy.

Mike: Chemotherapy, maybe should be called liquid hatred. It's like if you hate yourself, do chemo.

Ty: Yeah, and unfortunately—I laugh at that, but it's just kind of this absurd laughter because this treatment that is so absurd, that is so contradictory to what patients actually need to actually heal is the predominant theory, not only here, but across the globe today. As a matter of fact, I mentioned to you earlier off the camera that in Riga, Latvia, they're now calling oncologists chemotherapists. Because that's their only protocol.

Mike: That's right. That's right. It's absurd. Look, we live in a society where people inject themselves with all kinds of different things for different reasons. But when they're using recreational drugs, for example, like heroin, they say that heroin makes them feel great. I mean, I've never used it so I don't know, but they say it feels great. Well, they're destroying their health in exchange for feeling awesome.

Chemotherapy is even worse. You're destroying your health and you feel like crap at the same time that you're destroying your health. It's like the worst of all worlds. I'm not saying heroin is better than chemotherapy, but I'm just saying of all the crazy things that people inject into their bodies, why would you choose to inject yourself with a toxic poison. Why inject yourself with anything at all? You know, I mean, that's my approach. You know me. I don't take vaccines. I don't use drugs. I don't get medical interventions. I don't do chemo, and as a result, here I am, very vibrant, very creative. I just released a new music video a couple of weeks ago. I mean, you know.

Ty: By the way, the kids love your music video.

Mike: Great. I'm glad to hear it. You know, I'm inventing new things, I've invented things for 3D printers, the Food Rising System, the search engine. But when I tell people my brain is just a normal, healthy adult brain. That's it. Nothing special. Everybody has the same potential. Everybody has the same biology. We're genetically almost identical.

The truth is, most people damage their brain by doing drugs, or chemotherapy, or pharmaceuticals, or eating lead in their contaminated food. Drinking fluoride, exactly. People damage their brains and that's why they don't have the capabilities that they wish they had, but the good news is you can reverse that. Your brain can actually start to heal, and repair, and relearn if you stop poisoning it.

Ty: Good words. Good advice. Right, you can always turn it around.

Mike: Yes.

Ty: So what's your advice, what's your encouragement to someone that might have recently been diagnosed with cancer and they've gone into the white coat office and the oncologist says, "You're dead in three months. Get your stuff in order."

Mike: Number one most important thing is to don't give in to the fear. Recognize that you have the decision, that you have options, that that oncologist doesn't know about. That oncologist probably hasn't read Suzanne Somers' book for example. That oncologist hasn't watched this video series. That oncologist hasn't seen the cures that you've seen traveling around the world, and hearing true stories of people with amazing recoveries. And I've heard them face-to-face too, you know, people telling me how they've overcome Stage IV liver cancer just by changing their diet, changing their lifestyle.

Look, the truth is, discover your options, and then make a decision about what you want to do. Now, I know people, who rationally, after doing all the research, and learning what they needed to do to overcome cancer, they made a rational decision to say, "I don't want to do that. I don't want to stop smoking cigarettes, I don't want to stop drinking the beer. I don't want to stop eating hot dogs and barbecue. I don't want to do wheat grass juicing or this or that or whatever." And they've made a conscious decision and that's their right, man. That is their choice. I honor their choice, whatever they want to do as long as it doesn't harm someone else. So there's no judgment if you make that decision to die from cancer.

Ty: But at least it's an informed decision at that point.

Mike: It's got to be an informed decision. Other people say, "I want to live longer. I want to heal, and I'm willing to make a few changes," and they're actually simpler than you think. You don't have to go crazy and do wheat grass colon cleansing and all. You don't have to do all that stuff. You can have an anti-cancer lifestyle that's actually very friendly, that's very enjoyable and quite delicious in terms of fruit: red grapes, citrus fruits. They're all anti-cancer. You know all these amazing things that you can eat, they're anti-cancer. Fruits and vegetables and even nuts and seeds, so many things, and spices. Spices are anti-cancer. So you can have an enjoyable life and you can live an anti-cancerous lifestyle at the same time. You don't have to suffer through it. A lot of people think if you go natural, you're going to have to suffer, and you're going to have to give up everything that you enjoy in life. No, not at all. Look at us. I mean, would you go back to drinking soda and eating hot dogs like the way we both probably did as kids? Once you make it through the transition, you never want to go back to that.

Ty: Yeah. And I guess today we're so into the temporary pleasure of that bite that tastes so good, even though you feel like crap afterwards that we keep going back. So I mean, it's good advice. It's conscious decisions. It's not something that—you don't have to go overboard and be totally crazy, and you can still enjoy your food. I think that's important for people to focus on. You can still enjoy your food and when you cook really good healthy foods, healthy dishes, you can make them taste great.

Mike: Yes. Yes.

Ty: I mean we eat healthy, but Charlene cooks some fantastic dishes.

Mike: You know, the most delicious dishes are usually the most powerful anti-cancer meals because they have all the colors and all the different tastes of all the plants that have anti-cancer properties. You know, it's someone who eats a bland diet that is headed for diabetes, or cancer, or heart disease. Look at the processed food diet. It's high-fructose corn syrup, soybean oil and…

Interviewer: Sugar and salt.

Mike: Yeah, sugar and salt, just garbage processed ingredients. That's a diet of cancer, and that diet tastes horrible. But that's what people have been trained to think is okay. You know how the food companies make those foods taste good is they add toxic chemicals to them, MSG, taste enhancers, whatever. So if you eat real food, you're eating an anti-cancer diet just automatically.

Ty: Yeah, it's always a pleasure my friend. Thanks for allowing me to interview you.

Mike: Thank you Ty.

Ty: You keep up the good work.

Mike: All right. You too.

Ty: All right, man.

[end of transcript]

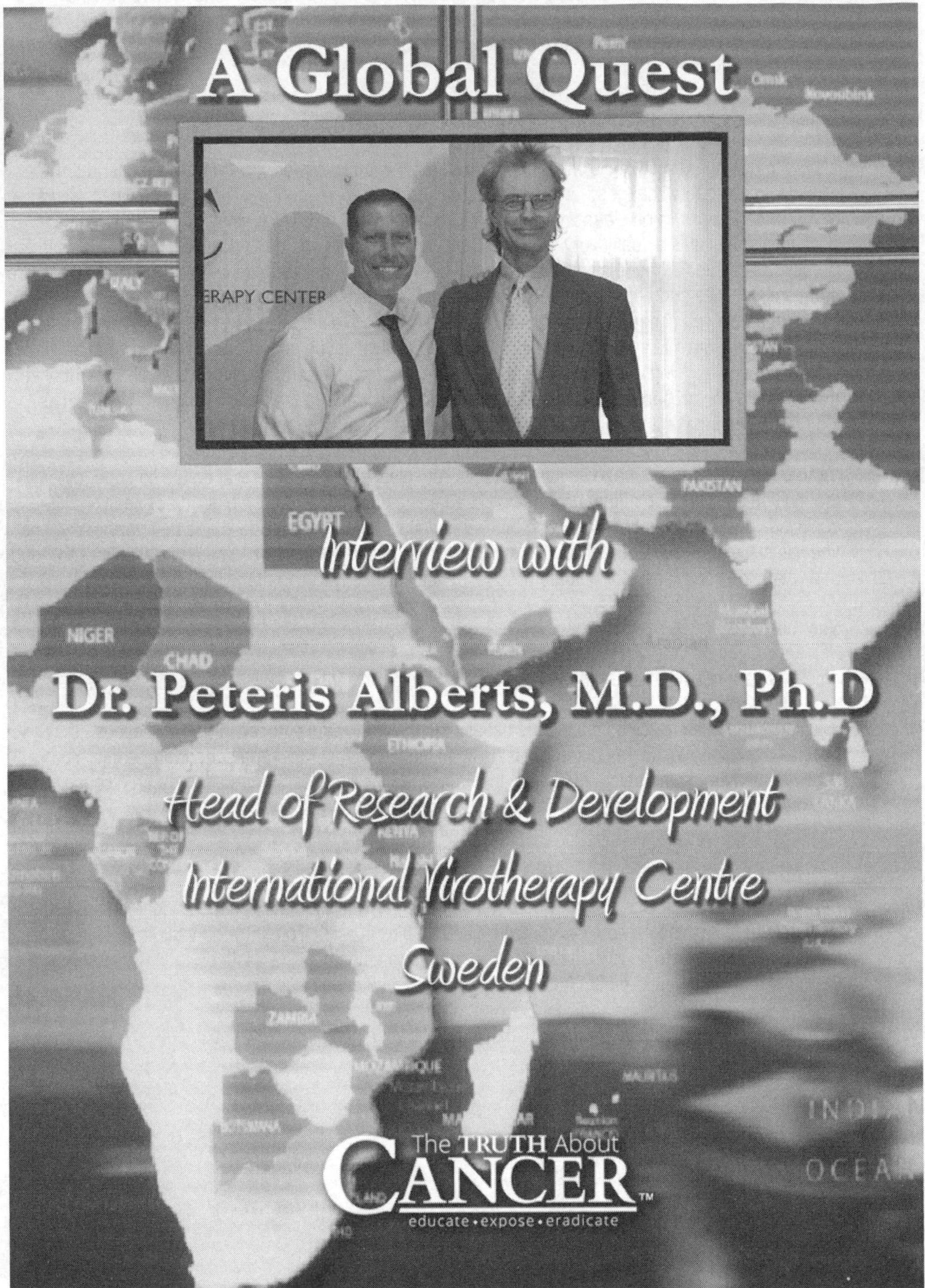
A Global Quest
ERAPY CENTER
Interview with
Dr. Peteris Alberts, M.D., Ph.D
Head of Research & Development
International Virotherapy Centre
Sweden
The TRUTH About
CANCER
educate • expose • eradicate

THE TRUTH ABOUT CANCER

Ty: I'm here at the International Virotherapy Center in Riga, Latvia. I'm sitting across the table from Professor Peteris Alberts. We'll call you Peter. Thank you for joining us today.

Dr. Alberts: Thank you for having me.

Ty: Yeah, and I'm really looking forward to getting your knowledge about RIGVIR. We've had interviews with scientists and doctors so far today about this amazing substance. But you're going to kind of put together the different missing pieces of the puzzle so that we can understand exactly what RIGVIR is, what it does, and how it works. So thank you for being here, and take it away.

By the way, what is your home country? Where are you from initially?

Dr. Alberts: I'm from Sweden.

Ty: From Sweden.

Dr. Alberts: I'm coming here.

Ty: Oh, so you're coming…

Dr. Alberts: I'm coming to Latvia.

Ty: Coming to Latvia from Sweden.

Dr. Alberts: Yes.

Ty: Great. Well, thank you for coming this distance.

Dr. Alberts: Yeah, well, thank my wife.

Ty: Thank you. Thank you Mrs. Alberts. Go ahead. Take it away and tell us a little bit about RIGVIR. It goes way back about a millennia actually.

Dr. Alberts: Usually, I talk about virotherapy and oncology. It sends you a promise of a decade of progress. It's not really true because the Catholics, they know that they have a patron called Peregrine Laziosi. That's for cancer patients. And he made an observation almost a thousand years ago that an infection made the amputation of leg with a tumor unnecessary. I don't know if they made the conclusion that it was due to bacteria or something like that, but they at least made the observation, which is a good thing I think.

A hundred fifty years ago, people were given all kinds of bacteria, and maybe viruses, which they didn't know about then, the patients, and trying to cure them. So, this thing has been in the air for some time. People have made all kinds of observation that look after infection, tumors, go down.

I usually state virotherapy is one kind of immunotherapy, which is grouped in three groups: active, passive, and indirect. The active comprises at least two things that we will talk about, or we think about, which is oncolytic virotherapy, which is the first, of course, and also about immune immodulators, because RIGVIR has two actions. It's dual-acting thing.

Ty: What do you mean when you say oncolytic?

Dr. Alberts: Good question. Next slide please. Look, what do I mean? Oncolytic and oncotropic go together sort of. I'm not sure they're the correct thing to do, but they at least tell you the observations. People have observed that viruses tend to attract to something. For example, cancer cells, then they call them oncotropic. If they destroy the cancer cells, then they call them oncolytic. RIGVIR is an oncolytic virus.

So this is a cartoon, but it shows how the cartoonist would display it. The virus infects tumor cell, it replicates within the tumor cell, and it just destroys it; blows it up. I think maybe it's a school book thing, but I think that's the way we can talk about it.

Ty: So the oncotropic is the attraction, and then oncolytic is the killing?

Dr. Alberts: Yes. And the specificity is that healthy cells are not usually affected, which can have two mechanisms of action. Either that the virus doesn't recognize anything on the cell to be able to get in, or that the healthy cell is able to get rid of the virus, somehow protect itself. I think it could be a balance maybe, and maybe yeah, it can be more. Virotherapy has been more and more interesting or en vogue last couple of decade or so. And there is a list of companies in academia that have been working with it. Maybe you know some of the—Mayo Clinic for example, which is renowned.

This is a paper showing clinical trials in virotherapy that we're on a couple of years back. And that shows you that a dozen of viruses have been tested, R&R tested. Some of them are pretty bad if they were to use them as is. And it also shows that there are a lot of indications. For a moment, there are two viruses registered. Maybe you heard the news, there is an American virus going to be registered and approved probably in this fall.

This is the short history of RIGVIR. The people around Aina Muceniece were working on polio virus in the 50s and they made it. They had to find something else to do. When working the polio virus, they were isolating other viruses. They were learning about them. And they isolated one from a healthy child's intestinal tract. You know how that is done. The child was healthy. The virus didn't do anything to him. But they found that if they take a tumor from a patient, put it into a hamster, then it will start to go on growing or something like that. If you put on the virus, it will just fade away. And you know who did that observation first? Ms. Gerklava, the lady you saw this morning.

Ty: Really?

Dr. Alberts: Yeah, she did that. Sometimes, the people who did it, you know, can't just get, you know, "I actually did that. It was me." But she did that, okay. Next, is 1965, Aina Muceniece founded. First we would set up a laboratory in the world in Riga, in the building next to the one where we interviewed Dr. Gerklava this morning. Okay. This was in '65. You look like you have been around 1968. You remember it was really a lot of things going on in the world. These people started clinical trials. And you know who was the one that brought the first trials to the first patient? Dr. Gerklava, again.

So she's been there, and they extended the clinical trials, not only in Riga, they extended it to other countries that we would say today, and other cities. So they did multinational and multicenter studies. Then came 1991, Latvia and Riga gain independence. So the structure and financial things were destroyed and couldn't continue in the way they had planned. They managed to sort of sort out the documentation and registered in 2004 in Latvia.

So that's the first sort of overall—just wanted to share with you so that you have the picture. Now, this would be the more specific part, I would say the interesting part for professionals. RIGVIR is the first cancer virotherapy. We have an oncolytic virus, which also has immunomodulating activities. That's the dual, that mode of action.

Ty: What does it mean to be immunomodulating?

Dr. Alberts: Well, you tell me. No, it activates the immune system. It doesn't only kill the cancer cell, it also activates the immune system. I'll show you a slide of that. This is the RIGVIR county—oh, sorry, it's Latvia. It's because it's the first county it's been registered in. If it's registered, it's reimbursable. It's for your charge to—what it's called? Residential Latvia by the manufacturer. That's nothing for you, but this is the pharmaco-therapeutic group for registration. It's registered as a immunomodulator. I don't think there is a class for oncolytic viruses. So you have to register for something that it is.

The virus belongs to the *Picornaviridae* family, Enterovirus genus, ECHO group, type 7, so ECHO type 7. RIGVIR is nine. It has been adapted to melanoma cells, meaning that it is more active in melanoma cells than it used to be without the adaption. And it has not been genetically modified. No GMO. That's probably important in some parts of the world. The vial that we sell contains virus and saline for injection and that's it. Nothing else. No stimulus, no toxic potentation, no toxic substances. No nothing.

It's a manufactured GNP. Some people ask me why I tell that, but some people ask. "So do you really manufacture GNP?" "Yes, of course we do." It can't do anything else. It's manufactured GNP. Has to be stored frozen.

What does it look like? If this would not been a small molecule, you would have been getting chemical structure here. It's tough to give a chemical structure a virus. So what we did, or people here did, they sent the vial to electron microscopist. Said, "Look, I guess you can guess what this is, but can you tell me, can you take a look, and can you tell me?" So she took a picture, couple of pictures. That's what it looks like and took her viral atlas and, you know, one page, second page. This is an antivirus. That's what she said and it doesn't contain anything else.

Viruses form crystals when they are in some kind of tissues. This is one of the heterotransplants and this is electron microscope. This is the crystal structure. It behaves like a virus as well. The nuclear sequence has been sequenced, and every virus has a prototype virus, which have been sequenced, and is publicly available. When we compare our virus nucleotide sequence in the library, it's 80 percent similar. So it's not the same one, but it's a similar one.

If you deduce the amino acid sequence—you know what that is? Because you know three nucleotides make one amino acid and then you can give back. That's the Watson and Crick thing, right. Then it's 96 percent similar. So it's pretty similar, so we say yeah, fine, it's ECHO 7.

This is a light microscopic picture showing that it's supposed to be inside the plasma and that's where the fluorescence is showing. There are nuclei here, and it's not in the nuclei, it's an RNA virus. It's supposed to be in the cytoplasm. We have to wait for ECHO-7 still someone.

This is efficacy in vitro pre-clinical. These are each line, are cells taken from human cancers, (inaudible - 00:11:46), and so on. The first column shows you what they look like at control zero hours. The second one is control if you don't do anything after 24 or 48 hours. And the third one is if you incubate with RIGVIR.

I'm told that any child can see that there is a difference here. That's what I say. This looks like that—you have to explain it. I don't have to explain it. I want to say is this effective in cancer patients? That's my primary goal. Even aspirin, people didn't know how that worked when it went into patients because it helped patients.

So here are similar slides for other cancer cells from other cancer patients, from lung cancer, stomach, pancreas, breast, monocytic leukemia. The same kind of story. The cells do not survive as good as on the control computations if you just add RIGVIR to the medium. That's the pre-clinical result. This is a summary of it, and this is oncotropic—this is what you're looking for. This is what you're asking. What is ECHO virus?

ECHO virus is a virus belonging to the enterovirus family. ECHO is short for enteric cytopathogenic human orphan, meaning that they got the viruses from the gastrointestinal tract, and that they do it. The people, the children they got it from were healthy. Now we know that there are ECHO viruses that are really bad, but they still are human viruses.

So why are they human? Meaning the host is the human being, not animals. No rats, no dogs will get it. Why? We don't really know, but we think that every virus needs some kind of receptor. You know receptors, the door lock and the key thing. They have to fit somehow to get them to the cell, and there are receptors that we think they would need—I mean, not we—in the literature. I mean nobody has said, "Look, this virus needs this receptor."

And these ones, we have compared. They're also published, the sequences of them. We have compared them. And the human receptors, these receptors are pretty different from those from any other animal. That could explain why these ECHO viruses are really aged here. They're human viruses. Why is the human specificity important? Why do I stress it? Because most things in cosmetics and absolutely all things in medicine need to be tested in some kind of species before they go to human. Why?

Because of course, you need to prove safety, some kind of safety because you can't have a drug that kill the patient. I'm sorry, I did my best. That's not good enough. And all the agencies, including FDA are very strict on safety. That's their job because everybody needs to prove that the drug or whatever you try to give to humans has some kind of balance because effect on safety. This is why it's important. Because toxicology is usually done in rats, mice, dogs. Why?

Because they should be predictive. They should be predictive for what you see in those species what you will find in humans. If the rats, dogs, mice are fine, we hope and we think that the logic would be that if they're in those respects, at least fairly, similar to the human being that will be fairly safe in man. This virus doesn't do anything in animals. So, fine, it's still not pathogenic in the normal human being.

Do reports on all kind of stuff. Other active ECHO viruses, for example, those that are pathogenic, people say "Look, we haven't found that they do anything during pregnancy to mother and child. It's circumstantial, but you're still fine. Clinical results. Would you like some clinical results as well?

Ty: Sure.

Dr. Alberts: Okay. Clinical studies were done before registration and about 2,000 patients were included. Fifty, fifty safety, 50/50 melanoma about, which is a pretty large number, even considering in those days. So some of the melanoma patients were eye melanoma, and most of the safety cancer patients were stomach, rectum and colorectal cancer patients, meaning not too many healthy volunteers were involved. Doesn't really matter. This still showed safety.

But 2,000 patients for (inaudible - 00:17:04) is pretty much even today. So how about adverse events? I have written down here there is no record of any untold side effects from the treatment or its discontinuation. Most common symptoms was sub febrile and temperature. The people that are working with a new generation or viruses, they would find the same about.

If you give—then the question is: Is it an adverse event if you give a live virus to human being that you see some, you know, increasing temperature. I don't think so. It's kind of effect-related because the immune system will try to do the best to get rid of the intruder.

So, I mentioned that the FDA—I don't remember which year they started, but increasingly, they ask for five year survival data in oncolytic medicines if you want to register in the United States of America, which is fine because if the patient doesn't survive, it's not that clear what the advantage is. These days, they also check for three and five year survival rates, and this is just a table of the melanoma results.

Five year results are not as complete as the three year. But the column most to the right, it says surgery only, and the three-year column says surgery and RIGVIR. I think those numbers actually speak for themselves.

Ty: Sure. You can tell it's markedly better with the RIGVIR.

Dr. Alberts: And you have statistical significances, which is not always the same as clinical significance, but it's good to have statistics on your side. These slides show you, also from those earlier experiments, these are not in vitro results. These are actually specimens from patients from surgery before treatment with RIGVIR and after treatments with RIGVIR. At least there is little to the left. At least you can see there is difference. There's not that many cells around.

And this is one I tried to answer your question. What the immune reaction, what those does, how do you look at it. Also, Dr. Garklava mentioned to you it's an immune system, it's a lymphocyte thing. Look, the lymphocytes just surrounding the melanoma cell. They round there, they go there, and they do their job. That's what I've seen. It's pretty amazing to me.

We have also results from the GI tract meaning stomach, rectum. There are not that many studies, but the numbers for—five year survival numbers and percentages between surgery and RIGVIR, and those numbers are also, to me large enough in order to say "Look there is a good reason to use this one." I mean, it's more than ten percent difference in twenty.

Now we go to post-marketing, meaning the previous results were those that were done before registration. There have not been that many studies post-marketing, and this is the one that has been published so far, and it shows time to progression in melanoma patients. It's a retrospective study, meaning they went to the registry and found out what happened, what did the patients get?

And these are Type II patients, meaning that these had—according to guideline, Type II patients really don't have that much treatment obligation. They have observation, clinical trial or whatever. Not that much. So, they gave RIGVIR to these patients because they have the freedom to do that in Latvia, otherwise, you not have to stick to the guidelines.

So the control group is observation here because the other ones, clinical trials, and anything else in that category was not included or they were too few to be. At least we're not in here. And this one says look, there is a big difference in these ones. Okay. This is plotted per patient when they had the progression, meaning every red line shows when you had progression, which is obviously here to the control group had more of it.

This is a study we have done, which has not been published, but I wanted to share it with you because what can I tell you. I mean, I'm not a clinician, I have not that lifelong experience in clinical trials, although I have did a couple. I've seen that when you see these kind of plots, they show you one group, they show you the control group, they show you the treatment group and they have 16,000 patients or 25,000 patients in each and they show you a minuscule difference between the groups.

I think in a way it's really—what can I tell you? The differences are—here are all the patients that we had. Stage IB or IIB, or II Stage. They're significantly difference. This is only Stage II. This is survival. They're retrospective still, but we go to five year and if we just take the IIB and IIC, it's a really big gap.

Ty: Yeah. Yeah, I noticed a little difference in the…

Dr. Alberts: They're all significant, statistically significant, and to me it's kind of more than encouraging. So, this is the recent TBEC study that was published last month. You know what that is? It's an American company going to FDA for a review and this is what they published. Okay, you can tell me this is not the same ballpark, but these guys apparently have to have Stage III and IV patients. So they're on a tough ground. But still, the virus was better than the control.

RIGVIR has been used in a lot of cancers. I don't think we have been able to have that many patients so we can say we have checked all these patients. That's good for them and it's good for them. And we have melanoma, we have GI tract, those we've seen. They're the ones we can say we have odd cases, we will do what we can. We asked our partners to give us data back—we call them CRFs—so that they can stockpile data and see: Is this good for this cancer, is this not good for this cancer. We do what we can.

Summary. We have a really unique mode of action, clinical cancer medicine. It's not an oncolytic virus, it's an immunomodulator. It's not been genetically modified. It's not pathogenic. It has clinical affect, it has little to no side effects. Can you prove something that is not there? It's tough, it's tough. So we say "No, that's little." And this is about the Virotherapy Center, and this isn't about the company that has its marketing authorization. And this is very nice photograph of Riga.

Ty: So what is it about RIGVIR that makes it selectively toxic to cancer cells, and it leaves the other cells alone? Any idea?

Dr. Alberts: Well, you can speculate

Ty: What are your speculations?

Dr. Alberts: Well, my speculations are, there are obviously differences between healthy cells and cancer cells. I guess one of them could be, it's not only my guess, that some of the protective mechanisms against viruses, bacteria may not be the same. I can only speculate. I think that also these things about the receptors on the surfaces. It's a lifetime project for a lot of scientists to find out which virus needs which receptor and maybe in which combination, and maybe differently between differently healthy cells and tumor cells. Can only be speculations in this point of time.

Ty: How does RIGVIR create an immunomodulatory response? What is the method of action by which it mobilizes the lymphocytes?

Dr. Alberts: The same as for every foreign agent, I guess.

Ty: Which is what?

Dr. Alberts: Well, you have cell mediated, you have non-cell mediated, all kinds of immune responses in the body. I guess it's a balance.

Ty: So, I'm just trying to get clarity for people that are going to be watching this. What is it about the RIGVIR virus that causes the immune system to react to it?

Dr. Alberts: I don't think I can tell you exactly what. That would be the safest, but it's still virus and all—but the body reacts to all kinds of viruses that gets close to you. I don't think there's anything unique about that. I mean viruses elicit an immune response.

Ty: Right. I guess whats I'm trying to get out of you is how does that happen in the body? How does the body mobilize lymphocytes to go attack something?

Dr. Alberts: Yeah, well, that would not be fair to me to go into details.

Ty: All right. Well thank you. It's been very interesting. I really appreciate it.

Dr. Alberts: Thank you for coming.

[end of transcript]

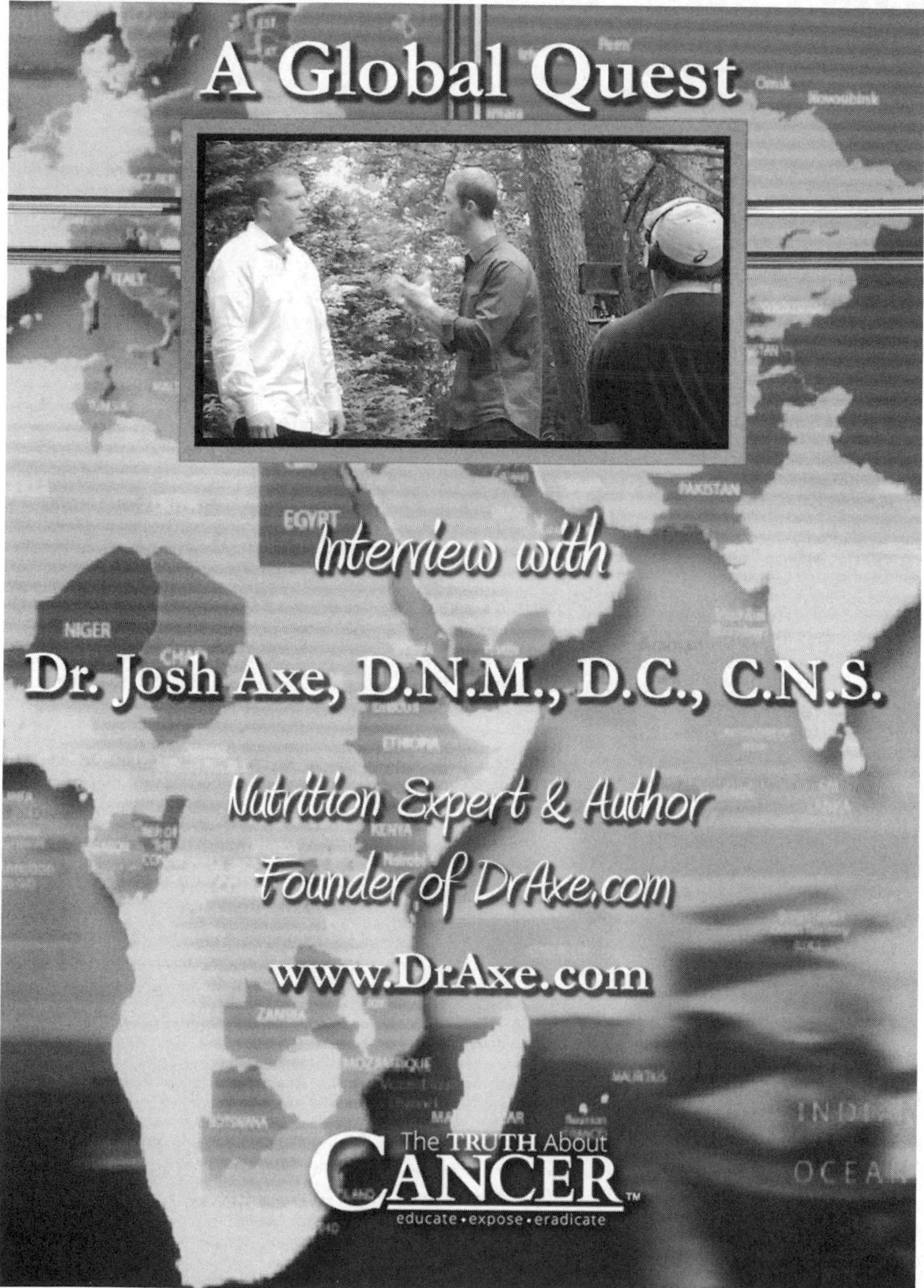
A Global Quest
Interview with
Dr. Josh Axe, D.N.M., D.C., C.N.S.
Nutrition Expert & Author
Founder of DrAxe.com
www.DrAxe.com
The TRUTH About CANCER
educate • expose • eradicate

Ty: Dr. Axe, so happy that you could join us today in sunny Nashville, Tennessee here.

Dr. Axe: Great to be here.

Ty: Beautiful place down here isn't it?

Dr. Axe: It is.

Ty: So tell us a little bit about your mother. You know, one of the reasons that I wanted to touch base with you today, was not only to learn about the essential oils, but to get your story about your mother that apparently had cancer, right?

Dr. Axe: You know, my mom's actually battled cancer twice. The first time a little over 20 years ago and it actually came as a shock to our family. My mom was diagnosed with breast cancer at 42. Growing up, my mom was my gym teacher at school. She was a swim instructor. So always really fit, active, and healthy, but yet diagnosed with cancer.

My family lived in, what I call, the medical model at the time. And we were always taking drugs, my mom was always taking some sort of medication, but she went and had a mastectomy. She went through rounds and rounds and rounds of chemotherapy. And Ty, I can still remember to this day seeing my mom's hair fall out. I remember looking at her after the chemo treatments and thinking she had aged 20 years in two weeks. And just saying to myself, "You know, I never want to see anyone have to go through that again." That's really what drove me into being a physician—is seeing how sick she was.

So she was diagnosed as being cancer free and healthy, but really, for the next ten years after she went through chemotherapy, she was really sicker than ever. She spent half of her days in bed. I remember she'd get home from work at 3:30 and sleep until 6:00 every night. She struggled with depression. She struggled with chronic fatigue, anxiety issues, and leaky gut, digestive issues, just sick all the time.

Ten years later, I was actually working as a nutritionist in Orlando and finishing up my doctorate and she called and said, "Hey, I've been diagnosed with cancer again. What do I do?" I flew home from Florida to Ohio and we sat down and prayed together. And I just said, "Mom, I think we need to take care of you all naturally."

So we started an all-natural treatment program and she started juicing vegetables every single day. We had her start doing antioxidant rich foods, loads of probiotics, and using things like essential oils in helping her body heal. We followed this treatment protocol for about four months, went back to the oncologist—and their first recommendation was surgery and radiation immediately—and we followed it for four months. After four months went back to the oncologist, got a CT scan, he called us two days later and he said, "This is incredible we don't see this." He said, "But the tumors have shrunk more than half." He said, "Keep doing whatever you're doing."

Ty: Whatever you're doing is working, right?

Dr. Axe: He said, "Come back in nine months." We went back nine months later and complete remission. And today my mom is in the best shape of her life. In fact, her and my dad just retired from Ohio down to Florida and she water skis every day. She's ran three 5Ks with me in the past few years and gotten second and third in her age group.

She says she actually feels better now in her 60s than she did when she was in her 30s. So she actually now teaches people how to use essential oils, and make healing smoothies, and juicing vegetables, and how to ferment their own food. So she just is a—she's doing amazing.

Ty: That's awesome. So Dr. Axe, that's awesome. So you just shared the story about your mother. She was diagnosed with stage four. They didn't, "Give her the terminal diagnosis," but stage four's pretty bad and now she's alive because of your intervention, really. I mean because of the fact that you put her on some oils. And you mentioned the essential oils—one of the things that you all did. What oils did you use?

Dr. Axe: The primary oil at the time—we started using was oil of oregano. Oil of oregano is packed with some incredible compounds, thymol, carvacrol. One of the things that she had chronic issues with is digestive issues. She had leaky gut, chronic constipation, and severe issues with yeast. So she was constantly craving sugar. She even developed a toenail fungus, major yeast and candida issues.

So we started doing oregano oil, three drops, three times a day internally, as well as topically on the toenail. It was amazing. When she had tried creams and all of these different things in the past, antifungals, and she started doing the oregano oil and after two months it completely cleared up that issue. So I mean, oregano oil was an incredible part of her treatment.

Now, today we also have her using frankincense oil on a regular basis. And frankincense oil, if you look at the research today, it is probably the most powerful essential oil, if not the most powerful supplement period when it comes to natural cancer treatment, in my opinion.

Ty: What's in frankincense that makes it so good?

Dr. Axe: You know, frankincense is really high in a compound called boswellia or boswellic acid and it's highly anti-inflammatory. It's also a very powerful anti-oxidant. There's a study that came out of the UK pretty recently showing that frankincense oil is effective at shrinking tumors. It's effective against ovarian cancer, colon cancer, and breast cancer. And so that boswellian in frankincense, very, very powerful compound at fighting and treating cancer.

Ty: So you mentioned the inflammation, it helps with inflammation. So could it be effective at—that's one of the reasons it's effective at brain cancer because of the inflammation of the brain.

Dr. Axe: Well, you got it. And one of the most incredible things about frankincense is that the essential oils themselves are very, very small molecular compounds. Most everybody knows this in cancer treatment, that chemotherapy is not effective at treating any sort of cancer of the brain because it can't pass through the blood brain barrier. Versus frankincense oil, those compounds are so small they can actually pass through the blood brain barrier and start to reduce that neural inflammation.

I'll tell you an incredible story. I was speaking recently and had somebody come up to me at the end after talking about essential oils and she said, "I can attest to what you're talking about with frankincense oils." She said, "My husband was diagnosed with a brain tumor six years ago and was given three months to live. We got turned on to frankincense oil, started using it every single day. We diffused it in the home, we rubbed it on the roof of his mouth." She says, "It's been six years and he's still alive and we really believe it's because of this use of frankincense oil."

But you look in the medical studies, it's effective against Alzheimer's, it's effective against any sort of brain inflammation. And again, four separate studies showing that it's effective at treating cancer.

Ty: That's amazing. So in the Bible, the wise men that gave baby Jesus the frankincense and the myrrh, maybe they weren't giving him just precious gifts, they were giving him medicine.

Dr. Axe: Absolutely. When you hear the story of the three wise men bringing the infant Jesus gold, frankincense, and myrrh—I remember years and years ago not really knowing—I mean, everyone knows what gold is, most people don't realize what frankincense and myrrh are. But those were the two main sources of medicine during that day.

And frankincense, actually, at the birth of Jesus would have been used. Because you look at children right after they're born, oftentimes there's bruising and sometimes it's a traumatic experience and so they would have actually rubbed frankincense oil on a child, which actually helps bring down that inflammation and swelling. Also, it's great for supporting and protecting the immune system. So if he was exposed to different types of pathogens at that time, frankincense oil really protects the body. So absolutely, Ty, I mean, frankincense oil was used as—it was more than just a sweet smelling fragrance, it was the biblically based medicine.

Ty: So your own private personal army, the immune system, frankincense helps with the immune system, it helps with inflammation. There's been studies in the UK that it directly fights four different types of cancer. So it's really an amazing substance, isn't' it?

Dr. Axe: It's something that I use on a regular basis. I just use it for wellness. It's also been shown to be effective at reducing scarring. It's been shown to be effective at evening out skin tone.

Ty: What about stress?

Dr. Axe: Well, that's the next thing I was going to bring up is that it's also been used for spiritual awareness and relieving stress. And if you go to even certain types of orthodox churches today they actually diffuse frankincense, incense, but frankincense specifically during those ceremonies. I believe the reason why people throughout history have really connected it with spiritual awareness is because it reduces that brain inflammation and allows you to have clearer thinking, reduces brain fog, which really, in turn, can help reduce stress.

Ty: That's a great connection. I did not know that they used frankincense, the scent. That they burn frankincense.

Dr. Axe: Eastern orthodox churches today. And actually it's part of something in the Bible. Frankincense was used along with something called the holy anointing oil, which actually had myrrh essential oils. So a lot of people when they hear frankincense also start thinking about myrrh. And myrrh is referenced over a 160 times in the Bible. Myrrh was also—actually there was a study in the journal of *Food and [Chemical] Toxicology* recently that found that myrrh, another essential oil that's referenced in the Bible, is also effective at treating cancer.

Ty: Really?

Dr. Axe: Yes.

Ty: Okay, because that was my next question, "What about myrrh?" Because you have the frankincense and the myrrh, so both were medicines, both were sweet-smelling fragrances. Here's something interesting that Dr. Sunil Pai told us last year, he believes that the gold wasn't actually gold, he thinks it was turmeric, the golden spice.

Dr. Axe: I mean, you could absolutely see that in that area in the Middle East. And turmeric today and cancer treatment, talk about a powerful compound, frankincense, myrrh, and turmeric.

Ty: You got a triple play there.

Dr. Axe: But you look at something like myrrh—and it's powerful because it really works on the hypothalamus and the liver. So it reduces liver inflammation and also balances hormones. And what happens a lot of times today—a lot of these cancers are estrogen-based cancers and so what myrrh can do is it really supports the body. Very similar—if people have heard of indole-3-carbinol or the benefits of cruciferous vegetables.

Ty: Broccoli, right?

Dr. Axe: It works in a very similar, but an even more potent way to where it really helps clear the body of excess estrogen or xenoestrogens that are found in things like soy and plastics and parabens today. And really helps detoxify the liver and also boost a very important antioxidant called glutathione, which supports detoxification. So that's the way that myrrh essential oil actually helps in fighting cancer.

Ty: It sounds like frankincense and myrrh oils would be like a good one-two punch.

Dr. Axe: Absolutely. You know one of the things that I've had my patients do, including my mom over time, is start creating an at-home frankincense and myrrh body butter and body lotion. So basically she takes 10 drops of frankincense, 10 drops of myrrh along with some coconut oil and shea butter and makes her own at-home body lotion. Rubs her entire body with that and really those oils—the great thing about essential oils is they've been used as aromatherapy. So those small compounds coming off the body are protecting the body. They're fighting cancer. They're doing some incredible things there even topically.

Ty: So that's what aromatherapy is then, is burning these essential oils?

Dr. Axe: Well, oftentimes—now traditionally, they were burned as incense. And, in fact, it's referenced in Egyptian medicine, Chinese medicine, and in biblical medicine it's diffused or, basically, burning them as incense. Now, today one of the ways you can do it is actually put it in a diffuser. So you can put it in a diffuser, you can simply smell the essential oils.

So all of my patients, or as I mentioned, my mom, take those essential oils and especially put it around the area of the neck. And when you put it on the neck and the back of the head, you're constantly also breathing in those beneficial compounds.

Ty: So you're not only absorbing it through your skin, you're breathing it in as well.

Dr. Axe: Absolutely. And that's a good point, your skin is your body's largest organ and this is why—this is the amazing thing about essential oils, we've talked about frankincense and myrrh. Other essential oils as well like lavender and sandalwood are so incredible at fighting cancer

But, you know, so many of these products people are using today, the body lotions, make-ups, moisturizers, shampoos, conditioners, they are loaded with carcinogens. You know, they're loaded with parabens and phthalates and sodium lauryl sulfate, and all these different chemicals that cause cancer. Versus if people make their own at-home personal care products with essential oils rather than causing cancer, they're fighting cancer.

Ty: That's a great point because that's one of the things that many people don't realize is the fact that your skin—you absorb anything that touches your skin, you're going to absorb it and so that's a great suggestion. Make your own personal care products with these essential oils. Where could they find a good essential oil to use? Is there a certain brand or type that works better than others?

Dr. Axe: There are several brands out there that are great. I think that, ideally, people are buying what's called therapeutic-grade or medicinal-grade essential oil. There are several companies that do that, but if people want to learn more they can check out my website. I've got several long-form articles on frankincense and cancer, on myrrh. And even some DIY recipes on how people can make these own essential oil recipes and so I've got a lot of recommendations on draxe.com.

Ty: Draxe.com, great. So let's shift gears real quickly, talk about the fact that people need to prioritize their nutrition. Because I did an interview a couple of weeks ago. I was up with Joel Salatin at Polyface Farms. And we shared some stories together and we both came to the conclusion that most people that say they can't afford to eat healthy or to do this or that, really they can, they just haven't prioritized that. So can you talk about the fact that we need to prioritize that?

Dr. Axe: Sure. I think a lot of times it comes down to money, but more so time. I'll give you an example. One of the things that I have my patients do especially—one of the things I specialize in, along with supporting cellular health, is really treating digestive issues. I teach my patients how to make at-home bone broth. And it's taking that time to do it and it's actually very simple and easy once you get started doing it. I think if you're going to beat cancer or prevent cancer, be healthy. Your health has to become a priority, but the biggest part of that I believe is time.

My wife and I wake up every Saturday morning and we go to the farmers market here, actually, around Franklin, Tennessee. That's a priority for us in the morning. We've blocked out time to exercise. We make a lot of our own meals at home.

I think priority is key and I think part of that is setting out a budget and looking—I think people would be surprised at what they can get for their money if they shop wisely. So many things now you can buy online or go to certain other stores and buy things in bulk. I'll give you an example, we've mentioned turmeric. Turmeric, an amazing healing herb and you can buy that if you buy it bulk online.

Ty: Yes, huge bag.

Dr. Axe: A huge bag of it. So I think it really comes down to planning ahead, actually looking at your budget. And I think people can buy and invest a lot more than they think into their health if they really set out a plan and budget to do so.

Ty: I like what you said about budgeting not only your finances, but your time like your priorities. It reminds me of a cartoon that I've seen. It's a big obese man standing with a doctor and the doctor says, "Well what does fit better into your schedule, exercising an hour a day or being dead 24/7?" You've got to prioritize exercise, you've got to prioritize your nutrition. I think that all goes hand-in-hand.

Dr. Axe: You know, one of the things we did when my mom had cancer is we really set up days and times where she would go shopping. So she would shop on Sunday afternoons, she would shop on Wednesdays and she made a lot of food in bulk ahead time. And so if she was making bone broth, she would make not one batch, she would make multiple batches that would last her a whole week, is so important. But planning ahead is crucial when it comes to overcoming cancers we've talked about.

Ty: And if that's your priority, if you want to stay alive, especially with certain types of cancers that are more aggressive. I did an interview last year with a young man that was 23 when he was diagnosed with terminal cancer and he used what's called the Gerson Therapy. I'm sure you've heard of it. He was doing 12 or 13 juices a day, several coffee enemas. This is a 23 year old. He prioritized that and 10 years later, he's alive because he made that a priority. So, I think that's good advice for everyone that's listening.

Dr. Axe: Absolutely, it's lifesaving stuff we're talking about here. Some of the things are obviously more time consuming, juicing your own vegetables, making bone broth and those types of things. But certain things don't have to take much time. We talked about essential oils, how hard is it to take a few drops of frankincense oil, rub it on your neck a few times a day? Some of these things are quick, but powerful and effective.

Ty: Right, absolutely. Great input Dr. Axe and great interview. I really appreciate all your input on the essential oils, the nutrition, sharing your mother's story with us has been great. I really appreciate you spending time with us.

Dr. Axe: Well, awesome, Ty. Thanks for the mission here. I'm so excited about your quest in taking on cancer. So thanks.

Ty: You bet, thanks. God bless you.

[end of transcript]

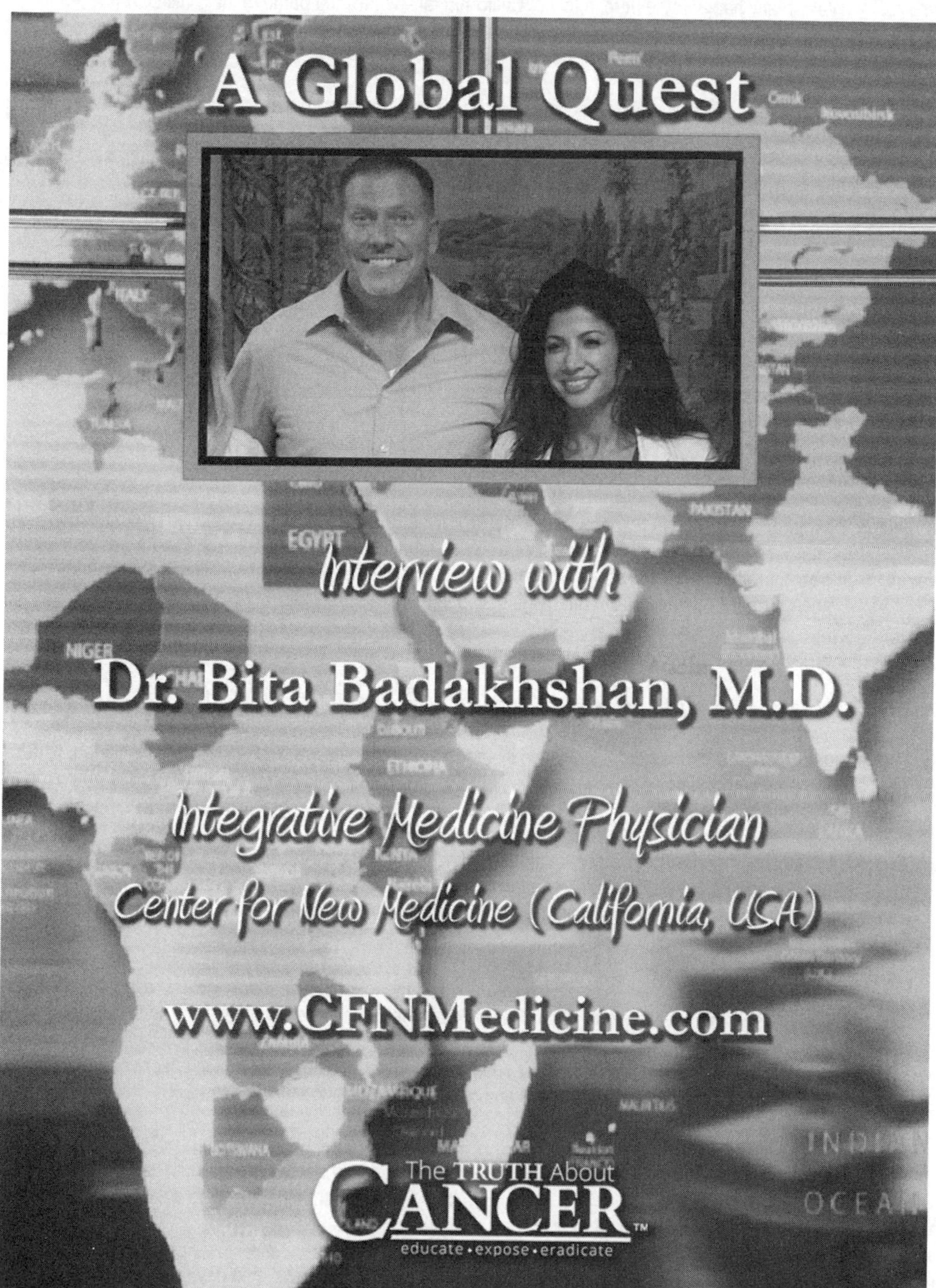
A Global Quest
Interview with
Dr. Bita Badakhshan, M.D.
Integrative Medicine Physician
Center for New Medicine (California, USA)
www.CFNMedicine.com
The TRUTH About CANCER
educate • expose • eradicate

Ty: We're really happy to be here in Irvine, California, at—what's the name of the clinic Dr. Bita?

Dr. Bita Badakhshan: Center for New Medicine.

Ty: Center for New Medicine. Dr. Connealy said there are a couple of different clinics here, but we're at the Center for New Medicine. We're really privileged to be talking to Dr. Bita here. We met for the first time in San Diego several months ago. She was speaking at a conference. And I'm really interested to get your perspective here on cancer treatments and really what got you into treating cancer.

So, first of all, thank you Dr. Bita for being here with us.

Dr. Bita Badakhshan: Thank you for having me here. It's a pleasure to be here.

Ty: Thank you.

Dr. Bita Badakhshan: It is a great opportunity to inform the general population about other ways of treating cancer. Other than the conventional way.

Ty: Other ways than the big three, right? So where did you grow up Dr. Bita?

Dr. Bita Badakhshan: I grew up in Sweden, Scandinavia. My parents are Persian. We moved out of the country when I was twenty days. They came first to the US and we lived here a little bit. Then it was revolution in Iran, then we moved out of the country. It was hard to live at that time. We lived in Spain, and France, and then Sweden. And after high school I moved to the US.

Ty: So you lived everywhere. You lived all over the place.

Dr. Bita Badakhshan: A lot of different countries, yeah.

Ty: I know there are a lot of people involved in cancer treatment, cancer research, myself included, who had some kind of a personal tragedy that got them involved in this line of research. What's your story as far as why are you doing what you're doing today? Treating cancer integratively.

Dr. Bita Badakhshan: So I started as a conventional doctor. Finishing family practice residency in New York and then moving back to California, I started working on different urgent cares and for Kaiser as well. And then at Kaiser and urgent care I was seeking the patients who were treating themselves or living their life in an integrated way.

Like pancreatic cancer, late stage. She said, "I was diagnosed a few years ago. I was told I'm going to die in a few months, but it's now almost three years I've been living doing great." And initially they would say—because they would see me as a conventional doctor—they said, "I know you won't believe in this stuff." I said, "No, I'm open to it, I'm very open to everything. I want to learn. I'm eager to learn." So much stuff out there that we could learn and give a better care to patients.

So anyways, to make a long story short, I just kept seeing patients like that and I got guided into that and then I started. And what hurt me was in Kaiser they would get the diagnosis of cancer—they didn't even have time to research. Within a few days they had to do chemo, otherwise the doctors would tell them they're going to die or it would spread everywhere.

So they would come—one patient I had she had urinary infection and next day she had to do chemo. I said, "No honey, you have to take care of your kidneys first. It's a urinary infection. Get rid of the bacteria and then do your research. There's no rush." You don't get cancer overnight, cancer is a process of 10 years, 12 years. I mean within eight years you get a tumor. Sometimes people don't get diagnoses until 10, 12 years.

So, they kind of tend to scare the patient and they get worried. They don't have time to research. Then they start the chemo.

Ty: So it's really almost a process of creating fear to get them on the treatments quickly.

Dr. Bita Badakhshan: Correct. Correct.

Ty: That would be considered your kind of "aha" moment where you realize what we're doing—its not working here.

Dr. Bita Badakhshan: Exactly. It's not working and we need to educate people. We need to tell them there's other ways to go. Going with the conventional surgery, radiation, chemo is not the way to go. There's other ways you could do. And also you could do surgery, but no, don't rush into it. Improve the immune system, boost your body before you do surgery because any cut, any kind of surgery in the body, it will suppress the immune system and also it will attract all the good white blood cells—all your good cells into that area, then what happens? All those cancer cells that are already floating in your body they keep growing.

Ty: So the surgery is a really bad impact on the immune system. A drastic effect.

Dr. Bita Badakhshan: It is, and sometimes we do have to do it and we do recommend it, but before doing that you want to boost the immune system before doing any kind of surgery.

Ty: You said that cancer sometimes is eight, 10 years in the making. What exactly is cancer?

Dr. Bita Badakhshan: Basically, cancer is abnormal growth of cell and basically they lose their apoptosis. Programmed cell death. They don't die, they become immortal. And your body's immune system usually takes care of the abnormal cells in your body. We do all have ten to a hundred thousand abnormal cells every day.

But our immune system's job is to get rid of those cells. If your immune system is perfect. If you don't have virus that it's already trying to fight, you don't have too much chemical or other stuff going on in your body.

So, then they keep growing and growing and are increasing in number and then you get a tumor.

Ty: And so the tumor is really a result of a lot of years of things going wrong.

Dr. Bita Badakhshan: Suppression of immune system, exactly. And I think one of the main things is the viruses. We do see a lot of different kind of viruses in patients with cancer. Not only HPV, herpes, you know, you see mono, Epstein Barr virus, even Lyme disease—which is not a virus—but Lyme disease even suppresses the immune system—and parasites. I have a handful of patients with breast cancer who have parasites. When they do coffee (inaudible) enema they actually see the worms coming out.

And what does parasite do to your body? It suppresses the immune system. So there are some doctors who believe you develop cancer because of the parasite, some believe candida, the fungus, yeast, but I believe everything has to do with that.

Ty: So the thing they all have in common is they suppress the immune system.

Dr. Bita Badakhshan: Exactly. It's all about suppression and there is a doctor who said cancer is a metabolic disease, has to do with mitochondrial dysfunctions. What is mitochondria? Mitochondria is the organelle in our cell that produces ATP—and other toxicity can affect it. What we call toxicity and all that can affect the mitochondria. Your mitochondria can become dysfunctional and that causes an anaerobic environment and then cancer cell grow, abnormal cells grow.

Ty: In an oxygen deprived environment.

Dr. Bita Badakhshan: Exactly. But we still have—the cancer cells are very smart. In some cancer they shift, they change their metabolism to utilize oxygen. I mean we do say most of the cancer do not survive in high oxygenated environment, but now we see some cancer they do survive even in a high oxygenated environment.

Ty: Okay, so some do.

Dr. Bita Badakhshan: Some do, yeah.

Ty: So one of the machines that we will see today is the hyperbaric oxygen chamber. Works for a lot of cancers, but for some, not, because they have adapted to use oxygen.

Dr. Bita Badakhshan: Yeah.

Ty: Very interesting.

Dr. Bita Badakhshan: One of the problems with chemo is—because when a new patient does chemo, those circulating tumor cells, cancer cells that you have once you have the primary tumor, they can mutate and they become more resistant to other treatments.

Ty: Okay, so it's the stem cells.

Dr. Bita Badakhshan: Stem cells or the tumor cells. So circulating tumor cells is formed from the primary tumor. And also circulating stem tumor cells. And those can become bad cells, cancer cells, or may not. But circulating tumor cell as well. Both of them will float in your body. That's why when you do surgery or chemo or radiation attacking one area, you not getting rid of the cancer—what happens? You have these circulating tumor cells floating in your body.

That's why I love the RGCC we have in Europe because I have patients who come, "Oh, I'm in remission." Two years ago I had a patient with lymphoma and she did chemo. She said, "Yeah, three, four years remission and now I'll just go and see my uncle." I said, "Oh, okay really? Let me do a circulating tumor cell on you."

So I did the test on her and it came eight. I said, "I know you don't have any symptoms, I know you feel great, but please, let me to do a PET scan on you because when the circulating tumor cell is eight it's pretty high." She already has somewhere else.

So I sent her, did a PET scan. It was into her bones. But she didn't have any bone pain, she didn't have any symptoms. So I told her, "You know what? Go back to your uncle and see what he has to offer." Then she went, but then she wanted to do our treatment. Her cancer responded very well to hyperbaric, PMF, pulsed electromagnetics, she did IV vitamin C, she was on supplements. But before we did all that, I made sure to change her diet, change her lifestyle.

I detoxed her because if you don't do that—let's say if she had leaky gut, and I don't fix her and I give her a bunch of supplements, it's not going to help her. It's not going to get absorbed. Let's say if I don't do the spectracell test, for example, which shows me what kind of mineral, amino acid deficiency that patient has. If I don't do that then I cannot really help her just by doing all these treatments. Because B12 and folate—there is the enzyme. I mean there is a gene called MTHFR gene which has to do with activation of B12 and folate and that is a very key component of DNA and all that.

So if you don't have active form of B12 and folate, genetic mutation happens. People do develop cancer, which I see usually a mutation of both of the MTHFR. You have two of them. If you have mutation of both there is more risk of cancer on those patients. A lot of cancer patients have that mutation. So if I don't fix that problem and give her an active form of B12—doesn't matter how much B12 from food she get—or inactive form of B12—it's not going to help her.

So we did all that on her. So I've been seeing her for a couple years now. She's been doing great. She lost weight. She had heart disease. I got her off of her medication. She was on blood thinner as well. I got her off of that and all of her blood pressure medicine is off. So until a few months ago, she was on a bunch of supplements, used to do a lot.

Her last scan—she had a PET scan when she went to an oncologist a few months ago he said, "Your cancer is stable. There is one tumor. One area is actually shrinking. You're doing great. Go back to whatever you're doing."

It is against the law in California for oncologists to recommend integrative medicine.

Ty: Is it really?

Dr. Bita Badakhshan: They cannot tell you, "Go do integrative medicine," not in California. But the oncologist said, "Go back to whatever you're doing. Come back in a year." Then when I saw her I kind of modified her program. I said, "Okay, I feel better now. You don't have to do this, this, that, but I still want you to do hyperbaric oxygen." I still want her to do the PMF, the pulsed electromagnetic. One of the reasons I love that is because when you have cancer, or any injury in your body, the voltage of the cell goes down. It becomes like 20, 30 millivoltage. Your healthy cell has 70 to a 110 millivoltage, so when you do PMF, you actually charge the body, the cell membrane.

Ty: You're plugging it in.

Dr. Bita Badakhshan: Exactly, and then I have her do hyperbaric and she responds better to the treatments. So it's always good to do pulsed PMF before any treatments, IVs, any.

Ty: What about the SOT treatment? The SOT?

Dr. Bita Badakhshan: Okay, SOT, Supportive Oligonucleotide Technique is done by RGCC Lab. So, similar to this technique—it's called antisense therapy, which has been used in Europe for over fifteen years. But it's not genetic therapy like antisense, and it's not a drug. It's not a chemotherapy.

So basically our cell in our body, good or bad, they are all led via your DNA. DNA tells them what to do. So then what RGCC does—they make a messenger RNA. They prepare a messenger RNA, which is genetically modulated to the patient's circulating tumor cell, cancer cell. So then, what it does is it causes apoptosis, which is programmed cancer cell death.

So what we do is we'll get a powder, like a tiny clear powder and make a solution out of it and give an IV to the patients. And then, within a few weeks, the patient usually has some symptoms. And once you have a tumor, they will have some tenderness. That tenderness will increase a little bit because—I usually tell people if the tumor is greater than three centimeters we don't want to do it because it can increase the size of the tumor initially.

The reason is it causes necrosis inside of the cancer cell. What is necrosis? Necrosis is cancer cell death. Basically it kills those cancer cells. So it can increase, cause obstruction if it is an area that it can cause obstruction.

So that's that. So we do that every four months. We give three treatments a year and it works in your body 24/7 for 12 to 16 weeks. But the efficacy of the treatment, I believe, goes down if someone is doing chemo right now, or radiation. And it doesn't work as well as—if people just had chemo and radiation.

But it may go down by 50 percent. It may slow down a little bit. But it still works, but not as well as someone who never had chemo or radiation.

Ty: Why do you think that is? Why do you think the chemo and the radiation might cause it to not work?

Dr. Bita Badakhshan: Because I think that it affects all your immune cells, all the cells in the body and then it will affect those, I think.

Ty: So that's the SOT treatment. It's something that you add to the other protocols?

Dr. Bita Badakhshan: Exactly. It's not like—even that patient I just talked to you about who's doing amazing, she's been doing SOT. And when I follow the prognosis—I don't follow the PET scan. I don't want her to do PET scans often—I say, "You know what? Let me follow your circulating tumor cell and the stem cells and let's see how you're doing." And I see that number going down.

So that's the best part with the SOT. We always do a baseline and after a couple of treatments—I don't do it right away. I say, "Let's do two treatments," depending what their circulating tumor cell is. Then I just follow that.

I have one patient with breast cancer. After a couple SOTs, three SOTs, her CTC has been stable. I'm like, "That's strange. It hasn't improved much at all." But stable is not a bad thing either. That means her cancer is not spreading. Because circulating tumor cells keep adding up, adding up, and then what do they do?

They go and metastasize, even regional, that area, recurrence, or they could go do distant metastasis. That is what happens. That is why patients are like, "But I removed the whole breast. I removed all this. Why is it somewhere else?" It's because of the CTC.

Even conventional doctors, oncologists, they do know about it, and there is a lot of research. If you look at the clinical oncology they do a lot of research and they measure the circulating tumor cell and they realize it is a worse prognosis the higher the number is. And also they see that chemo doesn't really affect those numbers. It doesn't bring the circulating tumor cell to zero.

Ty: That was my next question then. Do traditional oncologists know about the circulating tumor cells?

Dr. Bita Badakhshan: They should know.

Ty: And do the treatments that they use do anything to affect them?

Dr. Bita Badakhshan: There's a lot of clinical studies now in conventional oncologists. They do. But regular patients who go to their doctors—they don't measure it, no. And also circulating tumor cell and stem cell done in U.S lab is not as good as the one we're doing in RGCC.

Ty: And that's the lab in Greece?

Dr. Bita Badakhshan: Yeah. The lab in Greece.

Ty: Okay, for me it just make sense that you would measure the circulating tumor cells, the circulating stem cells, because that's the real measure of the cancer. Not, "Did you cut out a tumor?"

Dr. Bita Badakhshan: Exactly, and when I see a patient—a patient could have stage one triple negative breast cancer, both of them, but one may have worse prognosis. I check their CTCs. One of them may have an immune system very suppressed, CTC very high. She's not going to do as good as the other patient. That's what it tells me. I tell them, "PET scan this, that, it doesn't really help me much. I need to know the circulating tumor cells and nagalase level.

Nagalase level tells me where your immune system is at. In a healthy patient your nagalase level should be less than one. But if you have virus or cancer in your body the nagalase level tends to be higher. So I actually started on my regular healthy patients, who don't have the diagnosis of cancer, but have viruses in their body—measure the nagalase level. If it's high, or higher than one, I tell them, "Your immune system is being suppressed, and then you're going to develop cancer."

So I prevent them. I change their lifestyle. I put them on natural, like essiac tea, for viruses and other stuff and I measure their nagalase. Once it's normal I say, "Okay."

Ty: So essiac tea is one of the things that will get the nagalase levels down. Dr. Panelli mentioned GcMAF.

Dr. Bita Badakhshan: Yeah, GcMAF and Bravo suppositories we use, but essiac tea doesn't necessarily bring nagalase levels down, but it kills the viruses. Since viruses produces the nagalase level, indirectly you're right. You are right. Indirectly it will bring it down. But for our cancer patient, because we may have cancer patients who don't have virus who have elevated nagalase level.

And I have, sometimes, stage fours with lower circulating tumor cells and lower nagalase and I know they're doing better because their immune system is doing great compared to someone with stage two with high CTCs and high nagalase levels.

Ty: So these measurement tests, they really help you to get a better sense of if the patient is improving or not.

Dr. Bita Badakhshan: Exactly. We follow those and there is no radiation, no toxicity, and nagalase is only a hundred dollars. It's not too expensive either for them. CTC is a little bit more, about 450 Euro or, depending, 600 Euro.

Ty: So, Dr. Bita, last question. What would you say to somebody that's recently been diagnosed with cancer? What questions should they ask their oncologist to figure out if they are going to receive adequate treatment or not?

Dr. Bita Badakhshan: Okay, if someone got recently diagnosed with cancer, first of all you want to know why. Why did you get cancer? Going, rushing into doing chemo, radiation, surgery is not the way to go. And they shouldn't get scared. It's just a wake-up call for them to change their lifestyle, change everything and trying to have their body fight this.

Your body can handle anything as long as you don't hurt it. You have good sleep. You don't have stress. You make sure you drink water enough and all the basic stuff. And they should want to do different kind of labs to see what kind of nutritional deficiency they have, what they do, and boost their immune system before they do any surgery, any chemo, any other things.

Or look at the integrative part of it. See your other options. I mean chemo is good, for cancers like—some fast—like some testicular cancer, some leukemia lymphomas. Some cancers do respond to chemo. But some less solid tumor cancer, like breast, lung, melanomas, those you don't respond. And patients say, "Oh that's not true, because there are patients who have been living for 20 years after doing chemo." Yeah, because circulating tumor cells in your body can live 30 years.

I have a patient that was diagnosed with melanoma 30 years before and then died with seizure because the CTC end up going to his brain after 30 years. So we know circulating tumor cells, stem cells, can live forever, and it all depends on your immune system and how your body is handling it. If you have perfect immune system, you take care of your body well, you keep the circulating tumor cells in control.

I mean, I tell people—later stage, you could live with your cancer forever. Like diabetes, like hypertension, you just have to keep the immune system good.

Ty: So then your message to somebody who may have been diagnosed with what the oncologist says is terminal cancer is, "Don't give up."

Dr. Bita Badakhshan: Exactly. Don't give up. Don't give up. That's the thing, you have to be willing to fight. It's all you. If you give up, if you say, "Oh, that's it." That's it. You have to first be very strong, decide that you are going to fight it, and you can do it. You could fight it. That's the thing. You could do it if you really want to.

And you look at the other alternate, integrative ways. You don't rush into it. Do your own research. You have time. You don't get cancer overnight. You've been having this for years.

Ty: So take the time to make a good decision, maybe find a doctor like yourself.

Dr. Bita Badakhshan: Thank you.

Ty: Thank you Dr. Bita. I appreciate it.

Dr. Bita Badakhshan: Thank you, pleasure to be here.

[end of transcript]

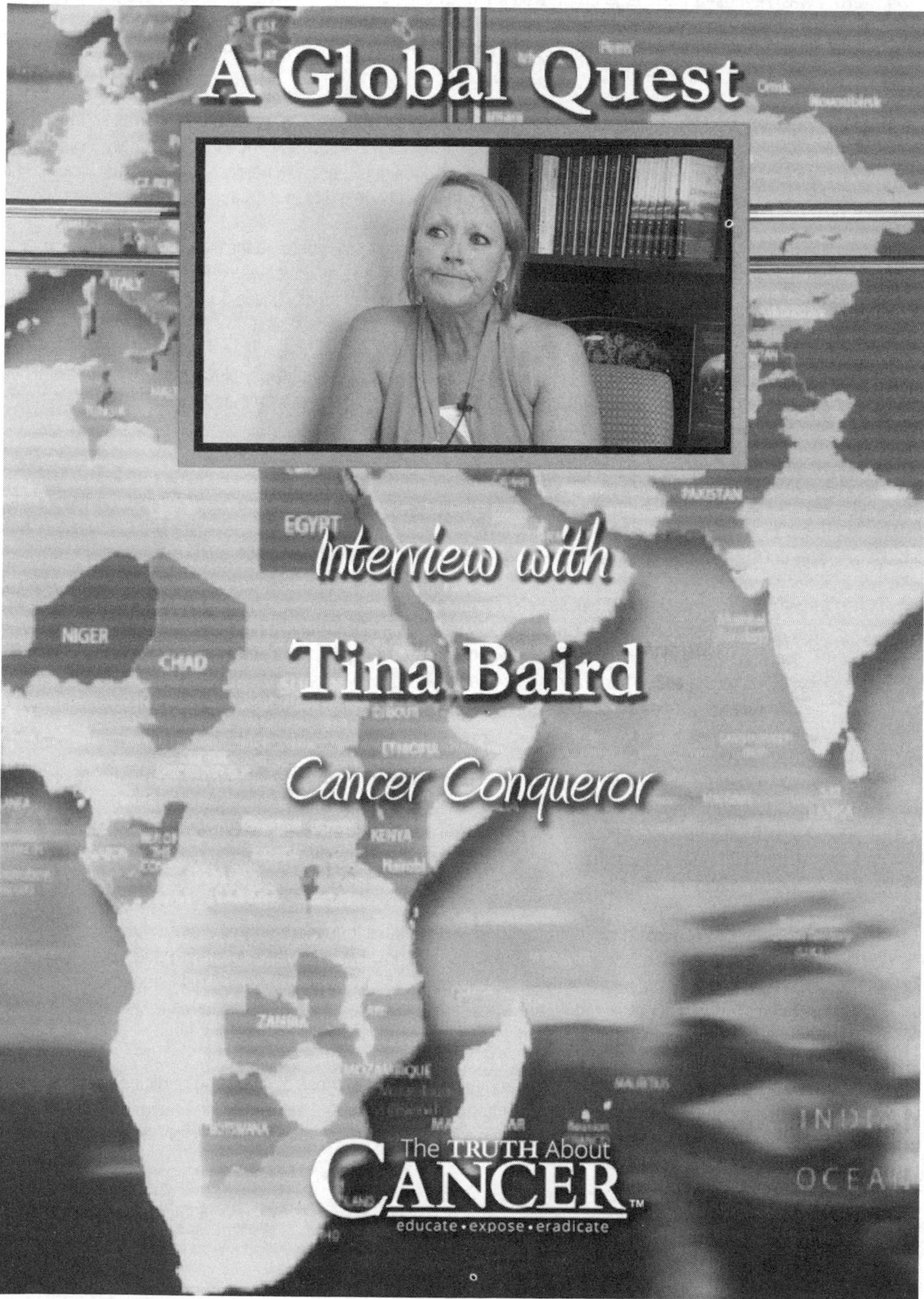
A Global Quest
Interview with
Tina Baird
Cancer Conqueror
The TRUTH About
CANCER
educate • expose • eradicate
EGYPT
NIGER
CHAD
ETHIOPIA
KENYA
ZAMBIA
MOZAMBIQUE
PAKISTAN
ITALY
INDIA
OCEA

Tina Baird: I was diagnosed with Stage 2A breast cancer December of 2010. I was 45. Then in 2011 I ended up doing chemo first, six rounds of chemo, starting the first of February 2011. Then after that, I had surgery, a double mastectomy in July of 2011 and then radiation in October/November 2011. So I had the full gamut of treatment.

I remember thinking, "I just want to close my eyes, and I just don't want to wake up." I was so mad at the world and the doctors. I just thought this isn't working and how can you feel so bad? My tongue was swollen, but I didn't know it was swollen. I had all kinds of issues, was hardly eating and just sick. I thought I just want to close my eyes and not wake up the next day and do this again.

Then when I woke up the next day I thought, "Well, darn it. I've got to go through this, I've got to go through another treatment." I wanted to quit but felt like it was a sign of weakness. And me being type A, we've got to go through it and just get to the finish line. I thought, "this is not really a way of living. This is being poisoned." I felt it and just didn't have the courage to stop it.

At the beginning of last year I was doing blood tests every six months. My blood tests came back elevated. So I went in for another bone scan, CT scan, PET scan this time and found it in sternum and a spot on my left hip.

I did one round of chemo and then at point that is where Ty Bollinger and Chris Wark and even Kelly Turner's book *Radical Remissions* had just come out and it was just released. I saw that the day I went in for my round and couldn't get the book in time so I had that first round of chemo and came home that day, got the book, started reading the book and then that's when I stopped the chemo.

In talking with Chris, I asked him who he recommended, if he knew of anybody here in the Charlotte area and he recommended Dr. Buttar. That's how I got to Dr. Buttar. I think it was God just saying, "There's another option for you." That's when I said "Okay, stop. I don't care what happens. I've got to look at something else. This is someone else speaking to me, someone else higher is speaking, and I need to listen." I just know I would not be here today, not at all. I wouldn't have made the 12 rounds, the 12 treatments.

When you get that diagnosis, you're shell shocked and you just—it just takes all the breath out of you and… sorry. It just takes you right down to your knees. When I talk to other people, I tell them you have other options. I tell them about Ty and I tell them about Bill Henderson or Chris Wark or Dr. Buttar or a thousand other doctors out there that are actually trying to get the message out that you don't have to go the conventional way.

I feel better today than I have in probably 10 years. I have tons more energy. I started running again and I ran three to five miles until I broke my arm and now I'm back down to square one. But I feel better today than I have in probably 10 years. Thank you to Ty and Chris and Bill Henderson. I've watched all of Ty's documentaries, the whole entire thing several times. I continue to watch some of his excerpts on Facebook when he'll bring some of those out every once in a while.

Dr. Gonzalez. And a big thank you to each and every one of those doctors who participated because they truly saved my life and I think Dr. Buttar definitely is one of those—if I didn't have that I wouldn't think I would have had another option. So it's just a huge thank you. Thank you for doing what they're doing.

[end of transcript]

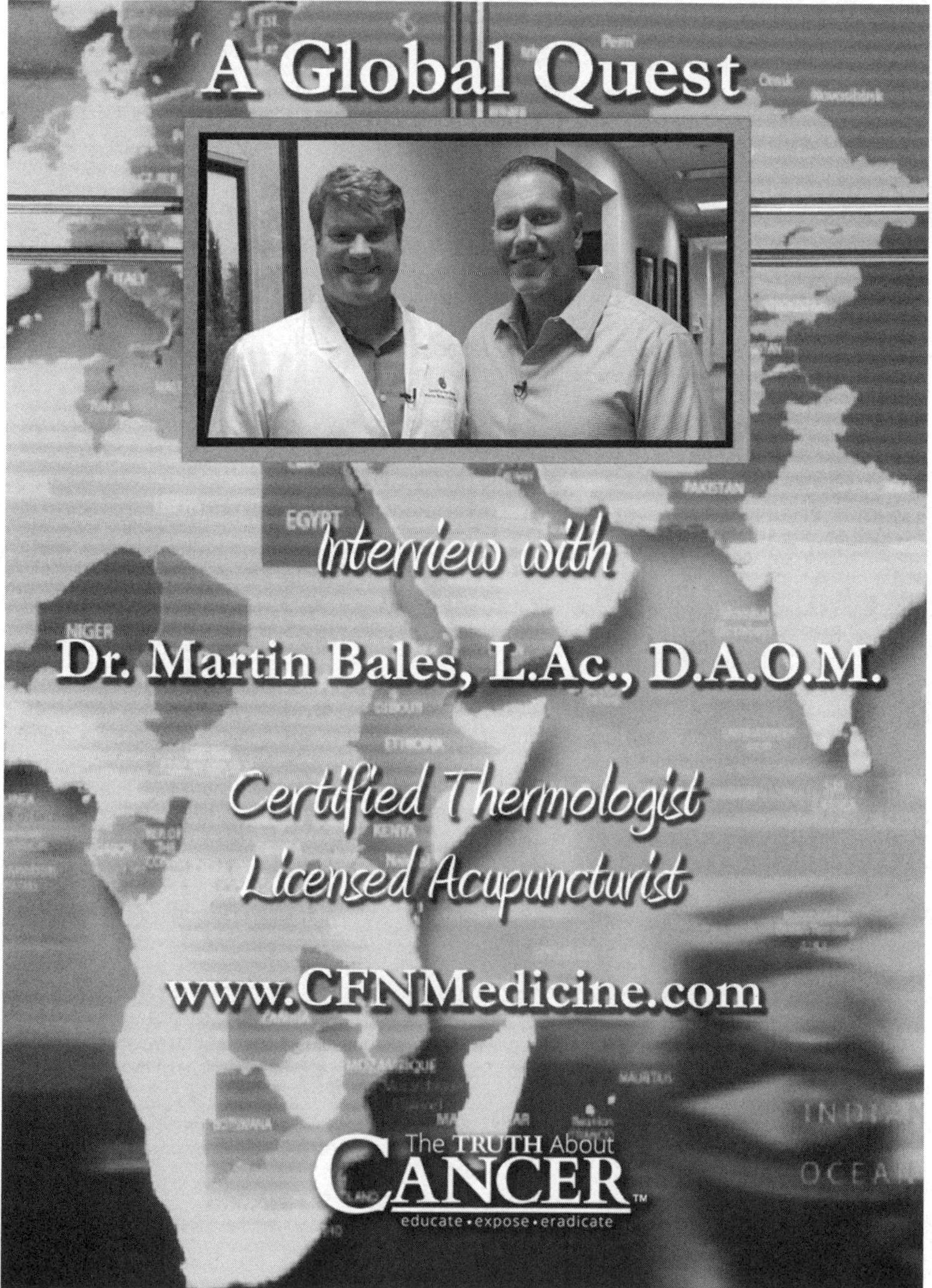
A Global Quest
Interview with
Dr. Martin Bales, L.Ac., D.A.O.M.
Certified Thermologist
Licensed Acupuncturist
www.CFNMedicine.com
The TRUTH About
CANCER
educate • expose • eradicate

Ty: We've heard about the PEMF machines, the PMF machines, pulsed electromagnetic fields—frequencies actually—and Dr. Martin Bales is here with me today to help explain that. Thank you for being with us.

Dr. Bales: You're welcome.

Ty: I'm not cracking my knuckles, that's actually one of the machines that's ticking here. But if you could explain to the viewers, what is a PEMF machine and how does it work? And also thank you to Coleen, who is actually going to be receiving a treatment.

Dr. Bales: She is actually undergoing active treatment right now. That's the sound that you hear. So Ty, as you mentioned, PEMF is pulsed electromagnetic field therapy. The therapy is not new, it was actually first described by Tesla in the 1880s and 1890s. If you consider that malignant cells and also damaged tissue run at a lot lower voltage, or electrical potential, this therapy is designed to up the potential, or increase the energy of the cells. So, that makes the cancer unhappy. In addition, here at Center for New Medicine, when patients have the IV therapies or the hyperbaric oxygen, it helps drive those therapies and those nutrients to the affected area.

So as we can see with Coleen here, we've placed the loop, which is one of the attachments, right over her affected area—so we'll run that for ten minutes. And then we'll also run the mat which she's currently lying on—the blue mat here—for ten minutes, to help the electrical pitch in all the cells in her body.

Ty: So this is actually pulsing good electricity, or good frequencies. Is that what it is doing to the body?

Dr. Bales: Yes, it is. You know, we hear a lot about EMF and we know the dangers of the very high frequency EMF. The very low frequency is actually beneficial. It's similar to the earth's magnetic pulse that we are actually losing the effect of.

Ty: Is that one of the reasons—let me ask the question because I don't know—is that one of the reasons that you hear about people that are earthing—it's so good because their feet are touching the earth and they're getting those frequencies?

Dr. Bales: Correct. Earthing, or grounding is actually being able to be in touch with the earth as human civilization has been for all of time—most of its existence—and now we wear shoes so we're immune to that throughout the day.

Ty: Right, and you also mentioned earlier that your father invented a couple machines that are over here behind me. Can you describe them?

Dr. Bales: That's true, we use those as well in there, our big machines here for cancer therapy. There's the Bales Photonic Stimulator. It is designed to increase blood circulation to the area. So, once again when we have a soft tissue type cancer, and the patient has undergone the IV therapy, the hyperbaric oxygen, or even the SOT or low does chemo, we can focus those therapies to the specific area by vasodilating, or opening up the blood vessels. So it's a great way to kind of focus. A little bit of a joke—we say when patients undergo our therapy, they probably don't need it in their big toe, they need it in the affected tumor site. So all the therapies here are painless and we see each patient every day that they have the IVs.

Ty: I ask most doctors what was your "aha" moment, but seeing that your father invented this I think you're a lifer, right? You've always understood this.

Dr. Bales: I've always understood the photon—we had a pulse electromagnet for four years now and right away when we started implementing it with the therapies we were already offering, I could see an improvement in the patients.

Ty: So Dr. Bales, one of the things that we've learned over the last couple of years with these interviews is that a mammogram is not necessarily the best way to detect breast cancer. There are other ways that are much better, that are superior, and one of them is thermography.

You're going to demonstrate a thermographic machine for us today and talk about that.

Dr. Bales: I will. My father actually invented the first all-digital infrared camera in 1979. But it wasn't for anything with body or health, it was actually for our defense. It was used in missile detection back in Afghanistan.

Ty: So it was looking for heat.

Dr. Bales: It was looking for heat, for missiles. It used to be you had to track the missiles going across the sky manually. Now on our warheads we have that it does it automatically. In the early 80s a group of doctors approached my father and said,
"You know, we've heard the body—obviously is circulation—we can diagnose a lot of diseases by seeing where there's hot spots and where there's cold." He said, "Okay, I'll make a medical version for you."

Ty: Really? That's fascinating. But the first one was missile detection?

Dr. Bales: First was missile detection. So basically, it can be used in any part of the body. Probably—as most people have heard—the breast thermography is the most popular. And it's really limited as far as cancer to breast, possibly some skin cancer because it is skin deep. It doesn't look, like, for liver or other organs. But it's a great way—it's completely painless. The ladies like it because it's no pancake smasher, as they say. There's no ionizing radiation, so it can be done as little or as often as one wants. It's just in a cooled room that it's performed.

Ty: Okay, great.

Dr. Bales: So here on the screen I've pulled up a couple examples. So on the left here we'd see this woman—we would say is very low risk for acquiring breast cancer. Because there is not a lot of etching, you see the red or that around the breast tissue. She does have some red up in these areas. That means she's alive. That's her carotid and jugular. So we hope we have a little bit of circulation there.

As opposed to this image here on the right where you can see there's quite a lot of activity. Now, thermography is not a diagnostic, so it can't say you have cancer, or you have this. It's just a screening. So after this we would do one of many things, we would either watch the patient, have them in for a recall—this being their baseline. Or perhaps to go on to an MRI. You mentioned some of the limitations. There's been at least two studies, very large, that have come out, on the limitations on mammography. One of them was a Canadian study, I believe, it was 20 or 25 years that they've watched in the past. They found no benefit.

Also *The Lancet*—which is a large British journal equivalent to our *Journal of the American Medical Association*, known as JAMA—in that it said there is really no benefit at all to doing and possibly some harm. The harm being it is ionizing radiation, which we know isn't the best for us. And also, again with the pancake smasher, if you do have a cancer and you smash that wall that the body has put around it, are you spreading the disease that way? I don't know, but I don't want to find out.

Ty: Yeah, and then that's *The Lancet* right? That's pretty reputable.

Dr. Bales: It's pretty reputable and also the BMJ, *The British Medical Journal*, I believe, did a write up as well. That's two or three very reputable internationally published articles.

Ty: Yeah, it is. So talk about thermography as opposed to mammograms. Mammograms—this will detect pre-cancer cells way before a mammogram would right?

Dr. Bales: Right. All cancers, not just breast, but all cancers go through a process called neoangiogenesis, which is new blood vessel growth. Because the cancers grow faster than the healthy tissue around them, they have to have their own discreet blood supply after they're a couple years older. Well, it turns out that when most breast cancers—not all, there's a few that are faster, but most of them are actually quite slow growing—to become the size of a pea, is between eight and ten years. So if we can catch them in year one or two when they're just getting that new blood vessel supply, when the blood vessels are warm—and that's how the thermography is picking them up.

The mammography is about two thirds accurate at finding them when they're pea sized so they're already eight years old. So we're going more from a prevention standpoint. If we find something early on we can change the diet and lifestyle, perhaps use some of the therapies we've discussed here. As opposed to, okay, you've already had something for a year, it's already in this bucket, what can we do?

Ty: Right, and that's a huge difference, the eight years of formation of the cancer. If this can detect—I've read anywhere from five to seven years before a mammogram you can get a thermogram that will show pre-cancerous, or cancers that are forming. Whereas you would never know that with a mammogram.

Dr. Bales: Exactly. And the other benefit of thermography is, especially here at Cancer Center for Healing, is when a breast cancer patient comes in we can take a baseline, a pre-image. And then after a couple weeks of our therapies we can take another image and oftentimes it will show reversal of neoangiogenesis. So you can actually see the blood vessels starting to not dilate into that area because the cancer is dying off.

Ty: And this is way before anyone would be treated for breast cancer.

Dr. Bales: Exactly.

Ty: We're talking about the early stages before any other techniques that we currently use would even know that you had cancer—this is able to detect it.

Dr. Bales: Right, and the cancer would be the end of our pinkie or the size of a small thimble as opposed to something that's larger.

Ty: Right, right. It makes sense that this would be used. Is this used in very many places?

Dr. Bales: More and more. I think, as the word gets out, it's becoming accepted, if you will. You have to be careful. Unfortunately, thermography is not regulated by the FDA. You know, if you were to go in for an X-ray or CT scan or MRI, anywhere in our country it would be relatively the same level of image quality and care by the radiologist. So you have to be careful and I can give you a website that shows some of those certified centers.

Ty: So you want to make sure you're getting the real deal.

Dr. Bales: Right. As opposed to someone who just bought a camera and thinks they know what they're doing. It's about a thousand hours of training to read these. So, it's quite a program, as it should be. He did want that level.

Ty: You should be proud that your father really—the father of thermography.

Dr. Bales: Exactly. I guess I'm the son of thermography.

Ty: It's been a pleasure interviewing you, the son of thermography, Dr. Bales.

Dr. Bales: Thank you so much.

[end of transcript]

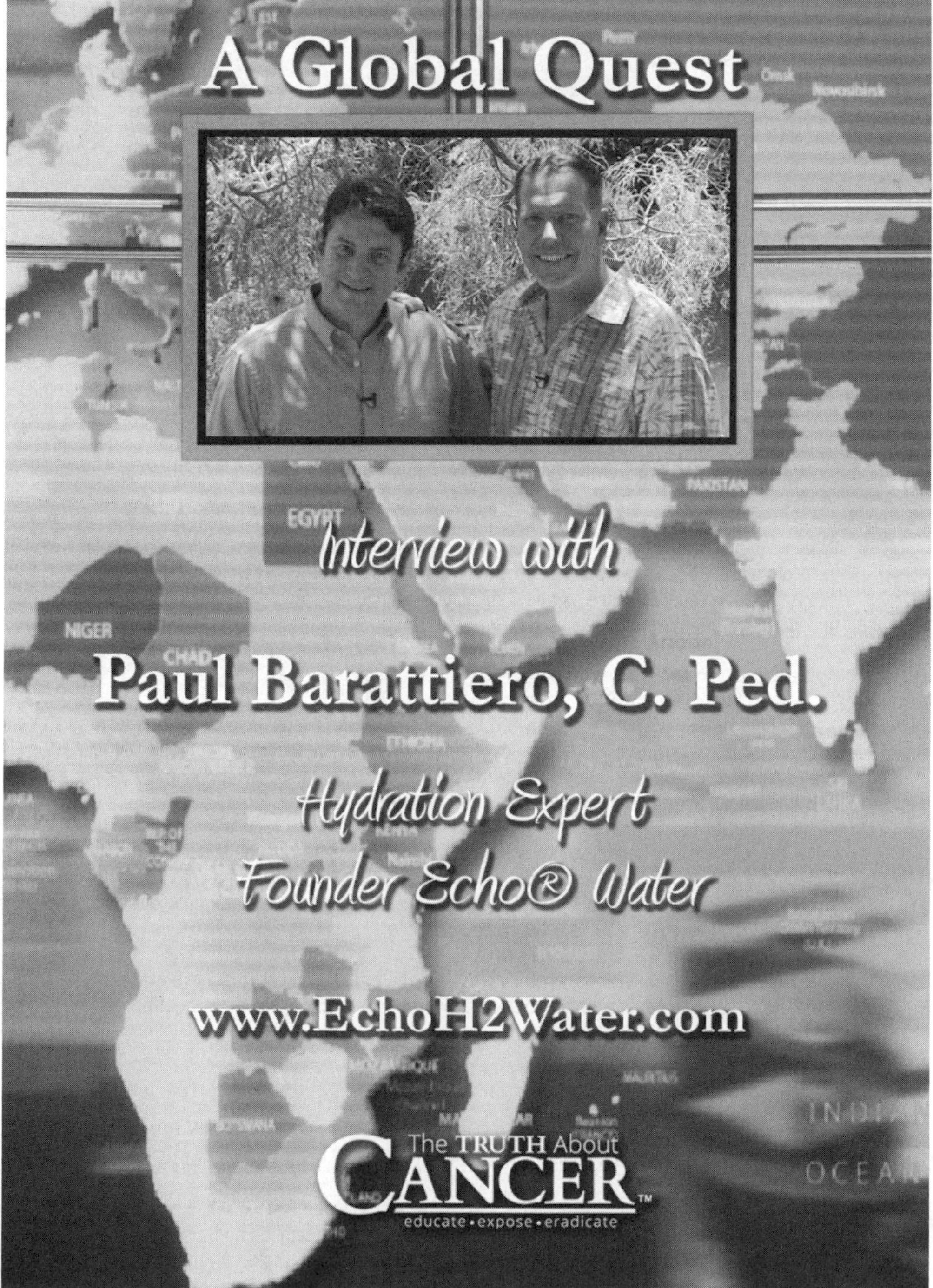
A Global Quest
Interview with
Paul Barattiero, C. Ped.
Hydration Expert
Founder Echo® Water
www.EchoH2Water.com
The TRUTH About
CANCER™
educate • expose • eradicate

Ty: I'm here at Shangri-La Resort in Naples, Florida, and I'm happy to have [with me] Paul Barattiero again.

Paul Barattiero: Nice to see you.

Ty: Paul, we talked last year, had a lot of great information that you shared about water. We're here so I thought it was appropriate to do the interview in front of water.

Paul Barattiero: That's right.

Ty: If you answer any of your questions wrong we're going to jump in together. So yeah, no right answers, no wrong answers. But what I want you to do this year is to get you to share a little bit more about the molecular hydrogen, because that's something that we didn't really get much of last year. And there's a lot of stuff, just in the last year that's come out, studies that have come out, that I want you to share with those that are watching.

Paul Barattiero: Absolutely. So, that's what it's all really about, even the water that we do. It's all about the molecular hydrogen. And we have over 400 studies, forty of which are human studies. So you've got double blind studies showing the therapeutic effects that molecular hydrogen has on 150 different human diseases and every organ in the body. So, very, very, very amazing breakthrough information is coming.

What we're also learning is that it has some cell signaling capabilities in the body. I was just in Japan at the Molecular Hydrogen Symposium, the medical symposium at Nagoya University, and they were showing that two hundred gene expressions can be changed; up regulated, down regulated, just from molecular hydrogen in the body.

Ty: Epigenetics.

Paul Barattiero: Yeah. So we have a very symbiotic relationship with the bacteria in our gut that produce hydrogen on a daily basis. You know, a lot of people, when they get cancer are told to eat a heavy fiber, healthy diet. Well, the fiber gets broken down by the bacteria and hydrogen is the bi-process that gets into the gut and into the body. So very, very powerful.

But what we're doing is, in the water we want to get as much concentration in parts per million of molecular hydrogen. Because we have a few studies on animals, a few human studies, and some cell studies, showing that molecular hydrogen benefits cancer. So there are therapeutic effects that, in preliminary studies, that it's actually beneficial for cancer.

And then, one of the main things, even for people that are taking chemo, that have made that decision, there are some huge benefits on the molecular hydrogen in stopping the negative effects on the body.

Ty: The negative effects of chemo. Great.

Paul Barattiero: Right.

Ty: So, how do you get molecular hydrogen into the water?

Paul Barattiero: Well, there are two main ways that we have. The water that we sell, the machine that produces it, in electrolysis. So, electrolysis, by virtue of having a cathode and a nanode, on that cathode produces hydrogen off of it. And so you have what's called molecular hydrogen, or diatomic. It's two hydrogen molecules together and then that gets into the body.

One of the main things it does is the most cytotoxic or cell damaging free radical in the body is called a hydroxyl radical. H2, or molecular hydrogen, combines with HO to create water in the cell. So, in the mitochondria, tremendous benefits. In the cells of the body, where you would have that free hydroxyl radical damaging the body, hydrogen gets in there, combines with it, and the bi-process is water. So you're converting the most cytotoxic free radical into water molecules. Very, very powerful.

Ty: And so it's actually converting something that could be really bad for you into something that's really good for you. Just with the molecular hydrogen combination.

Paul Barattiero: Right, right. And so the science of molecular hydrogen is—there are studies going on right now. We have over 400 now that we have found; there's more going on every day somewhere in the country. There are six right now in the US going on with prestigious universities. So, it will continue to advance, and they will continue to understand more and more the mechanisms of molecular hydrogen.

The other way is there are tablets on the market that we have that are elemental magnesium, a specific type of magnesium that, when you drop it in water, it produces significant amounts of hydrogen. And then there is inhalation. There are machines that produce hydrogen and people can inhale the hydrogen, which is another effective administration method.

Ty: Okay, so basic three methods. You can inhale it. And then there are the two methods that involve water. One is the pills, the drops in the water. Or the tablets in the water.

Paul Barattiero: That's right.

Ty: And then one is through an electrical machine.

Paul Barattiero: Right, electrolysis.

Ty: Electrolysis, okay.

Paul Barattiero: And so the studies on cancer particularly utilize a water ionizer that produces hydrogen and so that was what their studies used to produce the hydrogen. And one of the most effective methods of administration is dissolved molecular hydrogen in water and consuming it in that manner.

So, that is what most people do. They drink water with hydrogen in it for that reason, cause it's a very, very effective method of administration.

Ty: And that's what we do. Because we have one of the machines that you sell at our house. And so you sell the EcoWater system.

Paul Barattiero: Yes, I developed it, yeah.

Ty: You developed it too. Awesome, I didn't know you developed it as well, okay, awesome. So, that machine, I know there are different settings to the machine, but no matter which setting, on that machine, you're getting molecular hydrogen in the water?

Paul Barattiero: You are, as you move up the scale, there are four levels of the drinking water. The amount, or the concentration of molecular hydrogen increases. And so you can get more.

Ty: So it goes more alkaline? Are you getting more molecular hydrogen?

Paul Barattiero: It does. Well, you're getting more molecular hydrogen, you're also getting a higher pH, which is not beneficial. The pH itself is not therapeutic to the body, and what you can do is just put a few drops of lemon juice in that water to plummet the pH, cause there's very little buffering capacity in ionized water. You would have to drink ten thousand liters of a pH ten water to buffer the same amount of stomach acid as one teaspoon of baking soda.

Ty: Really?

Paul Barattiero: Yeah, no one's going to drink ten thousand liters of water any time soon. So, effectively there's very little buffering capacity. The pH is a bi-process of hydroxides being produced in the electrolysis.

Ty: So the real benefit then of this type of water is not the alkaline water, it's the molecular hydrogen that's produced and then the alkaline pH is a byproduct of that.

Paul Barattiero: Right, and the easy way, people could use vitamin C powder, a tiny bit, or they could use drops of lemon juice, it doesn't take very many. And that pH will be gone, but you'll still have the hydrogen in high concentration.

Ty: So, you say the pH will be gone, so you don't want the high alkaline water, is that what you're saying?

Paul Barattiero: No, really when you drink levels of pH more than ten on a regular basis, there can be potassium issues in about 15 percent of the population, certain individuals. So, drinking a high pH is not beneficial.

Ty: So, that may be a myth that's going around. High pH water is not necessarily beneficial.

Paul Barattiero: Completely. While most people cited Otto Warburg in saying that cancer can't live in an alkaline environment. That's actually false. He never said that. It's just misinformation from marketing people. And in fact, many cells don't actually duplicate in cancer until they accomplish alkalosis. So, it gets into the science of how a cancer cell functions.

Ty: So, what exactly did Warburg say in his Nobel Prize?

Paul Barattiero: He never even got his Nobel Prize having to do with cancer.

Ty: It wasn't about cancer?

Paul Barattiero: No. So many people think that because the ionizer company is promoting it. We have a whole page to right the wrong of Otto Warburg and say what he did actually get his Nobel Prize in. And we have all the stuff cited there so that you can actually understand it. So, we're happy to share that.

Ty: I'm happy to see that, awesome.

Paul Barattiero: So we do have studies. It's true science. It's not pseudo-science, which I think is important. It's good to be able to know what the mechanism is and it's good for people to be drinking hydrogen-enriched water and that's where we focus.

Ty: Great. Well, thank you for all your work in hydrogen-enriched water. My family thanks you because we drink it every time we take a drink of water from our kitchen. We're drinking the EcoWater. So, Paul, thank you for sharing today.

Paul Barattiero: Thank you very much. Appreciate it.

Ty: Okay.

[end of transcript]

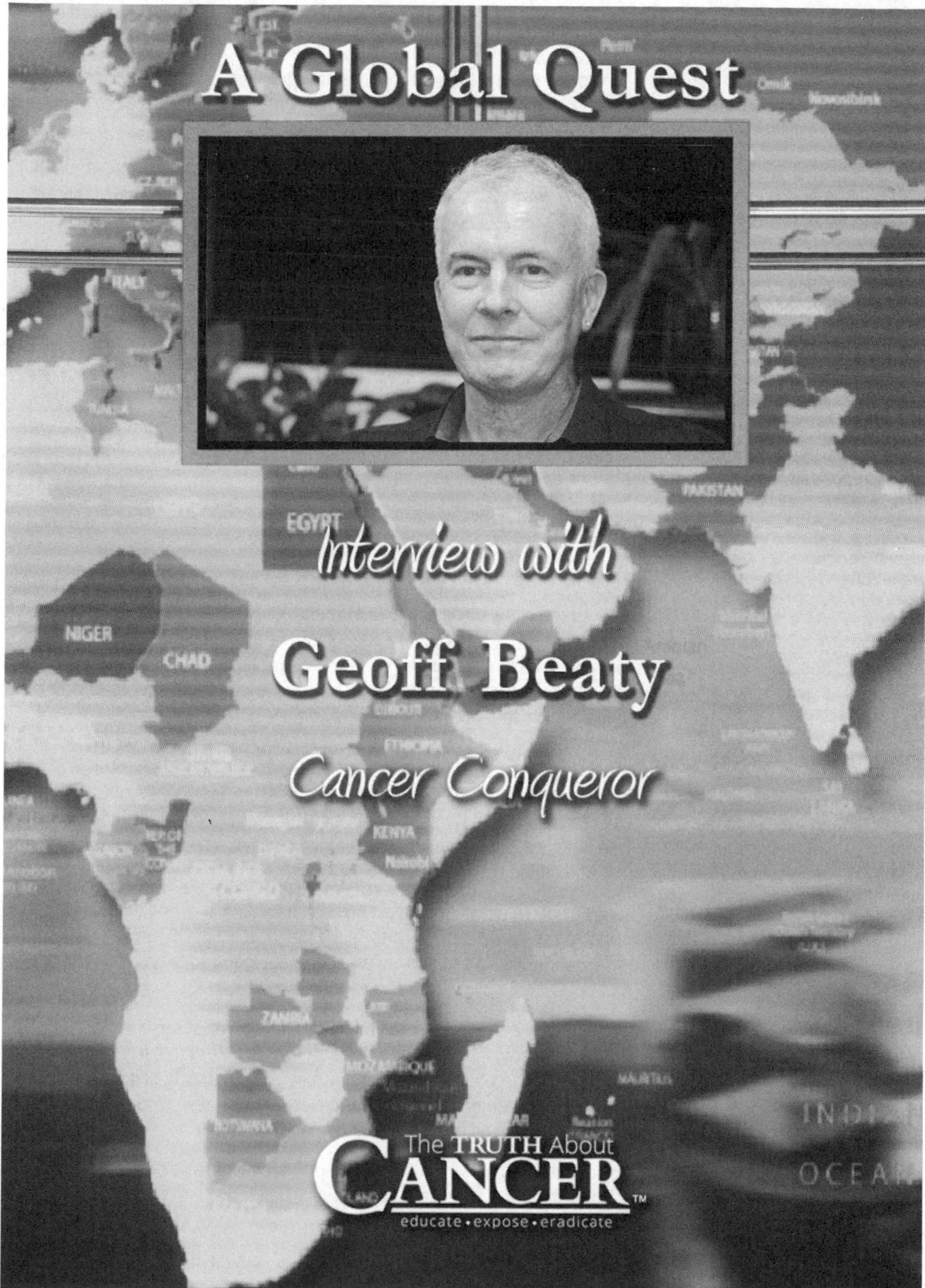
A Global Quest
Interview with
Geoff Beaty
Cancer Conqueror
The TRUTH About
CANCER
educate • expose • eradicate

Interviewer: I'm very interested to know as to how everything happened. Let's go back to the start with the diagnosis. That's obviously the biggest deal. What happened when you went in to see the doctor?

Every story is unique and that, obviously, would have meant something unique to you when that was happening. What was happening in your life at that time? And then when you got that diagnosis, what did that mean to you, what was being said? Take me back to that place.

Geoff: I had some big problems going on in a relationship, and that had been going on for some time. When I was coming up the stairs I felt very, very dizzy, and I didn't recover quickly. And when I didn't recover, and I had some bowel issues, it was clear I had to do something. I was severely disoriented and dizzy.

And when I went to the hospital they discovered quite quickly I had lost six pints of blood, which is half of my blood supply. So then the investigations began. There was a lot of stuff that went on in the hospital, to start off with, that wasn't really good and wasn't managed very well, but it took quite a lot of finding—endoscopies, and colonoscopies.

And eventually, after several of each of those, I swallowed a camera. And after it came out I got quite stressed because it took quite a while for them to find where it was, because it took a photo every two seconds or something, as it went along. And so, there were hundreds and hundreds of photos that they had to go through, and eventually they found it.

Interviewer: They found what?

Geoff: A gastrointestinal stromal tumor.

Interviewer: How did you feel when you got that news?

Geoff: Well, it was a hell of a shock, but they took me into surgery within a couple of days and took out a foot of my small intestine. And then, actually, it was kind of like another world at that time. It was difficult because I was not—my relationship was in such a bad way. So I was in hospital pretty much alone and trying to deal with this thing—this foot of small intestine that I lost, and a future that was up in the air. There's not a lot of people who survive that one.

Interviewer: Yes?

Geoff: Yes. And the Gleevec, I'm sure, did help—or Glivec it's called, and Gleevec in the US. It helped, but it also knocked the stuffing out of me, and yes, it was very difficult. And then I had a second one a couple of years later, a different type of tumor. Then investigations started so there were a whole lot of colonoscopies and endoscopies and they couldn't find it.

After multiple attempts then they put a—I swallowed a pill that had a camera in it, and that found it, and I had a gastrointestinal stromal tumor. So as soon as they found that, in a couple of days I was—oh, they did another endoscopy to try and get to it to see more about it, but they had to go down a long way, so that was a difficult one.

A couple of days later I was in surgery and they took out a foot of my small intestine, it was a gastrointestinal stromal tumor. It was about 10 cm so it was very—I'm very lucky that it bled. If it hadn't have bled and it had got much bigger, I probably wouldn't have survived. So they took it out, and I was put on chemotherapy—Glivec. I think in America it's called Gleevec. And that was hard. It just knocked the energy out of me. It was difficult, I stayed on it for a year.

And I think something about that affected me. I got a second tumor sometime later on. That was probably a few years, I can't remember, exactly, probably two years later, and that was in my neck. And it grew very rapidly.

And I decided that I want to approach this not just medically. So once I got the diagnosis for that I didn't have to think about it. Treatment would have been chemo and radiation, but I just didn't want it all coming back again. So I knew that if I just did straight medical stuff it was not necessarily—you know, this was the second time around.

So I then had the treatment that was involved but I went and approached Manuela. And Manuela put me on a regime of things that during the treatment—because I got Western medical treatment, but I also got Manuela's treatment.

There were a whole lot of people that I knew that were diagnosed at the same time and I watched us all go through, and the difference in me and the other people was amazing. I just coped with the treatments so much better. Less nausea—I didn't need to be fed by a tube, which nearly all of them did that were going through at the same time. And you could see just by looking at me that I was coping much better than the others. It was still not a lot of fun. It was difficult to go through. But I did cope much better.

I had much less of the burns from the radiation on my neck than the other people. But once the treatment stopped I just started picking up very quickly, and within six weeks I could go back to work. And because we were cycled in going back to the doctors at the same time through the hospital, I saw a number of the others and many of them four and five months later still were not back at work. They were still not in great shape.

So, what Manuela did for me made a huge difference. The herbs, and the nutrients, and the diet that I was on just made a huge difference in my recovery. And now, three and a half years on, I'm back to full strength. And I've been back to full strength for quite a while. Just amazing. Really, really good. Feels good. And I feel confident that it's not coming back, so I'm here to stay.

Interviewer: That's great, man. It's unique. What a cool recovery, what a cool journey.

Geoff: It was pretty intense, absolutely. What was remarkable was seeing the difference between myself and the others. And they hadn't been through two sets, they had only had the secondary one, the head and neck tumor.

Interviewer: Whereas you…

Geoff: I had been through—this was my second lot and I still recovered way better than any of the others. It was amazing to see the difference.

Interviewer: Why did you recover so well?

Geoff: What I was on—the herbs. And that was difficult, too, getting the medicos to accept that I wanted to do this. It took a lot of negotiation and Manuela supplied me with a lot of information that I could take to them and the testing—what do you call it? Research data, that I took to them, showed them. We argued over a few things, we gave in on a few things. But it made a big difference, a really big difference.

Interviewer: That's incredible, man. And in terms of what new things—you mentioned some of the things that you were struggling with before, what doors opened for you in terms of the things you have seen since—like what quality of life have you you seen?

Geoff: Well, after the first one I realized that my relationship was not okay and I ended that one. And the thing that I learned was that I was not cutting out dead wood. Things that are dead you need to remove from your life, and I wasn't doing that, and it was festering and causing a big problem. And I think that was a big part of my healing, learning to do that. I've always been a very positive person, but I wasn't good at ending stuff that wasn't okay. I just kept going.

Interviewer: I think it is an incredible contrast between the two groups. There was the one group that was declining, and in a competitive sense, it is like, "Well, cool—you won." But then in a relational sense, it's like, "Well, these are people that are really suffering." During that stage, did you know the people that were going through that?

Geoff: Not really. Initially, we were in the same wards at various times when we were getting treatment. But it was only conversational, I didn't know any of them personally. But you got to see them and their families. And a couple of them were quite a bit younger than myself and you'd expect that they would have done better, but they didn't. Those that were a little bit older than me, they took a lot longer, a lot longer. But these younger ones still took longer than I did, considerably, more than double.

Interviewer: Did you feel sorry for them?

Geoff: I felt frustrated that we weren't allowed to talk to them about the other options that they could possibly have. The medical machine had them, and sure, it was good that they had that, but there were many other things that could have helped them on their journey. But were not on offer, and it wasn't okay for us to talk about them.

A couple of the doctors were very interested in the progress I made and how quick I was recovering, and they wanted to know what was going on and how it was being achieved. But most didn't. A couple of the younger ones that were coming through were quite interested.

Interviewer: There's a real feeling when you feel like you have your hands tied, and there is something that you really want to share, and you've been all this time living in a free country where you could basically say whatever you thought on any subject to anyone and any time, almost, within reason. But here, you weren't able to say something that could have saved somebody's life. You weren't able to say that.

Geoff: No. No.

Interviewer: Is that okay?

Geoff: Not really. But it is what it is.

Interviewer: Are you content with that?

Geoff: I would really like to—the fact that we are getting out in this sort of way is really good.

Interviewer: It sounds like you couldn't be silent then.

Geoff: Oh no. And when there is an opportunity, I talk about it. But another person who is very close to me went through the same thing that I did, went through exactly the same treatment, and she has ended up with no saliva at all. I have a reduced saliva now, but hers—there's nothing. So she is never going to recover. And I think, again, some of the things that I took protected those organs from the possible damage that they would have.

Interviewer: You finding these natural treatments, you finding Manuela—what does that mean to you? What has she meant to you, to be able to help you like that?

Geoff: Well, it was a Godsend. How can I repay her, and how can I say enough about these things? I think she knows how much it has meant to me. I have a quality of life now that is great, and life ongoing. What do you say? It's worth everything isn't it?

Interviewer: That's a gift you give to her, that gratitude.

Geoff: It is a gift. It's a gift to me. I hope she knows how much it has meant to me.

Interviewer: Well, Geoff, your life is a precious gift, and it is a Godsend because your life is a gift from God and it wasn't your time, and…

Geoff: Yes.

Interviewer: And you obviously had the fight in you.

Geoff: Absolutely.

Interviewer: What do you think—if you were talking to a former version of yourself—imagine that is me—what would you say to me if I was in that battle right now, and confused, afraid, feeling that impending fear, that there isn't hope. And that this is all going home to an imminent end, and that's me right now, what would you say to me right now?

Geoff: There's always hope, healing is available but it's not always in the places that are promoted by the system. That many of the alternative things—you have to be careful, of course, and find someone who is really good and does know what they're talking about. And that is sometimes a bit challenging, but it's really important for your own healing to do that, to find a person who can really help you, or people, it's not always just one person. People who can help you mentally, psychologically, spiritually, and with substances and nutrition, that will help you survive.

And there's a lot—and from what Manuela tells me, there is more research going on all the time and it gives us more hope, more ways of doing this. The medical stuff—it does save lives, but also I think it costs lives as well, sometimes. And it's unnecessary. So, very hard to fight that, that's there. But I would encourage someone to look beyond, to look at herbs, to look at nutrition, look at diet, look at lifestyle, look at your spiritual status. Take a good look, and learn. Open yourself up to all the things that are available, because there is a lot.

Interviewer: If there is one thing that you would see, your success, and your recovery, and attribute that to—there are many—but let's rephrase the question. If there is one particular thing you would like to share with us that was very incredibly helpful for you, what was that? It seems like Manuela had shared with you some things and was there one particular thing, like this really helped me? I don't know, like the coffee enema, you know?

Geoff: I think it was the herbal formulas. I can feel them—the impact of them. They were very powerful and gave me more energy, cut down the nausea a lot. It was like superfood, and the superfoods that you get from the health food shop you don't really feel. They might be doing you good. This I felt. I felt the lift that it was giving me. So the herbal formulas were great.

Interviewer: That's great. And when you were taking those herbs, those superfoods, did you feel hope coming back into your life?

Geoff: The lift that they gave me certainly did give me a lift, a hope. But I knew, and I don't know how I knew, that I was going to beat this, whatever it took. But I wanted to also be as healthy as possible at the end of it. And I think that it was the herbs, particularly, because I could feel them making a difference, that really helped.

Interviewer: Thank you for sharing.

Geoff: Well, thank you.

[end of transcript]

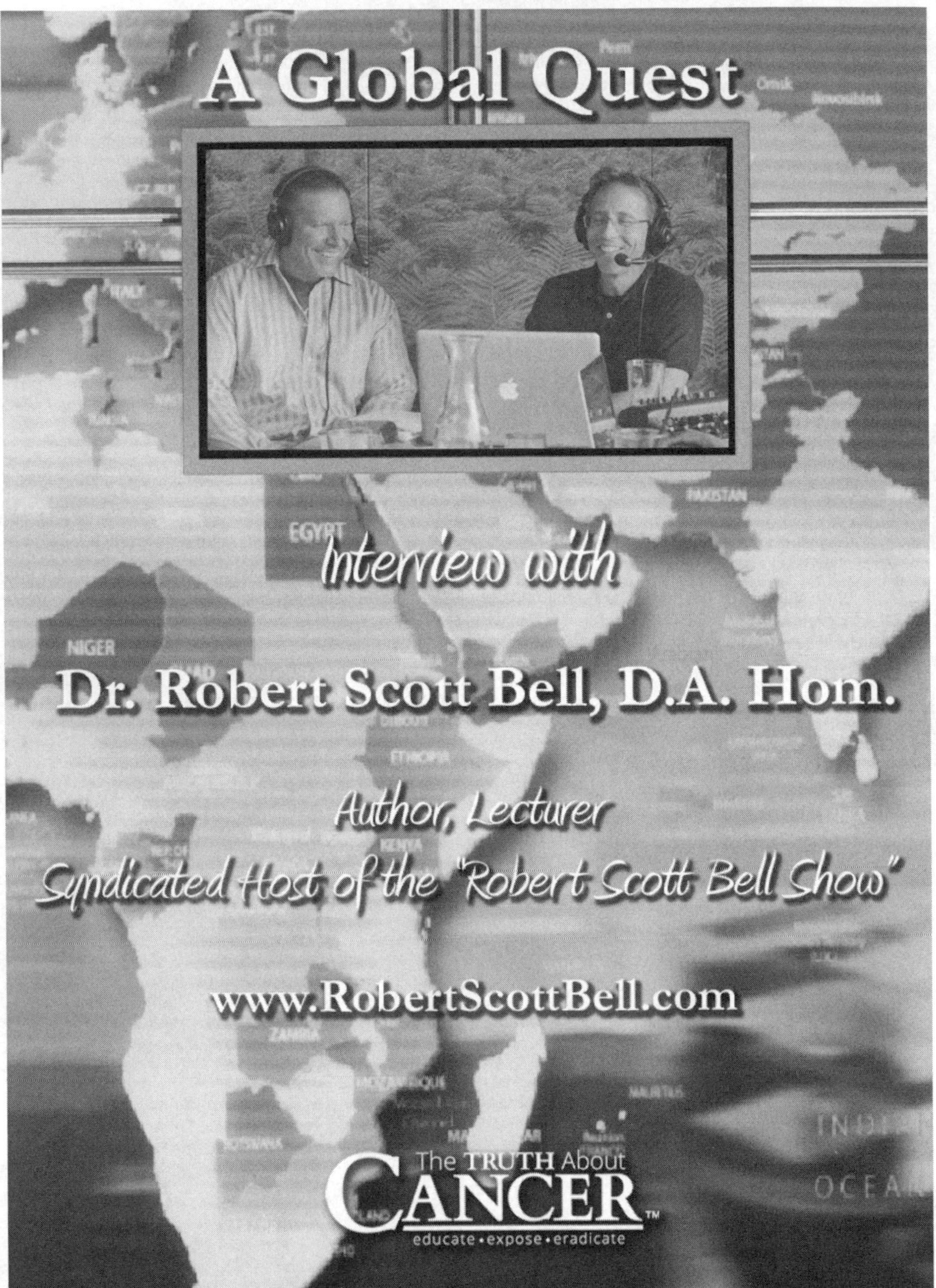
A Global Quest
Interview with
Dr. Robert Scott Bell, D.A. Hom.
Author, Lecturer
Syndicated Host of the "Robert Scott Bell Show"
www.RobertScottBell.com
The TRUTH About
CANCER™
educate • expose • eradicate

Ty: All right. Robert Scott Bell, we meet again, my friend.

Dr. Bell: Ty Bollinger, it is so good to be reunited with you.

Ty: I was really impressed with your interviews last year, got a lot of great feedback from people who saw the *The Quest for the Cure*, said we've got to have some more RSB, so got you back here. We're in Naples, Florida. Beautiful place here.

Dr. Bell: Yes.

Ty: It's a very historic place, Shangri-La, a lot of historical significance. So what I want get you to today is go back in time, give us a little history. You gave us some history last year on the Flexner Report. Let's talk about the history of food to start with. Over the last 100 years, how has food morphed into what it is today?

Dr. Bell: Well, I grew up in a pharmaceutical raised family and we went to the grocer's freezer to eat. So as a child, I didn't know where food came from. I heard about this thing called a farm and I heard about animals in the wild, but that wasn't anything other than what you've heard, stories about.

So the transformation of food happened prior to my coming on to this planet in the 1960s and the reality is the processing industry, the ability to ship food long distances, the ability to keep food fresh for days, months even or more meant the adding of synthetic chemistry—if you will. The organic chemist from Germany that imported this idea, we can color your food, we can make it last longer and these synthetic chemicals were thought to be benign at least initially and really cool because look what we can do with it. We can even make things taste differently, artificial flavors.

But at the time they didn't consider the unintended consequences of synthetic chemicals interacting with our own bodies' organic chemistry, it is organic as well, and altering it negatively. In other words having a negative impact—being let's say, toxin-burdened, if you will.

We don't know how to metabolize things if we don't know how to metabolize things, right? If it's been in the food supply for thousands or however many years, our body has adapted, it knows what to do, there are break down components, we combine, we can enzymatically break it down. We can then excrete.

If, however, you introduce something through a lab—a chemical, that has never before been in existence anywhere on the planet and then you introduce it into a biological system, the system looks at it and says, I don't know what you are. It might to our higher minds look like something we might recognize, but to the chemistry of the body itself, it's foreign. So it must be looked at almost an enemy and we must then relinquish certain things that will protect us, the antioxidants, the minerals. And in this way we begin the depletion process, not only the toxicological burden to the body, but we begin to diminish the very vital nutrients that keep all of the functions going—at a more accelerated rate. And then we don't replace them as much because those chemicals, those synthetic organic chemicals, begin to replace the minerals and things that would normally be in the food that we would eat that work actually from the farm or from your garden or from the wild. That is something I've had to learn of course later in my life from the city slicker kid to the country boy—that I like to pretend that I am.

Ty: What we've got then, now, are foods that while they make look like food and they taste sort of like food, they're really not recognized as pure foods by our body. So we're not getting the nourishment—we're not getting the nutrition from these foods. I guess maybe that's how food has changed over the last 100 years. They didn't have canned food before the 1940s.

Dr. Bell: Canning of course is benign compared to some things that are done, but certainly the addition of certain cans that contained lead or other things and now this phenol A with the plastifier is very disruptive of hormones, normal endocrine function—that becomes corrupting of a food that could still be viable in a canned stay. But even fresh frozen might be optimal, but then again, the idea of moving back to the food production at home is what I've been encouraging for so long and something that I desperately missed in my childhood.

When we talk about eating the chemically grown laden foods, the first response by the body should be rejection. I think we may have talked about this in the last series about how I projectile vomited the baby formula out of me as fast as mom put it in me, because it was not designed to be eaten.

Some things within food that is chemically altered that the body does recognize and will and must in order to survive if that's all you're going to be given. So you kind of modulate a little bit of defense with every meal, in other words your body goes into a state of fight or flight by defending against an assault from food, which it shouldn't—if it were just food, the chemicals that were added to it for instance and then you find a way to deal with something that's good in there for your own survival and again that's the adaptation principle. The adaptation for survival, that Hans Selye taught us all about.

Now we're dealing with the—how much of that food puts our body in a state of fight or flight defensive posture versus how much of that food puts us into a state of growth and healing? How much is actually nourishing to the body? It's this constant battle.

There was a recent study out of Sweden that was interesting. It was a two week analysis, very brief, but what it showed was just so profound. A family that was eating conventionally grown non-organic foods, pesticide laden, who thought it was too expensive to eat organic. They did a test, they said, alright, we're going to take urine samples when you start, eating your regular food, then we're going to switch the whole family, kids, parents, everybody, to organic. Over the course of even one day and ultimately two weeks, the pesticide levels in the urine was extraordinarily high in everything and each day it dropped to the point in two weeks it was almost undetectable.

Now that tells you how fast the body can adapt once you've stopped putting the onslaught in. In other words the things that you put in you a defensive posture. Now I'm not saying they're out of the woods in two weeks, but the reality is, as the body then regains that strength that it used to defend against and detoxify from most pesticides, now it's got to relinquish that energy to go after the synthetics that have been bio-accumulating in their bodies and that's the long term recovery that's not always pleasant, but it was a very powerful visual for people to recognize how fast—especially in children, you can reverse ill health by simply stopping the inflow of things that put your body in a state of defense instead of growth and healing.

Ty: Right. It also affirms the saying, "You are what you eat."

Dr. Bell: Oh, yeah, absolutely. And you are what you don't detoxify. But even the detoxification process takes a lot of energy and it saps that energy that could be utilized for other promotion type things—when we talk about growth and healing versus decaying, generating, and dying.

Ty: You mentioned endocrine system. Talk about the endocrine system because I've heard it referred to as the quarterback of the immune system. What exactly is the endocrine system?

Dr. Bell: The endocrine system is the hormonal system. It's a vital communication tool. It's related to almost everything in the body from digestion to immunity and everything in between. We talk about youth hormones like the most commonly known estrogen, testosterone and progesterone. And we covered more recently on the Robert Scott Bell Show, you and me too, we talked about this— the use of statin drugs to reduce cholesterol because they theorized initially that cholesterol was the cause of heart disease, so we must reduce it and prevent heart disease when in reality the cholesterol is very protective of the integrity of the lining of the arteries and veins that only over time if you don't correct the true cause of inflammation, which are these toxins, heavy metals, etc., you then can reverse something in this regard instead of chasing your cholesterol tail. The reality on a cholesterol is that they're finding that it correlates—higher cholesterol with longevity. In other words if your cholesterol levels are higher, you will live longer.

Now, another aspect of this—not only the protective factors for the brain and the nervous system because the mile and sheath—cholesterol. The brain, 25 percent cholesterol.

Ty: Right.

Dr. Bell: The critical component of the production of your youth hormones—cholesterol, without which we're in trouble. So it's another aspect of the chemical influence if you will, not only in the food, but the drugs that are presented as if they're vital nutrients, statin drugs are not vital nutrients, but they do a lot also interestingly to protect the cholesterol from cancer, cancerous growth.

Another new study came out recognizing that higher cholesterol tended to provide more protection because the membrane is so dependent upon fat and cholesterol. Think about metastasis of cancer. When your cholesterol is lower your cells are in a much less strong posture, if you will to defending against metastasis and cancer growth. This relates to the endocrine system because the vital sustenance for those hormonal substances, if you will, are targeted for attack by modern medicine—for people who end up giving you inadvertently cancer. I'm not saying that's what they're trying to do all of the time. Some of the time, you might argue in a bigger sense, but in reality, they're inadvertently creating a situation where you're more susceptible to not only cancer's growth, but spreading or metastasis.

Ty: You mentioned just now about drugs—many times. Let's talk about a drug that's not really a drug.

Dr. Bell: Yes.

Ty: It's a plant.

Dr. Bell: Yes.

Ty: And you know what I'm talking about.

Dr. Bell: Cannabis?

Ty: Let's talk about cannabis or hemp and it especially relates to cancer.

Dr. Bell: This is perhaps one of the most amazing rediscoveries as we abandon a plant that has been used for thousands of years as medicine and many other industrial uses, even in more recent history. We're learning what is known as—what we all have, an endocannabinoid system or endocannabinoid receptors within the body. There are certain foods that cannabinoids. There are certain abilities to produce some from within as well, but these receptors are present almost everywhere in the body, particularly heavily entrenched in the gastrointestinal system, the liver, the brain, the nervous system, interestingly enough.

And what we're finding the impact of the key cannabinoids, they're not the only ones, that cannabidiol, which is CBD, the non-psychoactive component it's considered and the THC, the Tetrahydrocannabinol, which you say, oh so well. Those two aspects—the THC is considered the psychoactive component alters the state of mind and that's been argued as the dangerous addictive drug, which now doctors like Sanjay Gupta and other say well, maybe it's not really that addictive at all, in fact it might have benefit. We're finding out in relation to certain cancers not just one or two, but many cancers, a tremendous benefit.

Some to stimulate the apoptosis, the cellular death, others to address protection of cells neurological cells, brain and nervous system cells from cancer, a lot of epithelial integrity relying on the impact of these cannabinoids, we've talked about gastrointestinal recovery—seizure disorders in children and adults—a lot of it is actually sourced right there in that second brain in the gut. These cases we're seeing the use of CBD, sometimes THC or both together are reversing these cancers and reversing even seizure activity seizure disorders.

Ty: Are there studies that have shown there is effectiveness with CBD and the THC against cancer?

Dr. Bell: Incredible amount and in fact, in a book you and I wrote together it's called, *Unlock The Power To Heal*, we went into depth on it and it's almost too much to go through if we talk about the references that we have here for breast cancer, colorectal cancer, prostate cancer, stomach cancer, skin cancer, leukemia, lymphoma, lung cancer, uterine cancer, thyroid cancer, pancreatic cancer, cervical cancer, mouth cancer, glioma brain cancer, biliary tract cancer. We've got tremendous amount of scientific research validated and linked up in our book and of course in the researchers they know about this in the world and America it's been suppressed because of the status as a Class One, what does that class they call it?

Ty: I believe that cannabis is Class One drug.

Dr. Bell: Yeah. Which is the worst.

Ty: Same category as…

Dr. Bell: Highly addictive as heroin, right all of that. And of course we know—is it the U.S. government actually holds patents as fascinating as well when you realize this, for the use of cannabis on cancer. Let me see if I can find that in our book here.

Yeah, to elaborate on one of the studies related to lung cancer—a 2007 Harvard Medical School Study, published in *Science Daily* showed that hemp's THC decreases lung cancer tumors by 50 percent, significantly reduces the ability of the cancer to metastasize.

This is huge again. This is just one of many things. Here it is, cannabinoids, this is directly from a United States patent. This is the shocker. "Cannabinoids including THC and cannabidiol, promote the re-emergence of apoptosis so that tumors will stop dividing and die." This is profound. I'm not one that says one panacea that does everything for everyone, but if there was a plant, to look at one plant that does so many extraordinary things, this cannabis plant which is wrongly referred to as marijuana as a slang or hemp as well, in many forms has so much from a nutritional value, but now we learn more and more about its specific value in reversing cancers that are active much less in their prevention.

Ty: Over the last several months, I don't know how many people I have been contacted by that have used cannabis to treat terminal cancer. And they're still alive so it wasn't necessarily terminal, but many people I've been contacted by that have been using cannabis all over the world.

Dr. Bell: It really is a crime against humanity and animals for that matter. The idea of making illegal a plant that God created is an affront if you will. I know some scientists get annoyed if you mention that kind of level of creation, but I don't apologize for it because there is much more than what you can look at in a peer review because it's another issue we cover on the air as well. The faultiness, if you will, of peer review the inability to determine what is real and what is not.

Duplicability is really more critical and what we're seeing is duplicability in all of these cannabis studies and we're seeing a lot of clinical evidence as young children are reversing cancers, brain cancers, and reversing seizure disorders. You typically eliminate the placebo effect when you deal with animals and children in that regard. That's one of the arguments against—oh it's just the placebo. An adult knows they're taking something good. Of course, I don't speak ill of placebo. I'm happy if nothing can get you well just your belief, for me I applaud that. That's a great thing. Not something to be denied.

Ty: Right. You mention children with cancer. Why the explosion recently with children with cancer? Any idea?

Dr. Bell: They're living longer than ever before. The children are older. The reality is if we have a bioaccumulation over the generations. This is a cross generational decline. What we're seeing, wards at children's hospitals dedicated to cancer popping up even today. It's not that we're beating cancer because we got more technology, we've got more science and more drugs and in fact, there is more cancer than ever because of the toxicological burden and the corresponding nutrient deficiencies that are associated with that.

So children are being born to parents that have been just hammered by these synthetic chemicals their entire life. Now I chose to change my life at the age of 24, having been raised chemically, I've been vaccinated—all of the things I chose to do differently for my children and similar with my wife. We were hammered by these chemicals and had a lot of health issues.

So, we made a switch like that family in that two week experiment, but I went for now at 25 years later, going organic, cleaning up, detoxifying actively bringing in minerals that I knew would prevent it. And here I am in my late 40s and I am more vital than I was at 24, doing things I couldn't do then.

And my relatives, much like yours, many of them had cancer and died of cancer or the treatment for cancer and they were in their 50s, 60s and 70s, not 40. So I realized that generationally I could see that the writing was on the wall for me if I didn't do something different. Wasn't sure what it was at the time until I learned homeopathy and different things to apply that I transformed my future and the point is at any point in time, you don't have to be 24 like I was, I don't recommend waiting until you're 48 or 58 or 68, but if you're there now, it's never too late to make that change. Never too late.

Ty: That's a good point. That's a good message for people. It's never too late. Even people that have been diagnosed with so called terminal cancer, never too late. You mentioned homeopathy. Are there certain homeopathic remedies that might be effective of treating cancer?

Dr. Bell: Yeah in fact, I was trained clinically—that is it's a very practical way dealing with the environmental toxins and even the deficiencies that impact organ systems' function. Now the origin of homeopathy was about identifying one single remedy to match up to as many of the symptoms of the patient as possible. So if you picked something like the cinchona, which is China, or the bark of the Peruvian bark of a tree that's used for malaria. That was the original homeopathy because it induced fevers that mimic malaria and they said cinchona is the remedy for malaria. Now you can use cinchona for other things. Even gastrointestinal distress and things like that so it's not just one thing for one thing.

You can do many things if you understand the broad expanse of any given remedy, but when we're dealing with cancer, we're not dealing with one isolated cause and one result. We're dealing with a multifactorial cause developed over many years, decades or even generations. This goes into something called inherited predispositions or miasmas as well. I don't want to discount that, but for the sake of simplicity first, we'll talk about restoring to function to systems.

What are we recognize in a cancer patient or just about any chronically ill patient or person alive today? The liver is congested. You don't even have to ask the question. People say how do you, if my liver is congested? I ask, are you breathing? It's that simple. Now you can go for a liver test, they'll take the enzyme levels, they'll say it's elevated or it's not, but very often the medical system is designed to detect elevated levels at a point where you're years in trouble, years, many years, decades, in trouble.

What I'm talking about is much more subtle. It's just the inflow is not matching the outflow like that family I mentioned that was eating conventionally, the pesticides were coming out in the urine, they stopped eating conventionally, they ate organically, oh my gosh no more pesticides in the urine. They're still going to have to deal with level of bioaccumulation, but the point is you're not getting all of it out and that's that backlog, that congestion, like a congested highway traffic. You're not getting anywhere very fast and you're often getting stuck, your car is breaking down on the side of the road, it never leaves and it becomes a mess. An absolute mess.

So what I do functionally is I will take remedies like bryonia alva, it's the common hops, or nux vomica, it's considered the poison nut or chelidonium, which is the celandine plant, and we convert those into homeopathic form by a serial dilution, and succession, so you're not taking anything that will cause a problem of a toxicological burden. Safely can ingest these and these all have an impact on the liver and other systems and there are others, dandelion, taraxacum, these things could affect the liver and the kidneys and we say alright how do we work or stimulate the production to function of those organs. It's a little different than chasing symptoms because you think about symptoms of fatigue or a headache, how many times will somebody will go to the doctor and say, I have a headache, can you prescribe for me a coffee enema? They're not going to—they're going to prescribe you Tylenol, something that kills your liver.

Ty: Suppress the symptom.

Dr. Bell: That completely negates the cause. Where did it originate and by and large, the liver. Not excluding all of the other excretory system, organs or the digestive system at large, but we can say, focus on it, liver, kidneys, colon. We have remedies that we know of. So I work with formulations, complexes, I tend to work with lower attenuations or potencies, so I don't want to hammer blow people. I work gently over time. I figure, if they're 45 years old, it took him 45 years to get there. So I'm working with these things on a daily gentle basis so they're not overwhelmed and begin to restore the elimination patterns homeopathically. Now, we've talked before about minerals and herbs for detox, so it doesn't go to the exclusion of any of those things. I talk about the metabolic interaction that we have at an energetic level. We talk about I'm out of energy, I'm not out of molecules. That's the concept we're working with energy here.

Now, on top of that, we got the elimination started again, the detox pathways opened up. We want to work homeopathically with the digestive system, little more broadly, so we might do something like a baptisia tinctoria. There are a number of remedies that address digestive function. Nux vomica works with the liver and the stomach interestingly. You have a little spill over into other systems, but we work and we figure out which of these things work well with restoring the function of digestion by simulation. We talked a little bit last time about restoring the gut integrity. That was where I got my start in homeopathy, and then we expanded it—last time. I believe we talked about the silver aloe recovery protocol and things that I do there. Homeopathy was that deeper level starting point. It's still a powerful adjunct. Then my third phase, again—I would do on a three times a day because you tend eat on that pattern three times a day so I look at that as a homeopathic support recovery of digestion that way too. Very simple.

The third aspect of this and this is not even addressing cancer directly, but phenomenally transforming the terrain of the body—would be to address the inflammation, the free radical, the systemic inflammation of not only the skeletal system, but the vascular system and any system that's impacted. We have a number of remedies that address that, that can Rhus toxicodendrun—one of my favorites, poison ivy. A lot of people will take it for arthritic pain, but they don't realize it will also work for inflammation of the circulatory system. Ruta, Pulsatilla. There are different things that will do that and I can go and everybody will glaze over with all of the Latin names. I wanted to share with you this system because maybe we can make it available for everybody to access because my whole goal as you know is to bring the power to heal back where it belongs.

This third concept is homeopathically working with systemic inflammation, which is damaging to cells chronically, long term and that facilitates growth where? Where the damage is most severe, most chronic, that's where we see the most cancer susceptibility—cancer grow. The cells lost their integrity and now we may find a tumor, which if you're lucky if it's a tumor because it's encapsulated, worst case scenario you've got the metastasis when the integrity is lost because of other deficiencies like silicon or silica—we talked about that last time.

Ty: So really what I'm hearing you say is that you're not really addressing cancer directly per se, what you're doing is you're getting rid of the things that your body needs to get rid of by unclogging the exits. And the entrance. Also then you're adding things that the body needs to run better. So what you're doing as you always say on your radio show—the power to heal is yours. You're giving the body what it needs so that it can heal itself.

Dr. Bell: Exactly and the thing is I haven't addressed cancer yet—directly—indirectly we—by clearing the terrain in this way in many cases you will see the manifestation of good health and cellular integrity return and cancer goes away. If you have specific tumors, like in the female's area, a tumor in the uterus or fibroids, things like that, you can direct homeopathic medicine to address that and a woman could dispel the fibroids naturally as opposed to having it grow and explode and cause problem everywhere.

Or breasts—you talk about the use of sarcodes. These are homeopathic preparations of cancerous cells. To stimulate the targeting of those cells by the immune system that has been corrupted. That is why we can't just do that because the immune system is shot. That's why cancer is there. How do we restore immunity? It's not just boosting immunity, it's modulating it, but it's correcting the imbalances underlying why you lost your immune system's full functionality.

That's why we did the liver elimination, digestion assimilation, inflammation, free radicals, systemic etc. Then in concert with this correction of the entire terrain, we now can target homeopathically those cancer cells by sensitizing the immune system that is now reactivated. We talked also about using silver hydrosol last time because of its ability to powerhouse through any cancer cell because it has no defense mechanism against the electrical charge of those little nano-particles of silver or the oxygen it brings in with it as well. Any approach holistically that you give or do will be enhanced by utilizing this homeopathic baseline. Even if you don't go after and target the cancer homeopathically directly.

Sarcodes are the specific homeopathic preparations of cancerous cells into a safe form that you can reintroduce to the body. It sensitizes the system to target and attack and go after it like we want it to.

Ty: Okay. Awesome, well, Robert, great additional information you shared with us today. I think we throw this on top of what we learned last year, people are going to have a really good grasp of homeopathically how they can use different homeopathic drugs to treat cancer, but not only that, they're going to have a little better understanding about hemp and the history of hemp and the way that we use hemp to treat cancer as well.

Dr. Bell: Beautiful, so important and remember all of the things we did in prior episodes in the *Quest for the Cure* is still valid. The replenishment of the mineral, selenium, silica, DDF chromium. All of that is building on and giving people more information that they're empowered to do that. And one more thing you may have already covered in this series, if you haven't I know there is some exciting information to be revealed on use of molecular hydrogen released from water. And that's been another area of interest and intrigue for me now for many years to say what is it about water? I'm a homeopath. I love water. It does some amazing things, but can we measure it and this molecular hydrogen released through electrolytic type processes can also go in with that free hydrogen available for the cells, it can combine with hydroxyl radicals—the most damaging of inflammatory components in the cells and convert them to water and run them right out of the body. That fits in with all of this protocol of restoring detox pathways, helping the body facilitate elimination.

Ty: Paul Barattiero shared that with us. Great information on that as well. We put all of this together, people will be really empowered with knowledge, aren't they?

Dr. Bell: Oh, man, it's so great. We get to do it each week together on the show, which is a blessing that this information just keeps on giving gifts and empowering people and they can go on and teach others. It's not just about you and me. It's about everybody else who gets this information that can actually put it into practice and you don't have to have a PhD to do it.

Ty: And what does everybody that's watching need to remember?

Dr. Bell: "The Power to Heal is Yours." ***[end of transcript]***

A Global Quest

Interview with

Al & Karen Berrios

The TRUTH About CANCER™

educate • expose • eradicate

Ty: I'm sitting here with Karen and Al Berrios. Thank you for joining us today.

Karen: Thank you, Ty.

Al: Thank you.

Ty: You bet. I talked to you last night. We're at the conference here in San Diego, the Integrative Health Conference. And you mentioned the fact that *The Quest for the Cures* has had a dramatic impact on your practice.

So tell us a little bit about who you are, what you do, and how did *The Quest for the Cures* change things for you?

Karen: Yes, certainly. My name is Karen. And I was diagnosed with thyroid cancer about six months ago. As you can imagine the diagnosis was really impacting, or shocking, but something in me said, "You know, we're not going to do the conventional approach, we're going to seek other alternatives." And I came across Hope for Cancer and I ended up going to Mexico.

Ty: Dr. Jimenez.

Karen: Yes, Dr. Tony. And he was such a blessing. So, while I was there I came across the *Truth for Cancer* documentary. And I had a lot of doubt, a lot of fear, which I think is normal considering that we were going against the flow. And watching the documentary really impacted me. It gave me a lot of hope, a lot of strength, watching testimony of cancer survivors, people that have done it, and gone through it—it was just amazing. And it really was a blessing. It was a blessing.

Ty: That's awesome. So it really impacted you personally. What did you change about your lifestyle at that time?

Karen: My diet, nutrition, lifestyle choices that I have made. It gave me a profound understanding of the choices that we were making, and the impact that that was generating in our children's lives. So we changed. We did a 180-degree change.

Ty: Okay.

Karen: Not that it was bad, but we didn't know a lot of things, so it's a whole new world for us. And we feel blessed and grateful in so many ways. And your documentary was just so comforting and it resonated with everything that Dr. Tony said and it was just a blessing, and we're so grateful for it. Thank you.

Ty: Thank you for sharing that and I'm humbled when I hear people say things like that because that's really our goal is to give people that knowledge, to give them that hope. Cancer is not a death sentence, it doesn't need to be, there are things that you can do. But not only did it impact your life in that way, you have a practice, correct?

Al: Yes, I'm a nurse practitioner. We've been in practice for a few years and we opened a practice in Fallbrook, California about four or five years ago. We practice conventional medicine and some nutrition, but the nutrition was never a focus—the main focus of the practice. Even though you recommend, you don't enforce it.

So when my wife was diagnosed with cancer that was eye-opening, not only for us, but for the people around us. So it really changed a lot of things. So we watched your docu-series and it was just great. It opened my eyes tremendously. I was like, "Okay, I'm doing a lot of things wrong."

Karen: He was so excited. He was posting it on our blog and our family circle, our friends, and on Facebook and sharing it, and we were just so excited. And everyone was interacting—what they learned from the documentary, how they agreed, and it was just amazing to see the dynamic, everything that started flowing from the documentary. And yes, cancer, you are right, is not a death sentence. It's life-changing.

Ty: Wow.

Karen: And so many blessings have come from all of this. And in practice, my husband has an opportunity to reach out to so many people.

Ty: And being a registered nurse you are working with medical doctors, I assume?

Al: Right, right. But, you know, as a nurse practitioner I am able to see patients, treat patients. I do family practice and urgent care and some internal medicine based on my experience. But it changed completely—a 360-degree change. My main focus right now is alternative. I know I have to use conventional medicine, but I'm trying to move my patients from conventional to alternative because that's the way to go.

You have to heal your body completely, and that's what I learned from you, from your docu-series and from other doctors that are here, and we learned about it and we did a lot of research. So I'm teaching that to my patients and a lot of them they follow and they do great. They don't have to take all these 20,000 pills. It's just great to see those changes. But there are some people that don't want to change and it's just a constant reinforcement and education and you have to do this, this is good for you. And we have proof—my wife is my proof.

Ty: That's awesome, and you know, like I'm saying to you, being that you are a medical professional, people listen to you.

Al: Right.

Ty: So when you've got your patients...

Karen: They might notice.

Ty: Yes, that lends more credibility than when I say it because I don't have a degree in medicine. But when a medical professional wakes up like this, and you see the importance of nutrition and all these other things on health, you have the ability to change the world. And so, that's why we are so happy.

I was so thrilled last night to get your story because I said, "We've got to get this on film," because we are partnering with you to spread this message far and wide. And so, when we get a medical clinic like this that is teaching, now, nutrition—one step closer to enlightening everyone with this. And so that's our goal.

Karen: Yes, it's happening. Even in our lobby we have a series of you speaking.

Ty: Oh, you've got the docu-series playing?

Al: Yes.

Ty: Oh, that's great.

Karen: And some of our patients are like, "Wow!" Enlightened on the whole reality. It's not known to many of us, because it's hidden. Like my husband said many times, it's not about just treating the illness, it's finding root causes.

Ty: The cause.

Karen: Yes. And it brings an awareness. And prevention—talking about prevention. It's such a blessing that our medical practice is now a vehicle to help many people.

Ty: That's awesome.

Karen: *Really* help.

Ty: What's the name of your practice, again?

Al: Fallbrook Medical Center.

Ty: Fallbrook Medical Center.

Al: Yes.

Ty: Here in California.

Al: California. Yes.

Ty: Okay, awesome. Well, this is a blessing to me, it's a real encouragement to me and to the whole team here, everybody that is filming. It's not just me, it's the whole team here—The Truth About Cancer team. When we see these stories, we hear these stories, it is encouraging to us because that feedback keeps us going.

Karen: Thank you, Ty, for your boldness and your courage to continue, and for taking the lead and doing this work because you really—you touch people's lives in a deep, deep way. And I know—I heard of your story, your background, your dad—and it was not for nothing, it had a purpose.

Ty: There was a reason.

Karen: There was a reason, yes.

Ty: Well, thank you, Karen, for sharing. Thank you, Al.

Karen: Thank you, Ty.

Al: Thank you for everything you do.

Ty: So nice of you to sit here with us today, and I wish you all the best in the future. I'm sure that your practice is going to grow by leaps and bounds, and I'm sure that you are going to continue to improve your healing process.

Karen: Thank you so much. God bless you.

Al: Thank you.

[end of transcript]

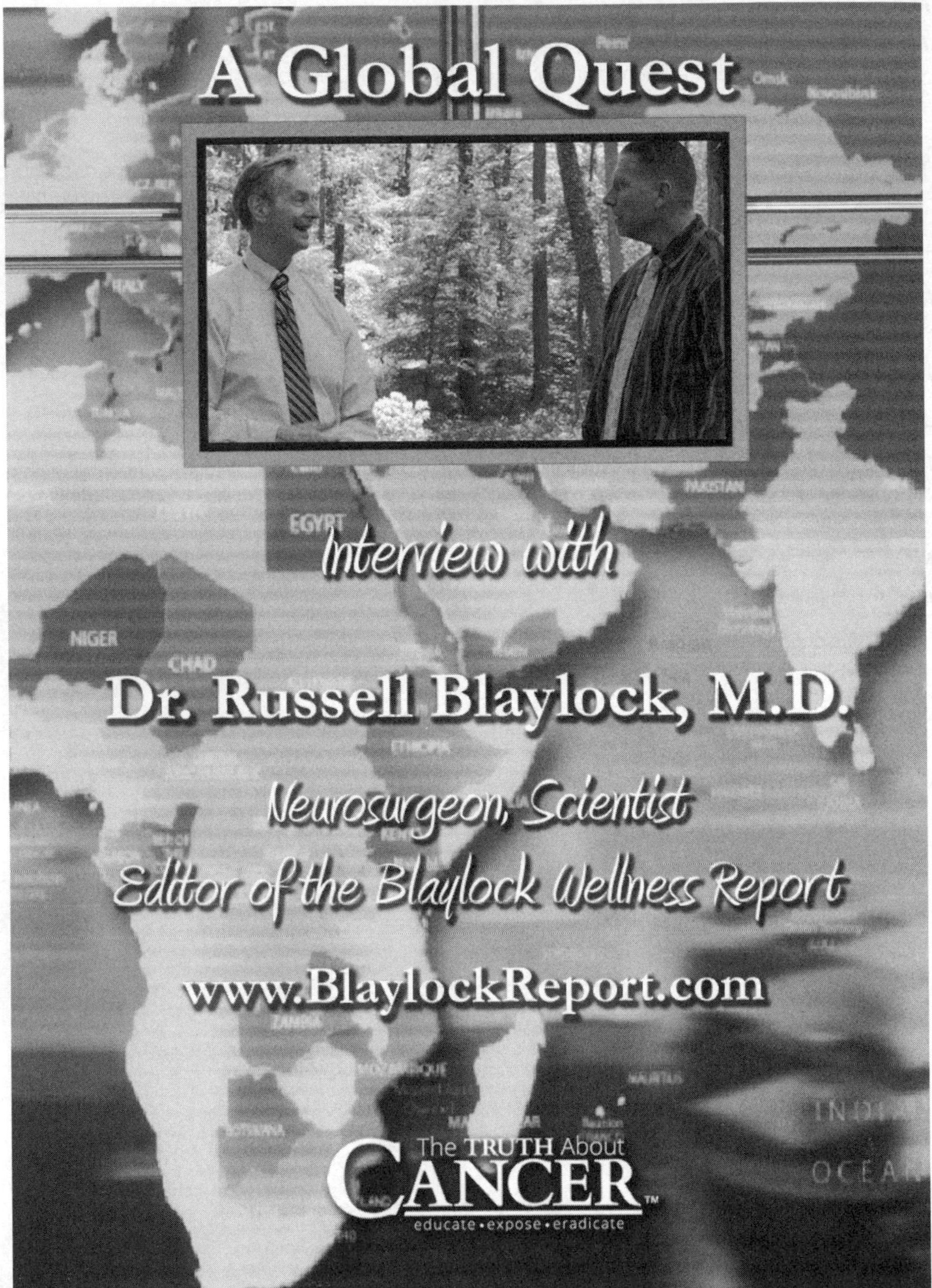
A Global Quest
Interview with
Dr. Russell Blaylock, M.D.
Neurosurgeon, Scientist
Editor of the Blaylock Wellness Report
www.BlaylockReport.com
The TRUTH About
CANCER
educate • expose • eradicate

Ty: Dr. Blaylock, I appreciate you joining us today.

Dr. Blaylock: Thank you, I appreciate it.

Ty: I'm really looking forward to getting your input on cancer for our documentary here, but I want to get your take on what got you interested in medicine to the begin with.

Dr. Blaylock: Well, I've always been interested in science and medicine, so I set my goal kind of early. And after medical school I became interested in neuroscience and particularly cancer as well. So I studied both of them in medical school. I met the cancer researcher there in the medical school and we worked together. My interest was more in how cancer occurs and what to do about it.

Neurosurgeons see a lot of cancer. Number one, we see a lot of brain tumors. And primary brain tumors are a very common cause of death in people with neurological diseases. But all of metastatic cancers, most of them go to the brain first. In fact, a lot of the time, for instance with breast cancer and colon cancer, we'll see the patient first because before they even know they have the cancer it's metastasized to the brain. And so we end up seeing them early before most people.

Ty: Why is that? Why do they metastasize to the brain first?

Dr. Blaylock: It has to do with a complex tagging mechanism in which the site the cancer is going to go is tagged. And the brain seems to be one of these tagging sites so it attracts the cancer to the brain, and also bone. And because of the metastasis—for instance with breast cancer to the spinal column, we see a lot of spinal injuries of the spinal cord from the cancer compression. So a lot of times we'll pick them up with paraplegia and they don't even know they have breast cancer.

And sometimes the primary tumor, like the breast cancer, is very, very small and undetectable but the metastases are much larger. We'll see that. But we see a lot of them so I became interested in it. And I had always been kind of interested in the biology of cancer, what makes a cancer cell a cancer cell, where they come from.

Ty: So what is a cancer cell and where does it come from?

Dr. Blaylock: Well, we used to think that any cell could become cancer except for a few limited ones. We thought that if you irritated a cell enough and damaged its DNA enough it would become immortal. Just keep growing. Now we find out that's not true. Only stem cells seem to be the source of cancers. And stem cells are the cells that haven't decided what they want to be yet.

They're very primitive cells so they could be anything, a heart cell, a brain cell, a lung cell. So these stem cells are all through your body just sitting quietly but if you damage the DNA of the stem cell enough, through free radicals or whatever, it'll become immortal. And then it just keeps producing more and more cells. It wakes up and it's producing lots and lots, thousands, millions, and billions of cells, and it becomes a cancer.

But it's the stem cell that's pouring it out. Kind of like a water hose is pouring all these droplets of water out. The trouble with chemotherapy and conventional treatments is that they have no effect on the cancer stem cells. They only kill the daughter cells, the cells that are produced by it. So the tumor will shrink and they'll claim success. But you haven't killed the stem cells so it all just comes right back. And what they found is when it comes back it comes back infinitely more aggressive than it did before.

Ty: And why would that be?

Dr. Blaylock: It's kind of complex chemistry but it has to do with the chemical changes and what we call the microenvironment of the stem cell. And what you're doing, you're producing a lot of cytokines around those stem cells—these are inflammatory chemicals.

Those inflammatory chemicals produce even greater DNA damage so the cancer that comes back is more malignant than the one that started. So what they're finding is that when you treat a patient with chemotherapy and radiation and you don't cure them, then you make the cancer infinitely more aggressive and patients usually die quicker.

Ty: That's a common thread that I hear from cancer patients all over the world. They'll email or call and say, "You know, I was diagnosed, my friend was diagnosed. And it was breast cancer. We did the chemo, radiation and now it's a year and a half later and it's back everywhere." And that's why. That explains it.

Dr. Blaylock: And that's well documented.

Ty: It's documented in the literature.

Dr. Blaylock: It's accepted in the oncology world that that's what happens. And this is why, it's because you're causing that microenvironment. What most people don't know, what oncologists don't seem to understand, is that chemotherapy, radiation, conventional treatments all are inflammatory.

The source of cancers is chronic inflammation. So once you change that microenvironment to even more inflammatory by pumping in these chemotherapeutic agents, or radiating it, you make it more inflammatory and that changes it to more malignance.

Ty: So it's adding fuel to the fire.

Dr. Blaylock: So if the chemotherapy and radiation doesn't kill everything, all the cancer cells, and wipe out the stem cells, you've really made things worse and not better. And that's what we're finding. In fact, I just wrote an article on that—it's going to be published real soon—about the effect of microenvironment and inflammation, microenvironment and cancer growth.

And invasion, particularly invasion, it makes the cancer more invasive. And that's because once you stimulate that cell with this inflammation it starts secreting what they call "metalloproteinases," which are enzymes that dissolve the blood vessel wall. So all these cancers start pouring into blood vessels and that makes the cancer spread. And that's what it's doing. The inflammation turns on these enzymes that make the cancer penetrate tissue, break through these barriers that the body tried to put around the cancer to keep it from spreading, and that makes it worse.

Ty: And that's what the tumor really is; that wall of the tumor is the body walling off those cells.

Dr. Blaylock: Right. Usually, it tries to form a capsule around it, a fibrous capsule. This is why vitamin C and things that increase that fibrous capsule's strength help out in cancer because it's helping contain it. And certain flavonoids, for instance, will suppress those proteinase enzymes. For instance, like curcumin, quercetin, ellagic acid, they suppress those enzymes so that the cancer can't penetrate. And then it's a localized cancer and then it's easy to get rid of.

Ty: Do we have medical literature that backs up the use of flavonoids? Are there studies where the literature shows—?

Dr. Blaylock: Numerous, numerous studies. This is one of the hottest fields of research in cancer. It's flavonoids, plant extracts, and their effect on cancer. The problem is is that clinician is not reading the journal articles in his own journal. All these—they're in there, the clinical journals, they're in the research for oncology journals. They're just not reading them because they don't understand it. It's a lot of biochemistry. It's a lot of mechanism they're not familiar with.

They're not familiar with the plants. They don't know how to give it. They don't know that these extracts are purified and available. For instance, you see in leukemia research, they have absolutely shown that leukemia is much more curable if you use quercetin. Most of the leukemias are very sensitive to quercetin. Lymphomas, all of these things, are curcumin, quercetin, ellagic acid, and resveratrol. All of these things inhibit the cancer stem cell. And that's what's interesting about this. For instance, curcumin actually kills the stem cell, this cancer stem cell. It doesn't bother normal stem cells but only cancer stem cells.

Ty: Curcumin?

Dr. Blaylock: Curcumin. And that's the other thing about flavonoids and these plant extracts is that they're very selective. They only damage, inhibit, and kill cancer cells. They have no effect on the normal cells except to make the normal cells stronger.

Ty: So that selective toxicity. That's a big thing because you don't want to kill the good cells. You want to kill only the cancerous.

Dr. Blaylock: That's what they always look for, what they call the "magic bullet." Something that will kill the cancer cell and not hurt the normal cell. Well, this does even more. It kills the cancer cell, but it makes the normal cell stronger.

And so what they found out, for instance, in radiation treatment of breast cancers, colon cancers, and lung cancers, is that it actually makes the radiation much more effective. And it protects the tissue that's being radiated that's normal around the cancer.

Ty: Really? And all of these do, the ellagic acid, the resveratrol, curcumin.

Dr. Blaylock: It's a long list of them. Orinogan and ellagic acid, and resveratrol.

Ty: And they affect the stem cells?

Dr. Blaylock: They kill the stem cells and suppress the stem cell growth. They kill the daughter cancer cells. They help encase the cancer. They suppress these invasion enzymes and reduce the metastasis. And they protect the tissue, the normal tissue, to help keep it from converting to the same process.

Because when they did this study to see if inflammation is the cause of cancer, most people who have cancer should have chronic inflammation. So they did this large study and that's exactly what they found. For instance, in certain people, 70 percent of them had definable inflammation—you know, arthritis, chronic atherosclerosis, some chronic infections. And that's what caused the cancer. If you stop inflammation you stop the cancer from ever forming.

Ty: So do these substances you're talking about, these flavonoids, do they have any effect on the inflammation?

Dr. Blaylock: They're powerful anti-inflammatories. They're very powerful anti-inflammatories. That's how they are preventing the cancer from occurring. And then they have other mechanisms that affect the cell signaling that kills the cancer, turns on the cancer suicide gene like p21, p53. And that'll make this cancer cell commit suicide –what we call apoptosis.

Ty: Dr. Blaylock, in light of the fact that these flavonoids are so beneficial why is not every oncologist using them to treat cancer?

Dr. Blaylock: Well, because they don't read their articles, and they don't know what these flavonoids are because they don't know the chemistry. They've never heard of it. They go to a meeting and the meeting is about the latest protocol and the latest chemotherapeutic drug.

And who sponsors the meeting? Makers of the chemotherapeutic drug. So you have a room full of oncologists listening to the latest drug and they'll say, "Oh, this one. We're getting incredible responses with this drug." Well, as I explained, what happens to that incredible response, it causes dramatic shrinkage of the tumor initially because it's just killing the daughter cells.

And some are not even malignant cells. But it's not affecting the stem cell so then the cancer grows tremendously. But they can say, "Oh, we get a good response from this chemotherapeutic drug."

Ty: And when they say "good response" they mean the tumor shrunk.

Dr. Blaylock: They mean initially it shrinks the tumor but they don't say, "well, six months later or less it's actually going to grow a lot faster. And it's more likely to metastasize."

Ty: So they're using the wrong measurement stick for success.

Dr. Blaylock: Yes. And what they don't do and what they don't tell most of the patients is that it depends on when you diagnose the cancers how long the cancer patient lives. For instance, if you go back to literature 50 years ago and you say well that patient normally will live about a year to two years with that cancer. Well, it depends on when you diagnose it. If the tumor had already grown for three or four months before you diagnose it and then they live another year that's really a year and three or four months.

So if you diagnose it earlier and they die, and in a year and a half or a year you say, "Gee, we've cut three months off to death rate," you didn't really. You just diagnosed it earlier but they died in the same length of time. The oncology research journals are looking at it and they say, "Well, that does seem to be what's happening." We're not really curing cancer or giving people longer lifetimes; we're actually diagnosing them earlier and it may be they're actually dying sooner than they would have. That's never explained to cancer patients.

I always tell cancer patients, I say, "when you go talk to your oncologist, number one, when they start talking about, 'oh we're getting really good response from this drug.' Ask them the most important question, 'what are the chances this will cure me? Not make me feel better. Not make the tumor shrink for a little while. What are the chances that it'll cure me?'" Then you'll see this blank look come on the oncologist's face and he'll say, "Well, most people will die of this cancer anyway."

This might make you feel better or live a month or two longer, or six months longer. So they're really being— it's deceptive, it's not being truthful when they talk to these cancer patients. So I tell them always ask that question.

Ty: Any other questions that cancer patients should ask their doctors?

Dr. Blaylock: Well, you want to know what are the complications of this? What is the known death rate from using this chemotherapy? Because a lot of patients don't understand that a significant number of cancer patients are dying from the treatment itself and not the cancer. So it can vary between one or two percent, or as much as 10 to 15 percent, that are dying from the treatment.

A lot of patients have to stop their treatment because their treatment makes them so sick. They die if you keep doing it and they find that if you have to interrupt the treatment, the cancer grows a lot faster and they're less likely to live. So all of these things patients need to ask their doctor and the doctor is not going to volunteer it because he's trying to sell a protocol. He's trying to sell you to take his 500,000 dollar treatment and if he says, "Well, there's a 15 percent chance you could die. It's probably not going to cure you. You'll only get a few months. It's really going to make you sick. It's going to destroy your immune system. And these are known to cause heart failure that's incurable. And this'll destroy your lungs."

These are all things known with chemotherapy; not many people would do it. Most people will say, "Well, I don't think I want to do that if it's going to going to destroy my lungs. If it's going to destroy my heart and I'll go into progressive heart failure. I don't think I want to do that."

Ty: So really the devil's in the details that they don't tell you?

Dr. Blaylock: And they're not going to volunteer them. You're going to have to do a little research and ask them. Now, if you ask them, by law they have to tell you.

Ty: That's good advice for cancer patients. It reminds me of a story from one of our favorite preachers. He tells a story about when he signed up for the army. He said, "They didn't lie to me. They just didn't tell me the whole truth. They told me that we'd have three hots and a cot but they didn't tell me it was going to be in Guantanamo Bay." So it's in the details that you don't know. So I think that's good advice.

Dr. Blaylock: And a lot is being left out of these interviews patients do when they first appear to their doctors. He's gotten this new drug in the mail. This information about this new drug. He's excited about it. The pharmaceutical company told him, "this is a real chance of a cure and we're getting great responses." So that's what he tells the patient. It's straight out of the literature from the pharmacology manufacturer. It's not from the scientific literature.

The other thing that's really scary—a lot of these articles that are written in these manuals were written by the pharmaceutical company. We call them "ghost articles." And what they'll do, they'll get this company that writes articles that look just like beautiful medical articles. It has all the graphs, and charts, and numbers, and references. And they'll write this article without any authors for the study because they wrote it. And then they'll go to an oncologists that's very well known and they say, "wouldn't you like to put your name on this article and if you do it's going to be in a very prestigious journal, *New England Journal of Medicine* or some oncology journal that's very prestigious."

A lot of these people are tempted because this puts their name even further out front. So they'll say," yes, put my name on there." So they'll put a string of names on the article who had nothing to do with writing it, had nothing to do with the study and they'll end up in a very prestigious journal.

Well, these journals they choose are the ones that affect how doctors behave; how they treat patients. So they'll read this article not knowing it's a ghost article and they'll say, "they've gotten tremendous responses and there are hardly any complications." So they'll order the drug and then they'll tell the patient the same thing they got out of that article, "There are hardly any complications. Patients are doing very well and there's a good chance that this could cure you."

Ty: And it's not an independent article.

Dr. Blaylock: It's not an independent article and the doctor has been tricked and the patient has been tricked. The doctor is not doing it on purpose, it's just that he believes the article because it's in this prestigious journal.

Ty: Right. I mean it does lend credibility to the article if it's published in a medical journal. Unfortunately for the patient, a lot of times they're tricked at the cost of their life.

Dr. Blaylock: Right, I mean this can cost your life if it turns out that, actually, there's a very high mortality. This can cause, as I said, progressive heart destruction or progressive destruction of the lungs or this causes brain damage. Now, this is one of the things I wrote in my cancer book years ago. I said, "there's a good possibility that chemotherapy is damaging the brain." At that time the literature was denying it.

They said, "no it can't damage the brain because it can't get pass the blood brain barrier." And I didn't believe that. Well, now it's been proven. They went back and they looked at cancer survivors and measured their cognitive ability; the ability to think and remember and learn language. And found that they were impaired. Virtually all of them were impaired.

Ty: From the chemo.

Dr. Blaylock: From the chemo. And then when they did it in animals, when they looked at their brain, yes it was destroying parts of the brain that had to do with those functions. So now it's well recognized that it produces— well, they have no way to protect the brain. These flavonoids like curcumin, quercetin, ellagic acid, resveratrol, naringenin, they powerfully protect the brain against damage by the chemotherapy.

Ty: They sound like miracle herbs.

Dr. Blaylock: They are. They're incredible but this is what you expect when God made something.

Ty: Yes. He didn't make any mistakes.

Dr. Blaylock: And when you look at what these things are doing—like curcumin, for instance, is one that's most researched. It does virtually everything that you want it to do. And the difference between it and a chemotherapeutic agent is that chemotherapy attacks one thing in the cancer cell.

The cancer cells finds a way to go around it very quickly. And that's why it escapes the treatment. Curcumin affects so many processes in the cancer cell it can't overcome it so it dies. So that's the advantage of these flavonoid things being used for cancer treatment versus chemotherapeutic agents.

Ty: Dr. Blaylock, I know you're an expert on excitotoxins; things that excite the brain cells. It excites cells to death actually. Can you talk specifically about aspartame and MSG? Two very well know excitotoxins.

Dr. Blaylock: Well, MSG is monosodium glutamate. It's just a salt of glutamate. The damaging element is the glutamate; not the monosodium. You forget that. Anything that's a glutamate is an excitotoxin. That means it can destroy brain cells. Now, when I did most of my research and writing about excitotoxins it had to do with the brain because that's where we thought all the glutamate receptors were.

Now we found out that there are actually glutamate receptors in every cell in the body. Not a single cell doesn't have glutamate receptors. What that means is that if you eat glutamate, now you don't have a blood brain barrier to even consider protecting you. Because glutamate goes to all these cells without any interference. And your blood level rises very rapidly and very high for over a prolonged period of time. Humans have a higher and more persisting level of glutamate in their blood than any animal that you experiment on.

Well, the second thing once they found out that glutamate receptors are everywhere is they found out that glutamate receptors trigger and stimulate the growth and invasions of cancers of every kind. First they thought it was brain tumors only. And they demonstrated that if you had high glutamate levels around the tumor, the tumor became highly invasive and grew twice as fast as a tumor that had low glutamate levels.

Then they started looking at other tumors; lung tumors, colon cancer, breast cancer, prostate cancer, thyroid cancers. Every cancer they looked at they found the same thing. Glutamate acted as a fertilizer, if you will, a stimulant for the growth of that cancer. It made it grow extremely fast, made it highly invasive, and less likely to be cured. Research has continued and we're finding that more and more.

Now, the second corollary is that if you block the glutamate receptor, the tumor starts slowing its growth. It becomes less invasive and the tumors will start dying; the cells start dying. It has no negative effect on normal cells. So if you block the glutamate normal cells reproduce and function just fine. It's only the cancer cells that start dying when you start blocking a glutamate receptor. And then they found, that if you take a patient who's getting chemotherapy and you give them these glutamate blockers, the chemotherapy works a lot better.

Ty: So you can take it along with the chemotherapy.

Dr. Blaylock: You can take it along with it.

Ty: Because I know a lot of people that are watching are on chemo now.

Dr. Blaylock: Right. So this is a really hot area of research. The big question is—you don't want to block all glutamate receptors because the brain needs them for its function. You wouldn't be able to remember you've fall into a coma. So you want to do a selective way to cut down that glutamate production. Well, there's an enzyme in your cells called glutaminase and its function is to convert glutamine into glutamate. And that's how that cancer cell starts producing lots of glutamate. And if you block that enzyme the tumor starts shrinking. The tumor becomes less invasive.

So there's a lot of research now focusing on ways to block the glutaminase enzyme as a cancer treatment. And it holds a lot of promise because when they do it in animals, even with human implanted tumors, the tumors start disappearing. They grow much less rapidly, they become less invasive, and they start shrinking.

Ty: So you've got—glutamine is converted by glutaminase into glutamate that fertilizes the cancer cell. So what are some sources of glutamine? You don't want glutamine then, apparently? At least not in excess.

Dr. Blaylock: No. Cancer cells use two major fuels. They use glucose and they use glutamine. Of the two—

Ty: Sugar.

Dr. Blaylock: —glutamine is a more powerful stimulant for cancer cell growth.

Ty: Okay, so we hear, "watch out for sugar, glucose, because cancer cells do feed on it." But you're saying glutamine is worse?

Dr. Blaylock: Yes, because the Warburg Effect is the fact that normal cells use both anaerobic and aerobic system, the Krebs cycle. Cancer cells only use the anaerobic system it was thought. Glutamine can work the aerobic system and produce a lot more energy. So if you are eating a lot of sugar and you're eating a lot of glutamine, you're really stimulating your cancer powerfully.

So the idea is you want to cut down on your glutamine intake. Well, a lot of people are promoting glutamine as a way to heal the gut; leaky gut syndrome. So they're saying take five, six, 10 grams of glutamine. That is a powerful stimulant for degenerative brain disorders. A powerful stimulant for cancer growth. So you don't want to do that. There are better ways to repair the GI tract that work better, are safer, and actually inhibit cancer.

Ty: But not glutamine.

Dr. Blaylock: But not glutamine. The other thing is foods. For instance beans, like black beans, are high in glutamine. Mushrooms are high in glutamine. So these foods that are high in glutamine, you don't want to eat either. You want to try to eat only low glutamine foods and a lot of those are your vegetables. And some cancer researchers think, "Well, this may be why people who are on vegetarian diets and juicing seem to have these spontaneous cures of cancer." It's because they have such a low glutamine intake and a low sugar intake. Both.

Ty: So, getting rid of the two fuels.

Dr. Blaylock: Getting rid of the two fuels. Now, cancer cannot use fat for its fuel so coconut oil is a good way to keep your energy up without having to resort to sugar. And cancer can't use it.

Ty: You've given us some sources of glutamine. MSG is one form of glutamate. What are some other sources of glutamate to avoid?

Dr. Blaylock: Well, the industry really got hammered when my book *Excitotoxins* came out and everybody was looking at glutamate. So they started taking MSG off the label and they even put on the label "contains no MSG." And then they put sources of glutamate in it like hydrolyzed protein, soy protein isolate, soy protein concentrate, idolized yeast, caseinate is a very common one. All of those are extremely high in glutamate. But the law allows them to put those in the foods and still put on the label "contains no MSG."

Ty: Because they're not monosodium glutamate.

Dr. Blaylock: They're not monosodium glutamate but they're just as dangerous and harmful as a monosodium glutamate.

Ty: So you want to watch out for all the forms of glutamate.

Dr. Blaylock: All the forms of glutamate and particularly soy. Soy is naturally high in glutamate and glutamine. As well as aluminum and fluoride and manganate. It has a lot of toxins in it.

Ty: So soy's high in aluminum—

Dr. Blaylock: Manganese and fluorides.

Ty: Fluorides as well as glutamine. So could that be one of the problems or one of the reason we're seeing these infant neurological problems?

Dr. Blaylock: Yes, I think so.

Ty: With a soy formula?

Dr. Blaylock: Sure. And that's been brought up. Some of the neurodevelopmental experts have said, "Well, this could lead to Parkinsonism when that child gets older, with a high manganese level in it." Also high fluoride and aluminum levels should do the same thing, Alzheimer's and developmental brain disorders of all kinds. ADHD could be worsened and ADD and those sort of things. So yes, soy is a very bad food and particularly a liquid food if you get it in milk and soy liquid products. It has very high glutamate levels, your blood level will rise as much as 24 to 54.

Ty: And that's even if it's organic soy right?

Dr. Blaylock: Doesn't make any difference. It's natural to the plant. In my estimation, people shouldn't be consuming soy products.

Ty: Let me ask you this, you mentioned ways to block glutamate. You mentioned glutamate blockers. Are there natural glutamate blockers that we should be familiar with?

Dr. Blaylock: Fortunately there's a lot of them. Virtually all of your flavonoids that I've discussed: curcumin, quercetin, ellagic acid, resveratrol, anthocyanins, they all reduce glutamate receptor activity. And that's their advantage and they do it safely. So the brain can function normally but the cancer can't use it.

Ty: So these things are powerhouses. They are selectively toxic the cancer cells. They reduce inflammation. They stop the uptake of glutamate. Everybody should be taking these things.

Dr. Blaylock: Yes, because most neurodegenerative diseases are caused by the same thing that cause cancer.

Ty: Inflammation.

Dr. Blaylock: Inflammation, chronic inflammation, which triggers excitotoxicity. I've coined the term immunoexcitotoxicity because they're linked. When you raise inflammation you get high levels of glutamate.

Ty: And that's immunoexcitotoxicity.

Dr. Blaylock: And I've introduced it into the scientific literature. It's a new term for the scientific literature but it's proven, it's not speculation, that this mechanism exists. And that it is responsible for Alzheimer's, Parkinson's, ALS, Huntington's. All of these neurological diseases, stroke, head injuries, this new chronic traumatic encephalopathy. In fact, I wrote an article on that for a journal about how that mechanism works to produce that chronic brain degeneration.

Ty: So you have the inflammation as being caused—I mean another source of inflammation—you're an expert on vaccines as well. Talk about the inflammation that could be created by vaccines and how that might play out with brain damage, cancer, and so forth.

Dr. Blaylock: Well, the interesting thing about vaccines is that experimentally you reproduce what you're doing with the vaccines which is that you're injecting an immune adjuvant stimulant, a powerful stimulant, into the muscle tissues. If you do that in an animal it produces intense inflammation where you injected it. But immediately the brain special immune system, called the microglia, become activated. If you do it again, then this produces a highly destructive release of glutamate. So if you are serially stimulating an immune system, say every month, every four or five months, you're producing this effect. We call it priming followed by full activation of microglia.

Well, that's exactly what you're doing in children. As soon as they're born you give them a Hepatitis B vaccine. And then a couple months later you give them an MMR vaccine. And a couple months late your give them more vaccines. And what they're doing is every two months or every month they're giving about five or six, to as many as nine, vaccines at each sitting. Combined, that's a powerful immune activation of your immune system. That's worse than a sickening. And it will produce what we call sickness behavior. That's why the babies scream and cry, are feverish, sleep a lot, are sick, and throw up. And it can last for months after their vaccine. And if you keep doing that you're interfering with the brain cell formations, the connections in the brain. It's pretty close to a full explanation of ADHD. Because that's just what you're doing and that's why now since the 1980s when they did so many vaccines, they just added a whole host of vaccines, we started seeing this exponential rise in Autism Spectrum Disorder.

And it makes since because you're producing this immunoexcitotoxicity in the brain anytime you over stimulate the immune system systemically. And we see this in aging. As people start getting older their immune system and their brain starts activating by itself. It's called priming. But it doesn't harm anything as long as it's just primed. But if you stimulate their immune system systemically they start getting degeneration of the brain. It starts wiping out synapses, (inaudible - 00:31:03). And if it keeps on they'll develop either Parkinson's Disease or Alzheimer's. And we know that if you vaccinate somebody with Alzheimer's or Parkinson's they get worse. And they progress much faster.

Ty: So it's not just the fact that these vaccines, they contain these heavy metals and these other dangerous toxins but it's the fact that they're actually causing that response in the brain.

Dr. Blaylock: Even if you took those out. But if you have mercury and aluminum in it, both of those are brain toxins by themselves, they accumulate in the brain and they produce high intensity inflammation in the brain. So if you keep giving these shots of aluminum, keep giving mercury, and it's accumulating in the brain and it's sitting in that brain for a lifetime, it's constantly keeping those immune microglia activated. So you have this constant pouring out of inflammatory chemicals. Constant pouring out of glutamate, excitotoxicity. And that's why they progress.

Ty: Is that one of the reasons maybe that we have this huge raise in childhood cancers now?

Dr. Blaylock: It could be. And it's also why we're seeing this enormous increase in neurological disease particularly in young people. And this is what most of the public don't know, there's this dramatic increase in these neurological diseases. It's affecting mostly young people. Where it used to be that you'd see diseases—Parkinson's, Alzheimer's —after age 65. Now you're seeing it in 30 and 40 year olds, 50 year olds.

Ty: Recently, I can't count the number of parents who've contacted me with kids, five, six, seven year olds with brain cancer. And it just seems like it's on the rise. I just thought maybe that's—it might be a link.

Dr. Blaylock: Yes. If the mother's not getting sufficient DHA in her diet through omega-3 fatty acids, if she's not getting the flavonoids she needs, if she's not breastfeeding, if she's exposed to certain pesticides, herbicides, chemicals—

Ty: Because they're coming through the umbilical cord right?

Dr. Blaylock: It will go through the umbilical cord and it will increase that child a risks of brain cancer.

Ty: If you didn't have a conscience or a moral compass, the business practices are superb. Because they are creating repeat customers, unfortunately, at the expense of the health, and lives, sometimes of the people that are the customers.

Dr. Blaylock: Well, it's been said that capitalism without morality is a monstrosity because murder incorporated is a capitalist enterprise. It is morality that makes business perform to the benefit of society. If you have a moral compass, like you say, or a moral imagination, you wouldn't do these things if you knew it was going to harm people. If you knew you were going to damage the brains of children and destroy a whole generation, you wouldn't do it. No matter how much profit you were making you'd say, "I'm just not going to do that."

Ty: And to the credit of Pepsi, they are removing aspartame. We were just talking about this.

Dr. Blaylock: But they're not doing it for moral reasons.

Ty: They're not?

Dr. Blaylock: They're doing it for financial reasons.

Ty: So let's talk about that. Talk about aspartame in the drinks and why might they be removing aspartame from their sodas at this point.

Dr. Blaylock: Aspartame has been studied for a long time. What a researcher did, he said, "I'm going to look at all the research that's been done. Those [studies] that are sponsored by the makers of aspartame versus independent studies." What he found, virtually, all the independent studies found harmful problems. None of the ones sponsored by the maker for it found any problems.

Ty: So you've got to look at who does the studies.

Dr. Blaylock: What the maker does is he goes out and he pays scientists to come up with articles, or ghost written articles, that say it's safe. And he fills the literature with it. And then when he goes before a camera and says, "Look, these are the pile of studies that show it's safe." So the news commentator looks at this and says, "Well, there's been hundreds and hundreds of studies that show it's safe." They don't even show the real studies that were done. The carefully done studies show it's not.

Now, the carefully done studies show that it's a carcinogenic agent and that it combines with other carcinogens, like nitrites, from your food to become even more carcinogenic. They found, in the original studies used to get approval for using NutraSweet, increased brain tumors. About a six-fold increase in brain tumors. They found increased lung tumors, breast cancers, breast tumors. All sort of tumors and thyroid cancers were found. But what the investigation did after the approval—because they approved it over all these findings—they found out that they were taking out the tumor from the experiment and throwing it away and writing down that it was normal.

Ty: Really?

Dr. Blaylock: Yes, all this was discovered. It's under oath in congressional hearings. A lot of these amoral shenanigans were done to get it approved in the first place. The guy who's head of the committee that approved it, after he approved it, within months he went to work for the company that was a promoter of aspartame. So that's sort of this revolving door we talked about between industry and government. Now, the studies have consistently shown that it's harmful. It does brain injuries, it produces abnormalities of the immune system, it affects the reproductive system, and it can cause cancer.

Ty: And wasn't there a study in Italy?

Dr. Blaylock: The Italian study was a study—I think his name was Rossini but he is one of the most respected researchers on carcinogenic agents. What he does is he tests these agents to see if they cause cancer. So they gave him this project. They said, "Look at this aspartame and see if it'll cause cancer in animals."

He did the largest animal study ever done. Now, his research is considered impeccable, almost unquestionable. Because he was so careful in doing it and so respected. He did it and he found that there seemed to be an increase in lymphoma and leukemia, and probably breast cancer, and maybe brain tumor. And they wouldn't accept it. So he redid it with a lifetime study of the animal, as you would in human, because the human will keep drinking this stuff for a lifetime. And he found that there's definitely an increase in leukemia and lymphoma, most likely increase in breast cancer, and brain tumor. So then it went to the United States. The CDC said, "We'll look at his study and give a final determination for the American audience." And everybody knew how it was going to turn out. Exactly what they said, "well, we've had some criticism about how the study was done." You know the criticism was? Well, "you did a lifetime study. We cut it off at two years." And he said, "of course you do. That's when the tumors start appearing." So they cut off the study before the tumor started showing up.

Ty: It's the same thing Monsanto did with the GMO studies.

Dr. Blaylock: Yes, exactly. They knew at which point you were going to see the problem with the GMO so they cut the study off before that appeared. And then they said, "we didn't find anything."

Ty: And they did the same thing with the aspartame.

Dr. Blaylock: Yes, I mean, it's just prestidigitation. It's a magic act. And, of course, the public doesn't know these things. The public doesn't understand these delayed effects and onsets. To them it's a mystery. But if you understand the science and that this tumor, or this destruction of kidneys, or this destruction of brain, is not going to occur until certain time and then they cut off the study before that would happen and claim safety. It's a farce.

Ty: It's kind of a crude analogy. But I've often referred to this—when it comes to the GMO study, I was not aware of the aspartame study—but it's really the equivalent of me grabbing somebody by the hair and dunking them underwater and then after five seconds you pull them up and you say, "see, water doesn't cause drowning."

Dr. Blaylock: Yes, they didn't drown.

Ty: Because you didn't do it long enough. And then they don't do the studies long enough mainly because they're only required to be self-authored studies.

Dr. Blaylock: Right. I mean, they do the study, they pay for the study, and they cut it off when they want to. But I couldn't believe that this was the criticism, it's that you carried the study on too long. Humans are taking it. They don't stop taking it at age 50 or age 30. They are taking it for a lifetime.

Ty: I literally see guys and gals at the Stop and Go's or 7-Eleven's with these 100 ounce, huge half gallons of diet sodas.

Dr. Blaylock: Right. What we used to call "belly washers." Huge drinks and they drink all of it.

Ty: And they drink all of it. Also, from what I understand about aspartame is that it has something to do with the release of leptin or ghrelin so that you don't feel satisfied. And you actually gain weight. So is there a link with obesity?

Dr. Blaylock: Yes. What they found is—the hypothalamus is where leptin operates to curb the appetite. There are receptors there—in this particular nucleus, the arcuate nucleus— unless that leptin can react with that receptor, it doesn't work. Well, glutamate is a transmitter for that receptor. And aspartame has aspartic acid which is also an excitotoxin just like glutamate. It burns out that nucleus. So now the leptin won't work. The leptin levels start rising, which is inflammatory, and you start gaining weight. Actually, what they found is that aspartame is not good for weight loss. It actually stimulates gaining of weight. The other thing is that the tyrosine in it, the phenylalanine, stimulates hypoglycemia which makes you hungry.

Ty: So you're going to eat more.

Dr. Blaylock: So you're going to eat more. They knew that. It's not that they didn't know it. They knew it.

Ty: You wonder if that was one of the reasons that they put it out there. You don't know. It's all speculation.

Dr. Blaylock: Yes. You can't prove it but I know that they knew that this research had been done.

Ty: And we know that it does cause obesity, it is linked to cancer. We know those things about aspartame.

Dr. Blaylock: Oh, yes. I would think that you would really be foolish with all we know about aspartame to keep using it. Particularly giving it to children. Because the child's brain is in its stage of formation. A child's brain—the more complex part of brains are not complete until age 27. So all these brain pathways are busy forming their connections. And you're pouring this toxin in, you're damaging it. So what happens is that the kid has a behavior problem. You find out you can't control him. He has these outbursts of anger, or he's depressed, or he has anxiety, has panic attacks.

All of these different things are happening because you fed this glutamate or aspartame from NutriSweet at this particular time. [It] damaged those parts of the brain and then when he got older he couldn't control his behavior. Particularly the front lobe. The front lobe is what gives you your judgment. It says, "Don't jump off that cliff, you'll probably die. Don't run out in the traffic or a car will hit you." If you don't have that frontal control system you practice a lot of risky behaviors.

Ty: Make bad decisions.

Dr. Blaylock: And that's what we're seeing today. The youth are making terrible decisions. They do these crazy things and get themselves killed. And that's exactly what you can do with excitotoxins and vaccines. If you're vaccinating these children at an age their brain is forming and those frontal connections don't form properly, you've got a problem. They're not going to have good judgment. They're not going to feel fear when they're doing something really risky. They don't feel the fear response. They can't look into the future and say, "that's probably going to be harmful" or, "I could fall and die, and break my neck." They have no thoughts of that because their frontal lobe connection is not completely fixed.

Ty: So they don't see the result, that actions have consequences.

Dr. Blaylock: Yes. They can't gauge the consequences of things because it takes that frontal lobe amygdala connection and that's very sensitive to this excitotoxicity.

Ty: Just what you shared today is enough for anyone that's watching this—should run away from glutamate and aspartame, if nothing else.

Dr. Blaylock: Oh, absolutely.

Ty: Last question, Dr. Blaylock. What would your message be to somebody out there that's watching that has cancer? What is your message to cancer patients?

Dr. Blaylock: Well, I think that what cancer patients need to do is, number one, ask their oncologist these critical questions. Do some research. Cancer patients today have an advantage that no cancer patient had in the past. They have an Internet full of really good information. Check it and make sure it's good, accurate information. Talk to people who survived cancer. People who were told they couldn't live and what they did. I found—going around the country talking to a lot of survivors of cancer that shouldn't be alive, according to conventional medicine. The one common denominator I found is that they did juicing of a lot of vegetables. And when you do that, you're pouring your body full of these powerful flavonoids that suppress cancer and they eliminate things like omega-6 fats which are cancer fuels. Corn oil, safflower oil, sunflower oil, peanut oil, canola oil, they all oxidize. They are all powerful inflammatories and they promote cancer grow. And that's been proven. It's all through the literature. They make cancer grow faster.

Ty: And so not only does the juicing help from that perspective but it also doesn't contain the sugar nor the glutamine that fuels the cancer cells, right?

Dr. Blaylock: Right.

Ty: So it's like a triple whammy for them.

Dr. Blaylock: Right. Best of our world.

Ty: Awesome. Well, Dr. Blaylock, thank you so much for being with us today.

Dr. Blaylock: Thank you, I appreciate it. ***[end of transcript]***

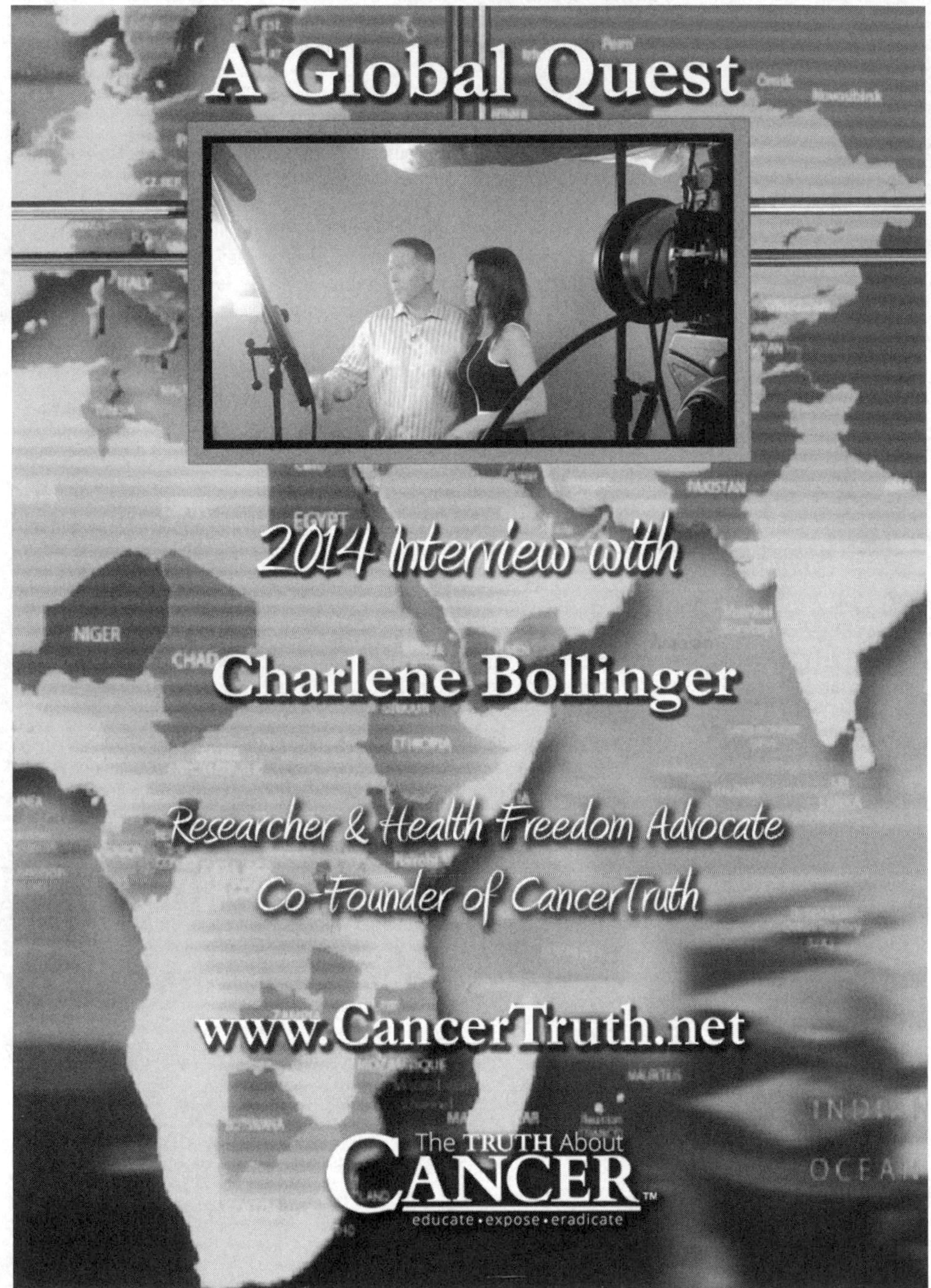
A Global Quest
2014 Interview with
Charlene Bollinger
Researcher & Health Freedom Advocate
Co-Founder of CancerTruth
www.CancerTruth.net
The TRUTH About
CANCER
educate • expose • eradicate

Charlene: Ty's a good daddy.

Interviewer: Yeah?

Charlene: Very good daddy. He loves the children and they love him, clearly. He's just like his father. Yeah, his father always took the time—always, no matter how tired he was—to play with him and as he got older, they shot baskets together and just did everything together. And his grandfather, too, his father's father. So it's been handed down now for generations—the attention and the time and the love. And so he's just naturally a good daddy because he had a really good daddy himself.

Interviewer: Yeah, he was really close to his dad.

Charlene: Yes, he and his father were very close. And when his father was diagnosed with cancer it was quite a shock. But we just were sure that we were going to find a cure and get him well. But unfortunately for us at the time, there was no time because in his case, he had stomach cancer. The tumor blew up in his stomach. And so we took him to the emergency room, he was in such pain. And the doctors came out halfway through the surgery and said—and they just looked rattled—they said, "It's cancer and he's so young and it's so advanced." And I don't remember, I don't think any of us remember anything they said beyond that because we were so shocked. We thought it was just gallstones.

And so they cut out, basically, his whole stomach and sewed him back up and we had the task of telling him—actually, Ty told him when he woke up—that he was diagnosed with cancer, which he was not surprised. Of course, the oncologist was the first to visit, offered chemotherapy and radiation, which, even at that time, we declined. His father was an outside-of-the-box kind of guy and so he wasn't interested in that. And we were looking at alternative treatments—the Hoxsey Clinic down in Tijuana, Mexico, because all that stuff has been outlawed, even back then for many years. But for us, we didn't have time to even find out what worked, and we didn't have the information that we have today.

Twenty-five days later, he died. And we didn't realize at the time but basically, he bled to death. They didn't sew him up properly so the surgery killed him. That's what killed him. It was not the cancer, it was the surgery. And it was heartbreaking, it was hard for Ty, it was hard for both of us. Ty was the glue that held the family together. His mother cried on his shoulder every day for a year, literally. They worked together, and he'd come and cry on my shoulder. And so yes, he and his father were very close and I was blessed to be his daughter-in-love. I was never an in-law. He was never an in-law to me, or his mother. We were in-love. And we miss him still and his mother and all of his family. And we are so grateful for the knowledge that God has given us today that many people, including even doctors and oncologists who don't know what to do when they get that dreaded diagnosis, get a hold of us, get the book, even the series that we're doing, are watching it and learning and doing one or more of the protocols. And contacting the doctors—many doctors out there—who are brilliant and helping and really curing. And that's our goal, to just get the message out there that cancer does not have to be a death sentence. And our children know their grandparents through the many stories, like you were saying earlier, that we've been able to share with them. And one day, because of Jesus, they'll get to see their grandparents again and we're very grateful for that. But yeah, Ty misses his parents and so do I. I was very close, especially with his mother.

Interviewer: Oh, really? You guys spent a lot of time together?

Charlene: Yes, actually, we did. We talked on the phone for hours every day, literally. She was just so dear to me. She just invested, as you saw today, Ty with the children. That was not only Ty's father, but it was also Ty's mother. And she invested her heart in me. I never felt like a daughter-in-law and I never felt like she was my mother-in-law either. She was just my mother-in-love. In fact, I was blessed. The family members called and asked me to write her obituary when she died, which I felt was a huge task because she was the most gracious, loving, kind woman that I had ever known. And I felt like how could I ever put together a summation of her life in a tiny little obituary? But the Lord helped me to do just that and I'm thankful for that. And all the memories that we have we carry with us. And we do what we do in her honor, too, as we remember all that she was. And if we knew then what we know today, I am certain she would still be here. She also did not die of the cancer but of the many conventional treatments that she had to undergo.

Interviewer: You really believe that she would be here today if she had known about natural cancer treatments?

Charlene: Yes, absolutely. Because when she had the surgery, they found cancer—the tumors. And now today, if we knew—you know, if it was today, we would have the knowledge. We would say, "Oh, no problem." We would have boosted her immune system through detox, we would've gotten her involved with one of the great doctors who we know, gotten protocols that would've killed the cancer, and she would've never even had to been cut on. But we didn't know and the doctor, he didn't know. And it wasn't that the doctor was a bad man. He was a good man. He was actually a personal friend of our family and he loved her. He just didn't know. So he came out, they thought it was just a couple of tumors, and he found that her stomach was covered—covered—with this cancer. And he was in tears. And he said, "She's just covered." And they did not know until they opened her up. And so the doctor said we could either just sew her back up or we could cut her stomach out. And of course, we didn't know either. We didn't have this information back then. And so Ty asked the doctor, "Well, if it was your mother, what would you do?" And he said, "Well, I would cut her stomach out." So he did. He cut her stomach out. And by God's grace, she was able to live a lot longer than they anticipated because she did do some alternative things like enzyme therapy to help to digest the food that she no longer had enzymes and other things.

But that was just like a death sentence for her. And of course, when you cut into cancer, that spreads it, and we didn't know that either. And neither did the doctors. Not that he was a bad man. He was not educated on the truth about cancer. And that's what we're trying to get out—the truth about cancer. It does not have to be a death sentence and people don't have to be afraid. We were afraid because we didn't have the knowledge. Knowledge is power and the truth sets us free. And so yes, I'm certain if we got that diagnosis and had the knowledge then that we have today, she would most definitely be here. Maybe she would've died of a car crash or something like that but it would not have been cancer. It would definitely not have been cancer.

Interviewer: I actually didn't know that your mother's stomach was removed. I thought it was your father, right?

Charlene: Yes, it was both of them.

Interviewer: I didn't know that.

Charlene: Yes, yes. They made a makeshift pouch for a stomach that basically, they cut it all out.

Interviewer: So yeah, it sounds like, you know, like most people that go through things like what you guys went through, they don't continue—they don't choose a path that would continually remind them of that. Like they look for things that would kind of stop that and so they can kind of escape that. And that's their way of dealing with the pain. And sometimes perhaps, I don't know, maybe it hurts them more or maybe it hurts them less, I don't know. But then you guys took it on and with it, I would suppose that it's hard for you guys to even hear the word "cancer" without thinking about your parents. Is that true?

Charlene: Well, things have been completely transformed from the way that they were back then simply because we have hope beyond this life, and that's a message we really want people to understand. It's included in our book, *Cancer: Step Outside the Box* that we're all going to die. And what we do with Jesus Christ is going to be where we spend eternity—two places, one or the other. And because my mother-in-love and father-in-love both were Christians, they're with him and we know that we'll see them again.

Also, too, we know that there's a purpose. I said this is just beauty from ashes earlier to you. It's a mess. I mean, humanly speaking, you look at this and think what is the hope in this? You've lost so many people.

Not only the mother and the father and all these grandparents, cousin, uncle, all these people in a pretty short span of time. Six months after we were married, one after the other. What is the hope?

Well, the first one was Ty's father and when he was in the hospital, he never complained. He knew where his hope was, he knew where he was going, and he was a good man, a good man. Just like when you look at Ty, that's who his father was—just a good, good man. Well, God was really working in my heart, as well as Ty's, during the time that his father was ill, showing us that the things that we were pursuing, that so many people in the world pursue, are transient, they're temporary. And one day, they'll be gone, just poof, gone. And we saw that Ty's father was living for what really mattered—for eternity.

And I was sharing these things—there's so much more—but I was sharing these things with Ty's father. He's a big, tall, strong man, beautiful smile. We're walking around the hospital, he's getting his exercise hooked up to all these machines. And he looks down at me after telling how God is really using him in my life and in my heart for good. And he just smiled that brilliant smile he has that you see in Ty and said, "If that's all that God does, is work in your heart with my cancer, then it's all worth it for you." If he could only see today all of the lives that have been spared, all of the souls that are still here enjoying their families and their families enjoying them, he just couldn't believe it. Maybe he knows in heaven, I don't know. But he said it was worth it for me. And to look at all the lives that we have been able to touch just simply by bringing this information into the mainstream. It's criminal that this information has been hidden from the mainstream media, that the information flow has been blocked. And so that's why we feel it is a matter of life and death, this message. The truth about cancer has got to be known.

And so that's what we do. When we hear "cancer," we know that it's easy to cure. We did not know that back then but today, we do know. From the first series, *The Truth About Cancer: The Quest for the Cures,* Webster Kerr, Ty asked him, "If you got cancer, what would you do?" And certain doctors and experts said what they would do, the protocol they would choose. Webster laughed and he said, "Oh, goody. I would say I get to experiment on myself." That's how confident he is. Because he has seen testimony after testimony, patient after patient, and so have we. We have seen patients sent home to die. Says who that they're going to die? We know somebody from Canada that the doctors said—years ago, "Get your affairs in order. You will be gone before Christmas." He got a hold of Ty, read the book. We got him hooked up with a brilliant doctor. The doctor walked through it with him and in his case, he took LifeOne. That's an immune boosting cancer killer. And he did a few other things and he's cancer free. He was so happy he got on his motorcycle and drove down to West Virginia to see this doctor to shake the man's hand that he attributed to saving his life. And he stayed with the doctor and the doctor was very happy to meet him, shake his hand, as well. And then he got back on his motorcycle and went back to Canada. And he said, "I was just so happy to have the energy to get on this bike and ride. I'm alive and completely cancer free." That's the joy that we think of when we hear the word "cancer" now. People like that.

A doctor from Norway who was also sent home to die, they thought he was going to die so many different times—a doctor got a hold of Ty. Today he's back at work, doing well. His wife is doing well. We keep in close contact with him. And we just have testimony after testimony. So today, it's not just theory. There are people out there today who are alive and cancer free because of this information and it's a joy. It's the purpose for which God placed us here on this earth. And Ty's parents, those precious souls, we'll see them again. We know that.

There's a lot of other families enjoying their family members—their fathers or their mothers—because of this information. So when we hear about cancers, hear the word "cancer," that's what we think. We just live to help people. I mean, this is just a passion that we both have and it's a joy.

Interviewer: That's amazing. Such a gift. I am going to ask you shortly about—so get back on some of these amazing success stories and seeing the cures and what that's been like for you to be a part of that. But before I do that, you talked about the closing moment to your father-in-love's life that you know, you obviously—I mean, that was 10 years ago, right?

Charlene: Actually, it was 18 or 19 years ago—18 years. It's been a while.

Interviewer: It can't be.

Charlene: Yes.

Interviewer: You're kidding me.

Charlene: Yes. That was in 1996, so right, yeah.

Interviewer: Twelve years.

Charlene: '96, yeah. Eighteen.

Interviewer: Yeah, you're right, okay.

Charlene: Yeah, 18. And then his mother was 2004 so that was 10. You're thinking about his mother because that was 10 years ago.

Interviewer: Yeah, okay.

Charlene: That's what it is. It was an eight-year span that we went through many deaths. And it was 18 years ago that his father died and 10 that his mother died. And so we had that eight years of tragedy.

Interviewer: Wow. And yeah, because what I was thinking about is with, in particular, zooming back to that unique relationship that you have with your father, that it was 18 years ago now. From the time that he was diagnosed on that day to the time when you said goodbye, it was only 25 days.

Charlene: Mm hmm.

Interviewer: And so it's like it's such a small window that you guys got to say goodbye and yet in that 25 days, you just talk about going through a change in your life that was something that meant so much to you and it meant so much to him to know that you had become a better person. And if it filled God's purpose in your life and God had used him to be a vehicle, a blessing, and that—and then, obviously, like it was the time to direct all our energies and our mind to the suffering—in his own mind to his suffering. That's what he could've chosen to do but it's like what did it mean to you to know that your life and your happiness was more important than his own life to him?

Charlene: That was the man. That's who he was, without a doubt. He was authentic, courageous, and good. Sacrificial. Everything good. During that time, the 25 days that we spent with him, we spent more quality time than some people spend in a lifetime with their father or with their mother, literally. Just to give you an example of what an amazing man he was during that time—I'm not sure if this is included. We included some of the details of what we went through in *Cancer: Step Outside the Box.* But he kept bleeding because they did not sew him up properly. And Ty and I were always there with them or at that time, we had a janitorial service so we had to leave. We were at their house and we left to go clean some buildings or something, and came back and we had maybe eight or so messages on our answering machine. And it was Ty's mother and family calling and saying, "He's back in the hospital. We found out that he had bled everywhere, just passed out and blood just came out both ends." It was terrible.

So he's back in ICU and this is his second or third time he's in the hospital with just major trauma after the surgery. And at this time, Kerith, she was in Abilene, that's Ty's sister, was able to come down and see him. So she was at the hospital when we first got there. And only two people could be in ICU and Ty's mother—beautiful, beautiful woman—was in there with him. And it was my turn to go in. It was just such a privilege to get to go see him. And Kerith had come out and she kind of slumped on the floor and her face was a pasty white and I said, "Are you okay?" And she said, "Dad just doesn't look good." And it was just really affecting her. She was just so shocked. But she didn't have all the time that we had spent with him, it was just a shock for her.

So I went in to see him and as I walked in, he just did not look like himself. If you didn't know him and you were just walking by and you would look in, he would look like maybe a monster. He was just all blown up because he had had I don't know how many blood transfusions. But his face had just swelled to the point where you couldn't even recognize him. And then when he spoke, it was just, you know, real rough. It wasn't his voice. And at this point, he couldn't drink water because of the extreme things going on in his stomach, and we know he was bleeding to death. He wasn't even sewn up properly. And Geri, his wife, his beautiful wife, my mother-in-law, was feeding him ice chips. And she gave me this cup of ice chips and I held it and I went him to feed him the ice chips and he looked at me and even though he didn't look like himself and he didn't sound like himself, his eyes, I could see him in his eyes. They were sparkling and they were just screaming goodness and joy and contentment. In this difficult situation, he never ever complained.

And I didn't say anything but I was thinking, "Wow, he's just beautiful." You know, and the world would say, "Oh, wow, what is that?" But this man was just beautiful. You know, the spirit is what lasts forever, not this outward body. We found that out clearly.

But when I was thinking that, Geri looked at me and she said, "He's beautiful, isn't he?" And I didn't say a word, she just knew. And I said, "Yes, he is." And at that time in my life, it was probably the closest I had ever been to Jesus ever. That's how much like him that Ty's father was. And now he's perfect. He's free from the pain and the suffering. So that's one of the instances that I got to see this man, this amazing man. There's just no one—there was no one on Earth like him. But then he's got this amazing son, Ty. And Ty is a reflection of his father and he's doing the work that would make his father proud. You know, Ty does this because, of course, he wants to honor his mother and father and with all of his heart, he wants to honor the Lord. And together, we know, we desire to help others not to have to suffer as we saw his father suffer and as we had to suffer when we said goodbye. That was very difficult and our lives were forever changed. But over the days and the weeks and the months and even the years now, we see God's goodness.

A question that we get asked is, "How could a loving God allow this to happen?" Well, this loving God cared for Ty's father. As he was going through this, we saw His grace more than than ever in our lives. And Ty's father is now free and we know that we're going to see him again. And we now have the joy to help people around the world. And Ty's father thought it was worth it for me and we can say it was worth it for all the people that we've had the joy of escaping tragedy early before their time.

Interviewer: That makes you feel happy.

Charlene: It does. It does more than most things in life, yes. Yes, it's something that God has put deeply in our hearts that we couldn't live without being able to help these suffering people. We know what it's like to suffer. We know what they're going through and we have the answers for them. And really, it's, I keep saying joy but that's what it is. It's a joy to be able to give them answers, hope, truth, and health. Beauty from ashes. There's just nothing like it.

Interviewer: Wow, that's amazing. Yeah, I mean, it all makes sense. Like it makes sense because it's a pain that you felt and it's a pain that you can still remember because it's part of human experience. It's one that brings–the memories bring so much joy and you know that your parents are holding the hands of God. And yet, at the time, like there's nothing that you wouldn't have done to trade that circumstance and had perfect health.

Charlene: Oh, yeah, yes.

Interviewer: And to have had them around and to have them playing with the children and being in the photographs and the videos this evening.

Charlene: Yeah, that's the hardest.

Interviewer: Why is that hard?

Charlene: Because they were so loving and these children are so sweet. We take turns. Sometimes we say, "Oh, if they were only here, if they were only here, they would be beating down our door to get to these children." Yeah, that's still difficult. We still both have a difficult time with that. And we have to remind each other that there is purpose, there is a reason. And we get to tell the children the wonderful stories that I'm telling you now about their amazing grandparents. And they miss them. They say all the time how they miss them, as if they know them. So that is a consolation to be able to give them these beautiful stories, to have it written in a book and many articles and interviews. They do have a connection so that's a consolation and it's also a consolation that others get to have grandparents, that that's a blessing.

Interviewer: Yeah, because I mean, when I was just chatting with Ty, you know, it makes sense. Because like Proverbs 17:6 says, "Children's children are the crown of old men and the glory of children is their father." So children's children, so that means like a child, my child has a child. So it's grandparents, children are the crown of old men. So it's like that is–it's like being crowned. And so like, it is special, so there's every reason why you guys feel the way that you do because God made it that way. He made those relationships so rich and you guys have every reason to desire that God put in your hearts and the desire that the children have in their hearts. You know, and so it makes sense that you guys would grieve that. And yeah, obviously, look at photographs of all these things, right?

Charlene: Yes, we show them pictures frequently, yes. They think their grammy is just so beautiful and she is. She was beautiful on the outward appearance but more so, in the heart. But yeah, we look at pictures, tell stories.

Interviewer: Yeah. And the kids will never know sorrow, yeah? They don't know about—they don't understand grief and loss, do they?

Charlene: Through the loss in the stories that they have—they've experienced grief that way but they've not dealt with it firsthand. The big kids—we have four, of course—and the two older ones were very little at the time that Grammy died. Brianna was three, Bryce was about eighteen months old. So Bryce says he has memories of that. He's a bright boy. I don't know, he may have a few. But they certainly, even if they had memories, would not understand grief at that age and loss. So no, not like we—it would be devastating for them to lose a parent or a sibling at this point. Or a grandparent now.

Interviewer: Yeah, yeah. Yeah, perhaps God, in his mercy, spared that loss, too, you know? Like that is—that's a hard one to look at both sides of that. And with that experience would come greater pain because you know, I had my granddad die when I was one and so I wasn't old enough for me to remember. He was a hero in the mind of the family. But I'd hate to go through that, you know?

Charlene, what's it like for you? You see—it's like every—it's like people have a mission to save lives for all different reasons. I admire anyone that's involved in something that they believe is contributing and helping to either enrich or rescue someone's life. But then the actual value and the gift of what life is, then that changes things again. It sounds like with you and Ty, like you value relationships so much, people are really important to you. Or like people that are your family, friends, loved ones that become like family. It sounds like with you guys, when you go out to reach out, like you do it because—yeah, it's almost like you guys are inviting people into having that richness and that—you know. I don't know if you can see in your mind's eye right now what it would be like for that family that did go through that book and they went through the documentary series, or the one that's just going to air. And you know, they might just be in their 50s or even, say, 60s, or whatever. But somebody has just watched and they suddenly had this full resolve and then they get hit with the news even a year later. And then all of a sudden they know exactly within their hidden emotion and they start the treatments right away with all the immune system boosting and the detoxification.

And then, you know, and so then you see this picture in your mind of this same person living 20 years past and enjoying all these precious moments that they have on this Earth and playing with their grandchildren. Not only seeing them when they're little but watching them kind of go through school and then graduating. What's that like for you seeing that image and knowing you're a part of it?

Charlene: There's just nothing else like it. When we first started, we got *Cancer: Step Outside the Box*, it was our intention to just get the information out here. We were just working so hard to get that book together because with all of our hearts, we wanted to get the information out to everyone. We thought it was criminal that this was not mainstream information. And so as I told you earlier, when we had that book—the proof in our hand, we just couldn't believe we had a book. And then it dawned on Ty, "Oh, wow, do you think we'll sell a copy?" And we talked to someone that we knew that was high up in one of the computer companies. And we told him we just wanted to charge the price of the book, or our cost. We wanted to just get the information out there. And he laughed at us and he said, "Are you kidding?" You do that and no one will take you seriously. If you want people to think this is a real book, you've got to put a real price on it. And we thought, "Oh, yeah."

So we went ahead and put a real price on the book but we put on our website, "Please, if you cannot afford this book, email us. We don't want you to not have the information because you cannot afford it. We will get this book to you. Tell us what you're going through." And so we got so many emails from people and they would make us just cry. One that I remember early on was from a man. He said that he had been through the conventional treatments—chemotherapy and all the rest of the things—and that he had no money left. And the doctor said, "Okay, but there's nothing left we can do." And he said, "I know this sounds terrible but I don't even have the money to buy your book. And I have a nine-year-old son and I want to see him grow up." Well, of course, I'm crying when I get that one. I mean, still, it makes me tear up every time I think of it. Of course, we give him the book. So many people we don't hear back from and we do pray for these people. But God, the great physician, would touch their bodies, would direct their steps, would give them wisdom and connect them to these amazing doctors that are all over the place helping with great protocols that really are curing cancer.

And some we do hear from. And it is, like you said, you know, not having our parents—grandparents for our children—and we get into moments. Like today, the amazing filming, the beautiful pictures that you got of Ty or the children in our family. Of course, we think, "Wow, if Grammy could only see this." You know, Ty's parents, but they're not here. And who knows what they can see in heaven? We don't know that. We like to think that there may be some glimpses, something. They probably know more than we do. But we don't know. You know, we don't have that physical connection. But yes, there are families out there that because of this information, have been able to see their grandchildren grow up, or will be able to see their grandchildren grow up. Or their children or their parents, whatever the case may be. For us, it was parents and grandparents that we don't have.

Interviewer: God has called you also to be sharing in this and I can see that and you've obviously been involved in sharing it because just the way you speak about it.

Charlene: I just want to say to you, you may have been diagnosed with cancer. You may be struggling with cancer right now and not know what to do. You may have a loved one that has just been diagnosed with cancer. You may be—or a loved one—may be diagnosed in the very near future. We've experienced it again and again in my family. And when we went through it, we didn't have these answers, but we have them today. We have them for you. There is a purpose right now for you watching this. There is a reason. And I'm so glad that you're watching it. And with all of our heart, we want you to be well. We want to give you the answers to be well, and your loved ones to be well. We want you to join us in this mission, share it with your friends. Share it with everyone that you know. This information should be everywhere. Everyone that you know should know this like the back of their hands.

Cancer does not have to be a death sentence. That is our message to you today. Life is a gift and we have the answers to abundant life beyond a cancer diagnosis. We pray that this is a blessing to you and that you watch it again and again. Share it with your loved ones. Learn the truth that will truly set you free. God bless you.

Interviewer: Well done. ***[end of transcript]***

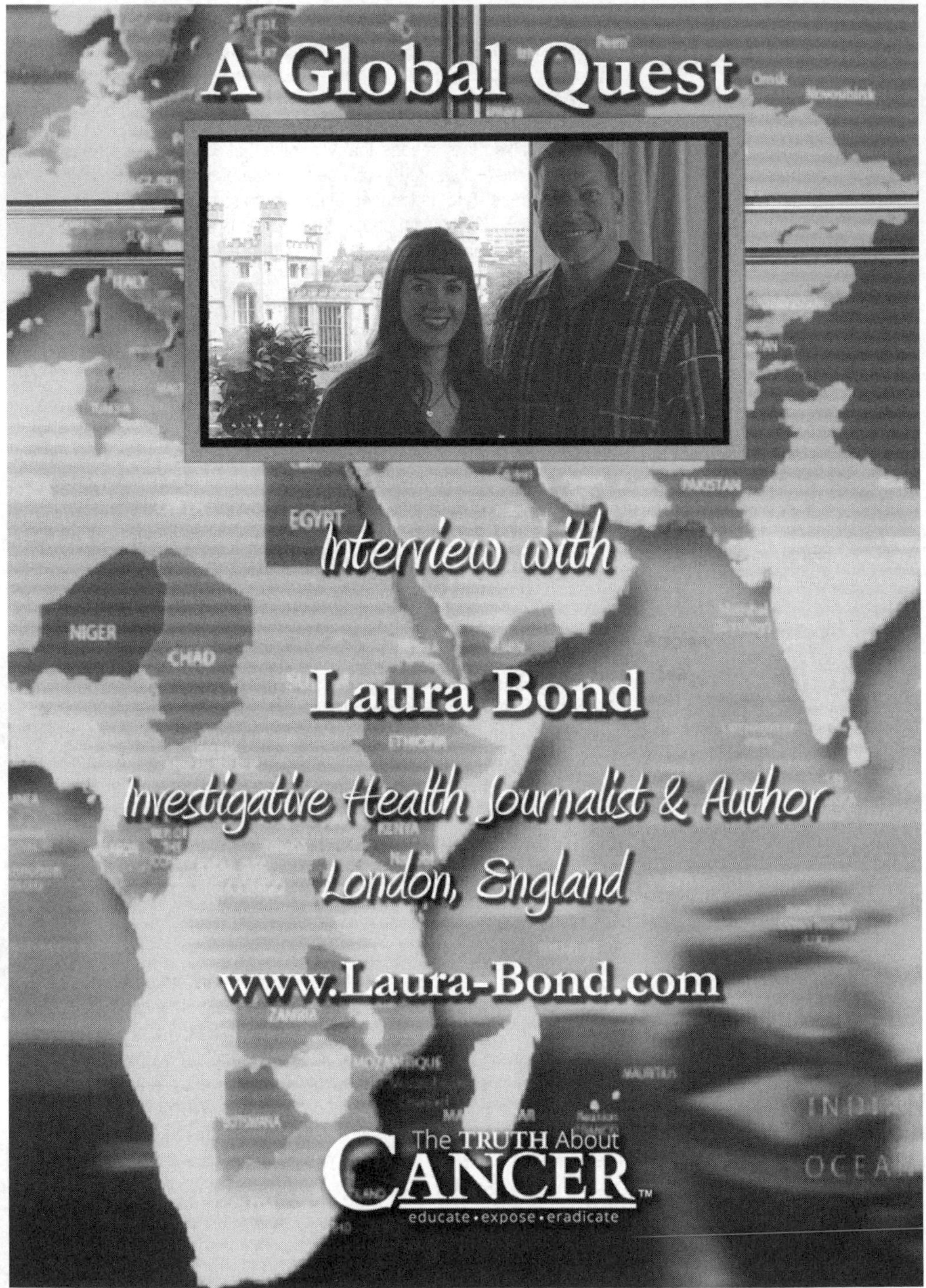
A Global Quest
Interview with
Laura Bond
Investigative Health Journalist & Author
London, England
www.Laura-Bond.com
The TRUTH About
CANCER
educate • expose • eradicate

Ty: I'm really honored to be here today in London, England. You can see we've got—in the background here—we've got Parliament Building, we've got Big Ben, and I'm sitting here with Laura Bond. Laura, thank you for joining me today.

Laura: It's an absolute pleasure, Ty.

Ty: So I'm really looking forward to getting onto the story that you wrote about in your book. And—as well as some other information—your perspective on cancer.

Laura: Well, it's a privilege to share it with you Ty, because me and my mom are both huge fans of *The Quest for the Cures*. She wanted to send her gratitude for having us on the show. She's in Australia at the moment, so sadly can't be here, but yeah, huge fan. So it's a big privilege.

Ty: You—were you born in Australia?

Laura: Born in London, actually.

Ty: But your mom lives in Australia now?

Laura: Exactly. Yeah, so she's coming over here in a couple weeks. We're going hiking in Romania together, so it's nice. From London, you're so close to the rest of Europe.

Ty: Okay, yeah, very nice. So tell her that we're sorry that we missed her. But we're glad that you could be here today to communicate her story.

Laura: Thank you.

Ty: Yeah, so let's go back in time to the impetus that caused you to write your book. You wrote a book on cancer and it was called—what?

Laura: It's called *You Can Say No to Chemo*. So in 2011, my mom was diagnosed with ovarian and uterine cancer, which is a pretty tough diagnosis. And people were shocked by her decision to say "no" to chemo, and to radiation. She didn't want to do any of that.

So part of the reason I started writing a blog and then the book was to bring to light some of the limitations of chemotherapy, but also to show what else is out there. And there's so much else out there, as you well know. From electrical fields for brain cancer—which is FDA approved—to turmeric, to cannabis oil, to high-dose vitamin C.

I'd already been a journalist for about six years. And so, as a journalist, I had access to doctors around the world. And I started interviewing them to find out what they were doing. And, you know, I'm indebted to these doctors, because they were so generous with their time and I wanted to share the information that they were sharing with me with other people.

So that's the whole point of the book. It's about choices. I'm not telling people what to do. Far from it. I'm simply opening their minds to the wide range of healing possibilities out there so people can make a decision based on information rather than fear.

Ty: Right, right. That's really our mission as well, is to put the information out there and to give people choices. Unfortunately—I don't know how it is here in the UK—but in the United States, people feel like they are—they're limited to only chemo and radiation, surgery, if they're diagnosed with cancer. What's the atmosphere like here in the UK?

Laura: It's pretty similar. I mean, I think you'll find the same thing in Australia as well. So unfortunately, doctors in America, Australia, the UK, they can risk losing their medical license if they recommend anything other than the gold standard, which is chemotherapy and radiotherapy. In my mind, those treatments are substandard.

So we know that chemotherapy and radiotherapy cause cancer, which is the very thing they're supposed to prevent. I mean, you look on the back of the chemo— certain chemotherapy drugs, like doxorubicin— and you'll see a listed side effect is leukemia.

Ty: And doxorubicin's a pretty popular chemo drug.

Laura: Yeah. Absolutely. And you know—you know as well as I do that the latest research from Harvard Medical School and UCLA is showing that chemotherapy actually stimulates cancer stem cells, which are the germ cells from which new tumors arise. So I wanted to make people aware of this, but also to bring them other options.

There are ways—if you are going to do chemotherapy, there are ways of doing it which are far more targeted, which don't devastate the immune system as much. You can avoid losing your hair, you can avoid feeling nauseous having chemotherapy, by doing so. Hyperthermia.

Ty: So things you can do while you're undergoing chemo?

Laura: Exactly.

Ty: Okay. Name some other things that you may have come across in your research that might help somebody that's watching right now—

Laura: Yeah, sure.

Ty: —that's doing chemo?

Laura: So, high-dose vitamin C. It boosts the immune system, and protects you against viruses, and it's said to reduce the toxicity of chemotherapy.

Ty: Which, by the way, I hate to interrupt you but if you're in Indonesia, you can just go into any clinic in Indonesia and get high-dose vitamin C.

Laura: That's amazing!

Ty: You can walk off the street, have $35 to 40 dollars—you can get high-dose vitamin C.

Laura: No way.

Ty: Yeah.

Laura: And I mean, vitamin C is a cheap substance, so it should be cheap. But unfortunately—because I suppose doctors have to, you know, legally cover themselves and all this other things—it is expensive privately. And that's the other thing my mom found.

She thought it was—it's so sad that people are punished financially for choosing alternatives, because, of course, you know, chemotherapy and radiotherapy, they are actually expensive, but mostly, you get them free on the National Health Service.

Ty: Right. So National Health Service here, in the United States—most of them are covered by insurance with a very, very low deductible. But one of the things that we've heard from countless patients is, "The reason that I went with chemo and radiation is because they were covered." Not because they worked the best, but because they were covered. So it's kind of the same here.

Laura: And that's why, in my book, I—the final chapter is *Overcoming Cancer on the Cheap*. And I wanted to talk about things like turmeric, things like cannabis oil—that there are other things out there that are more affordable.

Even—something my mom's recently started using, is this machine called the Pyro-Energen, which uses negative static electricity. And what it's supposed to do is to interfere with cancer cell division. And there's no published research reports on this particular machine, but in 2011, the FDA approved a machine using electrical fields for brain cancer. And the way that they describe the way that works is by interrupting cancer cell division. So it's kind of interesting.

And I think this area of electrical nutrition—that's what K. Scott-Mumby calls it—is really exciting. And these machines are becoming more and more affordable, which is great news.

Ty: Yeah it is. I was mentioning that I did not know that the FDA had actually approved a machine.

Laura: Yeah, absolutely. If you look up—and anyone can Google it—I think it's Bill Doyle. He talks about it on TED Talk actually. And there's some case studies on that sort of video, linked to the TED Talk. People can go and look it up. I think the company's name is Novocure.

Ty: Alright, great. So let's go back in time. You mentioned that you were a journalist for several years. Who did you work with?

Laura: I've written for *The Sunday Times*, *The Mail on Sundays*, *Psychologies*, different health magazines over here and in Australia. I've written a piece for *Sunday Times* about why sauerkraut is the new super food and pieces in Australia about high-dose vitamin C. So what kind of motivates me is bringing news about natural health to the public.

Ty: Right.

Laura: It's great to be able to do that. But I also love working one-on-one with health coaching clients. So I've been doing that for the last two years. So I work with people with everything from anxiety, to hormonal issues, to people who want a cancer-preventative diet

But the interesting thing is, Ty, the more research I've been doing on anxiety—because so many people are coming to me with that at the moment—is that there's so many links between foods you need to boost your mood, feel better about yourself, lower anxiety—these same foods are also anti-cancer. And so I know in your last series you had that great quote from Keith Scott-Mumby. I think he said that, "Any good health measure is an anti-cancer measure," which I love. I really liked that. And I'm finding that more and more that a lot of the anti-cancer measures are anti-anxiety measures.

So things like celery. We know that celery stimulates the parasympathetic nervous system, which is that calming part of the nervous system. So you know, a perfect snack is a bit of celery with some peanut butter or nut butter, make it a bit more tasty.

And the reason it does that, is because it contains this plant hormone called apigenin. And apigenin is powerfully anti-cancer. And anyone can Google apigenin and it will come up with a load of scientific references. And then the other thing, which I often recommend food-wise for people with stress is foods with B-6.

So sweet potato, pumpkin seed, seafood. B-6 improves or stimulates serotonin in the body, which is that feel-good neurotransmitter. But there's all these studies recently showing that high blood levels of B-6 are powerfully anti-cancer. So you can reduce your risk of cancer by up to 49 percent by eating a vitamin B-6 rich diet. Which is kind of cool.

Ty: That is very cool. It's fascinating how many foods contain anti-cancer properties. Really, they all do in some way or another.

Laura: Yeah, exactly.

Ty: All natural foods do.

Laura: Absolutely. And it's so exciting, you know, hearing about all these foods like broccoli sprouts and turmeric that can actually take on cancer stem cells.

Ty: Yeah, that's the big one, right? Because many people in the last few weeks—we've been interviewing all over the place—and we're getting that common thread that you want to take care of the stem cells. And there's certain foods that do that, and broccoli, broccoli sprouts, because of the sulforaphane is one of the foods that actually do that.

Laura: Yeah, absolutely. I mean, there's a study from Liverpool University here showing that, you know, a serving of broccoli a day reduces your risk of colon cancer 50 percent. Well, imagine then, if you're having broccoli sprouts, which contain up to 100 times more sulforaphane than normal broccoli.

And people are always a bit like, "Well, what do I do with the broccoli sprouts?" They've got a kind of mustard-y flavor. They are quite strong, but I find if you put them in your juicer with beet root, celery and carrot, kind of—if you're not mad about the flavor it does mask them a bit. Just sprinkle a few on salads.

Ty: Sure.

Laura: I mean, they're so potent that you only need a little bit of them. And they're so cheap, that's such an affordable super-food. If you go to an organic supermarket here, it's like a pound-fifty, which is probably like $3 or something.

Ty: Right.

Laura: And they last in your fridge for two weeks or something.

Ty: Right. Very inexpensive. You mentioned super-foods. I'm going to ask you a question. I hope you can answer this. Why is sauerkraut the new super-food?

Laura: Sauerkraut is the new super-food because it's wonderful. You get—a spoonful of sauerkraut delivers trillions of probiotics and enzymes, which are just so powerfully anti-cancer. So our gut health is the center of our immune system, 80 percent of our immune cells are in our gut.

So looking after the healthy bacteria there is just so important for whatever you're dealing with: digestion, stress, any immune sort of problem, which cancer, of course, is.

I came across an interesting article recently though, from the University of Michigan, and it was showing that healthy bacteria can help you get through chemo. And the—I think the article was titled *Gut Reaction: Mice Survive Lethal Doses of Chemotherapy*. And they're talking about how important this healthy bacteria is.

So great for people going through chemotherapy. Great for anyone. I mean, I have a lot of people that come to me and they get bloated all the time. They've got digestive issues. And they might have cut out dairy, they might have cut out gluten, but they're still sitting at their desks getting a horrible bloated feeling. And so often it's because of a lack of enzymes in their diet and too much stress.

But so having, you know, say a tablespoon of apple cider vinegar, or a scoop of sauerkraut before you start eating gets those digestive juices flowing.

Ty: So that's one of the—that's something that can be really practical for everybody that's watching this. Sometimes you go to buy enzymes or probiotics—they're very expensive. But you can make it on the cheap with sauerkraut.

So explain to somebody real quick how they might make some sauerkraut that has all of these enzymes and probiotics.

Laura: Okay, well, to be honest with you Ty, I'm a bit lazy. I make my own almond milk, I make my own juices, but there's only so much you can do, so I haven't actually. I've tried my own kimchi. I haven't made my own sauerkraut, but I do know that all it involves is salt and cabbage.

And you know, you can press it, the cabbage shrinks a little, and then you can just keep it for a couple—I think for about two and a half weeks is about how long you need to wait for all those healthy bacteria to start proliferating.

Ty: Right.

Laura: Because basically, cabbage contains those bacteria naturally on the cabbage leaves. And then when you're salting it and preserving it, you're bringing all those to the fore.

Ty: Right. Well, you just did a great job of explaining it even though you say you didn't understand how to make it. It's salt and cabbage. You let it sit for a couple weeks, you keep pressing it down, and you've got the sauerkraut.

Laura: Exactly, yeah.

Ty: It's very inexpensive.

Laura: It's very inexpensive. I mean, I guess I'm lazy with that one because my organic supermarket, for a pound-fifty—you're getting about the same price—for $3 you get a delicious jar. There's a brand I really like. So I have it with eggs, because it's got that sort of acidity that's quite nice. Put it on top of salads. It's a great thing. Have it daily.

Ty: Now the Germans eat it on top of hot dogs. I guess if you're getting a hot dog that's no nitrates and no preservatives that would be okay. If you don't want to put it on top of a hot dog from the supermarket.

Laura: No. But it's interesting you say that though, because the healthy bacteria in the sauerkraut—it's great if you are having a barbecue or whatever, because it's said to offset those cancer-causing compounds that you get from cooked meat.

Ty: The HCA.

Laura: Yes, exactly.

Ty: Right.

Laura: So it's great to have around at a barbecue. Any sort of pickled food—really, really good for that.

Ty: Yeah, it's funny that you mentioned that, because last week we were in Atlanta, Georgia. And we were sitting at a table with about 10 or 12 guys. And one of the men there was Dr. David Jockers, who we interviewed for *The Quest for the Cures*.

Laura: Oh, fantastic.

Ty: Now, we ordered—it was a completely organic restaurant, and so we ordered some hot wings. Now they came out, and some of them had the black on them, which is the HCA, heterocyclic amines. Now what we did before we ate them though, is we drank this shake that contained probiotics, enzymes, ginger and a bunch of other compounds that offset the heterocyclic amines. So you can actually eat it, without having the carcinogenic effect, if you drink the shake first.

Laura: First. Offset the guilt.

Ty: So there are things that you can do to offset it, right? Yeah.

Laura: I love hearing about these tips, because people want to live a normal life. They want to be able to enjoy their favorite things.

Ty: Right.

Laura: And actually, that's something that really surprised me in the research—and this is going off track a little—but it's how important pleasure is in the healing paradigm. You know, there's a study from the University of Pittsburgh showing that pleasure, or a sense of joy, is the second most important factor for predicting cancer recovery.

So I'd advise people not to cut out completely anything that provides them with a lot of pleasure, or—obviously if they're dealing with cancer, cutting out sugar is a must. Dairy, something that's probably quite advisable, especially if you've got hormonal cancers. But finding pleasure in other things.

Taking time out every day to do something that just makes you lose track of time, where you're completely absorbed in it.

Ty: Right.

Laura: Give yourself that rather than constantly being on this to-do list world of doing this and do that, and suddenly the day's gone, and you haven't squeezed out that joy.

Ty: You haven't enjoyed anything.

Laura: Yeah, absolutely.

Ty: No, I have to agree with you on that. That's really congruent to the information that we've gotten from a lot of other interviewees, is that the emotional, the mental state, is very important. And so, joy, happiness, pleasure, laughter, all these things actually not only make you feel good, but they help regulate your immune system.

Laura: Yeah. It's really, really interesting. And especially the stress thing. I think, you know, we know intuitively that when we're really, really stressed, we're more primed to get sick, you know? You come down with the flu, you get a breakout of acne, you get a throbbing headache.

And you might shrug your shoulders and say, "I'm under a lot of pressure right now." So we intuitively make that connection. But for so long we've been sort of reluctant to make this connection between stress and cancer. We'd rather attribute it to bad genes, bad luck, smoking.

But the latest research is telling us otherwise. I mean, there's a 2009 study from China showing that adrenaline, which is that fight-or-flight hormone, can actually make cancer resistant to treatment. When I interviewed Dr. Joan Borysenko for *You Can Say No to Chemo*—she's a Harvard-trained scientist and psychologist.

And she said, "Yeah, we never thought that there was a link between stress and cancer, but we now know that when you're stressed, the enzymes that repair breaks in DNA are damaged. So in essence, you can't repair damaged DNA as well." So I think it's good for us to know the impact that stress can have on disease.

Some people initially are frustrated by that. They're like, "Well, what do I do? Life's stressful. I've got elderly parents to look after. I've got kids. I've got a pressurized job." And it's not about avoiding stress so much as it's about changing your perception to it, building certain things into your day, quick things you can do which can dial down stress.

Ty: Right.

Laura: And—yeah.

Ty: So if you're a cancer patient and you go to your oncologist, and they say, "Laura, you have cancer. You're dead in three months." What does that do your stress level?

Laura: That totally triggers the amygdala in your brain, and you go on that panic—panic side, and of course, you know, everyone might have that immediate reaction.

But sort of stepping back—I mean, the first thing I recommend to patients is don't stare despairingly at statistics. Fill your mind with stories of survivors, because if they can do it, why can't you? Because I think that's the first thing that people do when they're diagnosed, is they go online and, "Oh my God. I've got three months," or whatever. You read the horrible prognosis. So I think it's taking your mind away from that and start researching all the wonderful possibilities that are there for you.

So, yeah. In terms of dialing down stress, there's lots of things my mom built into her life, especially in that first six months. Getting outside was one of them. Nature's a great relaxer. Just having a beautiful canopy of branches above your head, fresh air in your face, and just being able to actually look into the distance.

So often we get stuck against a phone screen or a computer screen, we're not looking into our peripheral vision, or distance. And just literally doing that can take you out of that rumination and can sort of give you a bit of perspective.

Ty: Right. What else did your mom do? Talking about your mother and her cancer. So she refused chemo?

Laura: Yeah, and radiotherapy.

Ty: What did she do? She refused chemo and radiation.

Laura: Yeah, despite much pressure—I mean, so much pressure—from her oncologist, and from doctors, and from family, and from friends. I mean, part of the reason was Mom's brother, Douglas, had leukemia in his 30s, and he died after a hellish year of chemo.

And that had obviously quite an impact on my mom, and she vowed that if she ever got cancer, she wouldn't do chemotherapy. So she had no idea how much pressure she'd be under.

Ty: So a lot of pressure from everyone?

Laura: Huge amount of pressure, but she stuck to her guns. She just—she knew intuitively, for her—she just didn't believe that you could heal yourself by poisoning the body. So thankfully she was already very interested in alternative health, so she knew about vitamin C injections and that was her start. That's where she started off. She had 60,000 mg of vitamin C injected twice a week.

Ty: Wow.

Laura: And we know from the National Institutes of Health in America—I think it was Mark Levine—studies in 2008 showing that over 50,000 mg of vitamin C can take on cancer and leave healthy cells intact.

Ty: Right.

Laura: It's wonderful. Exactly. So my mom did that. There's also studies from Japan showing that women with uterine cancer live 15 times longer when they have vitamin C. So it's a really great thing. Of course, that wasn't the only thing my mom did. She really focused on detoxing the body as well.

So she started having infrared saunas at least twice a week—so take off that toxic load of the body. It helps pull out heavy metals, which can compromise the immune system. She started taking different supplements with medicinal mushroom. She started doing ozone therapy. So she had quite a program in the end. She really looked after her emotional health. For her, that was a big thing. And she cut out dairy. That was huge.

Ty: Cut out dairy. Did she do this under the supervision of a medical doctor here in the UK, or was it on her own?

Laura: It was in Australia.

Ty: Oh, it was in Australia.

Laura: Yeah. It took her a few months to find, you know—she did have various sort of physicians and naturopaths that she was working with, but also—because I'd started being heavily interested in this research, I was interviewing. I interviewed 60 experts around the world in the course of writing the book.

So each time I'd speak to Dr. Johnathon Wright, or Dr. Gary Gordon, I'd be like, "Mom, I think we should start looking into this as well and you might want to try it." Or I'd speak to someone from Indian medicine about turmeric, "We have to start juicing that."

My mom did a lot of research herself as well. As I said, she's always been into holistic health, so a lot of these things I talk about in the book, it's been Mom pushing me. She's like, "You should look at this," and, "I don't think we can ignore energy healing in the healing paradigm." So it was a really collaborative effort.

Ty: Now, the book: was it a direct result of your mother being diagnosed, or was it something that you already had on your mind?

Laura: No, it was a direct result of that. Yeah, so prior to that I was actually doing a lot of research into prenatal nutrition. Looking at other things to do with that. So this was a completely different path.

But as I said, now I'm sort of—I'm dealing with health coaching clients with all sorts of problems. And what's been interesting for me, is that doing the research for the book—it's provided such a base knowledge for so many things.

So whether people are coming with arthritis, or anxiety, or hormonal issues, to me, they all boil down to about five factors which you look at. Which is too many toxins, missing minerals like magnesium, not enough enzymes, too much stress, and too much sugar.

So right now, in London, I run a lot of workshops on, like, how to beat stress and cut sugar cravings. Because that's something so many people are doing.

Ty: Oh yeah. Sugar's very addictive. You mentioned prenatal nutrition. So let me get your opinion on why we have this explosion in childhood cancer.

Laura: That's, yeah, it's interesting. I think toxins play a huge part in that. I mean, you look at how—you know, phones. I'm just thinking of phones in general, because I'm thinking of childhood brain cancer has really gone up. And the average person looks at their phone every six minutes.

And we know that the radiation from the phone can cause brain cancer. That was a World Health Organization report showing that. That just 10 minutes a day for 10 years ups your risk of glioma and certain deadly types of brain cancer by a huge amount. So I think, you know, having all this radiation around us. Of course, kids are much smaller, so they're much more susceptible to all these pesticides, toxins, mercury, that we're surrounded by in the air and the water, and everything else. So that's my opinion on why I think we have more childhood cancers.

Ty: Yeah, I think you're right on as far as the fact that they really are more susceptible to all this toxicity. You mentioned mercury. I'm not sure what the vaccine schedule is like here in the UK, but in the United States it's horrible. It's upwards of 50 vaccines now before they even start school.

Laura: Oh my God.

Ty: So, you know, you get these kids, and mercury does go through the blood-brain barrier.

Laura: Yep, absolutely.

Ty: So you're going to hit them as soon as they're born with all of these toxins. A couple of them, in most vaccines, are known carcinogens.

Laura: Yeah. Absolutely.

Ty: So it's no surprise.

Laura: I mean, if I—everyone's going to make their own decision about what's right for them, but certainly I don't know that—vaccinations are certainly something I would be not wanting to compromise my small—especially that first one they give you within 24 hours of the child being born, the hepatitis B. It's a sexually transmitted disease, why on earth do they need to give that to children within 24 hours of them being born?

Ty: Right.

Laura: It just seems crazy to me.

Ty: I've not yet known a newborn that's sexually active.

Laura: Yeah. I mean—

Ty: Or an intravenous drug user. That's the two biggies for Hep B.

Laura: And so—I read the other day also, it's not just children, but now doctors are being struck off the list if they don't have the full spectrum of these vaccinations.So it's pressure coming from every angle.

And I think what it really comes down to is health freedom. That's what it's eroding. And whatever your stance on vaccinations is, I think everyone would agree that if we live in a democracy, we should have the right to choose how we treat our body and what we put in it, and not be told, "You can't attend the elementary school unless your child has A, B, C, D, Zed vaccinations."

Ty: Yeah. And at the same token, with treatments for cancer, that's what we're all about as well.

Laura: Exactly.

Ty: It's just the choice.

Laura: And that's what people are being denied right now. I had a health coaching client the other day who—she'd had some lumps in her breasts, which turned out not to be cancerous, but she wanted to be proactive, and she asked her doctor, "What can I do to prevent cancer?" And he said, "Don't get fat and don't smoke."

And she said, "Well, what about diet? I heard dairy—there's some links between dairy and cancer." He's like, "Oh, no. There's nothing in the medical literature about that." There's a ton.

Ty: Yeah. There is.

Laura: And so, it's just—it leaves you so despondent, you know, if they can't even tell you to cut down on sugar. I mean, a 2009 review of over a million people found that your risk of cancer goes up for every extra unit of glucose in the blood.

So not only is it when you have cancer—because we know that cancer's a sugar guzzling machine—but in terms of prevention, it's very important to cut down the amount of sugar in your diet.

Ty: Yeah. And they're just now learning that sugar actually is oncogenic. It creates cancer. It not only feeds it—

Laura: Really?

Ty: —but is also—it gives rise to cancer.

Laura: Okay.

Ty: There's a recent study that I don't know the citation, but Sayer Ji—we just interviewed—he mentioned the fact that sugar is now known to be oncogenic. So it doesn't just feed it, it creates it.

Laura: He's a legend. He's always getting the latest.

Ty: He really is a good researcher, yeah. So Laura, what would your advice be, what would your message be to somebody that may be watching that's been recently diagnosed with cancer?

Laura: I'd say take a step back. I mean, give yourself a week to 10 days to just sit and think about what you want to do. Maybe get a second opinion. Do your research. Work out what's best for your cancer. Research as much as possible and find out what the right path is for you.

So sort of think slowly and then act quickly. And once you decide on a path, put your faith in it. Because faith is so important in the healing paradigm. So put your faith in healing and the fear behind you. That's what I'd say.

Ty: That's good advice. Now what—where are you at now? Where's your mom at now, how is she doing? Talk about the reaction maybe of her doctors to her healing process.

Laura: Yeah, okay, absolutely. So Mom, she looks and feels fantastic. As I said, she's over here in a couple weeks. We're going to go hiking in Romania. But she did—so she completely got rid of her ovarian and uterine cancer. So it's four and a half years on from that.

But in January 2014, my mom was actually diagnosed with pancreatic cancer which was a total shock. And it's adenocarcinoma, so the really tough one. So the typical survival time for advanced pancreatic cancer is three months. Well, we're 18 months on. Mom looks, feels fabulous. So she's under the care of Dr. Nicholas Gonzalez in New York.

Who—I'm so grateful that I interviewed him for the book, so I knew about him. He's been working with cancer patients for 25 years, has phenomenal success, and particularly with pancreatic cancer. So for him—the story—for patients that are under him, the story can be different. He has, you know—he had a patient that lived for 14 years and died after a car accident.

So his protocol involves enzymes, individualized diets, and coffee enemas daily. So Mom's doing all of that, she's taking about 60 enzymes a day with magnesium, because you need magnesium to activate the pancreatic enzymes. And yeah, she's feeling and looking really good.

Ty: Oh, she's going to do great under his care. We'd interviewed him for *The Quest for the Cure* last year. And he actually has one pancreatic cancer patient that's over 30 years out.

Laura: That's amazing.

Ty: Which is unheard of.

Laura: It is completely unheard of.

Ty: Yeah, and those enzymes are very important for pancreatic cancer patients because they're not producing them on their own.

Laura: It's so, so important. As Dr. Nicholas Gonzalez describes, you need the enzymes to break down the fibrin that creates cancer cells, so you can let the immune cells get in and do their job.

I also like Dr. Gary Gordon. He explains why enzymes are so important really well. He said, "The enzymes make the blood less like ketchup and more like red wine." And I said, "Well, what's that got to do with cancer?"

And he said, "Well, when the blood's really thick it actually moves cancer from one place to the other more easily. And so when you have blood that's more like red wine, and thinner thanks to the enzymes, you've got less chance of metastasis." So it's that kind of preventative reason as well.

Ty: That's great reasoning. And actually, what kills cancer patients many times—it's not the cancer, it's the spread of the cancer throughout the body.

Laura: Exactly.

Ty: It's not a localized tumor. It's when it starts to go everywhere.

Laura: And then, you know, that's when it gets pretty tough. But I mean, enzymes are great for everyone to include in their diet, because so much of our modern diet is lacking in enzymes. Anytime anything's heated or pasteurized, when it's heated to so many degrees, processed, you're denaturing all these enzymes.

So getting more sprouted foods into the diet—I think sprouts like broccoli sprouts are far, far—they've got about 100 times more enzymes than normal raw food. Sauerkraut again, any fermented food, packed with enzymes. So really, really important for anyone, whatever they're dealing with.

Ty: Right.

Laura: Because they're just so preventative and good for the immune system.

Ty: Yeah, so get them in, believe that they're going to work. And your mental state, along with taking all these nutrients—you've got a pretty good shot, don't you?

Laura: Exactly. And actually, one more thing on enzymes that's, you know—to stimulate your body to produce more enzymes, it's often in preparing food. So in the process of chopping and frying onions, all those things, they actually stimulate the digestive juices. So thinking about food, the aromas, all of that, is so important. I think a lot of us, we're living at breakneck speed and grab that takeaway, or whatever. And you miss that whole ritual part of it that is so important, too.

Ty: So actually the preparation of the food helps to produce the enzymes as well.

Laura: Yeah, exactly.

Ty: Before you eat it?

Laura: Yeah.

Ty: Okay. So if you're buying everything at the local fast food restaurant, you're missing that.

Laura: Yeah, or you know, working at the nightclub and sitting down watching TV and just nom-nom-nom—mindless eating.

Ty: So yeah, give it some thought. Give it some positive thought.

Laura: Yeah, exactly.

Ty: Well, Laura, this has been fascinating. I'm really impressed. I mean, this has been an incredible interview. The studies that you have cited to support these things that you're saying are really incredible.

Laura: And people can find them in the book, in *You Can Say No to Chemo*. It's fully referenced. So people can find that. It's also got physicians around the world, in the back resources section. It's got places where you can find coffee enema kit, wherever you live. So I hope people find it helpful.

Ty: Yeah, I mean, I'm looking forward to reading it now. I've not read it before, but thank you so much for spending time today.

Laura: Such a pleasure. Thank you.

Ty: It's been awesome. Thank you.

[end of transcript]

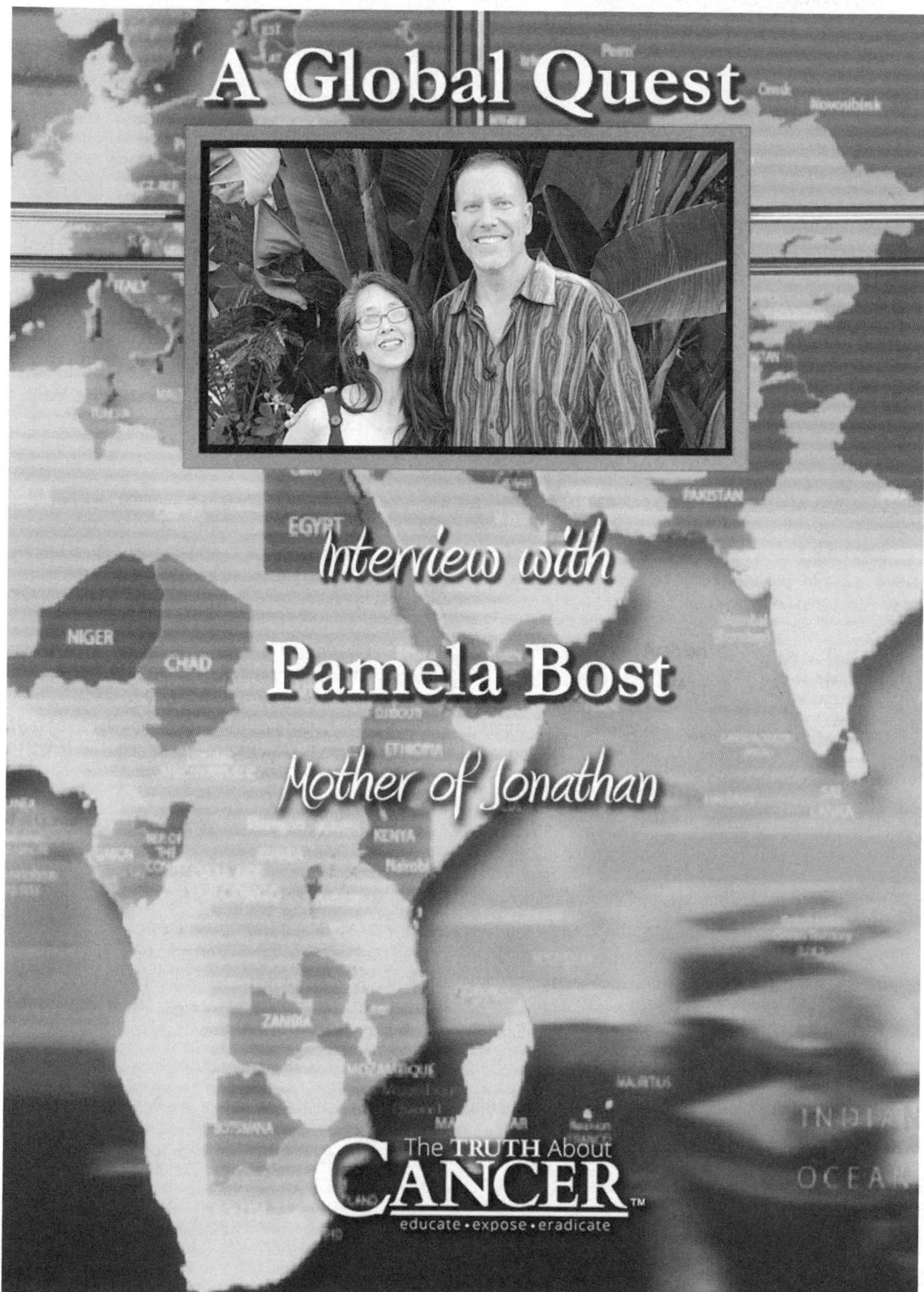
A Global Quest
Interview with
Pamela Bost
Mother of Jonathan
The TRUTH About CANCER
educate • expose • eradicate

Ty: I'm here in sunny San Diego this morning and I'm with Pamela Bost. And you approached me this morning as I was walking through the courtyard and you said, "Ty, last night you were talking about forced chemotherapy on children." And you've got a personal story that you wanted to share with us about your seven year old son. What's his name?

Pamela: I do. His name is Jonathan and, as you would suspect, any story about cancer is a pretty emotional story. This one doesn't concern me, but my son, and so you have a different bird's eye view there. I think cancer is different when you're talking about pediatric cancer.

People say in our integrative medicine world that we have choices. But Ty, I have to tell you that I don't agree with that when it comes to pediatric cancer. You're talking about a momma who's been out there. She's been teaching and moving and being that voice for integrative health and living the lifestyle. And what a humbling moment when you find out that your then five-year-old little boy was diagnosed with Leukemia.

It's a very humbling moment and it's a moment when you go back and question. All those things, all those tools, and all that information that I gave to so many others who had to walk the very same walk with their cancer. It was now my turn. But Ty, those tools were not available. They may say that you have a choice, but when you are there there's very little choice. I'm talking about things like supplements and things like his activity. And it's no longer you calling the shots.

But I have to tell you that Jonathan has become a very strong voice himself and sometimes we say that something wonderful comes out of something horrible. And Ty, truly, that's been what's happened in our case. I am so grateful to our Lord for allowing that to happen. Because truly many lives have been changed, many lives have been touched, and many options that others did not know about at the time have been revealed to them.

And so here we are, forced to carry on a protocol that is pretty much the same. It's standard protocol for what my son has which is Leukemia, pre-B cell Leukemia. There is a standardized protocol for that—very little deviation, only when there's maybe some alterations in their lab work. And what we've learned to do is we've learned to build immunity and really oversize detox. And when we over emphasize detox it takes a lot of time, but it has a great payoff and John has basically taken on that. He's become a crusader.

Ty: Tell us the story, or tell the viewers the story, that you were telling me this morning about the oncologist that will try to give him sweets and ice cream.

Pamela: Sure. Oftentimes when you take chemo, as you well know, your digestive system is nauseated and throwing up is something that is frequently associated with taking that chemo. So they offer them sodas and they offer them popsicles. And one very nice nurse practitioner came in and saw that Jonathan was struggling with his tummy at the moment and said, "Jonathan, can I get you something from the kitchen? A 7-Up or perhaps a—" what do they call them? An Otter Pop. And he says, "Didn't you just give me chemo? Don't I have cancer? Chemo is to kill a cancer you say. But now you're giving me sugar, don't you know that sugar feeds the cancer?"

It got her attention and it may have seemed a little bit disrespectful, but it's been his voice that has been so empowering to him. And I have to tell you, the staff, the medical community there, they've embraced us in such a way that they like the fact that Jonathan has his voice. It's been what's got us through. That and wonderful people like you paving the way.

Ty: Thank you.

Pamela: I appreciate it.

Ty: Do you have other children?

Pamela: I do. I am a momma of eight children. All from the same papa and momma, it's not a blended family. And we are a full-time Christian ministry. On the road 11 months out of the year and we are a family band. My husband is a minister and I go out and I speak about women's wellness and I am a health coach. But things changed.

Ty: When he was diagnosed, what were your first reactions? Was it just like a crushing blow?

Pamela: I could see the nurses and the doctor's mouth moving, but I couldn't hear anything. It was the most devastating contradiction in my life. The conflict was so enormous. I felt so powerless and I was rushed. Do you know that by the end of that evening he already a port and within less than 24 hours he already had his first chemo treatment.

Don't you think we need to have time to get used to the idea when a message so devastating and so grand that it can alter not only his life, but your life and that of your family? Don't you think we need to have a little bit of time to assimilate that? And here's this child who you as a parent up until this moment has been able to protect, to be his voice, to have influence on what he eats and what he does. Ty, I'm telling you, pediatric cancer has got to change. It is not the choice. We don't have that choice.

Ty: When he was diagnosed, after you regained your composure or began to hear the words or got a grip on what was going on, what was your reaction? Did you voice any kind of an opposition to the chemo?

Pamela: I asked. I said, "What choices do I have? Wait, I'm not sure if I want to take that route." I knew I didn't want to take that route. I teach that I don't want to take that route. But they said, "I'm sorry you don't have a choice in this matter" and that's how it was.

Ty: So they basically said, "This is what will happen."

Pamela: "This is what will happen." And I don't want to get into the "what ifs" if we didn't follow through, but you can read about it. So often we hear about it in our news reports of parents who are standing up and asking and seeing and pushing the boundaries and saying, "Can I have another option? Is there another way? Can we try it?"

It took six weeks before Jonathan was diagnosed. I was told during that time he couldn't have any supplements or alternative medications or anything that may interfere. Even now today, during his treatment, unless it's in a food source, he's not to be given anything. Doctor has to okay everything that comes through.

So little simple things like vitamin C or vitamin B12, some of these things that help to build the immunes, we cannot give them to our children. But the important part to know here is that in integrative medicines we do have that availability of building the immune and detoxing and that's what I would like to do. That's what Jonathan would like to do. Jonathan is working on getting his DVDs out there where he is talking to the children himself and he's saying, "We have to do this, therefore, we're going to fight like crazy to do this." And he has a very strong regiment and he won't miss a day of it.

Ty: How long has he been on chemo?

Pamela: He's been on for almost a year and a half and the protocol lasts three years and two months for boys, two years and nine months for girls.

Ty: So he's got another year plus, year and a half.

Pamela: He does. He's getting chemo every day. At this time, in maintenance. He only gets chemo in his spine once every three months, but he gets chemo orally every day and he gets it intravenously every month. Over time, no matter how much you and I detox and build immunity that is going to have its effects on tearing his body down. And how is it that I can help so many others Ty, but I'm helpless when it comes to my own?

And I want to be there to help so many other mommas who are unaware about this and who believe that when they're given the news that their child has a certain disease, that these are the only options. Ty, there are so many more options out there that so many don't know about and that's what Jonathan and I would like to do.

Ty: Well, you know, by sharing this today you are helping people to wake up to the fact that this is an issue and you're bringing awareness to this very big problem in pediatric oncology. This is a huge problem.

Pamela: It is a huge problem, Ty. I am so grateful for the work that you and your wife are doing and many countless others.

Ty: I'm thankful for people like you that are having the kind of strength that you have in a time that's, I know, very difficult for the family. I honestly can't imagine if I were in your shoes, I don't know how I would be feeling or reacting. But I can see that you've got the strength of the Lord that's holding you up.

Pamela: Truly, it's been the strength of the Lord. And Jonathan is an incredible young man who has been touched by the Lord. I could tell you stories that would just—you'd need another series for that. I could tell you stories, but truly in the face of this devastating news, the Lord has used it in an incredible way to reach so many others and to make a difference. You know, in pediatric cancer sometimes whatever is on that lab report, if that number doesn't change it can result in another something happening. "This is this number, therefore, we have to do this surgery or install this or give this or this round of series of antibiotics"

And so you can see how vitally and critically important it is to make those numbers go the right way so that our youngsters don't have to go through those things. And there are ways to do that.

Ty: It's very much—as we've talked to other people over the weekend—very much cookie-cutter medicine. It's not individualized at all.

Pamela: And our lifestyle is probably very similar to everybody, most everybody out there. Your children mean so much to you and they're the progeny and they're what we invest in. And from our lifestyle of being a large homeschooling family out there on the road always ministering together 24/7, we're close knit. But this monster that showed itself, it was really difficult. Everyone's learned different roles. Ninety percent of marriages fail during pediatric diseases.

Ty: Is that right?

Pamela: That's right. And it's been a tough strain. Jonathan was no longer something personal and unique, he was just another number. And albeit we have beautiful doctors and nurses that are out there doing what they know to do. Jonathan was only a standardized number. "Well, what happens next?" "Well, let me look. This is what happens next." "Well, what happens from this point?" "Well, let me see where his numbers fall. Oh, this is what happens next." "Yeah, but how about if he metabolizes it differently than kid A?" This is the protocol.

Ty: It's not part of the equation.

Pamela: It's not part of the equation. And could there be a place, could there be an opportunity where you could speak into that? Sometimes, depending on what doctor you have. It was constantly fluctuating. Does Jonathan have a say in any of that? Absolutely not, in no way.

Ty: But Jonathan is going to flourish.

Pamela: I receive those words. I tell you, Ty, he is on fire. And I don't motivate or push it because I want it to be his fire and I want it to be his voice and his message. But I'll tell you, that kid has touched a compassion that he's never known before. We'd be in the hospital and there'd be babies crying and it would be two or three in the morning and he'd say, "Momma, go pray for that momma or that baby because that baby needs help. Go talk to that momma."

So there are a lot of good things that are coming out in spite of this. And if each day we can embrace that, that's our motivation to carry on.

Ty: That's amazing for a six, seven-year-old kid to have that kind of maturity and that kind of compassion for other people, while he's sick.

Pamela: Ty, you know what was very big for me early on, very early, I'm talking weeks into the protocol of chemotherapy—not only do the dynamics and the cellular functions begin to change physically within him, but, Ty, his childhood was taken from him and almost overnight he turned into what they refer at the hospital as an old soul. He was far beyond his year within a short few weeks. Gratefully, he became someone who was empowered, but many don't.

And I long for those times when I could have my baby back again like he was. But those days are gone and all we can do is look forward. We have to, but I want mommies and daddies out there—you know, when we walk into the clinic, I don't let Jonathan go in, Ty. I make him stay outside.

The children look so differently. And when you walk in and you see the hopelessness in that momma's eyes and the giving up in that daddy's eyes and that child who's physically looking the part of the cancer patient, it's sad for that momma to behold Jonathan who looks very thriving. And it's very sad for Jonathan to look upon his peers in such a condition.

Ty: I bet it is.

Pamela: It really is.

Ty: Well, Pamela, the information that you shared, the personal story that you shared with us today about your family, about Jonathan, about the way that he's thriving, the kindness that he's exhibiting to these other cancer patients that are children, it's inspiring. It's saddening to me. It angers me that we are in a state of pediatric oncology in the United States when this is happening. But it does give me hope when I hear stories like yours because you've taken a lemon and made lemonade out of it.

Pamela: Thanks, Ty. I do want to say one thing. This weekend was the first weekend I've been away from John since his diagnosis and this weekend was all about self-care for momma. I made a promise to myself that I wasn't going to touch that element of anger in me, but you mentioned it and so I'll very briefly just kind of talk about it in a very generalized way.

Ty, I think when you're given the news that your baby has cancer and what's more than that, that you don't have any kind of influence on how you're going to proceed this journey of health with this news of having cancer, it is infuriating to have your position, your title, you strength, and your voice taken from you.

And I have to say it's very important and very healthy that you touch that and allow yourself to feel that anger. You can't let it take you over, most definitely can't, but I hope that it will take you to a place where then you can impart health and knowledge to other people.

Ty: Well, it has and it will and you've inspired me and I just pray for your family.

Pamela: Thanks, Ty.

Ty: And pray for little Jonathan. And thank you for sharing for with us.

Pamela: I appreciate it. God bless you and your ministry. ***[end of transcript]***

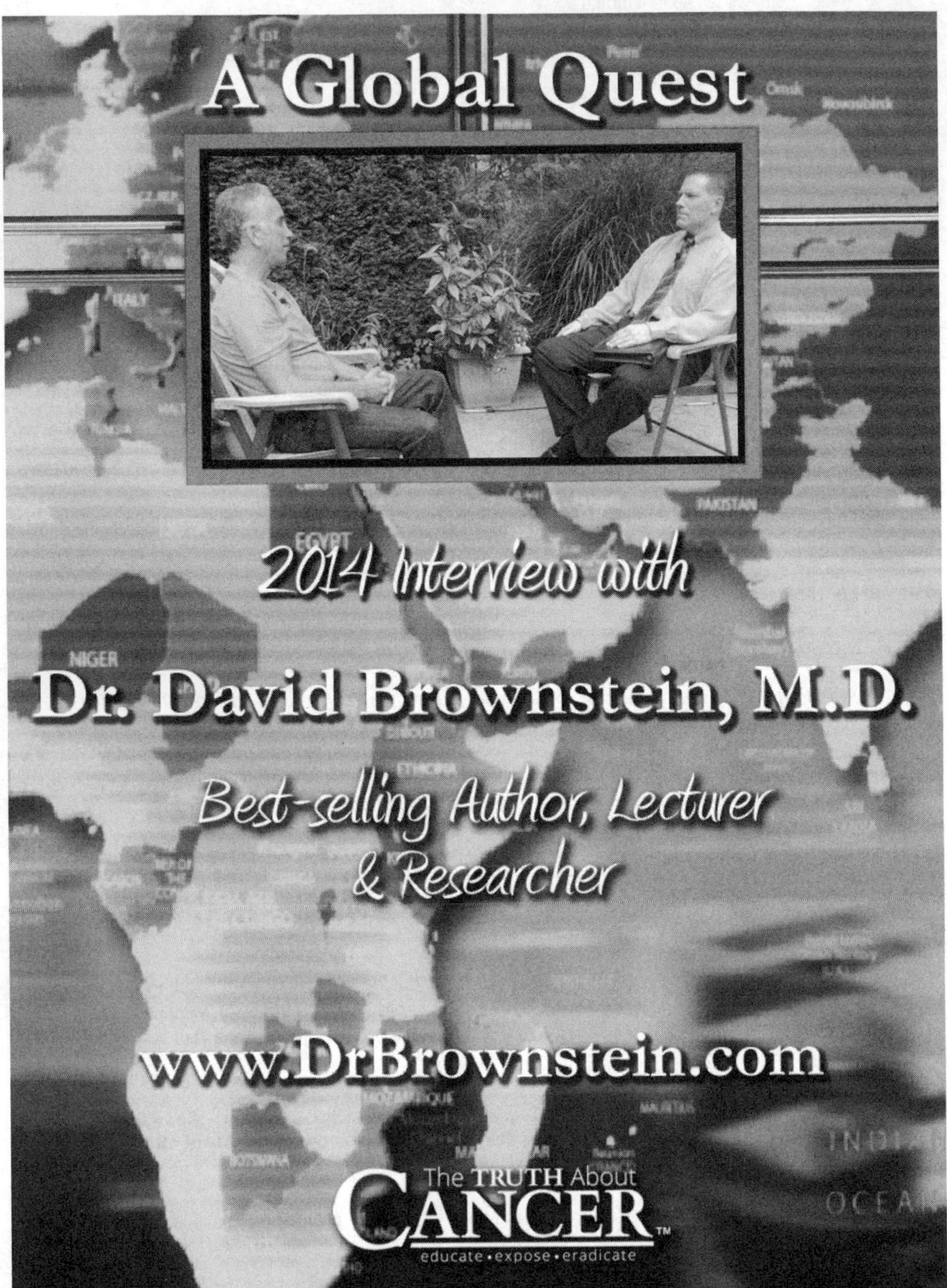
A Global Quest
2014 Interview with
Dr. David Brownstein, M.D.
Best-selling Author, Lecturer
& Researcher
www.DrBrownstein.com
The TRUTH About
CANCER
educate • expose • eradicate

Ty: I am honored to be sitting here today right by the swimming pool of Dr. David Brownstein. We're going to call him Dr. B in this interview, per his request. We're here outside of Detroit, Michigan. Dr. B, thanks for having, or being with us today.

Dr. Brownstein: Thank you for having me, Ty.

Ty: Good to be able to talk you. I've followed your work for a long time and I'm really thrilled to be able to pick your brain today about some of these issues relating to cancer and health and nutrition. So, first of all, if you could, Dr. B, just tell us about yourself. How did you get to be doing what you're doing?

Dr. Brownstein: Well, I had wanted to be a doctor since I was young. I went to the University of Michigan for my undergrad training and pre-med, and went to Wayne State University Medical School in Detroit. I wanted to be a family doctor modeled after my family doctor. During that time I wasn't interested in any alternative therapies. I just wanted to be a regular, conventional doctor. I went from my med school to family practice residency in the Detroit area, and then went into private practice, practicing conventional medicine. Around six months into that practice I started to just have some unhappy feelings about what I was doing. I didn't quite know what was wrong and I remember vividly getting up to go to work and my wife is getting up and we're both getting ready to go to work. I blurted out to her, "I don't want to be a doctor anymore." The first thing she says ... I'll leave that between her and I. We had $90,000 in student loans. But, the second thing she said was, "What are you going to do about it?" And I really had no idea. I just realized conventional medicine wasn't doing it for me. People weren't getting better from the therapies I was doing. I wasn't treating the underlying cause of their therapies, and I was using drugs that pretty much just treat symptoms of illness.

I started to look for alternatives to what I was doing, and I started to look at some natural therapies. I found that that's a better way to go, and it treats the underlying cause of the illness. I really started practicing alternative medicine shortly after that, and here I am 20 years later and 12 books later and a newsletter later, and very happy about what I'm doing.

Ty: Awesome. Let me kind of go through a little bit of your bio here I've written down. I'll have to read through it, because I can't remember all this stuff. You're a medical doctor, you're a board-certified family physician, author of 12 books. Two of the ones that I've read is *Iodine: Why You Need It, Why You Can't Live Without It* and *Overcoming Thyroid Disorders,* which we're going to talk a little bit about the thyroid today. You received the American Academy of Integrative Medicine's Distinguished Clinician Award for the advancements that you made in the diagnosis and treatment of chronic diseases, and that's just part of your bio and your resume.

Dr. Brownstein: I'm honored to do what I do. It's really a blessing to make a living trying to help people feel better and trying to improve their health.

Ty: Well, you're definitely helping people. You're definitely helping to spread the word, and we're going to get some of that information today. I was really impressed with what you just said. You were a classically trained medical doctor, but you began to realize that you weren't really healing. You were treating symptoms with drugs, became disenchanted, and wanted to find out if there were other ways. That right there sets you above most of the people I know because you realized that what you had been trained to do wasn't working, and you went for another way instead of just staying in the same path.

Dr. Brownstein: I couldn't stay in the same path, Ty. It wasn't working. I found I was just using more and more drugs to treat the symptoms from the other drugs, and more importantly, people weren't getting better. It just wasn't working for me, and either I was going to give up medicine or I had to find a different model to use. You know, looking at things from a biochemical model and a natural model to try and supply the body with what it needs so it can take care of itself is really a better way to go.

Ty: Talk about that then. How did you initially become involved in researching cancer, because this is "The Truth About Cancer: The Quest for the Cures" continues. That's what this documentary mini-series is being called, and so we're really focusing on cancer. How did you get involved with cancer research? Because you've done a lot.

Dr. Brownstein: Well, cancer wasn't hard to get involved in since so many people have it. We have one in seven women with breast cancer in the United States, one in three men with prostate cancer. We have got lung cancer and colon cancer more than we know what to do with, and really, the conventional therapies for most types of cancer are pretty bad. You know, if you look at the cancer statistics from 1930, which are being kept until the present day, our mortality rate is really unchanged for most of the hard tumors, which is breast, lung, prostate, colon. And, it's really sad, because we're spending these billions and trillions of dollars on therapies that aren't working. We really need a better model, and a better model is 1) searching for what's causing all this cancer, which nobody is doing. And, 2) then supplying the body with the underlying things that it needs in order to function normally and to fight this illness.

Ty: My next question was: Are we winning the cancer war that President Nixon declared in 1971?

Dr. Brownstein: Oh, we're not winning that cancer war. That's been a disaster. I'm seeing patients every day. I see a lot of patients with cancer. If you're going to see patients today, you're going to have to be involved with cancer because that's what's out there. And that's one of the chronic illnesses that we just need a better model for.

Ty: So talk about the model that you use to treat cancer.

Dr. Brownstein: Well, I sort of use the model I was taught in medical school. In medical school, I was taught to 1) take a history, listen to patients and hear their complaints, 2) to do a good physical exam to correlate what their complaints are, and try and figure out what the problem is, and 3) order laboratory tests to confirm or deny what you think might be going on and to guide you in a therapy. So I still follow that basic model, but what I do a little differently is, what I was taught in medical school was how to diagnose pathology. That was our first thing. So we could recognize when there was a problem in your body, and then what we were taught was how to prescribe that one drug to treat that problem. That would be a great model if that drug actually treated that problem. But 98 percent of the drugs out there, they don't treat the problem. They just treat the symptom of the problem. We really need to go back to work to figure out what's the underlying cause of these illnesses. I can tell you the underlying cause of cancer, it's multifactorial, there's not one single cause for everybody. But, I think that toxicity is part of the problem with it, poor nutrition is part of it, poor diet is part of it, dehydration is part of it, and lack of iodine is a big part of it. There's a whole bunch of things going on and either we start to treat these underlying causes that are part of the underlying cause of the problem of cancer or we're just going to continue going on with so many people suffering from it.

Ty: That's a common thread that I've heard from many different medical doctors that I've interviewed, is that what distinguishes what they're doing from the traditional model is they're actually looking for the causes and not just treating the symptoms. You're using the traditional model but you're getting to the bottom of what caused the problem.

Dr. Brownstein: You know, the analogy I'd use for you is someone with osteoporosis. I was taught in medical school that bone density reflects how thick the bones are. When the bones are too thin they have osteoporosis. Prescribe a drug to treat that osteoporosis. The drug builds bone density and then they won't have osteoporosis. Well they're not getting osteoporosis because of a bone drug deficiency problem. They're getting osteoporosis because they're eating badly, they're not exercising and they have toxicities. They're not drinking enough water. Those are the underlying causes of a problem that should be addressed. That's what really a holistic doctor should be doing—looking for that.

Ty: That makes sense. I've heard … I can't remember who it was in this series. I think it may have been Mike Adams said that, "Cancer is not a deficiency of chemotherapy."

Dr. Brownstein: I would amend Mike Adams' statement, "Not deficiency of chemotherapy, radiation or toxic drugs to treat it."

Ty: So, you're getting to the bottom. You mentioned several reasons, toxicities, bad nutrition, lack of iodine, dehydration. We'll get into those in a minute, but could you go into the detection techniques that you use initially? The typical detection for breast cancer is mammograms. If it's prostate cancer, it's PSA tests. What are you using to detect cancer?

Dr. Brownstein: Let's talk about breast cancer, since one in seven women have it. If we live in the United States, we've all been affected by this, either family members or friends. It's hard to not know anybody that doesn't have breast cancer or has died from breast cancer. In conventional medicine, women are supposed to go for their annual exams and annual mammograms. Mammograms can pick up breast cancer at an earlier stage than ever before. When you look at the mortality rate since 1930 from breast cancer, the age-adjusted mortality rate hasn't changed. So, yes, we're picking up cancer at an earlier stage, but women are living about the same amount of time with breast cancer as they were living with it 50 years ago. Yet here we are spending trillions of dollars with chemotherapy, radiation and hormone-modulating therapies, and they're really not working well. I think that definitely we need a better model for this. So, what do I suggest? I suggest 1) let's go back to the basics. I think one of my jobs as a doctor is to counsel people on how to eat appropriately. I can guarantee you most people are not eating appropriately. The standard American diet is nutrient depleting for people. It supplies them with toxic chemicals that set the stage for chronic illness like cancer and arthritis and other illnesses to appear. Unless they learn to eat appropriately, or eat better, I think that we're going to still suffer this cancer problem.

Ty: Let me ask you this. I want to get into what you mean by eating appropriately here shortly. So, breast cancer you're talking about ... do you think that mammograms are the best way to detect or are there better techniques that we can use today to detect it?

Dr. Brownstein: There's no question mammograms detect breast cancer at an earlier stage than ever before. So are they the best technique to detect cancer? I don't know if they're the best technique, but they're pretty good at doing it. But there are side effects with mammograms. They supply ionizing radiation to sensitive tissue in the body that can get cancer, in the one in seven women have cancer. One mammogram increases a woman's risk of breast cancer by one percent. After 10 years of mammograms, she's got a 10 percent increased risk of breast cancer. We already have one in seven women with breast cancer. Why do we want to increase their risk with doing this therapy? The problem is just early diagnosis in this case doesn't really matter. They live the same amount of time as if we diagnosed it later. I think mammograms should not be the primary mode of diagnosis used. I think we could use thermo scans. At least there is no radiation with it.

Ty: Thermography?

Dr. Brownstein: Thermography. They measure the heat off the breast, and they're looking for hot areas. Cancer cells are generally high metabolic areas of the body. They require a lot of blood flow, and a thermo scan of the breast can pick up a hot spot. From there you would go to a mammogram or an ultrasound or an MRI to try and figure out what that is. But, again, we're ahead of ourselves, because we're just talking about diagnosis now. We really need to focus on how to prevent getting it in the first place.

Ty: Let's focus on that.

Dr. Brownstein: Let's go back to diet. I think diet should be—you know, I call this the basics. The basic number one is let's eat a better diet. When we were growing up we learned in elementary school the food pyramid. The food pyramid showed that we should eat the majority of our food as grains. I remember there was a big loaf of bread there and crackers and grains were down in that big part of the food pyramid. Fats and oils were up on top and says, "Use sparingly." Well, I could tell you we followed that food pyramid since it was introduced, I believe, in the early 1970s or late 1960s. And the consequences of us, the American people, following this food pyramid was that we ate more grains, we limited fats and oils in our diet, we switched our fat intake from primarily animal fat products to using polyunsaturated vegetable oils like corn oil and soybean oil and some other oils that are commonly sold in the grocery stores. The consequences of that is we've become the most obese people on the face of the planet. We have more diabetes than we know what to do with. We have more metabolic syndrome than we know what to do with, and I say it's a direct result of following the USDA's recommendation of following the food pyramid.

Ty: Following the "SAD" American direct.

Dr. Brownstein: It makes people sad and it makes people fat and makes people diabetic. Certainly once diabetes comes into play, cancer and other illnesses follow suit as the blood sugar goes up, since cancer cells require blood sugar to function and to rev their metabolic rate.

Ty: So, Dr. B, you just mentioned the "SAD" American diet, the fact that we got the pyramid with the grains and the oils at the top, very few, use sparingly. What should a healthy food pyramid look like?

Dr. Brownstein: Well, in one sense, maybe we could flip the food pyramid on its axis and make the grains use sparingly, because grains turn into sugar very quickly. I frequently tell my patients to limit grains in a diet and to use a lot more fats in their diet because fats slowly releases into the body. So what should it look like? I say people should eat whole foods, free of pesticides, free of hormones, and organic food, absolutely. Organic animal products can be very healthy for people, such as organic eggs and organic meats and any organic product. It definitely needs to be free of pesticides, because we know pesticides are not metabolized well in the body. There are carcinogenic studies with pesticides. If we get enough of them in our body, and certainly with the hormones they're feeding the animals and the conventionally raised animals, that's a big problem. I think that's one of the things that's causing one in seven women to have breast cancer and one in three men to have prostate cancer.

Ty: Just off the top of my head, I'm thinking … so the hormones in the meats, the chickens … could that be one of the reasons that so many young girls are going into puberty so early?

Dr. Brownstein: Well, there's no question that's one of the reasons girls are going into puberty so early. There's no question that's why breast size has increased over the years, and there's no question that's why breast cancer has increased. For men it's prostate cancer. There's no reason they need to feed these hormones to the animals. They should be limited, and since they are going to feed them to conventionally raised animals, the only thing we can do is to eat a better diet.

Ty: Dr. B, I know you've written several books on diet and food and nutrition. Can you talk about this a little bit?

Dr. Brownstein: I've written these books trying to teach people not to eat that SAD diet and to eat a better diet. The first book that I wrote was *The Guide to Healthy Eating* and just gave an overview about how to eat better, like what we're talking about. My latest book is *The Skinny on Fats,* and I try and dispel the myths of eating fat and why we need to eat good fats in our diet and why we can't go on these low-fat diets. I think it stresses the body out and causes more problems, particularly more problems with people with chronic disorders like cancer.

Ty: Can you talk about good fats? When you say we need to be eating good fats, what are good fats?

Dr. Brownstein: Good fats can be from animals that are organically raised and organically fed.

Ty: Butter.

Dr. Brownstein: Absolutely, butter's a very good fat for the body. Organic eggs are the best pure protein source for the body.

Ty: I live on five acres in Texas and we have laying hens. So we get fresh eggs every day from our hens that free range. So I'm with you. I love organic eggs. What about other kinds of oils to cook with? What oils should we cook with? What oils should we be intaking? I know that one of the oils that's a staple in our diet is coconut oil.

Dr. Brownstein: We were taught in elementary school in that top of that food pyramid use fats and oils sparingly. We were also taught to switch to polyunsaturated vegetable oils like corn oil and soybean oil and those things. Those things are a disaster for the body. They're nutrient depleted, they're full of trans-fatty acids and they gum up the body's receptors. I think the single best cooking oil is coconut oil. Palm oil's a good choice. These things survive high-heat cooking very well. Olive oil's okay for low-heat cooking or just in cool foods. For high-heat cooking there's nothing better than coconut oil.

Ty: We love to cook up organic popcorn in coconut oil. The kids get popcorn that way.

Dr. Brownstein: Nothing better than using coconut oil, organic corn seeds and good salt, unrefined salt for that.

Ty: We like the pink Himalayan salt, is what we use. Great snack. While we're on the subject of fats, you mentioned good oils, you mentioned the butter, the eggs, what about nuts? What are some good sources of fats, because I know nuts are almost all fat? So, what are good sources of fats from nuts?

Dr. Brownstein: I think nuts make a great snack. They supply the right fatty acids for our bodies, but also Omega 6 and Omega 3 fatty acids. Nuts can be a healthy snack source, much better than a cracker or some kind of grain-based product.

Ty: Would you recommend with the nuts? Should they be raw nuts or roasted are okay, but not roasted in bad oils, of course, not cooked in bad oils?

Dr. Brownstein: What I tell my patients is that nuts do have some chemicals in them to inhibit some of the absorption of minerals in our body. They're called phytates. You can minimize that or disrupt that phytate formation by slow-roasting the nuts. In my book, *The Guide to Healthy Eating*, we describe how to slow-roast nuts. Basically, you just put them on a tray, cook at low heat for a few hours and it makes them much tastier and much healthier for our body. I do think raw nuts can be an okay snack as well.

Ty: Okay, but just watch out for the bad oils.

Dr. Brownstein: If you look on the container of the nuts, they'll tell you when they're made with soybean oil and they're roasted. If they're roasted in soybean oil or corn oil or something like that, they're not going to healthy because the oil's been hydrogenated at that point.

Ty: And, now the GMO factor as well, right, with soy and corn?

Dr. Brownstein: That's been a whole disaster, and we're paying the price for that as well.

Ty: That's another whole interview in and of itself, isn't it?

Dr. Brownstein: Absolutely.

Ty: So, talk about real quick—I've heard you mention the cancer medical complex. What do you mean when you talk about the cancer medical complex?

Dr. Brownstein: I've written about this, and I say the cancer medical complex is this whole monolith that's been set up to make money on cancer. Let's take the young woman who's been feeling a breast lump. She goes to her doctor, she goes for a mammogram, they pick up something. She's going to go for a biopsy, they pick up something. Now she's going to go for an excision, they tell her she's got cancer, she's going to get chemo and radiation. It's this whole system set up to treat cancer, and it's a multi-trillion dollar industry right now. The problem is people aren't living longer from these therapies. There're very few cancers that we've done well with. We've done well with some of the blood cancers, with some of the leukemias and lymphomas, and testicular cancer. The rest of them, the mortality rate has not changed much over the last 70 to 80 years.

Ty: So you have this whole system in place where people are, well, actually, the insurance companies are being milked for trillions of dollars and we're not really improving the life span of the cancer patients.

Dr. Brownstein: Well, I don't know if I'd use the term insurance companies being milked. The insurance companies milk us just fine to pay for all that stuff.

Ty: Well, you're right. We're being milked, yeah.

Dr. Brownstein: We're being milked in the end run, because what's not happening is that we're so focused on diagnosis and treatment that we've unfocused ourselves on why are so many people having cancer. Unless we refocus on that we're going to keep wasting all this money, really spinning our wheels and not making progress. We need to disengage from that. The Komen Foundation needs to disengage from that. The American Cancer Society needs to disengage from diagnosis and treatment. Really, what's causing all this problem? I think that it doesn't take a rocket scientist to realize what's causing it. It's pesticides, it's toxicity, it's poor diet, it's lack of iodine, you know, it's a whole thing that's happening, but nobody's really looking at that whole picture.

Ty: And, maybe one of the reasons is because there's so much money. It's a whole thing that has momentum in place. As you mentioned earlier, you got out of medical school. You're almost $100,000 in debt when you decided that what you were doing, the direction you were heading, wasn't for you. You were still in debt, and so potentially that's something that affects the decision of many people who get out of medical school. They're so in debt they just got to keep doing what they've been doing. Otherwise, they feel like they may never get out of debt.

Dr. Brownstein: You're hitting part of the nail on the head, exactly. Because, now I see medical students. They come and train at our office. They're two to three hundred thousand dollars in debt. And, you know, what are they going to do out there? Where's the money going to be? The money is in diagnosis and treatment, and unfortunately, that's where we've gone with things. I always tell people they should look twice before donating to charities like Komen Foundation and American Cancer Society, and really look—are they really searching for an underlying cause of these problems, or are they just perpetuating the same old model that's not working?

Ty: Right. We should be running for the cause.

Dr. Brownstein: Absolutely.

Ty: Let's talk about PSA tests real quick, and then I want to get into the thyroid. Talk about a little bit of iodine here because that's one of your sweet spots. I know you've written a lot on iodine and the thyroid, but let's talk about PSA tests. Are they a good diagnosis for prostate cancer? Do they ever create false positives? What's your take on the PSA and what does PSA test stand for?

Dr. Brownstein: PSA stands for prostate-specific antigen. It's a fabulous test to pick up prostate cancer, there's no doubt about it. It's a fabulous test to follow people with prostate cancer to see how they're doing. The problem is we haven't changed the age-adjusted mortality much for prostate cancer in the last 75 years, and we're spending all this money doing all these therapies. The founder of the PSA test has come up with a couple of articles recently saying that he didn't design that test for everybody to get it to diagnose prostate cancer. He thinks it's a wrong therapy that we're doing. Eighty percent false positives with the PSA testing and here we have the American Cancer Society and the powers that be recommending doing yearly PSA screenings.

Ty: Right.

Dr. Brownstein: They backed off a little bit from that recently. But basically, they're recommending yearly PSA testing for men over the age of 50. What happens is when the PSA elevates, which it can elevate from a lot of reasons besides cancer—prostatitis, if the prostate has been stimulated within 24 hours of the blood testing or anything that causes inflammation. They go into the whole cancer industrial complex themselves, where they're getting ultrasounds, biopsies, chemotherapy, surgery, radiation, and most men with prostate cancer can outlive it. If they don't do anything, they'll end up dying of something else. So, we've got a whole mess on that and, again, we need to search for the underlying cause of why one in three men have it, and we need to certainly do a lot less therapy on men with prostate cancer. We're not saving enough men from it and putting way too many men through too many toxic and traumatic therapies for it.

Ty: You mentioned that many men will outlive it. I think it was Dr. Dick Avland, or maybe it was Thomas Stayme, I can't remember who it—but, both of them have been involved with the PSA test for a long while—said that most men will die with prostate cancer but few will die from it.

Dr. Brownstein: That's right. I think the numbers are if you're over 80 years old, about 88 percent of men will have prostate cancer at the time of death if they do an autopsy. Three percent will die from it, 8 percent are affected by it. The rest are dying of something else.

Ty: They live with it and don't even know.

Dr. Brownstein: We're treating every man as if it's the same thing and it's just a disaster.

Ty: It is. Matter of fact, I think that's what happened to my granddad. He was diagnosed with prostate cancer and they went in and they did all of the biopsies and the radiation and the chemo, and I think he actually ended up dying from the treatment and not really the prostate cancer itself. This was back in the late '90s, but if I remember correctly, he wasn't sick at all. He went in and they diagnosed him with prostate cancer and they said, "You got to do aggressive treatment." And he died within a year of the time he started treatment.

Dr. Brownstein: When we graduate from medical school we take the Hippocratic Oath, which says in part, "above all, do no harm." I can tell you a lot of conventional therapies are harmful and toxic to the body, and they don't prolong life or improve the quality of life. So I'm not quite sure how we've gotten stuck into this rat hole. I think we've gotten stuck into it from what I've written about the cancer industrial complex that's set up to sort of feed itself with more and more money than it needs.

Ty: *Talk about iodine. What is iodine and do we need it to prevent cancer?*

Dr. Brownstein: I talk about—let's do the basics for people to help supply their body with the things it needs to function. How we were designed by our Maker. If we supply the body with the right nutrients it should do fine for a lifetime. I consider one of the basics iodine. Every cell in the body needs and requires iodine to function optimally. We can't function optimally in an iodine deficient environment. I've tested, along with my partners, over 6,000 patients. Over 96 percent were low on iodine, the mass majority significantly low on iodine. When I talked to clinicians around the country who are looking at this they find the same numbers that I'm finding.

Ty: Wow.

Dr. Brownstein: Iodine has a lot of jobs in the body. The immune system can't function without it. You can't fight infections without it. One of its main jobs is in the endocrine glands. The endocrine glands include the thyroid, the breasts, the ovaries, uterus and the prostate. What are we having problems with out there? The thyroid, the ovaries, the uterus, breasts, and prostate. I've mentioned the prostate, I've mentioned the breasts. The fastest-growing cancer in the United States is thyroid cancer. We have uterine and ovarian cancer growing at epidemic rates. We're having epidemic rates of problems with them. Iodine's main job is to maintain a normal architecture of those tissues. With iodine deficiency, the first thing that happens is you get cystic formation in the breasts, the ovaries, uterus, thyroid, prostate and, let's throw in the pancreas in here as well, which is also increasing at epidemic rates. Pancreatic cancer. Cysts start to form when iodine deficiency is there. If it goes on longer, they become nodular and hard. If it goes on longer, they become hyperplastic tissue, which is the precursor to cancer. I say that's the iodine deficiency continuum.

The good thing about iodine is, iodine has apoptotic properties, meaning it can stop a cancer cell from just continually dividing, dividing, dividing until it kills somebody. Iodine can stop this continuum wherever it catches it and hopefully reverse it, but at least put the brakes on what's happening. Over 80 percent of women suffer from fibrocystic breast disease. That's a precursor to breast cancer, which, as I said, one in seven women have. I say it's an iodine deficiency problem, period. That's what it is, and we either recognize this and start treating it, or we're still going to see one in seven women with breast cancer.

Ty: Wow. I didn't know that iodine was important. I did not know that it creates apoptosis in the cancer cells.

Dr. Brownstein: Iodine's been shown to have apoptotic properties for cancer cells. Iodine's been shown to be effective for treating a multitude of cancers ... all those tissues that I mentioned before, including pancreatic cancer, including some brain cancers. It's too bad that the cancer industrial complex isn't studying iodine as a good therapy for cancer because they should be. I think it should be studied, 1) as a therapy for cancer, and 2) as a prevention for cancer.

Ty: Okay. That makes sense, especially in light of the fact that you've shown the way that iodine affects the endocrine system and, the endocrine glands are the ones we're having the problems with.

Dr. Brownstein: You know, Ty, I've written about this extensively in my book, *Iodine: Why You Need It, Why You Can't Live Without It.* I did a study where I looked at 18 women. Nine had breast cancer, nine did not have breast cancer. I measured their iodine and bromide levels, and what I did was a test where we collected the urine. What I found was, before any therapy, the breast cancer women had half as much iodine as the non-breast cancer women. Now, they were all low on iodine, but the breast cancer women were lower than the non-breast cancer women. I gave them 50 mg of iodine for 30 days, and then I rechecked them. What I found at the end of 30 days, and there was one other check in the middle there, but what I found was that the breast cancer women had much more bromide, much less iodine than the non-breast cancer women. Iodine is part of the halide family, which includes iodine, bromide and fluoride. Now, out of those three, iodine is the only essential element that has therapeutic value in the body. Bromide and fluoride, as far we know, has no known therapeutic value in the body. Bromide, we're getting in toxic amounts in our environment. We're getting toxic amounts in our food supply from brominated vegetable oils. Many medicines contain bromide as part of their genetic or chemical makeup.

What I found in testing every breast cancer—well, I haven't tested every breast cancer patient—but, the ones that I've tested, 100 percent have high bromide levels and low iodine levels. I've tested over a thousand patients in general, some with cancer, some without. They all have high bromide levels. Cancer patients generally have higher amounts of bromide. Animal studies have shown bromide can push iodine out of the body. Bromide can bind where iodine binds to and bromide gums up the cells and does not work well. What we need is more iodine in our bodies. The only way we're going to get it right now is supplementation, just because we're getting too much in our food, in our drink and it's in a bunch of consumer goods such as computers and cars. You're probably wearing it in your clothing right now as a fire retardant. Iodine needs to be a continual supplement regimen for, I think, everybody.

Ty: Interesting. So, iodine and fluoride and bromide are all parts of the halide family. And so ...

Dr. Brownstein: Too much of one can put out the other one. What I'm seeing right now, we're getting too much bromide, not enough iodine, and we're getting too much fluoride from our water supply. That's another story, too. But, the good thing about iodine is … iodine can kick out both of these if we start ingesting it again.

Ty: Why do you think it is that so many people are deficient in iodine? I know one study that I read, or one article I read—I can't remember who it was, I think it may have been Dr. Blaylock, was writing about in the '70s, they took bromide out of the bread and started putting in…or they took iodine out of the bread and started putting in bromine.

Dr. Brownstein: Now, that was me who wrote about that.

Ty: Was that you? Okay.

Dr. Brownstein: That's in my iodine book, and I've written a bunch of articles on that. What happened was before the 1970s, iodine was used in bakery products as a conditioning agent. For some reason in the early 1970s, they substituted bromide for iodine. It's not clear why, but we started to get all this bromide now in our bakery products. Every slice of bread, cracker or cookie, cake, now had bromide instead of iodine. Well, if you look at the breast cancer rates, and the prostate cancer rates when they really took off was right about that time frame. I say that's when our iodine levels really fell off the cliff. What's also happened lately is our soil's become more deficient in iodine. I live in a nice suburb of Detroit, and in the Great Lakes area where I live, our soil's one of the most iodine deficient areas of the world. Now it's not just the Great Lakes area. If you draw a line down the center of the country, between the coasts, most of it is iodine deficient, except for the two coasts. Where you live is a very iodine-deficient area of the world. This has been going on for a long time. What's not been going on for a long time is this exposure to bromide and fluoride, which has exacerbated this iodine deficiency problem, and I think exacerbated the breast, prostate, thyroid, ovarian, uterine, pancreatic problems that we're seeing now.

Ty: Well, I'm even more honored to be talking to you today, because that had a big impact on the way that I've been communicating with people about iodine and the importance, and about the bread supply and the bakery supply back in the '70s. Thanks for sharing that again here with us.

Dr. Brownstein: My pleasure.

Ty: Is it possible to get enough iodine from eating and adding salt to your food? When you say supplement, do you mean salt your food? What do you mean when you say iodine supplementation?

Dr. Brownstein: The U.S. government recognized iodine deficiency was a big problem in 1920s, as goiter was in epidemic rates in women, especially in the Midwest area. I have a map on goiter around the whole country, north, south, east and west. There was a study done and the government recommended they could put a little bit of iodine in salt and take care of this goiter epidemic, which they did. It was a very effective treatment to prevent goiter, and it's still in salt now. It's in refined salts as we know it. The problem is only 10 percent of the iodine in that salt is bioavailable for the body. It's not a great way to get iodine in. Then you couple it with this bromide and fluoride overexposure that we're getting, and it's a recipe for disaster. So, salt is not the best way to get iodine in. At this point in our lives, I think with our overexposure to bromide and fluoride, we have to supplement with iodine. I think that the best way to supplement with it is either use Lugol's solution, which has been around for almost 200 years, or tablet of Lugol's solution. There is a form for Lugol's—Iodoral is one of them. Iodizyme-HP is another name for a tablet of Lugol's product. I've tested all of these products. They're all fine, they're all made from Lugol's Solution and I think that's a way to get it in.

I think it's impossible to get enough in through our diet right now in the world we live in. The best sources of iodine in the diet are sea vegetables such as seaweed, or ocean fish. Ocean fish do contain iodine. The problem is the longer that fish has been out of the ocean, the less iodine that fish has as it sublimates out into a gaseous phase, and fish have other problems such as high mercury levels to them. I still think a better way is we're going to need to supplement with iodine with the cancer epidemic that we're having right now. Average doses I find for people, 12 to 25 mgs for most people. If they have breast, lung, thyroid, prostate, ovarian, uterine problems, they may need more. A good holistic doctor can test your levels and the best way to test them is urinary levels. I describe all this in my book, *Iodine: Why You Need It, Why You Can't Live Without it.*

Ty: Yeah, great book, by the way. That's one of the ones that I've read of yours. I haven't read all dozen. That's good to know, because that's what my family takes is the Iodorol. I think one tablet is 13 mg ...

Dr. Brownstein: Twelve-and-a-half milligrams is one tablet.

Ty: That's right at the bottom end of what you say you need.

Dr. Brownstein: My testing has found most people need about 25 mg. If they have cancer or if they have fibrocystic breasts or cysts on their prostates or bumps on their prostate or something like that, or pancreatic lesions, they'll need a little bit more.

Ty: A little more, okay. Can you talk about the importance of Vitamin D in preventing and even treating cancer?

Dr. Brownstein: How about before we get to Vitamin D, I want to bring up salt and then we'll talk about Vitamin D?

Ty: Sure. What specifically about salt?

Dr. Brownstein: Salt, I think, is one of those basic things. You could say, "Hey, you wrote a book about salt, well, does have salt have any play in this?" And, I'll transition into that.

Ty: Dr. B, I know you have written a book about salt. What bearing does that have on our conversation here?

Dr. Brownstein: Well, Ty, we've been talking about sort of doing the basics, you know, eating a better diet. One of the other basics is making sure you maintain adequate hydration, drink enough water, taking iodine I consider one of the basics, and salt is one of the four basic things people need. Our bodies need and require adequate amounts of salt daily. Salt is the second major constituent next to water in our body. The immune system can't function well without salt. Our hormonal system can't function well without salt, and iodine can't work in the body without adequate amounts of salt. So, I consider salt one of the basics. I check salt levels in every patient that comes in the door. I can tell you the vast majority are salt deficient. As I write about in my book, *Salt Your Way to Health,* there is good and bad salt. I would say an inadequate form of salt is refined salt. It's the little white crystals that we're all used to. They fit in a salt shaker and they're real fine and they contain a little bit of iodine. But they only contain sodium and chloride, a little bit of iodine, and then toxic chemicals such as ferricyanide and they have some bleach chemicals in them to make them white. That's not a good product. A better produce is unrefined salt, which has over 80 minerals in it, lesser amounts of sodium and chloride. It doesn't have a lot of iodine in it, so therefore you need to supplement with iodine. But, this is a staple that people need in their diets. The adrenal system can't function well without salt, the thyroid system can't function well without salt, and the immune system can't function well without salt. And, iodine works better in the body with salt, as salt helps to usher out bromide and fluoride in the body while you take iodine.

Ty: Okay. So many diets that I've heard about, people that think they're getting healthy, they say, "Okay, I'm not eating any more salt." Not a good idea.

Dr. Brownstein: It is not a good idea. Not only is it not a good idea, it's a disastrous idea. Eventually, the adrenals get overstressed from this and don't function well. It's not good for the immune system and it's not good for fighting cancer. People need salt in their diet. It's a staple. Human beings have needed salt since the beginning of time. We were designed by our Maker to need salt.

Ty: How much salt?

Dr. Brownstein: About a teaspoon a day for most people. The latest studies that just came out, *New England Journal of Medicine,* verified what I've been saying for the last 15 years. You know, I blog about this. I write about it in my newsletter as those studies came out. You can look at the curves. It's very easy to look at them and you see high mortality rate and the low end of salt intake, and then it goes down. It doesn't really matter how much salt you use. Maybe at very high rates there are problems, but people aren't going to eat that amount of salt. They just need the right kind of salt, which is unrefined salt such as Celtic brand Sea Salt, Redmond's Real Salt, the Himalayan salt. I've tested all three versions of those four times. I didn't find toxic agents and I found adequate amounts of minerals. All of those kinds, I think those are very healthy forms of salt.

Ty: Awesome. That's good to know, too, because one of those Himalayan sea salt's what we use. So, good to know that we're doing the right thing, at least from that area. Question for you. You mentioned that sodium or salt is important in balanced hormones and the immune system. So, can you talk about how is it important in your hormones?

Dr. Brownstein: We need salt for our detox pathways to function optimally. If you don't have enough salt you can't detox from toxic chemicals such as what we were talking about before ... bromide and fluoride, plus other things. Low-salt diets depress the adrenal function, which eventually drops down the immune system function and then chronic illnesses start to develop, such as cancer and adrenal problems and arthritis and a whole bunch of other things. Salt just needs to be a basic in everyone's diet.

Ty: Talk about the importance of the immune system in fighting cancer, because one of the common threads that I'm hearing from most of the people who I interview is that good nutrition, avoiding toxicities, detoxing the body, all these things you've talked about, are what get the body's immune system to function the way it was supposed to by the Creator.

Dr. Brownstein: I assume you drove a car out to my house today to do this interview.

Ty: Well, our horses broke down, so, yes we did.

Dr. Brownstein: I also assume that when you take that car back to the airport, you're going to put gas in that car, because the car needs a certain kind of gas to run optimally. Let's say a gas station, maybe your own personal car, would be a better analogy for this. But, if there was a gas station that said 10 cents a gallon gas and you pull up there and you say, "Hey, I'm going to make a deal here. It's going to cost me less to fill up my car." Then you look at the gas and it's mud. Are you going to put that mud in your gas tank? No, because you know it's going to wreck your car. Well, I say the same thing. We need to put the right fuel in our bodies so our immune system functions optimally. We have a great design in the human body to fight infection, to stay healthy into old age, to keep brain function into old age, and if we treat the body right the immune system can work just fine. Treating that body right is doing the basics, like what we're talking about: supplying it with the right nutrients, maintaining hydration, keeping iodine levels up and maintaining adequate amounts of salt intake. The immune system can do its job—surveillance for foreign substances and foreign bodies and get rid of that. It can keep cancer at bay. It's when the immune system gets disrupted, I think that's when bad things start happening to us.

Ty: Let's say the immune system has been disrupted because of these toxicities that we're being exposed to on a daily basis. What's the best way to detoxify your body so that the immune system can function?

Dr. Brownstein: The best way to detoxify is to do those basics we talked about. Eat better, maintain hydration, iodine and salt. There is some specific testing you can do to try and figure out what are you toxic from. I hear people say, 'I'm going to detox." My question is, "Well, what are you detoxing from?" We're exposed to all this stuff. Are you detoxing from bromide, are you detoxing from pesticides, are you detoxing from whatever? I think it's good to do some testing, try and figure out what's disrupted the body, and then develop a plan for that. That's a better way to do it than to just say I'm detoxing without knowing exactly what you're trying to detox from.

Ty: I'm glad you said that. In an earlier interview, Dr. Butar from North Carolina, he said the word "detox" is kind of like the word "love." For instance, my 4-year-old daughter, Charity, a couple of weeks ago, she said, "There's two kind of love, Daddy. Love for food and love for Mommy." So, she realizes we say "I love my food," "I love the pizza," "I love my mommy," but they're different. And so I, I think it's good to distinguish that. We can't just say, "Well, I'm going to detox to treat my cancer," or to prevent cancer, because that can mean a whole variety of different things.

Dr. Brownstein: I do think, Ty, we would do better to search for what's causing all this stuff, and then develop a plan for that versus just diagnose and treat. Then you're trying to react to a situation that's already there. We're already behind the eight-ball when we're using even a holistic method. You're already reacting behind the eight-ball when you're trying to treat that cancer that's already there. You want to really get the body milieu in the correct mode so cancer doesn't develop in the first place.

Ty: So, famous quote. Last question, last topic for the day. Quote from Hippocrates, "Let food be thy medicine and medicine be thy food." What is an optimal diet that you would tell people, "You should eat this certain way to stay healthy?" What are some staples of what a good diet looks like?

Dr. Brownstein: Everyone's a unique biochemical individual who requires their own individual management of things. I don't know if there's one particular diet for everybody. However, I think most people would do well to eliminate all the refined food that's out there. Anything made with refined sugar, flour, salt and oil should be eliminated.

Ty: Because sugar feeds cancer cells, as you mentioned earlier.

Dr. Brownstein: Cancer cells feed sugar, so, a better way to do it is to keep grains low in the diet, even whole grains, because they turn into sugar very quickly and to eat good sources of protein, to eat fruits and vegetables made from organic sources without pesticides on them. If you're going to eat animal products, eat them hormone-free. A lot of this is common sense. I don't think it takes rocket science to realize this would be a better diet than the conventional stuff that's out there. But, it can be done. It is a little more expensive to eat this way, but in the long run you're going to save money because you're not going to be sick and spending money on pills and drugs that aren't treating the underlying cause of the illness. They're just treating the symptoms of you eating badly for so many years.

Ty: A quote from Joel Salatin. He said, "You think organic food's expensive, have you priced cancer lately?"

Dr. Brownstein: I like that quote.

Ty: I like that. A little bit of extra spending on the front end, getting clean foods into your body, can save you a lot of money on the back end.

Dr. Brownstein: That's why I've been writing all these books and newsletters and things, because I could see what works in people and what doesn't work in people and I write about what works. I see it every day in my practice and this stuff works.

Ty: When you're talking about eating good, clean foods and lots of organic vegetables, it reminds me—I did an interview with Patrick Quillen and he said, "Now, in the United States public education system in the schools, ketchup is considered a vegetable."

Dr. Brownstein: Ketchup is full of sugar. You look at how much sugar is in ketchup. It's a disaster. At least if they're going to eat ketchup, there is organic ketchup out there. It has much less sugar content than the regular conventional ketchup that's out there.

Ty: And no high-fructose corn syrup if it's organic.

Dr. Brownstein: High-fructose corn syrup is a disaster. It's in so many foods. It's in regular ketchup and that's what's making people fat and sick and feeding cancer.

Ty: How does high-fructose corn syrup affect people as far as the obesity epidemic? Because I've read doctors that have said the high fructose corn syrup, the way that it affects the insulin levels in the body creates diabetes and it creates obesity. Can you talk about that?

Dr. Brownstein: We can't metabolize high-fructose corn syrup as well as we can metabolize regular glucose that's in fruit and vegetables. What happens is the body stores it up as fat, and that's why one in three Americans are obese right now.

Ty: Right.

Dr. Brownstein: Two-thirds are overweight. We've got more diabetes and metabolic syndrome than we know what to do with. Remember, every time this blood sugar goes up it's feeding cancer cells. The only way you're going to treat cancer is to lower blood sugar levels, lower the obesity epidemic and then people have to eat better. Again, it's why I wrote my books, that's why I write my newsletter, that's why you're doing these interviews. It can be done, but people need to take a proactive way to improve their health and they need to eat better.

Ty: The way that we do that, as you said earlier, you take that food pyramid and you flip it over.

Dr. Brownstein: Absolutely.

Ty: Decrease grains, increase the fats, eat good proteins and the fats are great for cognitive function as well.

Dr. Brownstein: Absolutely.

Ty: Right. Well, Dr. B, this has been fascinating. I really enjoyed it. A lot of great information you've shared with us. I really appreciate you spending the time with us today.

Dr. Brownstein: Thank you, Ty. It was fun doing this.

Ty: All right. You take care.

Dr. Brownstein: Take care.

[end of transcript]

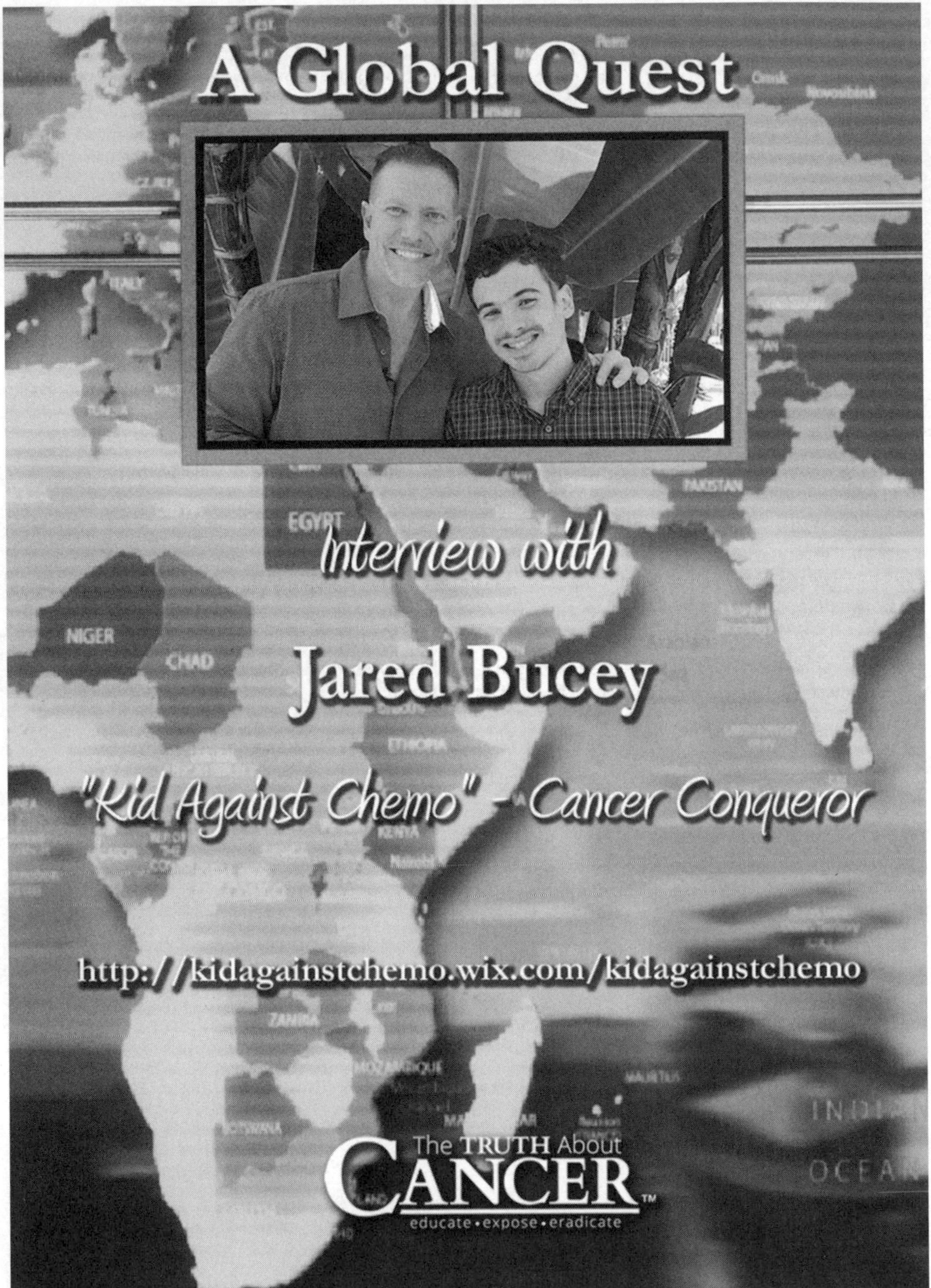
A Global Quest
Interview with
Jared Bucey
"Kid Against Chemo" - Cancer Conqueror
http://kidagainstchemo.wix.com/kidagainstchemo
The TRUTH About CANCER™
educate • expose • eradicate

Ty: So Jared, tell me a little bit about-- take yourself back in time about little over a year ago when you were diagnosed. You were diagnosed with cancer at the age of what?

Jared: At the age of 16.

Ty: Tell us about that.

Jared: Well, I had extremely bad pain in my stomach for probably about two weeks, a week or two, before we went into the ER. And they did a bunch of tests, stuff like that. And probably about another two, three weeks after I was in the hospital, they diagnosed me with cancer.

Ty: So, you went in you had a lot of pain, they did some tests, in a few weeks you're diagnosed with cancer?

Jared: Yeah.

Ty: So Jared, when you were diagnosed with cancer was it advanced, was it early? What was the stage of the cancer?

Jared: I had a late stage four Hodgkin's Lymphoma.

Ty: Stage four Hodgkin's Lymphoma: pretty serious diagnosis.

Jared: Yeah.

Ty: At that point, when you hear that you have-- you're 16, you find out you got cancer. How are you feeling at that point? How's your mom and dad feeling? What's the emotion in the family at that point?

Jared: I'm very upset, but I actually-- I didn't really know too much about cancer, or chemo, and I didn't think that there was much of a cure for cancer. I thought cancer pretty much just meant death right on the spot.

Ty: So, you thought, "Okay, I've got cancer. I'm going to die." That's what you're thinking. But what are your mom and dad telling you? What are they thinking? What's the emotion in the family at that point? I got a 14 year old daughter. If I can just place myself in that situation, I would be a wreck. We've met your mom, and she came to Austin. We met you there months ago. She's like Super Woman, right? She's like a rock. What was her emotion when you find this out?

Jared: They fell apart, started crying. But my parents said that I could do whatever--

Ty: Whatever treatment suited you?

Jared: Right.

Ty: So they've put that into your choice: it's your body. You have cancer, you can make that decision. And so, of course they're pushing chemo. The doctors want you to do chemo, right? Did you do chemo?

Jared: I did one round, one full cycle of chemo. And then all the side effects were just so severe. I had really bad mouth sores throughout my whole GI system. I had really bad bone pain. I couldn't stand. I couldn't walk. My parents had to help me walk to the bathroom and back. I could barely use my phone or the TV remote because my hands were almost cramping from the bone pain. I'm trying to think of the other side effects.

Ty: So, when you're doing the one cycle of chemo, the one round of chemotherapy, you're not feeling great.

Jared: No.

Ty: You're feeling pretty lousy. So at that point you said, what? "I'm not going to do this anymore"?

Well, it definitely took a while for me to think about it to see if I wanted to keep doing chemo or if I wanted to stop. Eventually, I just felt in my heart and soul that I was going to die in the next round, because all those side effects were killing me, so--

Ty: I've seen the videos that you shared on Facebook and the videos that you took during that time, and they're heart-wrenching. I mean, you were in bad shape. So, I think that decision to not do anymore chemo after that - that's what you chose - probably saved your life.

Jared: Yeah, definitely.

Ty: Because you may not have died of the cancer, but you sure might have died from the chemo. So you decided against chemo, and you're known now as Jared, the Kid Against Chemo. That's how we first learned about you; it was on Facebook, Kid Against Chemo. So, you decided not to do anymore chemo. And what did you do at the point you said, "I'm not going to do chemo, but I am going to do this"? What did you decide to do for your cancer at that point?

Jared: I just decided to do all alternative methods from vitamins, supplements, the infrared sauna; eating al organic, juicing and all raw vegetables.

Ty: Sounds kind of like Chris Work. That's what Chris did.

Jared: Yes, exactly.

Ty: He said, "Instead of overdosing on poison, I decided to overdose on nutrition." So that's what you did?

Jared: Exactly.

Ty: And now it's almost a year ago that you had the diagnosis. Tell me-- you shared this with us in Austin. We brought you to Austin and we were able to meet you and your family, and we were sitting at dinner one night and you told me the most insensitive thing that doctor said to you when you were diagnosed with cancer. What did he say?

Jared: Well, we went in to get the PICC line taken out and then I said I was done and I don't want to do chemo anymore. And they explained to me how it would be like to die if I didn't do chemo. They said that it would feel like I was drowning under water. They asked if I ever felt like I was holding my breath under water, and they said it would be like that, except I wouldn't come up for air.

Ty: So they're trying to-- it sounds like they're trying to scare you.

Jared: They're trying to bully me.

Ty: To bully you into doing chemo, after you told them you don't want to. Telling you if you don't, you're going to eventually--

Jared: Die.

Ty: --suffocate like you're drowning, if you don't do chemo. That is pretty insensitive to say to a 17 year old, at that time, right? You turned 17 by then?

Jared: No, I think I was still 16.

Ty: You're still 16. Regardless, whether you're 16 or 17, whether you're 80, that is something--

Jared: It doesn't matter.

Ty: --that should never be said to a cancer patient, to try to bully them into doing a treatment that they just told you that they're against. So, you're about a year out now. How are you feeling?

Jared: I feel great.

Ty: They told you you would be likely dead within six months, you found out later. Is that right?

Jared: Yeah.

Ty: You found that out later, but they're saying you would be dead in six months. So now we're getting close to a year later and you're doing great. Tell us about your latest reports, the markers your mom was sharing with me last night at dinner. The fact that there was an infection that they looked at the markers for the viral infection. What was that?

Jared: Well, the last blood test, all my cancer markers were normal. All my blood tests were normal. Everything was just normal.

Ty: So you're back to normal health right now.

Jared: Yeah.

Ty: I think you're probably excellent health compared to most people. I think compared to probably most kids that are 17, almost 18 years old - and actually by the time that this airs, you will be 18 years old - I think you're probably in exceptional health compared to most kids. I mean, you're out and you're walking and you're exercising and you're eating all organic and you're drinking all these juices. Your body's getting nourished. So you've gone from a place where they said you'd be dead within six months-- which I would contest that. I don't like when on call just play God.

Jared: Right, neither do I.

Ty: And they tell you you've got six months. But now you're at a point about a year later which you're in excellent health. Well, that's awesome, Jared. It's really great to get your story. It was great to meet you several months ago when you came to Austin with your mom.

Jared: Yeah, that was fun.

Ty: And my family just loves you. You're one of their heroes. You're becoming a lot of people's heroes out there. People are following you on Facebook, Kid Against Chemo. They're watching you. We're here in San Diego right now at the Integrative Health Conference and you're going to get to speak here. You're getting this huge following and you're almost 18 years old. I mean, that's great. I think the sky is the limit for what you have in the future, for the things that you're going to be able to do with this message. So, if you could share one message with people that are watching, that are looking at you - I mean, you're like a role model for people now - of how to treat cancer naturally and to do well, what would you share with them? What's one takeaway from this that you could people if you're diagnosed with cancer?

Jared: I would just tell people, don't always listen to your doctors and just go with your heart, mind, body, and soul. Everyone has a choice. You don't have to say what or do what other people say and tell you what to do. Just be yourself. Just heal how you want to heal, whether it be chemo or natural treatments or whatever. Just do it however you want to.

Ty: Jared here, I'm looking at a couple of things. I'm really proud of you here. Kid Against Chemo, Jared Story. So here's a book you've written. And then you were actually recently on the cover of Green Living Magazine. Had an article written about you, cover story. Man, this is awesome. I've never been on the front cover of a magazine. I'm a little jealous. That's awesome, Jared. I'm really proud of you. I'm really proud of you, man. You are going to be such a great role model for people in the future, for kids, because there is such an epidemic of kids that have cancer now. And I think that the way that you've treated your cancer, the way you've gone natural, the way that you've used nutrition and you've overdosed on vitamins and nutrition and juicing, I think that that's going to be a path that many children can follow and they can follow successfully because of you. So here, hold both of these up. I want you to just look at the camera. I'll give you a big hug here, man.

[end of transcript]

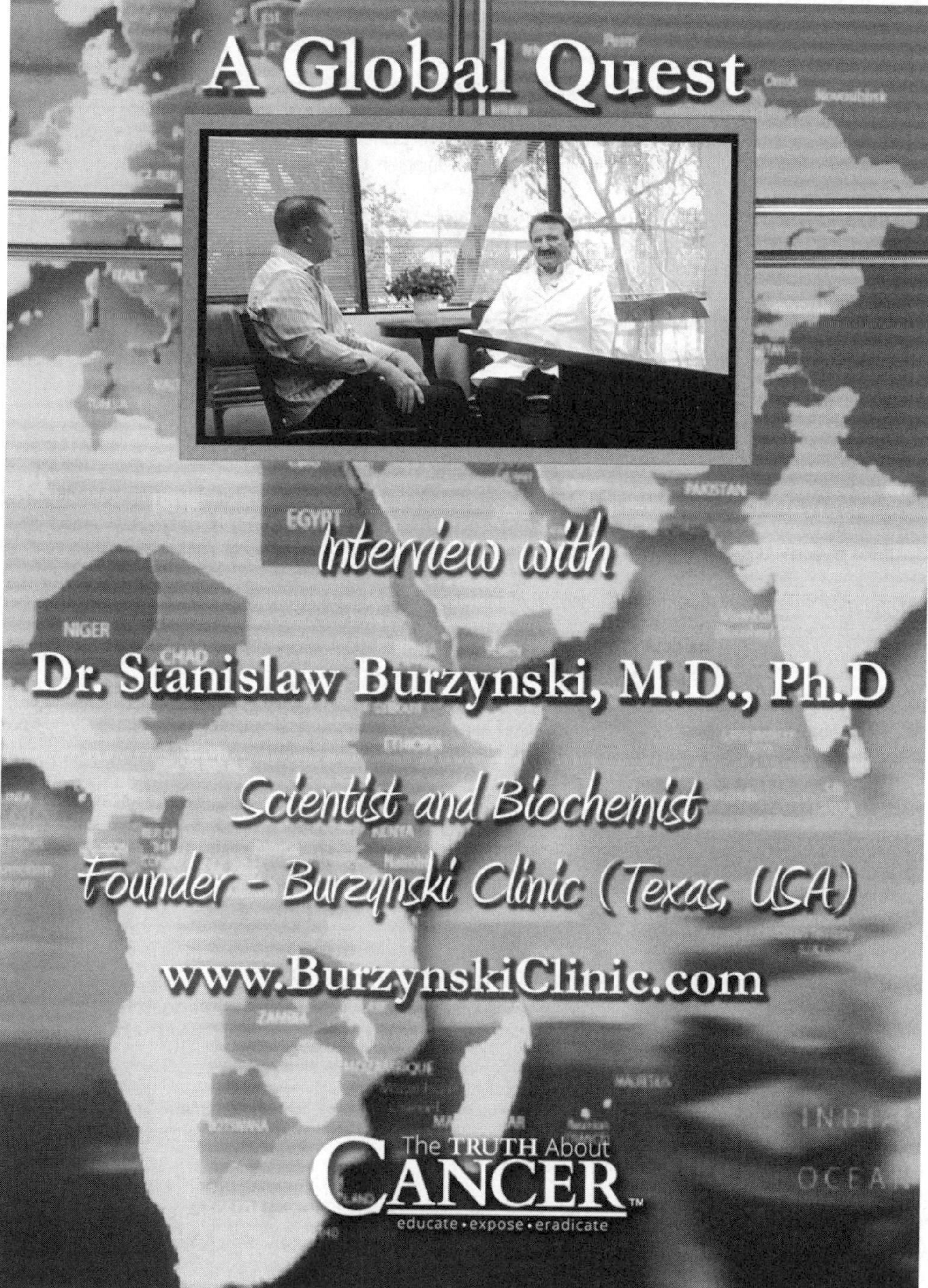
A Global Quest
Interview with
Dr. Stanislaw Burzynski, M.D., Ph.D
Scientist and Biochemist
Founder - Burzynski Clinic (Texas, USA)
www.BurzynskiClinic.com
The TRUTH About CANCER
educate • expose • eradicate

Ty: Well, I'm so excited to be back in Houston, Texas here at The Burzynski Clinic with Dr. Stanislaw Burzynski. Thank you.

Dr. Burzynski: My pleasure.

Ty: Thank you so much for having us in your office again. We were fortunate to interview you last year for *The Quest for The Cures* documentary and just had an enormous response. People loved seeing you. They loved what you had to share and a lot of the things that you shared angered people because of the abuse of power that we're seeing, discrimination against natural treatments.

Dr. Burzynski: That's unfortunate, but hopefully it can be corrected.

Ty: Yeah. Well, we're doing our best and you're doing your best.

Dr. Burzynski: Thank you very much, yes.

Ty: Yeah, working towards that goal.

Dr. Burzynski: That's right.

Ty: So one of the things that we were just talking about, I wanted you to share with the viewing audience, is I recently had the privilege to interview Dr. Gaston Cornu-Labat in Seattle. He's been working with you on your treatment, on the anti-neoplastons, and he shared with me that they're getting a lot of kick-back or push-back from the FDA on the NDI process.

Dr. Burzynski: Well, this has expanded access through the treatment, which has been discussed widely.

Ty: Expanded access.

Dr. Burzynski: That's correct. This was discussed widely in the news media and the impression was that the government is doing whatever is possible to make it easier for that patient. Well, unfortunately, it's not easy. This is the most difficult process you can find in entire world.

And by example, for instance, if the doctor in the UK or in Germany would like to have access to the new treatment, he does not need to ask the government for permission, he simply asks the manufacturer to provide the medication and he can use it in single patient investigational use. So that's pretty much his right and this is permitted in every European Union country.

Ty: Okay.

Dr. Burzynski: In Australia, initially the government in Canberra, in the capital of Australia, asked us to provide some documentation. We did it and after that, they made it very easy for patients and doctors in Australia to get access to our treatment. Simply the doctor needs to make a phone call to the agency, which is similar to FDA, and then he can go ahead with the treatment. That's it.

Then in Japan also, it's very easy. It's not even at a level of the central government. The doctor needs to simply notify the prefecture, the district government, that he is planning to use investigational treatment and he can do it—very easy process.

And in the other countries, it's even easier than that. The doctor can do it whenever the doctor feels this is the best for the patient because the doctor really has the best idea how to treat the patients personally because the doctor has very good experience.

Here, it became very complex because the process is similar to the pharmaceutical companies asking for permission to do a clinical trial. It's called, "Single Patient Investigational New Drug Application."

And in order to do it, the highly qualified specialist, like a consultant, needs to spend about 50 to 100 hours and these people are typically charging $300.00 per hour. These are highly qualified specialists. These are the people who are retained by pharmaceutical companies to put together the application to conduct clinical trials. And it's different to conduct clinical trials when you have 40 or 80 patients and it's different when you're asking to treat a patient who's dying from cancer and he needs the treatment right away.

So it takes time. It takes money to do it. And the doctors who would like to do it, he cannot charge for it. So the doctor has to go to the consultant firm, ask them, "Please prepare investigation for new drug application." "Okay, we'll be glad to do it, $100,000.00 and we'll do it." And it will take them probably four weeks or a month to prepare said application.

The doctor cannot charge for it so the doctor needs to take the money out of his pocket and pay for it. And then if he finds a stupid doctor who would like to do it for the patient who comes to him, well, it would be some challenge.

Ty: Right.

Dr. Burzynski: But anyway, once the application is filed, it goes to FDA and the FDA will look at this, will evaluate it, and will respond to the doctors. Usually they ask for a number of supporting documents. And in most cases, from what I know, they agree to it, which is nice. Well, I was told by Dr. Gaston that he checked this in about 1,400 cases of such applications, only two were rejected and this was his. Nobody else was rejected.

Ty: His?

Dr. Burzynski: Dr. Gaston.

Ty: Okay. And they were his applications for the anti-neoplastons. So this bureaucracy is killing people because they don't have access—

Dr. Burzynski: Yeah, people are dying because they have a deadly disease and we have a number of people who died needlessly because bureaucracy was really asking them for one document after another. Now, they respond promptly, but they usually reject. If they reject, then obviously these patients have nothing to try because they have a deadly disease. They die.

The explanation is, well, the risk of using the treatment does not justify the benefits. But Dr. Gaston proved that the risk is much lower than the risk of chemotherapy with any other treatments and the chances for risk were much greater.

But it doesn't matter. Who is shunting the law? People who are at the level of like retired nurses and there's perhaps one oncologist who did not see patients for the last 10 years, whatever, and they're making the decisions without seeing the patients. And they go ahead and they give permission, the patient lives. If they don't give permission, the patient dies. Many people die. And they will continue to die because that system exists. It doesn't exist in any other country. And this system has become very, very complex. It was introduced recently so despite of the facts that everywhere it's described, "Well, the government is trying to help the people to make it easy," it's extremely difficult.

And who is going to pay for it? Well, the doctor cannot charge for it and he is to prepare it. How should he know how to prepare it if he is simply in private practice? He has no idea about it.

Ty: Right.

Dr. Burzynski: This is the knowledge, which is just typical for consultant firms who are dealing with pharmaceutical companies and they're retained by pharmaceutical companies. They do it for them. Obviously, if you are asking for new clinical trials, it's the right thing to do. If you're asking for a single patient who's dying from cancer, that's a problem. Well, we did it for free for Dr. Gaston so he didn't need to spend any money of course…

Ty: But they still rejected it, right?

Dr. Burzynski: They rejected it. We spent a lot of time to do it. We used highly qualified specialists in our organization to do it. It was rejected not because there was something wrong with the application, but simply based on the fact, "Well, the risks are too great and the benefits are too little."

Well, it reminds me of what happened to me in the Communist system. I was trying to get a visa to get out of the Communist system and it was practically impossible because in the current system, it's like a big prison. Everybody stays in the country. Nobody leaves the country because if he leaves the country, he will find out that the other country is much better.

Ty: Right, right.

Dr. Burzynski: He will tell the other people and that's like a contagious disease. Finally, I was rejected like six times by the Communist government to give me the visa to visit the United States and every time I was like, "What are the reasons?" "The other reasons. Goodbye." Okay? I would never know what are the reasons – the other reasons. And that's all it took.

Ty: So they just basically arbitrarily rejected.

Dr. Burzynski: Well, it was their own judgment and that's what they do. And on the other hand, I am not permitted as a practicing physician to file such papers. Normally, I should have the same right as any other physician, but I am not permitted to do it. And the reason why I am not permitted to do it is because, "It would interfere with my involvement in clinical trials."

I have permission to run clinical trials, but we didn't start it yet because we don't have funding available so I'm not busy doing clinical trials because nobody is treated now. We finished one series of clinical trials. We are waiting for funding to start another one then we'll be busy, but not now. I am doing nothing regarding clinical trials.

So I can easily help the other patient using my experience. Nobody has such experience as our team in using this type of treatment, but we are not permitted to do it. The other doctor should do it who has never treated patients with anti-neoplastons, but we are not permitted to do it.

Ty: This seems like a system just of suppression and censorship that is being implemented here that is basically aimed at anybody that's doing anything outside of the norm.

Dr. Burzynski: Well, this is obviously against discoverers, against innovators, it's against American spirit. That's what I would say. It's got nothing to do with American liberty. It has nothing to do with the right of American people to make discovery to introduce something. It has nothing to do with the doctors to select the best treatment for his patient.

How the doctor can select the best treatment for his patient if the only thing that he can give is up to the lawyers, up to the nurses, who never treated such things? They don't have any idea how to treat advanced cancer.

This is a system, which is punishing the doctors to be inventors, to be discoverers. And the name of the game, it's big money because if you have many doctors who are inventors, it's no growth for the large institutions because they're getting better results than large institutions. And then the large institutions will not have as much business so it's not good for them.

So that's what developed and this is completely not according to American spirit. And it probably needs another new solidarity movement to really reprogram this because it's going in the wrong direction. The inventors should be awarded, not punished.

I am being punished now by Texas Medical Board for saving the lives of the worst cancers you can get. Pancreatic cancer—we have a patient who survives over six years, his pancreatic cancer, which spread to the liver. I am now investigated. I have to go to court. I may lose my license because the Texas Board is harassing me because I used my invention to save the life of this patient.

This patient obviously was sentenced to die. Everybody dies from pancreatic cancer. It's one out of a million cases, which lives a little longer. It is related. People who have pancreatic cancer spread to the liver, they're dead within a few months. This man is surviving 6 months. No tumors. He lives a normal life.

Ty: Six years?

Dr. Burzynski: Yes.

Ty: Six years. Okay.

Dr. Burzynski: Of course, he is too primitive to understand that this was the treatment, which he took for something like five weeks which got rid of his cancer. "If at all, I was praying, I was using the right diet, and I'm saved." Well, if this is praying, this is a miracle. Okay? I am not aware of any miracles of somebody surviving advanced pancreatic cancer this way. Perhaps he's the first one and maybe he'll go to sainthood, I don't know.

Ty: So your treatment is literally curing people that are deemed to be incurable.

Dr. Burzynski: Well, everybody dies from such cancer. Especially if pancreatic cancer spreads to the liver, then you're dead. The liver will get involved and then in a few months, there's nothing you can do.

Ty: Right

Dr. Burzynski: I mean, you can live a little longer, but it's inoperable. No treatment works on this. FDA approved the medication, which can do something in pancreatic cancer because it can increase survival by three weeks.

Ty: Three weeks.

Dr. Burzynski: Three weeks, yeah. It was approved for this. On the other hand, recently, randomized clinical trials have been completed by our Japanese colleagues on anti-neoplastons in colon cancer, which spread to the liver. They proved that they can increase the median survival by about three years.

Ty: Wow.

Dr. Burzynski: Three years versus three weeks or versus three months because the overall standard for FDA for approval for a new drug is to extend median survival from three weeks to three months. Here, you've got about three years.

Ty: And they're still having issues.

Dr. Burzynski: No, no. Know what I'm saying? Well, the risks…

Ty: The risks are too great.

Dr. Burzynski: The risks does not justify the benefits.

Ty: Well, my question is this—if you look at risk versus reward…

Dr. Burzynski: Oh, the risk is death because…

Ty: The risk is death.

Dr. Burzynski: Obviously colon cancer spread to the liver, practically everybody dies from it. Well, in some cases, this can be operated, but it comes back. Finally these people are dead, okay? Well, we are talking about survival over five years—median survival—which means some of these guys, they survive over ten years, some of these guys will survive four years, but the median is over five years.

And if you've got about substantial difference, we have quantum difference compared to the other drugs. But this is documented and I'm talking about it because this is published in good articles in peer-reviewed journals. Everybody can read it. So it's not advertisement, this is a true scientific fact.

Ty: Sure.

Dr. Burzynski: So the survival in the treatment group with anti-neoplastons has been increased by about 3 years—33 months which is close to 3 years—and it's not enough of course. It still didn't make such progress as it should, but of course it can be read by anybody. It's available.

Okay. So basically, I am referring to this thing that is merciless harassment by the authorities of doctors who are inventors. I'm now going through three years of harassment by Texas Medical Board and one of the reasons why I'm going through this is I used the treatment which is not standard treatment for pancreatic cancer. I use this for a type of incurable lung cancer like malignant mesothelioma.

This patient is also surviving over 5 years. He would have been dead a long time ago. These results were evaluated by our site oncologists, had amazing results and I have been harassed because Texas Board is saying, "You used a treatment which is not standard." There is no standard treatment for such patients.

Ty: Right. And to me, it seems there are certain areas of the world where if someone is dying and you do not offer help, it's a crime.

Dr. Burzynski: Yeah, it's a crime obviously.

Ty: But we see the same thing going on with these authorities. They are withholding treatment that could have helped.

Dr. Burzynski: Yeah, they're withholding treatment. They will provide the evidence that this treatment at least can offer a chance. And we know very well that we cannot save everybody. We can help some patients because we are dealing with different types of diseases. Every patient is somewhat different and they need a specific approach, but at least they may have a chance. Some of them make an amazing recovery.

And it's not just out of the blue because we already have documented cases. We already have published papers. Within the last year and a half, we already published about 20 articles in peer-reviewed journals so this evidence is available. Anybody can read it and it's scientific. It went through peer review so it's not advertisement.

I am permitted to present scientific facts. Of course, I am harassed for doing this because, according to Texas Board, the only thing which I can talk about is my address and phone number. So that's the degree of American liberties at this moment to practice in the state of Texas.

Ty: Right.

Dr. Burzynski: It makes you nauseated. And most of you don't have any idea about it. What happened to the freedom in America—the freedom of speech, the freedom of practicing your trade? So this is going down to hell unfortunately. The people need to be awakened because obviously this is killing people.

And I am presenting this to the other doctors. The other doctors can't do it. Everybody is afraid to touch it because the same thing may happen to him and this is a total war. Texas Medical Board is going after my doctors, is going after my assistants. They are suing everybody because of using the treatment which is non-conventional.

We actually have the right to use this treatment. We are using medication which is approved by the FDA and the results for some patients are very good and is scientifically valid. We are still harassed mercilessly and that's what is happening.

Ty: It's like a medical dictatorship.

Dr. Burzynski: Unfortunately, that's what it is. And it doesn't exist in any other country. This is the only country in which you can find it. So it's horrible.

Ty: That's what it is. Well, since we interviewed you last year, about a year ago, tell me some happy stories that you've had with the success on—I see the pictures on the wall out there—all these patients that are alive decades later. Tell me some positive movements.

Dr. Burzynski: We have a bunch of success stories. We have a number of patients who are very long term survivors, like over 20 years or approaching 20 years. And within the last year or two, we had a number of weddings to which we were invited. These are weddings of the patients who started as little children, now they grew up, they don't have cancer, they live normal lives. And they live highly productive lives. They don't have long term adverse reactions. They tolerated the treatment well. They live normal lives.

So that's what we see in various categories. You can see this of course in brain tumors in which we concentrated our efforts. You can see this in colon cancer. You can see this in malignant lymphoma, in various different types of cancer, malignant melanoma, you name it—because we had a number of tough cases.

But as far as within the last couple of years, we're concentrated on scientific documentations so we are trying to publish as much as possible. There is also our clinical trials. We've completed successfully 13 clinical trials, Phase 2 clinical trials. So now we're at the level of about 20 publications and we still need to publish probably another 10 so we are working step by step. It takes a lot of time.

Obviously it's not easy because we have a heavy burden by continuous harassment. So it's not easy to treat these advanced patients because you're continuously being harassed for doing this, which is incredible. We should be awarded. We should be set as an example. We are saving the lives of people who are sentenced to die. No. We are mentally harassed by lawyers, by people who know nothing about treatment, who are stupid puppets over the guys behind who knows very well what we can offer, but are directing these guys, like in Nazi Germany—they are simply obeying orders because they're programmed this way.

I think there will be a time when they use some type of Nuremberg trials so all of this white-collared, nicely-dressed lawyers and clerks who are treating the (inaudible 00:21:15) taxpayers may be held accountable for what they do because many people die because of directions and they do it secretly, they are not exposed. They feel they are beyond any punishment and they can continue to do this type of work.

I think your type is to expose these guys because these are some white-collar criminals. Because of them, many people will die. Because of them, the cancer will still continue to kill people because the doctors are afraid to really make inventions in medicine. They are afraid to practice what is called medical art. After many years of practice, doctors have something which is called, "Art of Practicing Medicine," and you can't really learn this in a medical school. You acquire this after years of practice.

But forget about practicing here because everybody is forced to use some stiff standards which obviously, in cancer, they work only for very few people, they don't work for most of them. If you're trying to do some innovation, forget it. You'll be punished. You will lose your license.

Ty: They tell you to practice medical Art, but they take away your paintbrush.

Dr. Burzynski: They take away your freedom. And you are under the dictatorship of the lawyers and these lawyers obviously are manipulated by big medical institutions. So that's what they do because big medical institutions realize they are too large to make innovations. It takes them years and years and years.

And practitioners, they can see what they can do because they have cancer patients all the time. Some of them who are bright can introduce innovation and they can help people. So I have nothing against the large medical institutions, they're fine. But these things, they should work together.

Ty: Right. And that's the problem, is that they're not working together. It's segregated.

Dr. Burzynski: And not only that. They are reactionary because they are destroying those individuals who can make discoveries because it's bad for the business.

Ty: Well, we've seen that throughout this documentary miniseries that it's about the money. The money is driving these decisions, but one of our purposes is to really expose this monster.

Dr. Burzynski: Absolutely, absolutely.

Ty: And so you're helping us to do that today with what you shared.

Dr. Burzynski: So anyway, another important advancement, which we had—of course, I mentioned about publishing by the Japanese doctors of controlled randomized clinical studies in advanced colon cancer. It included two groups of people. Both of them had colon cancer, which spread to the liver. And then one group was treated with chemotherapy, the other group was treated with anti-neoplastons plus chemotherapy. So there was the addition of chemotherapy, but a low dose of chemotherapy.

The results were very good. Thirty-three months increase of median survival compared to the control group, which is something unusual. And that's very good because this is a very important cancer. There are about 130 cases suffering in the United States from advanced colon cancer so it's very important.

But in brain tumors, we published a number of papers, especially in the area of treatment of highly malignant brain tumors like glioblastoma, which came back after starting radiation and chemotherapy. Again, the glioblastoma probably have about 50,000 population in the United States and most of these people are dying so only perhaps one or two percent will survive longer than five years. We have now some of these patients who are surviving close to 20 years as a result of treatment with anti-neoplastons.

We've published the results and now we decipher what kind of molecular signature is permitting these people to live so long. We have now a publication, which is under peer review and hopefully, it will be published soon. So it happens that the type of GBM which responds very well to the treatment with anti-neoplastons, is a very common type—it's called classical GBM. And at the same time, it's a deadly one. These people usually are dead within a year. So it's very good news and now we have a new clinical trial. We'll be concentrating on this type of GBM. Hopefully we'll get good results.

Ty: Thank you for spending the time with us today and shedding some new light on what's happened over the past year. You are a freedom fighter and we are supporting you 100 percent.

We really appreciate the fact that you've really, over the last 20 years, you've been the front runner, being heavily persecuted and attacked and you've really opened up the freedom pathways for a lot of other people to be able to open their minds to the possibility that there's a way to treat cancer that's outside of this box. And you've been really the front runner in this and so you've really made it possible for what we're doing so we thank you and keep up the good work.

Dr. Burzynski: Thanks a lot. Somebody has to do it. It was done in Poland by my friend, Lech Walesa, who is something like six months younger than me.

Ty: You're older than Lech Walesa.

Dr. Burzynski: Yeah. Well, he came to visit me a few times. He's a good man. So he did it in Poland so somebody has to fight for freedom somewhere else.

Ty: Well, you're doing it here and we appreciate you and rooting for you 100 percent. And keep up the good work.

Dr. Burzynski: Thank you.

Ty: Yeah, thank you.

[end of transcript]

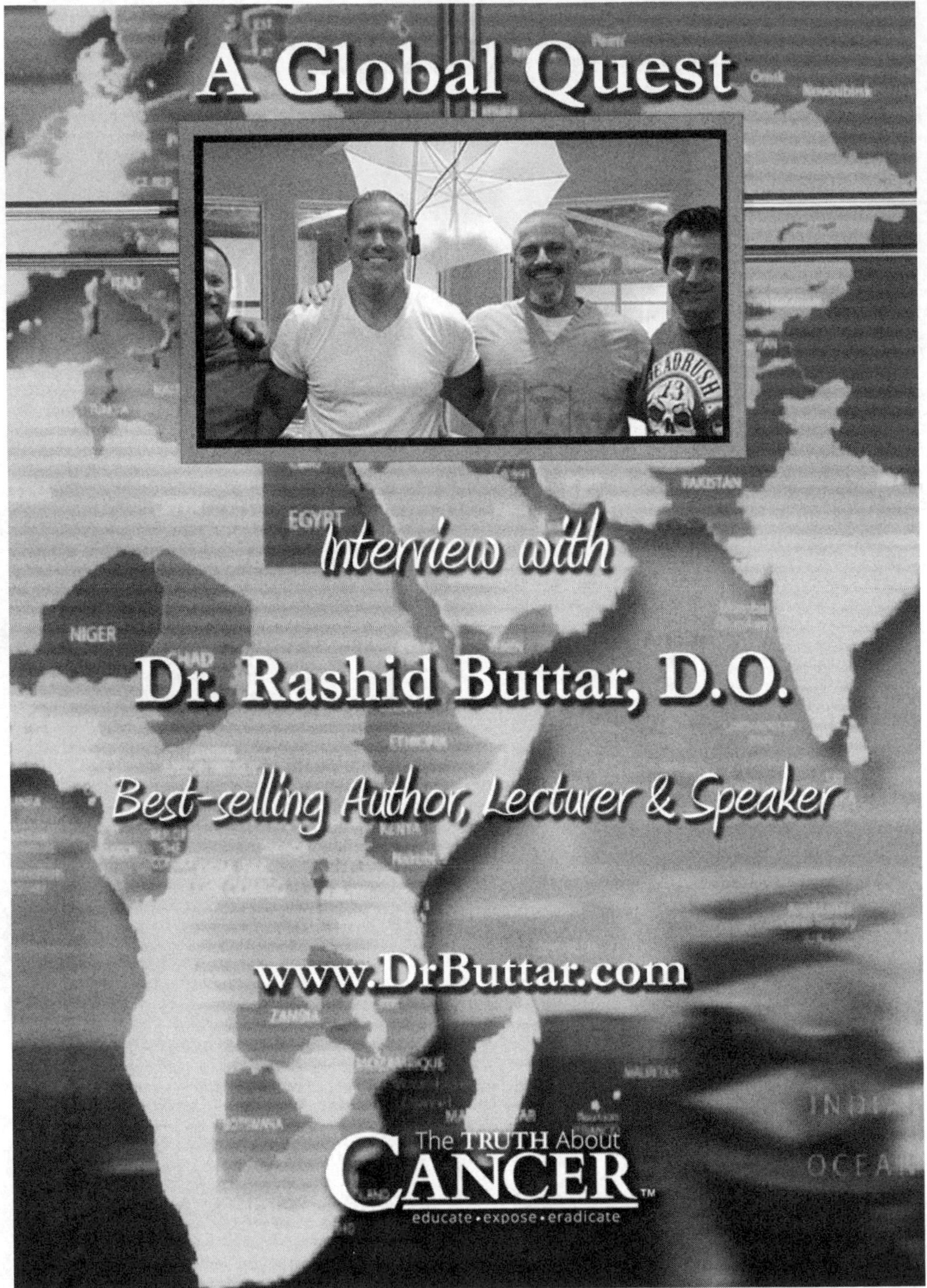
A Global Quest
Interview with
Dr. Rashid Buttar, D.O.
Best-selling Author, Lecturer & Speaker
www.DrButtar.com
The TRUTH About
CANCER
educate • expose • eradicate

Ty: Once again, I sit here with Dr. Rashid Buttar. We had a great conversation last year for *The Quest for The Cures* and thought we'd include you in this "*Global Quest* because we had a lot of response after we aired that documentary and they said, "Hey, we loved Dr. Buttar and the things that he said and we want to hear more." So thanks for joining us today.

Dr. Buttar: Thank you, Ty.

Ty: Yeah, yeah. So I want to get your take on a lot of new issues. I want to get you to explain your protocol again today, but the first thing I want to talk about is just recently, we had the scenario of an oncologist in Michigan who was recently sentenced to 45 years for treating patients with chemotherapy that did not have cancer and he milked Medicare for something like $93 million dollars. What is going on?

Dr. Buttar: Unfortunately, it's probably more prevalent than we know. In my own practice, I've had 12 or 13 patients that have come to me with a diagnosis of cancer who did not have a diagnosis of cancer. In fact, I introduced you to a friend of mine. Remember the Christmas present that I sent you once and it was Burton Goldberg who, after he read your book, said, "This is a good book."

Ty: Yeah.

Dr. Buttar: Burton was a perfect example of somebody who was diagnosed with cancer who did not have cancer. He had cancer, but not the cancer that they thought he had and it had been already treated and so that wasn't an issue for him. Now he ended up getting cancer later on in life, but when he came to me, he was told that he had an aggressive abdominal cancer that was growing at an unprecedented rate and he needed surgical resection and then chemo and radiation and he came to me. He was actually in Germany to get treatment and, it's a long story, but bottom line is, he did not have cancer. And so I think he ended up being the eighth or ninth patient—I've had a number of patients since then too—that did not have cancer.

Unfortunately, the way this whole thing works is that if they don't quite understand what's going on, they can't find the primary etiology, they're not sure, they'll just automatically assume that it's cancer because the thought process is, Cover your rear end—the CYA type aspect—that it's better to say that you had cancer and not have cancer rather than say, no, you don't have cancer and you had cancer and then somebody can of course come back and sue you and says, "I had cancer. You didn't diagnose me."

But what people don't understand is that it's not the cancer that really hurts people. Statistically, 42-46 percent of patients that have cancer will die of cachexia, which is basically wasting of protein. They basically lose all their lean body mass. So that leaves between 58 and 54 percent of patients that didn't die of cachexia. And the joke, which is only maybe half funny, is that the rest of them die from the treatment. In other words, really nobody dies from the cancer. If you think about it, when a patient gets immuno-suppressed and they have cancer, what actually takes them? Liver failure, kidney failure, pneumonia, sepsis. But all these things are usually associated with also the person getting chemo and radiation.

Now, how can a treatment actually kill a person? Well, it's almost like sending in napalm because you've got an ant problem. So, yes, you'll take care of the ants possibly, but then you've got to take care of every other form of life including the grass and you've got to level the site just to try to get the ants. So the collateral damage are the people that live there in the same house as the ants, meaning that the normal endogenous healthy cells are also going to get massacred.

And remember that cancer is an issue that starts at the DNA level, right? So for people that are maybe watching this and, just from a common sense standpoint, does it make any sense to take a therapy—let's use radiation as an example—to take a therapy that we know is dangerous under any circumstances—you break your leg, your break your hand, you go to the hospital, they take you in to get an x-ray, they've got the skull and cross bones, they've got the universal triangular radiation sign as a warning. Why is that warning there? You tell me.

Ty: Because it's known that it's harmful.

Dr. Buttar: And how is it harmful?

Ty: It damages DNA.

Dr. Buttar: It damages DNA. And what is the consequence of damaging DNA?

Ty: Potentially cancer.

Dr. Buttar: Bingo. So then why would we take something that we know has a very high propensity to create cancer and use that to treat cancer? It's really interesting that Einstein's definition of insanity was that, he said, "You cannot create a solution with the same mindset that created the problem in the first place." And that's exactly what we're doing.

Ty: Yeah.

Dr. Buttar: We're taking a situation, we're taking a thought process that caused the insanity in the first place, and trying to use that as a solution.

Ty: Yeah.

Dr. Buttar: It's absurd. Let's do the chemotherapy for example. Chemotherapy, yes, it can kill cancer cells possibly. It can kill any cell. Here's the issue that I have with chemotherapy. When I see somebody that's handling chemotherapy, making chemotherapy, and they have to wear hazmat suits and gloves and you can't touch it because it's toxic, then why are you going to give it to a person who's already sick? Does that make any sense? You ask a three-year-old child this question. I would bet you that 90 percent of the three-year-old children would get it. If that looks dangerous, then I shouldn't touch it. That's it.

Ty: Much less put it in my body.

Dr. Buttar: Exactly.

Ty: Well, we've seen the case over the last few years of the pharmacists that are actually making the chemotherapy that you mentioned that are now coming down with what they're calling secondhand chemo cancer because they've not actually even had the chemo, but they've got exposure to it from making it and now they're getting cancer from making the chemo.

Dr. Buttar: Look at that term—secondhand chemo cancer.

Ty: Yeah.

Dr. Buttar: That's like a double oxymoron, isn't it?

Ty: It is. It is.

Dr. Buttar: It's unbelievable.

Ty: Yeah. So this case of Dr. Fata, the oncologist in Michigan, it's bizarre to me—and I've asked other doctors about this—it's bizarre to me because we are, as you just said, we are using poisons to treat a disease that's caused by potentially exposure to too many poisons or chemicals.

And it's odd that we see these stories of these patients' families. They're being interviewed now. Patients have died and it's widely accepted even on the mainstream news now that the patient died from the chemo. They're saying, "My husband died from the chemo." They're admitting it in this case. But then, why, if there's somebody that actually has cancer and then they die, why don't we say, "Well, they died from the chemo too, but now it's actually the cancer." Right? It's because we double-think.

Dr. Buttar: Yes, exactly right. It's because it's the standard of care. It's the standard of care which is basically a stamp of approval that means it doesn't matter what you do, if you do it this way, it's accepted. It's an acceptable way of killing people.

Ty: Right.

Dr. Buttar: Now, let's look at the counterpoint. I don't want to talk about something off topic, but I want to bring that counterpoint. You remember my situation from 2007-2010? The Medical Board of North Carolina was coming after me since 1999 for multiple different things. Every time they tried, we won and every time, they postured and we had to go to court and ended up going to the Superior Court a number of times. In 2007, as you probably remember—we've discussed this off the air—in 2007, I was brought up on charges of ethical breach of conduct for doing treatments that were not effective in cancer patients and taking advantage of them.

And fast forward three and a half years, they committed *ex parte* which basically is that—we basically won, but then they tried to bleed me dry because they couldn't get anything so we had to do the whole thing again and my attorney told me that that's what their strategy was. But the interesting thing was that we had 42, I think it was, 42 patients that were ready to testify. The Medical Board gave us an opportunity to only pick five. So the five patients that we picked, all five—

By the way, just to go back for a second. There was never a complaint from a patient. All the people that made the complaints were people that had never been to my practice, never talked to me, no email. Two of them weren't even from the state of North Carolina. And then when the Medical Board started to put this out, they tried to basically character-assassinate me and then they had a couple of complaints that came in, "Well, yeah, I came to Dr. Buttar. My wife, my daughter, and myself came for mercury toxicity," that Boyd Haley had referred the patients to me. The wife got better in five weeks of treatment, the daughter got better in three weeks of treatment with 90 percent resolution of symptoms, but he didn't. And they were supposed to come for 20 weeks because it's one treatment per week. They only came for like five weeks and his complaint was, "Well, I didn't get better." 'Well, you weren't compliant." But that was all after the fact, after the Medical Board started creating the issues.

But the point was that there were five patients that testified—and this is the best part, Ty. One was a doctor who had cancer, one was an oncological nurse who had cancer—45 years, she was an oncological nurse, and then the other three were lay people. All five had been referred to hospice, all five had stage IV cancer, four out of the five had already had chemo and radiation and failed it, one refused it, all five were told to get their wills in order and that there was nothing else that was possible for them, and they were all given a prognosis between three and six months to live and that was it.

When they testified before the Medical Board, one was 8 years out from the cancer, one was five and a half years out from her cancer, and the remaining three were three years to three and a half years out from their cancer. So five patients that testified, that showed the PET scans, CT scans—14 hours of testimony. And guess what the Medical Board's response was?

Ty: I can't remember. You told me before.

Dr. Buttar: One word response and that response was, "Irrelevant."

Ty: Irrelevant.

Dr. Buttar: They brought me up on ethical breach of conduct for doing treatments that don't work in cancer in patients that were documented that they were supposedly going to die in hospice, but after we showed that that treatment did work, the results are the answer. No studies, this, that and the other garbage. The actual proof of the patient—their response was, "Irrelevant."

Ty: It doesn't matter.

Dr. Buttar: It doesn't matter. So if you do the standard of care and you give chemo and people die, it's okay. If you don't do the standard of care and people live, that's not okay. It's politically incorrect.

So this is the amazing thing. You take the poison, you give it to people, they die—it's part and parcel of the normal status quo, modus operandi. This is how it's supposed to be. Now you break that, you actually do something that's not toxic, you help patients, they live—"Hey, we don't care whether the patient lives or not, that's irrelevant. It's not part of the standard of care." And my response to the Medical Board was, "I haven't done a damn thing in my life standard and I'm not about to start now." But that kind of shows you the thought process.

And here's a testament to the universal consciousness and how people are evolving now, Ty. During that three and a half year period, I publicly stated that if I am guilty of even 0.01 percent of what the Medical Board has accused me of, it is their fiduciary and ethical responsibility to remove my license immediately because I'm a threat to the public. Then remove my license. Of course, they couldn't because they knew that they would've stepped into another bigger can of worms.

Ty: Right.

Dr. Buttar: Right? Because now they're violating constitutional—I was trying to get them to do something that would really be egregious but, they're not very smart, but they had some intelligence there.

But what was really interesting to me was the response of the public. Even though it was all over the Internet—and that's how patients were finding us—I probably had 35 to 40 new patients over that three and a half year period. And there was no obligation on my part, but I felt that it was necessary to let these new patients that were coming to me that had cancer—and you've got to remember, financially, we were being devastated. I had 29 employees, we were down to 14, we couldn't afford to pay them. I lost my office. All this stuff is going on over a three and a half year period.

But I felt that I should let them know that I've been brought up on these charges just so that they're fully aware. And do you know what the response was? Every single patient, except for one, had already known about it. And the one that didn't know about it, he said he didn't care. He said, "I don't listen to anything that the government says to me. Anything they say, I do the opposite." But every single patient—this is what was amazing to me—every single patient said to me the reason they came to me was because of what they read on the Internet and all the attacks.

And I was surprised by that the first couple of times, but they said that anybody who gets attacked like that, they must be doing something right. That's what the patients said. Because they said, "We've heard of doctors cutting off the wrong legs, leaving instruments in patients. You never hear about it. You can't find anything about them." But they've been sued and this and that. They said, "But here you are, you've never had a lawsuit from a medical malpractice case or anything and they're coming after you so hard. So we felt that you must be doing something right." Meaning, that it actually built my practice.

And I told the Medical Board that during one of the depositions and they hated that. I said, "By the way, I wanted to thank you for increasing our pull because, before this all started, I had patients from 30-something countries and now we have patients from 80"—at that time, it was like 60-something countries and now it's 84 countries. But they did not like that.

Ty: I bet they didn't. So that really helped. I mean, you've heard the old adage that there's no publicity that's bad publicity. I guess, in certain situations, there probably are like this Farid Fata thing.

Dr. Buttar: Right.

Ty: But for you, people could see through that.

Dr. Buttar: Well, I don't know whether everybody saw through it, but the ones that did—it reminds me of a quote that I have in my book from Confucius, I believe it was. He said, "For those people who understand, no explanation is necessary. For those people who don't understand, no explanation is possible."

Ty: Wouldn't work anyway. One more thing on topic—this medical tyranny topic or whatever we're talking about here, whatever you want to classify it—we interviewed earlier this week, a couple of days ago, a young lady from Connecticut who flew down and we interviewed her. She was 17 and diagnosed with Hodgkin's lymphoma. Cassandra from Connecticut.

Dr. Buttar: Yes.

Ty: And they took her, strapped her to a gurney, and forced chemotherapy on her. And the whole time, she was telling us in the interview, "I do not consent to this. I do not consent. I do not consent." And they put her under five months of chemo and, each day, she did not consent. She had been taken from her home, couldn't see Mom, couldn't talk to Mom or anything, sitting in a hospital room with an armed guard at the door. What's going on?

Dr. Buttar: Well, I would like to know, how is that any different from Nazi Germany when people were put into concentration camps and experimented on or forced to do certain things? I don't know what the difference is because we live in the United States—the land of the free, the home of the brave—so that makes a difference.

I mean, it's amazing to me that the entire population of the United States doesn't know about this. I mean, the reason they don't know about it is because it's shushed up by the media. Nobody wants to talk about it. But this is no different than what was done in Germany or when people are basically raped and pillaged.

To me, that's the same thing. It's probably more violent than rape because this is going to kill her eventually. It's going to reduce her immune system. It's going to have consequences down the stream from her life that she'll never be the same.

Ty: Yeah.

Dr. Buttar: I mean, to me, if somebody comes to me—if somebody pulls a gun on me and somebody tries to give me chemotherapy, pulling the gun is a safer option. And I'm not exaggerating. I'm not trying to be facetious here because at least with the gun, you've got a chance. They may miss you, you can disarm them, whatever.

With chemo, they are poisoning your essence. There is nothing left there. They're annihilating your immune system. They're getting rid of every natural God-given defense that your body was created with, what the master engineer created us with, and they are removing it. They are annihilating it. They are demolishing it. It's devastating to the system.

Ty: Yeah, I was speechless during the interview a few times. The things that she shared with us, it's just such a travesty. I mean, it's horrific what they did to her. But I can only imagine if that was one of my kids. I mean, I think the animal in me would want to come out at that point.

Dr. Buttar: I don't know how the animal in any parent could be restrained.

Ty: Yeah, it's horrible. And the thing was, they took her from her home when she was by herself. The cops surrounded her house, took her from her home by herself. She was hiding in a closet. And then they took her, did a couple of rounds of chemo on her, she ran away. And then they got in touch with her and somehow they found out where she was staying and they said, "If you don't come back, we're going to arrest your mother." And so then she went back and that's when she said, "I don't want chemo." And that's when, she said there's 12 people in the room to hold her down.

Dr. Buttar: So the criminal act here—because obviously the cops wouldn't have done this on their own.

Ty: It was the Child Protective Services.

Dr. Buttar: That's right. That's where the criminal act starts. And you and I have talked about this before. On the radio show, we talked about this once too. Because somebody at some point should have filed a lawsuit against the Child Protection Services and they didn't. And when we were talking about this—you remember we talked about this—about the mentality of a victim.

And when you were telling me this, I got very aggravated. I didn't get aggravated at Child Protection Services, I got aggravated with the parents and with the family, if you remember, because those that are swayed by honeyed words—this is a Supreme Court Justice. I think it's the Supreme Court Justice Aguilar who was quoted as saying that, "Those who are not belligerent and insist upon their rights, those that are swayed by honeyed words, give up their right for freedom."

And I think that that is a very important thing for people to remember. In fact, I think he goes on to say something about unless you defend your rights, your freedoms, through sustained combat and belligerent actions, you've basically given up your rights. And so I think that it's important for everybody to not be passive, not be a sheep. You have to stand up and say, like this girl was saying, she's 17, she's a minor. They're threatening her, they threatened her parents, and she's saying, "I don't consent to this. I don't want to get chemo." Somebody should have immediately done an injunction on some level.

I mean, I'm not a lawyer, but my point is they have emergency hearings and this and that, but obviously nobody did. They were too paralyzed like a victim, like a prey, the deer in the headlights type of thing. And people have to remember that you have to stand up for yourself. You cannot take that victim mentality because as soon as you become the victim, as soon as you take on that personality, as soon as you take on that persona, it will feed the predator. You have to punch that. It's like a bully. You've got to punch him in the face.

I'm not saying go around and punch everybody in the face. I'm saying if somebody steps on your foot, give them a chance to back off, but if they don't back off and you let them continue stepping on your foot, then how is that different from deserving that type of behavior? You need to punish that behavior. You need to reward desired behavior and you need to make sure the person that has infringed upon your child's life has to pay some kind of consequences.

I mean, for me, I can tell you, if somebody threatened my child like that, I would pull a gun. I would not hesitate and I would put a round in between their eyes. And if I was brought up in court and I was in front of a judge and I didn't get the person, I'd tell the judge, "You better put me in jail because if I get out, I'm going to kill that son of a bitch, whoever tried to hurt my child." I mean, there's no qualms about it. I'm defending my child. This is what our Constitution was based on—the right for life, liberty, and pursuit of happiness. This is life. This is the very first thing our founding fathers said.

If we don't defend our own life and our own child's life, then what the hell is the point of this whole thing, this thing that we call life?

Ty: Right.

Dr. Buttar: You have to defend life. It's part of the natural selection process. An animal is going to try to defend its own young. And if you allow your child to be taken by Child Protection or through—I'm not saying that what happened to them was a good thing. You understand that.

Ty: Sure.

Dr. Buttar: But I'm more aggravated that they would allow something like that to happen. Would you allow that to happen to your family?

Ty: No.

Dr. Buttar: I mean, would anybody? The camera people, would you guys allow that to happen to your family? So how can somebody stand back? This whole victim mentality, it takes your power away. You're letting your power go away. You can't do that. You've got to stand up.

Ty: Yeah, I agree because if we don't stand up for our rights, we lose them.

Dr. Buttar: That's exactly right.

Ty: Yeah.

Dr. Buttar: And the last thing I said to the Medical Board after the conclusion of this whole hearing—it was all kangaroo court. I told my attorney I want to say something. My attorney said, "No, this isn't the right time." And it didn't matter. They basically said they were going to fine me $250,000, I was going to have my license removed, blah-blah-blah—all this stuff that they said. And I stood up—and my attorney just put his head in his hand—and I told them that when people allow a government to dictate the foods they put in their mouth and the medicines to take into their bodies, their souls will soon be in the same sorry state as those who are ruled by tyranny. And as much as I would like to take credit for that phrase, that was uttered by Thomas Jefferson over 250 years ago.

Ty: Yeah.

Dr. Buttar: And I'm looking at the Medical Board saying this, "I only promise you one thing—that I will expose your witch hunt for what it is." Three and a half years, what I went through, it's not a big deal. To me, it's not a big deal. To me, it was no more different than sustained combat. But what they were doing was that they were signing the death certificates of these patients that had come to me.

At one point, it was only one day out of the three and a half years, my attorney, my second attorney, my dad who's a criminal attorney—they all were trying to tell me that I should go ahead and agree to a consent order. And the consent order was basically I would stop seeing cancer patients and they would drop all the charges. And they said that was a good offer. And in my heart, that's the only night that I did not sleep at all.

I couldn't sleep because all my advisors are telling me this and I said I can't do that. I asked the Medical Board—I mean, I'd be lying if I said I didn't entertain it, but I entertained it for about 15 seconds—and the question I asked them was, "What about my existing cancer patients, the ones that I see every year, two years, that are fully treated?" They told me I couldn't see those patients either. And my response was, "Then you need to bury me with them because I'm not going—you can kiss my blah-blah-blah."

I mean, my attorney now says to me the Medical Board sent me a number of letters since then about this, that, and the other and I tell them, "Look. Do whatever you've got to do and I'm going to do whatever I'm going to do." But I was told that I was like the porcupine or the skunk or whatever that they bit into and it was such a bad stench for them that they wouldn't deal with it. They could find better and easier prey somewhere else.

But the point is that if they had won—I mean, you could do anything to me, fine. But my family, my patients—if they had won, people would've died. The people that are alive today, and in fact, some of the patients that you're going to be interviewing, some of the newer ones just since the last year or two, stage 4 cancer patients, multiple cancers—not just metastasis, but two primaries that have been picked up—you're going to talk to these patients. Those patients today would be dead. I'm not saying that I saved them. I think God's the only healer. I mean, you and I both know that.

Ty: Yeah.

Dr. Buttar: But my point is that they would not have been able to get the treatment that we provided. I mean, certain things that we do, nobody else does them. But my point is that that was, to me, it wasn't like, "Do I give this up or do I not give this up?" People were saying, "Look. You built this office. You're losing the revenue. You're losing employees. You're losing your clinic that you built. You're losing all this stuff. Just sign it and be done with it." But at what price?

Ty: Right.

Dr. Buttar: The price was—even if it was one person's life—and this was multiple people's lives and all the patients coming in the future. So to me, it was like, "Okay, if I'm going to die"—and I honestly thought that this was going to be the end of it, but I was going to try to take as much as I could. I wasn't going to let them go easy.

Ty: Yeah.

Dr. Buttar: And with the grace of God, I guess I was still supposed to continue to practice unrestricted, which I am still.

Ty: You're still doing it, yeah. Talk about the protocol that these patients use to get well. You mentioned some of these unique things that you use in your practice. Talk about your cancer treatment protocol for those who are watching.

Dr. Buttar: Well, I'm probably a little bit jaded compared to most of the people you've talked to because I've gone through things that you hear about the aftermath and then those people are—I guess you know that there have been a couple of doctors that do similar things or try to do similar things. Some of them actually have come through my training program—three just in the last few weeks that have been killed under mysterious circumstances—and I'm not so worried about that part of it. I'm more sensitive, I guess you can say, to painting a target on my chest. And the one thing that nobody can—if I say that X, Y, and Z will help a patient with cancer or will cure their cancer, you understand that I am not protected by the First Amendment – Freedom of Speech. You are because you're not a doctor but, doctors, you have no rights.

Ty: Let me rephrase the question.

Dr. Buttar: Okay.

Ty: What protocol do you use to make the patients' bodies healthier so that their bodies can fight disease?

Dr. Buttar: That's good. The question, the way it's stated, can make a big difference. Well, I'm going to talk about it from a philosophical standpoint rather than specifics because it can attack a philosophy.

We have a five step program which has been evolving since 1997, so almost 20 years, 18 years right now. My first cancer patient that I saw, and from that point onwards, the evolutionary process has basically continued, but the five steps—it started off as three, then went to four, then five. But the five steps, I will outline.

The first is systemic detoxification. You have to clean up the body. If you don't detoxify the body, then there are too many things in the way for the body to function correctly and most of these toxicities are causing a detrimental effect in the body like increasing oxidative stress, etc., etc.

So what we know as poisons is different mechanisms of how these poisons affect the body. I know you're familiar with the 7 toxicities—my whole philosophy that I have all the different toxicities. And it goes from the heavy metals, the persistent organic pollutants, the opportunistics—that's the bacteria, viruses, spirochetes, mycoplasma, yeast. The fourth one is energetics like electromagnetic radiation, microwave energies, this, that, and the other—ambient cell phone radiation's a big one.

The fifth one is the most important, in my opinion, and that's the emotional psychological toxicity. The sixth one is foods—not what we're consuming because that falls into the first and second, middle, and persistent organic pollutant toxicity—but the sixth one is foods, what we do to the foods—which I know is near and dear to your heart. The irradiation, the homogenization, the pasteurization, the genetic modification of foods. All these things that we do to food and change the basic molecular structure of the things that we're taking into our body to sustain ourselves. These are severely, severely detrimental to the body, and the seventh toxicity is spiritual. So these toxicities that I'm talking about—that's the first step. We deal with all those things.

The second step is physiological optimization. What I mean by that, the best way of thinking about it—if you have two people and one has shortness of breath when he walks down the steps or up the steps and the other one runs three miles every day. Well, the one that's running three miles every day is more physiologically optimized. So I want to optimize a person so their bodies are functioning at the highest level.

And when you're dealing with cancer, the way you deal with that—and I'm not saying the people have to run although I have cancer patients, and one of them that you're going to talk to, does run three miles every other day and she's stage 4 with multiple metastatic disease. But the proudest thing that I am offering for her—if you see my patients, none of them look like they have cancer. That's the thing that…

Ty: That's a big thing.

Dr. Buttar: Yeah. That's the best way of being able to look at a patient.

Ty: Because that means they're not in cachexia cycle.

Dr. Buttar: Absolutely.

Ty: Yeah.

Dr. Buttar: So there's an old saying, "Where growth stops, decay steps in." And so, to me, this is not a static process. Either you're getting worse or you're getting better. There's no such thing as staying right there in the middle. So physiological optimization, when you're dealing with a cancer patient would be, for example, the use of oxygen. Oxygen is highly detrimental to cancer because cancer is an obligate anaerobic metabolizer. It likes an oxygen-free environment. So if you give oxygen, it's detrimental to the cancer.

Cancer is an obligate glucose metabolizer so it needs sugar to sustain itself. The brain needs sugar, the body needs sugar, but we reduce the amount of glucose that's coming to the body so that there's less fuel for the cancer.

So these are the types of techniques—and there's many different ways of doing this and we have some very evolved ways of dealing with that.

Ty: You don't have a candy jar in the office like most oncologists do?

Dr. Buttar: No. No, I don't. And if we did, it would be like something that would be a multivitamin type.

Ty: Okay.

Dr. Buttar: In fact, we're developing a gummy right now that's a multivitamin antioxidant so that would be my idea of a candy. But, yeah, it's amazing when you look at the standard oncology practices. When a person is becoming cachectic, they recommend Ensure. Are you familiar with Ensure?

Ty: Sugar.

Dr. Buttar: Yeah.

Ty: Sugar and cream.

Dr. Buttar: That's exactly right. Now, during my surgical residencies, I can tell you that Ensure was a precious commodity. Surgical residency, we'd go through the different wards and open up the refrigerators and find the Ensure and drink it because it is very tasty, I'm not going to deny that. But for a cancer patient, it's poison. It's literally poison. It is like pouring gasoline on a fire. It is like feeding that fire of cancer. So the first step—I'm trying to come back on point. Did you like that? I came back on point.

Ty: That was good.

Dr. Buttar: Yeah.

Ty: I'm surprised.

Dr. Buttar: Exactly. The first one is the systemic detoxification. The second one is the physiological optimization. And most doctors that are doing cancer treatments that are non-conventional, they're doing some of that in some way, fashion, or form. And everybody has a different way of doing it. People have refined some of those things. What distinguishes us, and I think this is one of the things that you were asking me just now is, What makes it different?

Ty: Yeah.

Dr. Buttar: It's probably the third and the fourth step and possibly even the fifth step. The third step is immune modulation. Now, immune modulation is an important component. Do you notice that I didn't say increasing the immune system or decreasing the immune system? I said modulating the immune system because each patient is going to be different.

Generally speaking, a person that has cancer has a suppressed immune system. Their immune system has been damaged and it's lower so we want to repair that immune system, we want to get it back up.

Now, a very fundamental component—I'm not talking about the research of what's going on right now. The newest therapy in cancer treatment is immune therapy. That's what they talked about.

Ty: Sure.

Dr. Buttar: And I had one of my patients ask me about two months ago, she had just been accepted into this new trial for immune therapy, and she's a patient of mine. She's been a patient for probably, I don't know, four or five years and she still keeps on getting these calls and she tells the doctor she has no interest in that, but she asked me, "Dr. Buttar, they're talking about this new immune therapy so how is that different than what you're doing?" I said, "Besides the fact that we've been doing it for 18 years or…?" She said, "Well, yes, besides the fact that—are they trying to make this like you're doing?"

And our way of modulating the immune system is different and I'll explain that here in a general standpoint. But they're just recognizing now that the immune system is important in cancer. I have had patients tell me that they've shown their doctors the natural killer cell profile that we do before and after, the lymphocyte cell population that we do before and after to measure our results, to see where the patient is at, how much further improved have we been able to help the immune system get to.

Ty: Yeah.

Dr. Buttar: And I've had patients tell me, including this particular patient, tell me that when they showed their oncologist this paperwork, these lab tests, the response that they got from more than half the doctors was—some of them said they didn't know what that meant or didn't know how to interpret it, but more than half of them said, "What relevance is this? What's the natural killer cells got to do with cancer?" For god's sake, that's why they're called natural killer cells because they naturally kill things that are not supposed to be in the body like cancer. So it's a really severe disconnect that the conventional side has.

And when I say conventional, there is only one medical science. It's just that you've got these different groups and some are open to innovation and some are not. So I consider myself in the category that are open to innovation and then the ones that are not, they're just too vested in the status quo, too ingrained in it, the way it is right now. So the modulation of the immune system is key because you cannot have cancer if you have an adequate and functioning immune system.

If you don't have a functioning immune system now, you can get cancer. But there is no such thing as, "Oh, my cancer has nothing to do with my immune system because my immune system's fine." There's no such thing. If you have cancer, you don't have an immune system. Your immune system's been damaged. That's it. So our focus is to get that immune system back up. And we do that through various techniques, things that we've developed ourselves. There's various immune modulating peptides and such that we use to stimulate.

Now, once the immune system is up—and we've got great results from 1997 till like 2000, 2001 time-frame—but there were still some patients that weren't responding the way we wanted them to respond or the way we expected them to respond. And I started realizing that there are certain commonalities in cancer and fetuses. When a woman is pregnant with a baby and a cancer, there are some similarities. The first initial response is probably, "How can you say there are similarities?" Well, a baby is uncontrolled cellular proliferation. Right? It's rapidly growing.

And to make my case even stronger, there are non-specific markers of cancer—alpha-fetoprotein and human chorionic gonadotropin. Alpha-fetoprotein is also used in pregnancy when they do amniocentesis to see if there's any type of genetic anomaly that the baby may have and human chorionic gonadotropin, the other non-specific mark of cancer, is also known as the pregnancy test.

Ty: HCG. I mean, everybody knows HCG.

Dr. Buttar: Yeah. When we do a pregnancy test—urine or blood pregnancy test—that's what we monitor, is HCG so these are non-specific markers of cancer. And our goal in this fourth step is target acquisition that we want to acquiesce the target. We want the body to identify the cancer as being formed because right now the cancer is mimicking a fetus and saying, "Hey, hey, I'm supposed to be here and that's why you see cancer secreting alpha-fetoprotein and human chorionic gonadotropin. Even though it may be a male, it doesn't matter because it's trying to show the body that, "I'm okay. You don't have to be worried about me. I'm supposed to be here."

So we want the body to identify the cancer as being foreign and the way we do that is through AARSOTA and that stands for autogenous antigen receptor specific oncogenic target acquisition. I can say that I don't care about whether the Medical Board hears me or not because when I signed that consent order, which by the way, all I did was I got a reprimand.

This is how the final case settled. Again, loose association—I'm diverting off topic, but I got a reprimand for a staff member dispensing a prescriptive item, which by the way, I developed and I testified in front of the US Congress for—the DMPS—across state lines for a child with appropriate lab work, but without a provider seeing the child. Not to mention the child was already on a similar type of thing, but not our version, and everything else was done right. But because a staff member sent it out without a prescription, I got the reprimand because they were working under my license. That was the whole thing after a three and a half year battle, by the way.

So this fourth step is to acquiesce the target, meaning having the body identify the cancer and being able to do what it needs to do to follow the way that the ultimate engineer designed our bodies. Our bodies were designed that when the body's immune system identifies cancer, it starts doing what it's supposed to do. But because the immune system first is defunct and not functioning, you can't do that, so we fixed that with the third step, which is immune modulation. And then with the fourth step, now the immune system may be strong and capable to fight, but it doesn't know what it's supposed to fight. It doesn't know who the enemy is.

So that fourth step, AARSOTA, is designed to allow the individual's immune system to identify the cancer as being foreign. And we actually had that put in the consent order that we signed, AARSOTA, so they cannot come after me for the AARSOTA, but basically, it's a fancy term for creating a vaccine specific to that individual's cancer, but it's not a vaccine. It's allowing the body to identify the cancer as being foreign and when we give those injections, then the person's body starts responding.

Ty: So it doesn't have any mercury or aluminum or…?

Dr. Buttar: No, no, no. We create it ourselves from the patient. We collect certain specimens from the patient and then we go into one of those little baking oven things and we bake the cookie for them and then create them.

Ty: Cool.

Dr. Buttar: It's our little, what do you call it? Easy-Bake Oven. That's what I was trying to say. It takes about three weeks to make one.

Ty: The reason you call it vaccine is because it's injected. But other than that, it has no other similarities to what we think of is a vaccine.

Dr. Buttar: Well, a true vaccine is something where you give the body a little bit of the substance that it's supposed to fight and the body sees that it's being formed and starts fighting it. The vaccines that we are against are not so much the vaccines. I'm not against the principle of vaccination at all. I'm against the stupidity, is what I'm against.

And to give the body a live virus at a time when the body can't even build an immune response—meaning the first six months of life because the immune system hasn't developed yet—along with certain substances that are acting as preservatives that suppress the immune system under the false pretense of building up the immune system. That's just hogwash. There's no validity to it. That's like me saying, "Ty, you need to move that couch and you need to fill up that water because that's going to affect the weather pattern in Congo right now." There's absolutely no correlation to that.

My goal, when I'm talking about a vaccine, is to give the body something where the body sees it as being formed and creates a reaction to the actual offending substance. So it's almost like you give the body a thimble of water because you know that a typhoon is coming down. So that thimble of water allows the body to say, "Ah, a storm is coming" and allows the body to prepare so that when the storm hits, the body is already prepared. That's what a vaccine is supposed to be.

So from the conventional definition of vaccine, actually, no, this has nothing to do with that. But from the philosophical principle of a vaccine, we are basically getting the proteins from the cancer, creating a treatment that is specific to the patient because where does cancer start from? It starts from the DNA, right? That's what's unique about the cancer. So it's specific to that individual's DNA. We give it back to them and the body now sees that as being foreign. And as soon as it sees that as being foreign, it sees anything but the same morphological characteristics as being foreign, and all of a sudden, the whole body lights up. Wherever the cancer is in the body, it lights up because we just introduced it in a way the body can see it as being foreign and "boom," it just snaps to it. That's what we call the shift. That's when a person gets sick because their body's responding.

So all of a sudden, the immune system, the way that God designed the system, now recognizes the substance that's cancer, that shouldn't be there, and the body is fixing the individual. Not me, not chemo, not radiation, not some other pill or vitamin. No, it's the body itself doing what the ultimate engineer created it to do to fight the cancer, to prevent the cancer from being an issue. Everything else we do—the supplements and the IV—that's not for the cancer, that's to support the immune system. That's to clean up the person. That's to get the body strong enough to be able to fight. But the actual mechanism is the body's own innate immune system.

Ty: Got it.

Dr. Buttar: So that's the fourth step. And then the fifth step is arguably the most difficult. That's maintenance, meaning that, once you've crossed that line, you have to live your life a certain way. And I think that probably the sub demographic that would probably understand this the best would be the athletic individuals that are watching this. As an athlete, you know that if you don't continue to work out, you're going to lose it. Right?

Ty: Yeah.

Dr. Buttar: No, I'm not saying anything about you, Ty, specifically.

Ty: I'm laughing because I used to be a competitive bodybuilder.

Dr. Buttar: I know, I know. That's what I'm saying. People like you and I understand this because you can get to a certain point, but if you don't maintain it, if you don't keep up with it—I mean, it's amazing to me. Two days without me doing my push-ups and I'm like, it feels like it's been three years since I did them.

Ty: It doesn't take long.

Dr. Buttar: No. And I think that when people say, "Oh, you're aging," that's a load of rubbish. What does happen when you age is that your ability to repair takes longer and your ability to get to that point of excellent health takes a little bit longer, but the ability to do it, there's no difference. I mean, I competed at the World level last year and the International level in martial arts. I never did that in my 30s. So your body can do things as long as you keep consistent with it.

And so the reason I said I think an athlete will understand that better is because they are more sensitive to that idea of maintenance. People that are not actively and regularly involved with exercise or an athletic program, they're not going to really appreciate it as much. But the maintenance aspect is so crucial—once difficult, now easy. You know if you keep on doing something over and over and over again, it becomes easy, but, originally, it was difficult.

So if there's one piece of advice that I could tell people that are listening to this—exercise. It's free. God gave us all the ability to do it. You don't need fancy equipment. I realized that I had a big hang-up because I had to have weights and this and that so I started eliminating everything. I have not touched a weight in over 10 years.

Ty: You do push-ups?

Dr. Buttar: I do body work. I do leg lifts, lunges. I do sprint on a treadmill or outside, depending on the weather, but it's all body work. And I'm telling you, for anybody that's listening to this, the most crucial thing you can do for yourself, it is absolutely free. People tend to think that if it's free, it's not valuable. Exercise, for god's sake. It's the cheapest and the most effective thing that anybody can do. I mean, tell me I'm wrong.

Ty: I agree. You have to because it not only keeps your musculature in order, but the oxygen that you intake and it gets into your blood system while you're exercising, especially aerobic exercise, you can't get it anywhere else.

Dr. Buttar: Absolutely. You've got the improvement in profusion. Everything starts to flow better so your body's able to eliminate certain things. You're able to get nutrition into certain other areas of your body because the heart's pumping harder. If you could describe cancer in one word—well, not one word, it would be two words—lymphatic stagnation. So when you are actually exercising, you are stimulating that lymphatic. You're getting all the stuff to start flowing.

Ty: What's the lymphatic?

Dr. Buttar: So you've got two types of circulation in the body. You've got typically the blood, which everybody recognizes as the circulation, but then you've got the little known cousin that a lot of people don't recognize and that's the lymphatics. The lymphatics are the lymph nodes and the drainage system in the body that is basically there to remove waste product. So when people get the lymph nodes enlarged and the doctors say, "Oh my god, lymph nodes. We've got to take them out." You're just taking out the oil filters.

Don't ever have your lymph nodes taken out because if a lymph node gets hard when you've got cancer, it means it's doing its job. It's filtering the cancer, it's holding on to that stuff, it's keeping it from disseminating out. You take that filter out, that's like having your car—you've got a filter that's blocked. What do you do? You take out the filter and say, "Okay, now I don't have a problem. Nothing's blocking it." But now you've got all that sludge that was going into the filter before, now going right into the engine. You don't want that to happen. So the lymph node is a part of the lymphatics drainage system.

Ty: Okay.

Dr. Buttar: So that's a very, very important part. So exercise does all that stuff. You're absolutely right. But there's one other thing that exercise does and you were right about the blood flow and the oxygenation and all that other stuff in the musculature, but exercise also breathes energy into you. It's that "chi" that they talk about in Eastern medicine.

Ty: Yeah, because after you finish working out, you feel better than you did before even though you're exhausted.

***Dr. Buttar*:** Exactly, exactly. Even though it's painful. In fact, I'm addicted to the feeling afterwards even though I hate it. To me, if I'm not hurting, I didn't exercise enough.

Ty: It's euphoria afterwards.

Dr. Buttar: Yeah, maybe it's just euphoria because you know that you're done exercising and not hurting anymore. Maybe that's what it is, I don't know, but whatever it is, it is an important aspect. The whole energetic of the body shifts. And exercise is the Creator's gift to us and, by not partaking in something that is available to every single person—I mean, I don't care if somebody says, "Well, I don't have two legs and I can't walk because I had my legs blown up in Afghanistan." "Fine, you can do things with your upper body." In fact, in my book, you remember the story I talked about Dan, the guy who was quadriplegic.

Ty: Yep.

Dr. Buttar: Okay, that's a perfect example. So read that story. If that doesn't motivate you, then maybe it's time for you to go back home where we all came from, where we all want to go because, to me, if that story doesn't motivate you, you're probably already halfway back to the Creator.

Ty: What happened? In two minutes, recap the story.

Dr. Buttar: Quadriplegic, broke his neck in a motorcycle accident, 23, 24-year-old guy in the gym. I meet him, we start talking. This is over a period of months. He couldn't strap the straps of the dumbbells because his feet were so weak so he would have us strap the straps on and he would lift. And he was told he'd never be able to walk. He was told he'd be a quadriplegic, but here he was driving. He could control a car through his mouth and he could move it with his hands. He had like little hooks on his wrist that he could hook in and steer. He'd get out of the car himself, get his wheelchair out—this is a guy that they said would never be able to walk.

And I asked him to come to one of my seminars. This is 15, 20 years ago, just a little community thing. And I was talking about the importance of exercise and this woman stands up and she starts going off on me and saying, "You don't seem to understand the importance of the fact that people have had surgery on their back. Every time I walk, it's painful. And you sitting here preaching about exercise and you don't even take into consideration people like us that can't this and that and the other, blah-blah-blah." And she's just really, really vicious and everybody's like looking at this woman like, Oh my god.

And I'm looking at this woman and I see Dan sitting in the back and I thought this is beautiful. I mean, how beautiful can this be? And I said, "Hey, Dan." And he just put his head down like, oh crap. He knew where this was going. He's shaking his head. I said, "Dan, can you come up here?" And he shakes his head no and I said, "Come on up here." And there are other people that are kind of pushing him so he kind of stands up and he's got his cane and he throws one leg forward and swings his leg around and he drags himself up there.

And I said, "Dan, you want to tell everybody what happened?" And he goes, "No, not really." I said, "Tell them anyway." And he told them, "I was in a motorcycle accident and I became quadriplegic." And I said, "What did the doctors tell you?" And he said, "They told me I'd never be able to walk." And I said, "And what did you say?" He said, "I told them to kiss my blah blah blah." And I said okay and so everybody's laughing.

And I said, "Dan, how did I meet you?" And he's just like—because he knew I was going to ruin this woman's life—I mean, her day, by doing this and he said, "At the gym." And I said, "How did I meet you at the gym?" And he goes, "Because I needed you to strap on my weights on my arms?" And I said, "Why is that? Why did you need me to strap on the weights to your wrists?" He goes, "Because I don't have a grip that I can actually grab the weights." And I said, "So once I strap the weights to your wrist, then what do you do?" He says, "I lift." I said, "Huh."

And so I turn to this woman and I said, "Have you broken your neck that you can't walk…"—and she was like totally red. She didn't know what to do. She just sat down and people were like laughing. And I wasn't trying to make fun of her. That wasn't my goal. My goal was to put her into a state of humility that she'll understand that, "Look, any excuse will do. You don't have to give me an excuse about your back or your this or that. I don't really care. I'm telling you this is what it is. Now if you don't want to do it, then fine. You pay the consequences. You reap the rewards, you pay the consequences, but don't make an excuse. You don't have to come up with an elaborate excuse that I had this surgery and that and my dog ate my homework. I don't care. I'm just telling you this is the answer. You don't want to take it, fine. But don't make BS excuses because here's a person that has 1,000 times more excuses possible and he didn't make an excuse."

Ty: Right.

Dr. Buttar: That's what I was trying to do. And it succeeded.

Ty: Take control, right?

Dr. Buttar: That's right.

Ty: Take control over things you have control over.

Dr. Buttar: Exactly.

Ty: As we say at the end of every radio show, the power to heal is yours.

Dr. Buttar: Absolutely.

Ty: And as Robert Scott Bell says, "Take control over the things where we are given control over."

Dr. Buttar: That's absolutely—in fact, it comes back to the Serenity Prayer. And the Serenity Prayer—I'll talk about that in the sixth—

Ty: We had that on our wall, growing up. I remember my mom had it framed.

Dr. Buttar: Right. And it's important that we say it out loud because I never realized how important it is to say it out loud. In fact, I'm going to put you on the spot. Do you remember?

Ty: It says something like, "God, give me the patience to..."

Dr. Buttar: See, this is the reason why it's so important to say it out loud because even though you grew up with it, we forget. And it's so important. Look at a mirror and say this out loud. Exercise and then say this prayer. "God, please give me the ability to change the things that I can change, the serenity to accept the things that I cannot change, and the wisdom to know the difference."

Ty: To know the difference. I remember that part, yeah.

Dr. Buttar: So say that out loud, whether you have cancer or not. Anybody that's watching this, say it out loud. You, too. I'm going to ask you next week aloud on the radio show.

Ty: I've got to practice.

Dr. Buttar: So you've got to practice. But the thing is, there is power to it when you say it aloud. The words have a lot of power.

Ty: Yeah.

Dr. Buttar: And even though we may not understand it, the subconscious versus the conscious—the conscious processes, 2,000 bits of information per second. So think of it as $2,000 dollars' worth of information per second. The subconscious processes 400 million bits of information per second or $400 million dollars' worth of information per second. So if you have $2,000 worth versus if you have $400 million worth, which is always going to win?

Ty: Yeah.

Dr. Buttar: The subconscious. So the words, when you say them out loud in repetition, your subconscious starts to ingrain it. The subconscious has no opinion, right or left. There's a thing called the RASCOM in your brain, the reticular activating system control mechanism. It's a goal-seeking mechanism. If you give it a direction and a goal, it will start to channel to that goal and eventually you can just program it to do it. So if you can just say that prayer and do exercise 21 days, they say, form a habit. Do it for 28 days. Do it for a month. It'll be a habit and just stay with it. Just those two things is going to make it. Those two things by themselves will probably decrease an individual's chance of getting cancer by 50 percent.

Ty: It reminds me of our high school basketball coach. He used to say, "Practice does not make perfect, but it does make permanent."

Dr. Buttar: Yes, exactly.

Ty: So if you're doing it, it becomes a permanent part of you.

Dr. Buttar: That's absolutely right. In fact, in our martial arts forms, that's one of the things that our master would have us do. There's certain motions, you just keep on doing it even though it may be like a 85-part kata, the thing is it's difficult to remember those things unless you keep on doing a repetition.

And I know that if I think about it, you get locked in, especially when you've got judges in the national or international competition. You freeze. And I always am not thinking of anything with martial arts. I'm always thinking of my kids or on a date with my wife while I'm doing it in front of the judges because my body takes over. It's just repetition. My body knows what it's supposed to do. I don't have to think about it. So as soon as I think, I get locked up, "But wait a sec."

Get rid of the mind. The mind is the cortical monkey. It's on top. Have you noticed that you can do something really, really smoothly and then as soon as somebody tells you to do it and you consciously come to it, you get frayed and you don't do it as well?

Ty: Yep. Same principle with basketball—shooting free throws.

Dr. Buttar: Exactly. Automatic.

Ty: You do it the same every time. And my son, Bryce, he gets kind of freaked out because we'll go out and shoot and I'll close my eyes and I'll still swish them.

Dr. Buttar: Yeah.

Ty: Because I've done it 100,000 times. It's part of you. You can see it without looking.

Dr. Buttar: Exactly, because your brain doesn't need any—you're on automatic. It's like, Do you think about breathing? Do you think about walking? Do you think about your heart beating? No. It's all subconscious.

Ty: Yeah.

Dr. Buttar: The subconscious part of the brain is taking over. And so that's one of the things you want to do. You want to incorporate and harness the power of that subconscious and so exercising that prayer and some of these other components that you can do to make it part and parcel of your habit in your body so your body doesn't know any different—that's the key.

Ty: And remember that if you're diagnosed with cancer and your oncologist tells you it's terminal, don't believe him. There's always hope. There's people like you that know how to treat it.

Dr. Buttar: Ty, let's forget about people like me. Let's forget about hope. Let's forget about everything like that. Just forget about the series. Let's say that you and I don't exist. Let's say there's no doctors out there that treat cancer the way we believe exists. Why would you give power to a person that doesn't know you that's telling you that you need poison or burning to get rid of something in your body? Why are you going to give them the power by believing them?

There's no reason to give your power away. And trust me, a doctor will say you have 6 months to live. Now, let's look at the market, the stock market. It can go up, it can go down, or it can stay the same. Can they predict that? If they can't predict up, down, or staying the same, then how the hell are they going to predict when a person's going to die? And if a person believes the doctor, then they're more foolish than the doctor for believing them.

Ty: Yes.

Dr. Buttar: You should never believe anybody that tells you anything that takes away your power because by doing that, you have just become a victim. You have just become the prey. You have just done what I told you aggravates me when the family didn't do something to protect their daughter. They just stood back like a deer in the headlights. Or maybe they did try to do something, maybe they didn't have resources, I don't know. But the point is, no matter what it is, you've got to do something so don't give up your power when some doctor says, "Oh, you've got this problem, you've got that problem." Whatever the problem is, that's his opinion. That's why they call that concept of second opinion and third opinion.

Think of Dan. Think of all these other patients that were told that they're going to die. I mean, the patients that you've interviewed like Chris. You remember Chris from the last series, I think it was? I mean, he went to Mayo Clinic. They told him that he had a year left. Then he went to Cleveland Clinic or maybe he went to Cleveland Clinic first and then Mayo Clinic—both are very, very well established, well reputed cancer centers and both of them said between nine months and a year, they want to take his leg off. He had melanoma end-stage blah-blah-blah, whatever it was

Ty: And what's it? Years later?

Dr. Buttar: I think he's six years out now.

Ty: Six years, okay.

Dr. Buttar: And there's no trace of cancer. He brought his sister to me who actually ended up having a cancer that we just took care of and his sister's actually working in the clinic now.

Ty: Really?

Dr. Buttar: Yeah.

Ty: Cool. Great guy, isn't he?

Dr. Buttar: Chris is a great guy. But many of these patients, the point that I'm making is, let's put the treatment aside. Just that thought process—do not become a victim. You talked about the power, right? You gain power through knowledge. You empower yourself and as soon as you empower yourself with knowledge, you are now at a better place so that you can't become that victim. That's the first step. And then don't give away your power.

Ty: Right.

Dr. Buttar: If you want to give away your power, give your power to somebody that needs more power, that needs help, because that gives you more power back. But if you give your power away to somebody by listening to whatever garbage they're going to spew, that's not good.

Ty: Right. So we'll conclude the interview with this. For our good friend, Robert Scott Bell, what do we need to remember?

Dr. Buttar: The power to heal is yours.

Ty: The power to heal is yours. Absolutely. Thanks, man. Appreciate it.

[end of transcript]

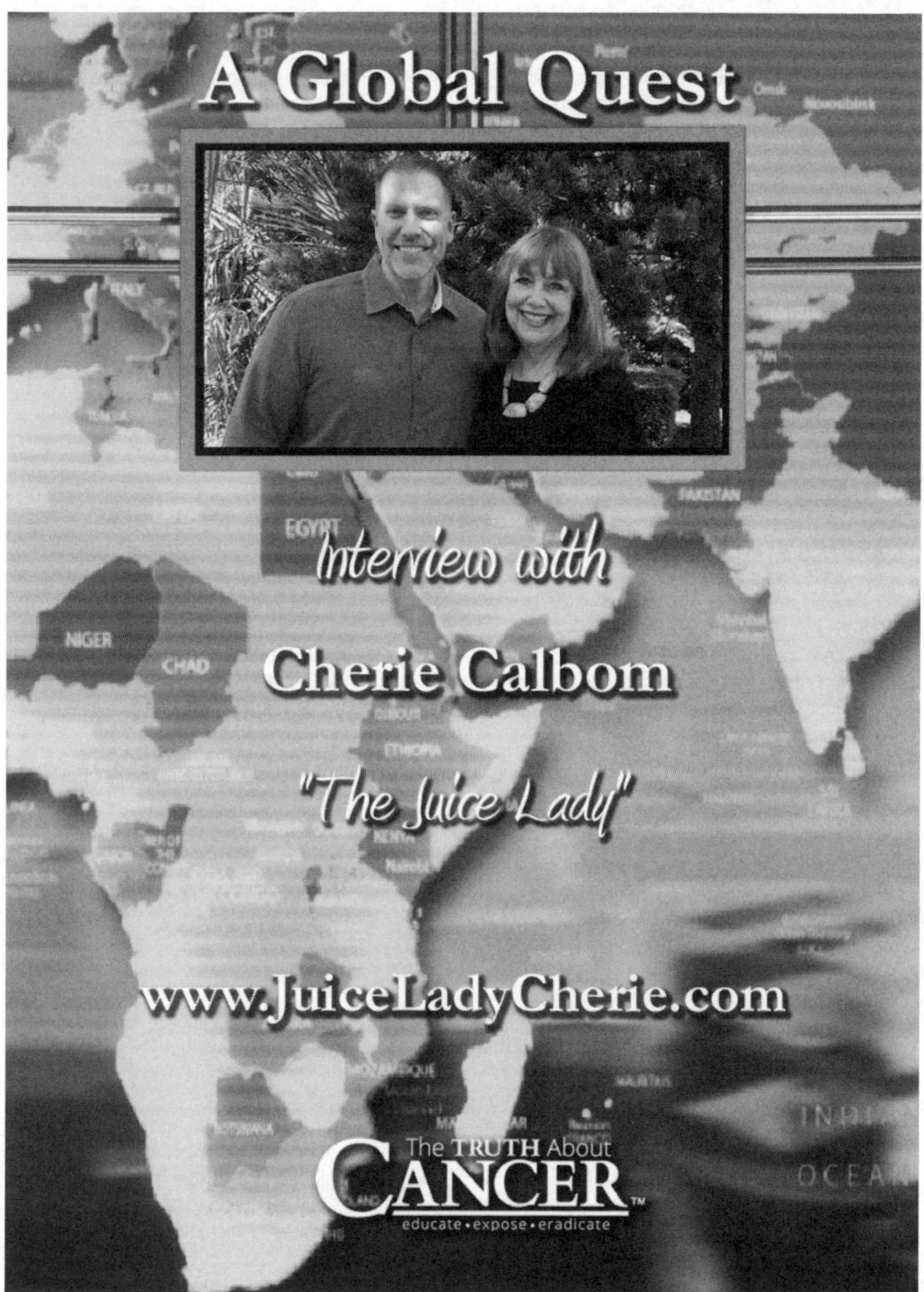
A Global Quest
Interview with
Cherie Calbom
"The Juice Lady"
www.JuiceLadyCherie.com
The TRUTH About CANCER
educate • expose • eradicate

Ty: Really excited to be here in Seattle, Washington with Cherie Calbom. The juice lady?

Cherie: Hi. Yes.

Ty: Three years ago we met in Atlanta, we spoke at a conference together. Really impressed with your knowledge of nutrition at that point. And I thought this would be a great addition to the quest on this cancer topic, to get your perspective on nutrition and cancer. And it only fits since you did do your Master's thesis on it, I just learned, right?

Cherie: I did. Nutrition cancer was my thesis at Baxter University two decades ago. And I've had such an interest ever since in helping people to know what to eat and drink when they have cancer because it is imperative to change one's diet.

What gets us sick, we want to get rid of. What's going to get us well is what we want to incorporate. So that's what my thesis was all about.

Ty: Well, what gets us sick is sometimes a really, really poor diet, right?

Cherie: Yes.

Ty: But we don't learn that from our doctors often times do we?

Cherie: No. And I've talked through the years to so many people who were told by their doctor, "it doesn't matter what you eat when you have cancer, when you're going through chemo it doesn't matter what you eat. Just get something that you can keep down."

That couldn't be further from the truth because what we know and what I know from all of my research is that we must get sugar out of our body. All the studies by Otto Warburg and cancer surviving on sugar, glycolytic fermentation, so we need to get the sugars out of our diet. But it goes way beyond that, way beyond just a sugar detox.

It goes to superior nutrition. Just flooding the body with all those wonderful nutrients to begin to feed our cells and bring them to life. That is what we want to bring into our bodies, live food.

Ty: And so one of the ways we do that is through juicing.

Cherie: That's why I am known as the Juice Lady.

Ty: So talk about juicing.

Cherie: Juicing is my passion because we take these beautiful fruits and vegetables, mostly vegetables is what I recommend, maybe just a little fruit for the flavor.

Ty: I apologize, because all I have here for props is a little bit of fruit.

Cherie: But imagine there are beautiful leafy greens here and maybe some carrots and cucumbers and celery and some ginger and a little lemon. That's what I have for breakfast almost every day. So you juice all that up. You've got everything broken down so well that your body can begin to absorb it right away. So everybody is into fiber, fiber, fiber, "oh you've got to have all this fiber in your juice."

But actually when it comes to juice as a supplement, like a liquid vitamin, mineral, enzyme, biophoton, phytonutrient glass of wonderful nutrients, it's even better when it doesn't have the fiber in there. The soluble yes, it's got soluble fiber, but not the insoluble because it's going to go right into your system.

It's guesstimated that it's at work in your system about twenty or thirty minutes. And that's bringing that life right into your body, all those anti-oxidants that are binding up toxins and carrying them out of the body. And when we're sick with cancer it's even more important to do these kinds of things to heal the body. Because as I see it, two primary reasons that people get sick, one is toxicity and number two is that we are undernourished in this country. People are not getting the vital nutrients that their bodies need. I just rattled all of those off really fast including biophotons and phytonutrients.

But we need all of these for all of the different reactions that our body has to do each day. If we don't have those, things are not going to happen. Repairs are not going to happen, cleansing isn't going to happen. So we must have them. So again back to the juice, broken down you can get a big concentrate of nutrients. A great big bowl that would take you maybe hours to eat, you can juice it all up pretty fast. It goes right into your system.

Ty: And it's so good, it's so good.

Cherie: It's delicious.

Ty: I mean before I left on this trip here to travel to Seattle I had juiced a couple of days before. We had apples, and beets, and carrots, and celery, and all the things that you just mentioned. And it is so good when it goes down. You can taste the goodness, right?

Cherie: You taste it and you feel it. You know within about twenty or thirty minutes after I have a big glass of juice—that's how I start my day and my husband's. People ask him if he juices, he says, "yeah, I reach out my hand and she puts it in there."

But you feel it. I feel life coming into my body. It's like, I might wake up a little tired, I drink my big glass of juice and in about thirty minutes I think, "ha I'm feeling a lot better. I've got a lot more energy." So it's energizing, it's healing, it's rejuvenating. It begins to bring that life into the body that people so desperately need. And if you're sick, you need that life more than at any other time or any other person. If you're ill you really need that life in your body.

Ty: Yes, especially if you have cancer. You have cancer because your body is sick. Cancer is the result of an already sick body so in order to get it well you need to give it that nutrition.

And when she says that it gives you energy we're not talking about the energy that you get from these temporary drinks in the stores that can give you heart attacks and whatever else. We're talking about energy that your body really can use. Not a quick fix.

Cherie: Not a quick fix. This is sustaining energy. It can keep you throughout the morning. Oftentimes I have this big glass of juice, and then I make a green smoothie with some of my juice. I do big batches of juice. I pour some in my Vitamix, add some chopped up greens to that and some supplements and avocado and then I eat a green smoothie. I say eat because it's thick and I put it in a bowl. Those are the two things I have in the morning and I'm not hungry. It's very sustaining, it's energizing. But it's a sustaining energy just like you mentioned. It isn't a spike up and then a big dip down like coffee would do or sugar would do.

Ty: I'm glad you mentioned that because that's something that, a lot of time when I'm talking to people about juicing they'll say, "I couldn't live on just juice." But you're not saying just juice. One of the things that people will say is that, "I'd be hungry if I just drank [juice]."

They don't realize that all the nutrition is what your body is searching for and when you juice you're getting it and you actually are satisfied. Whereas if you go up to the fast food joint down the street and you eat two thousand calories of empty food with no nutrition you're going to be hungry soon because your body didn't get nourished.

Talk about the difference between fake food and real food as far as nourishing your body.

Cherie: Fake food is where our country's at today. So much fake food and people are eating, and eating, and eating it. And gaining more and more weight and still hungry. And often people will say to me, "I'm hungry, like maybe a couple hours after dinner I want something more." So they have a bowl of ice cream or a couple of cookies or something. Your body is not needing that by any means. But people are very hungry in this nation. Overfed, as we say, and under nourished.

When it comes to juice it's just the opposite. We don't have a lot of calories but we have a huge amount of nutrients. It's very nutrient dense, and so people are getting a powerhouse of nutrients that are sustaining for the body.

I have a great story to tell of a lady who came to our juice and raw foods retreat, who had been through chemo and it had burned her esophagus. And really the whole pipe from top to bottom was very irritated. She had to use a feeding tube. She was very concerned about coming to our juice and raw foods retreat as to how this was going to work with the feeding tube and would she lose more weight. I'm going to make the story really short. She was able to start right with dinner. The juice cocktail that we served the first night had everything. She never had to use the feeding tube once and gained two pounds when everybody else was losing.

You know what I say? Your body is going to do what it's supposed to do when you give it the right nutrients. If you are really thin and really need to put on some weight, you start giving it the fresh juice and it's going to help your cells start communicating and your body is going to start doing what it's supposed to do.

And if you need to gain a pound or two you probably will. Just like she reported to me at the end of the week she felt like a brand new person and had put on two pounds. Everybody else had lost five to ten pounds.

Ty: Right. One of the things that you had mentioned about this is it's a lot of nutrition that's lower calories. It reminds me of something KC Craichy had said last year. He said the key to super health is super food nutrition, juice is definitely super food, coupled with calorie restriction. And throw those two together and all the studies show that those are the healthiest people. People who get the massive amount of nutrients with lower calories. And they've shown that in people, and they've also shown that in a lot of rat studies. Because we actually are the guinea pigs and a lot of times we don't know it.

Cherie: We're the lab rats, the big ones.

Ty: We are the lab rats. They've show in a lot of mouse studies, they've done different groups of mice with a lot of calories and no food value. And then they've done all the way down the line to the rats that got very low calories but a lot of nutrition. They always live four or five times as long.

Cherie: Yes, and that's what they've studied with people that are getting less calories and more nutrition, they live longer. And it's not just about living a long time. People say that to me, "I don't care how long I live." But one thing we do all care about is the days that we have here.

We want them to be good. We want to feel good. We don't want to feel sick. We want to have energy. We want to have a clear mind. And I've seen all of that happen for people who started juicing. They'll say that brain fog is starting to go away. And if you end up with chemo brain, which is that brain fog, I know nothing better than to get started on the vegetable juices.

Here's the thing too that I just want to clarify, that a lot of doctors would say, "don't juice because you don't want all that sugar." Well, they're talking about fruit juice. And just fruit juice, that is a lot of sugar and that's not what I recommend. I recommend all the beautiful vegetables, lovely greens, and maybe just a little fruit to sweeten and flavor like some apple in there, organic produce for sure. That isn't a lot of sugar, is it? It's very little sugar.

Ty: But isn't it disingenuous for them to say don't juice yet at the same time they got a candy drawer at the exit of their office.

Cherie: So true. And what are people given so often in hospitals? Popsicles, right after surgery. Candy, or yes, you're right, going through chemo give them candy to suck on or anything.

Ty: But don't juice.

Cherie: Don't juice because it's too much sugar. We have really gotten off track and lost our way when it comes to truth. And thank God you're doing what you're doing, Ty.. Because you're bringing truth and a light on the path. This is the way. This is the way to life. What we're talking about.

Ty: Thank you. I appreciate the kind words. Talk about your first five days of juicing a couple of decades ago. The story you told me.

Cherie: I was really sick in my late twenties and decided that I'd better do something. This was more than a couple of decades ago. I had better do something because no doctor knew what to do with chronic fatigue and fibromyalgia. And they still don't. So I got an old Norman Walker book. And if you've seen the old Norman Walker juice books it's not recipes, it's numbers, one to twenty something or whatever. And it just lists the vegetables that you should be juicing for that condition.

So I had to design my own recipes. The first I tasted looked like motor oil. You get too many greens in just the right mix and it looks pretty brown and nasty. But I didn't care. I was so desperate and I'm just a very determined person. When I'm going to go for it I'm going to go, completely jump in that pool and go for it.

So I decided, "I'm going to do a five day juice fast." On day number five, this is honest truth, my body expelled a tumor the size of a golf ball. About that big, with blue blood vessels attached to it. Looked like somebody just chopped them off. And that got my attention, like nothing else.

Ty: I bet it did. Five days.

Cherie: Five days on day number five. So I thought, "Okay, I should just get well after this." Whatever was making me sick is probably gone now and I should be well. No, I was detoxing. I had some good days and some bad days. I was climbing up that mountain but it seemed like a couple steps forward and then a couple steps back because my body was getting rid of a lot of toxins.

But there came a day when I woke up one morning and thought, "ah, somebody gave me a new body in the middle of the night." I felt like a brand new person. And it wasn't just that one day that I had turned the corner, I was turning the corner the whole time. My body was healing and healing and moving in the right direction. I just didn't see the manifestation of that.

And that's why I always say to everybody on their journey, "There is hope. I give you hope. As long as you're breathing there is hope and there is healing and there is so much that can be done. Don't give up." Because just about the moment you think, "Ah, this isn't working," you're probably about to turn the corner. And you could have a morning like I did, where you wake up and think, "Wow, I feel like a new person today."

Ty: I think that's great to share with people because a lot of times you have to detoxify when you're sick and that feels worse than you've ever felt before. And at that point a lot of people might think, "I should just give up." But you're getting rid of the bad stuff, you have to detoxify and this juice helps you do that doesn't it?

Cherie: It really does. The juice is very cleansing and detoxifying and especially when you aren't eating junk food and a lot of heavy foods. So I always recommend to people that they do a juice fast. Maybe start with one day and then go to two days after a few weeks and then maybe three days. So kind of work your way into it. You can work up to a five day juice fast. I just jumped in and went for it but you work your way up and when you're juice fasting you're not pouring all of these heavier foods that your body has to work so hard to digest. It can then concentrate on healing and getting rid of toxins.

It's like taking a vacation I always say to people. Say you took a week off and you've got it at home. You didn't go somewhere. You're going to clean your house. Alright, you've got extra time. You can dig into your closets and corners and drawers and you can begin to really deep clean your house. Your body is the same way. It can start deep cleaning into areas that it hasn't been able to work on because it spends so much time digesting the foods that we eat and it spends most of the day digesting all this food that we eat.

So that's why it's so powerful to do a juice fast. It gives your body a chance also to repair and rejuvenate and for your immune cells to go after what it should, cancer cells. That's what the immune system was designed to do, to go after cancer cells and attack them. And what if there is that protective coating around some of the cancer cells which some researchers have looked at, saying there is a coating on some on cancer cells that kind of deflect the immune system? I found a researcher in the U.K. that believed carrot juice helped to dissolve that protective coating.

Ty: I think she wrote a book on it.

Cherie: Yes.

Ty: I can't remember the name either.

Cherie: I can't remember it. Whether that's speculative or not, try it. I mean go for it. It's going to only help you and you and I both heard many stories.

Ty: Here's the thing. Give it a shot. It can't be any worse than your current diet, most likely. One of the absurd things to me is when you hear the advice given by a medical doctor that says, “Don’t take in too many fruits or vegetables or anti-oxidants because it will counter the chemo. So we're poisoning you. Don't take too much nutrition. Go eat your ice cream and your cakes and your whoppers.”

That's absurd to me, but that's the advice that people get. So we're really fighting an uphill battle to try to get nutrition into the picture because most doctors are just not taught about nutrition.

Cherie: No. In fact most medical doctors have maybe one course in nutrition. It might have changed, maybe they get two or three now.

Ty: Or less.

Cherie: Or less. Some get none. It depends on where they go to school. So they are not taught and I can't fault them in many ways because they just don't know.

Ty: You don't know what you don't know.

Cherie: No. So they don't tell you that you need to be very aware of what made you sick. How did you get here? What kinds of foods got you here? What kinds of chemicals or toxicity in your environment got you here? What kinds of mental toxicity and emotional toxicity got you here?

Let's look at all of this big picture and let's start unraveling this ball of yarn that's all in a knot and let's cleanse it all out so that you are then free. Your body is free to do what it is designed to do. Its God given design is to heal but we've got to give it the right tools. So that's where nutrition, and not just juicing, but the organic vegetables, and a little bit, small amounts of low sugar fruits like maybe the berries are really good, blue berries and blackberries, raspberries. Organic. I keep stressing that, organic.

And then tons of vegetables. Vegetables upon vegetables and seeds and nuts. And quinoa is a seed. So people can have that. You can have some cooked things. It doesn't have to be all raw. And you can do a vegetable fast along with your juice. I just completed one of those a couple of weeks ago. Plenty to eat. Stir fry, soups, salads.

Ty: But just veggies?

Cherie: Just veggies and seeds. And I had quinoa and it was a bed for my stir fried vegetables. And I put a little coconut aminos. Those are so delicious to cook your vegetables in, and cooked all those up and put them on top of a big bed of quinoa. Had a salad on the side. I could eat that way most of the time.

Ty: And you're stuffed. Because there's so much nutrition. We had a fellowship meeting after church this last Sunday and somebody brought this quinoa dish that had avocado, tomatoes, quinoa, and it was cooked in coconut oil. Incredible. And people don't realize how satisfying that is to eat just clean foods the way that our body was intended to. You are getting the nutrition that you need and that helps us to begin healing.

After my dad died in the mid-nineties, one of the first things I did was I began to learn about how toxic we are in the colon and I felt that I needed to do a juice fast. I was compared to a body builder at the time. I did a 21 day juice fast. Just juice for 20 days. Let me tell you something, and you've heard the story before, I didn't have hardly any body fat that time, I lost 20 pounds and it was all junk that was caught up in my intestines.

Cherie: The toxins.

Ty: I was so toxic I had no idea. And over the course of the three weeks it all came out. And I'll tell you what, one of the reasons I'll tell you is that you're not necessarily losing body fat. Sometimes when you're doing a detox you're getting rid of a lot of stuff that has been in your body a long time that can cause a lot of disease if you leave it in there. And that's why juice fasts are so good. One of the reasons.

Cherie: Absolutely. Oh, I've talked to people that have lost an amazing amount of toxicity from the colon. You'll know when you're losing it, everybody knows.

Ty: It's scary.

Cherie: It's scary. You're thinking, “oh my goodness, that was in my body?” Thank God we're getting rid of it, you know, because this is what's contributing to illness, to serious diseases.

Ty: Colon cancer, look at how high the colon cancer rates have gone.

Cherie: And they keep going up, they keep soaring. All the different cancer rates are going up and up and up. And it is because of all of the toxicity in our diet and in our world. Even if you eat quite well you still need to cleanse because we just have a toxic environment. Our air and soil and water are toxic too.

Ty: So when you juice, how long after you juice should you drink the juice?

Cherie: I get asked that all the time. So the sooner you drink it the better. However, it's the real world and I always say I'm a practical nutritionist and we've got to deal with what we've got. So if you're a busy person and running out the door in the morning and you do not have time to juice, then juice the night before and store it in the fridge covered. Fill the jar, or whatever you are storing it in, up to the top as close as you can.

I have other people that I've worked with that have to juice on the weekends and freeze some in individual jars because they just can't make it work if they don't do that. Do what's practical. You may lose some nutrients. It's still going to be one of the best things you could have on earth, is to have this juice. So just make it work.

Ty: Don't use the fact that maybe it's losing a little bit of nutritional value as an excuse to go back to the golden arches, in other words.

Cherie: Exactly. Or to just say, "I'm going to bag the whole thing, I just won't juice. I'll just eat a salad or something." No, no, no make it work. And yes, just do it, as the saying goes. It is so important to make these changes because it is truly many times for people life and death. And so there are lots of excuses of why it's not going to work. Or some people even said they don't like the taste. Well, find something then that you do. Try a little more apple or more ginger in there. Add a little lemon, spark up the taste for you, just to get your taste buds going in the right direction.

And then people ask me too about a juicer. It's so confusing out there, should I get a masticating, should I get a centrifugal, should I get a blender type. And everybody is selling you their product. So they're all going to, of course, tell you their product is the best and only theirs.

I always say, "You know what the best juicer is, on the face of the earth?"

Ty: The one that's in your kitchen that you're using.

Cherie: The one you'll use every day. If you won't use it, if it's too hard to clean, if it's too much trouble for you, it may be the most perfect one but it's going to go under your counter. You won't use it. Get one that you'll use.

Ty: I think that's great advice. Years ago we were reading about the debate and so if you want to do wheat grass juice you had to have a masticating. You can't use a centrifugal, you won't get anything from it. We bought one of the masticating, really expensive. It took so long to juice I never used it. So now at this point, I have four kids and busy, and want to get it done. We have things to do. My wife home educates so we're always busy. We use the centrifugal one because it's faster and you can get it in boom, boom, boom five minutes you're done. You have juice for the whole family. You go back to whatever you're doing. So I think that's great advice.

Cherie: I use a centrifugal. I've got about every type of juicer there is. I line them up in the garage all along the shelf. I use them at different times for different reasons or demos. But the one we use every day is a centrifugal and I do it for the same reason. I'm very, very busy. I want something I can clean in a minute. Just rinse off. And if I can clean it a minute then I can get my husband to clean it. One minute. He'll do that, he'll rinse it off.

But the one that you're scrubbing for five or ten minutes and you have to have a little brush in all the corners? I won't do it and my husband would never do that one. So make it work.

Ty: Right, be practical with it. Inflammation is very important in the cancer equation. So what types of juices would you recommend that would help to reduce inflammation? Or do they all?

Cherie: There are some specific ones that do. You don't know my latest book that came out is the anti-inflammation diet. Inflammation's at the root of every disease practically that there is, every condition. And we must get that inflammation under control. Ginger root is right up at the top. It's proven in scientific studies to be anti-inflammatory, and so juice a lot of ginger. You may have to work your way up. I've talked to so many people who say, "Oh boy, I just can't take the taste of that." So, have little bits. Work your way up. I'm up to giant pieces of ginger root and I love it.

Your greens. So important. The dark leafy greens, rotate them. Some people say, "I hear all these reports that greens can be toxic, or you can get too much of this or that." Don't worry about that. We were made for greens. But rotate them. It's a really good idea. Maybe one day you have kale or you used up your bunch of kale. Then you go to chard, and maybe you do some spinach, and some romaine lettuce and some parsley, or whatever. Just rotate your greens around.

Get lots of greens in your diet. Broccoli is wonderful and I use the big hard stems that normally we would throw away. I steam or stir fry the buds, the florets, and juice the base. There is good economy and you're getting all of those wonderful nutrients. And what are you going to do with that hard base anyway? So save it and juice it. All of those are wonderful anti-inflammatory nutrients in those foods. All your vegetables are going to be great.

Ty: It's hard to find a vegetable that's not anti-inflammatory and anti-cancer.

Cherie: It is, because God packaged them just right. They are our most important food in our fight against cancer. All the brightly colored vegetables. There are hardly any that aren't. There are a few and they're still good for us.

Ty: Eat the rainbow right?

Cherie: Yes, Absolutely.

Ty: One of our favorite juices—I need to get your approval here since you are the Juice Lady. But one of the ones that Charlene especially loves, my wife, is fresh orange juice, fresh lemon juice, and then garlic and ginger. And then we just put it in the Vitamix and blend it up. We put about ten cloves of garlic, couple of big things of ginger, and maybe half a thing full of juice. Blend it up with ice and it's a smoothie. It's so good.

Cherie: That sounds wonderful.

Ty: Oh, it's great.

Cherie: I've been one in the morning. This is a liver cleanse, a gentle, gentle liver cleanse.

Ty: Are you reading my notes? Because that's my next question.

Cherie: Was it?

Ty: Yeah, go ahead, hit me up.

Cherie: I didn't see that. Alright, here we go. I've been doing this one because I'm starting on my summer liver cleanse. Any time of year is a great time to cleanse but summer is just wonderful. Spring and summer when it's warmer and we can definitely eat lighter because it's just warmer. So I'm doing one.

But my morning shake is the juice of one lemon and one lime and you can add orange too if you want to. For me that's too much sugar. My body just does not like sugar at all, even orange juice. But you can put orange juice in there for sure. And then you add about a cup of water, a bunch of ice cubes, as many as you want to make it the temperature you want. A tablespoon of olive oil, one garlic clove, and a little chunk of ginger. And that's day one.

Day two, two cloves of garlic and two spoons of olive oil. And then day three, three and three. Four and four. Day five, five and five. Five garlic cloves, five table spoons of olive oil and the rest is the same. Don't breath on anyone that day.

Ty: Because the garlic.

Cherie: No. I'm just teasing you.

Ty: You need to make sure your husband or wife is drinking with you, right?

Cherie: Or chew on parsley. That takes away the garlic breath. Along with a carrot salad, a beet salad, and a potassium broth soup, and a beet juice drink, and a green juice drink, that is your liver cleanse. A gentle liver cleanse, program. And then you can add salads and soups and stir fries. It should be an all-vegetable week. And so this is my one day off. I'm not doing that today but I'm going to pick back up and complete my liver cleanse for the rest of the week,

Ty: You're in the middle of it then?

Cherie: Yeah, I took a day off. But it's a wonderful gentle, very gentle, liver cleanse. There are many others that are more heavy duty with herbs and different tinctures that you can add in. But if you want to do a gentle one, that is a great way to start working into it.

Beets are wonderful for the liver. They are known as a liver food, liver cleanse food, along with many others. The dark leafy greens, and carrots, and olive oil, lemon juice, all of that is just wonderful for a liver cleansing. And with my carrot salad and beat salad I make them with the pulp. So I juice a beet first and pull out the pulp. And then I juice all my carrots to get a cup of pulp.

And then add lemon juice and olive oil dressing to each of them, they're separate. I put cinnamon in there, in my dressing, because it just sparks up the flavor a whole lot. I love cinnamon. And then you eat your beet salad a couple of table spoons at a time throughout the day. Your carrot salad you can eat all at once. But it's done for you. It's so fast. It's all done for you.

Ty: And it really cleanses the liver? All these steps together.

Cherie: Yes. And if anyone has had chemo and radiation it's extremely important that you cleanse your liver. And I say to everyone who has cancer, who has had cancer, and has been through chemo and or radiation, you must, must, must cleanse your liver. Cleanse your whole body because those things are so toxic. And if you don't it's going to stay in your body and it could contribute to cancer coming back along with all the other toxicity that was there and contributed to cancer in the first place.

Ty: So really good advice to cleanse that liver. Because the things we are using, the conventional treatment, actually could be carcinogenic. They actually are known to be carcinogenic.

Cherie: Yes, and highly toxic for the body. But before you cleanse your liver, and we talked about it earlier, always cleanse your colon. Because we want that channel of elimination very open and as clean as possible so that when the liver starts dumping the toxins it can get on out, get through your body.

And I do want to say for everyone who does a cleanse, if you don't feel well don't worry. This too shall pass. It's going to come on through your system. You want it out. So if you end up with a headache or you feel tired or a little flu-ish or achy all over it's not going to hang around like the flu or a cold. It's going to move on through your body. And as those toxic things move out you're going to feel a whole lot better. And you're going to be preventing disease from coming back or coming to you down the line.

Ty: And this is a very personal issue with you because you were affected with cancer at a very early age, right in your family.

Cherie: Yes, my mother died of breast cancer when I was six years old and that had a major impact on me. That's, I know, one of the reasons I chose to do my master's thesis in nutrition and cancer. I wanted to understand what in the world had happened to my mother and why did she get cancer.

So I started interviewing family members. What was her diet like? Not good. She didn't like vegetables and she loved sweets. Lord have mercy, because that is a set-up for cancer. And along with emotions, she was not an expressive person, she tended to suppress them. Especially the ones that are considered sort of negative, the anger or, the non-positive responses she tended to keep inside. All of that is a set-up for cancer.

And I was following, most definitely in her footsteps. I loved sweets and I didn't like vegetables. So my whole life has done a complete turnabout. I don't eat any sweets at all, ever. And I now love vegetables. And there is a prescription for health.

Ty: That's the Juice Lady.

Cherie: Yes. And juice every day that you can.

Ty: Cherie, here's a question, we've had this explosion over the last couple of decades in childhood cancer. So if somebody is watching out there and they have cancer or they are parents, wondering what they should be feeding them. Is juicing an option for a child with cancer?

Cherie: Absolutely. And again I've worked with parents with children with cancer. I can't think of a better food for a child than juice, fresh vegetable juice. It's wonderful for that child. Just as it is for an adult.

You may be able to do a short juice fast with your child. It depends on the age. If they're really young, and really young, what do I mean by that? Maybe under six years old. I wouldn't do a prolonged juice fast by any means. And it's a little iffy as to what age, teenagers I know can, but you can start them juicing. I wouldn't say for a child juice fasting, but juicing the vegetables and the supplements and purees and green smoothies. And lots and lots of vegetables and then have lots of juice. That would be fabulous for any child. And you can give juice to babies as well.

Ty: And they love it too.

Cherie: They love it. That's right.

Ty: Last question, so what's your advice to somebody that might have recently been diagnosed with cancer?

Cherie: I have great hope for you that there is so much you can do to get well. Start juicing immediately. Go get a juicer. Get one that you'll use every day and drink lots of juice. Not just one glass, that's more preventative. You need many glasses, three or four at least. Some people say a couple of quarts of vegetable juice a day to start off with. Flood your system with these nutrients.

Cut out all sweets. Just don't eat one thing that is sweet. Read all labels and pretty much cut out everything in a package, a box, all junk food, all fast food. Don't eat in restaurants very much unless you can go to an organic restaurant or a wonderful juice bar. Places like that of course are wonderful. Raw foods restaurants are wonderful.

But get all the junk and the chemicals out of your diet. Buy organic foods. Try to get vegetables in as many meals as you possibly can. Quinoa is wonderful. Organic seeds and nuts are great. Make animals proteins a minimum or cut them out completely if you can for a while. Until you really get your system turned around. And there is great hope. And then do a colon cleanse and a liver cleanse. Minimum those two.

I would also add, if you can, do a kidney bladder cleanse. Do lung, do lymphatic system, and skin and blood. I like to take people through a four step process. It takes about a month and you've really covered it then if you can do all of that.

Ty: Hit us up real quickly with the details of the other cleanses. You know, you've told us about the liver cleanse, the juice, and the colon cleanse.

Cherie: It isn't dietary for the others. It is tinctures. Different tinctures that are used in different herbs. And I use some products that are already designed to do that. That is the program that begins to work on all systems of the body that are systems and organs of elimination. So, so important. And if you do that you're going to notice amazing things happening in your body. I already know it.

I hear from people from around the world, I know you do as well. People who are given no hope. People who are sent home. I'll just leave you with a story of a woman that got my book, *The Complete Cancer Cleanse*, years ago. And she was given no hope at all. Just told to go home, get your affairs in order and, "you're going to die." She had tumors throughout her body and she thought, "well, I've got Cherie's book. I'm just going to give it a try. Why not? I have nothing to lose."

She said about day eleven she felt this ripping sensation starting in her neck. And pain like this ripping, pulling sensation. All of a sudden a giant tumor fell out of her body. She said, almost cursing, "That Cherie Calbom." She was in so much pain as it came out and then, "boom," that cancerous tumor fell out of her body.

And she said from that day on her system took a major turn for the better. She healed completely. She said, years later, when she had contacted me again. She said she looked ten years younger than when she started the whole process and had her health completely back.

So I always say, "never accept a death sentence, you never know." Give this program, juicing and changing your diet and cleansing, give it a try. Give it your all because I know it's only going to help you.

Ty: Well, that's something that over the years I have been contacted by people that have given juicing a shot. I've never, not one time, been contacted by anybody that says, "Hey, I tried it, and it just didn't work."

Cherie: I know.

Ty: Everybody feels better, they look younger, their skin gets better, their physical condition gets better. It works for everybody. And so your answer is consistent with the very first. She said disease is a result of malnutrition, coupled with toxicity. Toxicity is coupled with a deficiency, yes?

Cherie: Yes.

Ty: Well, the answer you just gave is consistent with that. Get rid of the toxicity through all of these different body cleanses and give your body the nutrition that it is deficient in through juicing. I think that's the recipe for success isn't it?

Cherie: It is, yes. Everybody should do this, give it a try. And a great preventative too.

Ty: It is, isn't it? And that's what we do as a family, we juice as a preventative. Plus it tastes great, you can't beat that.

Cherie: I know. And it's energizing.

Ty: Thanks for spending time with us today. It's been really fascinating.

Cherie: Thanks, Ty.

Ty: Alright, appreciate it.

[end of transcript]

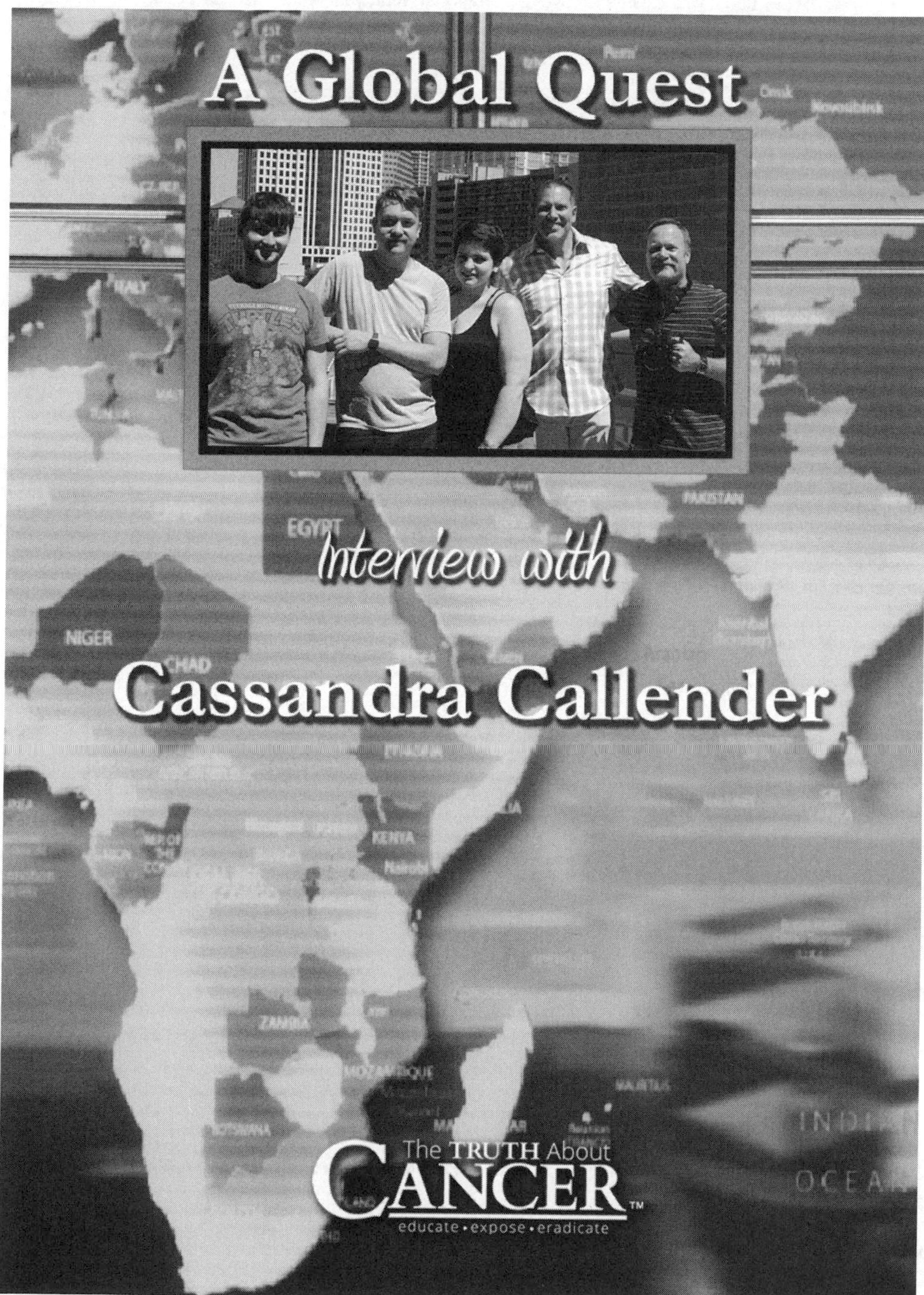
A Global Quest
Interview with
Cassandra Callender
The TRUTH About
CANCER
educate • expose • eradicate
EGYPT
NIGER
CHAD
KENYA
ZAMBIA
MOZAMBIQUE
BOTSWANA
PAKISTAN
ITALY
Omsk
Novosibirsk
INDIA
OCEA

Ty: I'm here in Austin, Texas with Cassandra Callender and I'm so happy to be able to talk to you today about your experience over the last, what, year, year and a half, has it been?

Cassandra: Yes.

Ty: With some interesting events that occurred up in Connecticut, right? Regarding cancer and then forced chemotherapy. Thank you for joining us here in Austin.

Cassandra: Thank you for having me.

Ty: You had a good flight last night?

Cassandra: I did. I'm tired.

Ty: Are you?

Cassandra: Yes.

Ty: Okay, but you slept well?

Cassandra: I did.

Ty: Okay. Tell us a little bit about yourself, Cassandra. You are how old?

Cassandra: I'm 17, turning 18 this fall.

Ty: All right, almost 18.

Cassandra: Yeah. Exciting.

Ty: Good deal. What do you like doing? What do you like to do?

Cassandra: I like being outside, going shopping, movies, hanging out with my friends, hanging with my cat.

Ty: With your cat? What's the cat's name?

Cassandra: Simba.

Ty: "The Lion King."

Cassandra: Yes.

Ty: All right. Cool. Tell us about your overall health that led you to go to the doctor and eventually be diagnosed with—was it Hodgkin's lymphoma?

Cassandra: Yes.

Ty: Talk about those days before you knew that you were diagnosed with cancer. What was going on with you?

Cassandra: It started with having severe stomach pain, like cramps, abdominal pain, so I had to go to the emergency room because it was so bad.

Ty: When was this? What year was this?

Cassandra: It was May of 2014. And when we went to the hospital they couldn't find anything wrong. They just sent me home and I had to do a follow up with my doctor. And there was a lump on my neck about the size of a golf ball and they weren't sure what it was.

They put me on antibiotics for months and they couldn't figure out what was going on because the lump wasn't going down. They wanted to start testing it and do biopsies. They were getting nowhere. They were poking me with needles and biopsies every week and they just said it was suspicious. We did an initial surgery to remove the lymph node and that's when they started questioning cancer. And that was in September 2014.

Ty: September 2014. So at that point they thought it might be cancer?

Cassandra: They were questioning it. When we talked to the oncologist they said, "It looks like Hodgkin's lymphoma." And from there that's when they immediately said we had to start chemotherapy. But my mom and I wanted a second opinion because "looking like cancer" isn't an actual answer for us.

Ty: Right. They thought it looked like Hodgkin's lymphoma, but they didn't do a biopsy. They didn't know for sure.

Cassandra: Yes, they did the biopsy but—

Ty: They did do a biopsy.

Cassandra: But they refused to do a second one.

Ty: Okay. At that point, that's when we started reading about this in the papers. That, "Cassandra C. in Connecticut is—"

Cassandra: We went up to Bay State Mass to a different doctor to get another biopsy and they refused to do it. They had talked to Hartford Hospital where I originally was and they said there was no need to do another biopsy. There was no need for any other surgical procedure.

They just wanted to immediately start the chemo. And my mom and I were researching chemo and I didn't want it. I wanted to look for an alternative. And considering they wouldn't test me again, I wasn't sure of everything.

Ty: Right. Basically, you didn't want to do chemo and you wanted a second opinion. And what were the reasons that you wanted to stay away from chemo that you had research?

Cassandra: The side effects, the long-term side effects that people potentially have—organ failure and problems with your health and digestive system and everything that goes with chemo. I mean, I did it for five months and it was horrible.

Ty: Okay, so you did do chemo.

Cassandra: Yeah, not willingly.

Ty: Was it your choice?

Cassandra: No.

Ty: The long-term side effects of chemo concerned you. Right? Being only 17.

Cassandra: Yeah, and I was reading into it and they were saying possible organ failures and difficulty doing physical activity the rest of your life and I didn't want that. Especially when I knew that there was homeopathic and natural ways of treating cancer. They told me chemo was my only option.

Ty: They told you chemo was your only option.

Cassandra: Yes.

Ty: Okay. At that point you wanted to get a second opinion. At some point, did the Child Protective Services get involved? What happened?

Cassandra: Yes. After we left Bay State with nothing because they refused to do another biopsy, the Department of Children and Families was called because we were wasting time, according to the doctors. They wanted me in for chemotherapy a week after my biopsy was done in Hartford. And they came in and they took me because they said that I had to get the chemo.

Ty: What do you mean, when you say they, "took you?"

Cassandra: They came into my house in October, around Halloween, and they said that I had to go with them.

Ty: And who is "they?"

Cassandra: The DCF workers.

Ty: Okay, the Division of Family and Child Services, or whatever it is.

Cassandra: Yes.

Ty: DCF. Okay. They actually came into your home and took you from your mom.

Cassandra: Yes, they had about 12 police squad cars surrounding my house and the block. And they basically just came into my house and said, "We have to go." My mom wasn't even home. I was hiding in my closet upstairs because I had no idea what was going on.

Ty: Were you the only one at the house?

Cassandra: Yes. I called my mom crying and she came home immediately to police and DCF workers surrounding our house.

Ty: That's unbelievable.

Cassandra: And they said I had no choice, but to go with them.

Ty: What were you feeling at that point?

Cassandra: I was scared.

Ty: With your house surrounded?

Cassandra: I had no idea what was going on and I was scared and I didn't understand why, because at the time I didn't know that I didn't have a choice. I didn't know that you couldn't refuse to do chemotherapy.

Ty: You didn't realize that they were going to force you.

Cassandra: Yeah, I didn't know because no one said anything. The doctors just said that it was in a timely manner and we had to do it and I was telling them no.

Ty: I assume then that you lived outside of Hartford, Connecticut.

Cassandra: I do.

Ty: I assume that there are never any crimes in Hartford because they took 12 policemen—police cars—away from things that they should be doing, keeping us safe, to go surround your house.

Cassandra: Yes. It was unnecessary to have that many people around my house. It wasn't necessary to have police there at all, but they did.

Ty: So Cassandra, DCF, how did they learn about your case?

Cassandra: The doctors contacted them because I wasn't starting the chemotherapy in the time period that they wanted. They initially wanted me to start the chemotherapy immediately after my surgery in September. And that's not what I wanted. I wanted to go to another doctor and I wanted to seek a different treatment besides chemotherapy.

Ty: You aren't a good patient to those doctors, you didn't do exactly what they said so they called DCF.

Cassandra: Yes. Doctors don't like when you don't do exactly what they say because they are the doctor. They're supposed to be right with everything. When you choose to do something that they don't want, they get mad.

Ty: Yes. Did your oncologist have a little bit of an attitude?

Cassandra: He was upset in the beginning when my mom was on my side because he believes that most parents, if their child doesn't want the chemotherapy, the parent, still talk them into doing it and makes them do it.

When both my mom and I were arguing with him, he was probably confused and angry with us. Because most oncologists take it as when you're diagnosed with cancer you'll do anything and take any medicine out there to cure it. And for me, I looked up chemotherapy and I did not want that. I wanted something that wasn't as harmful to the body.

Ty: Well, the initial chemotherapies were derived from the nitrogen based mustard gas in World Wars that they used to dump on the opponent, the enemies, to kill them.

Cassandra: That explains why I was so sick.

Ty: Yes. So at that point, they took you, they told your mom, "We're taking Cassandra. You don't have any options." And then at that point, did they tell you, "We're going to start you on chemotherapy?"

Cassandra: No, it was a longer process. They brought me to the hospital to get me evaluated and placed me in a foster home in the meantime because we had to go to court because they really didn't know what they could or couldn't do with me because this had never happened before. So I went from a foster home, in and out of the hospital, and eventually I ran away.

Ty: Did you?

Cassandra: Because I couldn't do it. I didn't want anything to do with this. They were ruining my life basically. They came in and they took me away because I didn't want chemo when there are other options out there. I just didn't understand why they were doing it.

Ty: When you say that they evaluated you, what do you mean, "they evaluated" you?

Cassandra: They brought me to the hospital, to the emergency department and basically they just give you a physical and just make sure you're well.

Ty: Okay. Any kind of psychological evaluations or evaluations of your family situation?

Cassandra: That came later on, after I was initially admitted to the hospital. They had psychs and other people coming and talking to me. But in the beginning there were no psychs talking to me.

Ty: Okay. You mentioned that you ran away. What happened?

Cassandra: They let me come home from the foster home through a judge ordering to still stay in custody, but I could be at my house, ordering that I had to do chemo though. And I did two days of it and that was because I was court ordered to do it and I was freaking out.

And basically, I did two days of it and it was horrible. I felt sick. I didn't feel myself and I didn't want it. I was being forced to do something that I wanted nothing to do with. So I ran away for about a week and when I started getting phone calls from people saying they were going to place my mom in jail and people thought I was dead, I came home.

And from there is when the court dates started coming up and they were talking about what they were going to do with me and I was admitted to the hospital in December.

Ty: Okay, and so in December, when you were admitted, what happened? More chemotherapy?

Cassandra: Yes. I was admitted December 9th directly from the courtroom. The judge ordered that I had to be hospitalized until further notice. It was never given exactly how long. It was just that I had to be hospitalized.

Ty: Okay. Why did the judge order that you had to be hospitalized immediately?

Cassandra: DCF ordered that. They stood before the judge and said it would be in my best interests to be hospitalized.

Ty: DCF?

Cassandra: Yes.

Ty: Are they medical doctors?

Cassandra: No.

Ty: But they ordered you to be hospitalized?

Cassandra: Yes.

Ty: And they are not doctors.

Cassandra: No.

Ty: Okay, that's bizarre. That's just weird that they have the authority to force you to go to the hospital and they don't have anything to do with medicine.

Cassandra: They had my doctor, my primary oncologist, talk to the judge and basically all the doctors were telling the judge that I was going to die. They said that they don't know when I'm going to die, but I'm going to die if I did not start the treatment immediately.

Ty: And this is on a diagnosis of cancer that they weren't even sure about.

Cassandra: To them, they were sure of it, but the refusing to do a second biopsy is what made me unsure of it. Why they refused to do it and why they were so anxious to start the chemotherapy immediately.

Ty: So then you began more chemo in December.

Cassandra: Yes. After about two weeks of being in the hospital, going through courts and judges, they got the order that they could force me to do the chemotherapy.

At that point I was in the hospital, I could not leave my room, there was a guard sitting outside of my door. I couldn't use my phone. I couldn't contact my mom. And basically it came down to one morning they came in and they strapped me to the bed and they said they sedated me for surgery.

Ty: Really?

Cassandra: Yes, because you have to have a port to have chemotherapy which is why I have a ***scar.***

Ty: And you didn't want a port.

Cassandra: No, because I didn't want the chemo. The idea of having an object inside of me grossed me out. And so they came in to insert it in my vein and I said no. They had to have the officer and the security guards and the staff come in and they brought in the bed bag straps and they had to tie me down by my wrists and my ankles. A woman came in and put a needle in my neck to knock me out. And the next thing I knew, I woke up and I was in the recovery room. It was horrible.

Ty: That's horrible. They literally strapped you to a bed and did a procedure against your wishes.

Cassandra: It took twelve people. Four of them lifted me up by my arms and my legs and had to hold me down. I wasn't going down without a fight at that point.

Ty: Well, good for you. But I'm at a loss for words that they literally did that to you.

Cassandra: At that point I didn't feel like a human anymore. I didn't feel like I was being treated like one. I didn't know what else to do. I just did not want the chemotherapy and they were telling me I had no other option.

Ty: Well, you weren't being treated like a human. Humans don't strap other humans down and do something against their wishes to them.

Cassandra: I told all of them. I told the doctors, I told the surgeon, I told everyone, "I don't want this. I'm not giving consent to this." I yelled it probably a dozen times and they said nothing. And the DCF workers just stood in the room and watched.

Ty: How did that make you feel at that point?

Cassandra: I was frustrated and annoyed and confused and mad and scared. It was a mix of everything because it's never happened before. And as a human, I think I have rights to choose what medicine I wanted. Whether it's natural or chemotherapy. Because there are people out there that do it and I wanted to be one of them.

Ty: And you had nobody there with you?

Cassandra: They wouldn't allow my mom to be there that day and they would not tell me why. She was supposed to come in that morning and at the last minute they said she wasn't allowed to be there.

Ty: So they did this to you by yourself? Seventeen years old. So what happened after this forced medical procedure where they put a port in you?

Cassandra: I woke up in the recovery room. They gave me heavy sedation so I couldn't freak out when I woke up. And basically they said, "This is what's going to happen every day that you receive chemo if you don't comply." And at that point it was traumatizing. I didn't want to be strapped to a bed every day in the hospital for five months so I just did it. There was nothing else I could do.

Ty: They threatened you, said, "If you don't comply, we will strap you down every day."

Cassandra: Yes, and the days that I had chemo, they wouldn't allow me to eat because the sedation medicine makes you sick and you could throw up and choke. Chemo lasted about six days a week once a month and then another eight days after that. It goes on a cycle.

So any day I had chemo, they wouldn't let me eat for 12 hours before in case they had to sedate me. So when it comes to that, you start complying with it because you don't want to starve. And it was horrible being strapped down.

Ty: They not only forced the chemo against your wishes, on the days that you did chemo, they basically starved you.

Cassandra: Yes, until I started complying with it and that stopped.

Ty: So let me get this right. Once you began to comply, then they fed you?

Cassandra: Yes.

Ty: It had nothing to do with the chemo you couldn't mix with food. They starved you to make you comply.

Cassandra: Yes, because if I didn't comply with it, they would have to sedate me and you can't eat when you take sedative medicine.

Ty: I see.

Cassandra: Like when you go into surgery you're not supposed to eat for 12 hours.

Ty: I see. Okay. So they said, "If you don't do it willingly, we're going to sedate you and starve you."

Cassandra: Yes.

Ty: I'm laughing, but it's an absurd laugh. It's something that I'm having a hard time believing that this actually happened. When were you allowed to talk to your mother and did she figure out that this had actually happened to you?

Cassandra: I was not allowed to talk to her on the phone by myself. Phone calls had to be supervised. Everything had to be supervised. If she were to come see me in the beginning, DCF workers had to be in the room with her and it was limited to two hour visits. Eventually they didn't allow her to come at all anymore.

Ty: Why?

Cassandra: After court, certain things happened and they were afraid that she would be a bad influence on me because she was fighting for me. She's my mom and she was taking my side. And if I didn't want the chemo, she was going to stand up for that. DCF looked at that as a bad influence. They didn't want us together and it came down to that's what they thought my best interest was.

Ty: Best interest was to be away from your mother because she was on your side. She might influence you to continue fighting them.

Cassandra: And my mother had a very strong opinion about this and she still does and she's very outspoken and DCF didn't like that. They came down to where they thought it would be better that she wasn't always around.

Ty: How did that make you feel, that you couldn't talk to your mother for so many months?

Cassandra: It bothered me because my mom is the only person I've ever had, along with her, DCF didn't allow anyone else to come see me except for a very small list of people that were approved.

It was basically sitting in a hospital alone for five months. And they would make comments in court saying how I wasn't alone because my DCF workers would come and see me and visit me and bring me food. But at the end of the day that's your DCF worker, not your friend that's your family, your mom, your pets, anything like that. It's just a DCF worker.

Ty: They made comments like that in court, that you weren't alone because you had the DCF that visited you.

Cassandra: Yes, because I would tell the judge that I was in there alone and they would stand up and say I wasn't alone because they would come and see me every week.

Ty: Well, people that are in jail for life aren't alone either. They have the guards bring them food and put it through the door. That sounds kind of like what happened to you.

Cassandra: DCF was nice to me. They'd bring me anything I wanted, but that doesn't make up for locking me in a hospital and forcing me to do the chemo.

Ty: Right. You underwent chemo for five months.

Cassandra: Yes.

Ty: From December 2014 through April?

Cassandra: Yes. The first the cycle was supposed to be in November when I had two days of it and I ran away. So then in December through April, they finished the remainder of the five months. I was in the hospital for a total of 140 days.

Ty: Against your will.

Cassandra: Yes.

Ty: And you couldn't leave.

Cassandra: No.

Ty: With a guard at your door.

Cassandra: Yes. After a few months they removed the guard and I was allowed to roam the halls of the hospital and use the kitchen and the game rooms and whatnot. But I was still there. I wasn't allowed to leave. I didn't have fresh air. I became pale. I lacked vitamin D. It was overall horrible. I felt unhealthy and I didn't feel like a person.

Ty: Did you ever voice these feelings to the DCF workers or anybody while you were in there?

Cassandra: I did. And they always told me that. "We're in and out of court" and they don't want to see me there, but it's what they have to do.

Ty: Right. Why did they stop the chemo at five months? That was just the regimen?

Cassandra: Yeah, that's just the regimen of the cycle that the doctor said that I should have.

Ty: When you stopped chemo—I guess in April of 2015?

Cassandra: Yes, April 27th was the last dose of chemo.

Ty: You remember the date.

Cassandra: Yes. That was the day I was released.

Ty: So they let you out of the prison at April 27th.

Cassandra: Yes.

Ty: And you were able to go home?

Cassandra: Yes.

Ty: What did that feel like at that point?

Cassandra: It was unbelievable because after five months you adapt to living in a room. And stepping outside, I could just smell everything. You could smell people down the street that were smoking. You could smell food in people's cars. It was just being in the world again.

Ty: A good feeling for you?

Cassandra: It was a good feeling. I didn't even know what to do with myself.

Ty: What was it like for you and your mother when you got reunited finally? Because she wasn't able to visit you in the hospital.

Cassandra: She was able to visit towards the end because I was done, per se. But actually, being back home with her and my family and my friends and, of course, my cat was a great feeling because you shouldn't have to be taken away from that for so long.

Ty: Right.

Cassandra: I didn't do anything wrong. I just simply didn't want to start medication. I wanted something else.

Ty: But you were treated like a criminal.

Cassandra: Yes.

Ty: They don't put armed guards at many people's hospital doors.

Cassandra: A lot of things that I tell people is, "Some people that are prison at least got to go outside for an hour a day. And I didn't get that."

Ty: Now that you're out of the hospital, you're back home free to do what you want to do. Have you had any further testing on the Hodgkin's lymphoma?

Cassandra: Yes, and that's what the problem is. My last PET scan that I received in July I believe didn't look good. And it came back that things were questionable and there's still activity in the still remaining tissue. So my doctor said that there could be a slight concern, but they'll worry about that in August.

Ty: That's bothersome that they forced this treatment on you that was supposed to cure the cancer and now there is still questionable—

Cassandra: There is still a questionable remainder of something in my abdomen. The PET scan didn't come up clear.

Ty: But they're not sure?

Cassandra: They're not sure.

Ty: Whatever happened to the lump? Is it gone?

Cassandra: It's gone. Most of the lumps and things that they claim that grew in my lymph nodes inside of me are gone. But it's the abdomen where they say there is something that is still lighting up. It's concerning and they're not sure what it is, but it's not a clear scan.

So to force me to go through the chemotherapy to save my life and then say, "Well, we're not sure" if they actually did or not, to me that's horrible. Because who is to say in August if they're going to make me do it again if I still have cancer.

Ty: What's your birthday?

Cassandra: September 30th. According to the judges, even in the Supreme Court, they claimed as a minor I can't make medical decisions like that. So in August, if they were to say that I have to do chemotherapy again, I'm still a minor. I'm closer to 18—

Ty: Until the end of September.

Cassandra: But I'm still a minor.

Ty: Right. At that point, what do you think you would want to do?

Cassandra: Get a really good lawyer. I mean, my lawyers fought from day one for me and it's really hard fighting the State and we were turned down in every way. And to be told that I have to go through this again when it didn't work the first time, I don't know what they could possibly do with that.

Ty: I think you could possibly have a good case right now for what they've already done, with a good attorney, to be honest with you. Because they did inhumane medical procedures to you against your will and it didn't have the result that they said it was going to have.

Cassandra: Yes. They claimed late February, early March that I was in remission, but just a few months later I get a PET scan and they are not so sure of it.

Ty: Well, the main problem with what they say is remission is they look at the tumor markers. And so the chemotherapy made the tumors shrink. But there are other issues that can arise from the chemo and they don't look at that eventually.

The good thing is, Cassandra, we can help you. We can help you with the direction on what you need to do in the future to be totally cancer free. The main problem is not can we help you. The main issue I see at this point is getting you to September 30th, when you turn 18 and you can make your own decisions.

So between now and then, do you think it is something that you would want any of this interview to be aired before that time or—

Cassandra: Yes. The world should know what's going on.

Ty: I agree. I just want to make sure that you're okay with that.

Cassandra: There are people out there that I've met personally that choose natural, homeopathic ways to treat their cancer and it works. And why I wasn't given the option in Connecticut, I don't understand.

Ty: That seems like a fundamental right to me. Every human should have the right, whether they choose natural or go with conventional cancer treatments. What do you think about that?

Cassandra: I think it's true. Either way, I'm still doing something to help my health. A lot of people in media have misinterpreted it, saying that I wanted to die of cancer instead of treatment. That's not true. I simply didn't want the chemotherapy. I wanted something that was less harmful to your body. Cancer is harmful enough to your body. Why would you want to add more to that?

Ty: Why would you want to add more—?

Cassandra: More harmful—

Ty: More harm to the body.

Cassandra: Yes.

Ty: Which is what chemotherapy is. Again, you've experienced that first hand, I'm sad to say, against your wishes. But chemotherapy is poison.

Cassandra: It is.

Ty: And it does kill cancer cells, but it also hurts you.

Cassandra: It hurts everything else. It kills the good and the bad cells. Chemotherapy doesn't know any different from a cell. It just knows it kills.

Ty: How are you feeling now?

Cassandra: I feel better now that I'm actually breathing fresh air and getting out and moving around. But emotionally it's hard to decide how okay I am after all of that.

Ty: Do you feel like you've been violated?

Cassandra: I do.

Ty: Well, the bottom line is that you have been. I think someone many people should be held accountable for that. But I think that legally you may have a case. So we'll let you figure that out, but I mean I think you might have a case against them for—I mean literally that's technically considered assault. If you physically touch someone against their wishes. If somebody comes up to you with a syringe and sticks you, that's assault and battery.

Cassandra: I had bruises on me to prove it.

Ty: You had bruises?

Cassandra: My ankles and my wrists and my hand were bruised.

Ty: When they strapped you down?

Cassandra: Yes, because I fought them. I wouldn't just let them do it.

Ty: So they assaulted you to get you down and then they assaulted you again when they forced a port in you. And then technically, I think legally, they assaulted you again every time they forced chemo on you against your wishes. Not that that does anything to help what you went through, but those people should be held accountable.

Cassandra: For the longest time, every day when they came in with the bags of the chemotherapy, I'd tell them, "I'm not giving consent to it." And the nurse would simply just say, "They're doing their job."

They were. That was their job. But I wasn't consenting to it. The DCF workers were the ones that came in and signed the consent forms and the paperwork and everything.

Ty: Did they have any compassion at all?

Cassandra: They did. They were nice. They were sweet. Anything I wanted or needed, they brought to me—food, clothes. I could ask for anything and they'd bring it to me. Partially, I feel like it's because they felt guilty and they knew what was going on was wrong. And also because I think they know it's a horrible situation. But like I said, that doesn't make up for what is going on.

Ty: Well, you know, Cassandra, the good news is that there is always hope with cancer. So the position you are in now, they see some activity in your abdomen, I don't think at this point that is something that you should be overly concerned with. Because there are things out there that we can help direct you towards that are going to get you completely healthy and live a long life.

Cassandra: That's what I wanted originally.

Ty: And that's what you wanted originally. And that's what is going to happen. I am confident that you are going to get healthy again. My concern is the month and a half period. Are they going to try to make you go back in August?

Cassandra: I have been receiving phone calls to set up the appointment for the PET scan in August, which I do have to do because I don't want DCF back involved for missing a doctor's appointment. So I will be going for the PET scan and I have no idea what those results will show. My previous results were not well, so I don't know what these ones are going to look like.

Ty: You go back in in August but you don't know what date yet.

Cassandra: No. My goal would be to try to push it as close to September as I can, to be as close to 18 as I can.

Ty: That would be my recommendation. Put it off as much as you can.

Cassandra: I can't see a judge saying that I'm three weeks away from being 18, but I have to do chemotherapy over again. Your statistics drop after you do chemo and then have to do it for a second time. I had an 85 percent survival rate and that won't be the same if I have to do it a second time. And if they couldn't cure me at 85, I have no hope that they could do it any less than that.

Ty: I think the main thing that we want to help you focus on now is getting your immune system strong again and getting your body healthy again. I know you are already getting there but just because you're out of the hospital, you're off the poison. You're able to get fresh air, get some vitamin D and just be happy. That's a big immune boost right there, is just laughing and having fun.

It's good to see you laughing and smiling. I know that will help you. But there are other things that we can do to help you. We can talk off-camera about that. So like I said, my concern is for that if they try to do it again. I don't think that when this video gets out and people see it, they're not going to—

Cassandra: There was controversy last year when the story went out. For this to go out again and say they are forcing me to do it again. I can't imagine what would happen.

Ty: No. To me, it's hard to believe that people were spreading the lie that you wanted to go ahead and die of cancer instead of doing chemo.

Cassandra: Everything gets misinterpreted in the media. And what people say and what they see on Facebook and what random blogs and websites say. I never wanted to die. I simply wanted to find a different way to live.

Ty: And you're going to live a long, healthy life. We'll help you do that. I'm glad that we have the connections with the best doctors and clinics and treatments and supplements and all that stuff, these natural remedies that people are using. I'll connect you with that without a problem.

But I'm really saddened by what they've done to you because, to me, it's criminal what they did to you. It makes me sad that you're only 17 and have had to go through that.

Cassandra: I made it through though. I wouldn't let them break me. They locked me away, but I'm still here.

Ty: That's clear that they haven't broken you and you've still got your happy spirit and you are glad to be alive and I'm just really glad that you've been able to share this with us today.

Cassandra: Thank you.

Ty: And I'm really proud of you.

Cassandra: Thank you.

Ty: Great job. Thank you, Cassandra.

Cassandra: You're welcome.

[end of transcript]

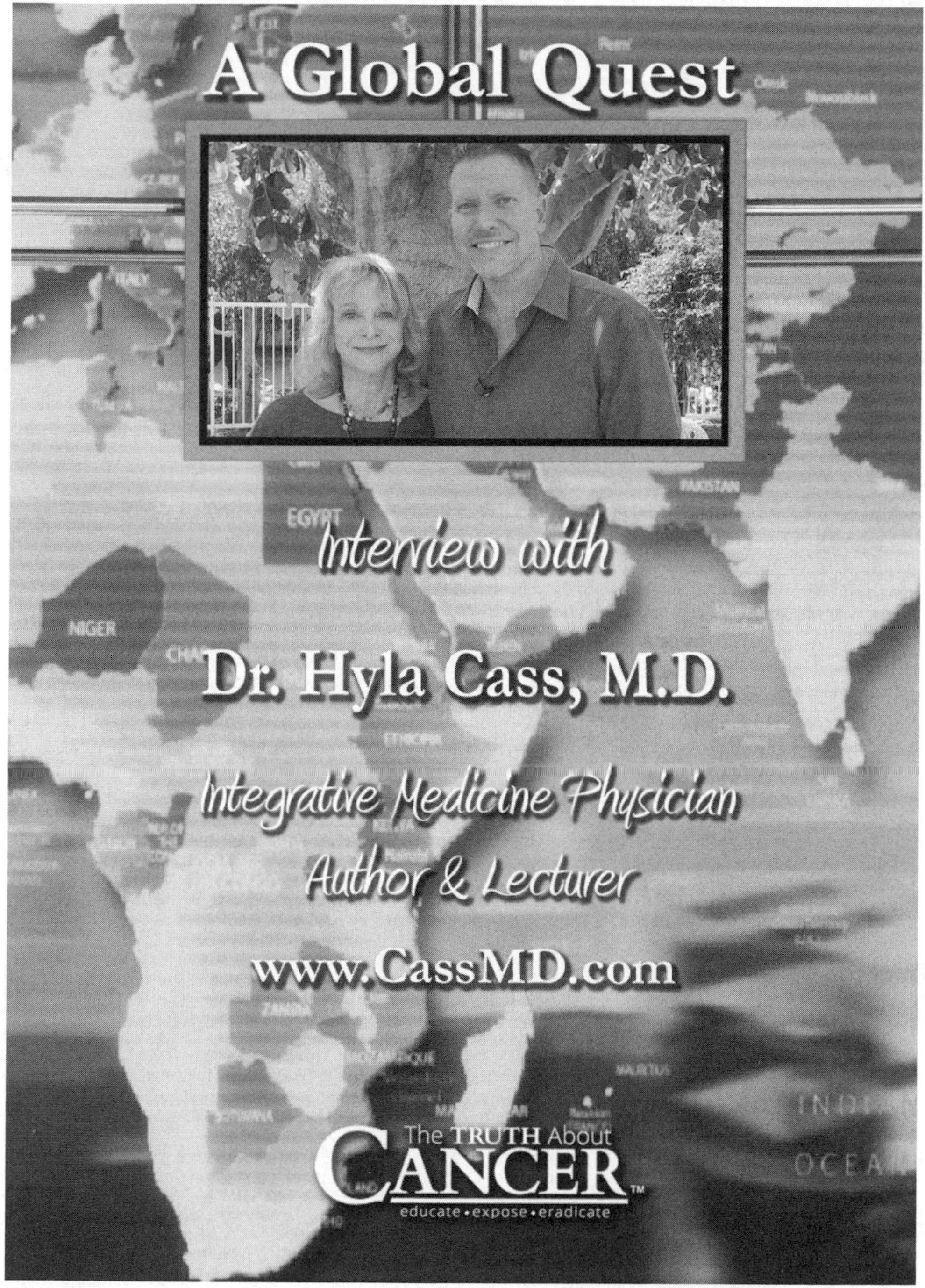
A Global Quest
Interview with
Dr. Hyla Cass, M.D.
Integrative Medicine Physician
Author & Lecturer
www.CassMD.com
The TRUTH About CANCER
educate • expose • eradicate

Ty: I'm here in a beautiful gazebo, sunny San Diego, California with Dr. Hyla Cass. Really appreciate you taking the time to talk to us today Dr. Cass.

Dr. Cass: Pleasure to be here.

Ty: Could you tell us a little bit about yourself? What you want the viewers to know about you.

Dr. Cass: Sure, I'm a holistic psychiatrist. I've been practicing medicine for over 25 years and my choice is always to use natural supplements and how the body's own healing processes operate rather than use medication or any other chemical intervention.

Ty: So Dr. Cass, tell us about what is chemo brain to start with and how can you—what natural treatments can you use to remedy this condition?

Dr. Cass: Well, here we are at a cancer conference talking about natural therapies and what I have found is many, many people who have undergone chemotherapy end up with this terrible condition called chemo brain where they can't think straight. They can't remember things. They can't remember where they put their keys or they can't remember—one woman she couldn't remember how to put dishes in the dishwasher.

I mean it's heart-breaking and what they're told by their oncologist is, A, be happy you're alive and B, it'll go away. It'll get better. It doesn't, it doesn't. It may wear off, usually not. And this is the same thing by the way, as—there's a kind of a brain fog that people get after any kind of surgery particularly if there's been heart, lung bypass. It really affects the brain and we need to do something about it and as a physician, I really want to help people.

So with chemo brain there are a number of things that I have found to be very helpful and one of them is neuro feedback, EEG feedback and I actually consult to a clinic called Chemo Brain Recovery, *chemobrainrecovery.com*. And what we do at this clinic is administer neuro feedback. We put electrodes here on the ears and put in earphones and some electrodes with paste on the head.

We don't stick them right into the scalp, just place them with some paste, electrode paste like a cardiogram and by giving a certain micro-current into the brain, it gives the brain a message to reform itself, to do what it needs to do to make it better and it's an amazing process because nature heals. We know how to heal ourselves. So when we give the right brainwave, when we put—and it's the right brainwave when it's just put in a position on your brain, your brain knows the right thing to do. We just give the right amount of current, very, very micro-current, very small. It's not a shock or anything.

Ty: Okay.

Dr. Cass: And the brain begins to find its own way and in a few sessions, people are thinking clearly, they have their memory back. We have this one woman Sherri who was unable to sleep so she came specifically for sleep and she went home, went to sleep, slept right through the night, right through—from when she came home and right through the night, got up the next morning and this is very unusual because she hadn't been able to sleep and she could remember all the things she couldn't do before. She was able to put the dishes in the dishwasher, make toast for her family. I mean this sounds simple and kind of silly like who can't do that, but when you have chemo brain, you can't do that.

Ty: That is so important for people to hear that are watching this because many folks, probably hundreds of thousands of people that are watching this now because we're going to have millions of viewers have undergone chemo and I guarantee that there's tens of thousands of people that are undergoing chemo that have chemo brain.

Before my grandmother died, she didn't undergo chemotherapy, but she was on so many prescription drugs that she would call me and she would say, "Ty I don't know how to turn on the TV." She couldn't remember, which button to push on the remote control.

Dr. Cass: Right.

Ty: So this is really important information for people to understand that they can detoxify their body, that they can cause their brain to not necessarily go through detoxification here, but that their brain can heal itself right? A mutual friend Robert Scott Bell, "The power to heal is yours."

Dr. Cass: Absolutely.

Ty: And it is, isn't it?

Dr. Cass: And not only that by the way you know you want to detox your body. You mentioned that's like a key word. You need to do a really good detox as well. So I'm not saying—

Ty: What does that mean? What's a good detox?

Dr. Cass: By the way using that neuro feedback is very useful, but I'm really looking at root cause. Let's go and fix the problem at its root. So we may have fixed the brain, but we still want to deal with any leftover toxicity. So antioxidants, oxygen therapies, all the different ways that people have that we have now that we didn't used to have for detoxing, saunas, infrared saunas and many, many—

Ty: I sit in one every night.

Dr. Cass: Many, many others, Epsom salts baths, on and on and on and some very sophisticated things with devices to take the toxins out and of course a clean diet and all of that is going to help to remove any residual chemo that should not be there. It's done its job, it needs to be eliminated from the body. Even after surgery when you have anesthesia and if you've had cancer surgery and anesthesia and then chemo, you've really had a shock to the body.

A lot of chemicals are circulating there so you really want to clean those up and then also for chemo brain, not everyone can get to neuro feedback and absolutely start on supplements and I have one called Brain Cell Support Plus that I love. My Brain Cell Support Plus it's good for chemo brain. It's good for aging brain. I've had some Alzheimer's patients who are doing so much better.

You can't cure Alzheimer's, but there's a lot you can do to give the body what it needs, give the brain what it needs in terms of what it can—raw materials to make neuro transmitters like phosphatidylcholine, phosphatidylserine, raw materials for building brain cell walls, vinpocetine and ginkgo, which helps the circulation in the brain.

So all of that are wonderful for helping chemo brain and people should know about this because their oncologists' not going to tell them. So take fish oil along with it, take fish oil, take Brain Cell Support Plus and then I have a few other things too when people have trouble sleeping.

I actually use my Nightly Calm because it has different amino acids and herbs in it that enhance what's called GABA, Gamma Aminobutyric Acid, which is the calming neuro transmitter. It's our natural built in chiller.

Ty: Chiller, I like that. So these are all great suggestions for people that may be undergoing or may be suffering from chemo brain because it is very real. The way that it's framed today is it sounds almost like a made up thing. Oh you have chemo brain, but it's real. It's very real to these people that are suffering from it.

Dr. Cass: Absolutely and by the way I can't give all the information here. This is a fairly short interview, I really appreciate the opportunity, but I have website, *cassmd.com* and I really want to encourage people to look at some of the programs I have and some of the supplements I have because I'm really out there trying to get people off of medication and on to the most natural products possible that work with the body's chemistry so that you can be the best you possible.

Ty: Well that's a noble goal. It's difficult in the United States and actually New Zealand specifically, because these are two countries that have what's called a DTCA, Direct-to-consumer advertising. So the pharmaceutical countries can run their drug ads on TV on radio—

Dr. Cass: And we can't.

Ty: And we can't, right. So that makes it kind of an uphill battle doesn't it?

Dr. Cass: Well, this is, I mean, it's crazy. Ask your doctor and then there's this whole big long list of you know—and you can get paralysis and this and this—and death, but ask your doctor if this is for you, "Well I'll take that death, that one—that death one."

Ty: Right.

Dr. Cass: Like are you serious?

Ty: Yeah you're taking a medication for a headache, but it may cause death.

Dr. Cass: I mean it's not funny, this is not funny.

Ty: It's really not.

Dr. Cass: But we can't make claims about supplements. I can't say you see this bottle of Brain Cell Support Plus, it will treat Alzheimer's disease. You can say that about the drugs that don't really do the job—

Ty: Right.

Dr. Cass: But we can't say that about something that actually does work or St. John's Wort for depression or SAMe for depression.

Ty: Right.

Dr. Cass: It's pretty crazy.

Ty: It really is.

Dr. Cass: And with the statins, people are given statins. They could use red rice yeast, they could use many other things for lowering cholesterol, tocotrienols, Vitamin E, many, many things and then take CoQ10 along with it if you're taking a statin. So if you're taking a statin and it's better not to, if you're taking a statin make sure you're taking coenzyme Q10 because otherwise you've become depleted. That's one aspect and the other is don't go on a statin in the first place and the other thing is, why is your cholesterol high. If you have high cholesterol, what's going on? You probably have metabolic syndrome because you're eating too many simple carbs. You're eating too much sugar and I just—

Ty: So you're going back to the root cause.

Dr. Cass: So I'm going back—I keep talking about, let's talk root cause, let's talk natural, let's get away from all the drugs and figure out what the body's message is. What's the body telling us? If we have high cholesterol, our body's telling us you're eating too many simple carbs. Eat fruits and vegetables, lots of veggies, high quality protein. Eat good food, your metabolic syndrome will go away, your blood pressure will come down.

Ty: Yeah.

Dr. Cass: Your cholesterol will come down. The weight off your middle will go away.

Ty: Well, you know one of the things that you said earlier was that we don't have a cure for Alzheimer's, but we want to get the brain what it needs so that really resonates with our message here because this is called, *The Quest for the Cures, The Global Quest for the Cures.* But really the cure is you. All we're doing is trying to give the body what it needs so that it works properly and when you give the body what it needs to work properly, when you give the brain what it needs to function properly, the body heals itself and so the real healer is in your own body, isn't that right?

Dr. Cass: Yep, we are our healer. The other thing is the big scourge of anti-depressants. Oh my heavens, I'm a psychiatrist and people come to me hooked on anti-depressants and when I say hooked it's because they're not doing well on them. They're not getting the anti-depressant, anti-anxiety effect. They may have at the beginning, they no longer are. So the side effects are worse than the actual effects, but they can't go off them.

Ty: Wow.

Dr. Cass: They can't get off them because of the terrible, terrible withdrawal effects, terrible.

Ty: And they're really not even side effects, they're really direct effects aren't they?

Dr. Cass: They are the effects and so what I have to do is help them very, very slowly to go off of that medication, very slowly because they've tried before. These people have tried before and their psychiatrists will say, "See look at that when you off of it, you really need it." No what they're going into is withdrawal, it's not that they really need it, but they really need it now.

So what I do is go off in very, very small increments and at the same time add in my own supplements that they can take to feed the brain what it really needs and it's—you add in more and more of a nutritional supplements as you lower the drug and then at the end you're just on the supplements and that's giving you the nutrition you need. You're getting the dopamine, the serotonin, serotonin from 5HTP. You're getting dopamine from tyrosine and phenylalanine. By the way if you have cancer you have to be careful about tyrosine and phenylalanine, that's another story. I mean everything is, it's all many-faceted.

Ty: Sure.

Dr. Cass: But we at least can get people off of the medication very gradually and very carefully and correctly.

Ty: You mentioned cancer, let's talk about electromagnetic pollution, EMF, there was a large study done in the late 80s that directly related cell phones to brain cancers. Talk about electromagnetic pollution, what is dirty electricity and what kind of effect could that have relating to cancer.

Dr. Cass: Well there's dirty electricity, which is a whole area, that's one whole big area. Magda Havas has done a great deal of work with that. So you can always look up her work. Magda Havas, H-A-V-A-S, and there are filters that you can put in your home to stop the dirty electricity, it's electricity that's not properly grounded and we all have electricity in our house where our houses are wired. That's one issue.

Then there's the Wi-Fi, that's a whole other, that's another level of radiation and that's affecting us terribly. It's absolutely increasing our cancer rate and when we think of children being exposed, babies in utero are exposed to cell phone radiation both by their mothers, but just because you're in a room with Wi-Fi. There's Wi-Fi everywhere, turn on your phone anywhere—

Ty: We're sitting right here in a Wi-Fi hotspot.

Dr. Cass: Turn on your phone and you're going to see a whole lot of Wi-Fi's show up, right? So we really do need to protect ourselves as much as we can. I read an article in the Huffington Post about it a while ago and these questions that are—devices that people have or little dots that they put on their phone and what I'd love to see is some really solid research on it so I can really say yes this is the thing to do, but we do notice that people that are very symptomatic when they use these various dots—dots that you wear around your neck, things you put on the phone.

Ty: I've seen them, you put them on the phone.

Dr. Cass: That they stop being symptomatic, that they stop having their headaches, dizziness whatever it is where they just could not use a cell phone or felt very sick around cell phones and Wi-Fi's.

Ty: What kind of advice would you have to parents that are—I read a statistic that's something like there's—in the United States alone there's something like 30 million children that are on their cell phones an average of four plus hours a day or something like that. I mean what advice can you give to parents? I mean you're already exposed to the Wi-Fi.

Dr. Cass: Kids should not be on cell phones and in some countries it's illegal. In China they just made it a crime to have a child under two hold a cell phone. So many countries are more enlightened than the US.

Ty: Well there was a big Swedish study that it was something like if you have an accumulated cell phone hour usage of like 20,000 hours, which really isn't that many hours when you look at the five years of use, it causes your brain cancer risk to explode like two or three times.

Dr. Cass: Well of course, if you look at photos you can see live cell exposures of cells of your brain when it's exposed or to cells when they're exposed to a cell phone field and when it's taken away. I mean clearly, it's clearly doing something. It's cooking our brain. A thermogram, you do a thermogram on the side of head—

Ty: I've seen the images.

Dr. Cass: Before and after, I mean the heating up, you are melting your brain cells. Not literally, but you're really making a mess and children should not be exposed and in schools in many countries they have removed Wi-Fi. They've removed it so this is something we have to think about and about cell towers near schools, I mean I know for example in Israel you can't have cell towers near schools and I believe they don't have Wi-Fi in the schools there anymore either.

Ty: They shouldn't.

Dr. Cass: So many countries are far more enlightened than we are.

Ty: And you know I agree with you, many countries are. It seems like we're way behind the eight ball.

Dr. Cass: Well it's not enlightened, it's—

Ty: Follow the money.

Dr. Cass: Follow the money.

Ty: I've got to agree with you. I'm looking at my notes here. Actually, it was the Swedish National Institute study, 2,000 hours of cell phone not 20, 2,000 hours of cell phone use cause a 250 percent increase in malignant brain cancer and if you look at 2,000 hours, the average on it four hours a day. It doesn't take long to get to that 2,000.

Dr. Cass: Yeah, and please don't hold the phone to your ear, please don't.

Ty: Use a Bluetooth speakerphone.

Dr. Cass: Speakerphone. I don't know that Bluetooth is much of mitigation.

Ty: Okay, well, there's a lot of things that we can do practically and I think what we are after in this "Global Quest for the Cure" is to give people practical advice that they can mitigate their risk, their exposures to these toxins that could cause DNA damage and eventually to cancer and other diseases. So the information that you've shared with us today is a real step in that direction so I really am grateful that you've taken the time to talk to us, Dr. Cass.

Dr. Cass: My pleasure and I also have some other books that people might be interested in.

Ty: Tell us about them.

Dr. Cass: I have, *Eight Weeks to Vibrant Health* that I am very proud of. It matches your shirt too. This book really is a summary of what I do in my practice and what it does is it empowers people to become their own doctor. Now not really, I'm not saying you have to totally be your own doctor, but that's where to start. Start by taking charge of your health, taking the questionnaire for example. There's a very cool questionnaire right at the beginning where you can figure out whether your issues have to do with thyroid, blood sugar, adrenals.

I mean who knows about like—you're not likely to go to your doctor and say, "I have a thyroid problem. I have an adrenal problem." People don't know, but once you've done this, for example do you have dizziness when you stand up quickly, do you crave sweets, do you have palpitations when you eat something sweet, mood swings, poor concentration, anyway with the different combinations that's all under the blood sugar imbalance issue. Do you have weight gain and difficulty losing it, dry skin, dry brittle hair, that's under the thyroid department?

By the time you've done the quiz and it takes you maybe 15 minutes to do it, you know what section of this book you need to focus on whether it's metabolic syndrome, which I was talking about earlier with cholesterol and weight around the middle and high blood pressure, thyroid adrenals, hormones, women's hormones, men's hormones. This is more focused on women's hormones than men's hormones, but a lot of the other things are in there.

Ty: It's a great book by the way, you gave me a copy of that about a year ago when we were speaking together in Asheville, great book and I highly recommend it and as Robert Scott Bell says, "The power to heal is yours." And just because you don't have a degree doesn't mean that you can't learn and that's a great tool.

Dr. Cass: Yeah, it's a great way to give you a vocabulary to talk to your doctor or your health care provider, to look up things online and have some education idea about it, about your own position vis-à-vis all of these issues because I know when you tend to read something, I know I have that and I have that, oh no I have that, everything you read you have, but here you can actually take a questionnaire and see if it really is so.

Ty: Very practical.

Dr. Cass: And what lab tests you can ask for and really figure out what's going on under the hood there.

Ty: Well, that's excellent advice and I just am very grateful for you taking the time to talk with us today.

Dr. Cass: Pleasure.

Ty: Thank you so much. ***[end of transcript]***

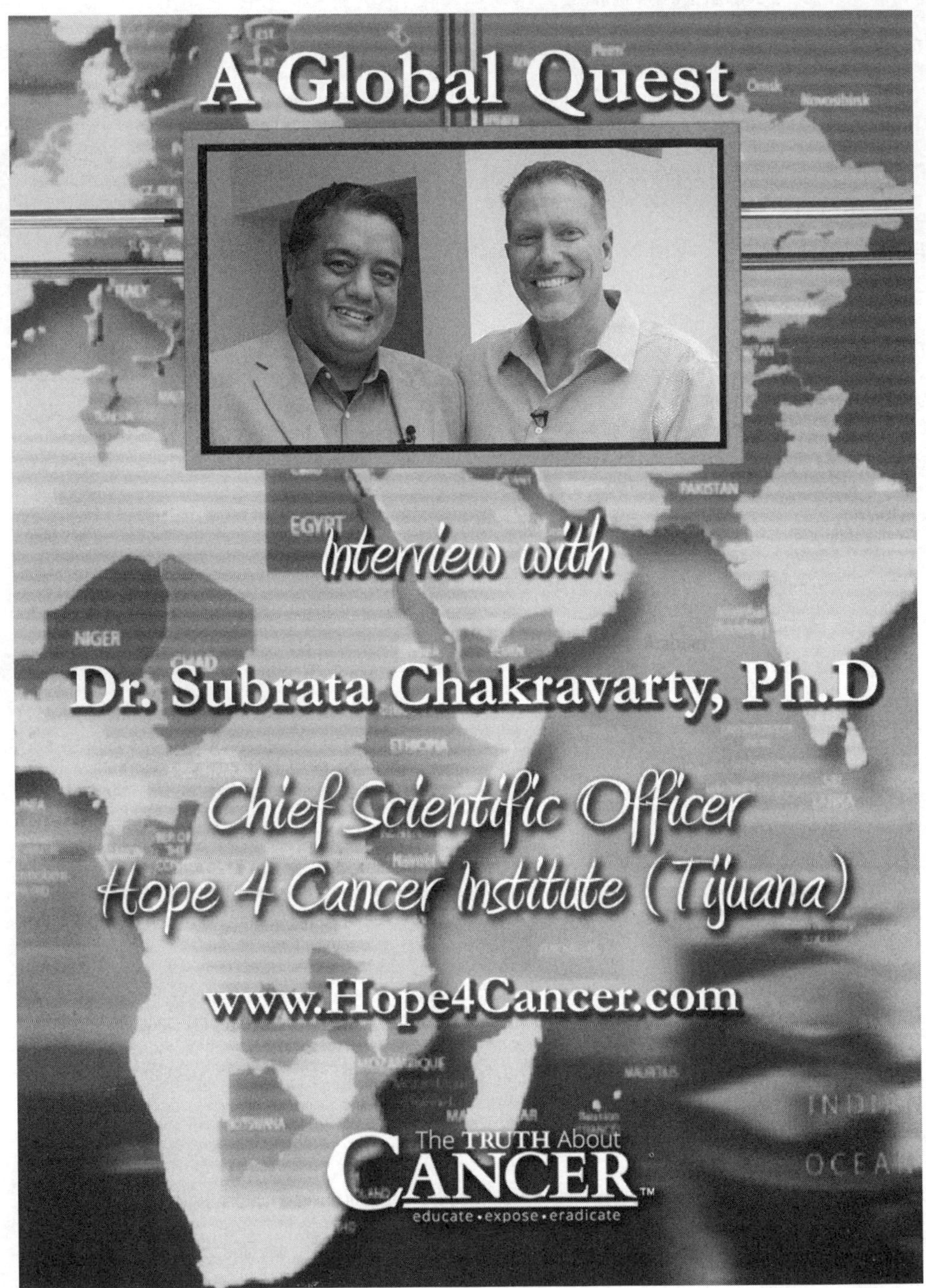
A Global Quest
Interview with
Dr. Subrata Chakravarty, Ph.D
Chief Scientific Officer
Hope 4 Cancer Institute (Tijuana)
www.Hope4Cancer.com
The TRUTH About
CANCER
educate • expose • eradicate

Ty: I am here with Dr. Dr. Chakravarty Chakravarty.

Dr. Chakravarty: That's right.

Ty: I am going to say it quickly before I screw it up. Thanks for joining me today.

Dr. Chakravarty: Thank you, Ty. It's a pleasure to be here.

Ty: We are here at Hope4Cancer in Tijuana. And I wanted to get your—a little bit about your background.

Dr. Chakravarty: Certainly. I'm the Chief Science and Technology Officer of Hope4Cancer Institute. I come from a background of conventional science. I'm a trained chemist. I got my PhD in organic, medicinal, and computational chemistry back in 1997. Since then I've been working in different research projects that involve cancer.

As a scientist, I was trained to work with a lot of chemotherapy agents. I did a lot of my doctoral work on Taxol. A lot of the work that I did after that was on kinase related anticancer agents as well. So that was where I was coming from.

Somewhere around the year 2000—about 2 years into my pharma career—I walked into a Wal-Mart and I find this gentleman with this little boy. And I was there with my son as well. We started talking and he introduced himself as Tony Jimenez. That's how we first met.

You have to understand that at that time I was a skeptical scientist who didn't know anything other than his science. And here I meet a person who is talking about healing cancer patients with alternative medicine. I was fascinated. I was really truly attracted to what he stood for. We struck up a friendship for a long time. It didn't stop me from being skeptical but it definitely kept me really fascinated for years.

So for about five or six years we maintained our friendship and we stayed in touch. One day he taps me on the shoulder and said, "You know what? Can you come and work with us for few writing projects that we have?" So that's how we started working together.

And then he said, "Well, we are opening a supplement company. Could you come and lead that company?" I said, "I don't know anything about leading a company. And I'll have to give up my pharma career to do that." He said, "Well, will you?" And I thought about it for five minutes and I said, "Okay. Yes, I will." And that's how we started working together.

Honestly, it was just the man that attracted me—you know, Tony. I knew that he was a great man doing great things and he was accomplishing something in life. And I was really at a point in time where, although I did enjoy what I was doing from a research point of view, I just felt that it was a dead-end and it wasn't getting me to where I wanted to go, not just from a career perspective but from doing something significant in life. I wanted to make a difference.

Most of the work that we were doing in pharma was very limiting in my mind. We weren't solving any problems. We were just creating more and more drugs that we are getting out there and going to the FDA and either getting rejected or approved.

When I started working with kinases, I kind of realized the problem. Most of the times when we are driving along a highway—if I can give an analogy—you know, you're driving on the roads and you hit a traffic light. You have choices. You can make a right, you can make a left, you can go straight and maybe you can make a u-turn at the worst-case scenario. In the case of when you're working with drugs, that is how scientists make decisions. You're going in there and saying, "You know what? With this drug we can either go right or we can go left." But the body is not like that.

When you study kinases, you study the way the body's biochemistry works. It is so many processes happening at the same time. It's like an accident waiting to happen. You can't control that with a drug that is built on a thought process of going, "Two choices: left and right." You have to be able to address the whole thing in one shot.

That just got me thinking that—how does the body not have more accidents doing what it does? It's an incredible beast. And that's when I realized that there has to be more to medicine than just creating drugs and trying to solve things by cause and effect. So I decided to take that leap and walk into the world of natural medicine with Dr. Tony.

One of the first assignments that I did for Hope4Cancer was to work on the home program in our Aftercare Department that needed to get strengthened. Working with patients directly for two years transformed my life because that's when I really understood what cancer was all about.

It wasn't about drugs. It wasn't about the treatments, but it was about the people who were suffering that needed the help and that needed the information that we could provide them. So that's what got me into that, working with Dr. Tony.

Ty: Well, that's interesting. So that was something that you felt, I guess, disillusioned in big pharma and you felt like that was not being discussed and that was not even in the picture.

Dr. Chakravarty: That was not in the picture and it had all become about money. It was all about disease management. It was not about curing the disease. It was about how long you can keep the disease going in fact. I would hear a lot in our meetings and in the town hall meetings that it was all about making the shareholders happy.

And I'm like, "You know what? I don't want to make the shareholders happy." That's not the point of what we are doing. We want to be able to solve bigger problems than to see how much money goes into the shareholders pockets.

Ty: Wow, that's really fascinating that in the shareholders meetings they are just talking about making money, really. So with a big pharmaceutical company, what's the way they make money? They sell more drugs.

Dr. Chakravarty: They sell more drugs, exactly. And they have to keep on selling more drugs, hopefully for them to the same people, over and over and over again.

I don't want to take away from that though because there are a lot of great people from the pharmaceutical industry who have devoted their lives and have discovered great things. There are a lot of things that we know today that we can apply into the work that we do here that has been developed based on strong science. And I rely a lot on that in being able to structure what we do here.

But at the same time I think we are missing the big picture there. That is where I wanted to make a difference. Get out of there and run towards the big picture. And that is what Dr. Jimenez is running towards.

Ty: And so now you are.

Dr. Chakravarty: And here I am.

Ty: Dr. C, I want you to elaborate now a little bit on one of the potentially most confusing aspects of cancer and nutrition and that's sugar. So we always hear, "Cancer cells feed on sugar."

So elaborate on sugar because we were talking last night at dinner with Dr. Tony and several other people and sugar is a word that's not specific in the English language. It's like, "Hey, I love my wife. I love pizza." Love is not specific there. You don't love your wife the same way you love pizza. It's the same with sugar. There are a lot of different types of sugars. But is it true that cancer feeds on sugar? And explain that please.

Dr. Chakravarty: Well, that's a great question. And it's such a huge question that we could do a whole conference on that and still not come to any conclusions because there will be so many different points of views. But for the sake of people who will be listening to this—and I would like to simplify it as much as possible, but at the same time not oversimplify it, too, so that people make wrong decisions.

Sugar metabolism in the body is probably the most complex process that happens in the body. It's something that without proper regulation, it can be the cause of so many different diseases. It can start from—of course cancer is implicated. You're looking at diabetes, you're looking at so many other chronic diseases that have a lot to do with the metabolism of sugars. I think that the lack of understanding of how that works has really made us all pay a huge price with regard to that.

Very recently I wrote an article about food addiction where sugar is one of the things that people get addicted to very easily. It's not just a question of it being a molecule. It's almost like a hormone that can impact the brain into wanting more and more of that.

So the question is, what is the reality of sugar and how does it actually impact cancer?

If you want to break it down into simple things, from a molecular standpoint sugar has got six carbon atoms. It's made up of carbon, hydrogen, and oxygen. And you're looking at sugar as not just one molecule, as you said. It's a multiple series of molecules.

You can think of little Lego pieces, glucose being one of them, the simplest form of sugar. Another one is fructose which you find in a lot of fruits. And there are several other little pieces that you can then join together. For example you can take a glucose Lego piece and you can join it to a fructose Lego piece and bond them together and there you have table sugar—sucrose.

So you have all these different forms. And you have the complex carbohydrates which involve many of those pieces that come together. The beauty about sugar is that they all look very similar to each other—all these Lego pieces—but they are all incredibly different from each other as well.

Glucose is essential for the body. If you look at how glucose works in the body—and this is a confusion that I hope a lot of people will—I want to clarify here. The body needs to have a minimum amount of glucose floating around in it. We need to have about between 5 to 10 micromoles per litre of glucose in the blood at all times. If we don't have that our brains will stop functioning. And our brain, of course, controls everything else. So without that sugar we don't have life.

So the question is, how do we deprive our body of sugar, hoping that we are going to kill the cancer cell, and yet hope that we are going to survive?

We can't do that. In fact the body has got compensatory systems set up so that if you do deprive it from sugar, it will find somewhere else where it can generate sugar from and it will boost up the sugar levels once again to the standard concentration that it expects. In the case of diabetics you will see a lot of variation in that sugar level and that's why their health becomes—why they have that risk factor that they are dealing with.

So the question then becomes, from a practical perspective, what is a cancer patient to do? Should they not eat sugar or should they eat sugar?

The good thing there is that the source of sugar matters. How you are eating the sugar makes a difference. But if you look at the patterns of sugar-eating back in the 1960s most of our sugar came from sugarcane. And that sugarcane—if you look at what it's made of, it is mostly sucrose. So it is 50 percent glucose and 50 percent fructose.

Over time what has happened is that high-fructose corn syrup has kind of caught up with it. If you look at the composition of high-fructose corn syrup it's again roughly 50/50 glucose and fructose. You have different varieties like the 42 or 55 which give you the percentage of the fructose. But essentially it is about the same in balance.

The only difference between fructose and regular sugar is that, in this case, the monomers are separate. They are not joined together like they are in sucrose. So the body has to go through a process of actually breaking down the sucrose into its subunits.

Does that make a difference? Research doesn't tell yet if it does, however there are a lot of indications to show that high-fructose corn syrup has got several negative health effects.

Part of the reason that we have to be cautious about high-fructose corn syrup is that there is a lot of sugar, glucose, being absorbed, too, in the body. So it's not just about fructose, it's also about glucose. So now the glucose level goes up and it goes through a spike.

If I really have to boil it down to the most important thing that we need to do is to control those spikes. If you think of cancer—inside cancer there is a processing center for glucose. Inside any cell there is always a processing center for glucose. They are what we call the hexokinase receptors, HK2—so to speak—in cancer cells and in normal cells as well. The only difference is that there are way more HK2s in cancer cells than they are in regular cells.

The problem that happens is that now you've got a hungry dog out here. And you've got a dog that is not so hungry, that will get satiated easily. And if you have a sudden spike of sugar—guess what? The hungry dog is going to overfeed on that sugar. So what we really are looking to do is to stop the spikes of sugar. That's why we are looking to give people diets that have got a low glycemic index.

A lot of people think, "Okay, fruits and vegetables." You know, that is something that we recommend for cancer and that a cancer patient should eat fruits and vegetables. A lot of people think, "Oh my god. Fruits and vegetables are so high in sugar. How is that going to affect our cancer cells?" The answer lies really in not so much the composition of the sugar itself, but in how it is delivered.

So in the case of sugars, if you look at the balance of what content most fruits have, it's different. Some fruits have got a higher level of fructose. Some fruits have got a higher level of glucose. Some of them have sucrose. So you have various varieties.

Apples, pears—they are pretty good to eat because they have got a relatively higher fraction of fructose to glucose, but they have both and they have sucrose as well. But they also have a lot of fiber with them. So when you're eating them what the fiber does is that it slows down the absorption of the sugars into the body.

And that makes sure that you are not going through those incredible spikes that are causing the absorption of the sugars into the cancer cells which then feeds into their mechanism of growth because the more sugar they get, the more they can grow and they can replicate themselves. So we try to avoid that.

Ty: That makes a lot of sense. So really what we are looking at is we want to avoid the spikes in the sugar or in the insulin. And the way that that is accomplished is by eating things that are natural. Because then you've got the glucose, the fructose, the sucrose or whatever it is, but it's coupled with fiber, that stops the insulin spikes. So then you don't have the problem with the cancer cells being fed by this because it's got the fiber attached.

Dr. Chakravarty: Well, the cancer cells would still be fed. It's not like they will—they will take nutrition whether you like it or not. The question is that you don't want to overfeed them. You don't want to give them too much fuel that they don't deserve.

Sometimes a lot of people ask this question that, "Why we don't just give a high-fructose diet because glucose goes into the path when that is the energy from that is used. Fructose itself cannot be directly used as energy. It can convert in the liver into glucose and then get to the cells. But it's an indirect route. Most of the fructose that we eat ends up as fat. And that causes other problems.

So now when you're looking at a high-fructose diet, now you've got your lipid levels going up, your triglycerides going up and all of a sudden your obesity is going up, so all those are connected together and cause different types of problems that we don't want to have.

I think the ideal is to have fruits and vegetables that are low in sugar, maybe a 1:1 balance of fructose and glucose, things that will absorb slowly in the body. Have complex carbs because we need carbohydrates. But make your body work to break it down so that it's absorbed at a slow rate. And that will make sure that the cancer is not being fed at an incredible pace.

Ty: What about juicing? So you got juicing where you're basically—you got a bunch of sugar in the juice, but you don't have the fiber. It's been removed.

Dr. Chakravarty: Well, juicing is again a slightly controversial topic. Very often—the way I would look at it in this case is that the proof is in the pudding. There are so many cancer patients who have done very well with juicing. So it makes sense that juicing is a good idea.

What I would definitely tell people to do though when they are juicing is to make sure that what they put in the juice—they have to be careful about that. If they are putting in too many fruits which are very high in sugar, their sugar levels are going to go up. You are going to go through a spike. And what you have to be careful about there is that you don't let that happen.

At the end of the day caloric intake is extremely important, whether it's through sugar or through different forms there has to be a balanced amount of calories that any patient is consuming during the day. That has been one of the big things.

If you really look at history—1960s we used to consume about a 100 pounds of sugar in all its various forms per year per person. Now it's somewhere around a 120 pounds per year per person. So that just tells you that that 20 pounds extra has to go somewhere and it's feeding things that don't need to be fed.

Ty: And a hundred years ago it was like five pounds.

Dr. Chakravarty: It was.

Ty: So it's really crazy the amount of sugar that we are intaking now, isn't it?

Dr. Chakravarty: Indeed.

Ty: So I guess maybe a good rule of thumb is that if you're going to eat foods that are high in sugar, eat the whole foods.

Dr. Chakravarty: Exactly.

Ty: So you've got the processed sugars that are not going to have the fiber, the man-made sugars, and the white sugars.

Dr. Chakravarty: Stay away from those, absolutely. And if you have to juice, lots of vegetables in your juice.

And once again it's about balance. For example with the potatoes you've got starch. Starch is a complex carbohydrate. It takes a lot to break it down. So that's why it may not cause massive spikes in the sugar. That's why eating potatoes, I personally think, is not such a bad idea.

But what I would definitely recommend people to do—and I think is an important point for anybody—is to seek advice of a good nutritionist, especially if you're dealing with a disease situation. Good nutritionists can really guide you very carefully because there are too many parameters associated with any one of these statements that I've made.

Sugar is something that we should not take lightly. It is—you know, how much of it should you take, how many of different sources? One of our scientists I was talking to recently said that, "If you're going to eat sugars, just make sure that you're eating it from a variety of different sources as opposed to any one source." I think that's a great advice to give as long as the total caloric intake is also in control.

Ty: So maybe a good rule of thumb would be sure you watch the glycemic index.

Dr. Chakravarty: Absolutely yes.

Ty: Eat things with a lower glycemic index.

Dr. Chakravarty: Exactly, yes.

Ty: Very good. Well, Dr. C, thank you for sharing with us today. I really appreciate it.

Dr. Chakravarty: It's my pleasure. Thank you.

Ty: You bet. Take care. ***[end of transcript]***

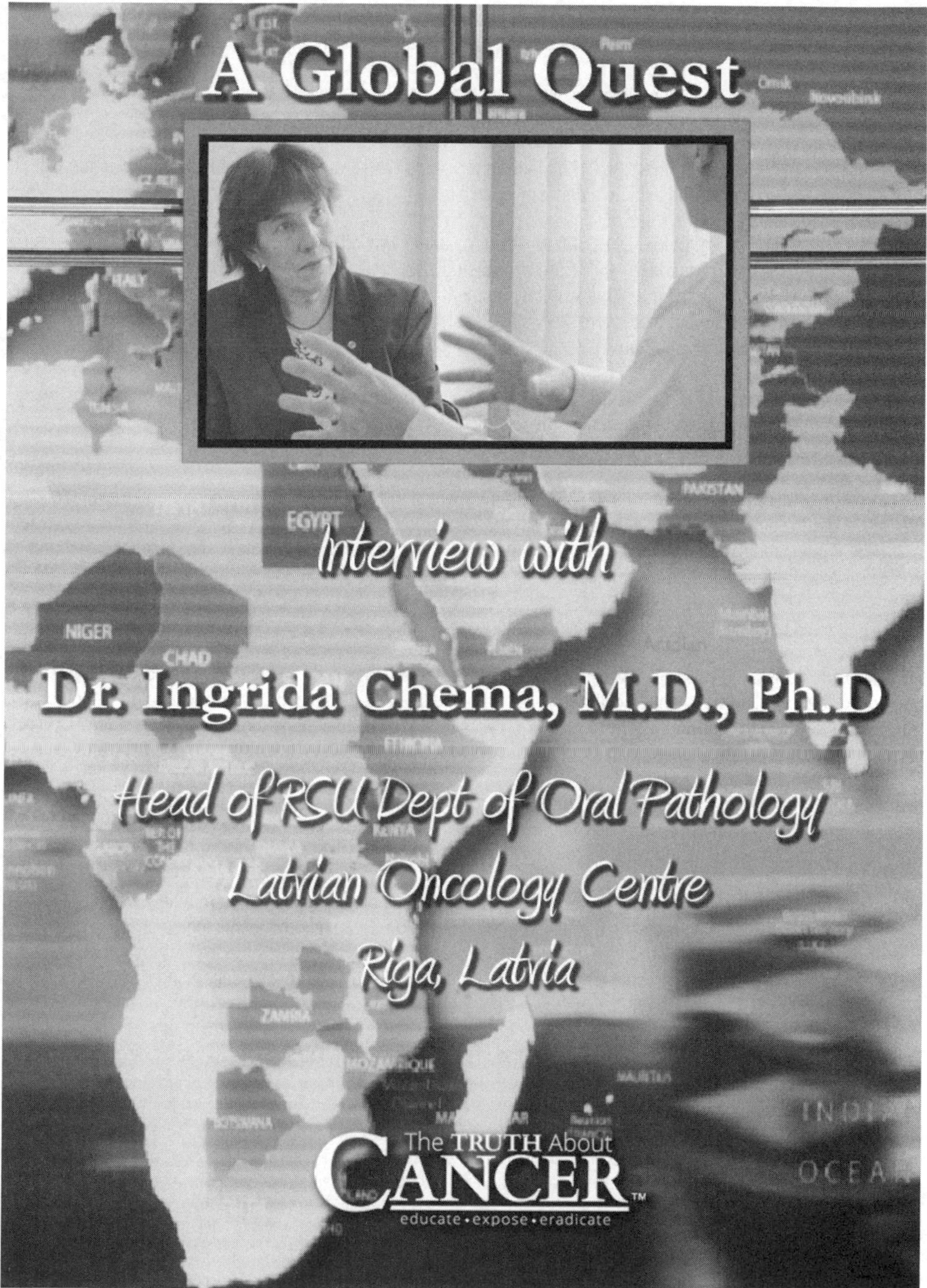
A Global Quest
Interview with
Dr. Ingrida Chema, M.D., Ph.D
Head of RSU Dept of Oral Pathology
Latvian Oncology Centre
Riga, Latvia
The TRUTH About
CANCER
educate • expose • eradicate

Ty: I'm really happy to be here today in Riga, Latvia at the Riga Stradins University with Dr. Ingrid Chema. Could you share with our viewers a little bit of your background in medicine?

Dr. Chema: [Translated 00:00:22 to 00:00:37] I have a credit from the Dentistry Faculty in 1979 but my way to oncology was a little bit not usual, it was a little bit unusual.

[Translated 00:00:50 to 00:01:01] More than ten years I have worked in a small town outside the big city as a surgeon and also as a dentistry specialist.

[Translated 00:01:12 to 00:01:28] And after ten years I was offered to come back to this premises here and to the clinic (inaudible - 00:01:34) and to study for the Dentistry Surgeon. [Translated 00:01:43 to 00:02:03] So it turned out at the very last moment that there were no places for students at the Dentistry Surgery but there were places in Oncology. So at the last moment I switched my thoughts and I entered the Oncology Faculty.

[Translated 00:02:20 to 00:02:35] I started to work actively, intensively in 1989 and I continued to work in this until 2004. And I still work in the Oncology Center, yes. And so I continued to work in the Oncology Center.

[Translated 00:02:57 to 00:03:26] Since the very beginning in 1989, I was working and I have started to get the patients with melanoma and with the cancer localized in the mouth. And that was the time when I got introduced to the Professor, Dr. (inaudible - 00:03:47) who you will meet, the next specialist and also Professor (inaudible - 00:03:26).

Ty: What treatments are you currently using to treat cancer here at the hospital?

Dr. Chema: [Translated 00:04:06 to 00:04:39] As a Dentist Methodology Institute still, we have some patients with cancer in the mouth and localizations but before with these patients, the On Point Center, Oncological Center. However here we have mostly patients that have cancer in the mouth. In the Oncology Center we have mostly patients with mouth cancer, and mostly these cancers are squamous cell carcinomas.

And of course, how do we treat? It depends on the pathology of course. We have to start with what is kind of morphology is it? Which kind of grade is it? Is this high? Is it graduated, is it more graduated or is it low graduated and which is the best cancer treatment?

And of course times change. And then I started to notice the style was mmm, maybe… The style was maybe to start with radiation therapy and then operation. But of course technologies cost more and more and the cost to start follow up, also the relevant standards and this means we have to see first the grade and then we can start with operation and then radiation therapy, so depending on squamous cell carcinoma (inaudible - 00:06:06).

Ty: Okay. So it depends upon the staging, the grade of the cancer, but you typically are going to start with radiation and surgery.

Dr. Chema: And of course, radiation, and surgery. Yeah. That's the main treatment. And we're learning hormone therapy, not so often, not so often. Of course it's possible to use also chemotherapy in squamous cell carcinomas but it's not usually. It depends; if it's a very advanced stage, yes. Then we advise to—we have special counseling and then we advise this chemotherapy. But some of that treatment regarding the histology, surgery, radical surgery plus radiation therapy.

Ty: Do you ever include Rigvir in your treatment protocol?

Dr. Chema: Yes. Regarding Rigvir, of course regarding the skin, the facial skin and the head and neck skin, they have melanomas and I think for advanced stages. And then if I have to say how many per year, probably… Of course I'm not the only maxillofacial surgeon. I have my colleagues also but maybe totally they per year 50 new patients, new patients we've seen on this other region.

Of course we have sometimes seen other therapy. They also have also melanoma but regarding the skin. Yes, regarding the skin, the official style is that when the patients come. We observe clinically. Then we do dermoscopy and of course we are advised to do it as a department and do a radical excision.

Before this of course if the patient put it that it was advised also to order some biopsy of the neck to exclude lymph nodes. The official style is that before going to the Department, one week before the operation, they can do injection with Rigvir to stimulate the immune system. Why one week before? It means that in your system, after Rigvir injections then we can see to work we need seven days and then how to see the result is the best course of operation.

Then follows operation and after this operation they advise to go to an immunologist and the immunologist asks two things. The first thing of course they have to know what is the conclusion of the histologists, which kind of blood and vessel, and second to do the lymphocyte calculations because you have to understand how it works the patient's immune system.

But I don't know what. Actually it was according to Advisor Professor [Montagna]. She once told me one thing. It was proved also in situ, in people it was proved that if you do injections around, or maybe directly in the tumor, you can get angiolysis of cells.

And knowing this, that Rigvir can cause direct angiolysis and knowing that seven days we need primary tumors began to start the lymphocyte and lymph node site reactions. Actually they were given both before the operation to do around the primary tumor injections. Changing the needle, we go around injections and saw during this week that lymphocytes began to form and they began to form like a wall around this primary tumor. Then it gives assurance also to the patient is doing in the next operation. Yeah?

But this wall will examine cells with something ran which lymphocytes will catch. Yeah? I'm sure that we will—very good to do this excision but no cells will run away and go around and there will be no metastasis. Actually it's like a wall which preserves us.

Ty: Okay. That's very interesting. So you say that the Rigvir injections one week before surgery cause angiolysis. Could you explain to the people watching, what is angiolysis?

Dr. Chema: Angiolysis is that big word for a solution that works directly on the melanoma cells and these melanoma cells already on the third day if I remember, according to the expert in the medical study, against localization. And the cells slowly will self-destruct. Shortly, this treatment destroys the cells.

Ty: So the Rigvir causes angiolysis, which is the cells are destroyed, and you said that it also forms like a protective wall around the tumor so there is no metastasis, no spreading.

Dr. Chema: No, we hope. You see it gives for us no such hope but maybe it is so. At first our cells were not examined with microscopes and we cannot say. But of course we cannot do the injection around very close. We do it in the distance about ten centimeters have to not … Actually again I have to state that every case we look at individually, what would be best.

But I have to say now one thing. They have not officially said and approved rules how to treat melanoma and non-melanoma cancers, and if rules are written. But for patients with melanoma we have to organize a counseling where there will participate immunologist, a maxillofacial surgeon, general oncologist, (inaudible - 00:13:21) therapists and actually to make solutions what will be best for this patient.

So it's not written in our rules. Of course because what we did before and of course it was not a solution of one person. Of course we are a small group of colleagues, one immunologist and also my colleague a general oncologist and we always come together and everybody states their thoughts and we all decide what will be best. But in general, actually yes, they do this in mass source injections all around the tumor.

Ty: So you have a team of experts that gets together and you decide more of an individualized approach for the patient.

Dr. Chema: Yes, it's actually very important. Every person is so different and they have to know how to speak to this person, how to explain things and explain what the risk is, what were the results we can get, maybe what problems. No, actually with Rigvir there are not problems maybe, maybe problems more with the disease, what we… Of course we always have to tell the patient, but the patient should be the force that is going to the department, be prepared to do this.

But patients which even couldn't understand what is melanoma and then they think it's very easy disease and other example have patients may come with other problems. A very simple woman saw a papilloma of the skin and they saw on the nose, was a very big… is was melanoma. I told the patient, "What do you mean it got on your nose?" "Oh I have some years already. No problem." But it is a big problem if you don't treat it.

Ty: You mentioned that with Rigvir—you mentioned that there is no problems. You mean there are no side effects to Rigvir?

Dr. Chema: No. It's rarely so, yeah. I've have for many years now I've had my own practice, this is oncology, let's calculate weekly since 1989 I never saw some side effects, rarely, never. Not some other after these injections or a week after the injections or even some (inaudible - 00:16:09) or ah, maybe it's only—I remember it was at the very beginning. It was I think this small other place, a small edema. But I remember only one such small case but never side effects. And what can be better. If you have medication and there is no side effects it will help, but it will never harm. You know?

Ty: Yeah. That sounds like the kind of medication you should be prescribing. So in 20 years I guess, 20 years… has it?

Dr. Chema: Twenty years ago.

Ty: Really no side effects, except an edema. I know a lot of people are watching this documentary are probably on chemotherapy and radiation right now. Is Rigvir something that could be prescribed while they are on chemo and radiation or do they need to get off first?

Dr. Chema: No actually, no. Radiation has no effect but I remember when I started in the end of the 90s, the end of the 80s and the beginning of the 90s it was of course advanced melanoma stages and metastasis, you can give some radiation therapy and may be some places first such it was prescribed, your advice will prescribe radiation therapy. But actually as far as I remember in our department it's really very rare and now it's a no no to give somebody recommendation regarding radiation therapy.

Yeah what I thought of chemotherapy of course I can speak only about myself. I never recommend it because I know one effect of one. No, actually I know side effects of chemotherapy and I know effects of Rigvir and of course my thoughts are only about Rigvir and I will always protect Rigvir.

But of course meanings are different and yeah, meanings are different and you know we have warnings and rules and there are some restrictions regarding some rules and chemo preparations, of course also.

But, again, I say only one thing. Very particular you will not interview other immunologists, Professor Dona Simona, she told me one case regarding one young girl. Half the melanoma it was not on the neck region. It was on her body and they recommended chemotherapy. And of course it was sad because it became forced and forced and forced, and what to do now, what to do now. The situation is very bad, and actually very, very bad.

And the woman started to think what she can do, they did it. And the woman decided Rigvir and she began to feel better and better and actually she is alive and feels better and she had actually also metastasis, but not there is none of it. But actually in the treatment with Rigvir, there was like a big jump to better side. Not what we finally have to say but…

Ty: So then you, from a personal perspective, you said you looked at chemotherapy versus Rigvir and you saw all the side effects of chemotherapy. Rigvir, no side effects. So you support Rigvir. And you mentioned the case of the young lady who was getting worse and worse and worse on chemotherapy; Rigvir got her better.

I guess maybe I didn't ask the question clear enough. For people that are watching, that their doctor has already prescribed chemo and radiation or one or the other, is Rigvir something that they might be able to consider even though they are undergoing these other treatments? Or are these treatments that they need to get off first before they might look into Rigvir?

Dr. Chema: [Translated 00:20:17 to 00:20:19] Yeah. I think it could be compared also but of course my thoughts are that when when we counsel on those thoughts really to work, they have to be patient. It will be honestly, if they could tell the patient more, the patient can also get his thoughts what he would like to do better.

But you know this is a very sensible question. It is very sensible question because there are colleagues which are very, how do you say, only on the side of chemotherapy of course. They believe only in chemotherapy.

But of course, yeah, to answer your question, of course I think it could be also combined but not together. First may be one and then we have to check the blood tests, what is growing and what is going with lymphocytes and maybe we can also add Rigvir. Yeah.

Ty: Okay.

Dr. Chema: The way I see it is not the problem, but that would be nice. What I do in my faculty, of course, I tell our students, dental faculty students about this Rigvir and what good things we can do and observe.

Of course it would be nice if such things could be taught also the medical faculty, that's many more. Rigvir is popular, but more and more may be popularized here also for students because students are the next generation. They are ready for other thoughts. They are not following thoughts strictly but then they saw that it's really good ethic and good move that I hope they will make the right solution. So that's my opinion.

Ty: So then you personally believe that educating the next generation of doctors about Rigvir is a step in the right direction.

Dr. Chema: Also examples one of the best because we have to think more about these new doctors who will come after us and who will work here; and they should be good prepared for this and they should know everything. Not a nice thing about chemotherapy but also about all the law (inaudible - 00:22:55).

Ty: So to be intellectually honest they need to teach the next generation not only about chemotherapy but about these other treatments like Rigvir that are virtually free of side effects.

Dr. Chema: Yeah. Exactly. Of course they can speak what they need more of hours so for students and all our software is of course limited. But it depends on the doctor who is given these practical classes. And Professor Dona is one of our best immunologists and she works in the Oncology Center and she works with the medical students and our dental students and I'm sure that she's speaking about Rigvir. So I hope in the future it will be good.

Ty: The last question. If you were to give advice to someone that's been recently diagnosed with cancer, what would you tell them, what question or questions should they ask their oncologist before beginning treatment?

Dr. Chema: [Translated 00:24:08 to 00:24:19] Yeah, what to ask. Of course every patient will ask, "What now will be with me and what will be the future?" And you know of course the patients cannot ask very clever questions but patients would ask simply of what now to do. We both know what to do and you know, what is more important? What's a doctor will answer because you know the doctor should be a very good psychologist and if the patient's in your shoes and they were admitted as a patient.

Not all patients will ask something. Some patients are not afraid. Yes, maybe they are afraid to ask some questions and maybe the doctor can understand to say the right words. And maybe it's not to force, maybe to encourage the patient that they have to start the treatment because the patients who tell, "No, I will not do, I understand, but no, I will not do." As a doctor you should tell you don't know the results of prognosis. Maybe you will be of the persons who answer the patient for a good face on prognosis, good in self-defense of person also.

So to give the thoughts, to give them the hopes that all will be okay and to encourage and to help to find the right way how to treat and do the treatment. And if the patient will do the treatment, only some results will be…

Ty: So you think one of the important messages from the doctor should be to give the patient hope.

Dr. Chema: Yeah, to give them hope and to…

Ty: Well you know I'm very grateful for you spending time with us today. I think that if the doctors are educated on Rigvir that they definitely can give them hope.

Dr. Chema: Thank you.

Ty: Thank you for spending the time with us.

Dr. Chema: Thank you. Same to you.

[end of transcript]

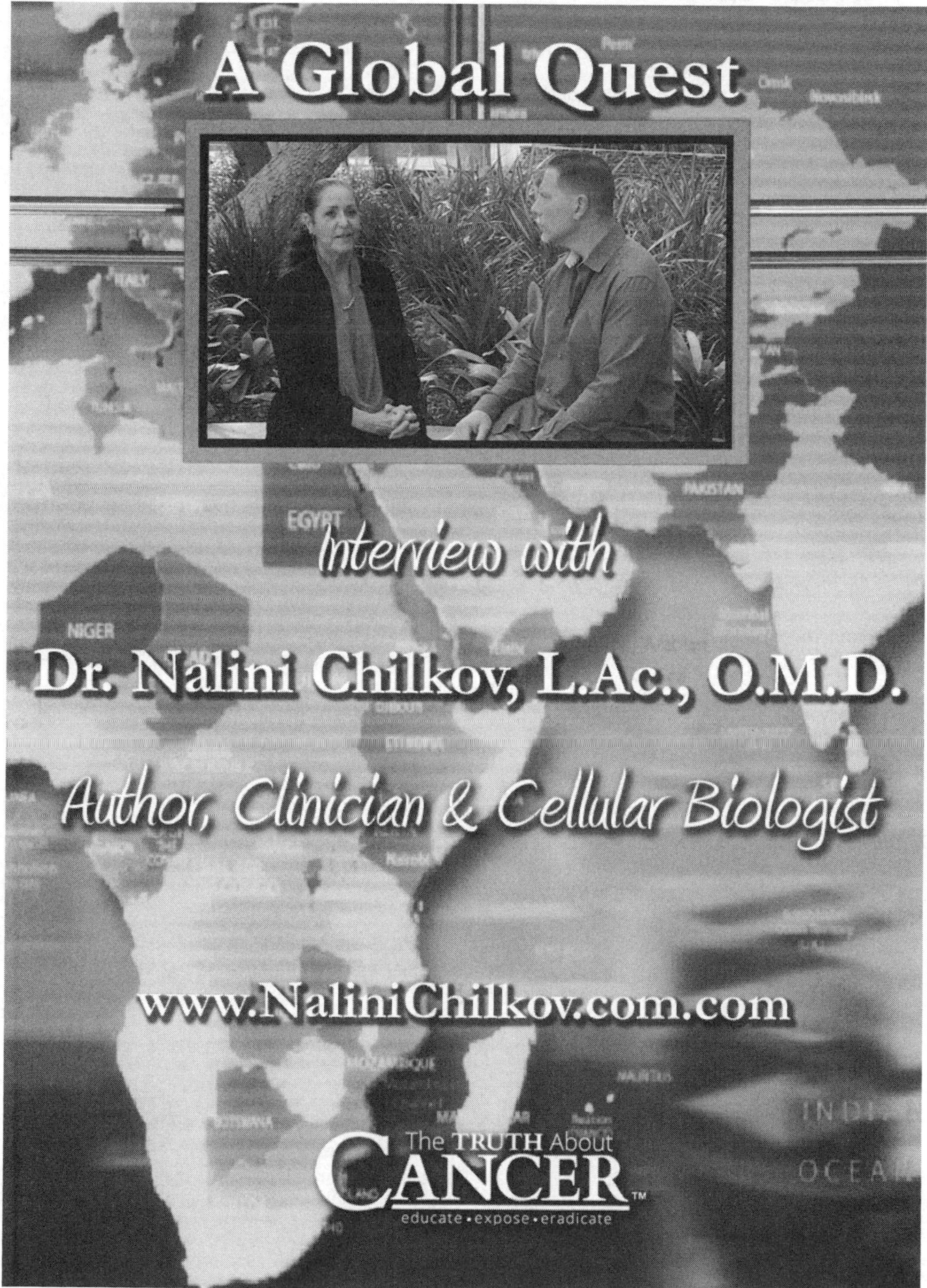
A Global Quest
Interview with
Dr. Nalini Chilkov, L.Ac., O.M.D.
Author, Clinician & Cellular Biologist
www.NaliniChilkov.com.com
The TRUTH About
CANCER™
educate • expose • eradicate

Ty: I'm really excited to be here tonight in Santa Monica, California, with Dr. Nalini Chilkov. Thank you for joining me Dr. Nalini.

Dr. Chilkov: Thank you for having me.

Ty: I'm really excited to talk to you tonight about integrative cancer, alternative cancer, whatever you want to call it. I've been sharing with you some of these stories that we've been getting. These patients that are choosing natural treatments for cancer, or integrative therapy, and they're alive to tell their story.

It's really rewarding to be able to affect peoples' lives that way, isn't it?

Dr. Chilkov: I have never done anything so meaningful in all my 30 years of practice. This is the most meaningful thing I've ever done.

Ty: Where were you educated, and what is your official title?

Dr. Chilkov: Well, my official title is Doctor of Oriental Medicine. In California that's almost the equivalent of being a Naturopathic Doctor, which means that I partner with nature in order to have solutions. Because we have a map of solutions in our own system. So if we partner with that, then we get to health.

And cancer—in conventional oncology, there's just a war on cancer. And it's all pathology-oriented but the patient wants health. So if there isn't a plan for health right from the beginning, how are you going to get there?

Ty: Right. What do you mean by pathology-oriented?

Dr. Chilkov: Well, in conventional medicine they're just interested in the problem, in the diagnosis, in the disease. And if you only focus on the disease, not the person, not the ecology of the whole cancer, then you're not going to have a long-term solution. You're going to have a quick, short fix that has some damage. So really, we have to be interested in what the patient wants which is a long, healthy life. That has to be the priority.

Ty: So with the Chinese medicine, the botanicals really—it's what you use? You use a lot of herbs?

Dr. Chilkov: Well, my first love is Botanic Medicine. Because in plants there are so many, what we call, plant chemicals, or phytochemicals. And molecules from nature bind to many different cells and receptors. So we get a lot of mileage out of using just a few things.

Many people know about curcumin from turmeric, it interacts with over 100 genes. So if that was a drug, that would be a blockbuster drug. Not only because it does that, but also because you can take it safely for long periods of time. So we don't have medications like that.

Ty: So curcumin, you mentioned curcumin. It interacts with 100 genes. So does it have an epigenetic effect on the person that takes it?

Dr. Chilkov: Absolutely. Epigenetics, if people don't know what that means, it means that something will act upon your genes. So your genetics is like your software. Something has to open it up and read it. And so you could have a toxic chemical in the environment that opens up some cancer genes and turns them on, but we could also turn those off with plant medicine. That's much more powerful than just trying to kill cancer cells. Right?

Ty: So here in Santa Monica, we're real close to Beverly Hills. Plastic surgery capitol of the world. One of the plastic surgeries, not really plastic surgery, but the surgery is being done so frequently—I can't imagine doing this—is preventative double mastectomies because somebody might get cancer.

Dr. Chilkov: So that's about fear, isn't it? You know, that's completely fear-based. And it's also because the media hypes that up, especially if a famous person like Angelina Jolie has a double mastectomy. But the kind of cancer that she had is less than five percent of all women with breast cancers. And so to remove your breasts is, I think, barbaric. It's really barbaric.

So you have to have an ecological plan. Cancer's really about the soil. It's about the whole system. If you transform that into an environment that's not supportive or permissive of the development and growth of cancer, then you have a long-term plan for health.

Ty: That's fascinating. So the soil, the milieu, as Antoine Bechamp called it, right? The internal terrain of the body.

Dr. Chilkov: Yes, exactly.

Ty: How do you get the internal terrain of a cancer patient's body back to where it is not a happy place for cancer to grow?

Dr. Chilkov: Well, there are a lot of factors. So a framework that I use, and the way I explain this to patients, is if you have a wheel with many spokes on it, those are all of the aspects of cancer physiology that we want to address. And in conventional oncology maybe they address one or two with some pretty toxic modalities.

But we want to look at vitamin D, at copper, at inflammation, at oxidative stress, hormone detoxification, at inflammation, at mineral status, blood sugar. So we want to look at all those things. So for an individual, one of those spokes might be more heavily weighted.

Let's say you're diabetic. Then sugar and insulin management is going to be more important for you. I have a prostate cancer patient, he's actually a nurse, and he didn't want to have traditional therapy. So I took his history, found out he's a poorly controlled diabetic, which means his insulin and his blood sugar are really high.

So it was my assessment that that was driving his cancer recurrence. As soon as we got his diabetes managed better, then that environment, that milieu, was not promoting cancer growth. Because tumor cells actually have more receptors for insulin and insulin-like growth factor.

So we have to look at the individual, see what's in the soil of their garden, and work with individuals. So you can't just do the same thing with everyone. But you want to look at all those factors in every single person.

Ty: I think that's really important. You mentioned you want to see what's driving the cancer. And is that not one of the places where the typical, the big three treatments, kind of fall short. It's that we see, okay, here's Jane with breast cancer, here's Linda with breast cancer. And it's the same type breast cancer, it's the same stage breast cancer, they're going to get the same drugs.

Dr. Chilkov: That's right.

Ty: They're different people.

Dr. Chilkov: That's right. One might be obese. So her fat tissue might be producing lots of estrogenic hormones and be full of inflammatory molecules. And that's a bigger risk for her than another patient who may be depressed, so her immune system is compromised. So you have to look at the individual.

Most of the therapies that are used in conventional oncology are interested in killing dividing cells. So if cells aren't dividing they don't work, which is why they only get partial results with a lot of toxicity.

So it's actually more powerful to turn on what we call the apoptotic switch, which is a signal, an intelligence, a wisdom in cells, that tells them they're not healthy cells, they should die and recycle themselves. That is lost in tumor cells. So not only are they growing, but they're failing to die.

So a better solution is over here, and there are so many botanicals and phytochemicals that turn that apoptotic switch back on. So that's really powerful. Resveratrol, curcumin, ECGC in green tea, those are examples of common phytochemicals used in cancer that do that. There aren't any drugs that do that.

Ty: The reason that I laughed is I was thinking back when we traveled to London. We got into our hotel rooms and I'm flipping all the switches in the room on and the lights don't work. And I realized that over there, you have to take your room card, your key with the strip on it, and put it into this little slot. And then the lights work.

Dr. Chilkov: Well, that saves energy. That's really smart. We should do that here.

Ty: It did, it saved energy. Because when you leave the room you can't leave the lights on.

Dr. Chilkov: That's right, that's great.

Ty: But I didn't know how to turn that switch on, right? These molecules that you mentioned, the resveratrol, the curcumin, the ECGC, which is from green tea. They are all molecules that turn on the apoptotic switch. And that is a switch that tells cancer cells, "You need to die."

Dr. Chilkov: That's right. So that's an example of partnering with nature, right? A solution that nature has for defective cells. So we have to turn that intelligence back on.

Ty: Are there ways to turn it on with not only botanicals, but through the foods that you eat as well?

Dr. Chilkov: Well, if you think about the color in foods, I always tell my patients to eat the rainbow. Because every pigment in fruits and vegetables actually enters the nucleus of the cell and interacts with your genes, which is why it matters what you eat, right?

So if you just eat the rainbow and half your plate is colorful fruits and vegetables, blueberries, spinach, kale, carrots, tomatoes, persimmons, pomegranates. If you eat color, you're going to also get these phytochemicals.

Also you have a medicine chest in your spice rack in your kitchen. Oregano, thyme, ginger, turmeric, all of the culinary spices not only aid your digestion but they also have these powerful chemicals. Carnosol is found in rosemary, for example. A very powerful anti-cancer chemical. So we can easily make our diets talk to our genes, really easy. Anybody can do it.

Ty: How did you learn all of these things about foods, and herbs, and the eating the rainbow, all of these botanicals that have these anti-cancer effects? Did you learn it in medical school?

Dr. Chilkov: No. Actually, I was originally a biochemist. So I'm interested in molecules and genes, and how they talk to each other. And when I started out 35 years ago, we did not have the science. We didn't have the human genome project. We didn't know enough about how cells work and how chemicals act on our cells as messengers.

Food and botanicals are information. They're actually telling the software what to do. You can determine what messages you're going to get. Say if you have chemical exposures, that's turning on a lot of negative properties in your cells, turns on inflammation, and turns on oxidative stress, turns on genes that promote cancer.

You don't want to have those signals. So you try to take toxins and chemicals out of your environment. And at the same time, if you're putting in all these plant chemicals from foods, and then if you also use medicinal herbs, then you have this powerful, overriding control over the environment.

Ty: What are your favorite top five medicinal herbs?

Dr. Chilkov: Well, I think I'm going to cheat and say more than five. So we already named curcumin. And resveratrol and EGCG. So there's irrefutable research on that.

Ty: And where do you get the curcumin?

Dr. Chilkov: Where do I get the curcumin?

Ty: Where would someone find curcumin? I mean, if they didn't want to go buy a bottle of curcumin, where does it come from?

Dr. Chilkov: Well, you can actually use turmeric in your diet. But remember, in traditional diets, when turmeric's in the food, it's also with some oil or fat.

So if you're going to use turmeric in cooking as a source of curcumin on a daily basis, then you have to have a little oil, like olive oil or coconut oil with it to really absorb it well. And a little black pepper, and then you'll really utilize it.

Ty: That's Dr. Sunil Pai, I don't know if you who he is. But he loves the curcumin with the black pepper.

Dr. Chilkov: Yes, I know Sunil. Yes. Well, there are a lot of studies that show that improves it. So I really am a fan of some of the great traditional Chinese herbs. All of the medicinal mushrooms are extraordinary immune modulators, signal cancer cells to turn their apoptotic switch on and to die, and also manage inflammation really well.

Also, the medicinal mushrooms are really good for managing insulin and blood sugar. And so are the ones you put in your salad, by the way. So that would be cordyceps mushroom, that would be reishi mushroom, ganoderma, shitake mushroom, you can add to your food, maitake mushroom, coriolus is one of the most powerful, that's turkey tail mushroom.

So those are very powerful and they can actually be used with chemo and radiation if a patient is actually having those therapies.

Ty: And they'll help? They'll help mitigate the side effects?

Dr. Chilkov: Well, they'll help mitigate the side effects, but they also keep you stronger so that your immunity is not pressed down. And in that same family—so all of the mushrooms have beta glucans and polysaccharides in them and that's what makes them medicine. They also have CLA, which is conjugated linoleic acid. That's anti-inflammatory and it also turns on a gene that regulates blood sugar and insulin, PPAR gamma.

And in the same family is one of my favorite herbs, astragalus. Astragalus is huang chi in Chinese medicine. Also an enormous amount of research. Also rich in polysaccharides and beta glucans, and really ramps up your white blood cells and your natural killer cells. So we're always looking for things that are going to increase natural killer cells. These are the army of our immune system that go after cancer cells and also viral cells. And astragalus is also one of these things you can take safely for long periods of time.

And for patients who've had their therapies like chemotherapy that depress their white blood cells and then they're vulnerable to infections, astragalus is one of the best things to increase white blood cells and be a natural killer to cells. And acupuncture also does that. Very powerful, I'm also an acupuncturist. So that's very, very powerful.

Ty: Astragalus, is that a root?

Dr. Chilkov: Astragalus is a root, yes. You'll see it in slices. It doesn't taste like much. So in China, they take some of these medicinal herbs like the mushrooms and astragalus, and they'll make soups out of it so that the food is medicinal food. And it's much more easy to assimilate. It's a lovely thing to do.

Ty: I'm laughing, it reminds me of Hippocrates, right? Let food by thy medicine. They're eating food that's medicine in China.

Dr. Chilkov: Yes. So then if you put all these colorful fruits and vegetables into the diet too, you make a soup with kale and spinach, and mushrooms, a little seaweed, put in the astragalus, and then you really have something that's really going to nourish you, that's easy to assimilate.

Ty: Absolutely. Are there herbs that you use to detoxify the body?

Dr. Chilkov: Absolutely. A lot of the herbs that are good for detoxification are either rich in essential aromatic oils, or they have alkaloids in them that stimulate us to excrete things, or they are rich in sulfur. So there are a lot of herbs and supplements that are rich in sulfur. I actually very much like garlic. That's a simple, simple herb that anybody can use.

I try to put into these resources things that anybody can get. It doesn't matter if you don't have a lot of money, or you do have a lot of money, everybody can do this. So garlic actually has some anti-tumor activity but it actually stimulates the excretion of a lot of toxic chemicals.

So do the radish and cabbage family of vegetables which are rich in sulfur. So the garlic family and the cabbage family have all this sulfur in them. A traditional remedy actually used to be cabbage juice. Before kale was so popular. And it's the sulfur that turns on your liver enzymes to start producing chemicals that detoxify.

Ty: Sulfur does?

Dr. Chilkov: Yes. Sulfur is one of the most detoxifying chemicals. So think about n-acetyl cysteine, lipoic acid, these are rich in sulfur. All the sulforaphanes, are chemicals in the cabbage family that not only interrupt the development, progression, and metastasis, travelling of cancer cells, the sulforaphanes interrupt every stage of cancer.

So they're very powerful, but they also promote detoxification, particularly of hormones. And for the hormone-driven cancers, I always add the sulforaphanes in for that.

Ty: And one of the things, I cannot remember who it was that mentioned this, the sulforaphanes in broccoli and cabbage, they also target stem cells as well.

Dr. Chilkov: Yes they do. Now, stem cells are a leading edge of research right now. Because it's now thought that the stem cells, which are what we call pluripotent cells—they can turn into anything. They are floating around in the bloodstream of cancer patients and chemo and radiation do not work on them. So it doesn't even touch them.

But there happen to be plant chemicals that actually do work on stem cells. So when we go back to some of our big levers, which are resveratrol, curcumin, and berberine, that's another one of my most favorite plant chemicals. There's a famous Chinese herb called huáng qín and that is scutellaria baicalensis. And in China today, modern Chinese herbal medicine, you'll find scutellaria baicalensis in almost every anti-tumor formula.

And it's got many, many phytochemicals, one of which is berberine. And berberine is very bitter, and it stimulates detoxification. Berberine also can control insulin so, again—because that's a driver of tumor cells. And because in the United States over 40 percent of people are diabetic or pre-diabetic, this is one of the great drivers of cancer in the United States today.

So look for plants and chemicals that do that as well. The scutellaria baicalensis also has bikalen, and baicalein, and wogonin, which are flavonols, a group of chemicals that turn cancer growth off, turn inflammation off, turn apoptosis on, act on stem cells. So you can see that plants are multi-taskers. We can do a lot with a handful of plants.

Ty: There are probably some anti-cancer plants in here somewhere.

Dr. Chilkov: I don't know. There's lots of grasses in here.

Ty: There are. But berberine—one funny thing you said about berberine, or not funny but it's unique—a friend of mine is a medicine man for the Cherokee Indians. And he has used berberine coupled with, I think it was, dong quai, angelica sinensis, to kill *Yersinia pestis*.

Dr. Chilkov: Yes, absolutely.

Ty: The bubonic plague.

Dr. Chilkov: Absolutely. These are powerful, powerful plants. And also, the scutellarias, there are many of them, they also promote detoxification as well.

Ty: Now where would you find the scutellarias?

Dr. Chilkov: Well, the Chinese scutellarias have the most research in cancer. So you would seek out someone who is a good herbalist and knows Chinese herbal medicine.

Ty: They're not going to grow here?

Dr. Chilkov: No. There are some herb farms that are starting to grow Chinese medicine in North America and Europe because there's a lot of contamination of toxins with herbs grown in China. So you have to be very careful with Chinese herbs.

I have a supplier that has relationships with organic farmers in China. But for the most part, a lot of Chinese herbs are contaminated with arsenic and lead,

Ty: I've read that.

Dr. Chilkov: You have to be very careful. So you want to find a knowledgeable herbalist.

Ty: The organic part that you just mentioned, really important with food and herbs?

Dr. Chilkov: Absolutely. Because we're not designed to be ingesting or be exposed to molecules that aren't from nature. And so some of those, we can't even excrete them. Or, some of those molecules that in food-growing—commercial food-growing, like the pesticides and the herbicides, they act like hormones. So they're turning on hormone-like activities which are proliferative which makes cells grow. So this is one of the reasons we have so much breast cancer and prostate cancer, hormone-driven cancers.

But people don't realize other cancers have estrogen receptors. Colon cancer, pancreatic cancer, and lung cancer, also have estrogen receptors. And so pesticides and herbicides will grow those cancers as well. So you don't want that kind of signaling. Plastics also have this hormone-like effect.

Ty: Pretend like you didn't see me drinking out of that bottle.

Dr. Chilkov: I didn't. That's actually a great point. We shouldn't actually drink out of plastic bottles if we have the option. We should store our food in glass containers.

Ty: And we typically do. When I'm on a long journey across the world, you get water where you can.

Dr. Chilkov: You have to do the best you can. We take control of the things we can take control of, so that we do the best we can.

Ty: What do you think about GMOs?

Dr. Chilkov: GMOs, I think, are misunderstood. Now remember, I'm a scientist. So the GMOs that are really bad are when you're mixing genetics from a virus or bacteria into a food. Those are the really, really bad ones. So if you put something into our food supply that kills the bacteria in our gut—it's used as a pesticide in agriculture, but then it kills the bacteria in our gut, then a huge part of our own immune system is damaged. So those are bad. But people don't realize, genetically modified foods are also hybrids. So we have to be careful how we use that word.

And understand that, when we're making plants that are like Frankenstein, that are not natural, that's where we get into trouble. Because then we're playing God with nature. And we don't know what kind of monsters we're actually going to create, or if our body can actually metabolize them, or if those combinations of genes are going to turn on other disease processes.

There are too many unknowns. So a lot of these are just for commercially producing more crops or making crops resistant to diseases. But if you have organic plants, they are stressed by having to fight off pests. And so they produce their own chemicals that do that, which makes them medicine.

And so actually growing organically makes our food more potent medicine, makes herbs more potent. And so we have to be careful to understand what we mean by genetically modified. For example, almost all the soy in America is genetically modified. We don't know what that's doing to our system. So I always err on the side of safety. If we don't know, let's pick non-genetically modified foods. We have to do that.

Ty: I'm glad that you just mentioned the fact that these plants, they mount—they're stressed, they mount a response against these pesticides. I think it was Dr. Patrick Quillin, we were at his house in Carlsbad, and he walked us through his garden. And he mentioned that these plants, when they're attacked, they produce these protective enzymes. That when we ingest them, they protect us.

Dr. Chilkov: That's right. So if we go back to the design of nature, and particularly food plants and medicinal plants, and herbs, and spices, that's a medicine chest right there. And remember, a lot of pharmaceuticals today are derived from plants.

Ty: Nature's medicine. Like 70 or 80 percent of pharmaceuticals, plants is what I've read.

Dr. Chilkov: That's right. Based on—you can't patent nature which is why we don't get a lot of money for research in plant medicine. But then they'll make a molecule that looks like the molecule from nature, and then a pharmaceutical company can own it. But that's not really the same animal.

Ty: But then they make the money on the patented drug.

Dr. Chilkov: That's right.

Ty: So why do you think there are so many kids getting cancer lately?

Dr. Chilkov: Well, think about a smaller body mass and the same amount of chemical exposure. So if an adult is in a room, and a little kid is in a room, just by body mass, that kid's overwhelmed with more chemical exposure in a smaller body. So it's a bigger dose.

Also, we don't know what chemicals are doing to the sperm and the egg. Certainly those are the most vulnerable cells. Anything that's dividing fast is more vulnerable. So the cells of the embryo and the fetus are dividing fast, so they're much more vulnerable to being damaged by chemicals.

So if we don't just talk about cancer, but we talk about all these kids with learning and attention disorders, we didn't have that decades ago. And so, this is changing how we develop as human beings. It's altering the software. It's altering our immunity. It's altering how our immune systems and our endocrine, hormonal systems, and our nervous systems, the regulatory systems of the body, where all this intelligence comes from, is being altered. And so the signals, the messages, are being altered.

So kids are really vulnerable and pregnant women should be extra careful with their exposures. Also, little kids should be protected and fed organic food, which is more dense in nutrients anyway. But kids are really much more vulnerable.

Ty: It's sad when you see—yesterday, we were in a clinic in Mexico and I saw a 14-year-old boy. It's sad to see that.

Dr. Chilkov: Yes. Oh, it's heartbreaking. It's just heartbreaking.

Ty: What do you think is probably the number one question that someone should ask if they're diagnosed with cancer? To know if the person, the doctor that they are going to use to treat them is the person they should use. Or maybe a couple questions.

Dr. Chilkov: Well, here's how I frame it. The doctor that any of us selects for any kind of health care should be person-focused. Is that doctor relational? Is the doctor respectful of your wishes and your values?

Because it's very important. You may be offered a treatment that the doctor believes in, but if it's not consistent with your values, if it's going to damage the quality of your life, and the quality of your life is the most important thing to you, then the doctor needs to respect that.

For example, I have patients in my practice that choose chemotherapy and radiation. I give them my opinion, but I also tell them, "I will respect your wishes, and I will take care of you no matter what you decide. I will take care of you. And we'll just manage the side effects of those things and then we'll keep you well afterwards."

It takes a person with a big spine to decline chemotherapy and radiation, and hormone therapy. So we have to really allow the patient to make their own decision. So are you with a doctor that allows you to make your own, intelligent decision, and doesn't manipulate you with fear, and tell you, "Oh, if you don't do this you'll die." That's not fair. So a doctor is respectful and fair, and will partner with you. Cancer is a complex illness, and you need a team. So is your doctor a team player?

And will you be the loudest voice on the team? That's really important. I always say you need a disease expert and you need a health expert. So at least, we need someone that's got a plan for your health during your treatments, and also afterwards. Because the patient wants health.

So is the doctor interested in health? That's really important. And then, is the doctor doing cookbook medicine, or individualized medicine? I think that's a really important question because we are all unique. Every tumor cell line is unique, and our genetics are unique, and then the environment as a soil in our body, are unique.

So does the doctor have an individualized approach, or do they do a standard cookbook kind of medicine? Because if you have a doctor that respects your wishes and will do individualized care with you, you're going to have a much better outcome. Much better outcome.

Ty: I agree. And I appreciate that about you. You mentioned that if your patients wanted to do chemo and radiation, you do the best you can with them. I think that's what this whole thing is about. It's just giving people information, letting them make their own choices.

Dr. Chilkov: Yes. Intelligent, informed choices. And the other thing I tell patients, "You get your diagnosis, and it's like your hair is on fire. You're freaked out. It's stressful. You're overwhelmed. You're not prepared for it. So in that emotional state, that's no state to be making a major life decision."

The doctor will say, "Okay, we're going to start your chemo and your radiation. We'll schedule your surgery." I tell people when they walk into my office, "Take a few breaths. Take some time. Get your life in order. Make sure whatever decision you make is your decision. It's not going to make or break your outcome if you wait a few weeks. Get other opinions. Do your homework. Make sure your kids are covered. Make sure you've got your job covered. Make sure you are at peace with the decision."

If your stress hormones are elevated, you can't think clearly, it alters your brain and your thinking. You're going to make an irrational decision. So I always tell people to slow it down, slow the process down. And then you want to see if your doctor will also allow you to do that. Because the doctor also knows, it's not going to change your outcome to wait a few weeks.

And be prepared for whatever you choose, be well prepared. And be psychologically in alignment, because that alters your immunity as well. And you have to have faith and confidence in your doctor and in the treatment. If you don't, you're not going to have the same kind of outcome. The mind is very powerful.

Ty: And you can't make your decision if you don't know all the choices.

Dr. Chilkov: That's right. I'm into people having choices. I think choices are like the main thing. So people should get opinions, and different opinions. Insurance will often pay for you to get multiple opinions. People don't know that.

And then make a choice or decide you're going to have an integrative plan. I think that's really super important. Because if you choose to have a plan that includes conventional care, then you also should have something that will protect you from the negative effects of that care.

Most patients who walk in my door are doing some version of that. People who fail that will often go looking outside of it. Even a patient who has a very strong feeling that they don't want to do conventional chemotherapy and radiation therapy, sometimes the pressure from the family is so huge that it's hard to go against that. So it takes a very strong person to do that and then to ask their family to support them during that. So it's complicated.

Cancer is a group experience. It's really multi-factorial how people arrive at their decisions. But it should be their decision. And they need a team, and a support system in their personal life as well.

Ty: I agree with you. And I agree with you that they shouldn't be rushed into it based on fear.

Dr. Chilkov: That's right.

Ty: I interviewed a man yesterday, I think it was, that had been misdiagnosed, or they had missed the cancer diagnosis for like three months. They diagnosed it on a Thursday and they said, "You need to come in Monday for treatment." They had missed it for three months and then they tell him in three days he needed to be treated. It's based on fear.

Dr. Chilkov: Yes. Well, and their fear that they messed up.

Ty: Their fear as well.

Dr. Chilkov: But that's actually very common. So let's talk about screening a little bit. Because it's really important to listen to our own bodies. Really important to listen to our own bodies.

An example is ovarian cancer. The symptoms of ovarian cancer are obtuse. You might just feel like you're a little bloated, or you have a little constipation, and maybe you feel congested in your pelvis. And many doctors will be dismissive of this and say that's all that it is. When ovarian cancer tends to be diagnosed, it's Stage 3, quite late. And then it's harder to treat because it's more systemic, there are more cancer cells.

So if you have a symptom that isn't right, then you also want a doctor that will follow up and ask lots of questions and make sure that what the doctor thinks it is, it actually is. So then you need an ultrasound to see what's going on. You need a blood test to see if you have tumor markers or if you're highly inflamed. You need to pursue that, because most women should have been diagnosed earlier, because they had these symptoms. They already had these symptoms. It doesn't come out of nowhere.

Ty: So that really is a good theory. This is going to be airing in October which is Breast Cancer Awareness month. Early detection is your best protection.

Dr. Chilkov: Always.

Ty: That is a good theory but a lot of the early detection methods aren't really early detection.

Dr. Chilkov: No they're not. One of the things I do in my practice, once a patient has a history of cancer, is I do a series of blood tests that actually look at the soil, look at the terrain. Because if we can see microscopic changes in the blood then we know we're tipping in a direction.

I'll give you an example. I had an ovarian cancer patient. She went through traditional therapy and she had a good result. And then about a year later her tumor markers started to go up. And the conventional treatment is brutal. It's really hard to go through.

So she called me up and she said, "I can't go through that again. I cannot go through that again." So I called her oncologist and I said, "Give me three months." We did a very aggressive botanical, nutraceutical protocol, with a very strict diet, and with acupuncture.

And, I can't remember exactly, her tumor markers were something like 60 something, and they should be below 35. We're talking about CA-125. They went down to six in less than three months, and stayed there.

So, we changed the ecology. We changed the ecology, we changed that soil. So when someone is just having little signs of recurrence, most oncologists aren't going to treat anyway. They're going to wait until you're worse because they can't give you that toxic therapy.

But we can intervene with less toxic therapies and actually turn the needle. And so if the patient is listening and if the patient knows they have choices and other resources—most people don't know they have choices. So hence this series. So that people know they have choices. Then you can reach out, get other opinions, and find something that makes sense to you or that is a good choice for what you're dealing with.

Ty: Yes. Well, thank you for all this information that you're sharing. Because this is information that many others have not shared, especially about the botanicals. I think that's fascinating.

Dr. Chilkov: Really powerful.

Ty: So last question for you, Dr. Chilkov. Is cancer a death sentence or is there always hope for someone who's been recently diagnosed?

Dr. Chilkov: Cancer is absolutely not a death sentence. In fact, one of the top surgeons here in LA, one of the breast surgeons—I love what she says, and I also say this to patients, "If you get diagnosed with breast cancer, you should just expect to live." How many doctors say that to cancer patients? So the big "C" word is never a death sentence.

There's always a path; there is always a path. Maybe your life will be shortened, but I always say to people, "How do I know if I'm cured?" I say, "What if you die of something else? So my wish for you is that we manage your cancer, and you live to be 98, and you have a heart attack." Then we know we did good.

But some people are living with cancer as a chronic illness. So that's fine, it's the same as living with diabetes, or high blood pressure, or high cholesterol. If we can manage it and keep it at a microscopic level, you carry on with your life.

It is not a death sentence. So that's my goal for a lot of patients with advanced cancer. Because we might not get to zero cancer cells but if we have good control, if we know how to put the brakes on, if we know how to keep the soil right where we want it, and we know how to monitor that, then you can just live with cancer at a low level. And keep taking your herbs, keep taking your supplements, change your lifestyle, change your diet, deal with your stress and your emotional issues.

Then you can have a very long life that is not about death. So I think that's where people's minds go immediately. It's a great question, because it shouldn't be about that. It should be, "How am I either going to solve this completely, or how am I going to take control of it?"

That's a better way to think about it. So that if we have a good plan to manage it, we have a plan, and we have a toolbox to do that with that's safe long term. That's what we want to do.

Ty: Well, you know what? You've given us a bunch more tools for our toolbox and I thank you Dr. Nalini. I really appreciate you.

Dr. Chilkov: Thank you so much.

[end of transcript]

A Global Quest

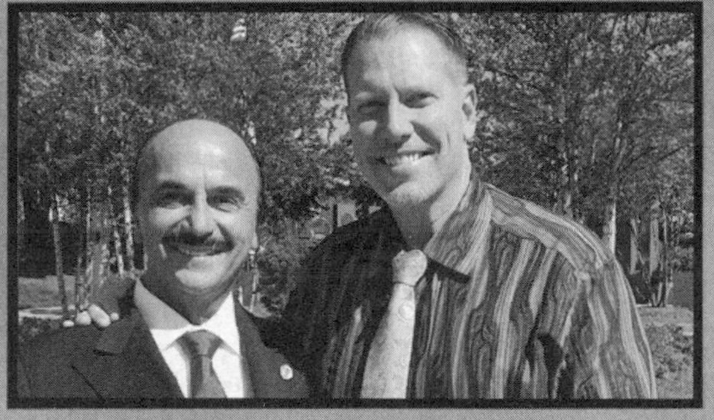

Interview with

Dr. Leonard Coldwell, N.M.D., Ph.D

Syndicated Radio Host & Best-selling Author

www.DrLeonardColdwell.com

The TRUTH About CANCER™
educate • expose • eradicate

Ty: Dr. C, so good to see you here today.

Dr. Coldwell: Oh, Ty, thank you so much for inviting me. It's a beautiful spot, a beautiful place.

Ty: Asheville, North Carolina.

Dr. Coldwell: And it's just wonderful.

Ty: Yes. I'm really glad that you could join us today because one of the things I wanted to get you to tell us, as well as your knowledge about cancer, is the story of your mother.

Dr. Coldwell: Yes.

Ty: I was on your radio show and you told me about her, and she had been diagnosed with cancer. So tell everyone that is listening the story about your mom.

Dr. Coldwell: Yes. It starts out, actually, with all seven siblings of my mom had cancer, my grandmother and grandfather on both sides of cancer, my father died of cancer, my sister had cancer.

Ty: Wow.

Dr. Coldwell: And when I 12 years old my mom was diagnosed with hepatitis C, liver cirrhosis, and terminal liver cancer with a maximum of 6 months to live. So basically, if you had a prognosis of six months to live, the good thing was that the medical profession didn't do anything anymore to her because they knew liver cancer, they drop a little bit of poison in there, like chemo, she is dead on the spot.

Ty: Right. So actually, that she was so unbelievably sick saved her life.

Dr. Coldwell: Right.

Ty: So Dr. C., in essence, it was really a blessing that your mom didn't receive any of the conventional treatments for cancer—no chemo or anything like that.

Dr. Coldwell: Absolutely, Ty, because they basically said with hepatitis C, liver cirrhosis, and terminal liver cancer, to drop a little bit of poison in, chemotherapy or anything, no matter what, she would be dead on the spot. So basically, we were really lucky that she was so unbelievably sick that nobody even wanted to deal with it and that really saved her life at the end of the day. When people really understand that there is one thing—my message is a message of hope. And my mom is a living example. I just came back from a book tour in Europe and had my mom, 80 years old today, 43 years later after she should be dead—for 42 and a half years she should be dead by now.

So I had her on stage and if you look up my website she is on there and I have an interview on stage, eight or nine minutes, where she is telling her story. And you will not see somebody that alive who is the age of 80, that life-loving, that good-looking. You know, people were just stunned, and nobody believed her age.

That is something where, most people, in my experience, Ty, die because they have no hope anymore. Many cancer patients—since I only work with cancer patients—I work with 66,000 patients personally, but 25,000 cancer patients. And they were all given up—they all had six months to live, nine months to live—by the medical profession. So basically, my mom is the best example that it doesn't really matter what they say. It doesn't matter if they say you will die of hepatitis—she didn't—if you will die of liver cirrhosis—she didn't—if you will die of terminal liver cancer—she didn't.

Because this is not really just a matter of treatment, it's a matter of hope, it's a matter of attitude. Because health—everything, as we know, Ty, is frequency and vibration. So if we vibrate on a higher level we are more positive, we are friendlier, we attract everything we are vibrating. So if you dial in on the radio, you dial a specific station, you dial a country western station in, that's what you are listening to. That's not opera coming out.

So, it is just really important that we really focus on what we want because people that are diagnosed—Dr. Bernie Siegle, a Yale professor, Dr. Bernie Siegle, said he found out with his cancer patients, the moment the cancer patient gets a diagnosis of cancer the immune system goes down over 90 percent, when they need it the most, actually.

Ty: So that leads to this question, then. Conventional treatments really don't offer hope when you go to be diagnosed and the doctor says, "You're going to be dead in three to six months." That is the opposite of hope. They offer *no* hope. And you just mentioned the fact that once you get that diagnosis your immune system goes through the floor, right?

Dr. Coldwell: Absolutely.

Ty: It completely devastates you. And then, not only the diagnosis, but then the words of the doctor, "You will be dead." They offer no solutions.

Dr. Coldwell: Absolutely not. And let me throw in, Ty, because it is really important, people that like their doctor die young. There is a study that has been done that stated when you like your doctor you don't want to prove your doctor wrong. So if their doctor says they have four months to live, and they really like their doctor, strangely enough, it is psychologically easy to explain, they die within this four months because they don't want to prove their doctor wrong that they like. So it's very, very dangerous.

Ty: Well, the mind has a lot to do with our health.

Dr. Coldwell: Absolutely, Ty. Cancer is caused, 86 percent, to mental and emotional stress. All illness is based on lack of energy. There is no other cause of illness. Now, we need to find out—where is this lack of energy coming from? And what happened from the moment when I was born—and of course we are born with pre—cancerous cells, potentially cancerous cells, atrophied mutated dead cells, and our little body, our immune function, our repair system, just gets rid of it from day one. So if this stops, and cancer is not even an illness, Ty, cancer is just really a symptom. So that means if there is something going wrong that did go right before, what happened?

Ty: Right.

Dr. Coldwell: Something must have happened. And in my opinion, my system is called instinct-based medicine system, because I believe our instinct, our soul, is God talking to us. I don't believe that our instinct can ever be wrong. The mother knows exactly what is going on with her baby. And so our instinct is absolutely perfect.

Ty: That leads me to the question, then, you mentioned the mother knows what is going on with her baby, and this is a question I am asking everybody because I, honestly, have theories about it but I don't know for sure—why the explosion in childhood cancer?

Dr. Coldwell: That's an issue, Ty. The main cause is vaccination. What people need to understand is, you cannot put heavy metals, you cannot put dioxin, you cannot put mercury, you cannot put live cancer viruses into a human body and hope that all will be well, we know every vaccination causes brain inflammation—every single vaccination. Every single vaccination has heavy metals in there. That is why we have the explosion of brain tumors because the mercury, the thimerosal, crosses the blood-brain barrier without a problem.

Ty: That's really interesting that you said that. I never thought about it, or made that connection before, but most of the childhood cancers that you hear about are brain cancers.

Dr. Coldwell: Yes.

Ty: And so you explained that. The mercury in the vaccines crosses the blood-brain barrier.

***Dr. Coldwell*:** And the other thing is, Ty, how scientifically we are able to explain that every autism case is caused by a vaccine. There is not one single child that has not been vaccinated that has autism. Every child that has autism has been vaccinated, or it grew up in an environment where there is mining going on, heavy metal mining. They are the only exceptions because I just talked to a good friend of mine who is a professor and really doing the research on that. He said the only exception is, literally, if they are next to a mining operation.

Ty: That is interesting. My cousin, their second child was vaccinated, and within 24 to 48 hours, completely regressed to not speaking anymore—a year or two previous to where they were from a functional standpoint. They go back to the doctor and the doctor says, "It was just coincidence."

Dr. Coldwell: Of course. But there are millions of coincidences now. There are people falling off the chair with the needle still in them from the vaccination.

Ty: Right.

Dr. Coldwell: It's like with Gardasil. Gardasil is this vaccine that has been created to supposedly protect women from cervical cancer because it supposedly protects you from the HPV virus.

Ty: Which, by the way, usually clears up on its own.

Dr. Coldwell: Yes. And it doesn't lead to cervical cancer. My sister had cervical cancer. I just had her do three douches with sodium bicarbonate, with baking soda, and it was gone within 24 hours—cervical cancer gone in 24 hours. Dr. Simoncini wrote a book called *Cancer is a Fungus*. I just spoke with him together on the same stage in Germany.

Ty: Talk about that. The theory that cancer is a fungus, because a good friend of mine, Doug Kaufmann, in Rockwell, Texas, he's written a book about fungal infections being misdiagnosed as cancer.

Dr. Coldwell: Yes. Dr. Simoncini explained it this way. He says that the mutated atrophied cells—the cells that multiply in the wrong way, or the wrong cells multiplying endlessly—have to be kept together to cause harm, otherwise they would just float around and the immune system would grab them and get rid of them. But to keep this together as a tumor, the fungus, actually—that's why cancer can only exist in an acidic environment because a fungus can only exist in an acidic environment. So, it's keeping the cancer cells together.

Dr. Simoncini has videotapes, where—he is an oncologist in Rome, Italy, he has this huge hospital—he opens up cancer patients, pours sodium bicarbonate in a liquid form onto the organ, onto the cancer. You see, on contact, the white—every cancer is white, the white is a fungus—going away and the tumor disappearing on contact. That is so phenomenal. And when you understand—see, there are two ways of looking at cancer. In my opinion, cancer is caused by mental and emotional stress—86 percent. So that only leaves 14 percent for toxemia, all the food preservatives, and basically, you get poisoned.

And since 1911 and 1936, when Otto Warburg and Max Planck won a Nobel prize in medicine proving that cancer can only exist in an acidic, toxic, oxygen-lacking environment, we know that since 1911, Ty, since 1911 we have needed just to focus on how do I get the body alkaline and how do I get oxygen in the system, both of which are extremely, extremely easy. And when we still had the former Soviet Union going and Professor Munford from Nandena did the oxygen molecule therapy—we did this later, too, you take off a quart of blood, put ionized oxygen in, it gets really pink, from nearly being black to pink, and you leave it back, and after eight times the body—it's like a baby.

Ty: I've read many instances of that.

Dr. Coldwell: Remember when the old Russians all got so old when the Soviet Union was there?

Ty: Yes.

Dr. Coldwell: All the politicians, everybody got kind of like 100 years old. The second the wall collapsed and the Soviet Union collapsed and they didn't have access anymore to Professor Munford from Nandena to the oxygen therapy, they all died within two years. Because oxygen is actually the only really healing energizing factor. And people can, of course, do a lot of green juices, everything that is green is chlorophyll and fills the body up with oxygen and helps you also to get alkaline, because there is more calcium in a little bit of parsley than you can get in any calcium supplement. So everything that is green will help you in that way.

So people really need to understand, the cure for cancer—I know 400 natural cures for cancer, from laetrile and B17, to turmeric, to oleander soup, we all know the Budwig diet, we know the Gerson diet, Hoxsey.

Ty: When you say cures for cancer, though, wouldn't you agree that most, if not all of these cures for cancer, really, what they do is they provide your body with what it needs so that is heals itself?

Dr. Coldwell: Yes, Ty, but here is where I am different from anybody else you might interview, because since I believe that cancer is caused by making compromises against yourself, living a life that is not congruent with who you truly are, hanging on to a relationship you know is wrong. That is why most deadly heart attacks happen Monday morning between eight and nine o'clock when people get ready for a work week that they cannot handle anymore.

Ty: They can't stand their job.

Dr. Coldwell: They can't stand their job. So for me, that's why the IBMS system is identifying and eliminating the root cause of every negative result in your life. So I am after what takes your energy away. Yes, of course, it might be the food. Yes, of course, it might be—but I can fill you up with silica and B17 and you eat apricot seeds and I put you on the Rife machine, and basically, in 21 days you have no tumors anymore, or 100 cc of vitamin C intravenously three times a day and in 11 days you might experience all tumors are gone. But they will come back, because you have never gotten addressed the root cause.

Ty: Because you are talking the root of that being the stress, or the emotional imbalance.

Dr. Coldwell: Yes. Living in constant worries, fears and doubt, lack of self-love, lack of self-respect, lack of social interaction, because we are social beings, Ty. See, we connected instantly when we talked the first time on the phone. We connected instantly because there are so many things that connect us. And that's what we need because nobody can exist on their own. And loneliness—I work with the richest people in the world and I figured out that most of them are extremely lonely.

And if you are lonely you create a stress, a social anxiety stress, that you cannot handle either. And there is no social net that is catching you. If I am down I just call somebody up. I call a friend up and say, "Tell me something nice." And they say, "You know, you've been through so much bad stuff, you're going to make this, too, so don't worry." And off I go again.

And this is what is so important, Ty, that we understand we need our social group, we need our herd, we need our tribe. And very often we are born into a family where we don't really connect, so we have to create our own family. And that is what I do all my life, I call them the open eight-percenters because…

Ty: Where were you born?

Dr. Coldwell: In Germany.

Ty: In Germany. Okay, so I want to ask you a question about that. I know you are a bit of a history buff, so I want to ask you about the history of chemotherapy.

Dr. Coldwell: Yes.

Ty: Because coming from Germany you will know this.

Dr. Coldwell: Yes, absolutely, because chemotherapy is based on mustard gas. Mustard gas was invented in the First and Second World War to murder soldiers on the battlefield. After the Second World War was over they didn't really know what to with it. It was like with aluminum, the fluoride, "Let's put it in the drinking water because it is too expensive to get rid of it otherwise." So what they did is, actually, they said, "Just let's put it into people. We'll just get rid of it by putting it into people." And the approach of chemotherapy—imagine you have a beautiful garden, Ty. And you have like here, you have flowers, you have trees, you have bushes, grass, everything. And a little bit of weeds. So now you take Agent Orange and you wipe it all out, and you kill the entire beauty of the entire back yard, the entire garden or park here. And then you hope only the flowers come back, and the trees.

Ty: It doesn't make sense, does it?

Dr. Coldwell: No, it doesn't make sense at all. The only thing that is coming back is weeds.

Ty: Right.

Dr. Coldwell: And since cancer is based on lack of energy, when you take the energy away with chemotherapy, chemotherapy is basically an assault with a deadly weapon. That is, literally, all it is. And radiation, everybody knows radiation causes cancer, it doesn't really matter what they try to tell you, how now all of a sudden radiation is good for you, and when you are pregnant it is never good. The absurdity—I cannot even follow that anymore.

Ty: It doesn't pass the smell test.

Dr. Coldwell: Not really. And then you talk to friends and people like us who really think about these issues, you will easily find out it is completely absurd. It is about the 300 billion dollars they make a year in the cancer industry. It is a 300 billion dollar a year industry. And that doesn't even include the prevention hoax, and the early detection hoax, which are all hoaxes.

Ty: So Dr. C., talk about these hoaxes, these detection hoaxes, because this month, October 2015, is Breast Cancer Awareness Month, and everybody is going to be urged to get their mammogram, to Run for the Cure. Can you elaborate on that?

Dr. Coldwell: They should run *from* the cure. So basically, what it really is, you have to understand, 50 pounds of pressure on the most granulated load of tissue of the human breast—50 pounds of pressure during the mammography. That cannot be good. Then the radiation—every mammography basically ups your risk of getting cancer two percent, just in general. Early detection just means early death because the earlier they find it the earlier they start cutting you, the earlier they start treating you with chemotherapy and radiation, and the earlier you die.

There is no such thing as early detection that will save your life. People, basically, virtually die within a certain amount of time, no matter what, after diagnosis. Breast cancer grows 7 to 12 years to a size in the breast that you can even diagnose it. So there is no rush—you know they find breast cancer, "Oh, you have to go and get surgery tomorrow morning!"

Ty: A lot of pressure.

Dr. Coldwell: A lot of pressure, because they don't want you to take the time to get educated, and educate yourself. So let's talk about this early detection. Imagine your lymph system. You have four times more lymph than blood. So your lymph system, your lymph nodes, are there to neutralize poison. It's like when you have tonsillitis, there are the big lymph nodes, and then there are just working hard. It's not a bad thing, it's a good thing, showing the tonsils caught all these poisons and basically they are just diluting it and neutralizing it and then getting rid of it. So when you have that, Ty, and imagine a pimple that is ready to burst. Now, the lymph node in the breast might be working hard and be inflamed, and looks like a pimple that's getting ready to burst. So now they put 50 pounds of pressure on it.

Ty: That makes sure it bursts.

Dr. Coldwell: That makes sure it bursts. And the worst thing is needle biopsy. Cancer is the cure. People don't understand that. Cancer is there to save your life. When your body is so toxic that you are going to die of the poison, the body builds a bag and stuffs all the poison in there and locks it up—the tumor. So now imagine, this tumor is full with poison. Imagine an air balloon filled with water—poison. So now you come with a needle biopsy. And you pinch into this balloon, or into this lymph node, or into this so-called tumor. What happens is that it explodes into the entire system.

Ty: Right.

Dr. Coldwell: And very soon you have a fast-growing, very aggressive form of cancer.

Ty: And that always happens, doesn't it? I mean, how many stories have you heard? Thousands of stories of people that said, "I had a tumor, they biopsied it, and now it's everywhere."

Dr. Coldwell: Absolutely, because they poured the poison back into the system. And now it is highly concentrated on top of it. So early detection is like colonoscopies. First of all, they don't even get high enough to even find anything important. Secondly, they poke holes into the colon. And third of all, they are unable to clean all their so-called sterile instruments the way that they don't present a harm to you, or a danger, anymore.

Ty: Yes.

Dr. Coldwell: So people really need to wake up to all of this. It's all about making money. It's not about curing you, it's not about helping you. There is not one medical doctor in the universe that can cure you. Ask your doctor, "Why am I sick? How did I get the cancer? What are you going to do to cure it? When will I be cured? How long will this take?" And this is basically, all you all get, "I don't know."

Ty: They don't know.

Dr. Coldwell: They don't know. And then they always believe, because you see, medicine is a religion, Ty, it's not a science. Because it is not based on science, it is based on "I believe." I believe in three weeks this could happen. I believe you have so-and-so long to live. It's always, I believe. And we give you this, and we hope, you know? It's all about...

Ty: You know, it's interesting that you mention it being a religion. Our mutual friend, Robert, Scott Bell, specifically of vaccines, he says that vaccines are the sacred cow of the Church of Biological Mysticism.

Dr. Coldwell: (laughs) That sounds perfect.

Ty: That's kind of what it is, right?

Dr. Coldwell: That's just what it is, Ty.

Ty: Because, you're right, if you ask any medical doctor, "Will this cure?" "I hope it will." "Why did I get the cancer?" "Well, we're not sure." So they don't know the cause, they're not sure if it will cure it, it really seems like a bunch of hocus-pocus at times, doesn't it?

Dr. Coldwell: That's what it is. It is basically quackery with a license. Here is what they do, Ty. They use science to trick us into believing medicine is science. So they use a blood test, they use x-rays, they use whatever they use, and that is science. Fine. But what do I do with the result of the science now that has nothing to do with science anymore?

Cutting something out—I explain it to my patients always the same way. Imagine you have a splinter in your finger, and you say, "Oh, it hurts." And the doctor says, "I'll just push it deeper in, it's gone, you don't see it anymore, no problem." Now it hurts, now you get a pain pill, now it gets inflamed, now you get an antibiotic, now it's really inflamed and hurts, and they cut it off, and they say, "See? No finger, no pain." And that is what they do with our soul. The splinter in the soul, they push it deeper in instead of identifying it and pulling it out.

Ty: Right. It's really a system of symptom management, as opposed to getting to the root cause.

Dr. Coldwell: Symptom suppression, actually.

Ty: Symptom suppression, yes.

Dr. Coldwell: Because they never even deal with the cause. They don't even know what it is. I still know doctors that tell you that health, wellness and vitality have nothing to do with food.

Ty: Right. And that is what we got last year, across the board, from every medical doctor we interviewed. "How much education did you get on nutrition while in medical school?" "None."

Dr. Coldwell: None. Yes.

Ty: How can that be?

Dr. Coldwell: See, there is no money in it. John D. Rockefeller, over a hundred years ago, invented the salesperson he needed for his chemicals and called it the medical doctor. So he wrote the entire curriculum for the medical education over a hundred years ago, and gave it for free to the universities, so now they all had the same medical curriculum overnight. Interestingly enough, only the chemicals he produced were the solutions, and the only licensed and lawful and legal solutions for any treatment.

Ty: Right. And we covered that last year with the Flexner report.

Dr. Coldwell: Yes.

Ty: So yes, the medical schools were monopolized.

Dr. Coldwell: Still are. Still are. It really hasn't changed since Rockefeller and Rothschild's control the entire pharmaceutical and medical industry.

Ty: Is this a worldwide control or mainly here in the United States?

Dr. Coldwell: No, it's really worldwide. First of all, I mean, I've been shot at, my car has been bombed, and I'm from Germany. When my first book came out, *Mama Please Don't Die*, after I cured my own mother from hepatitis C, liver cirrhosis and liver cancer, my book came out and it was over 40 years ago, they offered my $280,000 if it didn't come out. That was the first approach. And I said, "Uh-uh, under no circumstance. I have a deal with God, I will get it all out there, I want everybody to know curing cancer costs about $10. That's the end of it." So you just need to ask yourself the right questions and just follow your own answers. That's basically what I stand for.

And now you have this Bayer and Hurst, all the huge pharmaceutical industries are based in Germany, where I grew up. So now, the real problem is, Germany is the only country in the world that has in their constitution that the government has to license naturopathic physicians—the only country in the world. So for 2000 years naturopathy is a medical science in Germany, and there is nothing they can do about it. Hitler tried a little bit but it was trickery because he didn't want to have Jewish people being able to work as a doctor. The main thing is, Ty, that when you understand that seven people own the world, seven families own the entire world—that means they own the media, they own the pharmaceutical and medical industry, newspapers, TV and radios. So basically, if you owned a TV station and my product was better than yours, would you tell anybody?

Ty: No.

Dr. Coldwell: So the constant brainwashing is really—

Ty: They control the media, and then they control the medical schools, the medical education. So yes, it's a monopoly of information. And so, really, you're a medical doctor, it's not medical doctors' fault that they don't know these things, they're never educated.

Dr. Coldwell: Yes, I'm a doctor of naturopathic medicine, but I'm legally a medical doctor. So basically, it's never the fault of the medical doctor, Ty, because every doctor—first of all, most of my really close friends are medical doctors. Every doctor becomes a doctor because he is a good person, because they want to help, and then they get tricked into, "Oh, buy this machine, and buy that machine, and hire five more people." And then they get educated by the pharmaceutical reps, not anymore by the university. There are all these people coming with all these indirect bribes and these extremely good-looking young ladies that come on a weekly basis, and things like that. So the bribery factor is just really, really unbelievable.

But I want people to understand, every doctor becomes a doctor because they want to help. They are all good people. But then after five to seven years, reality kicks in. "I have to pay my rent, I have to pay the two million dollar loan off, I have to pay the interest on the two million dollar loan for all my machines. I just bought another machine for $800,000. If I don't have so-and-so may people or so-and-so many surgeries I cannot buy my food any longer."

Ty: It's pure economics at that point.

Dr. Coldwell: Yes. That's why the medical doctor, statistically, as far as I know, has the shortest lifespan of all professions, 56 years of age, highest suicide rate, and the highest abuse rate of alcohol and drugs, because these poor guys or girls get into this wanting to help. You don't become a doctor to go out there and say, "Oh, I want to just harm some people, I want to just murder people." You go in there because you want to help, and there are so many good people out there, believe me.

And when these people now see the reality that they cannot help, that all they do is murder people indirectly with vaccinations, with chemo, with radiation, with surgery—it's like back surgeries, I've never seen in 40 years a back surgery going well—ever—in 40 years.

And so, Ty, what we need to understand is, doctors are good people, and then they get corrupted by the debt, then they get corrupted by the pharmaceutical reps, and then everybody involved, and also by the insurance companies, because insurance companies tell them what they are going to pay for.

Ty: They will only pay for the things that are approved.

Dr. Coldwell: Yes. And not the things that help. Because it should be success-based medicine. If you look at it, practicing school medicine. Practicing? Shouldn't you be done practicing? Shouldn't you know what you're doing? And school medicine?

Shouldn't you be out of school? So basically, it is all trial and error and it always ends up bad.

Ty, imagine you have somebody's husband rapes and abuses her child, and you never address this issue. It doesn't matter how much Ritalin you give them, how much Valium you give them. All of this doesn't really help. The poor person has to be dealing with his past and find a way to deal with these issues. So the medicine is only…

It's like they invented ADHD and ADD, which doesn't really exist, it is like fibromyalgia doesn't really exist. There were all these neurotic people having all these muscle problems because they are just stressed out, and usually dehydrated, and they wanted to give it a name, and if you are really neurotic you want an illness, I mean you have the proof.

Ty: And then they can develop drugs to treat the illness.

Dr. Coldwell: Exactly.

Ty: Right. Really, what I'm hearing you say is a lot of—I'm glad you mentioned, you differentiated that doctors are not bad people, you're not indicting them.

Dr. Coldwell: No, absolutely not.

Ty: But, really, it's a broken system. It's a broken global system that pushes money and profits over people's health.

Dr. Coldwell: Absolutely, Ty, because they don't care. When you understand that the wealth accumulation is so tremendous that seven families own 99 percent of the entire wealth of the earth, there must be a reason for that, and there is something really wrong with this picture. So Ty, when you understand, and as I said, most of my close friends are medical doctors or naturopathic doctors, or Doctor of Naturopathic Medicine, like I am, when we sit together we are not talking about how we can harm somebody. We are sitting together and saying, "Oh, what can we do for that person?" Or we call each other up and say, "I have a patient, I just don't know what to do, do you have an idea?"

Ty: And I'm the same way. I'm not a medical doctor, but I have a lot of friends that are MDs and not one of them is a bad person.

Dr. Coldwell: Of course not.

Ty: They are caught in a broken system a lot of times.

Dr. Coldwell: The system is rigged, Ty. They don't even have a chance because they cannot legally—there was this licensed medical doctor in California who was on a talk show, live, presenting five cancers he cured with laetrile which is B17. He comes out of the show, he gets arrested, his license revoked, and he is still in jail years later. And he was a licensed medical doctor, for curing patients with about seven dollars' worth of apricot seeds.

Ty: Yes, I just spoke to a medical doctor a couple of days ago that said 20 plus years ago he was curing people with oleander.

Dr. Coldwell: Yes.

Ty: And he got a huge fine and a letter saying, "Stop using unapproved treatments." Even though they were working, they were unapproved, so he got fined, and he had to stop.

Dr. Coldwell: It's like with the Rife machine. Dr. Roy Rife cured with frequency, every tumor. In 100 percent of cases he cured every tumor. So, of course, they made the machine illegal, and it is still not legal to use it today. It is like Hoxsey. He watched his horses eating certain herbs. The horses were dying, and months later they were completely healthy. So he was looking into what herbs they ate.

Ty: Very effective treatment still today, the Hoxsey treatment.

Dr. Coldwell: Absolutely, Ty.

Ty: Yes. And you mentioned the Royal Rife frequency machine. I know there are still a few of those left, actually. I don't know where they are, but they are hidden, because they are afraid that if the location is disclosed, that the FDA will seize them, which is shame that we live in a situation that if you have something like that, which is a non-approved treatment for cancer, that you risk getting it confiscated by the government.

Dr. Coldwell: Ty, I have proven that I can cure, historically, every cancer in two to six weeks, as long as the people didn't have medical treatment before—chemoradiation or surgery. Every doctor that is in office for about 20 or 30 years has seen cases of spontaneous healing. Every doctor has seen what they call the placebo effect. So I went a different way. I said, "Wait a second, if this is possible, how can I make this happen?" I don't care if you call it placebo, I don't care if you call it spontaneous healing, I don't care if you say God cured you. It doesn't matter. It happened. See, all I need to know is that it is possible. Show me one case and I will find out how to make this happen. And I had a patient, Ms. Giller, who was four days before breast surgery. She had four tumors in her breast, and a friend of mine, Professor Doctor Rupert wanted to do the surgery. So they basically slice the breast off. So she came to me, never heard of me before, then came to me four days before. I worked with her a couple of times, she went in for the surgery, they did the x-rays so that they know exactly where the tumors are and he called me up and said, "The tumors are gone. What in the world did you do?"

And actually, see, a cancer cell is 13 hertz, a healthy cell is 70 hertz. The second the frequency vibration changes, the energy changes, it's not a cancerous cell anymore. We are just frequency and vibration. We are just molecules. Everything can change in an instant as soon as you get hope again, as soon as you change the energy level. We've all heard stories like some old person was dying, and they hear they just got a grandchild, and an hour later they are back out of the hospital, because the motivation was back. Most people that die give themselves—cancer is very often a suicide attempt, a suicide command, because Dr. Carl Simonton, in his work with his huge cancer clinic in Fort Worth, Texas, stated that most of his cancer patients, 18 to 26 months before the diagnosis of cancer—a traumatic event, losing a loved one through death, losing a child through death, getting a house foreclosed, losing a job after 30 years, these kinds of things. And they verbally said, "I don't want to live like this anymore." So basically, very often cancer can be a suicide attempt, or a suicide command, as I call it. So if I don't address it, if I don't find out where it is coming from, and pity and empathy just kills patients. That's why I have more success.

Dr. Hern conducted a study in Berlin, Germany that came to the conclusion with a cancer cure of 92.3 percent. Dr. Gary Allen and Dr. Simoncini say the medical profession has a cancer cure rate of two percent. We figured out, friends of mine, if you do nothing, 27 percent of all cancer patients recover without doing anything. You know, they get completely healthy. I believe, anyway, we all have cancer three, four, five, six times in our lives, and if you don't go to to these early detection hoaxes which is just a money-making tool, it is just getting customers.

Ty: What would you summarize your message to cancer patients as being? Because I know it is a message of hope.

Dr. Coldwell: First of all, there is always a solution, there is always hope, there is always a way to get out of it, to turn it around, because my mom, 43 years later, she should be dead for 42 years, is still alive and 100 percent healthy. My sister should be dead, she is 100 percent healthy. And then you understand that people just have to have self-motivation. It's like you say, "You can lead a horse to the water but you cannot make it drink."

And the same is with cancer patients. I am willing to poke you until you fight back. See, most doctors want to be the nice guy, and then that patient dies. But if I tell them, "Stop wallowing in self-pity. Yes, yes, your husband cheated on you, so what? Get a new husband." Just get them out of the self-pity, out of the self-destructive, "Oh, my life is over." This is the hardest part, to give them self-motivation again, the will to live and motivation to self-motivation. And then I have patients that have come and they say, "Oh, I have three months to live, and I say, "No, you need to leave, I have a near 100 percent cure rate. If you want to die in three months you really need to go." And then they stare at me and they say, "What do you mean?" And I say, "If you want to live you can stay, and let's work something out. What do you want to do in five years?"

Ty: Right.

Dr. Coldwell: So all of a sudden I'm focusing them toward a hope, toward a future. And it's not about—Ty, there is no such thing as false hope. I always hear from the medical profession this absurdity. If I have hope and I live one day longer with a high quality of life that day was worth it. There is no such thing as false hope. And so my message is, actually, you need to identify what's wrong. Why do you want to die? Directly, or indirectly. What changed since you were healthy? What traumatic event happened? Or how is your toxicity level? And why are you obese? You're not obese because you like to be obese, tell me why you are obese. Are you creating an armor of fat because you were abused as a child and now you want to be not attractive anymore? If we don't address this the problem doesn't go away.

Ty: Right.

Dr. Coldwell: And so every negative behavior, and every negative result, has a root cause in us. And even if we eat toxins, even if we eat bad food, it's that we don't value us enough. And in my opinion, since cancer is caused by lack of self-love, lack of self-respect, lack of hope, lack of future, lack of control, you can gain all of this. Just don't rely on anybody else. Let your friends help you, but don't hope the government is going to fix you, don't hope you eat for so many years to gain 300 pounds and then your poor doctor is supposed to cure you in a week. Or you're an alcoholic for 30 years and then you want to have a healthy liver in a week? It doesn't work that way.

Ty: So basically, take control over what you have been given control over.

Dr. Coldwell: Absolutely, because we are creators. See, Ty, we both believe in God without question. So for me, the Bible says we are created after the likeness of God. So if a dog gets a baby, it's a dog. If a cat gets a baby, it's a cat. If a god gets a baby, it's a god—not God overall, but we are creators in our own world, we are gods in our own life, because everything we contemplate, everything we intensively contemplate, visualize in an associative state, will come true. I know this from martial arts. If you hit something that is really, really big, and you are afraid you cannot break it, you will break your hand. But if you are sure, you see it breaking in your head first, it will break.

Ty: So your message is to cancer patients to believe you can be healed.

Dr. Coldwell: No. You *know* it, because it has nothing to do with belief. You can know you can be cured because God will not give you a challenge you cannot fix. That would be completely absurd. It would be like you go to school and the teacher says the very first day you come that you will fail. So why would you go?

Ty: Right.

Dr. Coldwell: That makes no sense. The purpose of living, Ty, is personal growth and development. That's the only reason for living—personal growth and development. And because we are all lazy, God says, "Hey, hey, if you don't do it on your own, I'm going to push you a little bit. You know, I'll apply here a little bit, I'll give you a little bit of problems, a little bit of pain, a little bit of illness. Start thinking about yourself."

Ty: You know what? I think that your interview today is going to be pushing people to start doing that, Dr. C. I really appreciate your time.

Dr. Coldwell: Ty, thank you so much. Keep up the good work, my friend. Thank you.

Ty: Thank you.

[end of transcript]

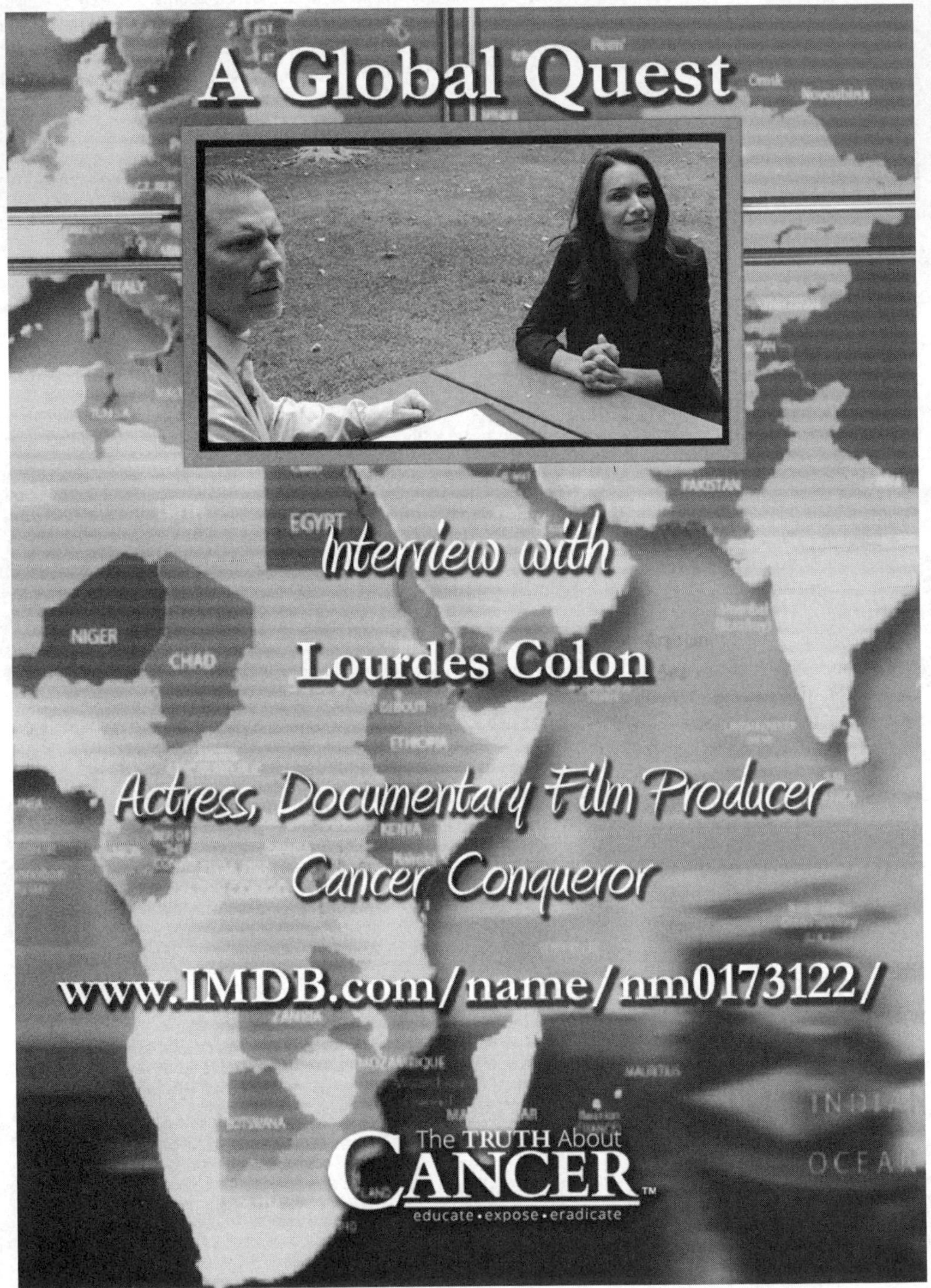
A Global Quest
Interview with
Lourdes Colon
Actress, Documentary Film Producer
Cancer Conqueror
www.IMDB.com/name/nm0173122/
The TRUTH About CANCER
educate • expose • eradicate

Ty: I'm really excited to be here in Orange, California today, with Lourdes Colon. Thank you for joining me.

Lourdes: Thank you.

Ty: Yeah, it's really nice to meet you, and I'm really excited to get your story of beating cancer. So first of all, you've got a documentary out.

Lourdes: Yes.

Ty: So tell us about it. It's called *Create Option C: My Journey with Cancer*. So tell us a little about your documentary, and then let's walk backwards to your cancer diagnosis.

Lourdes: Sure. Well, the documentary is really about my journey. I wanted to show people that there are things that you can do to not only prevent cancer, but once you have it, what you can do to avoid and get rid of it without having to do something so harsh like chemotherapy and radiation.

And I've always felt that there's always been a cure. We're just not taught that. So through the documentary—is what I did is, I started showing the cause and effect of things. Like, if I had something like a PET-CT scan, I would show them the before and after.

Like, here's this little tumor. I'm going to do this PET-CT scan, and show them how the radioactive sugar in that scan spreads the cancer. And so, within a week of doing the tests, it looked like a baby head was sticking out of my armpit from just the test.

And it started spreading, actually, immediately after the injection went in. So it's kind of that. Showing you: this is what happens when you do these kind of tests the doctor has you do. These are the things you can do to clean yourself out, to get rid of the stuff, and how to just shrink tumors and stuff, like with the stuff I was doing.

Ty: So you basically followed yourself through treatment?

Lourdes: Yes.

Ty: Okay, and in the documentary?

Lourdes: Correct.

Ty: Okay. That's interesting though. You say the PET scan, right, caused the tumors to grow?

Lourdes: Immediately. Like it was—I was fortunate enough that my cancer—because it was Hodgkin's Lymphoma, it was in the lymphatic system—it was very visual. Most people, when they have cancer, it's somewhere inside, so they don't see the results of what the PET-CT scan does, so when they get worse they just think it's the cancer.

It's all these other things, but they're not getting it's really the dye, it's the test they just did on you. And so, with the one I had, it was the greatest opportunity, because then I could show them. It's like, "See, look how it's growing."

Like my husband thought I was crazy. He's like, "You know you're getting rid of the cancer. Don't do this stuff that spreads it." And it was really important to me to do it, because I really wanted people to see how bad it is. Because I think most of the time—what happens if you tell somebody what it will do? To them it's your opinion, that's your own way of thinking.

So this way, it helped, showing them that it's not an opinion. It is a cause and effect, and that I did it with myself.

Ty: Right. And you're getting the visuals.

Lourdes: Absolutely.

Ty: And it's a great way to prove. A lot of visuals. Good.

Lourdes: Yes.

Ty: So, this documentary is out soon?

Lourdes: Yes, it is going out soon, with my DVD sale distributor, even though we have a couple people that are interested in distributing it for us.

Ty: Okay. Let's go back in time. Describe who you are—you're an actress—and so talk about your past, and then walk us up to the cancer diagnosis.

Lourdes: Sure. While I was an actress, I was always filming, always on set, always filming, and it was something I enjoyed. I had a deal with CBS, had a holding deal with them, which was great. I was put on the ballots to be considered to be a nominee for an Emmy in my role as Ana Rodriguez on *Without a Trace*.

I hosted a TV show called *The Movie Time Showcase*. I was doing a lot of independent films. I did a movie called *The Kiss*. And it was during that time that I started getting really exhausted. And I just thought it was because I'm filming all the time, and a lot of our shoots are at night, and maybe that's what's gotten me so drained.

But then when I stopped shooting, no matter what I was doing, I just wasn't getting back my energy. And so I knew something was off. And then I had, like, this lump that showed up on my neck. And I kind of knew, just by—because I have friends and family who had cancer.

My sister had had Hodgkin's Lymphoma, and hers started off with a lump on her neck. So for me it was an instant indication that I probably have Hodgkin's Lymphoma. And so, though I didn't tell my family, I just had to follow my gut.

Ty: What year was this?

Lourdes: That was 2010.

Ty: Okay.

Lourdes: And prior to that, I was consistently starting to feel and get things. Like a couple years before that, I really started getting lumps in the breast. And then I would immediately change my diet, and it would go away. So I would have documents from the doctors saying there's something fishy going on here, then I would do other nutrition, then would go back and they wouldn't find it. I'm like, "Okay, I'm fine." But then I'd go back to my bad habit. My habit was to eat sugar.

Ty: Okay.

Lourdes: And I loved sugar.

Ty: Who doesn't love sugar?

Lourdes: Oh my gosh. Mine was extreme. I would eat—95 percent of my intake was sugar. So it was like—if I had breakfast, I would eat 12 sandwich ice creams for breakfast.

Because I felt, "I'm skinny, I don't gain weight, I'm good." And not realizing the destruction I was doing to my body. And we'd go out for dinner and he would have a meal—and as my husband had his meal, I would have my brownie with ice cream on it and that's what I had for dinner. So that was like day in and day out, and then it really took a toll.

Ty: So Lourdes you had a real sugar addiction, didn't you?

Lourdes: A severe sugar addiction. It was—like literally 95 percent of my intake was sugar. And for me it was okay, because I couldn't put on weight. I didn't think about the destruction it was doing to my cells. For me it was like, "It's sugar." You don't think that something as simple as sugar that we put in almost everything is actually harmful to your health.

Ty: Right.

Lourdes: And so, I did it like—I don't put on weight. I'm okay. And so I ate like 12 sandwich ice creams every morning. I have a brownie, a nice warm brownie with ice cream on top for dinner. It was just cupcakes galore. It's all I wanted was just sweet—oh, rice pudding. So it was always—daily desserts is what I would have for breakfast, lunch, and dinner.

Ty: I can't believe you're eating like 12 ice cream sandwiches or whatever. I mean, you lived on sugar.

Lourdes: I lived on sugar. Yeah.

Ty: Literally, you weren't exaggerating.

Lourdes: No, I was not and I'm like—when somebody's like, "Oh yeah, I love sweets." I'm like, "No. You do not love sweets like I love sweets."

Ty: Okay.

Lourdes: And in fact, one of the things that, when I did get diagnosed with cancer, and I found out that sugar is one of the cancer feeders and you need to avoid it—that was like the toughest thing to do. I mean, I did it, but I'm like, "When is the craving going to go away?"

And I remember someone telling me, "Oh, you know, when you're doing this adventure, you don't have a craving for it." And I'm like, "Really? Because I could totally dive into sugar right now." And what I didn't get is that—once I was done with the cancer, where I was healthy again, I had something that someone gave me and it had some sugar in it and it was so repulsive to me. Because I wanted the sugar, but when I tasted it, I was like, "Whoa!" That was so strong that now I can't do sugar. And I'm like, they were right. You get to a point where you can't do the sugar, and I can't.

Ty: When you were diagnosed, did your oncologist suggest that one thing you might do is to give up this sugar?

Lourdes: My advice, when I was diagnosed with cancer—because I was really, really skinny. And again, I didn't know that I was losing so much weight because of the cancer—was, "Look, you're really skinny. Go out. Eat as much ice cream as you can. Enjoy yourself. Put on the weight."

And when she told me that, it was interesting, because I thought, "Well, no. Sugar feeds cancer, so I'm not going to do that." I didn't tell her that, but I was like, "Wow!"

Ty: That doesn't make sense.

Lourdes: No, and here they—they're not telling me get out there and start eating healthy. They're like, "Eat the sugar. Put on the weight."

Ty: So Lourdes, you learned that sugar is not really the food that you needed to be eating when you were diagnosed with cancer.

Lourdes: Right, absolutely.

Ty: Right?

Lourdes: Yes.

Ty: So at that point, did you have any kind of conversation with your doctor, with your oncologist, or did you kind of go out on your own and say, "Look, they don't know what's going on. I'm going to pursue my own path."

Lourdes: Well, I—this was where it was interesting, because before I was diagnosed, I wanted to be a difference in the world. And I was acting. I thought it was going to be through that, and I just couldn't figure out how. I'm like, "How can I be an inspiration to the world, to really inspire people in their life?"

And then, when I was diagnosed with cancer, as the doctor was telling me, "You have Hodgkin's Lymphoma," she went through this whole process of what they're going to do, and how they've got to put this port in me, and like, this whole process.

And as she was talking, I really didn't listen to her, because I was busy thinking, "Okay. So this is it. This is my opportunity to be an inspiration. I'm going to figure this out. I'm not going to do chemotherapy or radiation. I'm going to do it my way. And I'm going to do all the research."

And then there was my thought, "I'm going to get home. I'm going to start reading books. I'm going to start looking up who else fought cancer naturally." And there was the goal, and that's where I started learning what I learned, and I was like, "The doctors told me to eat sugar, and this thing's telling me it spreads cancer."

They're not telling me to go eat healthy. And there's all these other things I could do that is healthy and is anti-cancer, like berries, but to stay away from the fruit because of the sugar. There was just this whole set of rules.

And it dawned on me how not educated the medical field is when it comes to your health and cancer, and the things you should be doing when you're fighting cancer. Especially when they're telling me I should go out and eat ice cream and get back that weight.

Ty: Yeah. So at this point, you're beginning to do research. What did you learn in your research about the modern treatments for cancer? You said you didn't want to do chemo and radiation. Which treatments did you pursue?

Lourdes: I pursued completely non-toxic treatments. Anything that said it shrinks tumors or fights cancer, I took. And it had to make sense. If something—you had to add sugar to it, I'm like, "Nah, I won't do it." But if it was more like—it was all about detoxing, cleansing out the cells, getting the body back to normal.

When it started making sense to me, I'm like, "This makes sense. This is what I've got to do." Because one—and it's interesting because everything I searched out, every last one of them, was all about detox, you know, revamping your body, getting the stuff that's in there—that's been there forever—out. I read this book called *Kill Cancer, Not People*. I had so many books I read.

Ty: Is that Bob Wright?

Lourdes: I think so.

Ty: I think Bob Wright wrote that. Yeah.

Lourdes: And there's—I mean, I have so many books at home. And I did so much reading. That's all I did on a daily basis. There was one that talked about doing a colonics on a daily basis, so I went and got the Colema Board, and started doing the colonics every day.

Ty: Okay.

Lourdes: And I noticed—the moment I did that, I did start feeling a difference. Because before that, because they had did the PET-CT scan, it was still kind of—even though they say it's out of your body after 45 minutes or whatever, it was so not true. It continued. I continued feeling the process of the growth in the cancer.

So when I finally got the Colema Board, and started doing it daily, it started flushing things out, and I didn't feel so—I didn't feel the pain, I didn't feel the swelling, and I didn't feel the agony. I felt these— things did start shrinking.

Ty: Okay.

Lourdes: I learned about wheat grass.

Ty: Wheat grass, okay.

Lourdes: Yeah, wheat grass was a really big part of the things that I did in fighting cancer. And I found out that it has chlorophyll that's very similar to your blood, that's just one component away from what your blood is.

Ty: Right.

Lourdes: And they have iron that has amazing— I mean—and you've seen how it's built, I mean iron—it's a win-win. I learned that also vitamin B17—I knew that B17 fights cancer and shrinks tumors. So as much as I disliked the taste...

Ty: Yoah, bittcr.

Lourdes: Ugh. And I knew so many people that love it. It's so crazy. But I will say that when I started doing a lot of wheat grass, I would do between four to eight ounces a day. I did colonics every day. I would also do a coffee enema to detox the liver, which was very—it was immensely helpful in everything that I was doing.

And I would take the pulp of the wheat grass, and I'd dip it into the wheat grass juice, I'd place it on the tumors with—leave it on for an hour. I started seeing shrinkage that way. In fact, I did that for a couple days. And there was a time when I couldn't lay on my side because of the pressure, but doing that I was able to finally lay on my right side without any pressure. So it was that. It was wheat grass.

It was raw juicing. I did raw juicing for three straight weeks, where I saw an immense stuff that came out. I mean, there was this long—I can't tell you how long it was, but it was very, very long parasite that came out.

And this is just from doing the wheat grass shots and doing the colonics daily. But I was looking—like, "How is that possible? It was in my belly." It was just this very long parasite that came out.

Then you see, like, a lot of this dead cancer cell that came out. It looked like it was a web. And this stuff was coming out. It was tinted with the wheat grass when it came out. It was interesting. But it pulled all that out. So you got to see the results—

Ty: Yeah.

Lourdes: —of doing those things.

Ty: So Lourdes, when you were diagnosed with cancer and you were a sugar addict before—and now you changed the way you're eating. Give me kind of a typical day in the diet of Lourdes Colon.

Lourdes: If I ate—in the beginning I did a lot of raw. Because raw was very important because of the live enzymes. And I got used to where—I got that I was going to lose a lot of weight. And I was very thin already. But when you lose a lot of toxins, you lose weight.

So had to put in my head, "It's okay to lose weight as long as I'm healthy." And so, a lot of people tend to get wrapped in how skinny they get, that they forget about the point of it and it's to beat the cancer and get healthy. So, I had to get myself around back because I got down to 70 pounds, but I felt healthy. I felt like I could pick up a house. Because I was so healthy.

So it's really just—I would do wheat grass every morning and every afternoon. I didn't do it in the evening, because it gave you a lot of energy. I would do brown rice. I didn't do any more white rice. Because it's—I not only learned that it was not as healthy, but white rice breaks out into a more high sugar, just like potato does.

Ty: Right.

Lourdes: So I avoided those kind of things. I did a lot of avocado. When—after three weeks. At the beginning of the three weeks I didn't because it doesn't—even though avocado's amazing for you, because of the oil it slows down the detox process. And for me, it was really important to be detoxed. So avocado has good fats. I would put a lot of that in. I did that with a lot of the stuff that I would make. I planned everything with avocado. It all tastes good.

Ty: Yeah.

Lourdes: So I didn't do any animal products. No animal products. No dairy, none of that. I got real clear, after reading the China study, that it does help progress the cancer. So I was not going to give it anything. It didn't have a chance with me.

Ty: So you were like totally dedicated.

Lourdes: Very dedicated.

Ty: You changed. I mean, you have to, because as much sugar as you were eating—and sugar is more addictive than cocaine. So you were addicted to sugar and you broke that habit because you wanted to live.

Lourdes: Yes.

Ty: Right?

Lourdes: Yeah.

Ty: What advice would you have for somebody that's been recently diagnosed, and they go and, you know, they only get option A or B— and then we'll get you to say, to tell everybody what option C is, right?

So they only get these normal options, the standard protocol. What advice would you give to somebody that's been diagnosed? Where should they go for information and what questions should they ask their oncologist?

Lourdes: If they're diagnosed with cancer, this is their journey, this is their life, this is their health, and it's so important to educate yourself. I mean, start doing the research. Find out what other people have done. Find out what doctors they've seen.

Get questions from them, because a lot of times, when you go to—like the doctor I went to in the beginning, which I let go of, I thought was a great doctor, because he was so kind and very caring, and just listened. Until I said I wasn't going to do chemo. And then—

Ty: He got upset.

Lourdes: He was completely, like, a 180. And so I got clear at that moment that he was really for me, he was really Team Lourdes. He would listen to me, he would try to see how he could work with me.

Instead, it was more like, "Oh wait. You're not doing it my way?" And then it just became this other person. So I was like, "Oh, so you weren't being kind because you really care. You were being kind because I was going to do chemo."

Ty: Because you obeyed.

Lourdes: Yeah.

Ty: Right.

Lourdes: And in the moment I chose something different. So I looked at—I let go of that doctor, and I didn't see another doctor for a while because I decided I'm going to find the right doctor. And until then, I'm just not—I'm going to do it my way.

And I really advise people that they should educate themselves, find out other people that have done it naturally, who they saw, what were the questions they asked? What are the things that they need to know?

Because the more educated you are, the more educated decision you're going to make. Because doctors are going to put the fear in there, and because of fear, you're going to make the wrong decision, because fear does not let you think right.

Ty: Right.

Lourdes: And I got real clear on that, because they were telling me, at that time, I was stage 3B, almost stage 4. And then when I went to him again, he's like, "That's it. I'm done. There's no way of turning back."

But when you're at that stage, and they're putting this fear in you, like, "You have to do this, and this is the only way to do it, and I've had people that tried the other stuff and they died." I mean, you should have seen the conversation I had with him. I was like, "Wow!"

We are so not working as a team here. Because everything that came out of his mouth was very, very negative. And I feel that when you have a good doctor, everything that comes out of his mouth is optimistic. He's very positive. He's, "Let's see what works with you."

We can't just put everybody in the same little box and say, "Chemo for everybody, radiation." No. I think chemo has its place. I don't think it's to fight cancer, personally, myself. But I do think it has its place. But for me—I had an opening in my lung and the only thing that would seal it was going to be chemo.

Because it's so toxic that it scars your body from the inside out— that it would scar and seal it. So that made sense to do that. Because if I did surgery, that would cause more lung complications that I didn't want. So I think it does have its place. I don't think, for me personally, that it—

Ty: But as far as treating cancer, one of the top cancer treatments doesn't really have a place.

Lourdes: Yeah. Not for cancer. Because it causes cancer. That's what's funny. If you look at the book that they give you to read through and sign—but you never read through it—one of the side effects is to give you cancer again. It destroys your entire immune system. So your immune system—if something happens—it has nothing to fight with, because it's gone now.

Ty: Right.

Lourdes: So you know, it stays in your cells for so many years, and they tell people, "Oh no. When you're done, it's done." It's like, no, there's a reason why they call it remission. Because they couldn't get rid of that stem cell that's sitting in there from the cancer. It's not made to do that. So when you do chemotherapy and you do radiation, you have to know there's a reason why you have to go for the first five years, every three months to get checked. Because they know they didn't get rid of all of it.

They know that the treatments they give you is that—chances are, you're going to get it back. And you may get it back, not on the fifth year, but five years and two weeks later. They cut if off at five because they know that any time after that, for sure, you're going to end up with it again. They played it smart.

Ty: Well, you know, you're considered to be a success even if you die, after that period. Because you lived the five year period. Which is kind of crazy.

Lourdes: Yeah. And you've had the most depleted life. It's like—they know the process. And when you're doing chemotherapy, you have to understand that there's a reason why you get so sick; there's a reason why you get so weak; there's a reason why you lose your hair; there's a reason why your liver gets so taxed. And then it ends up going somewhere else. Because that's the destruction it's doing. And for me, it never made sense to use a treatment that's going to destroy my cells, when cancer's already destroying my cells. Why would I add to the fire? Like, it just doesn't make sense to me.

Ty: Right. How do you heal a sick body with something that will make it sicker?

Lourdes: Yeah. It doesn't make sense.

Ty: Right.

Lourdes: So, you know, I just think my advice to people is educate yourself, because when you educate yourself, and you listen to both sides—you don't want to listen to one side, because you get to one side, and you hear it, but when you see both sides, you go, "Oh. Yeah, but this does make sense." The moment you see the two sides, natural makes sense.

Ty: Right.

Lourdes: It's just that simple. It makes sense.

Ty: Right. I think that's good advice, too. It reminds me of—it's an anecdotal story at best, but it's the CIA. When they are studying counterfeit bills to determine if—to learn how to spot counterfeit bills, they don't study counterfeits. They study real bills. And so, once they know—they see the real bill. Then they can notice everything else is a counterfeit, because they already know the real bill. And so I think that's what you're saying.

Lourdes: Yeah.

Ty: You can see that these natural treatments work. And when you compare them with other things that will kill you, there's not really much of a comparison.

Lourdes: Exactly. And that's the thing. It's like, you know, you have to understand that when you go see an oncologist who is solely trained through the conventional way, they don't have much clue on natural. They don't.

Ty: Yeah.

Lourdes: And that's why I find it really interesting when they talk against it. It's like, "How can you talk against something that you yourself have not learned or educated yourself to know?" You know, for me, if a doctor wants to talk against it—learn it, and then tell me with all that knowledge why it doesn't work.

I get people who say, "Well, my doctor said that I shouldn't do this because then it will do this." I said, "He spoke about nutrition and he's not even trained in that? Wow! That's amazing that he spoke from a source of what he doesn't have knowledge of."

Ty: Right. And you know what's funny. A good friend of mine is a medical doctor down in San Antonio. He'll text me pictures sometimes from his hospital in the doctor's lounge. And in the doctor's lounge they're serving Twinkies and ice cream sandwiches. It's like, these are professionals who are supposed to be keeping us healthy and that's what they're eating. Why would we listen to that? You know?

Lourdes: And they don't see the damage that they're doing to themselves.

Ty: Right. Well, you can see it by looking at them. Because they're typically unhealthy people.

Lourdes: They are. They really are.

Ty: You know?

Lourdes: Yeah. It's like—in fact, I went to see my sister quite a few months ago, and she was sick with pneumonia. And usually, before I ever got diagnosed with cancer—that's what I always tell people. "No, I'm healthier now after cancer than I was before I ever had cancer."

Because my—if I would be around someone at that time, if they even had a slight cold, I don't care how minute it was, I always got severely sick, every single time. But the moment I got so healthy after cancer, I can be around someone who's sick. I don't get sick.

Ty: Because your immune system's working.

Lourdes: Oh my gosh. It's working like it needed to be working in the beginning.

Ty: Right.

Lourdes: It's not getting destroyed by sugar anymore and the terrible foods I had. But yeah, my sister was full blown coughing up a lung, and she just had this really bad case of pneumonia, and I never got sick. And I'm like, "Wow! There's testimony right there." I would get sick at the drop of a hat and I did not get sick. I felt great the whole time.

Ty: You're doing something right.

Okay. So the big mystery question now at this point. What exactly is option C?

Lourdes: Well, option C— you have to first know what option A and B is. Option A is to do solely everything that the doctor tells you to do.

Ty: Which is what most people do.

Lourdes: Yes. Most people just go to the doctor, the doctor tells him this, take this medicine, do this, and that's all they do. They don't do the research, they don't educate, and that's all they do. That's option A.

Option B is something like my dad did. And I met several people that did this. They get diagnosed with cancer and for them it's like, "It's what God wants. I'm not going to do anything. I'm just going to live my life without keeping it in mind."

Ty: Which a lot of times, the studies show they live longer than option A.

Lourdes: Absolutely.

Ty: If they aren't treated with conventional treatment.

Lourdes: Yes, absolutely. In fact, my grandfather had stomach cancer. Such a severe case that he ended up going to the hospital because he just bled that much. And he went home and he continued to live his life the way he lived. And he lived in Puerto Rico and he lived for an additional 10, 15 years—never ever did treatments. And he didn't have any problems. He didn't show any issues.

Ty: And yet he lived that long with stomach cancer?

Lourdes: Yeah.

Ty: And you can contrast that with my father, who had stomach cancer, and they cut his stomach out, and he died in 25 days.

Lourdes: See?

Ty: Yeah.

Lourdes: Yeah, my grandfather lived for an additional 10 to 15 years. And he didn't show any indication he was sick. And he had stomach cancer. Other than he was bleeding. He was strong. He was still picking up all that wood and doing his job. Like, he just didn't stop.

He was in his 70s. He was doing really good. So, you know—and then my dad, he didn't do anything, and he eventually died. But he did sugar. He craved—I think that's where I got the sugar from. My daddy. He craved sugar, so he was always eating sugar.

But so then, option C is doing the research, educating yourself, learning how your body works, and how it works with nature, with things that are out there. So option C is educating yourself, doing the research, and doing what's best for your body.

Ty: I like that. Well, that's what we're about with *The Truth About Cancer* is option C—is to educate people about cancer.

Lourdes: Yes.

Ty: And I think that one of the things that people need to realize is the power to heal is within your own body if you supply it with the right nutrients. And they also need to realize that we don't have to do everything that you do in option A. You don't have to just obey because it's a doctor, right?

Share with the listeners—the viewers—your story that you shared with me about your daughter, and the fish oil and all that—that happened. It's really fascinating. This is just proof that you're walking the walk, right?

Lourdes: Yes.

Ty: Because you're saying, "People, you don't have to do everything that the white coats tell you."

Lourdes: Right.

Ty: And so here's a real life example that you just shared with me that's really fascinating. So go ahead.

Lourdes: Through my research, I learned that the body fixes everything if we give the body the right tools, the right formula. It just does its job. It's got its own brain. It knows what to do. So my daughter had—last year—had this severe brain injury where she lost all the white matter.

And so they clinically considered her brain-dead. And so the doctor was going to keep my daughter alive until I got there. So I flew out to Chicago. And before I got there I did research. Because I got clear. They're not going to turn off the machines and I know this is going to be fixable.

So I started learning through all my research that fish oil—high doses of fish oil—rebuilds the brain. Because when you're in your mother's womb, the one thing that your brain is built from is omega-3 fatty acids. So if you saturate the body with omega-3 fatty acids, the body will then kick in high gear and start taking that and doing what it needs to rebuild whatever's missing.

And so I got there and I told the doctors—I even brought my fish oil with me. I went to a Whole Foods there, and got the fish oil, and I said, "Okay, you're going to give my daughter 20 grams of fish oil daily through her feeding tube. I'm not turning off the machines. I know this will work."

And you had to see the way they reacted. Because it was like five different doctors. They all thought I was crazy. They looked at me like, "Oh, wishful thinking. Oh, this one she's a little..." So I just said, "No this is what we've got to do." And one doctor's like, "What do you think fish oil's going to do for your daughter?"

And I was like, "Really? Like you don't know what it would do?" I said, "Look." I said, "When you're in your mother's womb, that's what your brain is built from, omega-3 fatty acids. So if that's what she's missing, we just need to add it. The body will do its job." I said—and I showed them, there's all these other facts that other people have done that it worked.

And the first three doctors wouldn't do it, and then I got the head doctor to do it, and he said, "You know what? We don't get taught this in medical school. I'll try it."

Ty: It's worth a shot.

Lourdes: Yeah. And he was the only one that was okay with giving the fish oil. Everybody else was so not— was so against it. And so they started giving her 20 grams of fish oil on a daily basis. And the first doctor's like, "You know, that's really high. It can cause bleeding."

And I'm thinking, "She's not going anywhere. She's bedridden. And I think she'll be fine. She needs that." So they went ahead and still did it. By the third day, she did wake up. And what they kept doing is they wanted to show me that she's still a vegetable.

And they would go and they'd get this little cotton ball-like thing, and they would touch her eyeball, because her eyes would stay open, and she wouldn't react. It's called doll eyes. And they would do this thing on her foot really hard and she wouldn't respond.

And I'm like, "I got it. It's only been three days. Give her a chance." And then they kept doing it. And then they stopped giving it to her because she's starting to get better.

Ty: They stopped when she started getting better?

Lourdes: Right. And I think it's because they were like—now I'm going to be right and they're going to be wrong. And so I noticed they weren't giving her the fish oil, so I told the nurse, "I didn't see them giving the fish oil today." And the nurse was very arrogant, because they all didn't like the fact that I had brought this whole natural thing into their realm.

Ty: Right.

Lourdes: And so she's like, "Yeah, the doctor discontinued that." I'm like, "Wait. What doctor discontinued it?" She's like, "I don't know. It's just on the thing." And I'm like... so I called my husband and let him know what they did, and I immediately stated that I was going to call my friend who was a state representative there, and I was going to get this hospital closed down, and I'm going to shake people's lives up.

And within five minutes of them listening to me tell this to my husband—because they were like, "Oh. Her friend is who?" They then brought in the fish oil. And I was like, "Oh, what's this?" She's like, "The fish oil." I'm like, "Oh." They continued it again.

And so she went—and by the third week, she no longer had doll eyes. She was responding. She couldn't speak yet, but she was responding. By the second month, she started finally speaking. By the third month, she started to go to therapy to walk.

And now, a year—ot even a year, because that happened in February, right, of 2014. And by November, she moved out already. And so—and here they are telling me that this is not going to work, and within months she was already walking. She's now moved out.

Ty: She's living on her own?

Lourdes: She lives on her own. She's doing great.

Ty: And they wanted to pull the plug.

Lourdes: And they wanted to pull the plug.

Ty: Wow. You know, the thing that's sad, which I shared with you earlier, is that—how many families have been in that same scenario and they haven't questioned the doctor and they just pulled the plug? And somebody has died that could have lived had they known that.

Lourdes: Yeah. They actually put an end to them. And they suffocate when they turn off the machines. They do suffocate. But because they can't tell you they're suffocating.

Ty: Right.

Lourdes: And actually, there were five people in the ICU where my daughter was, going through the same problem. Of course, they didn't get the fish oil. And five of them had passed away that week.

Ty: Well, I'm glad your daughter's doing well.

Lourdes: Yeah. Thank you.

Ty: That's awesome. And I think this is just more evidence that we should all choose option C, right?

Lourdes: Yes.

Ty: Do your research. Realize that you don't have to just obey—blindly obey—what the doctors say.

Lourdes: Exactly.

Ty: And I think that in the end, people get this information, they're going to be a lot better off from a health perspective long term.

Lourdes: Oh yeah. It's your life. You know? Your body, your health.

Ty: Yeah. Well, Lourdes, thank you for sharing this. This has been fascinating. And I understand option C now, and we're right in line with each other. Create option C. You have to. You've got to take control because the power to heal is yours, in your body, if you give it what it needs, and stop putting the sugar in it, right?

Lourdes: Yes. I don't touch sugar now.

Ty: Awesome. Well, Lourdes thank you so much. I really appreciate it.

Lourdes: Thank you so much. I appreciate it. Thanks.

Ty: Alright.

[end of transcript]

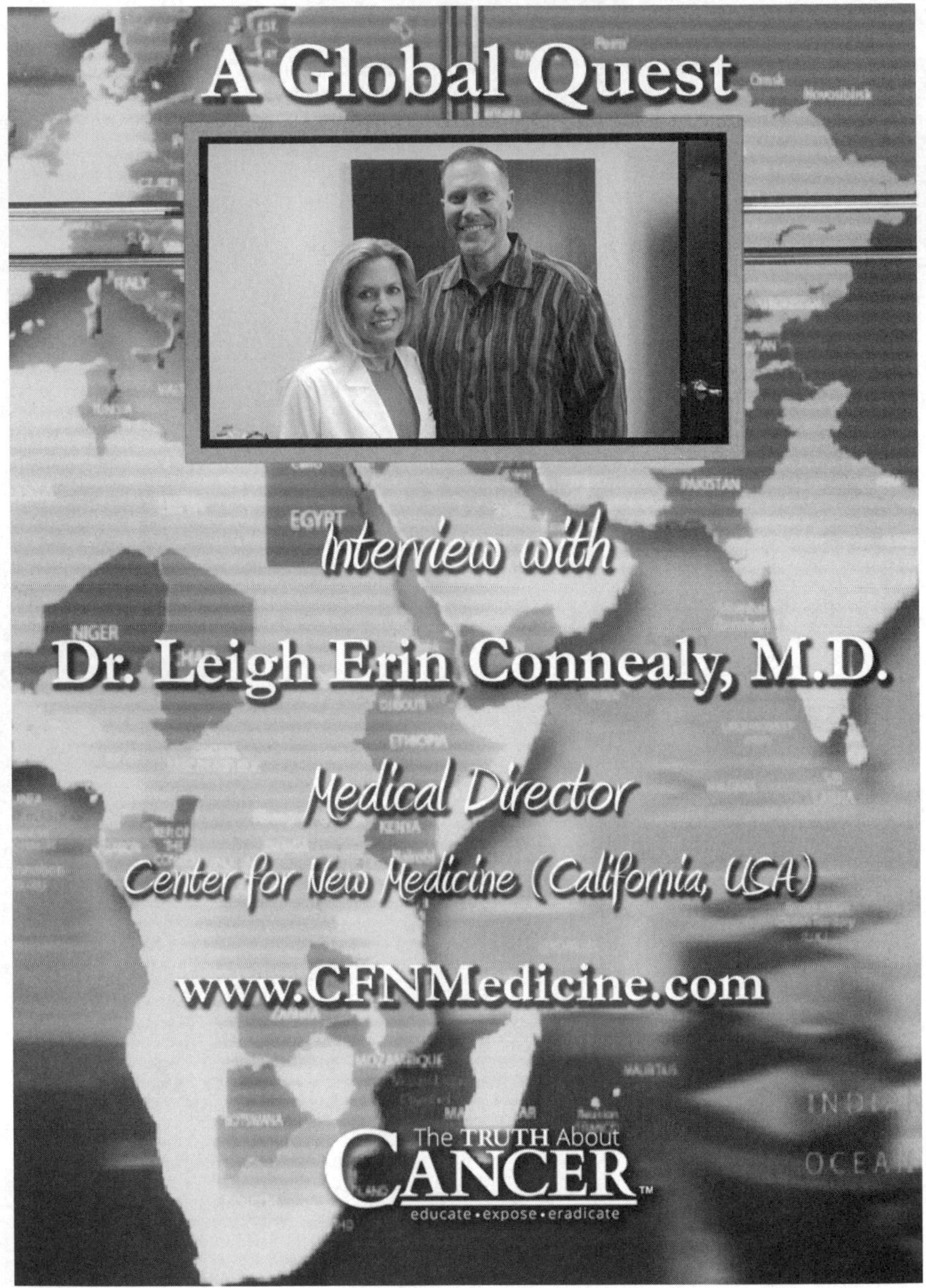
A Global Quest
Interview with
Dr. Leigh Erin Connealy, M.D.
Medical Director
Center for New Medicine (California, USA)
www.CFNMedicine.com
The TRUTH About CANCER
educate • expose • eradicate

Ty: Well, I'm really excited to be here with Dr. Leigh Erin Connealy again. I was able to interview her last year for our documentary mini-series. And now we're here at your office in Irvine, California. And you've got a couple of different offices here. First of all, thanks for being here at your office and inviting us.

Dr. Connealy: Thank you, Ty. It's so good to have you.

Ty: I know that you re-arranged your schedule today so you could be here. You're supposed to be speaking at a conference in Dallas. So thank you for being here.

Dr. Connealy: You're welcome.

Ty: Tell us about the two clinics that you have here.

Dr. Connealy: Okay. We have two clinics. We have the Center for New Medicine which takes care of general medicine patients which could be anything from cold, to diabetes, to heart disease, to chronic fatigue, to Lyme. And then we have, specifically for our cancer patients, The Cancer Center for Healing.

Ty: And Dana gave us a tour this morning and—just some incredible machinery and equipment here. Some of these chambers that you have, the hyperbaric oxygen, the baths, all of these things—I've never seen the quality of the equipment that you have here. Could you kind of go through this real briefly, maybe a synopsis of what you have here to treat disease, the different pieces of equipment that you've purchased?

Dr. Connealy: Yes. I tell people we have Disneyland for medicine here.

Ty: Yeah. It does look like.

Dr. Connealy: And it is. And I tell people, anyone coming here would absolutely feel wonderful, comfortable, and peaceful. Nothing we do hurts or invades you but everything is to restore balance and homeostasis to the human organism. And yes, we have multiple different devices. As you walk in, it's a place of comfort. And then there are different aspects to the clinic. We have the special IV room where we do IV infusions and everything from vitamin C to curcumin to brain restorations to immune system to healing of the liver and brain with phosphatidylcholine. We do glutathione drips. We have a complete menu of different IVs for different patients.

Then, we have a new device that we've been using called the Ultraviolet Light Rx.

Ty: Yeah, we saw that this morning.

Dr. Connealy: Yes. So basically what it is, it's—in your vein is infrared light, several different wavelengths of light that are designed to kill all the bugs in your body, but it also activates your immune system, increases your oxygen saturation and it's absolutely amazing.

So we've been using that for a couple of months. It's in a clinical trial, soon-to-be FDA approved. Then we have our ONDAMED machine. Basically, we can scan the body from head to toe. And what it is—we all are bioelectrical beings. Basically, it sets the electrical energy of your body. It's a machine from Germany. And it will tell me what is out of balance. And then we can put the electrical frequencies in to create balance in that organ or gland or system.

Then, we have our Infrared Sauna that's been utilized. We've had Infrared Sauna for over 15 years in our clinic. That's designed to detoxify the body and elevate the temperature of the system that—basically cancer cells don't like heat. But it's not just for them; it's for any chronic condition. It's an amazing way to detox.

We have our new Nano Oxygen Baths that are from Japan. And we're the first clinic in United States to have those—and actually this weekend will be optimized to a combination of two different technologies.

The Nano Bath is to create oxygenation to the tissue because, as we all know, the first and foremost thing we all need is oxygen to live and survive. And because you oxygenate your body, the body can detox better, the body's circulation can get better. If you have chronic pain, it's amazing, because pain, just like when you have a heart attack, is deficiency of oxygen.

And then we have our amazing hyperbaric chamber. Hyperbaric has been used all over the world for many, many years and growing. The interest in the hyperbaric is growing every single day in the United States. Around the world it is standard, but in the United States.

We can treat everything from cancer to wounds to diabetes to nitrogen bends and all kinds of medical problems that are approved for use for all kinds of different patients. Autism, we have brain injuries. We have a neurosurgeon that refers those patients who have that unusual brain tumor called glioblastoma. So, hyperbaric is a beautiful intervention for so many things.

Ty: And you also got that—Dana showed us a biological dentist on site.

Dr. Connealy: Yes, we have a biological dentist because as most people know, our mouth and head is connected to the rest of our body. And that all of our teeth—there's a whole macrocosm involved in our teeth, good or bad.

So for example, if you have a root canal that is actually an infection—if you have infections, it puts a drain on the body. And actually in breast cancer 97 percent they say are related to a root canal because your teeth drained into your body. But it is also a burden just like viruses are a burden to the body and increase the patient's risk of getting cancer.

Then, we have our whole body department where we do lymphatic drainage. We have the machine called the Light Beam Generator. And because your lymph removes the garbage from the bod—the blood delivers the groceries, the lymph removes the garbage. So we have the manual, we have the machine called The Lymph Star and then we have the Light Beam Generator with Ozone.

Speaking of ozone, we do all kinds of ozone. We do ozone IV. We treat autoimmune problems with ozone where we take the patient's blood out and combine it with oxygen and give it back to the patient. We use ozone—there's lots of different applications, for injury, for all kinds of bugs and everything that we use ozone for.

So you'll see we have an ozone generator which we make on site. We make individually for each patient and then we give it to the patient depending upon their clinical needs.

And then we have a star nutritionist on board that's been with me for 15 years. She knows everything and every diet and we try to customize the diet for each patient depending on what they have, whether it's diabetes, heart disease, or cancer. Every individual is unique, and so there isn't just this one-size-fits-all.

Then we have our PEMF, Pulsed Electromagnetic Field. You'll meet Dr. Bales. Dr. Bales is our expert in the Pulsed Electromagnetic Field. Again, we're an energetic being and when cells are sick they resonate at a lower hertz. The PEMF raises the hertz of every cell in your body and we also do targeted—whether you have a brain cancer, whether you have pancreatic cancer—we'll do the whole body and then targeted areas depending on the patient's illness.

Ty: Targeted PEMF?

Dr. Connealy: Target PEMF which you'll see today. So, we raise the energy hertz of the body so the body can heal itself. There are over a thousand PubMed studies on Pulsed Electromagnetic Field. It is actually FDA approved for the use of brain cancer. We will be showing you that today.

Then, we have our EVOX Therapy. "Vox" is the Latin word for voice. So we all have had trauma or unresolved emotional conflicts in our body and in our mind and in our spirit. And so what this does is it maps the brain. And you can tell—you'll see on the screen—you'll see the patient's brain-mapping and you would be able to know exactly what emotional conflict. And then we reframe that experience or that conflict or that emotion and resolve it depending on each patient, obviously. But it doesn't take, like, a lot of treatments. It could take just a few treatments.

Now, we do have expert psychologists here also. If a patient needs that one-on-one hand-holding, or maybe they've suffered something very serious or some very serious trauma and they need—we have Dr. McDonald here who will walk the patient through that issue.

Ty: Wow.

Dr. Connealy: I said it's Disneyland for medicine.

Ty: It is.

Dr. Connealy: You could just come here all day long and get well and feel amazing.

Ty: Well, I can't imagine being able to get in-depth on all of these different devices. Who scheduled us for only four hours here? Oh, that was me.

Dr. Connealy: The other thing that we do that is actually the emerging field of medicine and that's Energy Medicine. We do several different devices. We have the ZYTO device. And we'll have all of you experience that.

Basically, we have acupuncture points in our fingers and toes that correspond to every organ in our body. But it is impossible in a laboratory experience to find every single thing that is going on with Ty Bollinger today. But if we do energy testing we can see today what's going on in your system. What are the biggest toxins?

Let's say I want to fix your adrenal glands. I have 200 products that I can give you, but what is going to work best for Ty? We match the energy of the product with the patient. But we also—you come in here and you tell me you're fatigued, you can't sleep very well, you have joint pain, well, that can fit into many, many illnesses.

Do you have Lyme? Do you have rheumatoid arthritis? Do you have an autoimmune disease? Do you have cancer? So we can use the energy of the body, the biofield of the body to ascertain what is going on with you and how we can fix you.

We also do a machine called the Biomeridian. There is Dr. Voll and I don't know if you have ever heard of him. He taught all the courses, "Electro-acupuncture according to Voll." He was a physicist and a medical doctor from Germany. He taught the courses.

Many years ago I had an acupuncturist that came to interview with me. And he worked with me and he actually showed me the original manuals. And there were thousands of pages each on how to take every acupuncture point and then you can figure out what's wrong with the person and what to do about it.

So, that was all computerized in the 80s in a machine called the Biomeridian. What we can do now is—we do something called The Cancer Cascade because most people don't realize from one cancer cell to a tumor is 10 years. You just don't wake up and have cancer. You don't wake up and have heart disease. You don't wake up and have almost any illness unless you are exposed to someone with strep throat and, okay, you get strep throat. But these are chronic diseases.

So now we can figure out through your acupuncture points on your fingers and toes. And this was developed approximately 21 or 22 years ago by a gentleman who had osteosarcoma. As you know, osteosarcoma is a very serious cancer and usually the treatment is surgical removal of the tumor. Radiation and chemo is not favorable for that particular cancer.

He was 22 at that time. He was hit by a drunk driver and on Thanksgiving Day. I met him many years ago. I met him actually 18 years ago and he told me his life story and he became one of my mentors. They told him, "We need to amputate his leg." So, he said, "No, I'm not going to amputate my leg." He spent the next 11 years figuring out how to save his leg and cure himself of cancer. And so, that's what we developed as The Cancer Cascade. So I can determine in year one of the cancer timeline if you have cancer.

And this is what's so amazing, is when he was alive—he was diagnosed at 22 and lived till he was 69. So he lived a long time. And osteosarcoma people don't live for 5 years, most of them.

Anyway, he wanted to open up little minute cancer clinics all over the United States. Hopefully, that vision can be realized in our lifetime because, as everyone knows, cancer is pandemic and it is growing out of control. And we know now how to prevent cancer. I tell every patient, it is very easy to prevent cancer, but it is not easy to treat cancer. So if we can all learn how to find and detect—and now we have amazing science and technology to figure out and prevent cancer, but people just don't know.

That's why you're here because you are going to let the world know what is available all over the world and that is what we need to do because we are in an emergency crisis in health. Not only in the United States, but everywhere in the world.

And disease is only increasing in every category. We're talking about cancer now. But if you look at heart disease, if you look at diabetes, if you look at autoimmune diseases, if you look at diseases caused from conventional use of medication, they are all increasing.

So we all as a human race and a human organism are all interconnected, universally, all over. We need to change the world and allow people to know what they can do. A lot of it is what you can do yourself. That is what we're trying to do. We impart the knowledge to our patients and we tell them, "It is your job to be a good partner with us and do what we are recommending."

Ty: You mentioned it is relatively easy to prevent cancer, right?

Dr. Connealy: It is very easy to prevent cancer.

Ty: How would we communicate that to people that are watching?

Dr. Connealy: Well, I tell people prevention is priceless. It will save you lots of aggravation. I tell patients, "Look how comfortable you are, sitting here, enjoying your beautiful life. You're walking, you're talking, you're feeling, and you're enjoying your world. You go on a walk or you go and eat or you go out to a movie, and you're just having a wonderful life." But once you get the diagnosis of cancer, what happens, Ty? You know, you've talked to enough patients.

Ty: It changes quickly.

Dr. Connealy: Your world stops, okay. And once you enter into the system and you need a surgery or you need a chemo or radiation, you are losing your life. Because even surgery—just say you had a little lump, one centimeter—surgery is a major assault and attack on the body. It affects the nervous system, it affects your physiology, and it's outrageously stressful.

We do surgery all day long like it's no big deal. But no, you need to prepare the patients for two weeks for surgery, mentally and physically. Are their nutrients good? Are they eating well? Are they prepared to heal after surgery? So all of my patients before we even do surgery—because sometime surgery is necessary—I prepare them two weeks and get them nutritionally, physically, and mentally sound to be prepared so that surgery is easy and they can recover beautifully.

And the patients who do that recover significantly better when someone does.

Just like yesterday I had a patient. She just had a gallbladder surgery. And now, in a gallbladder they don't cut you from stem-to-stern, they just laparoscope. They put a little hose and they take—and she goes, "Dr. Connealy, it took me one year to recover from gallbladder surgery."

Ty: Yeah, you have, very frequently, people that are being operated on for cancerous tumors and they never recover from the surgery. That was my father. They took his stomach out and he died in 25 days. He never recovered from that surgery.

Dr. Connealy: That's interesting that you say that because I remember—this was about 12 years ago—I had a patient who came to see me for second opinion for her stomach cancer. And she was seeing another institution and they had removed her stomach. I did the consult, but I told the family and I said, "You removed the stomach, that's your gateway, your freeway to help your body to heal. You have to have your stomach." And so, the patient died in less than 30 days.

Ty: It sounds like my father.

Dr. Connealy: Exactly. There's a lot of literature on surgery, about health surgery. We have many, many patients. Dana, who is in charge of our patient services and she will hear all the stories. And if we just told all the stories that we hear everyday that in itself could be an exposition because these patients will tell me, "Okay, Dr. Connealy, I had surgery," and you know three months later it's everywhere.

Ty: Right. Yeah.

Dr. Connealy: Because surgery, once you've disturbed the natural milieu and the natural place and location of the homeostasis of the body, you've really opened up the spread of cancer cells. And there are scientific papers on this. And I know surgeons don't like to talk about it because it is obviously fearful for the patient.

But that is why if the patient is prepared and that they are taking the nutrients to make sure that doesn't happen. And then you have to follow those patients very carefully after, especially if they are young. If patients are young, their cancers used to be—because their metabolism is so much higher—it is a much more of an aggressive situation.

And so, all my young patients who were in their 20s and 30s, I watched them diligently. I tell them, "Unfortunately, in your situation, this is a non-negotiable program. You have to follow it."

Ty: Is that part of your—you mentioned and I love the quote, "Prevention is priceless." So, is that part of your prevention of cancer protocol, the nutritional aspect?

Dr. Connealy: Nutritional and a lot of things. I tell people illness boils down to five different things.

Sleep, if you don't sleep, how are you going to have a good immune system? It takes nine hours to restore your immune system.

Hormones, you have to have your hormones balanced. I'm not talking about female hormones and testosterone. I'm talking about all of your hormones. For example, if you have high insulin levels and your blood sugar is high, what do you do? Cancer likes sugar, right? Even though the doctors don't tell you that, the doctors will tell you "Oh, you can just eat anything."

First of all, it's all over the world about how you treat illness—whether it's a cancer or heart disease—you've got to get off sugar. Sugar is a poison for all of us. If you have a high hemoglobin A1C or high insulin levels, you're going to be predisposed to cancer.

If your adrenals—your adrenals are your stress, immune, and longevity glands. Well, if those are tapped out—which a lot of people's are, because people are in outrageous stress—so then, you are going to be pre-disposed to cancer.

And then the female—we can go through in the male. When do males get prostate cancer? They get prostate cancer 50 to 60 years old. What happens to your testosterone levels? It drops. But a lot of the cause of prostate cancer is the environmental estrogens, the xenoestrogen. "Xeno" is the Greek word for foreign. So the number one pollutant in men today is phthalates and then fungal infections, I find, are a big, big issue.

And then the female—why would God design the body to self-destruct with their hormones? All 25 year-olds—they are at low-risk actually for cancer even though we do have 25 year-olds with cancer. That means all young people would be getting cancer because their hormones are at the highest level. So it's all about the balance of the hormones. But when doctors see patients, they don't explore all that balance. But with us, we do a very expansive work-up on our patients to know every single, little detail.

Now, infections. If you have chronic infections, for example, HPV, herpes, HIV, you increase risk of cancer. We have multiple patients—head and neck, over 30% are related to HPV.

Then you have nutrition and it's not just that are you ingesting foods that have nutrients and power and potential, but are you absorbing them? Lots of us have gut compromise.

Ty: Why?

Dr. Connealy: Our gut is not good because they are loaded with chemicals, our food have GMOs. We have now, in the wheat, glycerophosphate. All of our food today is challenged and compromised. And then we're all stressed so our sufficiency of hydrochloric acid in our stomach, which is naturally there to deactivate all the bugs, whether it is viruses or parasites, is compromised. And then all of our food is laden with toxicity. We're eating dead food and we want to be alive. How's that possible? It's not possible.

Then next group is toxins. For toxins, we have emotional toxins and then the environmental pollutants. I have done thousands of heavy metal tests. I have never seen someone who has no heavy metals, never. Heavy metals interfere with the replication of DNA. So there's no way we can possibly—and I know the body was not designed—there is no safe level of heavy metals. Regardless of what the EPA says, the body is not designed to have heavy metals. Yes you can function and survive, but you are not surviving at the optimal.

Then we'll talk about the environmental pollutants, everything from phthalates to benzenes to fire-retardants. I mean chlorine, fluorine. The pharmaceuticals now that are in our body—you are not even taking.

Ty: They are in the water.

Dr. Connealy: They're in the water so we are getting them in another way.

Detoxification. We have every single patient, and it doesn't matter whether what you come in for, you're going to detox. We always fix those big five areas and get the body in homeostasis as much as possible. And then the patient has to do their part. I tell people I am only as good as you are. We're partners.

Ty: Right. So those five steps, that's part of the prevention. And then if you could hit all of those things you covered, the sleep, balancing hormones, the infections, nutrition, the toxins.

Dr. Connealy: The toxins, the environmental toxins.

Ty: Right. As well as the stress, right?

Dr. Connealy: Yeah, the toxic emotions is the stress.

Ty: Part of the emotional toxicity.

Dr. Connealy: So we teach our patients either with meditation—we do breathing. We give them CDs on how to do different things because you have to do things—you have to learn how to do it on your own. Yes, we'll hold your hand, but the bottom line is we want our patients to learn these self-help techniques on their own so they can survive themselves.

And you've got to have a doctor who is going to partner with you along the way because life is not going to be a cream puff. You're going to have blips. You're going to have roadblocks that you're going to have to deal with. So on a regular basis you are counteracting the challenges that someone is going through. They need help. We all need help.

Ty: That's why you are here?

Dr. Connealy: Yes.

Ty: Last question, Dr. Connealy because I got to get to the rest of the doctors. I could talk to you all day. One of the things that we got feedback from after our first documentary last year is that we want more of Dr. Connealy. Tell her that we want to hear her talk some more because you were very popular. Thanks for this interview.

One of the things they wanted to hear about was the GcMAF. So could you address GcMAF real briefly—and they have had some challenges with GcMAF in Europe if I heard correctly.

Dr. Connealy: Yes, right. Okay. So one of the key things in health is optimization of the immune system. I think it was in 1999, a doctor or several doctors—there was actually conflicting information about really who discovered it, but that's not my deal. But anyway, there is something called GcMAF, Macrophage Activating Factor.

What are macrophages? Macrophages are the packmen of your immune system. So we have to have a good immune system. Whether you have cancer, heart disease, diabetes, dementia, we need a good immune system to take care of ourselves.

When we make bad cells, cancer cells or viruses, they make an enzyme called nagalase. Nagalase poisons the macrophages inhibiting them attacking the bad cells. Now what you can actually do is you can actually measure nagalase.

It's not done in the United States. It's done in a laboratory in the Netherlands. So we send our patient's blood to the Netherlands to see what their nagalase is.

Now, most people we know who have cancer or viruses, we know they probably have high nagalase. Now, by the way though, GcMAF is used in everything from autism to Alzheimer's to heart disease to cancer to chronic, viral, bugs and infections.

We started utilizing it about two years ago. GcMAF was offered in a company in Belgium in injections. And then they made an advanced version of GcMAF called GOleic. Now there's been lots of different influences on the European company, on the laboratory, and I'm not really sure what the details are. We've heard some of the details.

But we have a relationship with a gentleman in Italy and he worked with GcMAF and GOleic. He actually was here. He's actually a doctor who has done tons and tons of research with GcMAF.

Now you can actually make GcMAF in a probiotic. You can actually make it in yogurt yourself. You have to buy the starter material and make the yogurt yourself that produces GcMAF. You can't just buy organic yogurt on the shelves at your local store. You've got to get the starter material and you can make your own GcMAF in a yogurt or what we use is a probiotic suppository called Bravo Probiotic.

Now I know it works because every single patient that I've used it on, their nagalase levels have decreased. So we know that an optimal level or somewhere— but between 0.3 and 0.9 and we try to get our patients to 0.6. And even if they get around 0.9 I'll tell them, "Look, it's time to get off, and your body is now taking care of itself. So let's see how you do and then I'll check your level in a couple of months."

Ty: So the way the GcMAF works is it targets the nagalase?

Dr. Connealy: Yes, so that your body now interferes with the nagalase so your body will activate the macrophages—exactly and attack.

Ty: Okay, that makes sense.

Dr. Connealy: Now there are lots of different things on the horizon that are coming out. There are lots of studies all over the world. I work with a doctor in China. They do immune assessments. So they check your T cells, your B cells, your Natural Killer cells and everything. And then they customize and design a protocol for each patient.

Let's talk about cancer. So there's something called dendritic cell therapy which activates your T cells. So what it basically does is it positions that cancer cell to be this antigen. When you have an antigen, boom, the immune system says, "You are not supposed to be here," and the activated T cell will go after the antigen, which is the foreign substance.

Then you have cytokine-induced killer cells. So these are all immune therapies that are coming on the horizon. They are not available here yet, but I would say in the next probably three to four months they will be coming because everybody is now working— it's all now about your immune system.

Your immune system has to be in the right order and in the right functionality for you to take care of these chronic illnesses. Rheumatoid arthritis, cancer— everything is related to your immune system. So now people are going, "Oh, okay. All these other things aren't quite working like we'd like them to and so we have to now employ and really get our immune system."

Because we know after 40 you start having something called immunosenescence. What does that mean? It's an old immune system. So we've got to now activate our immune system.

I've read a book that was written about 60 or 80 years ago by a doctor and it says— the book was called, *Your Body is Your Best Doctor*—and in the book he says we enter geriatrics at 40. What I tell my patients is you have a warranty until you're 40 and then from 40 on you've got to take care of your body.

Ty: Where might somebody get a hold of GcMAF that you could culture in yogurt?

Dr. Connealy: You can if you go to the website gcmaf.eu and you can order it from them.

Ty: And is there—you may not know this—instructions on how to do that?

Dr. Connealy: Oh yeah, they have very explicit instructions.

Ty: Okay, very good.

Dr. Connealy: But all my patients for the most part relate very positive. And we see positive changes in their systems and we see it working. I tell people there's not one magic bullet, because people will say, "Oh Dr. Connealy what do you think about this and what do you think about this?" I said, "They all have value, but we have to figure out what is best for you at this particular time. Because the person you are in a month is not the person you are today; you've changed."

And you don't live in a bubble. Everybody thinks you live in a bubble. If you have kids and you bought goldfish and if you don't check that—to have a goldfish live a long time is very unusual because that water has to be the perfect balance, perfect milieu for that organism to survive.

Ty: Oh yeah, I've killed many goldfish.

Dr. Connealy: Exactly. Your kids too have probably. So anyway, I tell patients if you walk outside you're exposed to lots of different challenges and we don't know. We talk about electro-smog. We don't know everybody—there's lots of stuff written on it, but we don't know exactly what our cellphones and EMF and cell towers and all of this electricity that is doing to our body. Some people think it's the single biggest threat we have to mankind.

But because people think that we are just this physical person that we are seeing—but no you have this bioenergetic electrical field that is probably more influential than what's just the 3D morphology that you see right now.

Ty: So we are kind of the guinea pigs at this point with that.

Dr. Connealy: We are. But we all need to take a stand, Ty. We need to take a stand for the survival of the human race. That's what I'm most concerned about. When you're young you think everything is going to be fine and forever. But now where I am today and working 29 years you see that we have a crisis in health and we have a crisis with human beings surviving. We all need to take a stand. We all need to inform and inspire each and every one of us to be better human beings.

Ty: Well, Dr. Connealy thank you for being willing to take a stand. We appreciate it. I know the viewers have learned some more from you. And they are going to be wanting more of Dr. Connealy after this. So thank you so much.

Dr. Connealy: Thank you. You're welcome Ty.

[end of transcript]

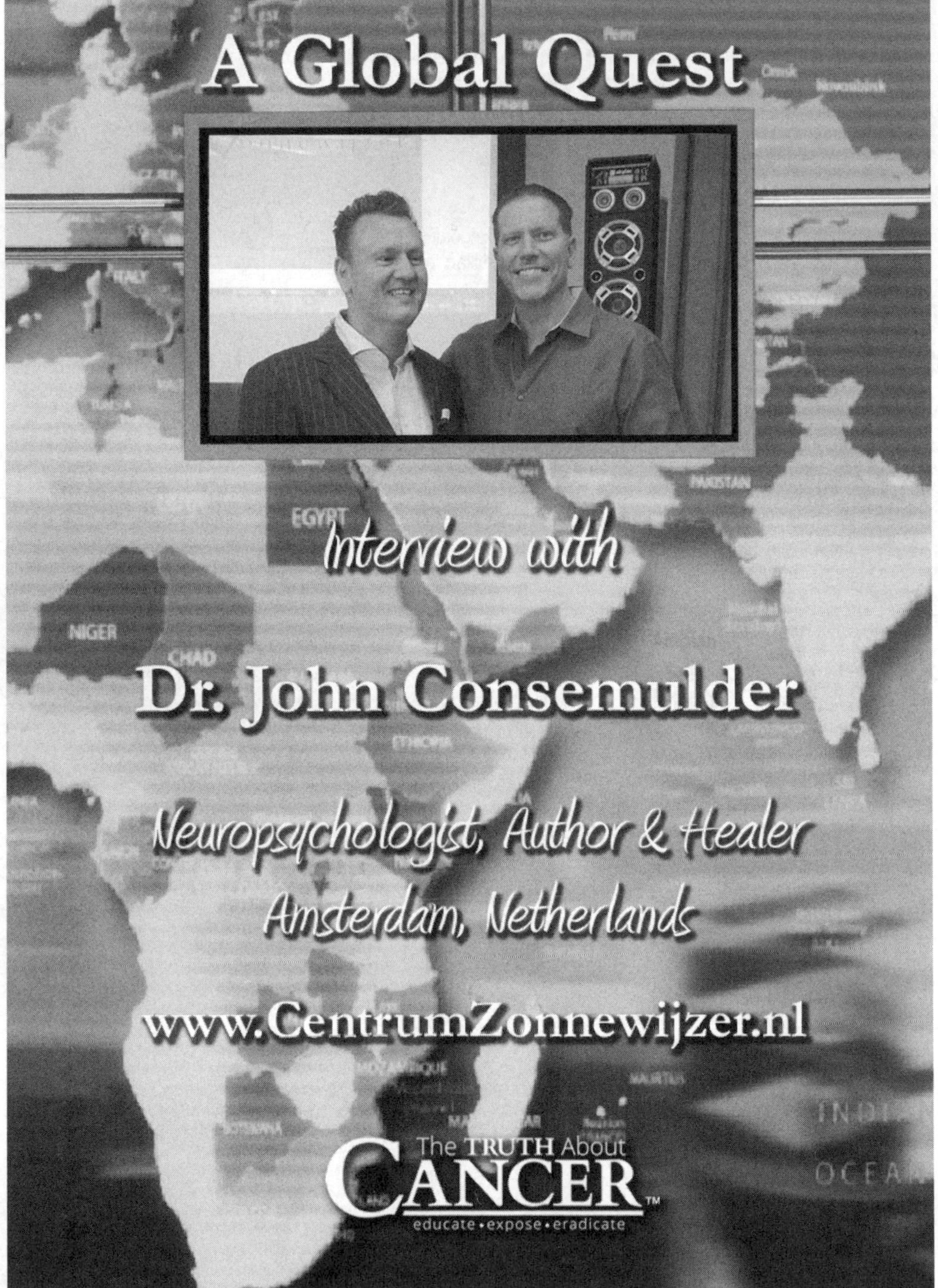
A Global Quest
Interview with
Dr. John Consemulder
Neuropsychologist, Author & Healer
Amsterdam, Netherlands
www.CentrumZonnewijzer.nl
The TRUTH About
CANCER
educate • expose • eradicate

Ty: Well, John Consemulder, finally we meet.

Dr. Consemulder: In the flesh.

Ty: In the flesh. We're here in Almere, Holland, right?

Dr. Consemulder: Yes. Netherlands.

Ty: Yes. Just right outside of Amsterdam.

Dr. Consemulder: Yes, half an hour.

Ty: We've been known to each other, since about 2008 I guess was the first time. But finally we meet in person.

Dr. Consemulder: Yes.

Ty: So, before we sat down here to interview, there was a dead mouse on the ground.

Dr. Consemulder: Yes, I thought it drank aspartame.

Ty: So, that's what I want to ask you about. So, talk about dead mice and aspartame. Tell us about aspartame and the sordid history and let us know if it's something we should be eating and drinking.

Dr. Consemulder: Sure. I would say no but then this is a very short interview.

Let me tell the story as it happened. As a neuropsychologist I knew that vaccines were safe and effective. Oh, that's the wrong answer for your audience.

And after some years of research after I studied, after I graduated, I found out it was the world upside down. So, vaccines are not safe and effective at all. And I couldn't believe that, of course. It couldn't be true that our health officials tell us lies, medical deceptions.

Ty: Let me interrupt you real quick. You say vaccines are not—we don't know that they are safe and effective. Haven't they been tested that they are safe?

Dr. Consemulder: They have been tested that they are safe. But if you test for only a few days while the immune response might be, after a month so to speak, and you haven't really tested all the groups, the ages, and you haven't checked for long term effects, you haven't tested for the cumulative effects, and the synergistic effects with all the other ingredients. Or all the other chemicals, all the other pharmaceuticals, and all the other drugs we have in store, then you haven't really, really tested effectiveness and safety.

Ty: Okay. I appreciate [it].

Dr. Consemulder: So that's the story.

Ty: That's right. So continue about aspartame.

Dr. Consemulder: I found out that there's like a real controversy, a real conspiracy. People say you're a conspiracy theorist when you talk about this. I found out it's like conspiracy practice. It's actually there not from the people who are talking that vaccines are not safe and effective.

But actually from the food industries and the pharmaceutical industries that are actually promoting and stating and saying they have the evidence that it's safe and effective, while this is not the case.

And what I found out, through the example of aspartame being the best example of how bad the situation actually is, the medical deception that it's neurotoxic, it's cancer promoting. It's ruining your immune system, your endocrine system. So it's a very dangerous substance we should not be drinking or eating in what way whatsoever.

I didn't believe this when I first heard it. So I researched it and I was like, this is the best example of how bad this industry is doing its job. How good it's actually doing to ruin our health.

And I found out more. I found out that there's not just conflict of interest, but there's actually a revolving door policy between the authorities that are supposed to be guarding the hen house – but the fox is guarding the hen house, so to speak.

So the scientists that are in authority that should be checking the safety and effectiveness are actually often working together with industry. Or later are being asked to work for them. And they work for the law firm for Monsanto or whatever.

So it's a conflict of interest in the highest degree even in the echelons of politics. So you can't really, really trust when regular science says it's safe and effective. You've got to look at the science and then you see it's being promoted through industry.

Or even the studies are been done by industry. We, the people, think that all the safety and effectiveness tests are being done by the regulating authorities. But it's the other way around.

It's the industry that's giving the authorities the summaries like, here are the good results. We've done six studies. Four were bad, but we don't show you. And the other two, they're quite good so here they are. So the FDA says, "oh it's proven safe and effective."

While the real true, effective, safe, and cost effective natural medicine is being arrested and suppressed, for I think already 100 years.

Ty: In the United States we have the FDA, the Food and Drug Administration. It's supposed to determine whether something is safe or not. If they give it the okay, it goes on the market. What is the similar body here in Netherlands or in the European Union?

Dr. Consemulder: I would say in English it would be RIVM. RIVM in Dutch.

The Rijksinstituut voor Volksgezondheid en Milieu. But also [name in Dutch]. So they're like a commission that's actually checking all the health issues of medicine. But over there you also see the conflict of interest.

The non-neutral positions regarding true effectiveness and safety of medicine. Also looking at cost effectiveness, they're suppressing the medicine that's actually very safe, very effective, and very cheap.

But they are natural remedies; you can't patent them so the industry is not interested. It's the same like the laetrile story. The vitamin B17. You're going to interview Hans Moolenburgh. I've worked with him on a few occasions. Also interviewed him. He knows a nice story. So it's nice to ask him as well also about vaccinations.

But we have the same position here like the FDA in America. Because the RIVM, like I mentioned, is also not open to discuss. Even just going to a dialogue about the non safe and non effective vaccines. I mean if we are crazy, show us. Give us the evidence.

Give us the independent evidence that vaccines are actually safe and effective. But if we show them the independent evidence that they're actually not safe and effective at all, they do not even want to discuss this menace. I'm like science is science, right? So this shouldn't be a double standard. But it is.

Ty: I think that's interesting that you said that because I think worldwide we have the same issue, whether it's in the United States, whether it's here in Europe, wherever it is. You've got bodies that are supposed to protect us are actually—the money. The money is influencing them to make decisions that are not in our best interests. They are in the best interests of the corporations that are the ones that are selling the remedies, the drugs, the pharmaceuticals, whatever it might be.

Dr. Consemulder: Absolutely.

Ty: So it's not really—I think worldwide we have the same issue. We have the fact that the money trail is what is influencing these decisions. Not whether it's good or whether it improves people's health.

Dr. Consemulder: Absolutely. Follow the money is a true story.

Ty: Yeah, follow the money.

Dr. Consemulder: Well, you are right. In another sense you said the body should protect us. Well, actually our bodies do protect us. But not the regulating bodies, but our bodies and the self-healing capacities we have.

For instance, as I just told you I had a car accident, a terrible one three weeks ago. And I'm sitting here with 13 broken ribs. So I'm supposed to be a medical miracle. But I have a feeling, well, I'm just trusting my self-healing capacities.

And of course I was very happy that I was able to get the painkillers because otherwise you can't even breathe; you'd die. So count your blessings of course and integrative medicine, great. But when you see through preventive medicine, then it goes wrong because we can prevent disease. And we don't have to fight disease.

We don't have to move around symptoms which is what allopathic medicine is doing, I think. We can just—it's a better suggestion to promote health and to activate the self-healing capacities and to maintain health.

Because that's the best way. Health is the best fast track bullet for not getting any disease. I mean we are on the wrong track of fighting cancer. It's like the war on cancer, the war on terror. Well, guess whose winning? Cancer. And if you see cancer, it was 1 in 10. One in two now.

But that's because the chemical substances, the pharmaceutical substances, are growing every year. The amount of stuff that gets in our environment, the outer environment and the inner environment, is staggering. And if you see the cumulative, if you look at the cumulative and synergistic effects.

So the building up of all that stuff in your brain especially, and even past the blood brain barrier, especially aspartame and monosodium glutamate—it is in your country, MSG? Both excitotoxins by the way. Both neurotoxic and cancer-promoting.

If you look at that, these things are in like 8,000-10,000 products from light drinks to health foods. Even vitamins sometimes contain them, chewing gum. People can't believe there are products like that...

Cancer-promoting, neurotoxic, immune system ravaging, [killing] glial cells, your immune system, in your brain… killing—is actually in the food. Because if it were not healthy it couldn't be in the food because we have the agencies that are protecting us.

But guess what? They really are not protecting us. So it's down to us to protect our own health and our own children.

Ty: I think you're right. It is up to us. As Burton Goldberg said last year in *The Quest for The Cures*, "the agencies that are supposed to be protecting us are actually protecting the interests they're supposed to protect us from."

Dr. Consemulder: Absolutely.

Ty: You know you mentioned something, and I'll end on this. This last comment and I'll let you remark on it. When we have topics like vaccines or aspartame or MSG or chemotherapy, all these different controversial topics, right? And we want to debate with the other side and they won't debate. Shouldn't that be a sign to us that they're not after the truth?

Dr. Consemulder: Maybe there's something wrong there. I asked all the health officials, up to the highest echelons. "Okay, if it's not true what others are saying, then let's do a TV dialogue because I'm doing that with different guests and themes." I invite them all the time.

They never—well, the first time—I'll tell you a nice story to wrap this story up. The first time I found out about the not safe and effective vaccines, I had the guts (I was a little bit afraid, but I still did it), I had the guts to send it to RIVM.

All the health officials, even the, how do you call it? The big company that goes about all the companies, they all knew about the article I wrote. And I was like, hell is going to break loose. What have I done? Oh my God forgive me because… And then it came. An ear deafening silence.

One hundred and fifty oncologists, virologists, immunologists, whatever-ologists, they didn't reply. Except one guy that said I was crazy. Should we go back to the times before Louis Pasteur? I would say yes by the way. And he was into HPV vaccines. Promoting and selling them. I was like, here we go.

But now I know this is a normal response. Back then I was like, this can't be happening. One hundred and fifty true scientists get an article from a neuropsychologist that went crazy and now says that actually vaccines are not safe and effective. And I want to share this with you. Here are the facts, here are the studies.

No replies. And then I started finding out about the conflicts of interest and the revolving door policies. Then I knew. Oh, it's better to silence that guy than to respond because then he will write a new article, make a radio interview with Ty Bollinger, produce a TV dialogue. And that's their greatest fear – publicity.

Ty: They want to slander and name call. But if they brought it to light, if they responded, then you would fight unfairly because you would go back to them with some more facts.

Dr. Consemulder: Absolutely, because you can you do character assassination. Of course they try. But then they know hey, he's actually making sense. He's a neuropsychologist. Hey, he's a TV producer. Hey, he does events. Maybe watch out here because if we kick him he might kick back and it's not good for publicity and for public opinion. Because actually they can't win on facts because the fact is those vaccines are not safe and effective. Aspartame and MSG are killing our bodies and the authorities are not promoting our health. These are the real facts which they do not want people to know.

Ty: Well, John it's been an honor. Keep kicking back. Keep spreading the truth. Together we'll change the world.

Dr. Consemulder: Thank you.

Ty: Thank you, John.

[end of transcript]

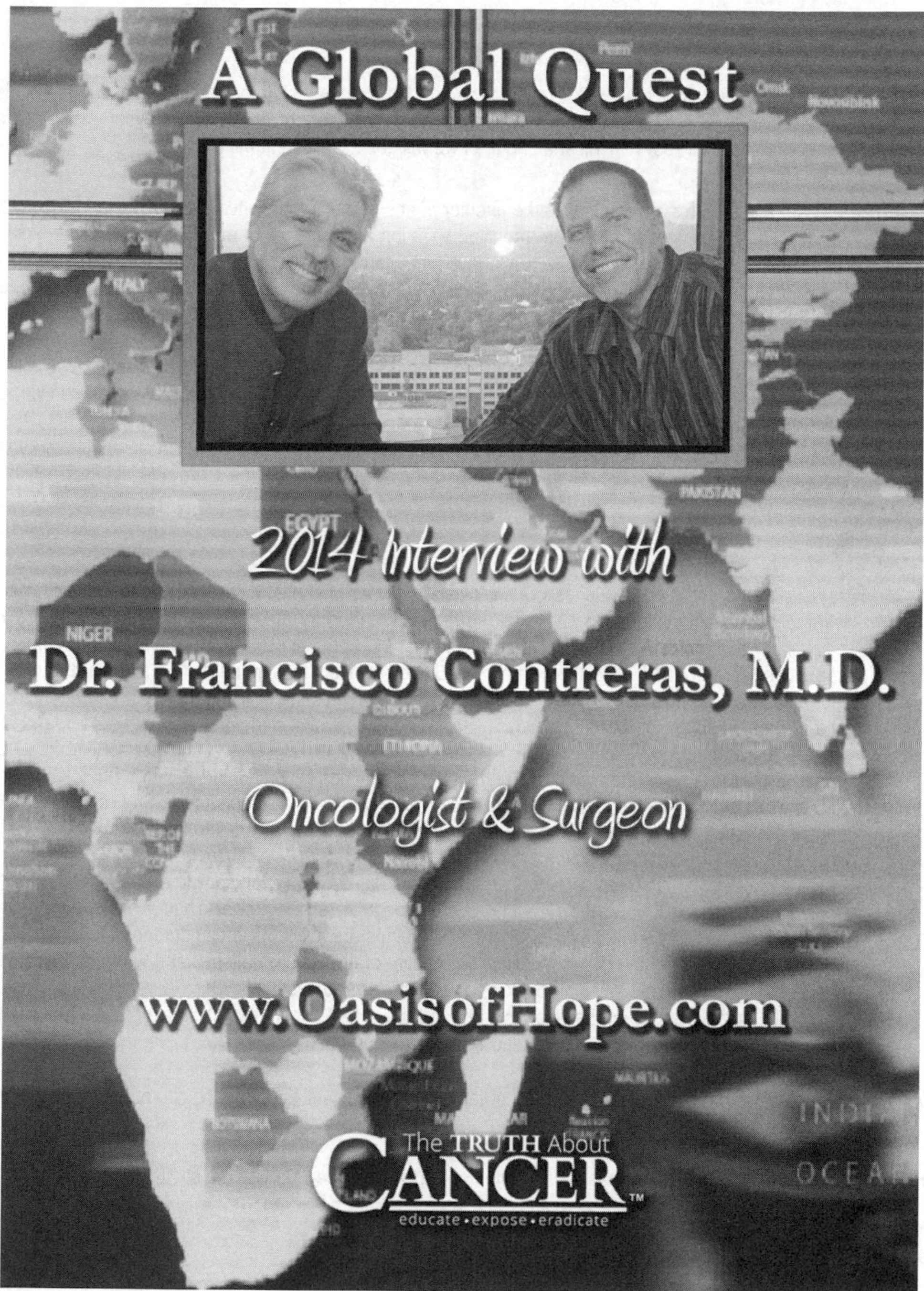
A Global Quest
2014 Interview with
Dr. Francisco Contreras, M.D.
Oncologist & Surgeon
www.OasisofHope.com
The TRUTH About CANCER
educate • expose • eradicate

Ty: I am thrilled today to be sitting here with a man that I have admired for many years, Dr. Francisco Contreras from the Oasis of Hope Hospital in Tijuana. Dr. Chris, thank you for joining us.

Dr. Contreras: Thank you. It is my honor.

Ty: I want to just pick your brain quickly about some of the treatments that you use, but first, if you could, share with our viewers here just what went into founding the Oasis of Hope and what your vision was for developing this clinic down in Tijuana and then we will get into the treatments.

Dr. Contreras: In the 60's, my father was the director of one of the biggest oncology centers in Mexico City. He was an army doctor. He went on a tour on vacation and visited one of the hospitals of the time of Hippocrates, 300 years before Christ. They gave him a tour and the tour guide told him that the hospital, at that time, was divided into three areas. The patients would come to the first area and be evaluated physically, the second area they would be evaluated emotionally and the third area was more or less a spiritual thing. There was a tunnel and they would go through the tunnel and somebody outside would be telling the guy that was going through the tunnel, unbeknownst to them, "You will be healed. You will be healed." They thought that it was the gods. After that experience, my father said that the reason we are failing in oncology so much is that we have become mechanics of the human body and we are not paying attention to the emotional and spiritual needs of our patients, so I am going to go back and change that. He went back, told the staff what they were going to do, and the next day they kicked him out.

Ty: Really? Oh wow!

Dr. Contreras: Yes, and that was the Genesis of the Oasis of Hope. My father said, "Well, if the system doesn't want to do it, I am going to do it." He began his work caring for the patients, not only physically, but emotionally and spiritually. He began singing with them, giving them Bible studies, laughter therapy and about three or four years later a lady from San Diego that went to Canada to do a study with a clinical trial with Laetrile came back to San Diego, and my father at that time was the only pathologist in Mexico and in San Diego. All of the oncologists in San Diego knew him, and when she came back and she wanted to continue with Laetrile nobody wanted to give it to her. One oncologist said, "I know an oncologist in Mexico and they are less stringent there. Why don't you go and see him?" She came to my dad and told him the problem and my father said, "I don't know anything about this." She was riddled with cancer. He said, "I see no problem. I will give it to you." He started giving it to her and six months later she was still alive, a year later no tumor activity, so my father said, "Well, there is something to this." This lady knew everybody that was going to Canada for the trial, brought everybody to my dad, and just a few years later the Oasis of Hope, that was a holistic approach to cancer, now also had alternative therapies. Our aim has always been to integrate whatever therapies are available to us from the conventional and the alternative that we can use to improve the quality of life for our patients, and we have been very successful. You can check our statistics on our website, oasisofhope.com. Our five-year survival rates in the most common tumors are between two and five times better than the national average in the United States of America, with this very combined whole body approach.

Ty: I would have to say the Oasis of Hope is potentially the most well-known of the alternative cancer clinics anywhere.

Dr. Contreras: Well, my father was the first one. He was the pioneer. He was the one that swam against the current. He was ostracized, persecuted ...

Ty: Which shows that he was doing something right, when he is persecuted.

Dr. Contreras: Yes. He paved the way for all of us; 15 or 20 years ago we were quacks and now we are alternative doctors, so we have some respect. We were very respected by the patients and really that is what counts the most. The patients knew everything that we do at the Oasis since my father—he was a very good scientist, Harvard graduated—everything that we do has a tremendous amount of science behind it.

Ty: One of the things, Dr. Contreras, that you mentioned was laughter and music. It is so ironic…the reason I am able to interview you today is because of Dr. Patrick Quillin. He spoke to you earlier today and said, "You should go interview with Ty." Dr. Quillin, on *The Quest for the Cures* back in the spring, mentioned two very important factors of any cancer treatment are music and laughter.

Dr. Contreras: They are the most potent immunostimulating agents available. There is no drug, there is no vaccine that is more potent to stimulate the immune system. There is a very interesting study that shows that for every minute of anger you will depress significantly and measurably the quality and quantity of your immune system. One minute of anger is six hours of depression. One minute of laughter will boost significantly your immune system for 24 hours. That is why children up to the age of five laugh around 400 times a day and adults only about 40. The reason why children can eat dirty and be dirty all the time is because they are laughing.

Ty: Laughter is the best medicine.

Dr. Contreras: They are protected. At the Oasis of Hope we have laughter sessions every day. Every time we get together with them, no matter how serious the thing is, we try to put in several jokes for them. They don't have to be. Sometimes we laugh at the people telling the joke—not the joke.

Ty: Sometimes you laugh at how bad the jokes were.

Dr. Contreras: Exactly. It is amazing how powerful things that cost nothing are. Meditation, colors…there are studies that show that the most immune depressing colors are white and blue. The typical hospital colors—imagine that. We painted all of our walls in mauve because there are studies that show it is the most immune-lifting color. We take into account all of those things. Those little things sometimes count for a lot.

Ty: The thing that strikes me about that, Dr. Contreras, is the difference between that approach and the traditional cancer approach today where you are diagnosed and the doctor says, "You are dead in three months." There is no hope. There is no joy. There is no laughter. There is nothing. What you just said about the fact that laughter stimulates the immune system and anger depresses it—what about the feeling of despair? Does that have any kind of effect?

Dr. Contreras: The Bible says that the power of life and death is in the tongue. If you pronounce somebody dead, they see the doctor as an authority and so they buy it and are dead no matter what. The truth is that not only doctors are not gods, we don't know, but nobody in this room knows if we are going to be alive tomorrow. By the same token, you can never say that a cancer patient is going to die. We have had patients that were told they were going to die in three months and then 20 years later, you met one—Burga Ratti—27 years later she is still alive. She is not cured. She is alive enjoying life. The first thing that I impress on a patient is that victory over cancer is a decision, not a happening. You don't have to be victorious for the tumor to go away. There are patients that have surgery and chemo and then the tumor goes away and they can't sleep. Why? Because they don't know when it is coming back. They are tumor free but not free of cancer. There are other patients that say, "Cancer is the best thing that ever happened to me. Before I had cancer I took everything for granted and now I see that life is beautiful and it is because of this cancer that I can see that and cancer is the best thing that ever happened to me." That person is riddled with cancer and is victorious over cancer. It is very important. If you have victory over cancer in your mind, everything follows. If you decide that you are going to die it is very difficult to bring you back. Victor Frankel could determine who was going to die within 24 hours in the concentration camp and it was when they smoked their cigarettes. You say, cigarettes cannot cause cancer in 24 hours. No. Cigarettes were their hope and they traded everything with cigarettes so when they had no more hope they started smoking their cigarettes like burning your money and they would die within 24 hours. The power of hope is incredible. That is why we are the Oasis of Hope.

We have been criticized enormously for selling false hope. My question is, if false hope is saying you are going to live, what is true hope? You are dead? No, there is no false or true hope. There is hope or no hope.

Ty: It reminds me, Dr. Contreras, of a quote from Charlotte Gerson, who was accused of spreading false hope much like yourself and she accused them of spreading false despair.

Dr. Contreras: Yeah. Well, really true despair, you're dead. You have to start chemotherapy now and you'll live six more months with no hair, vomiting, feeling terrible. At the Oasis of Hope we can do surgery, if radiation is necessary we give it, if chemotherapy is the best—we have all of those tools available, but it is not the only thing. For us, we are not fighting against the tumor. If anything would separate the Oasis of Hope from any other oncological center is that we are not fighting the tumor. We are rooting for the patient. We are providing resources for that patient to be able to fight off his or her disease. That is how you get rid of cancer, through your immune system and through systems that are already within you that have failed. What we have to do is get them to work again and that difference has made a tremendous difference in the results.

Ty: I bet it has. The whole body approach, not just treating the physical but the emotional and the spiritual but I would have to say the emotional/spiritual potentially is the most important.

Dr. Contreras: It is really one entity. You will react according to your spiritual fortitude. Depending on your spiritual fortitude your emotions can be functional for you or dysfunctional for you. We work very, very much on that aspect of patients because that is really what can change their lives.

Ty: Dr. Contreras, I know your time is precious but I have one last question for you. You mentioned Laetrile as one of the treatments. Can you name more of the therapies that you use?

Dr. Contreras: Laetrile has been our golden therapy for the last 50 years. It is a very innocuous anti-tumor agent that works for most common cancers. Then, for patients that do not respond well to Laetrile we have high dose vitamin C given in a very special way that actually converts the vitamin C virtually into chemotherapy without any of the side effects. We have hyperthermia available. We have all kinds of vaccines. Another major part of therapy is signaling transduction with foods to block the production of enzymes and proteins that are absolutely necessary for the tumors to grow. The combination of all of this is what we call the Contreras metabolic therapy or integrative therapy. We also use a number of immune stimulation agents, not only the laughter therapy and the emotional uplifting music and all of the things we mentioned before, but we have a product from Japan that has proven to be very effective and in at least 70 publications, AHCC. It has proven to improve significantly the quality and quantity of the immune system. Our therapeutic approach really has about 25 different things that we will integrate depending on the patient's needs and the patient's status.

Ty: I see, and by getting the immune system back to functioning you have given their body the fuel that it needs, the ability to fight off the cancer on its own.

Dr. Contreras: Correct. And for a long period of time. A lot of times you can give chemotherapy and the tumor goes away but you also destroy the immune system and then the cancer comes back with a vengeance.

Ty: Wow. Fascinating stuff. Dr. Contreras, thank you so much for being with us tonight.

Dr. Contreras: You are very welcome. Thank you very much.

[end of transcript]

A Global Quest

Interview with

Dr. Gaston Cornu-Labat, M.D.

Author, Holistic Physician & Surgeon

The TRUTH About CANCER™

educate • expose • eradicate

Ty: I'm here outside of Seattle, Washington with Dr. Gaston Cornu-Labat. A medical doctor out of Argentina originally, correct?

Dr. Cornu-Labat: Yes, sir.

Ty: Thank you for joining us today. We are here at the clinic of Dr. Jonathan Wright. He tells me great things about you. So I'm glad to be able to interview you in person here.

Tell us a little bit about your education initially and then I've got a couple of subjects that I want to broach with you.

Dr. Cornu-Labat: I'm a medical doctor graduated from the University of Buenos Aires. I graduated in 1991. When I came out of medical school at the time I was not sure what I was going to be doing. But my passion ended up being clearly in action. So I ended up going into general surgery. So I did a residency in general surgery.

I came to the US and I did all my residency training here in the US in Youngstown, Ohio. From there I moved to Seattle at that time to specialize in surgery of the liver and pancreas. I was not particularly interested in oncology at that time. Then I ended up practicing in rural Nebraska.

It was a very significant shift. I started my practice as a general surgeon and being exposed to a completely different world from what academic surgery was. At that time, my perspective in medicine started shifting, or maturing, significantly.

I started approaching it with a lot more of a holistic perspective. The natural progression of the holistic perspective was moving into natural medicine of which I didn't know anything until I crossed paths with Jonathan.

In between that transition, I had a fairly interesting run in with the system. I experienced what it is to be a whistle-blower and how the system retaliates and the significance of that.

I got quite well versed and educated on how all the structure of the medical industrial complex functions and how it impacts the bottom line, which is the relationship between doctors and people.

Ty: You said you got familiar with the whistle-blower. What happened?

Dr. Cornu-Labat: I was a surgeon in a small hospital in the east of Washington. At a small rural hospital. I had been brought in to start the surgery program from scratch. So I got that started.

At some point about a year into my tenure there in that hospital the CEO approaches me and says, "We need a new vision for the hospital. This is a small place and we want it to grow. But we need a new vision."

I had already been progressing significantly on consciousness, healing, and a holistic approach to health. And I said, "You want a new vision, the new vision is integrative health." That was a fantastic idea. Things were initiated. And with a consulting firm that came in to help in the process, a group very specialized in these types of structures, it became evident that the conditions were not there.

The hospital had a lot of deficiencies, particularly administrative deficiencies. Significant, probably quite ubiquitous in terms of the problems that are in all the health care facilities. Yet not conducive to the very serious project we had in mind. I said that we can't move forward. "No problem." And it immediately there was denial of the problem and pressuring me for that problem not to become evident.

I took it to the next step which was the group above the administration and the response was kind of similar. In the meantime, the straw that broke the camel's back happened because there was a state fire marshal inspection. And they found deficiencies throughout the hospital. So there was a widespread deficiency in the life safety code that kind of put in evidence the negligence that was present there.

They were asking me to continue with this and I said, "These conditions are impossible." And their efforts were really to keep everything under the carpet. And I said, "No, that is not possible." Then immediately what happened was, "oh, I think you're crazy." Literally. There were complaints filed about me having some kind of mental issues. So I said, "Okay, I'm not crazy and we'll prove it." And, "you have a problem, you're crazy."

Then I went to the next level. The board did the same as the administration. Then I went to the Department of Health. The Department of Health did the same as the administration, "I think there's something wrong with you."

I ended up continuously being put on the spot of being targeted and being questioned, on the defensive. And nobody really looking or attending or responding to the problem.

I kept going up. The Department of Health ended up—it became evident because I kept digging in it became evident that the problems in the hospital were related to lack of adequate inspections from the Department of Health.

Then I go to the State Auditor's Office. The State Auditor's Office said, "No, that's the problem of the Department of Health." They washed their hands off. In the meantime my license was being questioned. I go to hearings. I get suspended. I can't find a job anywhere.

I keep playing the game. I get analyzed like probably the most officially sane physician in the state of Washington by far because all the exams I went through were totally clean. However, that required a lot of effort and a lot of investment and downtime in terms of me not being able to work.

From the State Auditor's Office I took it to the legislature. There's a Health Care and Wellness Committee in the legislature. I took all the paperwork and presented it to them, had an acknowledged copy and never heard from them.

Then I went to the Governor. Again, I took everything to the Governor and I got an acknowledgement in writing that the Governor received the paper from them and never heard.

I always would hear back from the Department of Health doing something to make the process difficult or put me through hearings. There are videos on You Tube because I used unconventional strategies to address these. So at all the hearing I just filmed them. I couldn't afford a lawyer so I took a filming crew, friends. And put all the videos on YouTube and was doing an explanation of what was going on.

Eventually, at some point they suspended my license. And after everything was cleared my license was fully reinstated with no issues whatsoever or no restrictions whatsoever because there had never been any problem with me.

Yet to this day there has not been a single answer about all the problems that apply in the hospital that I dared to bring up. And because of that I was accused of all these things that dragged me through the mud. Me and my family, for two years. And financially, of course, that affected us deeply.

Yet neither the Governor, nor the State Auditor's Office, nor the Department of Health, nor the Washington State Patrol, which has to do with this too, not a single agency ever answered anything. And it's in writing. There's paper trail of absolutely everything. I have boxes with everything totally documented.

As soon as you put pressure, pressure, pressure, the technique is to answer with some kind of nonsense. And then when you call them on the nonsense, they try to pull something else. And when you call them on that other nonsense thing, in the end they say, "Oh, I'm not answering anymore."

The only option you have is to sue them, to initiate legal action. The problem is that either you have a lot o money to initiate legal actions or you won't find a single lawyer that will take on the government on a contingency basis.

Ty: Well, it sounds like basically the technique that they used is that they are going to run you through the mud. They are going to make you charge up a lot of legal bills and eventually you are just going to give up.

Dr. Cornu-Labat: In 99 percent of the cases that's what happens. The one percent that succeeds going through these tangled ways, it's all out of reach for the great majority that they become insignificant. The technique is actually very effective and universal because pretty much every corrupt system uses the same technique.

Ty: When you are speaking of corruption, one person that we are both familiar with is Dr. Burzynski. He's been in a run through the mud and he's been forced to pay lots and lots of legal bills to defend himself. Can you address that because I know that you've got some information that will be very interesting to share about?

Dr. Cornu-Labat: Yes, well I have some experience with Dr. Burzynski. I've had the pleasure of starting to work with him. I started last year. When he contacted us, the original contact was with Dr. Wright. And Dr. Wright entrusted me on this because he knows I'm particularly interested in these things.

They were restricted by the FDA. They were starting to get some kind of—it's very unclear exactly what's going on between the FDA and Burzynski. Except that every step he tries to take with the antineoplaston Therapy there's some kind of roadblock.

At that time, the roadblock in my understanding was that the FDA was looking into the Burzynski Clinic who started clinical trials. However, any patients outside the conditions of the clinical trial that needed treatment could not be done in the clinic. So they needed somebody outside the clinic to run antineoplaston Therapy. I said, "Okay, I'll do it."

I went to Houston and I spent a couple of days there. I started getting acquainted with the therapy. From then on I started developing all the necessary knowledge to be able to start implementing the therapy in our clinic.

Now, each patient that was referred to me for antineoplaston Therapy needed to go through a process of approval of investigation on a new drug application expanded access. So that's and IND application.

The initial patient I got was a two year old girl with a very advanced brain tumor. When I went through the application it took about 30 hours of work to get all the paperwork going. For that first patient the FDA gave the okay. Unfortunately, the family had issues that were beyond any of us and the treatment never got initiated.

Within two weeks of this patient I got a second patient who was a four year old kid from Florida with what is known as a DIPG, which is an advanced brain stem tumor. Diffuse Intrinsic Pontine Glioma. When DIPG is well established, it doesn't respond to anything. So it's common in children and these kids die from it.

Burzynski has documented cases. Not every tumor responds, that's for sure. But he has documented cases of complete response, of significant response, of significant prolongation of life. And documented cases of cure, of complete response, complete remission of the tumor with DIPG, which is the only therapy right now that can claim some some percentage of total response.

There's no other therapy that can claim it. Period. Nothing in the literature that says, "Oh, we have cured one patient or two patients." Nothing. Actually Burzynski is the only one that can claim that.

When I moved ahead with the application for the second case, they spent about four weeks back and forth picking on little things like, "oh, this word here doesn't fit, this word here doesn't fit. What are these charges?" So it was picking on nuisance, if the expression is correct.

For about a month and a half this kid, a very advanced case, was deteriorating on a daily basis almost. Then about after a month and a half they said, "Okay, the request is on clinical hold." Which means it's in limbo because we are not denying it but you can't do it because it's on hold. And okay, why? "Why, because we think the risks outweigh the benefits." And this kid is going to die.

Ty: This is with a terminal brain cancer patient that has no options.

Dr. Cornu-Labat: But the kid's going to die. We've really come this close with the information we have to complete this.

Ty: So the risks are greater than the risk of death? How can you have something that's more risky than death?

Dr. Cornu-Labat: I have no explanation whatsoever. We could not make sense. The family was totally devastated. My participation in this was to tell them I think it's absurd. I think you're responsible if this kid dies. You're responsible for this kid's death, not because he was going to be saved for sure with antineoplaston but because he had a possibility.

And the best evidence that we have and Burzynski has collected a lot of scientific—he's is by no means esoteric, natural, nothing. He's tremendously scientific. And all the evidence that was collected pointed out to the fact that antineoplaston is the only therapy available today that could give a possibility to this child of having an improvement or even a small chance, but a chance nonetheless, of a cure.

Now the FDA considered, in writing, that the risks of doing this therapy outweigh the benefits. I don't know. I can't wrap my head around it. It is very profoundly absurd.

Now that was a disheartening experience. There had been a lot of work. I'm not the significant one on this. This kid ended up dying. The family was totally devastated. I don't think the family ever initiated any kind of legal action or anything on this. They were running, getting into that with everything they could and trying to collect money to treat this little kid that was dying. And they were so broken down afterwards that they just hushed it. And it went into a kind of oblivion, it gets forgotten.

Ty: I can't understand that the FDA, who is supposed to protect us, and there is a little four-year-old that can be saved possibly, no assurance, but could be saved and they will not allow the treatment because it's too risky. I don't get that.

So if we are on the street here and someone gets hit by a car and there's an ambulance that comes up and one of the emergency workers refuses to give life support or to do the chest compression or whatever it might be, they can be charged with manslaughter because they withheld treatment and that's their job to treat. This is criminal.

Dr. Cornu-Labat: That's my understanding, yes. Actually, I think one thing that needs to happen is that these people need to be held accountable. I made sure in the process to get exactly the first and the last name of every person that was involved in making this decision. And I have it.

Unfortunately, I'm not in a position to initiate those actions. That's something that corresponds to the family or the support group of the family or any group that is looking into supporting these. And that's the way to go.

Ty: I honestly don't know how that if somebody works for the FDA and they are responsible for that and how they can even sleep at night.

Dr. Cornu-Labat: My impression, and I don't know these people except for the very little interaction I had with them, they seem to be heartless. To me they seem so callused. I don't know if they assume that they are dealing with a number or a piece of paper or something.

How do they sleep at night after condemning a four-year-old to die? Probably the kid had the highest chances of dying anyhow, but we don't know how things play on. But the chance was there.

Ty: But the treatment, the antineoplaston was too risky.

Dr. Cornu-Labat: It's worth clarifying the fact that there are side effects from antineoplaston. Antineoplaston is a very taxing treatment in terms of what is required for the treatment. It's a continuous infusion. Every four hours you get each dose and it's 24 hours a day. And it goes on for months. So it takes a lot of effort.

However, the biggest side effect that we have to remember is that we are using as a ruler or as a measure chemotherapy and radiation therapy. In kids, there are studies showing that 20 years later their brains are fried.

Although they may have survived that particular tumor that was treated, but 20 years down the line they are almost useless because their brains are fried. So that is the measure for side effects. The approved treatments. Antineoplaston, they raise your sodium. You get really thirsty. If you're a kid it can become a significant issue. Hypernatremia can be life threatening. But that's why 24/7 these kids in treatment have continuous supervision. And the labs are being done almost daily up to weekly once the treatment is very well established and things are safe. But there's very close monitoring.

There are other side effects that have shown up throughout the treatment that we can clearly establish if it is the antineoplaston or not. There's been five deaths during treatment that have been documented. However, if you look in detail into each one of those events, you're hard pressed to say, "Oh, they died because of antineoplastons" because there's no evidence. It's safe. You have err of the margin of safety and you have to assume until proven otherwise, "hey, let's be careful with this." But there's nothing pointing out to the fact that antineoplaston was the cause of death in any of these patients.

There is nothing in all the collected evidence that shows any significant major side effects. Nothing that as soon as the liver enzymes start creeping up or the white cell counts start coming down, you stop the medication and it goes away. And then you re-initiate the treatment and its okay. So really the risks of the treatment are not— compared to the old standard which we are using which is chemotherapy and radiation therapy, there is nothing. There is very little.

So I don't know what they are referring to. But interestingly enough, six months later we re-initiated the relationship with Burzynski. And I get a referral for another patient. In this case it's a 60 year old woman. This woman has a grade four astrocytoma which is a very advanced, and a very aggressive type of brain tumor for which, again, there is no possibility of a cure with standard therapies.

We initiated the process requesting the FDA for the approval for antineoplaston. And this time it took only a week. They received the papers and a week later they were telling me that it's on clinical hold. Why?

I recorded it, they told me they were going to send it in writing but they told me all this over the phone. So I had my recording there and recorded the whole conversation. "Well, the risks outweigh the benefits."

And I said, "Sorry this brings me back memories." And remembering the little kid, "you remember so and so six months ago. I couldn't figure out what you were referring to when you told me that the risk— the risk of what, of dying?" What risk can outweigh dying from the disease? "Well, we can't disclose the information." This is what they were referring to.

To the best of my knowledge what they were referring to is the fact that when the FDA starts looking into a new drug, it is common that the pharmaceutical industry and the manufacturer will share proprietary information. With the understanding that the FDA cannot disclose, unless the manufacturer is the one disclosing the information. So they are bound by that relationship with the manufacturer not to disclose certain information.

Here, the only logical thing is that if you have information that allowed you to reach your decision that whatever risk antineoplaston has is greater than dying, it has to be, I have to assume, that Burzynski has not shared with me all the information.

So as soon as I finish the conversation with them I said, "Please send all this in writing." I called Burzynski and asked him, "Listen, this is what just happened. Have you not shared information with me?" He said, "of course all the information we have we have shared it with you." I don't know. We are still puzzled.

I had long conversations with the head of clinical research at the Burzynski Clinic. On top of discussing this with Burzynski I discussed it with Sheldon Brookman who was the guy in charge of all the research. He had no idea what they were referring to.

We theorized so many possibilities of what kind of rationale they would have. They don't want to disclose to me, supposedly protecting the manufacturer. The manufacturer has no idea what they are talking about.

So there's a disconnect here, something doesn't fit. The only explanation that makes sense is that they are trying to derail antineoplaston. Somebody is trying to derail antineoplaston. Somebody is trying for this not to succeed or for this to be very difficult to move forward into a successful thing.

There is a ton of research and development that still needs to be done with antineoplaston because we still need to find what the exact role for antineoplaston is. We still need to be able to define what the niche where those patients where nothing else worked were totally cured. There are patients 20 years ago that are still running around.

Ty: I've seen the pictures on his walls.

Dr. Cornu-Labat: Right. And that requires work. And that requires an opportunity for this to be able to be properly tested.

Ty: They have been after this for 30 years. Since the mid-80s.

Dr. Cornu-Labat: And they have been persecuted for most of that time.

Ty: What happened to the elderly lady, to the 60 year old lady?

Dr. Cornu-Labat: Well, right now we are on hold. This is fresh. This is fresh out of the oven, it happened last week. The remarkable thing is in January—and I have it printed out. In January of this year *The New England Journal of Medicine* published a paper, a kind of a review article about IND applications expanded access. And I want to read one paragraph, it's very brief and very significant because it's talking about regulation of expanded access. And it's giving a little bit of history of how the FDA started this process.

It started with the AIDS epidemic in the 80s and how the FDA started considering and allowing the use, the off-label use, of certain drugs that were still trying to be determined if they were good to be used in the market or not. But since there were no other cures, "well, if I'm going to die from this let's give it a shot." That was a principle that started all these expanded accesses.

The paragraph says, "The FDA has permitted almost all expanded access requests regardless of category." And it gives a couple of citations. "The FDA estimated that by 2006, approximately 100 thousand patients had obtained the expanded access to experimental drugs."

Another citation here. "Between 2010 and 2013 the FDA imposed clinical holds on only two of 2,472 individuals, non-emergent protocols. On one of the 66 intermediate size requests and on none of the 41 widespread expanded access protocols that it received." So between 2010 and 2013 the FDA said no or put on hold two out of almost 2,500. Our record represented three requests to the FDA and got two on hold.

Ty: You got as much as they had totaled for the three years.

Dr. Cornu-Labat: In total for the three year period. The authors Darrow and Sarpatwari. I don't want to chop his name, *The New England Journal of Medicine*, January 2015. The title of the article is "Practical, Legal, and Ethical Issues in Expanded Access to Investigational Drugs."

Ty: So in reality the FDA almost never puts a hold on those but they did for you, for the antineoplaston. So you'd almost think that they were trying to derail the treatment.

Dr. Cornu-Labat: Well, let's not overreach in our conclusions, right. But let the facts speak for themselves.

So there's something going on. And for me I see Burzynski, I see how he dedicated his life to this and he should have all the support we can give him. He is isolated with a bunch of bullies to go after him for whatever interest or reasons they have. They have reasons, I have no question about it. They go after him and then the rest just watch and say, "Wow, how unfair. Wow, this shouldn't happen. Wow, how sad." And they don't do anything. And it's rare that somebody steps up and says, "Okay, I'll do whatever I can."

Ty: I think that if nothing else we should learn that based on these stories we should do everything we can to expose this corruption.

Dr. Cornu-Labat: I think the work you're doing is extraordinary.

Ty: Well, thank you.

Dr. Cornu-Labat: I think it's extraordinary because you're nailing, let me see if I get the expression in English correctly, the nail in the head. You're hitting the nail on the head. Because the core of what you're doing is empowerment. You are gathering up the information and you're bringing it forward. That process of empowerment is really the key to health. And that is the piece that's missing.

Eventually, medicine will come to terms, and humanity will come to terms, with the fact that healing comes from within. And that we, the doctors, the clinics, and the medications are the ones that facilitate that process of healing. So it doesn't belong to us. It belongs to you as a patient. My true role as a practitioner is to empower and facilitate that healing within.

Now, the downside of this is that once humanity grows into this understanding, I will have to go and open a restaurant or do something else because I won't be needed.

Ty: I can tell by talking to you that that would be a happy transition.

Dr. Cornu-Labat: I'd be okay with it.

Ty: You would be okay with that if you weren't needed.

Dr. Cornu-Labat: I would be okay certainly.

Ty: Well, thank you for the kind words. I appreciate that.

Dr. Cornu-Labat: So your work is very important. And at this stage we are in as a whole, as a society, humanity we deserve information. It's very important.

Ty: Well, thank you for sharing the story about Dr. Bruzynski. And the real tragedies that are happening with the FDA putting these treatments on hold. Because I think you're right, they look at it as a number. They don't realize that they are real people, these are real children. These are real people that are being affected and that are dying from this. These are real families that are being affected that their lives will never be the same because they put a hold on a treatment that could have saved their life. To me that's criminal. I don't know how it's not criminal but I guess according to them that that's okay. One more question. I want to talk to you about BEC5. I talked to Dr. Jonathan Wright about this extract from eggplant and the Devil's Weed in Australia. Share a little bit with our viewers about BEC5.

Dr. Cornu-Labat: Well, BEC5 is a very interesting compound. It's a natural compound. It's extracted, as you mentioned, from the Solanaceae family. I don't want to chop the scientific name of the family of plants. Eggplant belongs to this family. The Devil's Apple is the plant from where the original idea came from. Essentially, it's a couple of glycoalkaloids that when combined have a very selective receptor emolliated, anti-cancer affect. What it means is that these two compounds, because of the carbohydrate residue they have, trigger a response with very specific receptors that happen to be over expressed in cancer cells and under expressed, or not expressed at all, in normal cells.

When this compound hits the receptor and joins in, it is internalized into the cell and it triggers what is known as apoptosis. It has programmed that cell. Characteristically cancer cells have this concept of immortality where this programmed apoptosis is supposed to leave room for the next generation so they die. Well, that doesn't happen with cancer cells. So they keep going and going and going and going. BEC5 triggers that apoptosis and tumor cells die. And it selectively does that with tumor cells. And so far, in all the animal studies and on the online studies that have been done, have shown that it has a very broad spectrum.

Ty: So it works on lots of different cancers.

Dr. Cornu-Labat: So far the evidence is showing up that it works on a very broad variety of cancers. In sarcomas, in adenocarcinomas, in squamous cell, and basal cell. So BEC5 went through a very interesting development phase with using it on skin cancers.

Actually, it's still being used on skin cancers. This is a cream that's over the counter in those jurisdictions where it's legal. It can be bought over the counter. You apply the cream and it starts killing layer by layer the cancer cells of the skin cancer. You know, skin cancer is the most common cancer. And it just eliminates the cancer.

Ty: But just the cancer.

Dr. Cornu-Labat: At the beginning it's very impressive because the characteristic for this early cancer is that the cancer cells are quite a bit more spread than what is evident. So you start applying it and suddenly redness starts spreading out. There is a rough reaction. There is a little bit of an open wound in the first week or two that is a lot bigger and scary because it's bigger than what you thought it was.

After the second or third week, then you start seeing normal skin coming in and covering it up. The majority of times there's not even a scar left because there's no destruction of the tissue structures. If the cancer did not alter the skin layers and it was only superficial, all the cancer cells are kicked out and the normal cells go back into place. You can react to the vehicles used in the cream which is salicylate and urea, I believe. Which are the carriers for the medication. You may be allergic to the glycoalkaloids and may have a reaction to the glycoalkaloids. But per se, it has almost no toxicity.

I say almost because at some point there was one clinical trial, a phase one clinical trial that was run on very advanced stage three and stage four cancers, renal carcinoma and another one, where intravenous BEC5 was used. What was found out is that at high dose intravenously, it can increase the liver enzymes. So there's a suggestion that it produces some kind of liver toxicity.

When that happened the drug was immediately stopped. The medication was stopped and the liver was normalized. The liver enzyme count went back to normal. So other than that, there are no known side effects or toxicity from this medication. So it's a fantastic cure for an estimation which is like three million Americans right now with some form of skin cancer. This is an easy over-the-counter solution for them. They just have to apply a cream for a few weeks until all the cancer is gone. What I've seen is that it works consistently every time.

Of course, if you have a very advanced cancer and you have a rate, the cream is limited. So if it's growing really fast, the cream can kill so many layers but underneath it's growing a lot faster. Then you may get into a negative equation there. But otherwise it works systematically every time I've seen it in action.

Ty: That's pretty fascinating. So it is selectively toxic to just cancer cells and doesn't really have side effects, comparatively to the standards.

Dr. Cornu-Labat: To the standards that we were discussing, yes very minimal. Nothing.

Ty: Just real basic, you mentioned sarcomas, lymphomas, carcinomas. Describe the different types of cancers. Just really the basics. What is a sarcoma?

Dr. Cornu-Labat: Well, different types of cancers relate to the cell that gives origin to the cancer. So mucus membranes give origin to adenocarcinomas. Then connective tissue, muscle cells, cartilage bone, they are the sarcomas. And then it's a special type of, you can say of the adenocarcinomas, but it's more that the squamous cell which is another type, is the tumors that are derived from a special type of epithelium which is different from the mucosal cell surface that forms adenocarcinomas. Then you have lymphomas which are a type of cancers that are derived from the white blood cells.

Ty: Blood cancers. And are they the same as Leukemia?

Dr. Cornu-Labat: Same with Leukemia, correct. That's just the very basic.

Ty: Sure, but it's interesting. So the type is based upon where the original cancer cells come from?

Dr. Cornu-Labat: Right, exactly.

Ty: Okay, that's interesting. I think that's a good primer because a lot of times people hear, lymphoma, leukemia, basal cell carcinoma, squamous cell carcinoma, what is it? And pretty much if it ends in "oma", then it's some kind of a cancer.

You went to medical school in Argentina. First of all, how much training did you receive on nutrition when you were in medical school? Because I know here in the States it's almost none.

Dr. Cornu-Labat: Not much. It's very little.

Ty: Close to none?

Dr. Cornu-Labat: Yes. The medical school is a conventional medical school. The University of Buenos Aires is the most well established medical school in Argentina. It's totally biochemical. When I started it was very interesting in my opening to natural medicine. Things like energy, and biophysics, functional structure, those types of concepts were totally new for me. I started, "oh, that makes sense." And that makes scientific sense.

For example, for part of my initial training I went to Denver and I sat down with a very peculiar, very interesting character and a good friend too, in Denver who is Stephen Kaufman. Stephen Kaufman is a Chiropractor. He developed an extraordinary and a totally revolutionary technique for pain management that is based on neuromuscular reflexes. Literally, if you have a pain in your shoulder, in a few minutes they shut it off you don't have any pain. Literally, it's something that is absolutely remarkable.

Actually, I got so close to him and I had a chance to get a book out on pain neutralization. It's in print right now. It's going to come out because the world needs to know about this because nobody knows about this. But there's a history of people with 20 years of back pain that in one treatment they are suddenly pain free for the first time in 20 years.

Ty: But these techniques are not known because—

Dr. Cornu-Labat: Good, thank you. Because I was pointing to the fact that pain neutralization technique used on muscular skeletal pains but it barely hurts too. I have reflux and I'm short of breath because I have COPD and asthma. And for those that are short of breath, the respiratory system is a very good example for this. There are a lot of trigger points under the diaphragm than what you know of. If I do PNT, I neutralize those points the patient is breathing better.

So with these types of things there was not even a hint of these in medical school. Not even a hint of the complexity of the human being. There was a lot of information about the complexity of the biochemistry of the human body. Well, biochemistry is for the pharmaceutical industry you can say.

Ty: So you had to be basically re-educated once you got out of medical school?

Dr. Cornu-Labat: Pretty much. I think if we are smart enough and if we really love what we are doing, we have to be continuously in the alert to be re-educated.

Ty: Well, I commend you for that because I know a lot of doctors who are not re-educated. They are staying in the same model that's not working.

Dr. Cornu-Labat: Well, it's working for them. Right now, if you take a hard look at the core of the health care system, the patient is at the service of the system. It's not the other way around.

Ty: But it should be.

Dr. Cornu-Labat: It should. Unfortunately, that's not what's happening. It's completely the opposite. The reason why I congratulated you on what you are doing is because at the very core dis-empowerment is what maintains the system the way it is.

Ty: Well, what we want to do is to educate and that's what you're doing. And we want to give people hope. No matter what the diagnosis is, we want to let people know that they have options and that there's always hope. Until your last breath no one can tell you that you're going to die at a certain time. It's not their job.

Dr. Cornu-Labat: And even when we consider that process of disease, diagnosis, and then an end to that path, there's still the path. Even though there is a beginning where there is diagnosis and then there's an end path, maybe death is the end path, there's still a process. And a tremendous amount of things that happen in that process that when we look at disease and when we look at health and when we look at well-being, it's a very complex process where a lot of things happen at the same time. It's not just medication and symptoms and control or no control of dying or not dying. There's a lot more to the human experience. We have to take into account all of the human experiences when we are doing medicine. And that's what holistic medicine is about, its understanding and taking into account the whole experience.

If I tell you, "you have to do this", which is very typical of conventional medicine, "you have to do this." There's a degree of arrogance in that statement. "This is what you need." Given the complexity of the human experience, for me to presume that I know what you need, that is a tremendous arrogance. That's common. In medicine it's very common. That's a heavy load to carry on your shoulders. "I know what you need. I know that for this specific condition in this specific circumstance this is likely what's going to happen and this is the way of avoiding that which is likely to happen." That's the way we should state things. Not, "this is what you need to do. And if you don't do it, I'll force you or I'll have somebody force you." That happens and we know that.

We know that when somebody doesn't choose for their kids the exact path, "oh, we'll have somebody enforcing that so they choose that because that's what they need." Oh my God, what arrogance. What a humongous arrogance. It's very unfortunate how medicine is right now.

Ty: It is. We've had the privilege of interviewing several parents of children that have been forced into the conventional model, forced chemotherapy, forced radiation, which is really total arrogance on the part of the doctor.

Dr. Cornu-Labat: I walked away from that many years ago. I shifted away from that model. I don't want to be in their shoes when they have go to sleep at night. There is a degree of self-delusion.

Ty: Self-delusion, sure. Delusions of grandeur.

Dr. Cornu-Labat: I didn't want to take it on that side. I wanted to take it on this, keep convincing yourself that you're doing the right thing.

Ty: Oh, rationalization.

Dr. Cornu-Labat: Rationalization. But at some point it's going to dawn on you. And at some point you are going to be confronted with all those faces, and that's a law of life. You don't walk away from the consequences of your actions. You will pay the price.

Ty: You walked away from a medical system that wasn't working. You walked towards the path of light. And that's where you are now. I see you as one of the people that are helping to spread the truth about this holistic medicine.

Dr. Cornu-Labat: Maybe it makes me a little uncomfortable to use such terms but I'm definitely walking where I believe is the truth of health and well-being is.

Ty: Well, you didn't use the terms, I did.

Dr. Cornu-Labat: I know. I got a little uncomfortable.

Ty: I can tell from this interview that you're one of the good guys. I appreciate you doing that because it takes some intestinal fortitude to do what you're doing. And I appreciate it. And the guys here, our camera crew appreciates it. We weren't expecting to be able to interview you tonight but I'm glad that we did. So thank you so much for your time.

Dr. Cornu-Labat: Thank you. Thank you for doing what you're doing.

Ty: You keep up the good work too.

Dr. Cornu-Labat: I'm planning to.

Ty: Alright. ***[end of transcript]***

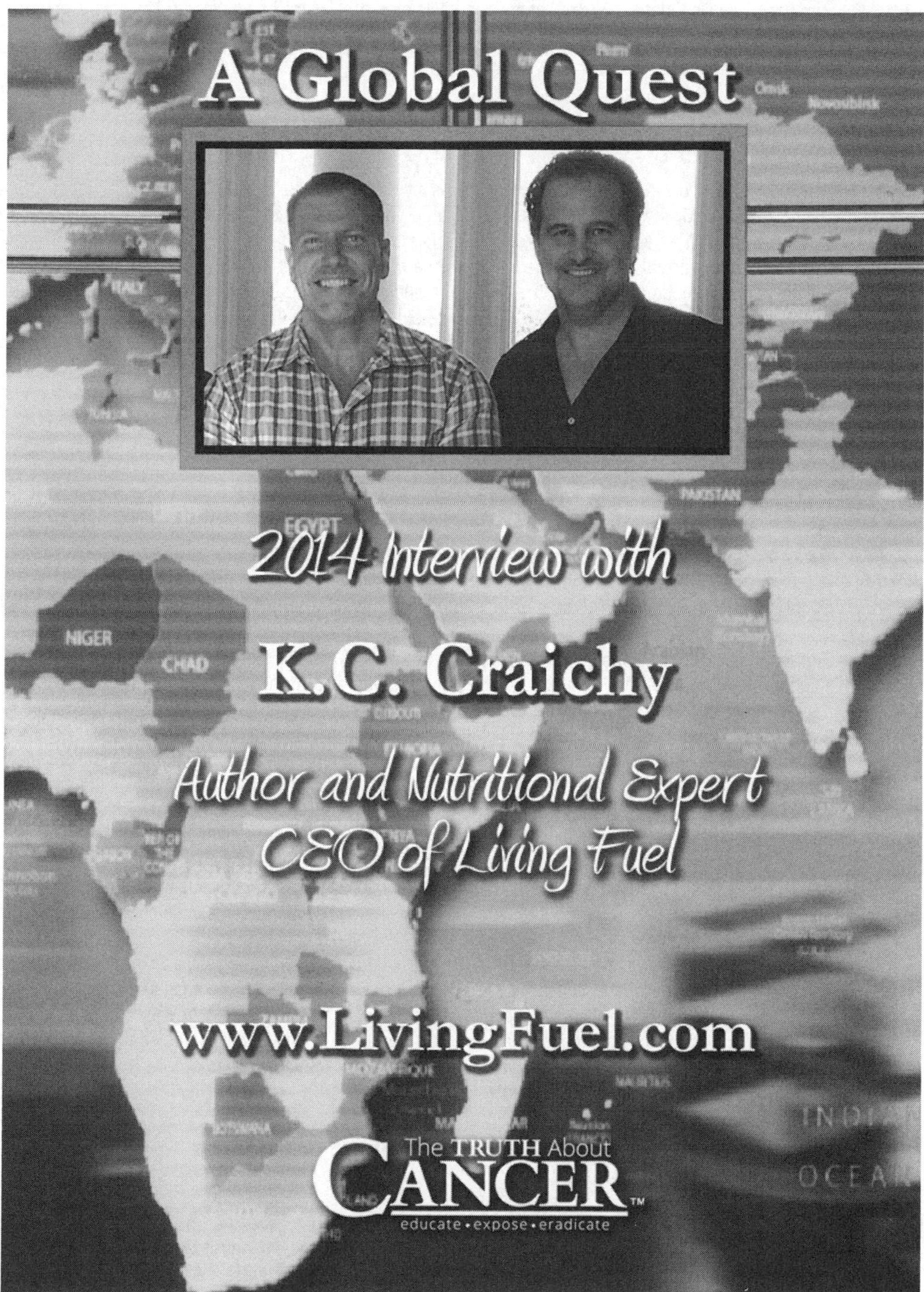
A Global Quest
2014 Interview with
K.C. Craichy
Author and Nutritional Expert
CEO of Living Fuel
www.LivingFuel.com
The TRUTH About CANCER
educate • expose • eradicate

Ty: I am here today in Orlando, Florida, at the beautiful home of KC Craichy, my friend. Thank you so much for spending time with us today.

KC: Great to see you, Ty.

Ty: So KC, tell us a little bit about yourself.

KC: Well, how I got involved in nutrition and health was my wife, who was Miss Florida and Miss Florida USA and competed in Miss America and Miss USA. I know you know the story but I am telling it for the benefit of the viewers. When we were married for a couple of years she came in with panic attacks, clinical depression and suicidal thoughts. The doctors were screwing her up really with Xanax and Zoloft and psychotherapy and it really wasn't much time at all when we realized she was basically personality-less. She was flat lined. It flattened her personally. Before, she would go anywhere at any time and now she wouldn't even leave her room. At that point we decided that drugs and the patient-for-life scenario couldn't have been God's will for her. So we decided we were going to dive into literature and weren't coming out without an answer. Over a 10-year period of research with trial and error, our company was born, our first bestselling book was born and all of our books and philosophies that we deal with and Monica hasn't had a drug in 20 years.

Ty: That's awesome.

KC: We've been able to help thousands of people overcome their own situations.

Ty: So talk about the company. You specialize in superfood nutrition, so talk about that.

KC: Superfood nutrition is a concept I started working on in the '90's, and I wrote my first white paper on the subject, which I called "The Four Corners of Optimum Nutrition" at that point. I now refer to it as "The Four Corners of Superfood Nutrition" because the piece of superfood nutrition that is so interesting is that, as we have defined it ,is that we know in health that there are something on the order of 50-53, it depends on how you slice them and by that I mean—some people will argue about how many essential vitamins there are or how many essential minerals there are. Some people say there are nine essential amino acids where others will say there are 10 and you add conditioner essentials there might be 12 so, depending on how you slice it, the things called dietary essentials means you have to get them from your diet in order to get them. The body can make the non-essentials. Technically, they are all essential, but the dietary essentials you must consume for the body to use that as raw material to make the other things that your body needs. If you are not getting those 50-plus essential nutrients in your diet then you are going to have physiologic consequences as a result. We also know, after many years of clinical study, what are the best forms of these nutrients. In the form of minerals you have seen iron oxide and calcium carbonate and those kinds of things. Those are cheap nutrients and say...vitamin D or D2's might be more toxic...a lot of the literature suggests those are toxic, or you might say that you have vitamin B12 would be methylcobalamin is accepted as the best form of vitamin B12 but cyanocobalamin is in most things that you find on the market and that doesn't match. You want to really match the Krebs Cycle. The Krebs Cycle should recognize the nutrients.

Ty: Real quick...what is the Krebs Cycle? Let's remember to get into that. Continue your thought but I want to get to Krebs.

KC: Dr. Krebs discovered the cycle of converting food to energy and oxygen...the whole process in the body called the Krebs Cycle. With the Krebs Cycle, the body will recognize things like citrates, malates, alpha ketogluterates and things along those lines. When your body sees these carriers for the nutrients it recognizes those have a message and what to do with it, so to speak. The net of it is, the best forms of these 50-plus essential nutrients are known. We feel like we have a pretty good handle on what those best ones are, but when you find most vitamins and minerals or supplements or foods, you usually find oftentimes the cheaper versions…that there are another one or two steps required by the body in order to make it into what you actually need. I am really going a little off course here but what I am trying to suggest is that since we know what you need and we also know, if you are honest, that there are things that you need that we don't know about. I call those the unknown essentials.

We have the essentials, conditioner essentials, unknown essentials, and unknown conditioner essentials. When you combine the 51…we have the best form of all the nutrients and you combine it with things like broccoli, spinach, kale, spirulina, barley grass, chlorella, blueberries, strawberry, raspberry and cranberry—now you are combining what is known with what we know—there are tons of studies to tell you those other things are exceptionally good for you in avoiding disease, being healthy and so on, but you hear, eat your vitamins with food. How often do you hear that? Why is that? There is a synergy that goes on when you combine nutrients with foods. When you combine all of these nutrients together the body recognizes and uses them and that is how superfood nutrition should work. That is our concept of superfood nutrition—getting what you need from known sources, combined with things that are exceptionally good for you, natural foods, and that gives you everything you know you need and everything you don't know you need.

We have broken that down a little farther and said, Wow, what does the literature say about the best approach to nutrition for weight optimization or life extension or delay in disease and so on? In 2002, my first white paper was called "The Four Corners of Optimal Nutrition," and now we call it, "The Four Corners of Superfood Nutrition," to bring in the concept I just described to you of the superfood nutrition. As long as you recognize you have superfood nutrition and you are getting optimal amounts of things including micro and macro—you have the protein, carbs, fiber and fats and so on—now you break it out in a way that is extraordinarily powerful.

This is the four corners where we start with calorie restriction with optimal nutrition. Years ago, you may remember the Biosphere project with Dr. Roy Walford at UCLA. They were in the Biosphere and the whole thing was about they were going to grow the food that they used. It was going to be a self-sustained environment and they weren't getting anything in or out of it—they would have to grow what they needed. They had something go wrong and they couldn't grow enough food for them so they had to ration what they ate to have less food. While they were hungry and all, they found remarkable physiological and psychological changes that were very positive and that really spawned the whole calorie-restriction movement—the calorie-restriction/fasting movement and so on. For calorie restriction and optimum nutrition there has now been more than 2,000 studies in virtually every single celled organism all the way up to primates and even in humans now that suggests that this is positive for physiology and that it actually—kind of like if you say there was a fountain of youth it would be to extend life, delay disease, enhance performance, optimize weight, increase mental clarity, and start going down the list of things that were beneficial from doing this approach.
There are always outlier studies along the way where this one didn't quite work or that one didn't quite work and so on, but the preponderance of the evidence from study after study showed, first of all, that just cutting calories of bad food was really good for you so instead of eating this much garbage you only ate this much garbage. That is really a cool concept when you think about it but if that really was the answer, then people starving in Africa or somewhere else would be the healthiest people in the world. That obviously isn't the answer but there is something to it.

The thing about calorie restriction is that it didn't catch on in the United States because in the last 10 years the average calorie intake has increased about 500 calories a day in the United States. Nobody likes to be hungry here in the United States in the land of plenty for sure. The people that got hold of this concept and really cut their calories by 40 to 50 percent literally looked like they were in concentration camps. They were so unhealthy looking, but somehow they were convinced that was healthy for them. There is this thing about optimal nutrition where you now take calorie restriction and you add optimal nutrition, most people would agree that if you eat less calories but you max out the nutrients and get all these 51 that we are talking about at the same time that it has got to be better for you than either eating a lot of calorically dense food or a little teeny bit of calorically dense food. Do you see what I'm saying?

Ty: Yes.

KC: That piece is a very important piece of the puzzle. Now we have enough people, there is one outlier study that is recent that a lot of people are saying has completely discredited the calorie-restriction movement, but it is going to take them 10 years really to sort it out because there was a 25-year study with Rhesus monkeys where they didn't get the results they were expecting on extending the life of these monkeys. But along the time of this 25-year study there was a 10-year study done with a similar kind of monkey that did get the results that they were looking for, so it is not going to be definitive. The net of it is we know, we know, we know that if you eat less high-quality food that is maximized in nutrient density, it is better for you than what people are doing out there. Of course, people still don't want to be hungry. The scientific argument then became, well, why does this work? So, the group over here we will call the Free Radical Theory of Aging Group. They are basically saying that the reason that you cut the calories and the reason that works is because less food equals less internal combustion, therefore less oxidation, therefore fewer calories equals low oxidative stress. Conversely, if we add back antioxidants to the diet you can increase the calories and get the same results as low calorie just by giving a broad spectrum of antioxidants. Broad-spectrum being hydroxyl, peroxyl, peroxide nitrites, superoxide anum and singlet oxygen are the five classes that are common in everybody and people think of antioxidants—I'm just going to take a vitamin C or something, where you are going to get one or two of those classes and you really need to address all of them. Really, the point is, they were able to mimic the results of calorie restriction by bringing in this antioxidant bouquet, if you will.

What are antioxidants? When you think about it and you think about how it affects health and in this particular case cancer—antioxidants are by nature anti-inflammatory and by nature anti-glycatin. In other words, anti-glycation.

Ty: What would that mean?

KC: Glycation is basically caramelization of a protein. Instead of having oxidation with oxygen oxidizing a fat or lipid it is like having a sugar caramelize on top of a protein and make the protein irrelevant. Advanced glycated end product—A-G-E—age. Really when you see crosslinked old skin what you are seeing is collagen cross linking or advanced glycated end products or glycation. I wrote about this in my book in 2005 and I said there, In five years glycation is going to be as well-known as oxidation. Well, here it is 10 years later and nobody still knows about it, but the point is simple. It is a foundational root of disease, including cancer. Oxidation, inflammation, glycation, and angiogenesis. Angiogenesis is basically getting a blood supply to an area. Say, if you twist your ankle, you are going to get a massive inflammation, and the inflammation is going to draw the angiogenesis to the area where the body will release new blood flow to the area, and then when the acute situation is over with, it will pull back the vessels and you are fine. It is the chronic angiogenesis that is the problem. In a cancer cell—most cancer cells will hide and get a blood supply through an angiogenesis which is chronic angiogenesis which is a big problem.

The point I am making here is this corner, the anti-oxidant corner, when you are addressing all five of these classes. Those things actually address and regulate these four major processes that underlie the disease. If you control oxidation, inflammation, glycation and angiogenesis then disease cannot progress. I am oversimplifying it but if you take these foundational root powers of a disease away, it is going to really stunt the growth of whatever that disease is trying to do. You can do that through nutrition, we have seen that. Dr. Li did an excellent TED Talk program if you ever want to go look up TED Talks. Dr. Li on angiogenesis, it is absolutely fascinating. He names the foods, some of which I have already mentioned, that regulate angiogenesis. I am staying a long time in that corner because it is so important when you talk about all the bright-colored vegetables and the bright-colored fruits and berries and all of those things—they have such power in these phytochemicals to combat disease and the underlying processes of which the disease actually operates and flourishes. Oxidative stress or high antioxidants, the free radical theory of aging group, has been shown to be able to mimic the calorie restriction.

The other piece that has been shown to mimic calorie restriction is if you cut the sugar and you cut the glycemic response. This is an area now that they have done plenty of studies on. In fact, the *Grain Brain* book that is out right now, the doctor shows and, gosh, this has been reported now for 15 years, that if your blood sugar is in the 90's, your chance of dementia is greatly increased. If your blood sugar is in the 90's, your chance of glycation is greatly increased. If there is more sugar around, there are more things that can be caramelized with that sugar and so 90-something blood sugar, while it is in a normal range, is not healthy or normal because all-cause mortality rises as blood sugar rises. If we realize that if you are reducing the sugar and glycemic response of foods—and they actually did a study which showed they can give 150 percent of the calories of a calorie restricted diet on a low-glycemic diet and they were able to mimic the results of calorie restriction with 150 oe of the calories saying greens instead of grains.

The sugar thing is a big deal. We have been talking about this a long time but one century ago sugar was a delicacy. Mom would make an apple pie or you would go to the store and get a little treat or something like that. Five pounds a year, it is estimated, would be the intake of sugar per year per person on the average. Today, it is a whopping 150-plus pounds per person per year on the average. The average is pretty high. The point is, people are eating their weight in sugar a year. When you think about the wisdom of incorporating this particular corner of the four corners of reducing the sugar and the glycemic response, all-cause mortality goes down as blood sugar goes down so now your blood sugars are in the 80's or even the 70's and it is a better case for you. Also, the chance of dementia goes up. In fact, in the *Grain Brain*, he talks about how the blood sugar in the 90's is asking for dementia and Alzheimer's later in life. That is a pretty cool thing. When you think about a lot of the ketogenics stuff, you actually can reverse some levels of dementia through going ketogenic. The same thing has been shown in cancer, that if you go ketogenic they have said some of these doctors—and I read this story recently—one of the doctors was able to starve his own cancer. I think it was a pancreatic cancer in some areas. It is fascinating the possibilities here—so there are three of the four corners.

The fourth one is healthy fats—primarily marine oil. I call it antioxidant fish oil and I always have to add antioxidant fish oil because if you are just taking fish oil and you are not talking fat soluble antioxidants alongside of it, you are asking for lipid peroxidation. Fish oil is a delicate oil and you expose it to oxygen. People say, Well, it has one IU of vitamin E in it. Well, vitamin E or alpha tocopheral, one IU is not enough to keep from spoiling in your body. It may keep from spoiling in the gel cap but not in your body. You need to broaden that out. Fish oil, we know, is anti-inflammatory. Again, we are coming back to some of these underlying processes of the disease states. Fish oil is a very powerful thing. We are seeing studies have shown that certain cancer rates with fish oil are lower and we are talking about including your fish oil. If you have vitamin E, alpha beta gamma delta tocotrienal and alpha beta gamma delta tocopheral you are now adding some oxidation protection to the oils and giving antioxidant benefit to the body itself. We like it when you have EPA and DHA to include borage seed or primrose oil because the GLA from those combined with the EPA from fish magnifies the anti-inflammatory property, according to the research, of the fish oil. Instead of getting prostaglandin E2 you get prostaglandins 1 and 3 which are more anti-inflammatory. So, then adding vitamin D and vitamin A at the levels of cod liver oil and then the amazing nutrient astaxanthin. If you want to know about a nutrient, go out there and do a web search on astaxanthin and look at all the benefits ascribed to this nutrient that is a small molecule antioxidant that has been shown to be able to cross the blood brain barrier and also into the eyes as an eye antioxidant and so on, and it is said to increase your tolerance to sun radiation or external radiation sources. For instance, gamma radiation when you are flying on a plane and so on. There are so many benefits to adding that in.

These are the four corners of SuperFood Nutrition that we have been talking about for so long. I got into a lot of detail on each one of them but there is a really cool study in *The Journal of Nutrition* in 2001. There are four groups of mice, genetically altered mice—altered to be more susceptible to disease. The first group of mice they called the all-you-can-eat group. They gave it all the food it can eat all the time so it grazed all the time. They also added corn oil to the situation. These mice lived an average of 232 days. So, 232 on the average. The second group, same kind of mice, same feeding method, but all they did was instead of corn oil they gave fish oil and they lived an average of 100 days longer just adding the fish oil. It was still garbage food underneath if you think about it. The third group was the calorie restriction group. They took the same food, same feeding method but actually cut the calories of the food by 40 percent and they lived an average of 200 days longer than the 232 day control just by eating less of the unhealthy food they were eating. The last of the four groups was the calorie-restriction group combined with fish oil and this group lived an average of 400 days longer than the 232 day control. So 600 something days versus 200 something days. That is a fascinating little study. I always say, if you are mouse, you really ought to be thinking about this kind of nutrition.

Anyway, this does translate in a lot of ways. It just shows the high impact that nutrition could actually be. You cannot ignore if you take the four corners and all the research that has shown positive benefits on each of these four corners and added it together, you are looking at more than 3,000 research studies, which would make this among the most studied approach. Add it together and integrate these four together—of anything that has ever been put forth. You have a lot of people talking about nutritional approaches but if you look at the body of literature behind what they are talking about it isn't that substantial.

Ty: That is substantial. Where do I go from here? There are so many notes that I have taken here over this first few minutes of the interview. One of the things that I really appreciate is the fact that you are not giving us conjecture. You are talking about the studies and what the literature has shown. I have seen the studies and the literature does show what you are talking about. It does verify this. One of the things that is interesting is within the last couple of weeks you spoke to a group of medical doctors in Miami, I believe…

KC: Yes.

Ty: …and you told me that they were using your lecture to begin to tweak their protocols for their own patients.

KC: That is what they were telling me. That is the feedback that I am getting, is that the way that I talked about the integrating of these things—you know most doctors have heard about calorie restriction on some level and about antioxidants on some level and about low sugar on another level and about fish oils and so on. When you put it all together, that you can actually integrate these approaches to where you actually don't have to choose one and you can do them all and let that be the way you actually guide yourself in your nutritional choices, they found that to be a very simplistic… I know it doesn't sound simplistic, but I guess to the doctor it was simplistic, compared to what they were… When you have an aha! and your understanding comes forth, it is really awesome.

Ty: Yeah.

KC: Instead of saying, go follow the food pyramid and eat grains and whatever else. It is a very powerful approach. I would say when people start doing this they will realize that you can bring in enough fiber and protein with all of these micronutrients and you don't need anywhere near the food that people put in their body. Calorie restriction—is it really calorie restriction if you cut your calories back to what our parents were eating 15-20 years ago? What our diets are now, if we cut it back some of the percentages in some of these studies we are just getting back to where they were, because it has been growing on a daily basis.

Ty: Yes and the epidemic of obesity here in the USA is unfathomable.

KC: Absolutely amazing. Again, that is a chronic inflammatory situation. This whole thing of obesity—if you say that people are overeating—now, calorie does not equal overweight. It is calorie distribution, and we can get into a whole interview on that one alone. Really, the point is that people are getting fatter. The fat is a factory. The fat, particularly the belly fat, becomes the largest endocrine organ in the body essentially. The fat produces TNF alpha interleukin 6 and aromatase. These are inflammatory cytokines. We are getting back to inflammation, inflammation, inflammation. So, inflammatory cytokines and then aromatase. They are worried about the T-levels, if you will. Testosterone levels are dropping a large portion as a result of the belly fat. Aromatase is an enzyme that converts whatever testosterone is floating around the male bloodstream and converts it to estrogen. What makes a man a man has turned into what makes a woman a woman. There are so many health problem with low testosterone, it is a terrible thing.

Ty: Interesting you mention aromatase, because a doctor that I know uses a product called dearomatase that stops that conversion with cancer patients. That is a big issue with cancer patients as well.

KC: That would seem to make sense. LifeExtension makes Super MiraForte or something like that, which is an aromatase inhibitor. It is an area to consider. You have to inhibit the aromatase, but the best way to inhibit the aromatase is to conquer the belly fat, which becomes an enemy that is working to your detriment because these situations that it creates makes people heavier, less likely to have activity and therefore more fat, producing more of these things that are bringing about death.

Ty: It is an endless cycle really.

KC: It is an endless cycle.

Ty: So KC, let's talk about sugar. You mentioned low-glycemic index, low-sugar diets and the positive effect that has on folk's health. That is also a keystone that I am finding throughout this investigative miniseries that I am doing. Almost every doctor that I have talked to that treats cancer says that one of the first things they tell their patients to do is to eliminate refined sugars because of the fact that sugar is the fuel for cancer cells.

KC: One of the presentations, I believe it was by Dr. Block, this weekend while I was in Florida, he suggested that cancer cells consume glucose at the rate—he might have said 20 percent or he might have said 40 percent more so than typical cells. It is a vacuum sound with sugar in the cancer cells. All this time you can see these cancer centers giving ice cream to patients and it is like, what are they thinking about?

Ty: I cannot remember who it was that mentioned that and said to me that when an oncologist tells the cancer patient, who may be wasting away with cachexia (wasting syndrome) to go eat ice cream and cake, whatever it takes to put on the weight, that they really sentence them to death. They don't know that, but the cancer feeding on the sugar that—you couldn't have a worse recommendation than that. The sweets, for somebody who is wasting away, because it will feed the cancer. It won't feed their body. You don't get nutrition from sugar but you do feed the cancer.

KC: The terrible thing is that people are getting this bad advice. It isn't just sugar, it is things that turn to sugar. We talk about sugar as a big problem. Yes, it is a big problem. Sugar is wonderful. Everybody likes sugar. I like sugar, but I choose not to thrive on sugar. Sugar should have been in our fun foods. Building blocks, fuel and fun. Fun foods. Every now and then you have sugar. But sugar—100 grams of carbohydrates. I saw a study that it was either 100 grams or 200 grams, recently, where it said if you had a pizza meal, or a pasta meal, within 15 minutes of eating that meal your leukocytic index, which is essentially white blood cells—how many bad guys can they eat in an hour... The study was suggesting that it should be about 16 per white blood cell in an hour. Within eating this carbohydrate meal within 15 minutes you drop from 16 to 1.9 and hold that for hours.

Ty: You have 10% capacity that you used to.

KC: Ten percent capacity and basically these patients are often in an immunocompromised state to start with. Some of the treatments they are getting are taking their immunity down to almost nothing and then they are throwing sugar in on top of that, which directly feeds the problem but it also directly takes a whack at the immunity. It is a terrible cycle that people need to consider.

Ty: It is.

KC: The other piece is that even in this weekend's presentation down in Miami they were showing research that said... Now, first of all, patients do not die of cancer. Seldom do they die of cancer. They die of complications from cancer treatment. That is just what happens. The wasting and some other things are complications from cancer treatments, as you well know.

We want to talk about antioxidants as a piece of this thing. Most cancer centers you go to today will tell you that you are not to take antioxidants during cancer treatment because the process which we are using, they tell you, is an oxidative process and our goal is to use that process for your benefit to try and bring about the killing of cancer cells, so if you used antioxidants, it would essentially quench what we are trying to do. But the research does not back that up. I have now seen multiple studies in this particular presentation say that taking antioxidants during cancer treatment extends the patient life outcome dramatically than those who do not receive antioxidants during treatment.

It is kind of like this. You take a Coumadin or aspirin—this is an analogy—it is called irreversible platelet aggregation. That means that if you cut yourself you are going to bleed for a good while before your blood stops, if ever. If you take fish oil, that is called reversible platelet aggregation. Dr. Stoll, from Harvard, 15-20 years ago, wrote a book called *The Omega-3 Connection* and he showed in the book that you can take fish oil and cut yourself and the body will reverse that and clot the blood. When you take natural things—all these vital chemicals and antioxidants and so on—the body is a signaling system. It is an amazing thing. We now know that a lot of times, even resveratrol has been shown to release positive genetic expression not just biochemical combustion. It is not just a biochemical response. It is a biochemical and genetic response, a positive genetic response. The body is an incredibly smart vehicle and if you give the body foods in forms which it can use or recognize then the body can do things that it needs to do for your benefit. A simple little test of this would be if you were to mix up some eggs in a bowl. Let's just say you mixed up a dozen eggs in that bowl and you scrambled them up. How many could you eat? How much of that could you eat? How many eggs?

Ty: As far as a quantity?

KC: Come on Ty, you can eat…

Ty: A couple dozen.

KC: OK, you could eat a dozen at least. A couple dozen? I don't know. That would have to be on a bet. The point is, if you take the same egg and you get hard boiled eggs and you line them up on the table, you are not getting anywhere near a dozen. You may stop at three or four, because there is a thing called CCK—cholecystokinin enzyme—some people say leptin is involved but the point is there is a signaling system in your brain and when you take a few bites of that egg you are going to get to two or three or four before your body will send a signal for you to throw up. You now are going to get nauseous. It is not because the digestion has gone to your brain, but if you eat carbohydrates, it is going to take you the time to chew, digest, 20 minutes, sugar hits the brain and the brain says—Okay, we're done. When you eat the foods I am talking about that have this CCK signaling system, you eat, and by the time you chew it your body knows what you have on board and makes appropriation for stopping you before you overeat. It is a fascinating concept. I believe the same thing. When you take these natural antioxidants during these times of treatments or whatever it is that you are going to do, the body recognizes what it is and what it is trying to do. The research seems to be bearing that out.

Ty: I have done numerous interviews with cancer patients that increased antioxidants while they were doing chemo and had much better success than folks that had the same type cancer that did not use antioxidants.

KC: If these researchers were being honest and looked in their own journals they would find the same thing. It is not like it is hidden. It is in their own journals.

Ty: Hidden in plain sight.

KC: A lot of times that is the best place to hide things.

Ty: Yeah, it is. You mentioned inflammation. A doctor that I know down in South Texas has used C reactive protein, which is a measured inflammation marker to stage cancer. He is able to use the levels of inflammation in that marker alone to determine if somebody has cancer cells or not. It is fascinating. I have been able to interview him on this project but the mention of inflammation rings true that cancer and a lot of other degenerative diseases are greatly affected by the amount of inflammation in the body.

KC: I would say that if you start asking your experts what role does oxidation play? It plays a big role. What role does inflammation play? It plays a big role. What role does glycation play? It plays a big role. What role does angiogenesis play? It plays a big role. It is amazing when you start seeing that these are really foundational principles. These are not just for cancer. You want to regulate these things for good health. Even if you don't have cancer and you have a diet that gives you longer health you would want to try and eat foods that help you regulate these processes in the body.

Ty: It is interesting the role that foods can have in your overall health. It is interesting that many of the medical doctors haven't been taught enough about nutrition while they are in school. I have a friend down in South Texas that is a medical doctor. He said in the decade of school he only had two hours of nutrition. That's it.

KC: I have never found doctor who has had more than six hours. I ask that question frequently because I find it very interesting. How many hours of nutrition training have you had? Their answer is, I think I took a class when I was in pre-med. When you really dig down into what they were learning, it was how warm the peas should be in the hospital for patients. It is nothing to do with clinical nutrition. This is no disservice. I am not dissing doctors. Doctors are not trained in this area and this has to be by design somewhere. You have dieticians who are trained based on—there are some dieticians who are brilliant nutritionists but they have taken it on themselves to take clinical nutrition protocols and learn it themselves but the typical dietician training to learn how to serve patients in the hospital and when you think about it—places like schools, hospitals and these kind of places—look at the food that is being given in these places. This cannot be based on nutrition science.

You talk about nutrition training for doctors but nurses have no nutrition training. Dieticians really don't have nutrition training. You have to start defining what does nutrition training mean? Well for many years dietician training came from the food pyramid which, as you know, was invalidated 10 or more years ago. I think it was the Physicians for Responsible Medicine group sued and they were able to show that the whole food pyramid thing was put together by lobbyists and lawyers and not nutritionists. This was the basis for nutrition in this land for many years in the schools and in hospitals and public places. When you think about that—if you ever sat in the hospital to see them hand somebody a plate what they are going to feed them while they are in the hospital, you look at that lifeless food and you really have to shake your head and say, "Okay, what place in the world would I really sit down and pay money for that or even eat it if somebody paid for it for me, or have my kid eat it?" The one saving grace of the food brought in the hospital, from what I have seen, is that they give garbage food a lot of times but there really just isn't much of it so it comes back to the calorie restriction theory that we were talking about earlier that if you cut the calories of the same garbage food it is actually better for you than eating a lot of it so there are some physiologic benefits for that.

It is pretty sad when you think that dietician training is not clinical nutrition. Now, I know some dieticians who are really nutritionists. There are a lot of them who have taken it on themselves to understand sports science or understand clinical nutrition and taken clinical nutrition courses, but what the medical schools don't offer as part of their curriculum is clinical nutrition. Dietetics is not the same thing as nutrition, although the dietician lobby is the one that has the power to make their title with the AMA and that sort of thing—they have the power to have themselves called nutritionists, when the truth is there should be a category that is a dietician, because there is a place for that, and there should be a category that is a nutritionist. If they both take the same kind of course they can both be nutritionists, or something like that. As you know, many of the brilliant nutritionists that you have interviewed with this thing aren't even licensed in their own state to practice nutrition because "clinical nutrition" is not recognized as an art and licensable in most states.

Ty: Earlier in the interview you mentioned that sometimes we will have people that are patients for life. I think, based on what you are telling me, if the focus would shift from treating symptoms with drugs to treating the whole body and giving the body fuel that it can run properly on the way God made it then a lot of those patients for life would not be patients for life anymore.

KC: Very true. It is funny. Jeffrey Bland gave a talk this weekend. He is the founder of functional medicine. The guy is brilliant. He was saying that he has always been blasted about—"Your stuff is not double-blind, placebo controlled." I only practice scientific medicine. He finally said he got to the point where he said to the doctor, "Answer this question. You'll be honest with me, right? We'll agree that I'm a little bit on the outskirts of what you are talking about as scientific medicine, but let me ask you this question. Have you ever prescribed a patient a drug that was already on four other drugs? Oh, of course. Could you point me to a study that showed a patient population on those five drugs?" "Well, I have the study for this drug and this drug—" "No, that isn't what I said. Could you show me a patient population that has been studied on those five drugs?" And the answer is, of course not. In fact, I was told by Dr. Scott Hannon about a study recently that says if you are on five or more medications it is impossible to predict the clinical response of the five drugs. That is when it is all a guessing game. You give a drug for this, a drug for that and then you end up giving drugs for the symptoms caused by drugs and it is an awful spiral. Now, there is a place for some drugs sometimes but I generally think of them as a Band Aid to get people over a hump before they can figure out how to get the body to respond like it is supposed to.

Ty: I like that thought…a Band Aid. It is not a fix. It is not a long-term fix; it is just a temporary Band Aid.

KC: There will never be a drug cure. I don't see it happening. Nobody has a drug deficiency to start with.

Ty: Sickness is not a deficiency of drugs.

KC: Right.

Ty: A lot of times it is a deficiency of nutrition.

KC: It is a confluence of symptoms absolutely. A confluence of symptoms from all kinds of reasons. Some people are exposed to radiation. Some people are exposed to toxins. Some people are exposed to viruses. There are a lot of interesting studies out there about viruses being associated with certain cancers. There is a lot more than we know. The biggest problem as I see it with medicine the way it is practiced today is that medicine is a business. It is the business of taking pseudo-science and selling it to the public. When I say pseudo-science—Jeffrey Bland talks about in 1962 they took a course on genetics seven years after the discovery of the gene. He says they took a course and they all passed the course. They had a meeting recently with the group of people that were in that class, and they said that if they were to take that same test today and answer it the same way, instead of getting an A they would have gotten an F because science changes over time. Does it really? No. Our understanding of science changes over time. Science has never changed. The truth has always been the truth. It is our understanding of truth and how we apply it. Unfortunately, the way we work things as the standard of care is a vehicle to keep people from getting sued, if you will. The standard of care gets implemented after things have been studied and studied and studied and people have a fair amount of comfort level that we are going to treat things this way and if you don't treat things this way then you open yourself up to lawsuits. Then it takes years of new stuff coming out before we can say that we are going to go away from that standard onto a new standard. If you would actually look at the standard of care over the last five decades you would be shocked. If you try to do some of the things today that were done five, four, three, two and even one decade ago you would be in malpractice just from doing what was standard care. Again, truth does not change but our understanding of it does.

Ty: Well put. I agree with that. One of the things that is interesting that you mention about drugs and the symptoms that drugs cause—my grandmother died a few years ago. She was 92 when she died. Before she died she was on about 12 or 13 drugs and if I remember correctly only two or three of those drugs that she was on were for the original problems symptoms. The other 10, a1 drugs that she was taking were drugs that had been produced to mitigate the symptoms that the first couple of drugs caused.

KC: It happens all the time. I remember my mom always complaining that her back hurt. It wasn't her back—it was her kidneys. If you ever read the side effects of the drugs she was on it was causing that problem. My dad died about three weeks ago. I can remember about three years ago it was to the point, or maybe four, my wife and I went to see him and he was so spaced out that my wife said, I am not sure we will see him again. He is in pretty bad shape. I thought, I need to go check his drug register, so I had them show me his drug books. He was on 13 different meds for all kinds of different things. There is a clinical condition now referred to as drug-induced dementia. If you are on a number of drugs and the condition of the patient is changing where they are just not themselves, sometimes it is prudent to have the doctors back way off these drugs and just use core necessary medication to see if they come back. My dad came back fully when we took him off half of those meds and he came back fully.

Ty: Wow.

KC: His brain was very sharp until the end.

Ty: That rings true, KC, because my grandmother who was on the 13 meds—we took her off the meds the same way that you did your dad and she came back as well. I think she did have drug-induced dementia. I would call her on the way home from work and say, "Grandma, how are you doing?" She would say, "Ty, you have to come get me." She was in a rehab center. She had broken her hip. She was on so many drugs it was unbelievable. "You have to come get me, Ty. The lady next door is staring at me. She is staring at me. She won't talk to me but she is staring at me all day long and she won't stop staring at me." I go to see her and she is staring at herself in the mirror. She didn't even realize it was her. We took her off all of the drugs. We just finally told her doctor, we're done with all this. She is not herself and she has been this way ever since you prescribed all of these drugs. We took her off and she did come back. Now, she eventually died but she was all there mentally until she died. At that point we knew that it was time.

KC: Praise God. There are a lot of people hopefully hearing this that can say, Wow, I am going to check into that. Have the doctors take a look at what that list of drugs is and see. Let's go down to just the critical few and see what happens. It is a detox. There are a lot of toxins in drugs and the combination of drugs.

Ty: Talking about drugs, real quickly, we have a little bit of time left and then we will let you go. I know that your time is precious here. Does modern medicine pays too much attention to drugs and not enough attention to nutrition? It is a loaded question.

KC: You've really got to ask that question?

Ty: You've already answered it.

KC: I promise you that no one has a drug deficiency. I really don't think there are very many drugs—most people are on drugs that they really shouldn't be on. You see things like drugs to bring down cholesterol levels. Cholesterol is really not a difficult thing to bring down nutritionally if you understand how nutrition works and how blood sugar works. The problem with cholesterol to start with is people think they are not eating cholesterol because they are trying to keep their cholesterol from going up. When you talk about what causes high cholesterol—this is just an example. High cholesterol, people think, is caused by eating fat or eating cholesterol. That is the preponderance. If you interviewed on the street 100 people you are going to get that the vast majority of the times. Very few people understand it is the carbohydrates that they are eating, the overfueling, that is causing the high cholesterol level.

First thing is just when you drive up the gas station, open the gas tank, and put the nozzle in there and you start filling the car and then it clicks a few times and then runs down the side of the car. Then do you roll the back window down and fill the back seat? That is what we are doing. We are overfueling to the point where the body is having to figure out it has no better capacity to deal with the gas in the back seat of the car then the body does. You really only have a teaspoon of sugar in the blood. That is what your body regulates. Then you have 500 grams of sugar stored in muscles as glycogen and such and maybe 100 in the liver. When you are full, like most people are already and they drink one soft drink that has 17 teaspoons of sugar in it depending on the size they have—what is your body going to do with that if you have already got one in the blood and your muscles are full? Your body is going to basically—it is called post-prandial hyperlipidemia. That means after you eat the body is going to quickly change it into a fat of some kind. That fat will be a triglyceride or an LDL cholesterol. That is where your cholesterol levels are jumping. It is not because of the eating fat or eating something with cholesterol in it. That has no relevance what-so-ever.

When you think about it people say 200 mg/dl is the perfect cholesterol level. Okay, if you accept that then eating 400 mg of cholesterol must be bad, right? You have to say how many dl of blood are in the body? Say 200 times what? Two hundred perfect level times what? It is times 50-70 dl. That means there are 14,000 roughly mg of cholesterol in the body at all times and if you eat 400 grams it is nothing. It is a drop in the pool. It cannot be coming from that area. There are people that have familial high cholesterol and that sort of thing and it is a different issue potentially but still—they need to stop the sweet drinks and the grains and white carbohydrates. This is not a cholesterol lesson but I am just trying to suggest that nutrition is super high impact. You can stop doing the things that cause it and you are going to reverse it. It sounds too simple but it really is.

Things like fiber. Fiber goes in the stomach and pulls/soaks up bile acid. The body goes into the bloodstream to get cholesterol to make more bile acid. It is like, Oh, that is a good way to use fiber to bring down cholesterol levels. It is pretty simple but yet complex. It is an incredible machine that the body is but dealing with nutrition before drugs by a long shot. If somebody doesn't have a pancreas they are going to need insulin but that is technically not really a drug. It is a hormone that is necessary for life.

Ty: Right. It is interesting that we had a very similar conversation yesterday at dinner about cholesterol, carbohydrates and sugar.

KC: Did you really?

Ty: Yes, that is another topic altogether. I think the mantra that we should eat to live instead of live to eat. If we applied that and we thought about, "Okay, is this food or this drink that I am about to ingest, is it going to give me life or am I just eating it because it tastes good?" If we can flip that switch to where we are thinking cognitively all the time, I want to be putting things in my body that give me life. Live foods. Living fuel. One of your products, LivingFuel, has changed the life of me and my family. It is one of the staples of our everyday nutritional regimen. We have living Fuel Shakes every day.

KC: Awesome.

Ty: I love the LivingFuel.

KC: Me too. All of us. If you were at my house and you are having breakfast and you don't have a LivingFuel you are going to be hungry.

Ty: You even have a fuel station where you have every kind of LivingFuel and they just go and get the nutrition they need.

KC: That's right.

Ty: I have heard this from different doctors thus far on this docu-series that I have been doing, that cancer is a nutritional deficiency. It is a disease that is caused by improper fuel getting to the body, the body's immune system is compromised because it is not eating enough of the good foods or it is eating too much of the bad foods or a combination of the two. At that point, the immune system gets overloaded, the amount of sugars that we are ingesting is unreal compared to 20 or 30 years ago—just the amount of sugar in our diets. As a matter of fact, I used to be a competitive body-builder. Low-fat diet was the king in the early 90's but what did they replace the fats with?

KC: Carbohydrates.

Ty: Carbohydrates, sugar. We were eating a diet that may have kept us lean for a while but not a healthy diet. One of the things that I appreciate about what you shared about the LivingFuel is that you are including not just the greens but the healthy fats—the probiotics. All of the different spectrum. All of the amino acids that we need. It is a complete food.

KC: It is a food. The thing about cancer is it is really an oversimplification to say that it is all nutritional disorder. Nutrition is a piece of the puzzle. In my first book I talk about how with my wife's health problems we went to clinical nutrition as, that has got to be the answer, and I buried myself in clinical nutrition. That is why over a long period of time I learned some incredibly high impact things in nutrition of which fuel is the result of this whole concept of nutrition we talked about which is completely embodied in LivingFuel. There is no food that accomplishes that system better than the LivingFuel system, no doubt. But to say nutrition is the problem—it doesn't give enough credit to environmental factors. If you think about the abuse of radiating scanning out there.

You are giving kids 16 frame x-rays for dental and you give them x-rays for this, and CT scans and all these things. Dr. Ron Golf wrote a textbook that talks about the radiation output and how he compares it to Hiroshima—the amount of radiation that was put out in Hiroshima, and mammograms and all of these other things. There are so many things that people are doing to themselves. Ground-up chemicals and not eating organic foods and eating processed meats like sausages and things along those lines. There have been plenty of studies to show that that stuff will cause cancer but people are eating it by the droves. Fast food and fake pink slime. There are a lot of things that are causing people's health problems including cancer out there and most of them are lifestyle- induced. Nutrition is a mega part of that. I didn't want to leave it oversimplified that it is a nutrition problem. In my first book I wrote I figured out it wasn't just nutrition. It was hydration, nutrition, exercise, stress, sleep, environmental hazards, meditation and prayer and all of these have a profound impact on your health and nutrition is a mega one for sure.

Ty: I appreciate you clarifying that. If I insinuated that doctors said that it was only nutrition, that wasn't it.

KC: I didn't think you did. I just wanted to make sure the listening audience or viewers were clear on that.

Ty: KC, I appreciate you mentioning that and clarifying that. I agree completely with that. I believe the doctors that I have interviewed would agree with that too. Cancer has a huge nutritional piece but there are a lot of other environmental factors. You mention toxins, radiation and so forth. I think we would all agree on that.

KC: I knew that is where you are coming from but I know that for viewers out there, for some of them it is the first time they are hearing some of this stuff and to say nutrition is my cure for cancer—it may well be a huge part of your getting through the cancer but it also may be a huge reason you had the cancer in the first place. There are so many of these things. In my first book in 2005, I wrote about hydration, nutrition, exercise and stress and sleep and environmental hazards, meditation and prayer. All of these things have a profound effect on whether you are going to get it in the first place and if you are going to get through it also. Nutrition is a mega aspect and a mega portion of that but stress—think about stress. What factor does stress play? If you have marital problems and financial problems and a special needs kid—their stress levels could literally cause your immunity to go into the dump and then you are basically a sitting duck for immune problems and cancer and all kinds of other things. This is a large problem with a lot of potential areas but if you manage these seven keys like I am talking about you really are guarding yourself against the eventuality and possibility of getting that kind of thing.

Ty: Great information and great clarification. So KC, tell me. Go through the seven keys one more time for us.

KC: The seven keys, from my book in 2005—*Super Health: The 7 Golden Keys to Unlock Lifelong Vitality* are hydration, nutrition, exercise, stress, sleep, environmental hazards and meditation and prayer. When you think about that, most people watching right now are deficient in at least four of those seven and I have seen it time and time and time again and just one of them has dramatic physiologic consequences as a result.

Ty: Right now I am deficient in the sleep one.

KC: Well, hopefully that is just for this four weeks.

Ty: Just temporarily though. KC, last question. If you were diagnosed with prostate cancer what would you do?

KC: hat is a scary thought for anyone because people when they hear about it directed at them it is a very scary thing. If it were directed at me, first of all—you have to understand that the diagnosis oftentimes is made on a test like prostate specific antigen that really has no bearing on whether it is real or not. If I were ever diagnosed with that I would say, "Doctor, thank you for your medical opinion but I am going to go find out the truth." First of all, is it really prostate cancer? That is a big question that has not been answered. Do I have inflammatory markers that look like that? Is the PSA out of whack? Are there other things that look like this? I will not rush to a biopsy because when you think about it, the biopsy goes through the anus, to the prostate and the chance of getting infection as a result of just doing that test is a very real possibility. There are other scans like thermal scans and things like that where you can get a thermal scan and see if the heat produced there is indicative of disease or something like that. I have these seven things which I advise people all the time.

People call me up and say, "I have just been diagnosed with this kind of cancer. What should I do?" I will go through these seven, and it goes something like this. First of all, stop all sugar and starch carbohydrates. I say of carbohydrates, if it's white it ain't right. The net of it is, first stop that. Stop feeding the problem and whacking your immunity like I was talking about. It is a double-edged sword. It is a terrible thing. Get your vegetables and eat tons of them. Vegetables primarily, fruits not so much. Vegetables, eat a lot of fibrous vegetables. If you are going to get a carbohydrate it should come from a fibrous vegetable. Then follow the four corners of superfood nutrition that I talked about.

Get all the nutrients that your body needs and get the four corners: low calorie, nutrient dense, high broad-spectrum antioxidants and taken in all five classes of antioxidants and as I talked about reducing the sugar and glycemic response and increasing the health fats—fish oil fats. I go to antioxidant fish oil. We have a lot of people out there touting shellfish oils like krill oil or green lipid muscle and that sort of thing. It is still omega-3 so it does have omega-3 benefit but the touting of that instead of fish oil is not appropriate according to the literature the way I have reviewed it. Yes, you can get benefit from those things but you talk about the krill oil has a lot of astaxanthin it and therefore it can keep it from spoiling—some of the things we talked about and keeping the oils from spoiling, but when I looked at how much astaxanthin was actually in a krill pill it was so minute it was unbelievable. You want to try to get 1 mg of astaxanthin in addition to all the trials and so on to get the fish oil. It is really important. All of these things I have talked about already are reducing inflammation and reducing the glycation, oxidation and angiogenesis.

I personally would go on a fuel fast. I would have LivingFuel for breakfast, lunch and dinner until I decided what path I was going to take to deal with this diagnosis and whether it was real or not. Then things like resveratrol is a very powerful antioxidant and that is one of the ones that you ought to be taking and then curcumin. Curcumin has been shown to be so anticancer. There is a lot of research on that now and recently a doctor sent me a photo which I showed you about this squamous cell carcinoma on the lip of this patient. It was just terrible. He put this paste with curcumin and coconut oil and in two weeks it was gone. I don't know what the biopsies looked like but the point is this: nutrition is powerful. It is extraordinarily powerful. If you start pointing in the right direction and doing some of the things that the research suggests it has to be good for you.

Another thing that is critically important is vitamin D. Vitamin D levels. I would make sure that if I was in that particular situation, I would make sure my 25 hydroxy vitamin D level was in the 70-90 range in a test. That is one of the first tests I would get. I would get all the tests including the inflammatory markers and so on but I would get a 25 hydroxy vitamin D test to see where it is. Vitamin D is the immune modulator of the body. Having your vitamin D level at the right level is imperative in this particular case. Another thing I would do is take significant amounts of vitamin A because it is also an immune enhancer and then there are some well-known mushroom extracts that enhance immunity too. This is not a treatment protocol I am giving to anybody. What I am saying is this is what I tell people—do these things while you are figuring out what it is that you are going to do. This business called medicine, or the business called cancer care, does a lot of fear to patients. You have this problem and we need to deal with it now. The truth is that it most likely is not that level of emergency. Now, it can be. Most likely you have some time to get a second opinion, to get your brain working and go to somebody like Ralph Moss or somebody else and buy a report. He has a great report which I always send people to get this report. It tells you what are the types of care used for that particular kind of cancer out there and what are the success rates of the various ones and who are the practitioners that are doing it and what are the alternatives. That kind of information is incredibly powerful because it is put in a way that you can literally hand that to the doctor and it is scientific documentation and they have to go, Yeah, I guess that does make sense. If your doctor refuses to work with you or tells you that you should not take antioxidants during cancer care you might want to consider a different doctor because the literature is not backing it up.

Ty: I think that is very wise advice KC. To do your research, take your time…

KC: Take some extreme steps with nutrition, like I talked about, but then focus in and figure out what the answers are.

Ty: Sure. I think the knowledge that you have shared with us today—this information—is going to allow people to be able to do that if they face that cancer diagnosis. Get the nutrition coming in, take your time to research, and don't be bullied into a treatment that you don't know anything about. I think that is key because one of the common threads that I have gotten from cancer patients over the years is that the doctor tells them that it is urgent and you have to do this now and they feel they have been forced into doing something they didn't know anything about. In the Bible it says "*My people perish for lack of knowledge*." I think you have provided some excellent knowledge here today and I pray that the folks that are listening to this have been empowered with it and that it helps them to change their lives. Thank you so much, brother.

KC: I want to tell you it also says in Jeremiah *"Call upon me and I will answer and show you great and mighty things you do not know."*

Ty: Thank you for your time today.

KC: God bless you, brother.

Ty: God bless you, too.

[end of transcript]

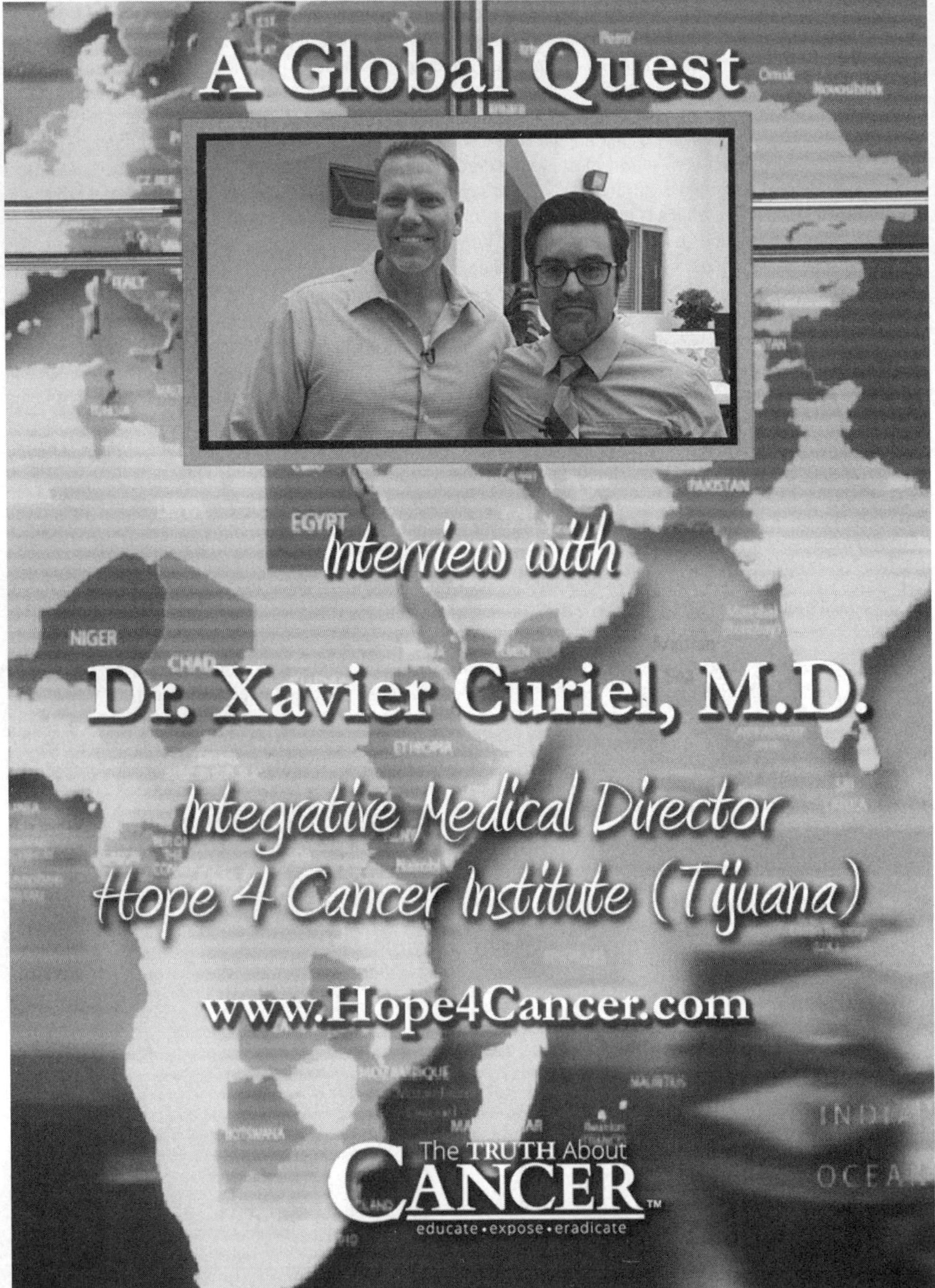
A Global Quest
Interview with
Dr. Xavier Curiel, M.D.
Integrative Medical Director
Hope 4 Cancer Institute (Tijuana)
www.Hope4Cancer.com
The TRUTH About CANCER
educate • expose • eradicate
EGYPT
NIGER
CHAD
PAKISTAN
INDIAN
OCEAN

Ty: Hi, I'm sitting with Dr. Xavier Curiel. He is a medical doctor here at the Hope4Cancer Clinic in Tijuana, Mexico. Thank you for joining us today.

Dr. Curiel: Thank you for having me here.

Ty: I really want to get your perspective on the emotional aspect of cancer because one of the most frequent things we hear from people that have been diagnosed is that their oncologist says, "Hey, you're going to die in three months." From an emotional aspect, that's got to crush someone. So share with us about the emotional aspect of cancer and what do you do here at Hope4Cancer to help people.

Dr. Curiel: Well, we use a system here and—I got trained in Recall Healing Therapy. My mentor is Gilbert Renaud. He is French Canadian. He was a student of Dr. Claude Sabbah in other methods.

Recall Healing is basically a system that has put together different knowledge to the benefit of the patient in emotional healing. The importance of emotion in cancer, in my opinion, is fundamental and is crucial. Especially in the last four to five years, I started to pay a lot of attention to that. Before that, I would considered it important, be stress free or whatever. But I did not really understand the deepness of the importance that that is.

I believe today, I'm convinced, that probably that's the main trigger, the main factor that can actually codify and program certain information at a genetic and cellular level.

What we do is not a one-size-fits-all. Every person is different. The way you're going to work with each person is very different. Because where they are, where they come from and what kind of perceptions they have and what kind of traumatic experience they might be going through plus the diagnosis experience can be very different.

What I do, personally, is I take them first of all on how to educate them. Knowledge is very important. If there is a lot of unknown it always generates concern, it generates fear and you don't know know. So that's always a little bit scary. Especially when we are talking about cancer and what's going to happen and how am I going to feel and what are the odds of me staying alive.

So all these kinds of things start happening and we start to build—imagine this baseball where you have the core inside and you start building all this ball around. And it's like an onion where you start making peels and peels on top of it. The way our nervous system now reacts to that is physiologically very stressful. Inside you feel like these guys are just running constantly from a lion. For our healing that's not good.

Now, when it comes to Recall Healing specifically, research today fortunately has been able to teach us that there are specific conflicts that relate to specific types of illnesses. For example, if you have women with breast cancer you may have breast cancer that originates in the breast milk gland and breast cancer that originates in the milk ducts. Each of them will relate to certain types of conflicts that are specific.

Ductal carcinoma has been noted that it is related to certain type of conflicts. Cancer of the milk glands is also related to a specific type of conflict.

Ty: So for instance, ductal carcinoma—

Dr. Curiel: Well, let's say breast first because we have to start from there. If we take a breast, the breast symbolizes the nest. What is a nest in a woman? So imagine little birds building their nest, it's the same thing. Whatever is for the woman, their nest. This will include their home, their marriage, their kids, their family, their mother, their father, and even animals could be in there.

But the way the brain works is very interesting. Let's say you build a business and you get so emotionally attached to the way you built that business and your achievements, and all the time you call that your baby. To the brain that will be like a real baby.

I've seen this in my clinical practice. When you talk to women with breast cancer very frequently it's not just an issue with the kids, or the husband, or the family, or the house, it also can be the business. And they tell me that that has been my baby and I built it. And the animal can be the same thing. So that's how the brain works.

Now when we talk about, let's say,ductal carcinoma, this is type of cancer that is related emotionally to conflicts when there is a perception of a fragmented nest, the feeling that there is a separation in the nest. You can even be sleeping in the same bed with the person but feel disconnected. So emotionally this brings the not loved feeling.

Ductal also is not just about the separation within the nest. There is also a lack of communication usually. You can be saying a lot of things but there is no real feeling that we are connected in a deep communication. So those are some examples of ductal.

Milk gland is different. Milk Gland normally has a sense of some kind of danger or threat or that something might be happening to the nest, whether that would be the home, the marriage, the kids or whatever. Either one part or the whole thing of the nest. And there's usually some kind of drama being involved. So that's an example about breast. But each organ is coded with certain type of feeling, certain type of experiences that we have.

At the beginning, when we started looking into this and then studying and researching this and I got trained and everything, the literature, the theory, sounded very interesting. I'll say that even 10 years ago I did not even believe in vitamins. Somebody would come to me and they would think vitamins, "Okay. Alright, I'll give in to them." I was like, "hmm."

I thought my mom was not making sense going to a homeopathy doctor because I was in medical school I knew it all back then. Eventually I grew up. I started reading more and I started understanding more. So I realized that there is more to it.

I got convinced because in the last four years that I have been practicing this, it's a 100 percent that this factor is always there. There has not been one single person that this factor is not there.

And not just that they have emotional issues, like I said, if it's a ductal carcinoma, every single time there is issues of the perception. There is a fragmented nest or there is a lack of communication. There is an inability of the expression of love and things like that. We mentioned breast but if we would say lungs it's the same thing. There's a certain group of conflicts.

Ty: There's specific conflicts and trauma that trigger different types of cancer.

Dr. Curiel: Exactly. And not just cancers, even other illnesses. Because I have had friends sometimes call me or ask me something. And I'll look into the physical aspects, the nutritional aspects, but I always ask them the question, "How are you emotionally?" I have found that it's also right on target every time.

Ty: And this healing is called Recall Healing.

Dr. Curiel: This system is called Recall Healing.

Ty: And why is it called Recall? So you are forced to recall these things and to get rid of them?

Dr. Curiel: There are some systems that we utilize where we go back into time. It's funny because numbers are very interesting. Things happen in cycles in life. There are systems that we utilize and when the patient sees the evidence of how something is going on in their lives and it tends to repeat or life tends to confront you with that. It's like an awakening moment for them.

I've seen that to be very liberating because you have the evidence there. And you can see that there is a cause. So you have the knowledge and it's up to you now to make a choice about how you want to act upon that. It varies, how you can work with each patient. But it is a beautiful thing when you see the impact that that can have.

Ty: And you've seen that in patients here at Hope4Cancer?

Dr. Curiel Yes.

Ty: Do all the patients here undergo the Emotional Healing?

Dr. Curiel: Yes, everyone. It's a must. It's part of our therapy.

Ty: And it makes sense that if that were part of the reason that you had this issue, you would have to resolve that before you could be totally cured.

Dr. Curiel: Yes. If you research on the Internet and if you go into websites that have extensive research, not just in alternative medicine but even in conventional medicine, there's a lot of research that demonstrates the impact of psychological social stress and emotional [stress].

At the University of Berkeley, I like an article they have by the Department of Psychology. It's called "Emotional expression cancer onset and progression." The article at the end mentions that research needs to continue. But I think it's very clear and very evident. To me it is because I've been doing this emotional therapy for the last four years. So it has been very evident.

It's too much of a coincidence for me to say someone with, let's say, colon cancer— someone could eat red meat and someone could not eat red meat. Someone might have had genetic factors for cancer and someone might have not. Even people who eat very well, organic, exercise and do all the right things that you're supposed to do to not get cancer and still you get it. So why is that?

The factor that's always there that I have seen clinically in my experience is this part, this aspect. And it's not just like I said, "Yeah, I have issues." No. There is a specific type of trauma related to a specific type of illness.

Ty: That makes sense. One question that I have, and I've not been able to ask anybody this before that has your knowledge, but we have this huge resurgence, or huge rise, in childhood cancers over the last couple of decades, how could emotional trauma be linked to any kind of childhood cancer?

Dr. Curiel: Well, first we have to consider that emotional trauma as a trigger can be the cause of up to 90 percent of illnesses. There are certain things that can be caused by a toxin, venom, radiation, and things like that. But, nevertheless, I've given a lot of thought to this, why would children have cancers if they are not really exposed to things like they don't go to work, they don't go to school, they don't have a boyfriend, or a girlfriend, or are not married, or anything like that. So what would really worry them? They are not worrying about money and things like that.

But the thing is that genetics is the answer because everything gets codified in our genetics. Everything gets printed in our genetics. And information like that can be transmitted generation after generation.

Even, for example, you've probably heard when you have someone donate an organ—unfortunately if someone dies and they donate an organ that the person who has received the organ, let's say for example before the operation they didn't like coffee and after the operation all of a sudden they love coffee. And you find out that the person who donated the organ loved coffee. So that's a very simple example.

But there are many cases like this where you can see that information can be transferred in this way. So imagine how much is now going to be transferred genetically from mom and dad or even siblings that we may have it's been said that up to three generations up.

We know by science, even today, that whatever happens during the development of the baby influences the psyche of that baby, whether or not their neurological system has been apparently developed for it.

In cases of children I don't yet consider myself an expert in that field. But I think the answers come not just at the point of when the baby is born but probably before that.

Ty: That makes a lot of sense. I've asked that question to others. Not from the emotional perspective but just from the perspective that they've done tests even on umbilical cord blood and found 200 plus chemicals in it. So the things the mother is eating are passing through to the child. Maybe the emotions and the trauma are passing through as well.

Dr. Curiel: They get through, we have seen that. I can give you examples of that. Let's say for example, a lady works surrounded by men. And she's not married. So in her mind she belongs to a group of men. She's a woman but she belongs to a group of men. All of sudden she gets pregnant and she's not married. And to her that's embarrassing. So for four to five months she tries to hide the pregnancy.

Her daughter, when she becomes 13, 14, 15, or 16 years old, starts developing anorexia and bulimia and starts eating and throwing up after that. The psychological programming underneath that was like, "I must not be fat. I need to hide the belly." Why? Because, the mom had to hide the belly, so this is a way that this can be transmitted into a child. So that's a very simple example. But there is the ability to research more into this area to start helping these kids more.

Ty: Well, that explanation does make a lot of sense. I think that the more that I learn, the more—I was with you five years ago, and I thought, "There's no emotional aspect to disease, that's ridiculous."

Dr. Curiel: That's hard. I was not eliminating completely that factor from the importance on a person's health. But I was like you five years ago. I would say, "Well, yes, (inaudible 17:15)." It's important that we don't feel stress. But I think consider that that was a real trigger and say, "This could be a cause of my cancer." Honestly, I was not in that mental state. But because there's so much coincidence in the last four years that I have seen. A hundred percent of people have proven to me that this is real.

And not just that, I've seen the benefit of people healing emotionally from it. The impact that this has not just at a mental level but at a brain, at an immunological, hormonal, neurological, brain chemistry. I mean, your whole body responds dramatically in a positive way to you the way they are going to respond to treatments. It's healing. But the simple fact that you are not in a constant survival or danger mode inside of you, and that how your nervous system behaves is going from catabolic, which is destructive, to anabolic, which is constructive growth and healing.

Ty: So pretty much every successful cancer protocol is going to need to include some kind of emotional healing.

Dr. Curiel: In my opinion, yes. Now, you can tell me, "Well, there are people that have not done that and they have healed." Yes, but if you analyze their lives maybe cancer turnaround was the way the whole family interaction was taken, the relationship between the marriage. You will need to do a very diligent analysis of each person's life and see the coincidences that are going on.

Ty: Maybe they healed emotionally and didn't know it.

Dr. Curiel: It's very common. We do that all the time. Even you and I, we do that. That's how the body works. When a person experiences a trauma and we have levelled out different levels of stress—because again, not every stress is also going to create an illness, that's a fact also. Not every single bad thing emotionally that happens to you is going to create a physical ailment or a disease. No.

What makes a difference is the level of intensity of when something happens and how long it lasts. How do you got through it? It's not the same to go through an experience that is hurtful, and go through that emotionally and lonely, than to have support or be able to talk about it. Because the emotional expression here is a crucial thing. Awareness and emotional expression is a crucial thing.

So it's not the same to lose my car keys. It's not the same to get a flat tire than to lose a loved one, for example. Emotionally, the level of trauma is very different. But also, at a physical level, the way the brain deals with it is very different. And here's where we are talking about now the electrical charge of things.

For example, if you have a TV and let's say the TV needs 110 volts of power and you give it 1000 volts all of a sudden. What happens to it? You blow it up. You fry the thing. The brain uses electricity. Your heart uses electricity. Your nervous system uses electric impulses throughout all your body.

Normally, your brain uses about 20 percent of all of your body's energy. When you go into high stress situations like losing a loved one or a severe danger, your brain may require up to 90 percent of all your body's energy. Electrically speaking, also this is a huge overcharge going on. So when people experience this trauma or this shock it's really generating an overload of electricity at the brain level.

So if you have a laptop that is overwhelmed, it freezes. What happens? You cannot use it the same way. The brain is kind of the same thing, although it's completely more advanced that than what would be a laptop.

Ty: You can reboot the laptop.

Dr. Curiel: We just turn it off and turn it on again. We can just go clean it and things. But the brain is always for survival. The number one priority the brain has is always to keep us alive and in the best optimal functioning conditions that are possible to its reach. So we need proper nutrition and all those things

But if at a given moment I'm going through a trauma that I'm not really able to process well at that moment, I cannot be completely overwhelmed or distracted because I could be walking down the stairs and if I'm all distracted I can fall and that's not good for my well-being. Or I can go cross a street and I can get hit by a car and I can die from that. So the brain is always on top of all these possible risks.

So what happens is that the brain redirects that stress, that impact or that information and then literally downloads it from your brain and stores it somewhere else. It sends that signal somewhere else. And there is a lot of research about this and it's available today.

So where, and what part of your body it's going to go to and what organ is not random. There is a specific reason why it will go into your breast or your liver or your prostate and things like that.

And like I said at the beginning, this is a very nice theory. But once you start to see it daily, that this is real, it's really amazing.

Ty: Dr. Curiel, thank you for sharing today with us. We really appreciate your time.

Dr. Curiel: Thank you.

[end of transcript]

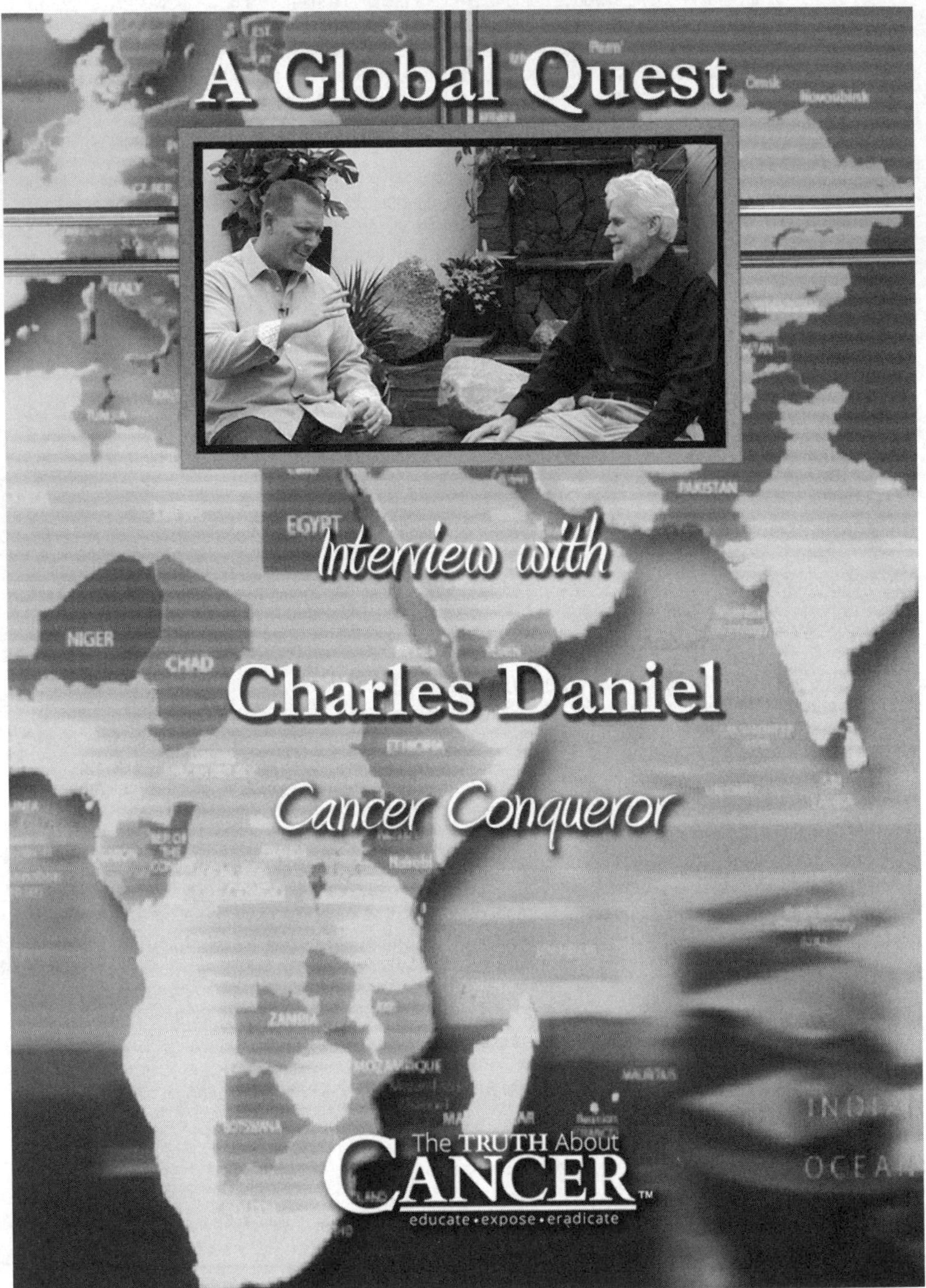
A Global Quest
Interview with
Charles Daniel
Cancer Conqueror
The TRUTH About
CANCER
educate • expose • eradicate

Ty: Yes, everyone, the Hope for Cancer Institute here in Tijuana, Mexico, is the setting, as you probably recognize from the background here. We've done a couple of other interviews here today and I'm really thrilled to be able to talk to Charles here, and to get your story about your healing from cancer.

Charles: Good to be here, Ty.

Ty: Now, we talked a little bit briefly before and you're not from New York, you're not from London, you're from Georgia.

Charles: From Georgia. Central Georgia.

Ty: Central Georgia. Very good. I'm from the Tennessee area, so I recognize the accent. I thought it might be Alabama, but your wife told me, "No, it's not Alabama, it's Georgia."

Charles: We're close to Alabama.

Ty: "Close," that's what she said. But you're a Bulldog through and through, right?

Charles: Absolutely.

Ty: All right. Very good. So tell us, Charles, about your cancer diagnosis. How many years ago was it?

Charles: In January of 2007, I was diagnosed with invasive bladder cancer.

Ty: At that point, what was the prognosis? What was the stage?

Charles: Well, initially, the test indicated that the cancer was confined to my bladder. However, being invasive, that meant that the cancer was in the muscle wall of my bladder and had the potential to spread to other organs and systems throughout my body.

Ty: So at that point, what was the recommendation from your docs?

Charles: The recommendation in the mainstream medical treatment for invasive bladder cancer is to remove the bladder, prostate, and surrounding lymph nodes. This treatment had a cure rate of about 90 percent, and would not require chemo or radiation.

Ty: So that's what you went with?

Charles: Yes. My daughter was 11 years old at the time of surgery, and I wanted—with a 90 percent shot at a cure, that's pretty good odds, so I went with the surgery.

Ty: And so you had good success with the surgery at that point in 2007?

Charles: I had a great surgeon. The surgery went wonderful, however, when they did the surgery they found that the cancer was also in my lymph nodes. This was previously undetected on my initial test. So suddenly, I went from a possible cure rate of about 90 percent down to about 40 percent. And I was going to have to have chemo. The initial procedure, when they thought it was just confined to my bladder, I was only going to have to have surgery and no chemo and no radiation.

Ty: So Charles, you had to add some things to the protocol because the prognosis was a little bit worse than you initially thought?

Charles: Yes. A good bit worse. Down from a cure rate of about 90 percent down to about 40 percent, and I mentioned I was going to need chemo. I didn't even have an oncologist at the time, so my surgeon set me up with an oncologist. One of the best around.

When I met with the oncologist, he requested another scan. So the scan results came back, I had three tumors in my liver that were previously undetected on the initial scan.

At that time, I asked my oncologist, was there was a chance of a cure? He said, "Not really." He added that with bladder cancer metastasized to the liver, the average life expectancy was nine months, some people die in four months. And he had never seen anyone last longer than 12 months. And he was a specialist in urological cancers.

Ty: So not a great prognosis at that point. How were you feeling? You were saying you did the initial treatment, your little girl is 11, you want to see her grow up. How are you feeling thinking about possibly not seeing her grow up at that point?

Charles: Well, even with that prognosis I wanted to live as long as possible, so I went ahead and went through with the chemo. At the end of the chemo, two of the tumors had gone away on the CAT scans. The largest tumor had shrunk. And after that, I had a liver surgery to remove that tumor. After that, I tried some infusions and some supplements to try to prevent the cancer from coming back. However, in March of 2008, a CAT scan revealed that the cancer had returned to my liver.

In April of 2008, I had another liver surgery, which was an ablation procedure to remove that tumor. My oncologist told me at that time that I couldn't take any more chemo. I had had even more than the standard protocol just trying to get a response earlier.

Then my brother, his wife, my wife, and I really started researching alternative cancer treatments, clinics, and so forth. We researched from the Bahamas to the West Coast, from New York to Mexico.

After about three weeks of this research, emails, phone calls, interviews, I had almost settled on a place in the United States. My sister-in-law got an email from a doctor in New York and he said, "I can't help you, but you should give Hope for Cancer a call."

I called Hope for Cancer, had several interviews with the patient liaison and with Dr. Tony, the Director. I was very encouraged by the information that I received from them. And in May of 2008, I came to Hope for Cancer. I completed an inpatient program and continued with their home program. And I'm proud to say that since then all of my tests and scans have indicated I am cancer free.

Ty: That's awesome.

Charles: It is awesome. It's a great day to be alive.

Ty: It is. Seven years.

Charles: Seven years and counting. I count every day, every minute.

Ty: I tell you what—and that's from a pretty bleak prognosis, right? Less than a year. You're alive eight years later.

Charles: Yes. My urologist who did the initial surgery says that I'm a miracle. My oncologist says that he has never seen anyone with bladder cancer metastasized to the liver live this long.

Ty: I'm glad you're the first.

Charles: It's good to be in that group of one.

Ty: It is, isn't it?

Charles: It's wonderful.

Ty: And now your 11-year-old girl is 19?

Charles: At the time of that initial prognosis of a maximum 12 months to live, I didn't think that I would see her even through middle school. Now she has graduated from high school and just completed her first year of college.

Ty: That's so awesome.

Charles: It is awesome.

Ty: Where is she going to school?

Charles: She's going to school at Georgia Southwestern [State University] in Emeritus, Georgia.

Ty: Just making sure you didn't send her somewhere in Alabama.

Charles: Wherever she wants to go.

Ty: I hear you. I hear you. Well, what an encouraging story. I mean, you know, from a really bleak prognosis. You were in the hands of some really good medical doctors, though.

Charles: I had great doctors all along the way. I feel like I give credit to each one of them for getting me to the next point.

You know, before I came to Hope for Cancer, it had been almost a year since that original prognosis of a maximum of 12 months to live. So each one of the—I mean, my urologist who did the surgery on me, my oncologist. I mean, I felt like I had great doctors all along the way. And of course, when I got here at Hope for Cancer I had great doctors here.

Everyone here at Hope for Cancer—I felt like everyone cared about me. Everyone had a smile, the custodians, everybody—they would greet me. And the nurses and the doctors, everyone. I felt like everyone really cared about me.

Ty: That's a common thread that we've heard today from other people that have been treated here.

Charles: I'm not surprised.

***Ty*:** Everybody says they're just kind. You're not a number, you're a person, they love you. And when they left they had a cry fest, right? They didn't want to see you leave. Happy that you were well, but didn't want to see you leave because you've made friends with these people.

***Charles*:** Right.

***Ty*:** Yes. So I guess the next thing in line for you is the wedding. Not ready for that yet, Dad?

***Charles*:** Sandy and I? Brenda's wedding.

***Ty*:** For your daughter's wedding.

***Charles*:** Well, she's not talking that now so we're not rushing.

Ty: I've got a 14-year-old, I don't want to talk about it either. You know what? I'm confident that whenever that happens you're going to be alive and well to see it.

Charles: I hope so.

Ty: Yes. Well, Charles it's a great story. A great encouragement to people that are watching. I really appreciate you taking the time today to share with us.

Charles: I'd like to add a couple of things if you don't mind.

Ty: Absolutely.

Charles: There were a couple of things that really sold me on Hope for Cancer. And as I mentioned, I researched for three weeks, interviewing, emailing, phone calls. I had pages of questions. When I presented those questions to the patient liaison and Dr. Tony they had all the time in the world for me, to answer all of my questions. First and foremost on my list was, "Your success getting cancer out of people's livers."

With the other places, the answer was always vague. But when I asked that question—I'm not sure if it was the patient liaison or Dr. Tony—there was no hesitation. "We've had real good luck getting cancer out of people's livers."

And the second thing that really sold me on Hope for Cancer was their strong home program. A lot of the other places I interviewed had an intensive inpatient program, but the home program seemed relatively weak. The home program at Hope for Cancer actually enabled me to continue a lot of the therapies that I was doing here, at home.

I was here for two weeks, but I knew two weeks wasn't going to be enough. But with a strong home program I really felt like I had a chance. Hope for Cancer I feel has given me a second chance on life and a lot of people don't get a second chance on life.

Ty: Well, you're a blessed man to have it.

Charles: Yes, I am.

Ty: Yes. Charles, thank you.

Charles: Thank you, Ty.

Ty: Appreciate it.

Charles: Thank you. ***[end of transcript]***

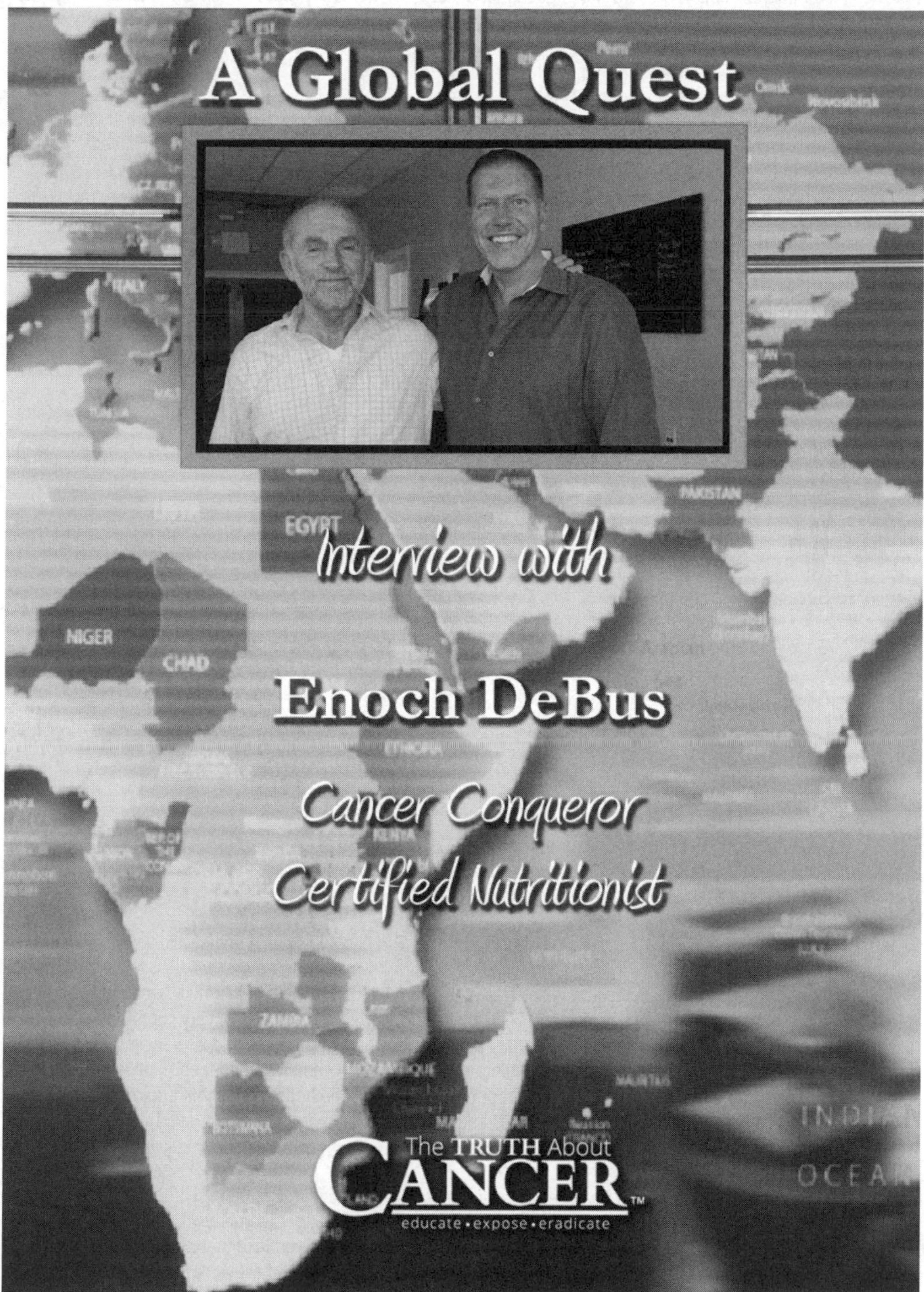
A Global Quest
Interview with
Enoch DeBus
Cancer Conqueror
Certified Nutritionist
The TRUTH About CANCER
educate • expose • eradicate

Ty: I'm really excited to be here with a good friend that I just met today, but I've heard about for a long time from Reggie at Better Way Health. Enoch DeBus, thank you so much for joining us today, brother.

Enoch: My pleasure Ty, definitely. I've been looking forward to meet you, too.

Ty: I say you're a good friend, even though we've only met today, because we have so much in common. And I know that one of the things that Reggie tells me about you is that you're just so focused on helping people, and helping them to get healthy. And you're really influencing this office to be healthy.

And so I'm going to start off the conversation a little bit differently than other interviews, because I want to guess your age.

Enoch: Alright.

Ty: You're like 58.

Enoch: Who told you? That's pretty close, you're pretty close.

Ty: How old are you Enoch?

Enoch: Seventy-one.

Ty: You're 71 years old.

Enoch: Seventy-two September 18th.

Ty: So, by the time this documentary airs in October 2015, you're going to be 72.

Enoch: Alright. Seventy-two young.

Ty: Seventy-two years young. And you are pretty much the health nutrition guru for this office at this point?

Enoch: I am.

Ty: As a matter of fact I'm drinking here, this is your Kick 'Em juice.

Enoch: My Kick 'Em juice.

Ty: So tell everybody that's watching what's in your Kick 'Em juice. I'll have a drink while you're telling me.

Enoch: I got a variety of ingredients that I use. This batch here was made kind of in a rush because I had a few other things to do. But I've got ginger, and I try to use everything organic. It's very important, especially like your root products, you know—ginger, turmeric, they're root products and it's very important to get the organic on that. But I've got a lot of ginger in there, and I'll chop it up and then I'll take the hottest peppers I can find—habaneros, cherry peppers, jalapeños—the hottest ones that are available that are in good shape. Clean everything up good. And I'll take those, chop them all up, and I'll take my ginger and I'll brew it for about 30 minutes.

And not boil, but I'll bring it to a boil, let it simmer for around 30 minutes, then I'll drop in my hot peppers for another 10 minutes. And then I'll take and I'll put some raw ginger, some raw turmeric, put it in, and I'll put it in a blender, and I'll blend it. You got to stand back when you take that top off; it'll knock you back. I'm serious. First time I did it, the fumes were so powerful it's unbelievable. And then I'll take and put that in a large glass jar. Again, everything I use, I use glass. For storing things, for cooking things, for eating off of. Because I don't need any petroleum products. I've had enough poison in my life. Since

I was a young boy I experienced a lot of poisonings, rat poison, lead poison, asbestos poisoning, lacquers. You name it, I've been poisoned. And so your body doesn't handle it too well.

Ty: Talk about that, Enoch. As a young boy being poisoned.

Enoch: Actually, I was about 14 years old, and I went to have my teeth fixed. I had very bad teeth. Went and had them fixed, and, of course, we didn't know back then the problems that would arise from it, the products they used. And I started getting acne shortly after that.

Ty: When you say you had to get your teeth fixed, what happened?

Enoch: Oh, I had about 14 fillings. And it was the fillings, the metal fillings.

Ty: The mercury.

Enoch: The mercury, exactly. And, of course, we didn't know back then, this was back in the '50s. And I was happy, first time in my life I had a toothbrush, and I was able to get my teeth fixed. But shortly after that I broke out with acne and I couldn't understand why. Because at this time now I was with my grandparents who ate fairly well. Grandma had a garden and we grew everything there.

And Grandma was the best there was, I'm still in love with her. She lived to be 89 and she was the finest person I ever met in my life. So, I started going to a dermatologist, tried to see if they could help me. Went to several different kinds. They tried all kinds of treatments, nothing happened. So I had this for several years. I graduated from high school at 17 and I wasn't college material, I didn't prep for it, you know, so I wanted to go into the Marine Corps. I went to sign up for Marine Corps and they turned me down because of my back. It was scarred up pretty bad from the acne. They said, "You would never be able to make it because you couldn't carry a pack. It'll just tear the scars open." And so I said, "Okay." So I went back looking for doctors that could help me. I found this lab that they did radiation.

They said it would shrink my oil glands, and by doing that it would hopefully stop the acne from happening. So I went to them for about six months, and they said that by the end of this, whatever you do, don't get any more radiation. I was 18. Since then I spent four years in the Marine Corps—much radiation there, and ever since then, for examinations, x-rays, just had a ton of it. So, at 15, it was mercury poison that I had, then radiation, then after I got out of the Marine Corps—also in those four years that I spent overseas I had some chemicals there that got me, and I started breaking out. And so they put me on tetracycline. And I was on tetracycline, it would hold things back and they had to change the type from time to time, of the antibiotics. Mainly it was tetracycline, but then I got out of the Marine Corps after four years and still had to use it.

And I went to a doctor and he did tests and he said, "You know, this is military-connected, you need to contact your Congressman on that." So he wrote a letter, I wrote a letter, and they sent back and took it to the military, they attached it, he said it was military connection. So they gave me a 10-percent discount to cover all the medications and that. After about 11 years from the first time I had tetracycline, I went to the dentist, and he said, "Are you on any antibiotics?" I said, "Yeah."

He said, "How long?" I said, "Eleven years." He said "Eleven years and you're still alive?" I said, "What do you think?" He said, "I can't believe it; you got to get off." Well, at 15 years old, what happened was, I forgot to mention, I got poison ivy real bad, from head to toe. And I went to the doctor to be treated and he gave me Calamine lotion. I had already gotten some of that, I had tried it, it didn't help a bit.

I said, "This doesn't work for me; what else have you got, doc?" He said, "Nothing else." And he seemed like a very good doctor. I remember his name was Dr. Boyd John; I respected him. But I lost respect for the medical field that day at that age, because I thought, "If he can't help poison ivy, my goodness it's ridiculous." So I started going into medical journals, trying to find out. I figure I was either lacking something or had too much of something.

Ty: At the age of 14?

Enoch: At the age of 14 I lost confidence in the medical field in medication. And I knew medication couldn't be good for you. But then when I got out of the Marine Corps, and a dentist told me about the tetracycline I've been taking for all those years. I said, "I have to get off." So I got hold of a book by Paul Bray, and he suggested, in the writings, try using dates and pecans to go off this tetracycline thing.

So I did it, and it worked, and I got to tell you the results for six months were—you wouldn't want to be around me, it was unbelievable. The toxins that my body had, and it was flushing it out, and you could tell if I was around, for six months. But it helped me then I started going to organic. I started picking up books. I picked up a book, I remember it was called, *You Are What You Eat*. At first I read it and thought, "That doesn't make sense," because we weren't taught that, you know. And today you're not taught that either by the orthodox way.

Ty: The medical doctors aren't taught that in medical school either.

Enoch: Exactly. I've found out, and you've probably known for a long time to get about five hours of six or eight years unhealthy eating. Pretty sad isn't it?

Ty: Yeah.

Enoch: And they depend on drugs. And I knew that drugs weren't good. When I was in the Marine Corps they had to use drugs on me for something for some ailment from overseas. It never had good results. It always had side effects.

Ty: They all have side effects.

Enoch: Side effects. In fact, if I can interject this, around three weeks ago, one of my tenants called me and there was a problem, and I went over there and she wasn't getting on too good. I said, "Gerry, what's wrong with Mavis?" And I said, "Are you on any medication?" She says, "Yeah, high blood pressure." "Anything else?"

"Yeah, a couple of others." I said, "Why don't you send me a copy of what you got and I said I'll check it out." So she did. Monday I went online there and checked it out. She had four medications for high blood pressure, one had 26 side effects, the second one had 41, the third had 81, the fourth had 90. She could hardly walk.

And each one of them said the side effect could have joint problems, swelling. He was giving her medication for her joints, which was caused by the high blood pressure. And I found out from many doctors and from my own experience, that you go into a doctor's office and you get checked for high blood pressure, you're going to have it; I don't care who you are. If you wait about 20, 30 minutes, it's going to calm down, and you're going to come back to normal.

I'd say probably 75 percent of people who have high blood pressure do not need the medication. In fact there's herbs, there's spices that can take care of it, and which I recommended to her. I gave her some information, I said, "Mavis, consider these things." I said, "Let your doctor know, he's probably going to argue against it, but you don't need it, there'll be no side effects to this." And I also mentioned a product that I'm a firm believer in; is it okay to mention the product?

Ty: Of course.

Enoch: It's a product I take, beta glucan, and I found out that it enables the immune system to fight off anything that your body has to fight off—cancer, sugar diabetes, you name it.

Ty: I just took it this morning.

Enoch: Really?

Ty: Me and the whole camera team.

Enoch: It's the first thing I took. I take it every morning about a half an hour before and I'm very grateful to the Good Lord, very grateful to the man who invented it, and it's a fantastic product. I happened to get mine through a company called Better Way Health, plus they've got fantastic service there. Maybe I shouldn't say that out loud.

Ty: That's absolutely fine.

Enoch: I'm a firm believer. When I find something that I can believe in that really works, I'm not afraid to announce it to the people.

Ty: Right.

Enoch: In fact, I have been a proponent of good eating since I was a teenager.

Ty: What does good eating mean to you, Enoch?

Enoch: Good eating. It's changed a lot over the years. But back when I got out of the Marine Corps—when I was a teenager, good eating was my Grandma's food and hers is all from the garden. And it was delicious. She had three meals a day that was like a feast every meal. Healthy eating is lots of vegetables, organic if you can get them. And even if you can't afford the organic vegetables themselves, just clean them real good.

Ty: Kind of like what we see over here, you can't see on the camera here but you were kind enough to make up a big spread for us. And today it's over there behind the cameras and we have peppers, and carrots, and cucumbers, and squash, and your homemade guacamole. And everything is organic.

Enoch: Exactly. And if you notice the peppers I got green peppers, yellow peppers, red peppers, and orange peppers. Each one has different nutrients that it's going to give you. The sharper colors, those are fantastic, your reds, your greens are so powerful. So it's not about color, it' s not about decoration; it's about getting those healthy nutrients from the creation that God has given us in the earth and the food that we grow, if it's not tampered with by man. I found out that God knows what he's doing, He doesn't need our help. When we mangle with his stuff there are side effects.

Do you realize when you take watermelon that doesn't have the seeds there's a side effect to it because the body does not recognize it as healthy? I will not eat anything that doesn't have its seeds. If it can't reproduce of its own kind it's lacking in the nutrients that you need, and it's not balanced. So your body is going to have to fight it. So I recommend to anybody—watermelon, take the seeds out, in fact I even eat the seeds.

Ty: A lot of the nutrients are in the seeds. As a matter of fact, if you look into the book of Genesis in the Bible, 1:29 talks about the fruit-bearing seed.

Enoch: Exactly, brother. The Bible tells us that the leaves of the trees are for you the nations, the seeds, the grains—they're all healing. God in His almighty wisdom knew what He was doing—he created us, he knew what we needed. Drugs a no-no, they bring good to no one. You might have a temporary relief but you could have a side effect that's going to be 10 times worse than what you had eventually.

Ty: They're at best a symptom Band Aid, yes?

Enoch: Oh my goodness, yes—a symptom Band Aid that's going to increase the problem tenfold eventually if you stay on it. I mean it pretty near killed me, the antibiotics. And also, when I was a young man I started my own business in construction, then I went into painting. I got a painting (inaudible - 13:10) license and I sprayed a lot of lacquer; that almost killed me.

And then I went back into my general construction, which I enjoyed more. And then I did a lot of sheet work with a lot of asbestos in it. That pretty near killed me. And we did a lot of sanding in the Victorian homes in California, where I lived, and they were all lead-based. And we'd spend weeks grinding at stuff when I was just a beginner at it, you know.

Ty: You've been exposed to everything.

Enoch: I really have. Radiation, lead, mercury. An ex-friend of mine fed me rat poison, but we won't go into that.

Ty: Not the aspartame rat poison but another rat poison?

Enoch: Not the aspartame, but the real rat poison.

Ty: The real rat poison. Okay.

Enoch: I don't know which one is worse.

Ty: They're both pretty bad.

Enoch: Aspartame would kill you, too. And, of course, for a while there I drank Coke, we all loved that Coke came from Georgia until we find out that it causes cancer, that is pathetic. You know, I've traveled all over the world. I've been to 45 countries. I've been to nine countries in Africa.

When I was in Africa, I did missionary time there, and I traveled all over, through the bush and what not. Wherever I was, if I'd stop all of a sudden there'd be an African pop-up, and you wouldn't believe what he had to sell you. I mean there is nothing around. Just trees, and he'd have a little cooler with Coke. Seriously. Coke, sir? Coke, sir? I mean it's saturated throughout the world. In 1963 we had McDonald's in Okinawa. Back in '63 we were already poisoning the people there. Isn't that pathetic?

Ty: Now, what you see across the board with people who are indigenous, they're healthy. And when they move, or we move to them, and they start eating our diet, they get sick.

Enoch: Exactly.

Ty: That should tell us something.

Enoch: Exactly, brother. When I lived in Fiji, I lived with some different families there, they took me in. I went to share the Gospel and when they found out what I was there for, they wouldn't let me pay for anything. They took me in, they treated me right, and they were eating western diet, I told them, I said, "Don't eat this." I said, "What was your main staple?" I said, "That's what you want to eat."

They look at me like I was crazy. And they had sugar diabetes, they had beautiful teeth but they were starting to rot. I said, "Get off of our diet." They thought it was like the gold standard, the stuff in the cans or whatever. I said, "It's no good for you," and they began to listen to me, you know; it's so sad. Africa, too, they got beautiful teeth. Their variety of food is very limited.

Ty: In Africa.

Enoch: Africa. But if they just eat their food, their teeth stay beautiful and they eat sugar cane—doesn't hurt it a bit. It's not processed. Sugar cane is healthy. I used to walk all day going from village to village sharing the good news of the love of God, and a brother joined me later—Larry Rawlings, fantastic brother in Christ, he lives in Missouri—and we used to share the Gospel and we'd share healthy eating all over.

I started back in the early '70s, I started promoting healthy eating. I think it might have even been '69—'69 or '70. But we would walk all day with a sugar cane, chewing on that. It gave us energy. It didn't give us any breakouts; it didn't give us any lapse. Like you take sugar here, it gives you a high, and all of a sudden you're let down. You know why that is don't you?

Ty: No.

Enoch: When they refine sugar, and it becomes white sugar, there are about 14 main elements that are taken out, vitamins and minerals. And the moment you put that in your body, God designs things so when it's out of balance and it has an opportunity to come back into balance, it will do that.

And those chemicals in your body it draws those elements. Those elements that are missing in it and it sucks it right to it and that's why you get the rush and then it goes through your urine. And it goes out with your nutrients and then you have a letdown.

Ty: So that's where you got your sugar high.

Enoch: That's where you get your sugar high and then you're let down. And that's your candy, everything does that. So when you eat things that are in balance, you get instant energy. I can tell within five minutes of eating. I just feel the energy flow from the healthy foods that I eat, and I eat them all the time.

And if I feel a little tired, I can just eat a cucumber or a tomato and instantly I'm charged up if it's organic. If it's not GMO—GMO the worst thing that ever hit this earth, GMO.

Ty: GMO some people say it stands for genetically modified organisms. What it really stands for is God Move Over, right? We think we're wiser than God who made the food and so we try to change it.

Enoch: Brother, there's a scripture that says, "The wisdom of man is but foolishness to God." People say God Move Over in every aspect of their life. God Move Over; I've never really heard that like that and that's fantastic; that's exactly what it means.

Ty: Let's fast-forward to your car wreck, because you were telling me about a car wreck that really changed you, and a certain type of fast or cleansing that you did, so could you share that with us?

Enoch: Yes, definitely. Back in 2011, it was December 1st, I was doing a job, me and my ex-business partner, we were doing a job by the lake in Woodstock, Georgia. And I got there about six in the morning and my partner didn't get there until about two o' clock in the afternoon, and he was pretty good at coming in late.

And I was going to leave at three o' clock. I said, "My friend," I'm not going to mention his name, "I'm going to leave now." He would stay the weekends at my house because he lives in Lawrenceville and he would stay a couple nights a week. I said, "I'm going to go off have dinner ready when you get here; you just got here, I'm tired." Usually I'd leave a little later but I'm tired.

He talked me into staying. I knew I shouldn't have. We left about seven o' clock, and coming home, he was driving his truck, I was driving mine, I turned off of Bells Ferry on to 92 going east, towards Roswell into Woodstock. And I made the turn and all of a sudden, I'm driving and I kind of get up to a speed, you know, I don't peel but I don't wait until the light's going to change again, I like to get up to speed. So I get up to the speed limit and I notice there's somebody alongside me did the same thing, which I don't see very much in Georgia, not easy to see people get up to the speed limit. And I thought, "Nice, he's pretty good a driver." And all of a sudden he steps on that gas and he shot up and all of a sudden he crossed in front of me, and he hit his brakes.

And it was a big truck, he just had a big old frame there. And I was driving my Dakota, I was driving my 150, which is a big one, probably wouldn't have hurt so bad. But I hit him and my truck kind of turned into an accordion, knocked me out, messed up my left leg real bad, tore up the cartilage there, my stomach real bad, concussion.

When I came to they were trying to get my door open to get me out. The police arrived even before they were able to pull me out of the car, took that long to open the door. And they thought I was on fire inside because when the bag opened up they saw a powder and it looks like smoke. So the guys finally got it opened, and they're pulling me out. And I said, "Let me get my seat-belt off first." They're breaking me in two, and I couldn't stand up on my left leg, it was hurt real bad, I just felt a mess. And what happened is, I'll fast-forward a little bit, for six weeks I couldn't lay down, because of my stomach, and I couldn't bend my left leg, and I couldn't eat.

And I started going to, I don't really care for GPs, general practitioners. I've had a lot of challenges with them when I was a young man, so I avoided going to the doctors. I would find a healthy way to do it. I figure if I would eat the right food, take the time, my body would heal. I always believed that. And that's what I would do because I didn't believe in medication. So, I couldn't eat. I did go to a chiropractor, I had my friend take me the next day, and they agreed to take care of me.

And I said, "I can pay cash or we can wait until after I recover." They said they would wait, which they did. And, so I'd go there almost every day, they worked on me, I didn't get much better. They wanted me to go to the surgeon and I went to her, and she was a woman from Germany, she was supposed to be one of the best. She has me take out my shirt, lay out on the table, and she taps me.

And she says, "You need surgery." And I said, "You can tell by that?" She says, "Yeah." She says, "What we are going to do, we're going to take out your appendix, and we're going to take out your gall bladder, and we're going to do exploratory surgery." She said, "The MRI is so blurry, all we see is inflammation, so we can't tell what it is." I said, "You can't tell what it is, so you're going to take out my appendix, which had no problem before, and you're going to take out my gall bladder, and then you're going to explore?" "That's right." I said, "I never need to see you again, I will heal without your help."

"You'll be in here. You're going to have surgery." I said, "No, I won't." That was in 2011, it took me about three years to completely recover. What happened was I couldn't eat, so I had tried 2004 I had come down with some kind of respiratory infection from doing a finishing over a garage. We restored the whole house and over the garage they had a lot of mold in there and mildew and I breathed it and I got an infection. I went to a chiropractor, I went to acupuncture, I didn't go to a GP. And finally a friend of mine says, "Hey, why don't you try this master cleanse?" I said, "I never heard of it." He gives me a book, a little yellow book with about 50 pages in it. I read it, I did it right then and there, and I was hacking. I hacked for three weeks straight, coughing and still kept working.

So I went on that; instantly I started that Sunday, and the next morning, I didn't have any hack. I did that for 12 days, the first time I did it. I worked six days a week, 12, 13 hours a day. Didn't hack any. I didn't do anything but drink that master cleanse, which is lemon or lime, with organic maple syrup, about a tenth of teaspoon per serving of cayenne powder. And then in the morning, you take that throughout the day; I'd drink about 12 glasses of it a day while I was working. It kept my energy up great. In the morning I'd do the salt-water flush.

One tablespoon of hot water and a quarter of warm water, you drink that and it cleans you out. I did that for 12 days. I had no more trouble with that respiratory thing. But the thing I had gotten from the time I was 14, I told you about the poison ivy earlier.

And when I moved to California from Michigan after the Marine Corps, I had poison oak continuously—years and years and years. Until three and a half years ago. When I couldn't eat from that accident, I had a 48-days fast, just taking master cleanse and since then I have not had any poison ivy or poison oak. And, evidently, even though I was eating healthy and all that, that had lingered in my system but it got cleaned out.

A good friend of mine, Dr. Selenski, Eric Selenski, who is like a son to me, I had the privilege to lead him to the Lord 13 years ago and love him and his precious family. He gets it, he doesn't normally get it, but I was helping him do some work on his house, he got it, I didn't get it, and I can pick it up and everything now. So that master cleanse, is a hundred percent. And then there's the Kick 'Em juice.

Ty: Kick 'Em juice is fantastic. I'm going to have another drink here.

Enoch: That is, I should mention, I had come down in 2009, that was actually before the accident—2009 I came down with basal cancer.

Ty: You had basal cell carcinoma?

Enoch: Yes I did, on my cheek, between my eyes, and under my arms. They did a biopsy that came back positive. When I went to the dermatologist, I knew I had it in 2009. I didn't go until 2010. The one in between my eyes would not stop bleeding. So I went to my chiropractor friend, Linda Force, fantastic woman, I've known her for many years, precious woman of God, and she's one of the best chiropractors that I've ever been to.

She's got a big practice in Canton and her name is Linda Force. She's got the force, I tell you, to work with people in chiropractic and the she loves the Lord, she says that's where the force comes from and I agree with her. I'm sure you do, too. But she says, "Enoch, you need to get that checked up, I think you have cancer." I can't imagine me getting cancer but I said I've had so many poisons all throughout my life all these toxins, you know, so it probably hit me, because I was going through a stressful time; 2008 the bottom dropped out.

I had been audited with the IRS. They did some things to me that we won't repeat. I had a number of homes and I had made quite a bit of money that I had put away and I end up spending a ton of money to keep these homes going. Because all of a sudden a brother was in it, he couldn't afford it. I bought my mother a home, taking care of mine, and one of the other homes were empty, that I had. So it all brought stress on. Work kind of dropped off in 2008. I had 55 guys working for me, it went from that to nothing, so you know, it was a lot of stress.

Ty: That could have been like the, those chain of events is what really kicked the cancer into gear.

Enoch: That was the straw that broke the camel's back, as they would say. And I saw that in myself, Ty, and that's exactly what happened.

Ty: What'd you use to treat it?

Enoch: Well this is what happened, I went to the dermatologist that Linda recommended, it was a friend of hers. And she looked at me, and she had me take my shirt off, check my body over. She says, "Normally I have my clients come in once every quarter." She says, "You are going to be coming in once every three weeks." I said, "I'm that bad?"

She said, "You're that bad." I said, "Wow"; that caught me by surprise. She got the results, let me see what it is. And I went back, the test was positive, and I say, "What can I do to help?" She says, "Not a thing." She says, "Basically this is from all the sun that you got over the years."

Ty: She said nothing you could do?

Enoch: She said there is nothing that *I* could do. She said the damage is done. And I said, "What happens if I don't get the surgery?" She looked at me very seriously, she was a young girl, itty bitty thing, you know, and she had a nurse in there, and she said, "If you don't get this done in six months you'll be totally blind, and 12 months from that you'll be a dead man." I said, "For sure?" She says, "Yeah." I said, "Thank you."

And she set up an appointment for the next day with the surgeon. I said I would go see him. I walked out of there and I shook my head, I said, "I'm not buying it." I went home, I got on my knees. I said, "Father, you know the results of the test and everything; you're in charge, you created me; I am not going to have them cut up my face; I'm ready if you're ready—if it is my time." I said, "I've been ready for a long time. I enjoy living and I enjoy sharing the Good News and I love people; you know that; but I'm not going to be cut up. So please, either give me the wisdom what I can do on my part so you can do your part." Right after that prayer, all of a sudden ginger came to my mind. Ginger and hot peppers and all that you know.

And nobody has ever told me about it. So I went and I got a bunch of organic ginger, I got habaneros, jalapeños, there a couple other hot peppers at the time. Tabasco pepper and another one. And I cleaned them, chopped up the ginger, had no directions, no recipe and I put that in to boil, turned it down to brew you know, just simmer. After 30 minutes I found myself putting these peppers in there.

I cleaned them and I chopped them off, seeds and all, after about 10 minutes and then I stopped and let it cool off. I put it in the blender and I ground them all up. I took off the lid and it blew me back. It did really take my breath away, it was powerful. So I put that in a jug and I had about a half a gallon of it. And I filled it up with filtered water and I tried it, it about burned my tongue off. And I cut it, and I added some other stuff to it, I put cilantro in it and as I did so I drank it. And I kind of had that as a stock and I'd take it and cut it each day when I used it. And basically I would take it for my workout. I'd take it to the gym, and I notice that it gave me a kick, you know.

Ty: Kick 'Em juice.

Enoch: And I named it right there! I said, "Man this is Kick 'Em Juice!" I said, "I'm going to bottle this to sell." So I tried it with a bunch of friends at the gym. They all loved it.

Ty: So, this Kick 'Em Juice—is this what you attribute to curing your cancer?

Enoch: This Kick 'Em Juice is what I felt the Holy Spirit inspired me to make and the bleeding stopped within days. It healed and filled up completely. I just started taking it, within two days, and I went to the surgeon because I was scheduled to go there, and he was tall, about six foot eight, young Jewish man. I really respected him and he was very respectful. He came and he said he'll be right back. The nurse came and I said, "What a doctor; he's really fantastic." She says his wife is just like him, precious people. So he came back in, he measured me and he tried to prepare me in a gentle way, you know, he says, "We'll do this at first, maybe we won't have to do radiation or chemo with that." And I said, "How long do I have—that I can wait before we start to do this?"

He says, "Well, I wouldn't go more than a month." I said, "Okay, I'm going to take that month; I'm trying something new." He said, "Okay; you'll survive for a month." And I said to him, "What's the chance of praying for you and your family?" He said, "Go ahead!" I just felt led to you. I've got a great (inaudible - 32:26) for the Jewish people, I'm part Jewish, I lived in Israel, my ex-wife she was an Israeli and I love everybody but God's given me a special love for the Jewish people.

And so I prayed over him and then I gave him a hug. He says, "I like a good hug now and then." And so he said, "We'll contact you in about a month." So, sure enough, they contacted me, a little after a month and I said, "I won't be coming in, I don't think I need it." I said, "It's all calmed down, I don't have any problems, I think the Good Lord touched me and healed me." I said, "I made up this stuff I call Kick 'Em Juice, you know. And so I've been using that, I use it when I work out. I've turned many people on to it."

Ty: And your cancer's gone.

Enoch: Well, as far as I know—I did have a breakout. I'm not saying it's cancer but last Friday I'm settled into my home, I was having it re-roofed on Saturday, last Saturday. So I went and I should have hired somebody else, but I left work, I went there, I worked from 4:30 to 9 o'clock at night, and sprayed this chemical all over it.

And I knew I should have jumped in the shower. Ty, I was worn out. I worked all day, I got up at three in the morning and I come to the job, I was here about four thirty in the morning and I left and I worked until late at night. And I should have jumped in the shower, but I just collapsed and fell asleep. I woke up in the morning, Saturday morning, and I had hives, like my whole face is all burned with welts all over it, and it itched all over. I jumped in the shower, washed, put coconut oil on there. Then I went, took some essential oils. I'm a great believer in essential oils, been involved in essential oils for many years. I've been aware of them for 27 years but I've really been heavily involved in them since (inaudible - 33:14) got involved. In fact I shared a lot with them over the years.

Ty: It sounds like what you had was a breakout from chemical.

Enoch: A chemical break out. And I thought, it was a chemical breakout, definitely. At 71, I've recovered rapidly, it just happened Friday night, and I didn't shower until Saturday—how stupid of me, not showering—but I would have had some reaction anyway, but it was peeling the last couple of days, there's still a little peeling but the swelling's all gone now.

Ty: It's less than a week.

Enoch: What's today?

Ty: Thursday.

Enoch: Thursday, yeah, less than a week. It happened Friday night, but by putting coconut oil, essential oils, drinking my Kick 'Em juice like crazy, my beta glucan, that helped a little bit, and prayer—the Good Lord touched me. And last night my back went out, I was trying to get the house ready cause the girls are coming in. Actually the women were coming Tuesday to take pictures and so Monday I'm taking everything down to the basement, the heavy stuff.

So my back went out on Monday, I'm recovering from the chemical breakout. My back hasn't gone out but when you push yourself beyond limits so my back went out. And I usually go to the gym every other day, I didn't go since that happened, and I can't believe it, I feel like an old man, and "old" isn't in my vocabulary, I don't believe in that. I mean you put 71 next to eternity, it doesn't even show. And I don't hang around with older people. I talk about life.

Ty: You said you go to the gym, right?

Enoch: I go to the gym. And guess who works out with me? Guys in their 20s and 30s, and I'm an inspiration to them.

Ty: Talk about that. This would be the last topic for this interview. I want to get your take at 71 years old. I want you to tell people that are watching this what some of the things you can do in the gym at 71, with eating and living healthy.

Enoch: Well, I'll tell you what I did last night, okay, after recovering from the back problem and this other. I said, "Lord, I got to start doing these exercises again, you know." So I started doing the pushups.

Ty: How many pushups?

Enoch: I did about six sets of pushups last night and I did 50, 50, 75, 50, 50. Normally I do 100 every morning. And then I did 50 between chairs all the way down, you know. And I did probably five, six sets of that, okay. But every morning I would do a bunch of calisthenics, a bunch of stretches. I would do pushups, 100 pushups, I do 100 crunches, I do three sets of 25 to 45 chin ups. When I do I'll put 25 pounds on me, and I do three sets of 25.

Ty: You can do 25 chin ups with 25 pounds hanging on you?

Enoch: Easy. Yeah, three sets of them. That's after I do my pushups. That's the last thing I do.

Ty: I don't think I know anybody else that can do three sets of 25 chin ups with 25 pounds hanging on them.

Enoch: Well, I know somebody who does 45 at the gym. This guy is huge. He's powerful. He's a lot younger than me, too. And he takes a lot of things. He takes all kinds—his son's got a—health, well they say "It's All About Health"—that's the name of the business, but they got all these products for building the body up. But there's side effects to that stuff. So, he's got all this stuff in him, but he's like Superman.

Ty: You sound like Superman to me.

Enoch: But he's going to suffer from it when he stops taking that stuff. It'll all turn into flab. Where I don't have the bulk that he's got, but I've got endurance.

Ty: Talk about your bench press.

Enoch: I was doing 225, five times.

Ty: Okay. I don't think I know another 71-year-old that can do 225, five times. That's pretty incredible.

Enoch: Yeah. I'm not that heavy, okay. I've lost a lot of weight the last month or so. Actually the last two and a half months. I was about 185, and I'm probably down to about 170 now. But I've been doing new things, a lot of things.

Ty: I think, Enoch, if nothing else, people that are watching this, especially elderly people, they can see you that you can overcome a whole host of troubles.

Enoch: Amen.

Ty: You've been exposed to chemicals, you've fallen off and broken your back, you've been in car wrecks. I mean, there's almost nothing that seems that it hasn't happened to you. And here you are, 71 years old healthier than probably 95 percent of 20-year-olds, and so I think that this interview, if nothing else, is going to be an inspiration to the people that are watching. And I just want to thank you for spending time with us today to share your testimony.

Enoch: Thank you, Ty, for having me, and my goal is to touch people to, number one, put their faith in the Good Lord, He is the answer, the ultimate, and eat healthy, exercise, you find something that works, Kick 'Em juice,beta glucan, and by the grace of God you're going to live. If the Lord tarries, I look at a 120 as no surprise; I'm serious.

Ty: I don't doubt you a bit and I wouldn't be surprised to see you at a 120, Enoch.

Enoch: Alright, and we'll have another interview.

Ty: We'll have another interview, but I'm not going to get into a bench press contest with you. You have a great day, brother.

Enoch: You too. I appreciate you and love you, brother.

Ty: Love you, too.

Enoch: It was great.

[end of transcript]

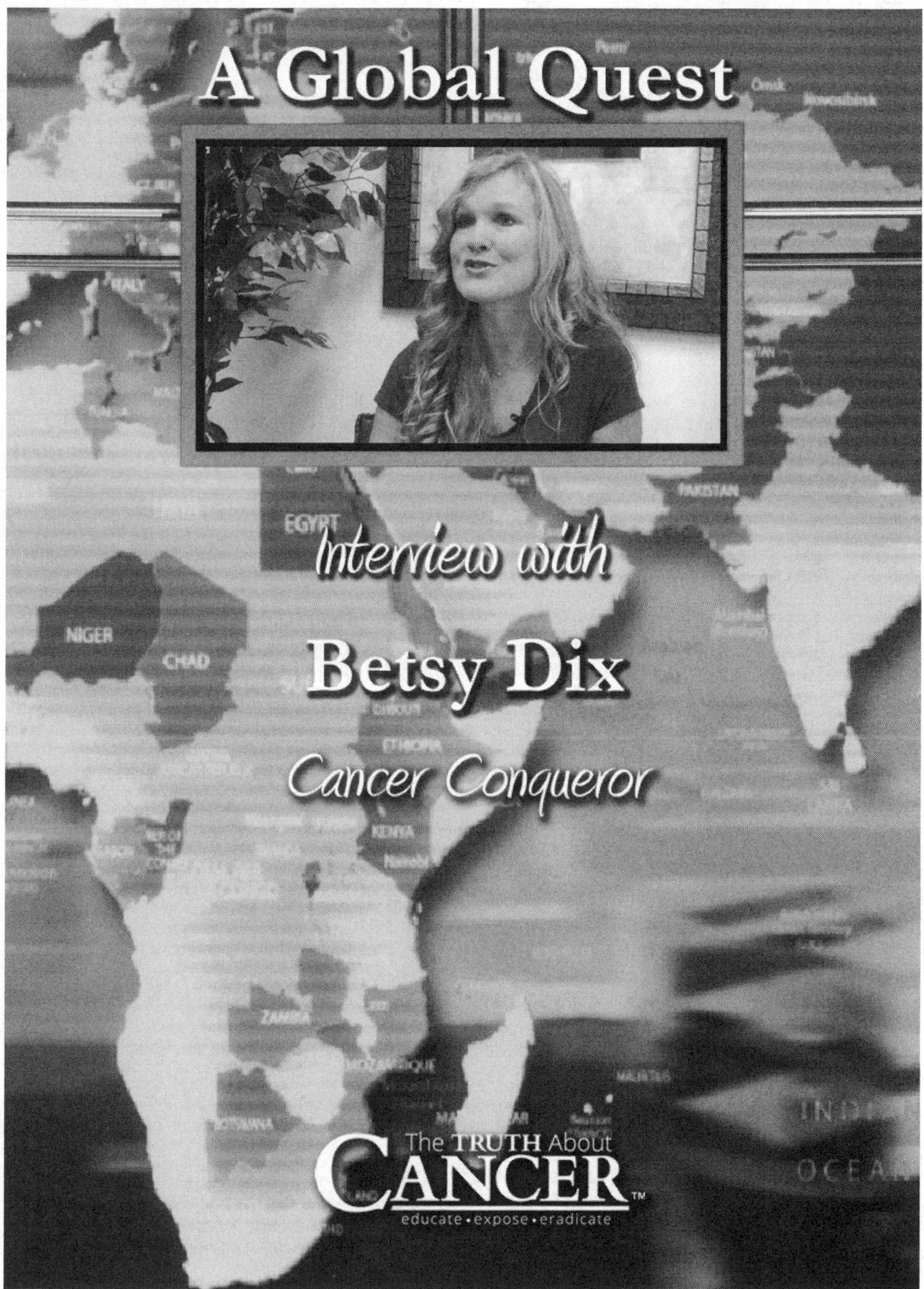
A Global Quest
Interview with
Betsy Dix
Cancer Conqueror
The TRUTH About
CANCER
educate • expose • eradicate

Betsy: I was diagnosed with cancer the first time in 2014 by an oncologist here in Charlotte, NC. It was Stage 2 ovarian cancer. Then five-and-a-half months later, unfortunately for myself, my family and also for Dr. Buttar, I was diagnosed with this secondary primary breast cancer that was also developing at the same time, unaware to my oncologist.

The conventional treatments in my case, the only conventional treatment I did was surgery. I was one of the fortunate few that had a cancer, primary cancer, and organs that were not necessary for life. I had a full hysterectomy. It did work in that it did remove the cancer, a primary portion of the cancer, and it had not spread and it was not in my lymph system yet.

However it was the treatment that the oncologist wanted to do – the chemotherapy – and it was not just plain "use one port and put chemotherapy" – administer it up here. They also wanted to put a second port on my rib cage, and they wanted to do something called intraperitoneal chemo where they would have been giving me chemo, blowing out my abdomen like I'm pregnant every Monday and blowing out my veins with a second chemo.

It was the over the top, aggressive chemotherapy they wanted to do that made me cringe. I lost 20 pounds after the surgery just thinking about the chemotherapy. I dropped to 106 pounds and was in menopause and was just a mess. My oncologist was ready to put poison in my body. I was like, "I can't do this."

It was during a trip to Atlanta my husband and I took to Cancer Treatment Centers of America to get a second opinion from an oncologist there that we realized *The Truth About Cancer* series was playing free that weekend online and we didn't have any children with us that weekend.

I was very conflicted. I had been a pharmaceutical rep for 14 years and had known the medical industry. That had been my career. We were able to watch seven to eight episodes of Ty Bollinger's *The Truth About Cancer.* It was during these seminars online that we watched that gave us the courage and the confidence that many other individuals and survivors had gone through natural treatments and were living.

Dr. Buttar, I believe, hits cancer from many angles. You've heard or may have read his book about the seven toxicities that he mentions in his book, *The Nine Steps to Keep the Doctor Away.* I believe I had many of these toxicities. Not only was my body toxic with metals, it was also toxic with pollutants and, I also believe, emotionally and psychologically. I had gone through three miscarriages trying to conceive our second and third daughter. And during these times of grief, that really contributed, I believe, to the ovarian cancer and breast cancer diagnoses that I received that year.

His treatment hits all three of these toxicities. There is chelation and many different IVs that Dr. Buttar gives that help your body get rid of toxins. And I have seen my body get rid of so many toxins through the protocol at home, which is very aggressive, as well as through the chelation in the office.

Also the things that Dr. Buttar gives to build up your immune system are phenomenal. I can literally go to treatment and be in treatment all day, have six or seven bags of various great things that I believe God made to heal our bodies that my body even makes, just not in enough—I didn't have enough of those substances in my body to heal. I can go home and cook dinner and take care of my little ones.

The cancer that I had in my body is definitely going away. I hope to be cancer-free any day or any month now. We are doing some of those tests as we speak and all of my parameters, my blood work is of a healthy 30-something-year-old. This is really great news. My energy, my color, all of those things, my liver, my kidneys are all functioning at 100 percent and like a healthy individual would be.

So we are very grateful that the cancer markers are so very low and I may be cancer free today, but I hope to be cancer free soon if I'm not. Dr. Buttar has brought something to my family we thought we wouldn't have.

After the diagnosis last year, psychologically, mentally I just thought I was on my way out. I'm usually a positive person, but all I could see was myself laying in a bed after doing chemo treatments and being 85 pounds. Having my daughters, my little ones, not even know me, grow up without a mother as well as my eight-year-old just watch me die, not to mention my husband.

What *The Quest for the Cures* gave us and also Dr. Buttar, was hope that you can heal naturally, that there are so many things that I believe God has given us in the world that can build up your immune system, can remove toxicities, and can also just increase your vitality and your overall health. I believe that I've experienced all of those through the unconventional treatment that we chose and this path.

I have to be honest. We thought, because I was a drug rep as I mentioned for 14 years, we thought, "Okay, if this doesn't work, then we'll go back and we can always do chemo." That was kind of our fall-back scenario that we gave to friends and family because they were horrified that we were not going through with conventional treatment.

There is a lot of pressure after a diagnosis to start treatment immediately – start the chemo tomorrow. I think I've done so well with the therapy there is no reason to ever compromise my body and my GI tract with the only thing I had going for me at the time of diagnosis. That would have been wiped out after one chemo treatment. We are just so grateful and thankful that we had this option, and we hope that many others will also be brave enough to travel the road less traveled, so to speak.

[end of transcript]

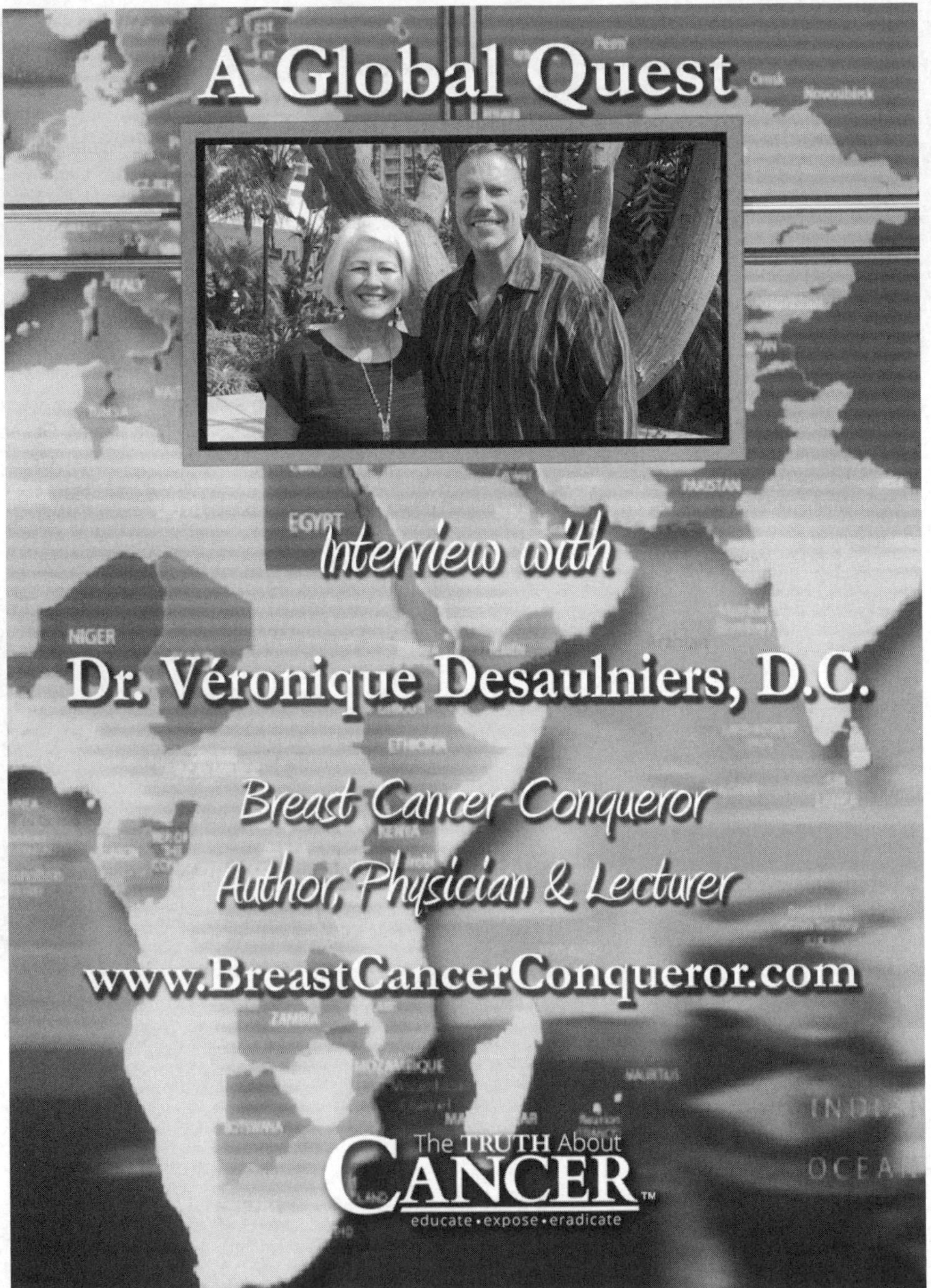
A Global Quest
Interview with
Dr. Véronique Desaulniers, D.C.
Breast Cancer Conqueror
Author, Physician & Lecturer
www.BreastCancerConqueror.com
The TRUTH About CANCER
educate • expose • eradicate

Ty: Dr. Véronique Desaulniers, thank you for being with us again.

Dr. Desaulniers: Thanks. Nice to meet you here again, Ty.

Ty: Yes, you were a big hit in *The Quest for the Cures* last year.

Dr. Desaulniers: Thank you.

Ty: And we're out here in San Diego and glad to be able to get another interview with you again, and this time I want to focus, specifically, on breast cancer. Talk about the difference in rates of breast cancer between the 1950s and now. In the 1950s it was—what? One in 40?

Dr. Desaulniers: So, 50 years ago, a woman's chances of developing breast cancer were 1 in 40, and now it's 1 in 8, so, obviously, this war on cancer has not succeeded.

Ty: Yes. If there is a real war on cancer—that's debatable. Sometimes people say there is a war on the cancer treatments that are natural.

Dr. Desaulniers: Exactly, right.

Ty: But, if there is a war that is being waged on cancer, we are losing it terribly, aren't we?

Dr. Desaulniers: Absolutely. Absolutely.

Ty: Why is your focus—your particular focus—on breast cancer?

Dr. Desaulniers: Well, my particular healing journey was, specifically, with breast cancer. So, I've walked in women's shoes. I know what it's like to go through the breast cancer journey. I understand the fears, I understand what it's like to wake up at three in the morning in hot sweats and wonder, "Am I really going to be able to survive this? Are my kids going to be okay?" And I had been in practice for 25 years, and I was helping people reverse diseases like cancer and autoimmune diseases. And, yet, I still had those feelings. So when I went through my healing journey and I put the pieces of the puzzle together, I just said, "How can I keep this to myself?" I had to share this, it's like a fire within me, that I had to let other women know that they don't need to live in fear when it comes to breast cancer.

Ty: It's not on the camera, but you've got some really neon-pink tennis shoes on. What about the Pink Movement? Right? The Breast Cancer Pink Movement. What is your take on the October "get your mammograms?"

Dr. Desaulniers: Well, its focus is on breast cancer awareness, instead of breast health awareness. And the Pink Movement has really caused so much fear and so much misinformation when it comes to breast cancer in women. There are so many myths involving breast cancer. Breast cancer Myth Number One is that women's hormones cause cancer. That is the biggest fallacy ever. First of all, if our hormones caused cancer, then every 20 year old on the planet would have cancer. So it's not our hormones, it's what we're exposed to. Look at the xenoestrogens and the chemical estrogens in the environment—the chemicals, the pesticides, the herbicides, the metals in our teeth, the antiperspirants. Those metals are actually classified as metalloestrogens and mimic and stimulate estrogen production in the body. So that's one aspect. Secondly, if a woman has a problem metabolizing or breaking down her estrogens properly, then the more aggressive estrogens will circulate in the body. So there is a way to support that methylation process, which doctors don't even talk about.

Ty: Talk about estrogens in food. Soy has what is called phytoestrogens, right?

Dr. Desaulniers: Right?

Ty: Talk about plant estrogens.

Dr. Desaulniers: Okay. Food has been around since we've been around. Plant estrogens do not act like aggressive estrogens. They are very protective. The don't—they protect against DNA damage, they block the estrogen receptor sites. They actually reduce the level of circulating estrogens in the body. Flax, for example—a study that I like to quote—there was a study done at the University of Toronto where they took women who were getting ready to have surgery, they measured their cancer markers and their tumor levels, and for a month they gave them five teaspoons of ground flax seed in a muffin, which probably was made with white flour and sugar, but, anyway, the ground flax seed was in there. And in 30 days their markers went down by 30 to 71 percent, just with ground flax seed. Fermented soy—if you use non-GMO, organic, whole fermented soy, it has a very protective effect. It turns on the P53 suppressor gene, it reduces the circulating estrogens. It is a protective food. Look at the Asian society. They have used soy in their diet for thousands of years and their breast cancer rates are much lower.

Ty: But the keys are that it is non-GMO and fermented.

Dr. Desaulniers: Absolutely.

Ty: It is interesting, isn't it, that we have to say non-GMO. Soy, by nature—corn, by nature—cottonseed, by nature—all of these things that are genetically modified—they are actually not GMO by nature, right?

Dr. Desaulniers: Correct.

Ty: And so when you genetically modify them, they're not really any longer *that substance anymore.*

Dr. Desaulniers: The real food.

Ty: They're something else.

Dr. Desaulniers: They're frankenfoods. They're foreign foods so your body doesn't recognize what they are.

Ty: Yes. You mentioned surgery. What is your take on preventative surgery? We see stories of people like Angelina Jolie that has both of her breasts removed in case she might sometime down the road get cancer.

Dr. Desaulniers: Well, that refers to the BRCA gene scare. It really was quite a Hollywood hype last year. And I'm not judging her; she saw her mother die a very horrible death. But there was a lot of misinformation. The BRCA genes are actually cancer-protective genes. They help to repair DNA damage. And so the BRCA gene, if it mutates, then it can cause a problem, possibly. But what causes it to mutate? Look at the foods, look at the radiation. So BRCA genes are tumor-suppressive protective genes.

Ty: So do you inherit breast cancer genes? Is it inherited? Is it genetic?

Dr. Desaulniers: That's the big thing. Well, my mother had breast cancer so I'm probably going to have breast cancer. But we now know through the study of epigenetics, which is the science of looking at gene expression, and nutrigenomics, which is the study of food, we know that we can change our gene expression by what we eat, how we sleep or don't sleep, how we manage or don't manage our stress. The foods that we eat—so something as simple as curcumin can help to really turn on the cancer-protective genes and change those gene expressions.

Ty: I interviewed Dr. Sunil Pai again and he mentioned that, specifically, that curcumin has an epigenetic effect. It can switch on or switch off the things that need to be switched on and off to keep you healthy.

Dr. Desaulniers: Yes. And that's just one of the foods. Things like broccoli sprouts, and ginger, and boswellia—all those things are anti-inflammatory and turn on those protective genes.

Ty: What about treating breast cancer or any kind of cancer, for that matter, with toxic drugs?

Dr. Desaulniers: Let's talk about aromatase inhibitors or drugs like Tamoxifen. Tamoxifen is a drug that most women are put on when they have breast cancer, but they don't tell them that it is classified as a carcinogen by the American Cancer Society and the World Health Organization. So does it make sense to give a woman a carcinogenic drug that will cause cancers in other parts of her body to prevent cancer? Again, it goes back to what we can do to support the body and support the immune system. And things like fermented soy and ground flax seed can have a very similar effect to drugs like Tamoxifen.

Ty: Is there a connection? You mentioned some good foods. Is there a connection between the foods you eat and breast cancer?

Dr. Desaulniers: Absolutely. You go to a chemotherapy suite, or you go to a hospital, and what do you see? Sugar everywhere. And if there is one food that women need to avoid if they are on a breast cancer healing journey it's sugar, because we know that sugar feeds cancer. Cancer cells have more insulin receptor sites than a healthy cell. So the first cell that gets fed the sugar is the cancer cells. So any type of GMO food, the sugars, anything that is packaged, can certainly lower the immune system and increase the risk for cancer.

Ty: During October of each year we "Run for the Cure," and "Race for the Cure," and all these other events to try to raise money because we are trying to find a cure because there is no cure for breast cancer, right?

Dr. Desaulniers: Well, I'm living proof. And thousands of women around the globe, and hundreds of thousands of people who have healed cancer, in general. We know there is a cure. The cure lies in our food, in detoxifying our body properly, balancing our energy, in dealing with our stress and our emotional wounds, making sure that we don't have dental toxicities, using food and plants to repair our body. And then staying on top of everything, making sure that you can prevent cancer in the future, because traditional medicine will use certain markers, but they are very, very gross and very ineffective markers. But there are markers like the PHI enzyme, or the Cancer Profile, or the ONCOblot test that can determine cancer when it is only a few million cells in the body instead of a tumor, because it takes five to eight years for a tumor to develop. Thermography is also a great tool to be able to access the physiological changes that are going on in the body. So, yes, there is a cure, and, yes, you can prevent it.

Ty: And if you want to detect it, what you are saying is that there are better detection methods than getting your mammogram. You're saying thermography is better?

Dr. Desaulniers: Absolutely. Thermography cannot diagnose cancer, but it can detect physiological changes going on in the body. And we know that mammograms, according to a 25-year Canadian study that was just published last year, mammograms are just as effective as a self-breast exam. And mammograms have not decreased breast cancer mortality rate, not even by one percent.

Ty: Wow. Well, you mentioned one other thing that you can do is to de-stress. And I highly recommend sitting out in the sun on a nice, sunny San Diego day to de-stress.

Dr. Desaulniers: Absolutely. Deep breaths, beautiful sunshine—it can't get better than this.

Ty: That's right. Well, Dr. V., very informative today. I really appreciate your input.

Dr. Desaulniers: Okay, thanks so much, Ty. ***[end of transcript]***

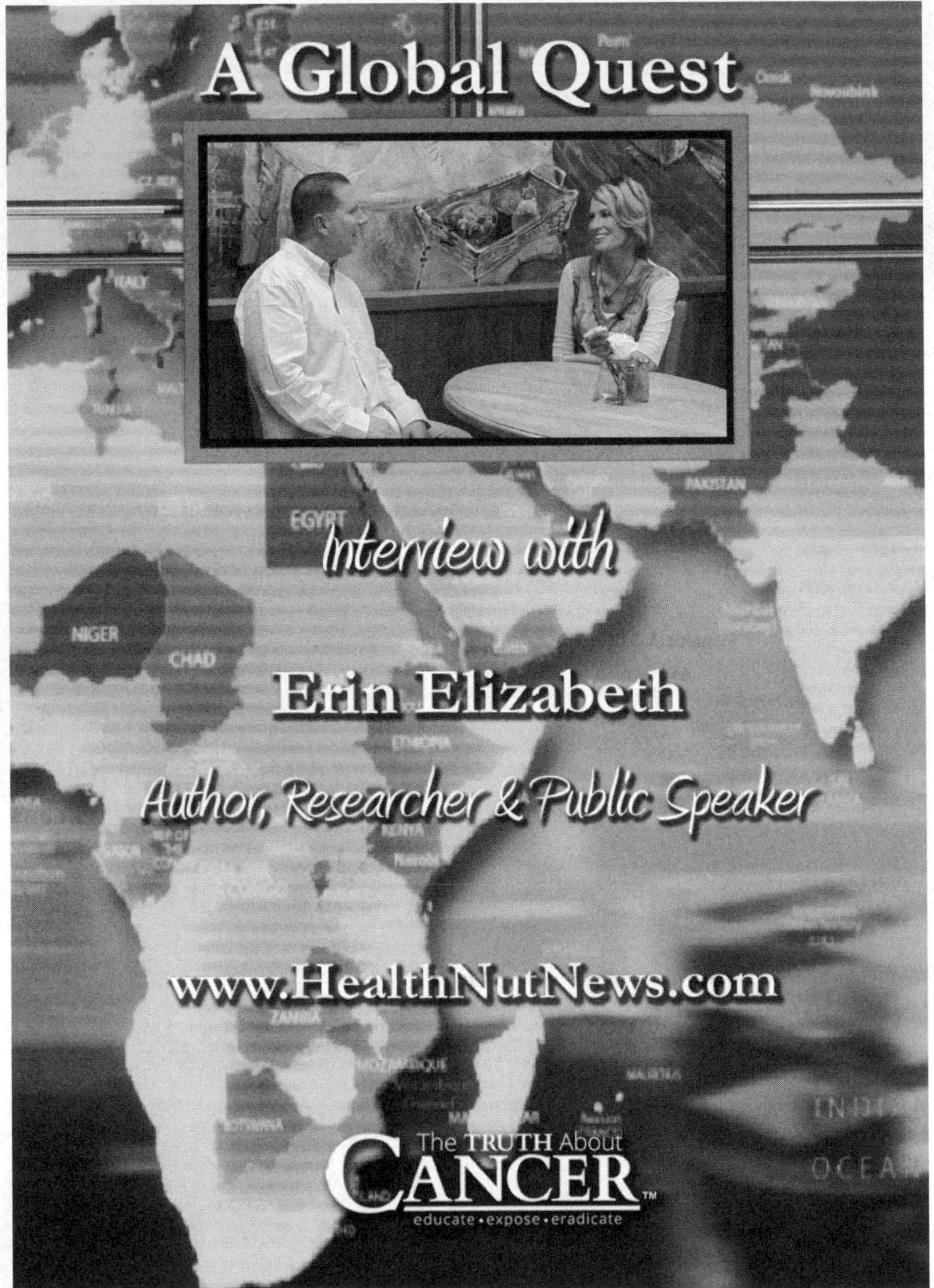
A Global Quest
Interview with
Erin Elizabeth
Author, Researcher & Public Speaker
www.HealthNutNews.com
The TRUTH About
CANCER™
educate • expose • eradicate

Ty: So I'm really honored tonight to be with Erin Elizabeth here in Naples, Florida. Thank you for joining us.

Erin: Thank you. Great to be here. Thanks, Ty.

Ty: I know you had a long drive.

Erin: Yes, had a long drive but it was worth it.

Ty: Good. Good. We're so glad to have you here.

We are really looking forward to getting your story about your life story, about being vaccine-damaged and overcoming serious health challenges.

So let's kind of rewind several decades to when the problems began for you and kind of share some solutions.

Erin: I would love to. Well, I am adopted and I know my birth mother. I was fortunate enough to find her through a book she'd written about the process of placing me up for adoption.

Back in 1970, I'm open [about] when I was born, abortion was illegal. She went to Mexico to have an abortion. As far as we know, she was put under. Thought they did the procedure and then a couple of months later when she came back to States, she found out that she was still pregnant.

So at which point there were still options that she could have, but she realized it was really my birth father who sent her down there and didn't want to take responsibility. And she realized at that point that it was meant to be, you know, she wasn't going to do that and she was going to have this child. But she was young and so she placed me for adoption.

I was born pretty sick with severe thrush. So for two months they couldn't place me for adoption. They had to keep me in this adoption agency, a kind of ward for sick babies, and treat me with strong antibiotics. We don't know if I was vaccinated there, but then after my parents adopted me—my mom and dad whom I love, they are still married and they are great parents—they just did what the doctor told them. And then in three months I got my vaccine, first vaccination which I knew included DPT and we think that was the culprit.

After I received the DPT, which would be better known, I guess, as the DTaPH or Tdap if it were a booster shot including the pertussis which can often times be the culprit in the vaccination. I started seizing, had a 104 fever for a week. So they were very worried. They did a spinal tap, couple of spinal taps, I think. No anesthesia. So I'm sure it was not fun as a child to be going through that, but I don't have any memory of it.

After the vomiting began and seizing, they had me in the hospital, and then it was almost another miracle. At only three months that I—the fever broke and they thought I may had spinal meningitis. So they were testing me for encephalitis from the vaccine, but it broke. I was pretty okay. I'm able to joke that I am okay but I did have some problems with attention-deficit disorder as a child. I don't think really a learning disability but problems with concentration and I still have those as an adult once in a while.

So that's kind of the beginning of the story. Not only that, but the pediatrician said that it was a coincidence initially with the vaccines so they kept vaccinating me after that.

I had severe allergies as a kid.

Ty: Isn't that bizarre though, you have something like that, you were vaccinated and you have these symptoms that begin to happen almost immediately. And this happens thousands and tens of thousands of times every year with different children. And the physicians always say it was a coincidence. Isn't that odd?

Erin: Oh yes, I know. Still to this day you read articles about that where right after the vaccines, a child will have some, I mean, I'm one of the fortunate ones. Or whatever might happen, including death, and still they'll tell them it was a coincidence.

Ty: A coincidence.

Erin: Yeah, I know. It's really sad.

Ty: Right. But for a thinking person, that doesn't make sense. Doesn't pass the smell test.

Erin: Right. Exactly. So I think the problem is—I guess it is a problem that we put so much trust into our doctors. That my parents said, "But the doctor said." They are educated, wonderful people, but we blindly sometimes trust those doctors because that's just what's ingrained in us, is what I think. But now people are waking up. I think they are seeing the light. So that's a good thing.

Ty: Yeah. So walk us forward from there. You're a child...

Erin: I'll skip a few years. I had a great childhood and have a brother who was adopted as well. And then at 8th grade, since I was born in 70, that was 83 or 84, I think it would had been 84 since I am graduating in 8th grade at 13. I was born late in the year at 13. We went on a trip to like a state part with all the 8th grade and I had a tick bite on my leg. And it was stuck on me, on the back of my leg for two days because we're kids, you know, you go out there and for the two days you don't shower, you shower when you get home, you know, you're a kid.

So I didn't notice that it was on there and it had to have been on me for at least one day. And then finally a counsellor—somebody helped tried to take the tick off. We wore long pants to try to avoid them but I didn't realize it was on me.

After that point, my Lyme-literate medical doctor now, who is from the same area I grew up in the Midwest, believes that it was that tick that probably caused the initial Lyme infection. But I didn't know this until two years ago. I finally got a blood test and it wasn't the cheap ELISA test, it was a western blot done through IGeneX and it was positive. So there's no denying it.

I was in denial for a while. I think when they said—I've had all these symptoms for years, I mean, since I was like 13, and they said it was growing pains or because I was getting taller that my joints just hurt because they're growing. I had all these excuses all these years, but I realize it was definitely the Lyme that was causing that.

Ty: What were the symptoms of the Lyme? Is it joint pain?

Erin: A lot of joint pain, almost like arthritic pain in the hands and feet and tingling and numbness. And I would say some cognitive stuff, like neurological. I would be forgetful, and weight gain, adrenal fatigue, a lot of weight gain. Because the thing about Lyme, you learn a lot because it affects everything. It affects your thyroid, you know, I was hypothyroid. Sluggish thyroid. Affects your adrenals.

I was gaining weight and it just got worse and worse. But then just two years ago, once I got that positive blood test. It took me a few weeks and five doctors, because I'm fortunate to know a lot of doctors that I work with and my better half.

So they all looked and said, "Yes, this is a positive test. There's no denying it." Once I accepted it, okay, at least I have a name for it and I have always been into kind of—I like solving mysteries. Finding my birth parents, knowing who they are, knowing my story and background, now knowing what I had. After

I accepted it, and it took a while, then I said, "Alright, well now we're going to solve the mystery of getting better."

And that's where I begin my journey two years ago with losing the weight. But it wasn't really—the weight was just the physical symptom that people could see—but to feel better and to get better.

Ty: So Erin, I've seen the before and after. Right, two years ago?

Erin: Yes.

Ty: And now, you're really healthy. So walk us forward. How did you get healthy, you know, from this diagnosis of Lyme's? You were much heavier then and now you're the picture of health. How did you do it?

Erin: Thank you. I was fortunate to know Lyme MDs around the country and I like to get a second opinion. And I realized right off the bat that antibiotics really weren't for me. I know people who have had—they'll get better and then kind of relapse again if they're doing the antibiotics. And if I had been—since I was late stage Lyme, I hadn't just had a tick bite or a bullseye.

If it had been years ago, that might be the route to go for someone just infected. I went with more of a natural protocol. So I wrote a book which I just give away for free to help people about that.

Ty: What's it called?

Erin: With the protocol. It's called *In the Lyme Light*. L-Y-M-E.

Ty: Okay, I like it. Nice title.

Erin: So I developed kind of my own protocol with a little bit from each doctor and then especially the ones who agreed on this particular protocol that I did. And the weight began to come off and I slept better for the first time in years where I could just feel like I could get a decent night's rest. Because one of the things with Lyme is you just have trouble sleeping, and insomnia.

The joke is that the little spirochete, the little Lyme bugs, go to sleep at night and then you get your energy and you can't rest. So finally I was able to get rest and to feel better and to lose weight as well.

So it was really life changing and I have energy, too. That was the hardest part because I just had so low energy where I felt like at days I couldn't even get out of bed. And just to be able to sleep well and get up in the morning and go out there and feel like I could take on the world was a really beautiful thing that I hadn't felt for a long time.

Having things like—I broke my foot traveling in Chicago, we were there over holidays. It's a set-back. There's always going to be obstacles, we're always going to have set-backs. But that I can just go with it even with a broken foot, it kept me down for a little bit, but I can get back up again. So yeah, that was really important.

Ty: So you went to treat the Lyme and to get healthy. Describe your diet. Describe the foods that you've been eating.

Erin: Well, that was a big part of it. The first thing was the foods that I stopped eating. I was definitely eating all organic, even if it was home-made or at an organic deli or stuff that I made myself. I was eating organic, non-GMO, organic grains, some sweets that were organic, sugar—everything organic. But still it was some refined sugar and grains. And because I had no energy, I had cravings because the adrenal fatigue, I crave grains and sugar.

So it was really that I stopped eating the—I say to people "fewer treats" and what is the other one? "Less wheat and treats and sweets" but I just really cut out almost the grains all together. And immediately there was a difference for me.

I don't like to just to say one particular thing you can do that will help. And then I added more fruits and vegetables and even though I used to do, still do, raw food treats. I knew that to heal my gut, which is where the health begins, that I had to do something a little more gentle than just raw vegetables. So I would cook and make a lot of vegetable soups. I think it is partly what I ate, but what I took out of my diet. I think that played a big part in it. Cutting out those.

When I was reading about for Lyme diet or for anyone, that I needed to cut out those sugars and grains. But I did eat fruit. I will say that I ate some fruit, not a high quantity, but would have a little fruit in the diet. But whole organic fruit, not fruit juice or anything like that.

Ty: Removing the sugar and the grains is a good idea, not only for Lyme but for cancer as well, because they both produce the glycemic response. And so then you've got the issue that these foods that you're eating, the sugar and the grains, are actually fueling the cancer cells. So a wise choice for cancer patients as well.

You say you do raw foods. Give me a couple of your favorite raw food recipes.

Erin: Let's see, I'm put on the spot here. There are so many. When I'm going to—something quick, you know, we all need quick and easy things to make. One of my favourite things are like the almond—we call them Red Ants On a Log. I don't know why I just thought of this, but sometimes when I go to a raw food potluck and I don't have a lot of time, I'll do something simple like organic celery, a little almond butter. If I said milk before I meant butter. A few little goji berries on there and that that will be a quick snack for me, something that I feel is nutritious.

Also, as far as food combining, when you're combining—like if someone eats a sandwich with meat and bread, that's one of the worst combinations if you're doing a protein and carbs together. So, I think I worked a little bit on food combing and also intermittent fasting helped me as well. I would not immediately get up and have a big breakfast; that I would go 12 hours without eating and kind of allow the gut to heal.

But yeah, there are a lot of—as far as raw recipes that I like. There are a few raw soups that I'm not sure ingredients off the top of my head. There's a raw sweet potato soup which is one of the few. You know, I don't eat a ton of carbs except vegetables, something like sweet potatoes or celery soup. I ate a lot of soups. It was easy on the gut just to help me heal it. Because my gut was in bad shape, but definitely it got better.

Ty: I got a question for you. You, being vaccine-injured. A lot of the vaccines that we're putting in the bodies of children today, and adults as well, they contain known carcinogens. Known substances that we know cause cancer, such as formaldehyde, mercury, aluminum. I mean the list is endless.

In your opinion, how wise is this to be injecting people with toxins that we know cause cancer?

Erin: I think it's frightening. It's really scary. I don't think it's wise. I don't understand why people can't see that. It seems so transparent to me, yet it happens and you see the rise in children's cancers, yet we're still doing that. Continually increasing the vaccine schedule with kids. More and more vaccines being added to their schedule.

And yeah, I don't think it's smart at all and I think that there's probably a correlation. There is a correlation there, I feel, but yet people don't seem to see that or they're in denial. It's almost like they are in some kind of denial. With the amount of vaccines children are given today it's really frightening, compared to when we were kids.

Ty: Oh yes. It's tripled or more, or maybe quadrupled. What do you think? I mean this is just a theory, but your opinion. We've got a huge rise in children's cancers over the last 20 years. What is causing this increase in children's cancer?

Erin: I think a part of it would be the vaccines. The amount of vaccines, the additives in the vaccines, the known carcinogens. Also our food; we're eating genetically modified foods. I believe in eating all organic. And even if it's organic if the kids are drinking organic juice boxes all day long, it's still—if they are drinking fruit juice that's probably too much sugar.

And just the diet. Also the environmental factors comes in to play. It is a number of things. I just don't blame it on vaccinations but I think that's a big part of it. But there are other things that I feel that we have to change before things are going to change as far as the number of kids with cancer, or adults as well.

Ty: Even with infants with cancer, we're talking about infants that are born, that on day one they have cancer.

Erin: Oh yes.

Ty: The reason being potentially the toxins that are coming through the umbilical cord from the mother, right?

Erin: Yeah. What the mother's eating. Of course now they're saying like—the MMR shot. Now, Merck is being sued by their own virologists because they're saying at least the mumps part of the MMR Vaccine might not be that effective. But now with the DPT, they're saying that the Tdap, the booster shot that they get, that the pertussis part it could be 34 percent or more chance it could wear off.

"So it's 50-50, but you should get it anyway. Just keep getting those vaccinations," the one that injured me. But so what they're saying now is, "You need even more vaccinations. And be sure if you are a pregnant mom to get that shot." The last thing that a mother needs for her unborn baby is to be getting the Flu vacs and everything else.

Ty: Because the baby is going to get all the toxins from the shot through the chord.

Erin: Oh yes. They're still in the womb and yet they're telling the mothers, the pregnant mothers, to get more and more vaccinations during pregnancy, which I think that's got to play a factor.

Ty: Yeah, I'm sure it does. Do you think that the—what's driving these decisions to push vaccines so hard, to push all these toxins so hard? What is driving it?

Erin: I think a big part of it is the pharmaceutical companies. And then as soon as you say that somehow you're a conspiracy theorist, you know, how there are the people out there who say, "Oh yeah, don't say big pharmaceutical because then you just put on the tinfoil hat." But yet, if people would just look, just use common sense to connect the dots here. I think that we have...

When I was a child, the MMR—I think it was the measles vacs before that—the MMR 44 years ago or 45 years ago, was just being developed. So we don't know. It hasn't been enough years or even a gener—my mom and my birth mom, they both had measles and were fine. My mom, she had eight brothers and sisters, they're all fine. But I don't think they've been around long enough for us to understand the detrimental effects.

I think science is going to take a while to catch up. I don't think that we're anti-science just because we might be a little bit ahead of the curve.

I think it's Big Pharma. Also, I think it might be a little bit of fear. We're using germ shampoos to kill—or hand-sanitizers to kill the germs, body soap to kill all the germs.

Ty: And all that bacteria, even the good bacteria, right?

Erin: Good bacteria, sure.

Ty: You mention the gut, you mention the antibiotics.

Erin: We need that good bacteria. Yeah.

Ty: Erin, does it make sense to be giving people round after round of antibiotics in light of the fact that it's destroying the good bacteria in the gut?

Erin: I don't believe so. I was given antibiotics as a child and then also, big surprise, I had terrible allergies. We had to go out of state to allergists and specialists. So I was given antibiotics even through teenage years into my 20s before I finally realized this isn't helping. Every time I have, whether it's allergies or upper-respiratory infection to be put on antibiotics, it left my gut in bad shape where I had to repair it.

I don't think it was just the Lyme. It was a number of things. So I don't think it's wise. And now we have the antibiotic-resistant illnesses.

Ty: Sure. The MRSA.

Erin: The MRSA. More people are antibiotic resistant. I think we're in serious trouble if we don't do something. So again, people still seem to defend those antibiotics after what they're doing to us. It's definitely not good for the gut. I will avoid antibiotics at all costs, unless it's like a life-threatening kind of thing. I really will avoid them even if I feel I have something respiratory.

Ty: You can use silver.

Erin: Yeah, I use silver. It was Robert who told me to put it in the nebulizer. He was the first one to tell me that. And within a day, because I was traveling and just broke my foot, within a day. I put that silver in the nebulizer, used it and boom, I was better. It was gone. You don't need antibiotics and then wreak havoc in your gut, too.

Ty: Yeah, absolutely. Erin, this has been fascinating. I really am thankful that you took the time to travel all the way down here.

Erin: Thanks, Ty.

Ty: This interview and your story is inspiring to me and I know it will be to everybody that is watching. Thank you so much.

Erin: Thank you. Thanks, Ty.

Ty: All right. God Bless you.

Erin: You, too. Thank you.

[end of transcript]

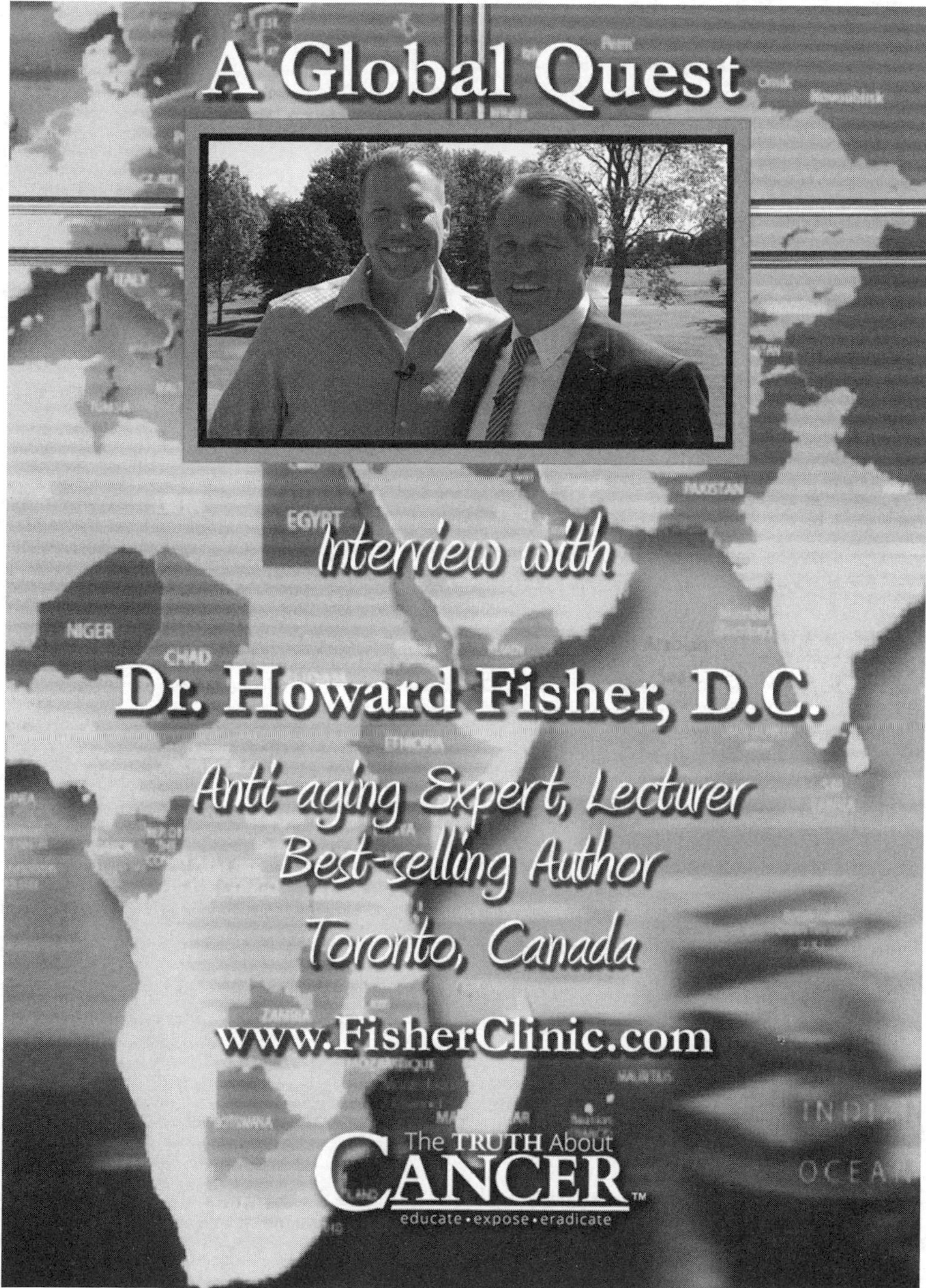
A Global Quest
Interview with
Dr. Howard Fisher, D.C.
Anti-aging Expert, Lecturer
Best-selling Author
Toronto, Canada
www.FisherClinic.com
The TRUTH About
CANCER
educate • expose • eradicate

THE TRUTH ABOUT CANCER

Ty: I'm here in beautiful Station Creek Golf Club in Gormley, Ontario just north of Toronto with Dr. Howard Fisher. Howie, thanks for joining me today.

Dr. Fisher: Ty, always a pleasure.

Ty: Beautiful setting we have here. I thought it only [appropriate] to do an interview with you here since you're such an avid golfer. Did you already play today?

Dr. Fisher: Absolutely.

Ty: Alright, how'd you do?

Dr. Fisher: I was even today.

Ty: Even? Okay, that's par for those of us in the US. You call it even here. I guess if you're an avid golfer it's even.

Dr. Fisher: Yes. It's up or down, you should look at above or below, couple over, couple under, you know? Even.

Ty: What do you call it if you're like 40 over par?

Dr. Fisher: Recreation.

Ty: That'd be me. So Howie, I want to talk to you today about a very important topic of cancer as well as nutrition, detoxification. So let's just get rolling. To begin with, what exactly is cancer?

Dr. Fisher: Cancer is a cell that's gone out of control, growth in the body. And it starts to either space occupy or it starts to kill off other cells. Simply put, it's being out of control with no limitation on what it can do to the body. And therefore, it changes the physiological function to something that is not conducive to life.

Ty: Before we go any further, one of the questions that I should have asked you to start with, give us a little background on yourself and your education.

Dr. Fisher: I've got a number of degrees. I've got three degrees from North America. I've got a degree from Asia, a medical degree. And basically, I've got a chiropractic degree from Canadian Memorial Chiropractic College. I have two undergrad degrees from University of Toronto.

I've written seventeen books. I've lectured in 30 countries, been to about 95. And I try to save the world by giving them information and hoping that they will be compliant to the information.

Ty: Before we started the interview you started to talk about some statistics, really alarming statistics about cancer. Talk about the amount of cancers that are actually caused by toxicity versus genetic. Can you share some of those statistics?

Dr. Fisher: Absolutely. Anyone who looks at the research will realize that we're looking at a high incidence of cancer right now. They just changed the prediction for that. It was at North American males 50 percent will have an incidence and 24 percent will succumb to it.

And basically they just changed that, so in the next five years 57 percent more incidents will occur. When you start to look at some other numbers—18 percent of all cancers are caused by infection. No one talks about that.

Ty: Eighteen percent?

Dr. Fisher: Eighteen percent. Twenty three percent of all cancers are related to obesity. No one ever talks about that because obesity is running amuck right now. This year overweight and obesity in the US alone will hit 75 percent with 41 percent being obese. And they've already (inaudible - 03:02)the numbers, the body mass index, for declaration of that.

Then we look at the other environmental factors and that's—they lump that into 41 percent of all cancers are due to environmental factors. So then we're looking at an unknown 18 percent, and this 18 percent that we're looking at, it could be genetics.

Genetics is small, 5 to 10 percent percent. Just other factors whether it's an ambient environmental radiation, non-ionizing, unlikely it's ionizing. But that can all be lumped in there into these same factors.

Ty: Right. So when you mention obesity, how would obesity impact cancer? Why would there be a link between obesity and cancer? Before you answer that by the way, we just got back from some interviews in Latvia, in Europe. In Riga, Latvia.

There wasn't an obese person in the country that we saw. Literally, in four days I saw two obese women and two obese men. And they were both from either England or the US. But the people there, because of their diet, they eat farm-to-table. No obesity.

Dr. Fisher: I have a program rationale to stop obesity now and that's something else just trying to give the information for people to that. It's basically what you're consuming with obesity.

And obesity changes physiological function. The things that we see, we see—Obese people are they diabetics? Sure, absolutely they are. Obese people do they have high blood pressure? Sure they do. Obese people do they have high triglycerides? Yes, and that's not even getting into any of the less frequent factors about obesity.

So anytime we can change normal—that's a scary word—physiological function by an onset of symptomatology, obesity, well we don't know what's going to happen. We can't predict that and that's why traditionally we do such a poor job of dealing with this disorder.

Ty: Does the fact that when you're obese you have a disruption in your hormone balance, could that have anything to do with the link to cancer?

Dr. Fisher: Everything is involved. Absolutely. Do we know? We don't have a lot of answers to the questions. We just know relationships. And right now relationships are good enough because it's getting to be out of control. And the fact that the relationships are good enough to say, "This, then that," mechanisms cease to be important.

Maybe at some point we can get to the mechanisms and fine tune it. But the reality is if we know that A does B, let's try and stop A. If we can stop A, then we can stop B. If there are some other factors involved in the mechanisms, well, we'll get to them. It may not be soon, but we'll get to them.

I mean they still sell cigarettes. There was a big case in Quebec where they just won a fifteen billion dollar reward, just in the news today. Because cigarette makers were less concerned about health than money. You might find that as something that you see a little bit of.

Ty: Well, we do see that. It's pervasive in the industry. It's pervasive in the medical industry. And ironically, 60 years ago you would see ads from doctors that cigarettes were good for your health. Now we know that they cause cancer, we knew back then that they were carcinogenic.

But we see the same thing with our food supply today, don't we? Look at genetically modified foods that are ubiquitous in North America. Talk about the toxicity of our food and how that might impact our health and cancer.

Dr. Fisher: Well, the liver is the boss of your body. No matter what you think. It's not your brain, it's not your heart, it's not your lungs, it's your liver. Because the liver carries predominantly the bulk of metabolism in your body.

Everything's got to go through the liver. So when your liver becomes overworked, overly toxic from all the environmental toxic factors, it shuts down. So your metabolism slows down, or doesn't work exactly in that manner. And when we're examining reasons for physiology breaking down—and that's all it is—it's proper physiology breaking down.

We can see that it's absolutely everywhere. And so we don't even have to realize what the actual factors are because it's so overwhelming, that we know about the whites. How many people eat white sugar, eat white rice, eat white flour, eat it every day?

Well, we know there's relationships between that and a number of diseases, yet people are still doing it. So getting the word out in your series, getting the word out is more important than having the actual activities take place. Why? Because it offers them the choice of being compliant or not.

Ty: So Dr. Fisher you mentioned the whites. I like that. The white flour, the white rice, the white sugar, all these processed foods that actually convert to sugar in the body and they damage the liver. How can we detoxify the liver?

Dr. Fisher: Well, I know you thought that your previous question escaped me because we were talking about GMO foods. But in the finding by Professor Seralini, who ran his same study that Monsanto ran, that recently came out—it was supposed to be for six months, but it actually went only for three months. In that study, when he ran it for two years on the same rodents. What did he find? Well, he found liver and kidney damage beyond control group.

He found 50 percent shorter life for males, 70 percent shorter life for females, beyond the control group. This is GMO corn. And he found 200-300 percent increase in tumors.

Now, in the United States, in Canada, they don't have to mark GMO foods. So what's happened is the non-GMO growers, producers, are marking theirs. So people have a chance. Because if you don't know and we have these incidents—we don't have to know the mechanism, we have the incidents. A then B, we don't have to know how or why, just that.

So yes, we're overwhelming the liver, we're having liver damage, the liver has to take care of everything, the liver has to metabolize everything. The reason so many people are obese is the fact that the liver has to store toxins somewhere. It's storing them in the fat. Liver will not break down fat, it cannot break down fat to overwhelm itself. Your body wants to survive.

Ty: So it puts it in the fat cells.

Dr. Fisher: Stores it in the fat. Why? It's nice insulating. It's good.

Ty: So if we want to detoxify the livers that are clogged, that are toxified, what's a good way to do it?

Dr. Fisher: Well, we go greens, lots of greens in your diet. There are a number of herbal tea formulations that can do that. And stop putting it into your body.

Ty: That's a good first step.

Dr. Fisher: That's a great first step. I'm approaching my third decade of being a vegetarian.

Ty: How old are you by the way?

Dr. Fisher: I'm 64 and I'll be 65. But I've been in anti-aging medicine for 30 years, and no it's not nips and tucks. I do it preventively. So yes, I get to collect a pension if I choose.

Ty: I honestly find it hard to believe that you're almost 65.

Dr. Fisher: In two months. In two months. It's nuts that people think, "What are you, 45, 48, 50?" I start chuckling. I get asked to prove—when I tell people my age I get, "Can you show me some ID?" I go, "Why? Do you think I would lie about being older?" It doesn't happen.

So, the reality is if you start to watch what goes in, well that becomes preventive anti-aging. There are seven areas that I look at that change the chronological clock that goes, "tick, tick, tick, tick" to a physiological clock. And you can control the physiological clocks it goes, "ticktick, ticktick."

And your buddy Mike Adams, he's all over food. I'm all over food, so my first factor is diet. Watch what you eat. And people go, "Why?" I go, "So you don't hurt yourself." And I use Mike's quote about the food chain being perhaps intentionally designed to end humanity. I like that one.

So watch what you eat. Two, find a nutritional source. Find something that's going to give you nutrition because it's not in the food chain. We can see that from the incidence of disease. So for me, my primary source of nutrition is moringa oleifera. I've written three books on it and I think it's a wonderful plant?

Three, exercise. Now, you used to lift in the big time. So you understand exercise. Exercise is important for your entire body. Absolutely necessary.

Fourth point, meditation. I don't care if it's religion. Any form of spirituality. For me it's walking around this beautiful golf course right here thinking of nothing but that little white dimpled ball. And the next time I hit it, I am generating a different brain wave.

Fifth [sic], good quality air. How many people sit inside where everything is off gassing all the time and never get out?

Ty: Most people.

Dr. Fisher: Most people.

Six, good quality water. Well, you're in Canada now. We have more water than anybody and we still have to make sure it's good quality.

And seven, protection from electromagnetic radiation which is everywhere. And I should quickly point out—because you'll be attacked for this, for me even making that statement as I am. If they're listening—cell phones, it's not like there's not enough ambient electromagnetic radiation everywhere because we're transmitting information. I'll get to that in a second

But if you examine what a cell phone is, a little battery powered device is not really dangerous. What it can do, some of the functions, can lead to danger. It's like a car parked in a parking lot never gets into an accident that's its fault. But it can be involved in an accident if someone hits it.

So a cell phone, a little battery powered device, doesn't really do much from that perspective. Now the carrier wave, I don't think our body can understand that. So what factor is it? The information that we are transmitting. That's the thing that's coming in between 0 and 100 hertz, that our body is being affected by. That's where the problem comes in.

So who's doing that? You are, I am, we are. We're all doing that. Information, data, information, all affecting us. So is it the cell phone provider? No. Are they allowing us to do that? That's like saying you got drunk and crashed your car because someone manufactured alcohol. No. You drank the alcohol. So the reality is we're responsible, we have to take responsibility.

And there's things we can do about all that anyway. There's things we can do about all of everything. You don't exercise? Well, exercise. You don't meditate? Well, meditate. You don't find nutrition in your food? Find some. So, if you follow those factors, we can get to a physiological clock which is anti-aging. Literally, anti-aging.

Otherwise you'd have a date stamped on the bottom of your foot. "You were born here and you're going to do here," so best before. Got it on milk, has it on orange juice. Has it in the supermarket. No "best before" date on humans.

Ty: So, in light of what you just said Dr. Fisher about the date stamp. Isn't that what an oncologist does when a cancer patient is diagnosed and they say, "You got advanced liver cancer, you got three months to live." I mean they just date stamp them. Is that wise and is that not the same thing in as, in effect, as giving them a death sentence?

Dr. Fisher: Well, it is a death sentence. But understand, on a previous episode of the "The Truth About Cancer," I believe that you had someone espousing what most oncologists would do if they had cancer. What was it 90 percent? Over 90 percent?

Ty: Right around that, yes.

Dr. Fisher: Around 90 percent would not follow their own protocols.

Ty: Right.

Dr. Fisher: So, the doctors are being honest. That's all. Because they understand that given certain parameters there's very little we can do by the parameters that they're using. So I don't hold it against the doctors. I think it's a system that people are inclined to follow. And I don't want to point fingers.

I just want people to be more compliant about dealing with their own health. I was fortunate enough to sit down with the head of biological research with Samsung. Very small company in Korea.

Ty: Very small company.

Dr. Fisher: Very small company. And he told me, "Listen, we understand that there is an issue. We can't figure out the issue because it's not coming from our phone. The research would take twenty years to try and break down and figure out is it one percent cell phone, is it three percent carrier wave, is it 96 percent people using it, is it two percent cell phone tower? We can't figure this out. It says in the manuals, 'Don't hold them next to your body.' Alright."

Ty: That's a smart first step, isn't it?

Dr. Fisher: There you go. Why would you eat food—it's the same thing, all the areas, it's the same thing. Would you go drink out of that pond? I wouldn't. I don't know what's in there, but I don't think it's clean enough to drink. But some people are doing that with their diets.

The food they put in their body is no better for them than drinking out of a puddle, or a pond, or your toilet. Not the clean water in the toilet, the other, which may be even better than a lot of the other things. You just get a lot of e-coli that kind of lives where that is. Take the steps that you need to move in the right direction.

Ty: Right. Dr. Fisher, I think that's good advice. To take control over what we've been given control over, which is our food, water, what we put into our body, the amount of exposure that we get to those cell phones next to our body. Keep them away.

It's just little wise steps like that can make a world of difference. I also appreciate what you said. It's not really the fact that doctors are bad, it's the system that's broken. It's not the individual doctors. We're working in a medical system, specifically with cancer, that's broken, right?

Dr. Fisher: Well, why is it that some protocols have a lot more success than other protocols? Why is it that some protocols that are extremely successful you've never heard of?

I worked with Dr. Igor Smirnov. Dr. Igor Smirnov in 1986 when Chernobyl blew up was one of the teams of scientists that came in to determine not, "why are there three million cases of cancer in this area," [but] why these people didn't have it.

And you never heard of that. Igor Smirnov went down and found that there's this group of people that didn't have cancer. And they didn't seek the reason to help the others, they wanted to know why these people didn't. And they found it was related to the water. It gets really interesting here for everybody.

The fact of the matter is, the mechanism was if you can super hydrate a cell, i.e. if you can get enough water into the cell so it functions optimally, it can basically take on almost anything.

So what was happening was the structure of this water was changing by coming over the Caucausus Mountains and coming instead of being iso-tetrahedral or pyramidal, it was coming in a linear format. That in itself doesn't mean much but it can access something called aquaporins [that] go into every cell, carry nutrition into every cell, bring toxins out of every cell, but still that doesn't matter.

It's allowing the cell, allowing the physiological function to be increased. Once again, not a cure, just enabling the body to do that. No one ever heard of it, called molecular resonance effect technology. You didn't hear that.

Ty: And that's where you determined that the people who had lived, that had not gotten cancer, they were drinking more of this water?

Dr. Fisher: They were just drinking this water—this water was allowing them to hydrate. And they gave a Nobel Prize to Dr. Peter Agre in 2003 for discovering aquaporins. When he found the water he didn't know the reason.

We kind of figured it out after. There are these openings that are one water molecule wide in every cell. We knew that if you hydrated a cell properly—for example, viruses in a dehydrated cell can multiply easily and a hydrated cannot.

So that lends itself to understanding that if you give the body what it needs to function optimally, we can defeat it with following compliant protocols. Not chemo trying to kill everything. Although sometimes it works.

Not radiation trying to kill everything. But, of course, we know if you radiate something, doesn't it cause a tumor? Oh, I'm being silly. But the reality of that is we know that we just have to enable the body.

Ty: Which reminds me of the story that we heard about Dr. Batmanghelidj. In Iran, I think it was, giving prisoners water and being miraculously cured of all these different diseases just because they were being hydrated.

Dr. Fisher: Frank. Yes.

Ty: In the past they were all dehydration. And his theory was that we're not sick, we're thirsty.

Dr. Fisher: Correct. He has a few books on that and I've read them. It's interesting because it's not volume of water, it's accessibility to the actual cells. So how can we get into it? So I actually was part of an experiment. We wanted to determine how the water was getting into the cell. Was there any difference?

We didn't know it was access through the aquaporin. So it's osmosis versus aquaporin. Well, it's one third of the time. So, in other words, you can get water in, it will function, the cell will function, so you need less water. Needing less and getting more.

Ty: And how does that happen?

Dr. Fisher: By restructuring the water. He uses a magnetic field to restructure, to change from an iso-tetrahedral structure, pyramidal structure to make it linear in sheets. And it's all documented. There are some books that were so heavy into the physics of this written in Russia by Vysotsky. It was like if you ever needed something to put you to sleep, by page three you're out cold on a desk. Read that one.

I wrote one on that trying to translate it so people could understand it. Because I think that Dr. Smirnov's technologies are something everyone should use. Is it a cure? No. Does it help your body? Absolutely.

Ty: Well, when you mentioned the word "cure"—we're on the global quest here and then last year was the quest for the cures. But really in reality when we talk about curing cancer or any other disease, do you feel the same that I do that really our efforts should be to focus on giving the body what it needs so that it treats itself as opposed to finding a silver bullet cure?

Dr. Fisher: You're the cure. Giving your body optimal function, or even enhanced function. Because we all function in such lower levels. Look at the fact—the statistic I gave earlier about 75 percent of the population being overweight or obese in the United States. I mean, that's not optimal function.

So look at the correlation to disease. That's not optimal function. So I totally agree with you. I don't even slightly agree or moderately agree. I totally agree that we should be able to theoretically overcome most factors. If you live in a radioactive waste site, you got some problems. If you keep putting toxins into your body—we only have four channels of detoxification. You can breathe it out, you can sweat it out, urine, and feces. These are the only ways things come out of your body. So if we're putting more in, then we're going to be toxic.

Ty: So stop putting in what's killing you and start putting in what will heal you. So talk about what we can put in that will heal us. You mentioned greens earlier. What's so good about greens?

Dr. Fisher: Well, first off, let's get down to chlorophyll. The best part about chlorophyll is the magnesium is the core element. Same molecule as hemoglobin. Hemoglobin has iron, chlorophyll has magnesium easily accepted by the body. In the reactivity series this will start to kick out other metals.

Are there toxic metals in our environment? You bet. Are they everywhere? Absolutely. They also provide nutrition, i.e., vitamins, minerals, a little glucose—plant-based glucose, not sugar, or GMO corn, sugar, high fructose.

Real nutrition that goes into your body. So love the greens. And you can live on just greens. My particular green is (inaudible - 25:18). I used to love spirulina back in the 90s when that was the best one going that was being cultivated, and chlorella, also very good. Mixed greens, fabulous. I just constantly seek best.

That's what I found that works best for me. So you need green food. Body is meant to function on it.

Ty: Right. What would you tell a cancer patient that's been recently diagnosed? What are a couple of good questions they should ask their oncologist to see if they are in the right hands?

Dr. Fisher: "What has your success rate been with my particular cancer at this particular stage?" And if they start to—"Well, you know, everyone's different"—that's not what you're asking. You want to ask what they know.

Why? Because the literature dictates now that doing nothing may be more effective than following certain protocols. Why else would the 90 percent of oncologists not want to follow their protocol?

I would also want to get a second opinion if you're not happy with the first opinion. And I would also ask are they using common sense, the person with cancer. Are they using common sense? Most are not. Most go to choose paths that are toxic to the body and it's, "can we kill the tumor before we kill the host?"

Well, apparently we're not so good at that. We do it sometimes. It happens sometimes, but it doesn't happen often enough.

Ty: I like your focus on logic. Just to a lay person, not a doctor, it just doesn't seem logical that you can heal a sick body by poisoning it.

Dr. Fisher: It's, "Can we kill the cancer before we kill the host?" And the answer is, how often does the host die before the cancer dies? You don't want to be the hero on the battlefield, "Yeah, we got it but I'm dying." You don't want that to happen. You don't want that to be you.

Ty: It reminds me of a quote by a Dr. Philip Binzel who was a doctor 50-75 years ago. I don't think he's still alive. But he remarked about just the absurdity of looking at shrinking tumors as a marker for success and how that oftentimes at the autopsy the oncologist would be thrilled that the tumor had shrunk. But the patient was dead. So we're really measuring the wrong things.

So talk about tumors and cancer being a symptom of a sick body as opposed to the cancer itself.

Dr. Fisher: It brings me back to one of the studies with MRET water, the activated water, where they took a group of rats, actually it was mice, sorry. They took a group of mice, they gave it Ehrlich's Sarcoma. They started some of the mice on this water so their cells were super hydrated and they were functioning properly, they put the tumor in and the tumor didn't take. The tumor could not survive in a body that was functioning well.

It took in the ones that they just put it into. But yet when administering the water, it allowed the body, whether it's via the hydration in the cells, improving the immune system function, or the nutrition it allowed to get in there, it allowed the body to defeat the cancer in over 50 percent of the cases.

So let's just look at statistics. Rodents—mice, rats—in the GMO study are 99 percent the same as humans with genetic codons. That's what you should be asking your doctor. "How did they do in the studies on mice and rats? Oh, 50 percent died." I would say 50 percent lived and that's still a lot better than the statistics that we're seeing now. You can ask—and you will and you have—a lot of other doctors what they're finding. So we have to clean it up. We have to give the body the opportunity to function optimally.

Ty: Change the environment right? I mean look,we're here at this beautiful golf course and let's say that you smoked, which you don't, but you smoked, you took a cigarette and you throw it here. There is zero percent chance that this is going to start a fire, because it's concrete. Concrete doesn't light, but if you throw it on the grass, it might start a fire. Right?

And so, don't we want to change our body's environment to where it's like concrete for a fire when the fire's cancer. We don't want to make it hospitable to grow the cancer.

Dr. Fisher: Well, that's interesting that you chose cigarettes because that is a great value, isn't it? You get four thousand different chemicals, two hundred known poisons, forty plus carcinogens, and it's really inexpensive. And you're now living in tobacco country so, you know, it's interesting.

How they still sell them, I don't know. You want to limit any chance that cancer or a tumor has of taking and growing.

It's difficult enough with the incidence that we have right now, but you want to cut that down, you want to virtually eliminate. You want to make it concrete. You want to give it zero chance. Can we do that? No we can't. Can we come close? Sure we can.

Ty: And we do it by the methods that you've listed.

Dr. Fisher: It's common sense. It's common sense. Why allow your body to have less than what it needs?

Ty: I think they're after us.

Dr. Fisher: I think they are. However, that, in fact, is the clarion and it came at an amazing time. Give your body what it needs. Try to avoid, to the best you can, toxicity and environmental toxins and you'll do better.

Ty: Dr. Fisher, obviously you are aware of what's going on today with medicine really not working properly as far as degenerative disease. What was the "aha moment that really woke [you] up?

Dr. Fisher: It's just statistics. It's what's not working. I mean, I had a few "aha" moments. Obviously, there are "aha" moments because I've gotten everything and quit everything on a number of occasions. And I have a fabulous wife who's stood by me for me having these "aha" moments and she realizes that I don't listen to what they say. I look for the answers and the reality is if it's not working, fix it.

Fix it. If it's not working, find out why it's not working, if you can. If you have the cerebral capacity to do that, do that. If you do not, find someone who does, listen to what they're saying.

Ty: Seems like what we do today is if the system's not working and somebody says that it's not working you call them a name for recognizing that it's not working as opposed to trying to fix it.

Dr. Fisher: You've been around I see, Ty. Because that's exactly what happens. They will call you names. I'll just give you a little incident. I've written seventeen books. Someone tried to buy one of my books on Amazon, but there's a certain group that is trying to hammer that. So they couldn't find it for under two hundred dollars.

I said, "I didn't even put any of my books on Amazon." So there are factors that be. If it doesn't make sense, then it's nonsense. Don't listen to nonsense. Listen to common sense.

Ty: Common sense. Use some logic.

Dr. Fisher: Wouldn't you rather be breathing and playing golf? Absolutely.

Ty: Just not against you.

Dr. Fisher: I don't play people as competition. The competition is within me for hitting the ball.

Ty: Why do you think we have so many kids today, Dr. Fisher, that are being diagnosed with cancer—even infants, newborns—with cancer?

Dr. Fisher: I think the food chain has been destroyed. I think the food chain has been absolutely destroyed. I think the toxic levels in our environment are so high right now with the billions of pounds every day that are being dumped into the environment. I think the body is overwhelmed.

I don't think we are giving them a chance. Why do you think they say it takes you a month of detox every year you've been alive, if you undergo a heavy protocol?

I don't understand the whys for what people are doing. It's becoming an individual thing. You can hear it, "Yeah I'm going to stop smoking." I have been on record, and I used to do this with patients—when I told them don't smoke, "Yeah, I will." Sometimes I would give them a spoon. Just a little teaspoon, actually it was a plastic teaspoon, so it wasn't the best thing. It was toxic because it was plastic. I said, "Every time you have a cigarette, go in your back yard, pick up a spoonful of dirt. When the hole is big enough for you to fit in it, you'll be in it." It's toxic. It's toxic. You don't go drinking gasoline. Why? It's poison. It's toxic.

But you smoke a cigarette. It's toxic. You'd eat food that you know is bad for you. "It tastes good." Okay, but understand that it's quid pro quo. Something for something. Always has to be there. Always has to be a trade-off. If you don't understand that then you're not using common sense. You're using nonsense.

Ty: Do you think that the childhood epidemic of cancer could have anything to do with vaccines?

Dr. Fisher: It's hard to say because we don't know enough. If we don't know enough that means we don't know much about it at all. Do we know that the attenuated virus that they're putting in is a bad thing to do? No. Attenuated viruses make sense if your immune system could fight it and beat it. What we're putting in otherwise as carriers may not be effective.

I'm one of six children, so when someone got Chicken Pox, we were all getting Chicken Pox. It was just going through the house. Some of us had it worse than others. But in getting Chicken Pox, if you stay healthy—they're now talking about shingles, one in three are getting shingles. Well, I had Chicken Pox, I'm not worried about shingles. So because I had a real case, there was no vaccination in my day for any of that.

So the reality is, your body's an amazing machine if you treat it relatively properly, most people don't. I won't make the standard comment that I usually make. But when I'm ninety and walking up that big hill—there's a big hill right out there on the 18th—you know what? People who didn't listen won't be walking up the hill with me. That's all.

Ty: So Dr. Fisher, last question for you and this is a tough one. Not really, but it's just your opinion. So somebody's been diagnosed with cancer and they've been told they're terminal, is there always hope for somebody who's been diagnosed with a late stage cancer?

Dr. Fisher: Always. Always! 100 percent. I'm glad you asked the question. Because if you give someone an extra hour, an extra day, an extra week, an extra month, an extra year, by changing their lifestyle, is it worth it? I believe it is.

Ty: It's a choice isn't it?

Dr. Fisher: It's a choice. It's a choice. The bottom line is, I deal with that all the time, as you know. I do consultations around the world all the time and we hear that same question. And I have to let them know that when there's been metastatic development, the numbers don't represent a long term survival rate. But longer is still better than shorter.

Have we seen that vanish? Yes we have, so we don't know. We can never know. But we can still go through the steps and make the efforts to bring about change that we know the body will like, and the body will be able to utilize and the body will be able to optimize. You keep hearing me say that word, optimization of physiological function. If we're not looking for that, what are we looking for?

Ty: And if we do that, we got a shot don't we?

Dr. Fisher: We do, don't we?

Ty: Thanks for sharing. This is awesome. Appreciate it.

Dr. Fisher: My pleasure, Ty. Always. ***[end of transcript]***

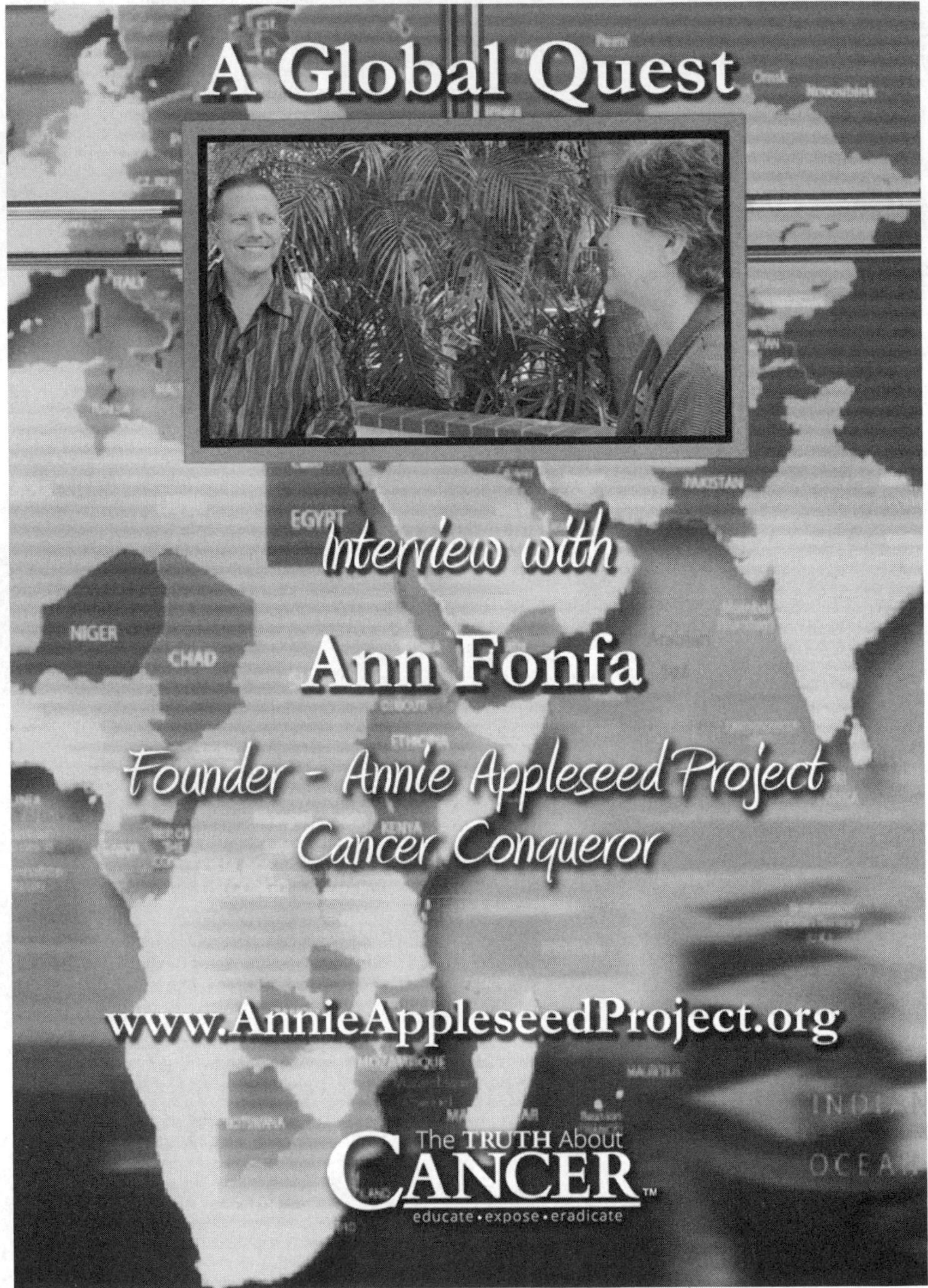
A Global Quest
Interview with
Ann Fonfa
Founder - Annie Appleseed Project
Cancer Conqueror
www.AnnieAppleseedProject.org
The TRUTH About
CANCER
educate • expose • eradicate

Ty: Ann Fonfa, Annie Appleseed Project. So glad to meet you this weekend, and so glad to get an interview with you here.

Ann: I feel that way, too.

Ty: I would really like to get you to share with us something that happened 22 years ago.

Ann: I was diagnosed with breast cancer when I was 44 years old. I didn't know a single person living with cancer. I, of course, got a professional diagnosis, had a lumpectomy before I even knew my name.

When I woke up from that and found out that the doctor had removed 18 lymph nodes from my left arm without my expressed or informed consent, I just felt really uncomfortable with the way they were doing it.

And they had told me on a Thursday that they had an opening for surgery on Monday. Which I understood to mean, "Uh-oh, you have the worst cancer in the universe," and you know. I didn't know that that is what they did with all women or men with breast cancer—rush us into treatment.

So I saw an oncologist, and the oncologist said to me as I walked in, "Oh, we'll start you on chemo next week." And I said, "You know, Doc, I have a problem." And he said, immediately, "Oh, it doesn't matter." And I said, "No, I just have to tell you what it is. I'm chemically sensitive. I respond badly to every kind of cleaning product, anything people are wearing on their neck or their hair, their laundry detergent. Everything's bothering me. Wet paint will cause me to fall to the ground." And he said, "Oh, doesn't matter." "Oh, goodbye, Doc."

Ty: You're still going to do it.

Ann: Have to go. It was great, you know, I walked out and I decided that's not for me and I started to explore what else I could do. And I was astonished.

Ty: You fired your doctor at that point.

Ann: Exactly. He probably would have fired me but, he was an idiot. I mean, "It doesn't matter?" It was my life. It mattered to me. But what I've found—I was looking for alternative medicine, and I was going to used bookstores. I actually thought it was old stuff. Well it was, in a sense, the ancient traditions. And trying to find more and more.

But luckily for me, a very good friend of mine was an acupuncturist and she was already treating me for a while. She had stopped my menstrual cramps in the past and I thought that was astounding.

So I was seeking information. And my nature was to share that information immediately and I began to do that. Of course, I cleaned up my diet and became 100 percent organic. I was much more physically active than I had been before. I started taking some dietary supplements, I started to detox, and I got a recurrence.

"What?" So then I began doing coffee enemas and I went through the Gerson program. I was there for two weeks because I was much healthier than everyone else. I hadn't done chemo, I hadn't done radiation. So I was well, compared to the people who were there. In those days, people went to Mexico when they were clearly at their last prayers.

When I got home, I did the Gerson Program for 18 months, but I continued to have all sorts of issues. My second surgeon, the one who didn't take lymph nodes without talking to me, told me that this was really the same cancer, but it was now growing so slowly that it was slower than normal cells.

I said to the doctor who told me that, "Wow, this must be good, I must be slowing things down. I'm doing a good job." And they said to me, "Well, you didn't do chemo so we can't tell you how you're doing." So no support at all. But I didn't need their support. And I just went forward with my program and I tried a lot of things.

So now I had so many tumors that I decided I'd better have a mastectomy. With no support. So I have a mastectomy and what do you know, I get tumors on the chest wall—I'm Stage IV. This was 1997. And I said to the doctor, "I am not Stage IV, you are not speaking to me." And I just pushed the entire thing away. It was absolutely inconceivable that they thought I was Stage IV. I wasn't, in my own head and in my body I wasn't.

Then I began doing Maitake mushroom extract, and that reduced a tumor. And then I got another tumor. I did high-dose vitamin A, and that reduced four tumors. I had them removed and they said, "Oh, they are well-differentiated. There is barely any cancer left and is very high estrogen-receptor and progesterone-receptor," which is supposedly a good thing. I didn't know much of what I knew. And then I got more tumors. It was very shocking.

I started going to conventional medical conferences and I met a Chinese herbalist at the San Antonio Breast Cancer Symposium in 1998, December. And he said, "I think I can help you." So by April of the next year I said, "I need help." And I went to see him, and in the first prescription that he gave me—I made a tea and when I drank that tea, my entire body turned into a hive, a giant hive, every inch.

So, of course, that was scary. But three days later, I realized my chemical sensitivity symptoms had completely changed and the intensity had reduced by about 65 percent. So now, I have a normal life. I can function like everyone else. I'm not going to pass out if you are a wearing fragrance 40 feet away from me, which was what my life was like.

And in addition to that, over time I never got any more tumors. I'd had an MRI when I started the herbs because I wanted to prove something. And at the end of the time I had another MRI and by then I was completely proven cancer free. That was September 2001. Ironically, I got that diagnosis September 12, 2001 in New York City.

There was no traffic—no cars, no buses, no taxis. I walked to the hospital. And my doctor came from New Jersey and she said to me, "We can't find anything of cancer. We're going to call you 'no discernible disease.'" So they didn't give me NED, which is the usual diagnosis because I didn't do chemo, I didn't do radiation. "We don't know how you're really doing." I knew how I was doing, I was going to live.

That was a long time ago. That was September 2001. I've never had any more tests after that. Very occasionally I think, "Oh, something hurts, maybe it's an issue." But you know what? I just live, and I just give other people information.

Ty: What you are doing is awesome with the Annie Appleseed Project. We appreciate all of that, the information that you share. I want to ask you a question about what was in the herbal tea?

Ann: It was a Chinese prescription, so it was about 20 or 25 different herbs. And it changed over time. Every couple of weeks I would visit him—and we stayed friends by the way—and he would give me a new prescription and I would try that. In about ten months he said, "You're done." But I said, "I don't know, I think I should go a little longer." So at the end of 14 months he said, "You're done."

But it was interesting. He had said to me when we started, "You've got to give up all your supplements and just do my herbs." And I said, "No can do. It's kept me alive these seven or eight years and I just don't want to give it up." So then he agreed with me—I won—and so I did it on top of. And I'm sure that is why I had such a very strong reaction the first time out. It made my whole immune system jump into well-being.

And it changed my life, really, because my life was about chemical sensitivity, not cancer. I was just so, so uncomfortable every single day. I often spent two or three days in bed with—although, after I started taking the supplements, I began to be healthier, but I still couldn't overcome it until the first dose of the herbs. So, what herbs they were? They were Chinese words, I don't really know. And it doesn't really matter because Chinese medicine was about me, at the time that I needed it. So the prescription he gave me was just for me and no one else.

Ty: Right. It's not cookie-cutter medicine.

Ann: Correct. And that's what I really liked about it. Because from the beginning, I wanted it to be about me, and conventional medicine absolutely is not. It's, "Well, everybody gets this because you have the type of cancer you have," which has nothing to do with the person at all.

Ty: Not individualized at all. Well, what I've really gotten out of this interview is, there is not one thing that works for everyone, whether it is conventional or whether it is natural. Because you tried certain treatments that are natural that worked well for some people, but didn't work for you. So I think that your story is not only a story of encouragement, but also to be persistent. Don't give up. Find the treatment that will work for you because there are treatments that will work for everyone, but they are not all the same.

Ann: I totally agree.

Ty: So you need to find out what works for your body. Stay strong, keep the faith, don't let fear take advantage of you, or take hold of you, right?

Ann: Right.

Ty: And eventually you'll find that treatment, or that combination of treatments that will work for you. So I think this is an encouraging story for people who are watching. Because maybe there are people that are watching that have tried this natural treatment and they want to give up on it and they say, "Natural treatments are quackery." Don't do that. Find another that resonates with your body and eventually you are going to be able to overcome the cancer

Ann: The thing is, we don't yet know how to personalize. So, you have to go with what you believe in your heart and what your brain is guided to.

Ty: The mind is a big thing, isn't it?

Ann: The combination has to be there. If you are doing something that you hate—like to me, wheatgrass is the worst thing on earth, for me. I never want to do it. But obviously there are many paths to wellness so you choose another one. And that works.

Ty: Well, I think you are right. The combination of the treatment with the mental attitude. And, to be quite honest, there are a lot of people that I've read about that have been cured with placebos. We've all heard of the placebo effect.

Ann: Yes, it's one of the best treatments we have.

Ty: And all of this is mental. Well, Ann, thank you for sharing with us.

Ann: My pleasure.

Ty: Your story is empowering, and what you are doing with the Annie Appleseed Project is fantastic. We really appreciate it. Thank you.

Ann: Thank you so much. I appreciate that. ***[end of transcript]***

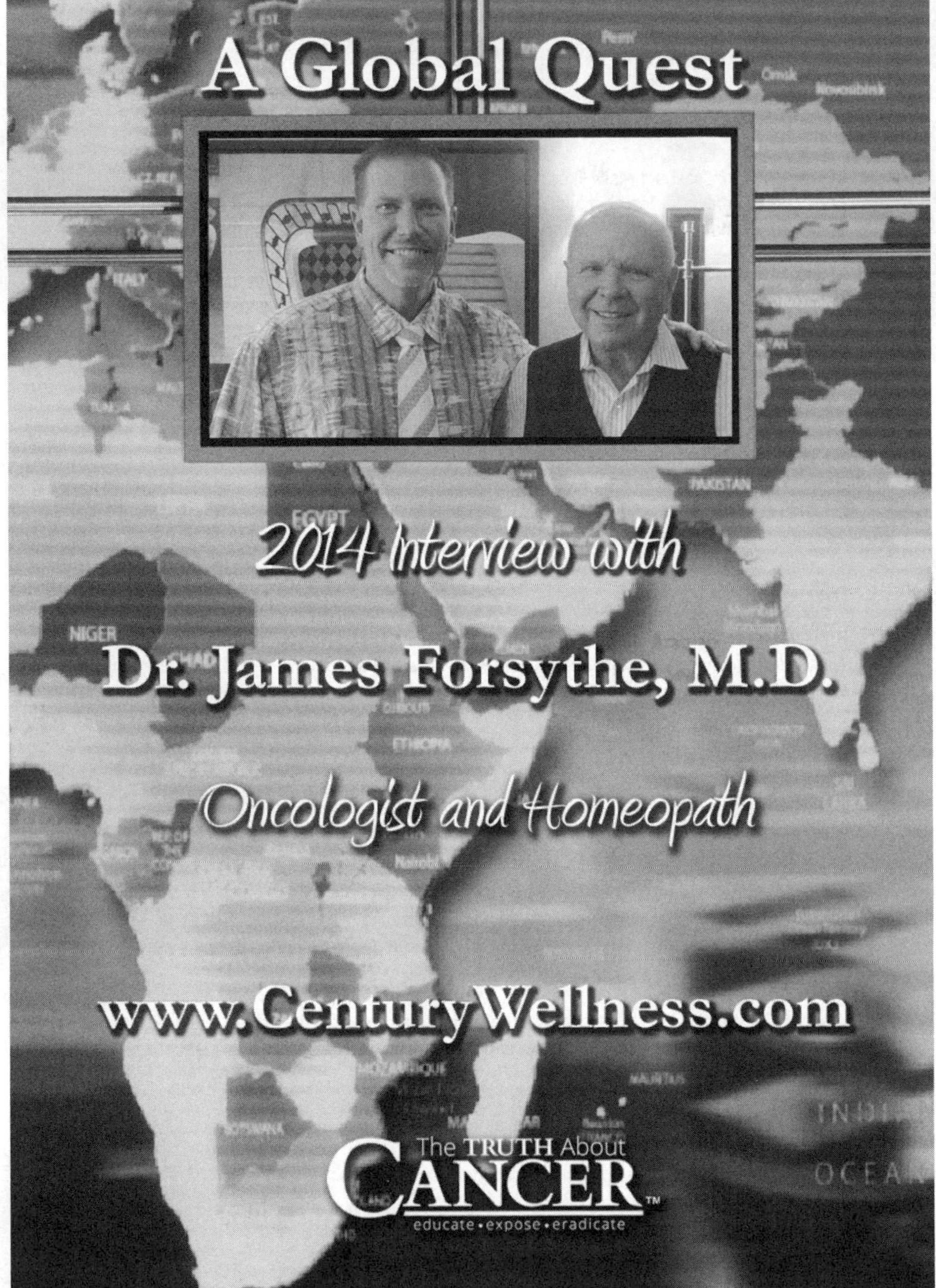
A Global Quest
2014 Interview with
Dr. James Forsythe, M.D.
Oncologist and Homeopath
www.CenturyWellness.com
The TRUTH About CANCER
educate • expose • eradicate

Ty: I'm really happy today to be sitting here with Dr. James Forsythe. I've been following Dr. Forsythe for many years. He is the Medical Doctor at the Century Wellness Clinic, in Reno Nevada, and you've got—how many MD's you have working with you there?

Dr. Forsythe: We have two other MD's. One is a Russian trained doctor. The other is a doctor who was trained at M.D. Anderson Hospital and was the Chief Researcher of the year there.

Ty: Okay.

Dr. Forsythe: So he's very well trained. And we have a couple of nurse practitioners and we have a staff of about sixteen people on the staff. We see it run, 40 to 50 patients a day through our clinic.

Ty: Yeah, I knew—and it's a big clinic. It's one of the clinics that I researched years and years ago when I first published my book on cancer, and I've been recommending that clinic to people for a lot of years.

Dr. Forsythe: Thank you.

Ty: So, I'm really honored to be sitting here with you.

Dr. Forsythe: Thank you.

Ty: And be able to talk to you today and get some of your knowledge on cancer. So how long have you been involved with cancer research and treating cancer as a medical doctor?

Dr. Forsythe: Well, I did my undergraduate at U.C. of Berkeley and then went to med school at U.C. San Francisco, just across the bay. And then I graduated in the top 20 percent of my class. After that I was running out of money so I joined the Army and it was about the time that Vietnam was heating up anyway, so I figured I better be in and have some rank rather than be drafted as a doctor.

Ty: Drafted later.

Dr. Forsythe: So after my internship on the Presidio at San Francisco, I was shipped to Hawaii to Tripp Army Hospital where I did a pathology residency. I kind of felt, at the time, I really was not interested in going to Vietnam, and I thought that pathology might be a good place to be because they did not need a lot of pathologists in the war zone. However, that was not to be the case. After my residency, I was shipped to North Carolina where I was part of the 82nd Airborne Special Forces Units, rather than the pathology laboratories at the hospital. And then after two years there, I got shipped—orders to Vietnam. And when I got to Vietnam, it was the second major Tet Offensive, which was in '69. And our plane, a 707, we came in full of soldiers, was fired upon so we had to circle the airport for about an hour until they cleaned out the Viet Cong that were trying to bring us down.

And from there we went to bunkers, because they were attacking the base at the time. And so our base—we spent the next couple of weeks in a bunker, they brought us food of course, but no weapons. But we could not really leave the bunker because we were getting bombarded every day. And then I got shipped up north to Chu Lai which is in the southern part of ICORP, right on the South China Sea, beautiful location, there is probably a Hilton Hotel there now. But anyway, it was a nice coral reef and I ran the laboratories there, and I was in charge of malaria control, blood banking, and forensic medicine, forensic autopsies, and also did emergency room work there.

After a year then, I came home and finished out my Army career at Letterman Army Hospital in the Presidio again, and then went into an Internal Medicine Residency in San Francisco where I got my internal medicine degree, and then from there went to oncology fellowship tie which was another two years. I kind of over trained actually, but finished that up in '73 and then went into practice in San Francisco as an oncologist with a group of oncologists. Starting to see first cases of AIDS there, because our clinic there, in San Francisco, on Bush and Hyde Street, was right above the gay area of San Francisco, where there were AIDS patients coming to us, and we had no idea what was going on, because there was no tests for AIDS at that time. Nobody even knew what it was until the early 80's. But we were seeing some very mysterious illnesses, let's put it that way.

Ty: Immune diseases.

Dr. Forsythe: Yeah, young men died of wasting diseases and neuropathies and—for no apparent reason. After a couple of years in San Francisco I decided I wanted to be in a smaller town so I moved to Reno and have been there ever since.

Ty: Okay.

Dr. Forsythe: Forty years ago. First 20 years of my practice there I was doing everything just cookbook style, Betty Crocker—

Ty: Conventional?

Dr. Forsythe: Conventional.

Ty: Okay.

Dr. Forsythe: Doing their protocols just like the book said. Then I began to notice that my long-term survivor list was pretty short. In reading the literature that everyone was, that after five years of chemo, in their own literature, they recorded only 2.1 percent survival rate, so any adult undergoing chemo for stage four disease, two out of hundred would be alive at five years. You wouldn't hire a baseball player with a 2 percent batting average. Not a real good—so I finally realized that I couldn't participate in this act for very long, so I decided to get my homeopathic degree. And under homeopathic boards, which they have in Nevada, they don't have it in every state, but I was fortunate to get my degree from the British Institute of Homeopathy. And so then I was under two boards that would allow me to do studies, outcome based studies on natural things.

So over the years and since the early 2000's, I have done studies on pawpaw, from the pawpaw tree, which that is a natural sunshine product, and that causes cancer cells to go into program celltive [PH]. And then I did a study for the Sanchez family on poly MVA, which is a complex of, like, boric acid and palladium. And that also hyper energized the cancer cell and triggers through the mitochondria the process of apoptosis. So the cancer cells which don't know how to die, and they don't have enough energy to go into a death spiral, they basically now, can die off and so that was effective.

Then I did the Forsythe Immune Protocol, FIP, which is a number of agents and started to use in genomic testing then, and some IPT, and that program lasted about five years, and they got about a 45 percent survival rate, which was 22 percent higher than the conventional guys.

Ty: Yeah.

Dr. Forsythe: Not 22 percent, but 22 times higher I should say.

Ty: Yeah, 22 times higher.

Dr. Forsythe: And then the last study I've engaged in started in June of 2010, and it's now 15 months old, that's what my paper was presented to here at the conference, was 15 months, 650 patients showing a 67 percent higher, which was now making the survival rate 33 times higher.

Ty: And what is that protocol that you've been testing?

Dr. Forsythe: That protocol basically is one in which we do genomic testing, gene testing on every patient. We send their blood off, we look for circulating tumor cells and thanks to the MN Genome Project, we're able to tell the patient what that result—what drugs, what hormones, and what supplements work best. So now, God forbid you had a prostate cancer, you came to me with stage four disease, I'd be able to give you a report showing what are the best hormones for you, what are the best supplements, and what are the best drugs. And that's unique to you and your genes, Ty. It's not for every patient with prostate cancer, because your genes are only yours and no one else's, you're going to respond differently to different drugs. Before, on the other side of the fence, it was a guessing game. I would be guessing what would help you, and as I tell all my patients, if I guess wrong, I'm giving you a poison, hurting you. And it's as simple as that, I don't want to do that anymore.

Ty: Well that's— that would be violating the Hippocratic Oath.

Dr. Forsythe: Yes, that's right.

Ty: You'd be harming patients.

Dr. Forsythe: So basically, by getting a blueprint, I run on track. That is why our survival rate is better than most. We compared ourselves with the NCI National Cancer Institute and Cancer Treatment Centers of America, say for in breast cancer, their survival rate, after two years, stage four disease, was 43 percent, Cancer Treatment Centers was 64 percent and ours was 85 percent. So you know, we beat them both significantly.

Ty: Yeah, now you said one of the treatments that you—I guess you've studied is—or you've been using is the FIP, the immune protocol.

Dr. Forsythe: Forsythe Immune Protocol, yeah.

Ty: Forsythe Immune Protocol, can you describe that a little bit?

Dr. Forsythe: Well, it's like what we call a Myers Cocktail, sort of immune stimulant, it has DMSO in it, it has selenium, it has important immune stimulants, vitamins, minerals, amino acids. And that's one of the immune therapies. We use high dose C, we go from 50 to 75 grams on C twice a week.

Ty: Intravenous?

Dr. Forsythe: Intravenous, oh yeah, you can't give that much orally.

Ty: Yeah, I thought it probably caused them severe intestinal problems.

Dr. Forsythe: Diarrhea, yeah, you're not going to handle that very well. Hydrogen peroxide, which is a bio oxidative therapy, that's given intravenously. And then poly MVA which is the lipoic acid palladium complex which is very effective. And then the alkaline nifio [PH] amino acid IV. So basically, what happens, Ty, is they're getting immune therapies three days a week, Monday, Wednesday, Friday. They're getting IPT, and I've modified the IPT program from what was originally started 40 years ago in South America by giving—putting the insulin right in with the chemo right from the start, so you could get less of a reaction, so you're not going to get the severe hypoglycemic reactions.

Ty: And you're using the IPT, it's low-dose chemo—

Dr. Forsythe: 10 percent dose—10 percent to 15 percent max.

Ty: So you have very—very little side effects with that, right?

Dr. Forsythe: Our patients don't lose hair, they don't get sick, they don't have rashes, don't get organ toxins, chemo brain, none of that happens.

Ty: Hmm.

Dr. Forsythe: So they're happy patients. We have a happy population.

Ty: I bet you do.

Dr. Forsythe: Yeah.

Ty: Everything that I hear from patients that have been there over the years is, it's always positive.

Dr. Forsythe: Yeah, they do well, and they're happy and of course it's a—we don't take any Medicare/Medicaid or—we do take some private insurance, but we try and—and they understand that when they come there is a global fee, but we do have a foundation that can help patients who have a financial need. So we have about $500,000 in that foundation money that can be used for them.

Ty: That's awesome.

Dr. Forsythe: Yeah.

Ty: Able to help people that can't help themselves.

Dr. Forsythe: Yeah.

Ty: Do you have any kind of a particular dietary regimen that you put folks on as they come in, is a nutritional regimen a big part of the treatment or not?

Dr. Forsythe: Absolutely, yeah, diet is extremely important. And I've written a book called "The Forsythe Anti-Cancer Diet." And we give examples. There's no one specific diet for every cancer patient. Any like an Atkins Diet, which is mainly a ketogenic diet, or Mediterranean Diet, or the Zone Diet, Paleo Diet, they're all good to a certain extent. Like the Bud—some of the diets are very, very stringent, like the Budwig Diet, which is cottage cheese, flaxseed oil, a few berries. And then the Gerson Diet which means no grains, no fruits, plus six colonics a day. Not too many folks want to be wed to a colonic tube six times a day, it could be habit forming.

Ty: We interviewed a patient that used Gerson and was successful, but it's a very stringent protocol, not just the colonics but the juicing twelve times a day as well.

Dr. Forsythe: Yeah, I know it's—

Ty: Very strange.

Dr. Forsythe: Compliance with that program is extremely low, as you can imagine.

Ty: I can imagine it would be.

Dr. Forsythe: Yes, yes, but—so there's no one doing that. I always tell patients, every cancer diet is a weight loss diet. Because anytime you're cutting out simple sugars and high glycemic foods, you're going to lose weight, simple as that.

Ty: Hmm, any anti-cancer diet is low in sugar because we don't want to fuel the cells, the cancer cells, right?

Dr. Forsythe: Cancer cells, Otto Warburg told us in 1932 that cancer cells only thrive on simple sugars, not complex carbohydrates, not fats or protein, and he was right then. But conventional oncologists completely ignored that. In fact, if you go into any infusion center in any hospital in the country, you'll see a big bowl of candy usually and soft drinks.

Ty: Yeah.

Dr. Forsythe: And so they totally ignore the properties of the cancer cell.

Ty: Yeah, that's almost like putting a bottle of vodka in a halfway house, right.

Dr. Forsythe: That's right.
Ty: You're trying to clean up an alcoholic.
Dr. Forsythe: An AA house, yeah.

Ty: Okay, last question Dr. Forsythe, the immune system.

Dr. Forsythe: Yes.

Ty: You know you talked about you have got the Forsythe Immune Protocol. Can we stress the importance of the immune system enough in fighting cancer?

Dr. Forsythe: No we can't, because as you know, with the AIDS epidemic, which was finally defined in the early '80's, Ty, we know that if your T-cells are depleted, your helper cells are depleted, you're going to be susceptible to a number of cancers, which ordinarily would not hit young men or women. Like CNS lymphoma, like in neck cancers, like Kaposi's sarcoma, like Hodgkin's disease, Non-Hodgkin's Lymphoma, A-O general cancers, those are all much more common in the AIDS population. But anytime your immune system, if you've had a liver transplant or kidney transplant, bone marrow transplant, you're going to be susceptible to a malignancy. So building your immune system, keeping it strong, very important. We do an immune competency test to see what your B&T cell populations look like, your natural killer cell population, we want to know those things. We do a lot of other things to look for triggers like hormone balancing, balance your—in women, even though they are estrogen positive, we want them to be on progesterone or testosterone, DHA, cortisone if necessary. And men, even though they are, sometimes the prostate cancer could be testosterone driven, we like to have their DHA normal, we like to have their cortisone level normal. So growth hormone, we stay away from, just because the FDA thinks that growth hormone promotes cancer. We don't really think so, but it's one of those things that's red flagged for the FDA.

Ty: You'd rather not cross that line. Pick your battles, right.

Dr. Forsythe: I have already done that, I've already been in battle with the FDA and I won the court case.

Ty: Yeah.

Dr. Forsythe: So.

Ty: You know, one of the things I appreciate about what you've shared is the fact that you look at the immune system, you look at hormone testing, the genomic testing, the diet. So you're looking at each patient as an individual, they come to you, and you find out what would be proper for them.

Dr. Forsythe: Yeah.

Ty: Would help them individually as opposed to having kind of a one size fits all.

Dr. Forsythe: It's not a one-size fits all as you know. Cancer is very individual, and everyone's different. Even the same cancer, the same stage of cancer, is different in different people.

Ty: Yeah, well you've been a hero of mine for a long time, I'm really honored to have been able to interview you today Dr. Forsythe, and I really appreciate your time today.

Dr. Forsythe: Well thank you, thank you Ty, it's good to see you. Thank you.

Ty: Thank you and take care.

Dr. Forsythe: Thank you ***[end of transcript]***

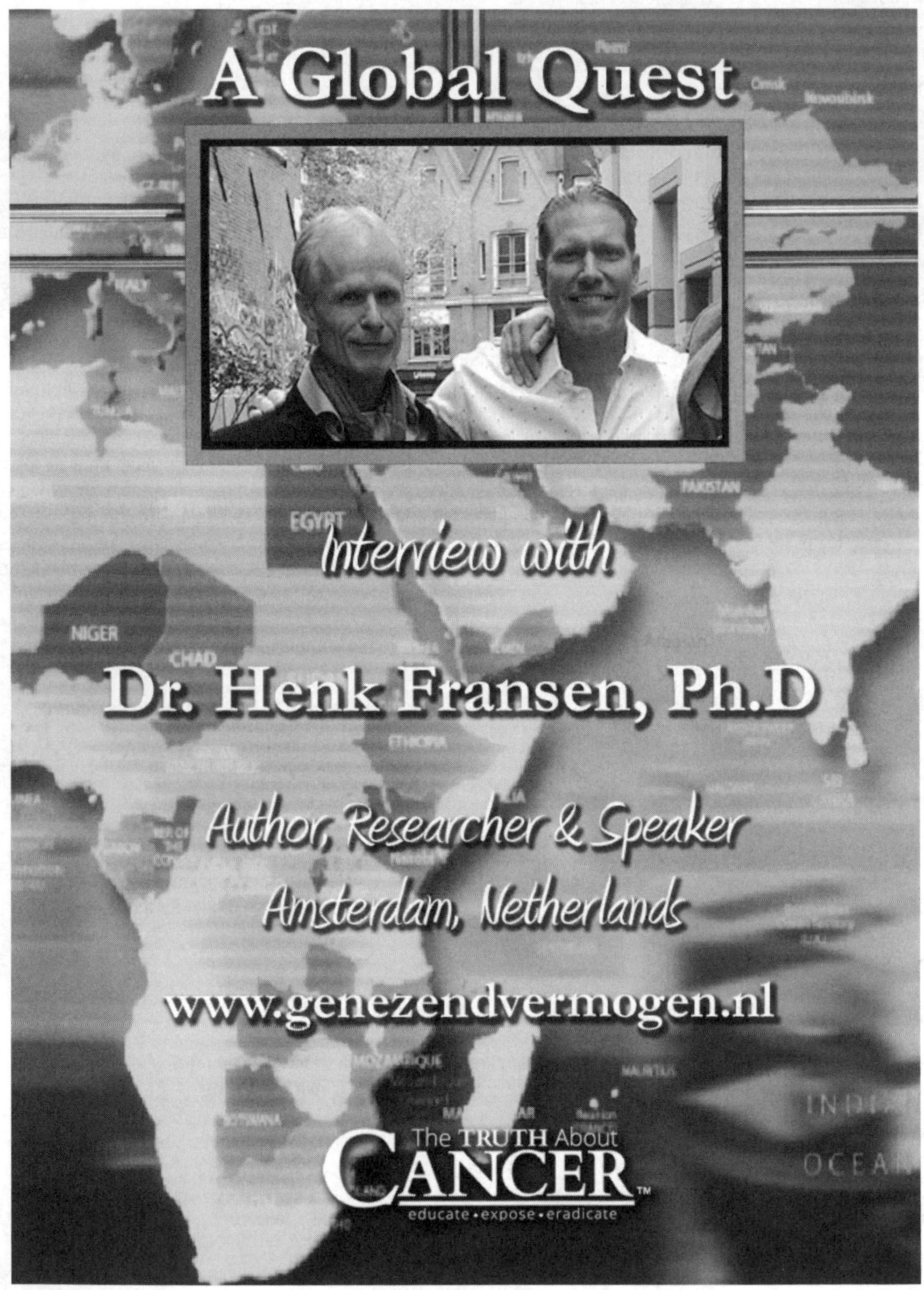
A Global Quest
Interview with
Dr. Henk Fransen, Ph.D
Author, Researcher & Speaker
Amsterdam, Netherlands
www.genezendvermogen.nl
The TRUTH About CANCER
educate • expose • eradicate

Ty: I'm here in Amsterdam, standing with Dr. Henk Fransen. Thank you for joining us today.

Dr. Fransen: Thank you for the invitation, Ty.

Ty: You travelled quite a ways to get down to Amsterdam, didn't you?

Dr. Fransen: No, Netherlands is small. But in Netherlands I travelled far.

Ty: Okay. What's your hometown here in Netherlands?

Dr. Fransen: Apeldoorn.

Ty: Apeldoorn, okay. Well, tell us a little bit about your history, your education, and how you became a medical doctor.

Dr. Fransen: I studied medicine. I ended my study in 1985. But during my study I missed many things. I saw that medicine made human beings too much like only a body, even a machine, which can go faulty and then you can restore it from the outside.

I was really curious about the human being that lives inside this machine and plays a role in health and disease. Also, what I really liked was when I heard about self-healing – that the human body is designed to restore and regenerate itself all the time. But we learn not much about it. And that set me on the alternative path.

At the same time my father got cancer. They couldn't help him anymore. He found alternative ways to treat himself and he lived more than 10 years. So that really interested me and put me on this path.

Ty: So, was that kind of your "aha" or you wake-up moment when your father was diagnosed with cancer and he was able to use natural treatments and lived a lot longer than he was supposed to?

Was that when you said, "there's more to this?"

Dr. Fransen: It was a process. So, after 10 years you could see 10 more years and it's really interesting. But I saw him all the time and it really interested me that there are alternative ways besides the conventional medicine.

Ty: Did you go to medical school here in the Netherlands?

Dr. Fransen: Yes, right.

Ty: When you were in medical school here what did you learn about nutrition and self-healing? How much did they focus on that?

Dr. Fransen: What I was surprised about is we learned a lot about nutrition in a way that the functioning of a cell is all about nutrition. But then at the same time it stops. So it's only about medicine but not much about nutrition anymore. But at the same time we learn all the time that nutrition is the basis of the functioning of a healthy cell.

Ty: Okay. So you did get a little bit of education here as far as nutrition. It sounds like you got more than they do in the United States about nutrition.

Dr. Fransen: Yes, maybe.

THE TRUTH ABOUT CANCER

Ty: Dr. Henk, you mentioned that nutrition is vital in healthy cells. We see cancer as a disease that the cells have changed. They have mutated and they have been damaged. So what is cancer? How would you define a cancerous cell?

Dr. Fransen: The way I look at it, let's say my way of treating cancer resembles most metro cancer therapists. What they say is we have to detoxify the body and also give it good nutrition. But we should not only do this on the physical level. I mean, we should also let go of toxic emotions and nourish the spirit in a good way. And then we have to take care of the environment and heal the relationships that we have.

But most cancer therapists focus on this nutrition. I think something is prior to nutrition. What do I mean with that? A healthy cell, we have equipment to measure that at the moment. It's full of light and it radiates a little bit of this light. This light filters through the DNA into all these millions of miracles of chemical processes.

But a diseased cell, it contains less light. It's like it loses light; it leaks light. A cancerous cell is almost dark. It can't contain hardly any light. So the intelligence cannot filter through the DNA in healthy processes in this cell. So I think prior to nutrition, the body, the cells must be flooded with light. That's the first priority of this cancer treatment.

Ty: Do you have a particular treatment that you use that will push light into the cells?

Dr. Fransen: It's exactly what you said. We teach cancer patients to flood their bodies with light. The most well-known way to do this is by taking fresh organic foods. You could say that sunlight is accumulated in the food, in greens, in fruits. When we eat this it's like the body can open this present, take the light out of it, and then this light resonates with the light of the cell itself and makes it stronger and more vital.

Ty: So Dr. Henk, how might somebody fill their cells with light?

Dr. Fransen: There are many ways to do this but the most well-known way is by eating fresh organic foods. You can say that the sunshine accumulates in greens and in fruits. So if we take this in it's like a present. The body can open it, take the light from it and it bio-resonates with the light in the cell itself and it strengthens it and makes it more vital.

And because the cancer cell is so dark and can hold so little light, we really literally have to flood this cell with light. So the normal amount of food is not enough for cancer patients. This is reflected in the Gerson Diet where cancer patients can take up to 30 or 40 kilograms of organic food each week, which you cannot digest that.

Especially when you are ill, when you have less energy and the digestive system is not so strong. So we have to juice this food. There are two things that are very important. When we juice with the normal juicers all the light goes out of the food too fast and it destroys the light. So we need slow juicing to protect the light in the food.

The second thing is we have to drink it within 15 minutes. Otherwise when we wait for half an hour or longer all the light has gone out of the food. The nutrients are still there, but first we need this amount of light. So this is one way to do it.

Another way, which is not so known in the West, but in Eastern Medicine, and in Yoga practices. The disciples learn certain breathing techniques which they combine with their concentration to take the Prana, the life force, the Qi or the Chi energy directly from the breath into the body.

In western culture we don't call it life force, but Holy Ghost. The Holy Ghost is really the spirit, the inspiration. We take the spirit, the life force in.

And an even more potent way to do this is directly looking into the sun. You can say the sun emanates many very small light particles. When we look directly in the sun we can absorb with the retina directly these light particles in our nervous system. This is very powerful, but not without danger or risk. So we should not look straight in the sun during the day. But it's possible in the first half an hour after sunrise and the first half an hour with sunset.

Ty: So you absorb it through your retina in your eye?

Dr. Fransen: Right. But there are some more restrictions even when you look at it [during] that time. So people should not try this at home, at least not before reading a book about it or looking at the Internet, what exactly is the protocol to do it. But it's very strong.

If we use all these techniques, we teach our cancer patients all these techniques to flood the body with light, then it filters through the DNA into those processes and there the nutrients are needed.

You can say the beauty of fresh organic foods is that with the light they bring all the vitamins, all the minerals, all the enzymes – everything necessary for the human body.

What I say [about] natural food is, "nature is God's laboratory." We have evolved as human beings millions of years in a close relationship to nature. The food and the human body are almost perfectly attuned to each other. No laboratory can match this and that's important.

If someone gets chronically ill there can be a depletion of the reserves in the body. So minerals, vitamins and all kinds of substances can be so low that we need extra supplementation with the nutrition for some time.

I think that just giving cancer patients a lot of supplements in high dosage is not good to do. With every individual patient we should test what exactly the nutrients are that are missing.

So we get first the light. Then we get the normal nutrition. And then we get some supplements that are tested for each individual. If we do this, it's so potent that the cell regains its full potential of self-healing and starts to regenerate. And the first step in regeneration is that it starts to detoxify.

Therapies like the Gerson Diet show that this is so potent, that there are so many waste products coming into the blood stream that people can get sick from these waste products. Or Gerson even says some people can even die from it, from a liver coma. So we should assist the body in detoxification.

Ty: And how would you do that? How would you assist the liver to detoxify?

Dr. Fransen: In the Gerson Diet and in the Gonzalez therapy and many other cancer therapies the best way to do this is with coffee enemas. Up to five or more each day during the healing crisis, but during the healing process at least two times a day.

There are many other ways to support the liver, the kidneys, the skin, the breathing, to help the body get rid of its toxic substances.

In my opinion we should understand that the body and the spirit are one. They are two sides of one coin. When the body starts to detoxify this also happens on the emotional and spiritual plane. When the body starts to heal itself you can see that all emotional wounds and spiritual pain comes to the surface to be released also.

But like we have to assist the body in this detoxification process, most cancer patients also need help in this process. We have many techniques like EFT, Emotional Trauma Therapy, and others, to help assist people to let go of their emotional pain.

Ty: What is EFT?

Dr. Fransen: EFT is a way of using affirmations while we tap certain acupuncture points to release old pain and to substitute them for new ideas and a new mindset.

Ty: So you're detoxifying not only the body but also the toxic emotions and the toxic feelings, I guess. The baggage that you might have.

Dr. Fransen: And it's very important that if we only focus on the physical and we don't assist the patient in the emotional and spiritual level and they cannot let go here of the toxic emotions, then all the energy in the physical body can really create friction on the other levels. That the tumor can even grow faster. We have seen this many times with patients. So this detoxification of the emotional and spiritual level with the physical level should go hand-in-hand.

Ty: I see. So is that one of the places where maybe the conventional model doesn't work as well, because they don't look at the emotional side of cancer? Maybe only treating the physical?

Dr. Fransen: Yes. And even at a physical plane they are more restoring from the outside. They are not working on the light, on the nutrition, and on all this support and detoxification. So I think that's also a lot missing in cancer therapies.

What we observed is if we do all this with cancer patients most patients do remarkably well, but not all of them. And we were triggered by this and we really did some research and we found out two other factors that are often forgotten.

The first is that the person can become whole or very strong by all these measures. But people have relationships and many relationships are stressful or they are even dis-easing the patient. And we have to look at that as well.

We saw that relations of a patient in this present time, like the partner, the children, they are often only a reflection of deeper wounds in the family system. So that is when our therapy, the Family Constellation work, comes in place. We look deeply with patients in their family constellation to find where the wounds are that stress the person itself.

Another thing we found is that the sleeping place is crucial for regeneration. You can say the oldest healing processes. They work out optimum during the night if someone goes to rest. So that's where the regeneration happens.

But in nature there are many places. Some places, they give power and energy. We really call them Power Places. But there are also places in nature that suck energy and where energy is taken away. We build our homes on every place. Many chronically ill patients sleep on a sleeping place that's not healthy.

So even if we do all these things that we were talking about and they sleep on such a place, they cannot create the momentum for complete healing. We have some experts on family constellation work, on testing the sleeping places, and making them healthy or correct them in anyway.

Ty: You mentioned one of the things that is important with sleep is the regeneration. Could it be anything to do with the fact that when you sleep well your body secretes melatonin?

Dr. Fransen: I think the body is very complex and this is just a small part of the whole. What I call a healthy body is a symphony of tens of thousands of processes and the hormones are very vital in that. And there's still one thing I want to add if that's possible?

Ty: Sure, of course.

Dr. Fransen: It's like what is light in the body, it has a parallel in the spirit for love. I think love and light are very closely related. And in the end we have to look with every cancer patient how they share and receive love.

I follow you and I see you sharing your love in the Ty Bollinger way. And I'm sharing it my unique Henk Fransen's way. I think using your talents, developing them, and contributing them to your society and to your community in a way they can be received is a lot of healing also.

We have observed that very often the way a cancer patient wants to express his love but is not capable of. The theme of this is closely related to the organ where the tumor is. So every organ in other medicine like Traditional Chinese Medicine, every organ is also a theme in emotion. And if this emotion is blocked in our life and if we cannot share it like we want to, it really stresses the organ also.

So on all these levels we have to work. And that makes clear that there is not standard therapy with cancer. We cannot say everybody should do everything. We should look with every cancer patient like what is missing in this patient and what needs to be the emphasis in this patient. So we make like a painter that has a palette. We create a treatment for every patient.

Ty: So it's an individualized approach based upon where that person is deficient?

Dr. Fransen: Right, on these many levels.

Ty: On many levels. One of the questions I was going to ask you is why does certain cancer manifest in different organs? And you just kind of answered that. Maybe it's because of the different emotional blockages that relate to that particular part of the body. Very interesting.

Dr. Fransen: And like some experts say, it's about oxygen, the oxygen in the cell, the cell breathing. You can say if we have a blockage on a certain organ, emotional, it will restrict the blood stream a little bit in that organ. If the circumstances in the body are on the edge, that organ will feel it first.

Ty: Dr. Henk, why do you think that there are so many children getting cancer today?

Dr. Fransen: That's a completely different topic with many layers which are quite sensitive to share, because it often creates guilt feelings with the parents. But to address a few, you could say children are grown up souls in a small body. And they lived almost as long as a grown up person.

Especially if you understand that in pregnancy in nine months we develop like millions of years the evolution of mankind. So this is such a long time and such a sensitive period that children can get deformities from medicines and the mother doesn't have any problem with it. So it's a very sensitive period in which many of the pollutions, many of the stresses in normal day life can affect the child more than the grown up people.

Ty: More sensitive.

Dr. Fransen: Yes. And then you have a part of the family constellation work where wounds in the family, in the generations even, they can stress especially the most sensitive elements of that family and that are often sensitive children. So that can also be a link of extra stress which makes the body break down.

There are also some spiritual factors. But I think you should make a follow-up theory, then I'll come and explain on that because that's a whole topic by itself.

Ty: Sure. Thank you for sharing what you did because it makes a lot of sense. One of the things that a lot of medical doctors in the United States have told me is that they think it's vaccine related because of all the vaccines in the United States. I know here in Holland you don't vaccinate to the extent we do in the United States.

We are number one in the world in vaccines. We give more vaccines to children than any other country. So that's what a lot of medical doctors said there. Fortunate for your children here you don't vaccinate to that same extent.

Dr. Fransen: Yes, it's getting more and more and they are clustered together. And it's one of the examples, what I say that the stresses that a grown up person can handle is too much for a child because it's much more sensitive. This world is full of these things. And of course it's not one drop in their bucket, but it's half a bucket.

Ty: Right. So Dr. Henk what would your advice be to someone that's recently been diagnosed with cancer? What should they ask their doctor? What questions should they ask to make sure they are being treated properly?

Dr. Fransen: I think it's more important than what they ask their doctor. I would advise them to take all their possibilities, both conventional and alternative, to really orient and find the best doctors in both fields. To be informed and to find out what might be most helpful for them.

I would really advise them, like I get a little bit sad that most cancer patients that come to me they are already a long time on their way, and they are really kind of self-help patients. They have found out by themselves. I think that's one of the values of your series, that we inform people better, because people get very confused on the Internet by all the information.

I think with a cold you can treat yourself, but with cancer you should take that very seriously and find the best doctors in both fields to help you. I would really advise that. Because to a certain extent you can help yourself and understand, but then you need really an expert on this.

Ty: Right. I think that's good advice. You use the best that we have to offer. Not all conventional medicine is bad. Not all alternative medicine is good. Find the best of both. Find a doctor or practitioner that can help guide you along the way and get rid of the toxicities, get rid of the emotional toxicities. I think that's good advice.

Well, thank you for what you're doing. We really are on the same mission to help inform and educate everyone. I really appreciate the time that you spent with us today. This has been fascinating.

Dr. Fransen: Thanks, Ty.

[end of transcript]

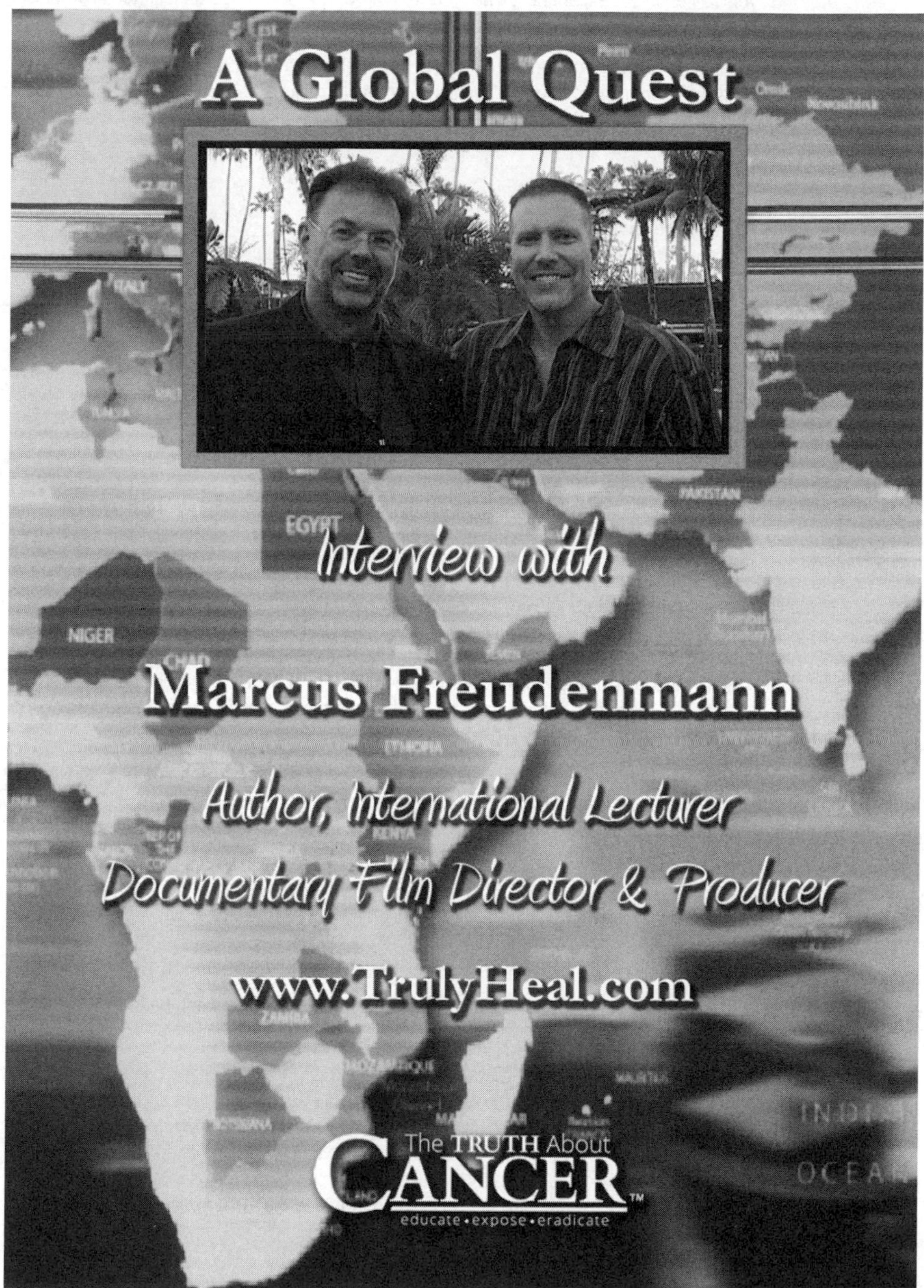
A Global Quest
Interview with
Marcus Freudenmann
Author, International Lecturer
Documentary Film Director & Producer
www.TrulyHeal.com
The TRUTH About
CANCER
educate • expose • eradicate

Ty: Marcus, thank you for being here with me today, and if you could, tell the viewers a little bit about yourself and your experience, what you've done with your documentaries, and then we'll get into the treatment protocols.

Marcus: Well, the main thing is we started to research cancer treatments in a very big way. I packed up my family and we traveled from clinic to clinic, and stayed in every clinic, and learned with all the doctors. And that turned into the first documentary, *Cancer is Curable Now*. But during that time I was on the quest to find the cure, you know, like—I recommend you buy it.

Ty: I like that name.

Marcus: And that's why also the name, *Cancer is Curable*.

Ty: Right.

Marcus: And we released the movie, and put it out, and the first feedback I got was not very positive—snake oil and everything. And the second part that was really big in that concern was that when you do something like that you don't have long-term experience, you rely on word of mouth. And five years down the track I realized that many of the things that we had put into the documentary didn't really work that consistently, or weren't that successful, or didn't work for everybody.

So I was kind of disillusioned and disenchanted. And I went back to the drawing board, and I was looking for that missing piece. What is it that makes Gerson therapy work for some, but not for all? And what is that helps with pancreatic enzymes, or hypothermia? So we really started to dig very, very deep into every treatment and what it does and why it works for some doctors but not for all.

And that's when I had an interview with Dr. Rao and he just really knocked me. He said, "Marcus, you shouldn't be asking what treatments I do, you should be asking what is wrong, how do you find the cause for that client, why does that person have cancer?" So I said, "Okay, if I ask that, what do you do?" And he said, "Well, then I tell you exactly that we approach it by finding the problem that suppressed the immune system, by finding the system that is out of balance, by finding the toxicity levels. And as soon as we know that and we balance that out, then we add a cancer treatment on top and it works."

And I was like, "Okay." And it really rattled my cage. I went home, started to learn about it, change, and edit, and then I thought, "Instead of making a new movie, I can't sell my old one anymore, there are so many things in there which aren't correct, I can't do that." So I dumped 10,000 DVDs, I dumped all my books. You know, you call Amazon and say, "Flush it."

Ty: Which is actually admirable to do because that was a big financial hit.

Marcus: It was, but on the other side, I can't sleep if I send people to a clinic and then they call me, and if you have 20 calls saying it didn't work, or it doesn't work, it's not very positive.

Ty: What that tells me about you, Marcus, is that you're a man of integrity. You want the truth to get out there.

Marcus: And I want to find the truth. So what we did is we changed our protocol, we developed a massive mind map to outline why do certain treatments work? Why does GcMAF work with him but not with all the others? What did I do differently? So we really outlined all of that and put that together. And once we had that protocol I presented that to a board of oncologists. I didn't want to go alternative doctors, I really wanted to have that reviewed by doctors—I almost said proper doctors—not that I discredit, but people that I respected in the community. So I presented that, and the most exciting thing. I was so nervous. You wouldn't believe, I was really freaking out, to present. I'm an architect.

Ty: You were presenting to oncologists.

Marcus: Yes, and I certainly don't have the medical background so I presented my research. They all sat there and wrote notes and put their hands up like school, you know. I shouldn't say that, but they put their hands up and asked questions, very polite. In the end all of them signed up for the protocol, signed up to become a test group. They established funds for a clinic to run our protocol for three years to check out how it works. The whole thing turned around. And all of a sudden we got peer review, we got research funding, we got everything to make it work.

And we are now three years in that trial, three years that the clinic has incorporated, step-by-step, all the different things. Because you know, yourself, from your studies, Germans do it different than Americans do it. Everybody has their specialties. What we've done with our protocol, we packed that all together with reasoning why each of the treatments work and how they work.

So it's now three years and yesterday was actually the official launch of our protocol because it's cleared. We can now sign up doctors, we can sign up practitioners, we have a three-year education program, a one-year education program, where doctors can learn how to implement that treatment, or how to look at all factors. And I just showed it to some of the doctors here at the show. Dr. [Cornely] has sent two doctors up to the show. Dr. Tony— so it's going to be something that we slowly integrate into the American market, as well.

Ty: That's awesome. That's really unique, I've not heard of anything like that, especially if medical doctors are now hopping on board wanting to learn about it.

Marcus: Sixteen standard conventional oncologists are now in our program, and I'll tell you what, they are having a hard time.

Ty: Tell me about the program.

Marcus: The program is actually an online program. It is about a 500-page book and it covers all the different protocols. And it's really divided into the main problems. We have seven areas. Like inflammation—we've heard that today in almost every talk. Every doctor spoke about inflammation. We need to reduce inflammation because it promotes cancer growth and it actually causes cancer in the first place. We have toxicity, we have deficiencies, we have organ failures or organ problems like liver detoxification problems, phase I, phase II.

So it's really broken into many different areas so when you work through with the client you can't forget anything. You cannot overlook hormones because it's not a pet treatment or you don't like it. You still have to look at some of the main tests and at least exclude it. And if you find in those tests that that is completely out of whack you have to at least find an expert that works with it because, let's be very honest, I think that's one of the main problems that has driven me: depending on the pet protocol a doctor has. They will follow that and ignore all the rest. Some of them have no interest in diet. You get macaroni and cheese and whatever in their clinic to eat and they tell you don't eat sugar but they don't care for it. In other clinics you are going to have no interest in hormones. Another clinic has not the slightest interest in mind, or psychology, or support. Others don't want to educate.

Now, when you go, as a patient, and you miss out on the most important area for you just because the doctor doesn't like it, you lose probably a lot of money and have no success with your treatments. And that was my main concern that we integrate everything. And you don't need to do everything, but at least when you find out that this is a contributing factor, that you then call in an expert or someone else to work with you.

Ty: So this protocol you developed, is it available for the general public to see online, or to purchase online so that they can learn, or is it just available for medical doctors?

Marcus: At the moment it's only available for health practitioners, which is naturopaths, nutritionists, everybody who has already a title who can work with clients, with patients. Our next step would be coaches, because I know exactly a doctor will always be limited in what they do. Coaches can help patients to work through, like you help a lot of people to find their way through. So if you have someone that is fully educated, knows the whole protocol, they can guide people.

And in October or November we are going to release a free app online for iPad, iPhone, for Android, for everything, which gives you step-by-step, what to do when diagnosed, what tests you need, what things your doctor should check, how he should check it, what kind of relevant—like blood serum tests, or urine test, or hormone—which ones are the most reliable, so that you can go through and really get a full-on education. Then you can work with your own oncologist, or with your own doctor. And it's been my challenge to the system. I've rattled a lot of cages with that.

Ty: That's awesome because when this is going to be airing, this "Global Quest for the Cures" it's going to be October.

Marcus: We could do that together, yes.

Ty: So how can they get the free app?

Marcus: Well, it will be online on iTunes and everything. We do it for 24 hours free, so we just use all our networks. We have massive networks.

Ty: Where would they go, what would they look for? What would be the keywords that would find it? Or would they go to your website that would have a link through to it? How can they find it?

Marcus: That would be on our website and through all our partners that will send out the email. We build it up and then we launch it all in one day because we have one goal. We need to get it all downloaded within one day, you know that.

Ty: Right.

Marcus: So that we get into the hit charts and iTunes and everywhere so that we really hit the market, and then it will stay there. So we'll just try to do that within 24 hours in October, and everybody who is on our website, on our newsletter, on your newsletter, they will learn about that.

Ty: What is your website?

Marcus: trulyhealed.com.

Ty: trulyhealed.com.

Marcus: Yes.

Ty: Marcus, that's fascinating information. It's almost like you just took everything and you put it into the full meal deal, right?

Marcus: That's it.

Ty: Except it's not McDonald's full meal deal, it's an organic full meal deal, right? But you put it all together.

Marcus: It took us, in total now, 15 years to put that all together and it's come, really, to the conclusion in the last four years since we have the funding and the support to really make it concrete. Every treatment, everything is referenced, it has Pub Med, it has research studies, everything included. And in the practitioner app they have everything at their fingertips. They just type through—every disease, every protocol, client management, all included.

Ty: Wow. This is truly evidence-based medicine right here because you have the links to the studies.

Marcus: I told you I've moved away from alternative into holistic. And holistic includes the mind, it includes the diet, includes everything in one package.

Ty: And it's all supported by medical studies.

Marcus: Exactly.

Ty: Yes. Marcus, you are a hero to many people. I'm really thrilled to be able to meet you here.

Marcus: I'm likewise happy to be here.

Ty: We just kind of ran into each other today. I really am a big fan of what you are doing, and I know that your heart, your goal, is to help people, the same as ours is. And so for that I am thankful, and I'm really thankful for the time that you spent tonight to share this with us. Thank you so much.
[end of transcript]

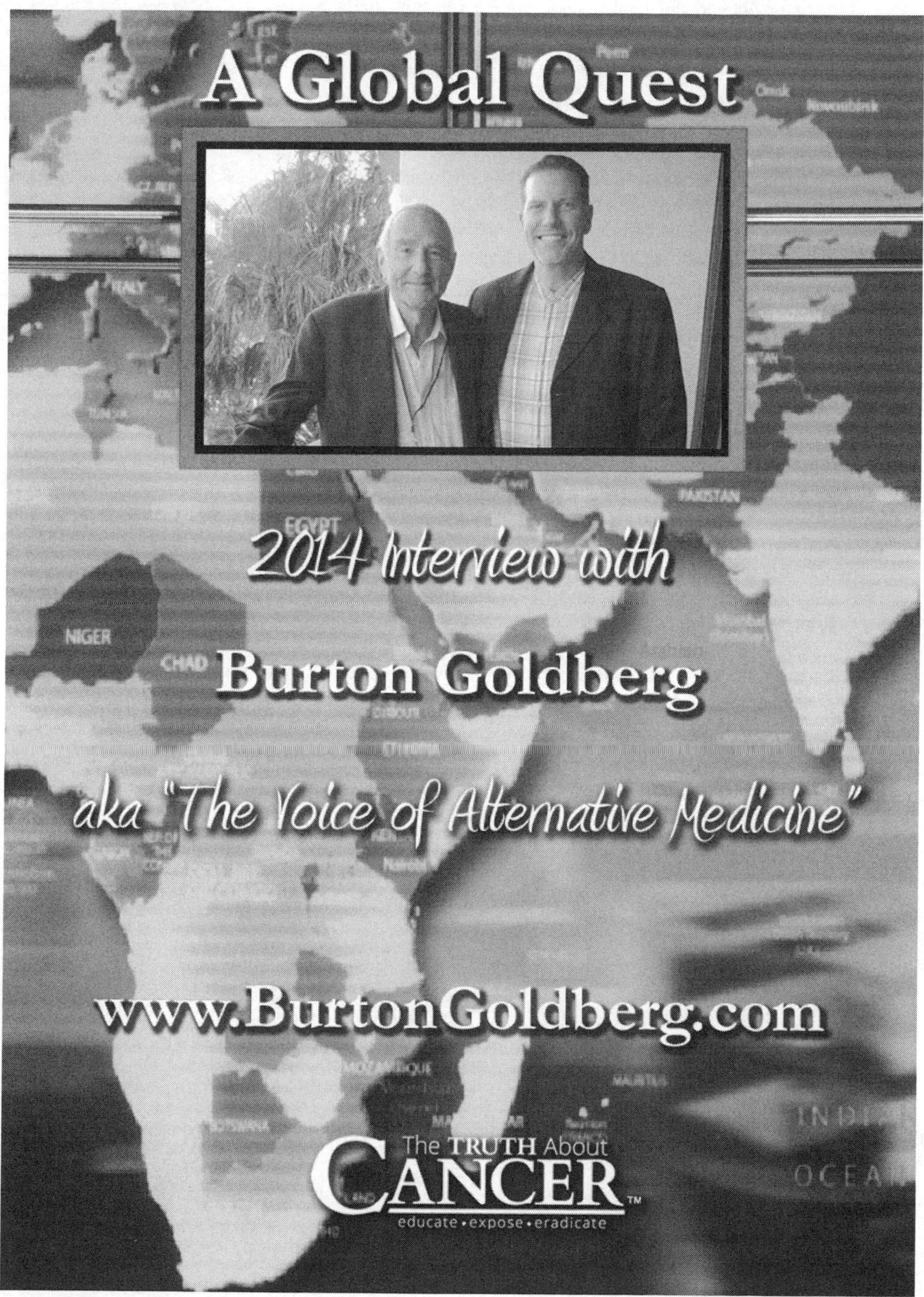
A Global Quest
2014 Interview with
Burton Goldberg
aka "The Voice of Alternative Medicine"
www.BurtonGoldberg.com
The TRUTH About
CANCER™
educate • expose • eradicate

Ty: Well, today I'm honored to have Burton Goldberg here with me -"The voice of alternative medicine" - and I just want to say thank you for taking the time out of your busy schedule to come talk to us today Burton, thank you so much. Let me ask you something, Burton, how did you get into health research? You've written several books on health and we'll talk about those but what got you interested in doing research on health?

Burton: About 45 years ago the woman that I was in love with, lived in Miami, had a daughter who at the age of 19 slit her wrists. She was depressed, anxiety, panic, and it was a holistic physician in California who did a five hour glucose tolerance test and she shook like a leaf and she was hypoglycemic. Simply a bleture of balance and when he treated her with diet and nutrition she got well from mental illness and that put me on the road to studying medicine. I was business man. I had no concept of medicine in any way, shape or form. I ran a night club/restaurant/hotel. I started the California Pizza Kitchen chain with two lawyers. I had no knowledge of medicine. But I kept reading books and the more I read the more I realized the corruption that exists in medicine.

Ty: I had no idea that you were one of the founders of the California Pizza Kitchen. Wow, so you have a business background.

Burton: I have a business background and so I approached medicine on a business basis. I'm not a practicing physician. I don't know anything about healing people except I know who does and who does the best job. And so and then I ended up doing a book called *Alternative Medicine: The Definitive Guide*. Which earned me a doctorate from a little medical school called Capital University. There I covered the entire school of alternative medicine. Therapies and how the doctors who practice the therapies use them for various health conditions. It was an 1100 page book and sold very, very well and it put me right up there. After that, I became a center for information and doctors would contact me and one thing would lead to another. Then I did an 1100 page book on cancer back in 1997, which is somewhat ancient history because the world's changed since then, but it's saved a lot of lives. I just enjoy learning from the physicians who successfully reverse these health conditions.

Ty: Those books are no small books believe me we interviewed Dr. Rashid Buttar whom you know. He's got both of those books on his bookshelf in his office and each of them about that wide, so they're big books. Lots of information in those books.

Burton: They are very, very important books. The definitive guide took four years because it had never been done before. Then the cancer book took me two years. But you remember everyone in that book is a physician who successfully reverses these health conditions.

Ty: Those books, they've sold what, a million plus copies?

Burton: Over a million copies all together but the big book which sold for $65 sold about 750,000 copies. Costco and the discount stores and television commercials and so forth and it became the bible and so almost every physician at that era has one on their library.

Ty: That's impressive. That's something to be proud of because through that information in that book you've probably influenced thousands, millions of lives.

Burton: I can't tell you how many physicians today tell me that book was a turning point for them and had them go into medicine and into the integrative aspect, or alternative aspect of medicine.

Ty: Was that your goal when you wrote the books?

Burton: Absolutely. My goal was to make a change in a very corrupt system.

Ty: Talk about corruption, you mentioned that now twice thus far, what about the current medical paradigm do you see as being corrupt?

Burton: You've got to separate medicine. There's preventative medicine. There's the emergency room and trauma and there's degenerative disease. You can't beat mainstream medicine in the emergency room and trauma. For preventions, they're ignorant. For degenerative disease they're guilty of crimes against humanity. The medical profession does not tell the truth and many of the systems that they use are truly not healthy. For instance, cancer. The oncologist uses sugar to carry the radiologic molecule into the cancer cell to show up on the x-ray, the PET scan. The oncologists knows that sugar feeds cancer because that's why he uses that as a Trojan horse. When you finish your chemo, in a conventional setting, they give you cookies and ice cream or candy. That is tantamount to putting gasoline on a fire. That means these oncologists are guilty of crimes against humanity. They are killing their patients. How else do you explain it? Would you call it ignorance? Would you call it stupidity? I don't know what to call it. You come up with a term. Feeding sugar to cancer patients when we all know that in order to have 7.4 saliva to make your body inhospitable to the critters, cancer cells, viruses and bacteria. Before you brush your teeth in the morning you should have a 7.4 and you can't do it with sugar. Sugar acidifies the body.

Ty: That does seem to be tantamount to crimes against humanity. Because being a medical doctor they know. Talk about sugar. Why is it? What is it about sugar that feeds the cancer?

Burton: Well cancer subsides on sugar. It loves sugar. And in order to reverse cancer you have to remove all the poisons and toxins and diet plays an enormous role and you can't do it with food alone you need to use certain products. When I guide people with cancer as a consultant I put all of them on a very special diet and you can find that diet free of charge on my website, BurtonGoldberg.com, under research, and it's Dr. Bernardo Majalca alkaline diet. It's 22 double pages. Plenty to eat. There's meats you can eat. Very special buffalo, lamb, goat, deer. There's rice you can eat. Certain rice. There's potatoes. Only bread you can have is Ezekiel bread and lots of juicing. Lots of raw food. I've used this test for years. It was given to me by Dr. Bernardo who passed away, god rest his soul, and it works. So diet plays an enormous role. Dentistry plays an enormous role, 95 percent of females with breast cancer have a dental involvement. Truman University study. As much as 50 percent in the remission of cancer can be in the oral cavity on ordinary cancers other than breast. But in breast cancer it's 95 percent. So everyone one of my clients are sent to a biologic dentist and all of these things that I recommend through trial and error and learning from the masters, the physicians are important. You can't leave anything out. You have to go to the cause, remove the thorn and god will heal. There's no easy way out you've got to do the work. Diet, nutrition, lifestyle, so cancer feeds on sugar.

Ty: I like that quote. Remove the thorn and god will heal. You remove the thing that's in the way of your health and your body's going to heal itself. That's the way god made it.

Burton: If you feed the immune system. If you take away every insult to the immune system. Whether it's plastic breast implants, or dentistry, or even geopathic stress. These noxious rays on everything from omnisphere down to the ground. I learned this in Germany back in the 80's when I went to school with doctors there. You must remove every insult to the immune system. Get rid of all the heavy metals. These are not easy things to do. They are not simple, but they can be done with a competent physician and you do need help. You do need a physician. Who is experienced in putting cancer in remission. At this conference where we have many doctors talking about no chemotherapy. I also agree. No chemotherapy the way conventional uses it. It is truly needed evil. Can you imagine, you lose your hair and vomit? Is the treatment they give you? But you can use chemotherapy. And since 2002 after Human *Genome Project* that the U.S. government performed, my mentor Albert Shellar went to a clinic, a laboratory in Germany, and said, why don't we use the genome project and find out what products will knock out the cancer in a patient's blood.

And so if you send your blood to Germany or Greece or some of the good laboratories. There are only a few in the world. None in the United States you can know which natural substance or chemotherapeutic agent will target the cells. So when all these people talk about no chemo, they're ancient history, because you can use targeting chemo. And what you're targeting is not only the primary, but the minute you put a needle in the cancer tumor or a knife it spreads and it can spread without the knife or the needle. Contrary to what your oncologists say. That's another form of crimes against humanity.

Ty: Spreading the cancer via biopsy.

Burton: And saying it doesn't happen. The biopsy doesn't spread it. It does whether its prostate or breasts, wherever. So you're looking for the circulating tumor cells. These are the ones that metastasize. That's why, John Wayne, died 12 years after his first cancer. Because they paid no attention to the circulating tumor cells. They knocked out the primary, but the primary is a piece of junk according to our doctors. It is the circulating cells that go to the kidney and the brain and the lungs. So you have to pay attention to both. In this country it's not available.

The man who developed this was Dr. Albert Shellar, went to the National Cancer Institute and said, this is what I find with the genome project, I developed this system. We can tell which chemotherapeutic agent will work on that person's circulating tumor cells and what natural substances, Vitamin C, or you name it. And it's done in Greece and it's done in Germany. I use a company called Biofocus in Germany. So that you know in advance. I've had cancer twice. I'm 87 years of age. Give you a perspective, I was in the Second World War. I am the same age as the Queen. I am a year older than the pope that retired. I've had cancer twice and I've had the best skiing of my life two weeks ago up in Aspen, Colorado. I've been on some special stem cells, unbelievable. Works fantastic. Anyway, cancer must be checked constantly. Once you have cancer and it goes in remission you must constantly, every year or two check and see that these circulating tumor cells are no longer present. Which I do, I sent my blood to Germany. And then they tell me. Now the purpose of knowing which chemo will work allows the doctor to use micros amounts of chemo. In other words it's never the full amount, because it does destroy the immune system. But if you use five, seven, ten percent fractionalized doses of the targeted chemos, and it can be one or two. Because the minute it leaves the primary it mutates and what works on a primary will not work on the circulating tumor cells.

So Biofocus has this test, it's pricey and they have a less expensive one that says you have cancer or you don't. But, the expensive one tells you which chemo or natural substances will target that cell. So the doctor then will use insulin potentiated carrying using sugar to carry the chemotherapy into the tumor, and then if you use full body hypothermia you have a 14 times better effect of killing the cancer than not having the full body hypothermia. Hypothermia, they put you in a chamber, your head's outside, you're in for an hour a day for two weeks. If you need more it's every other day because the heat shock. And it opens up the body and allows the chemo to go into the cancer cell and kill it. Remember it's five, 10 percent. You're not killing the healthy cells.

Ty: So it's a fractional dose of what the normal chemotherapy would be.

Burton: Fractional dose targeted with insulin potentiated.

Ty: To my knowledge that's called IPTLD, insulin potentiated low dose.

Burton: Exactly, targeted low dose.

Ty: Okay.

Burton: And with full body hypothermia, a temperature of 105, 107 unbelievable results.

Ty: And probably very nominal side effects because of the lower dose.

Burton: Minimal, you have very few violent side effects and that is what I believe. But you have to do the dentistry, you have to do the mental. Some people don't want to live, and the mind-body plays a role.

Ty: Yeah.

Burton: Look, have you ever heard an oncologist give up and say what's causing cancer? I have never heard an oncologist say, "what's causing cancer?" You ask them they'll say cigarette smoking and the sun, and we don't know. That's why their success rate is so miserable. When my daddy was born in 1900 one in 33 Americans had cancer of any kind, shape or form. When I was born in 1926 cancer was the tenth cause of death in children. Today it's the first cause of death before accidents. What's going on? There's a holocaust. It's not a question of will I have cancer, it's a question of when. And the oncologists are keeping their mouth shut. They use the chemo, they use the radiation. And radiation causes cancer. Mammograms cause cancer, we know that. Medical research, the medical journals prove it. And yet they still do it. Whereas stenography and ultrasound can be very beneficial without the violent side effects of annual mammograms and squeezing the breast. That's what happens if there is a tumor there. You're squeezing it through the body. It's insanity.

So the medical profession in my opinion is corrupt as any third world nation and this country is allowing it. And the reason it's allowing it is because subsequent to the Roosevelt administration the agencies that were designed to protect humanity are protecting the industry they're supposed to protect us from. The FDA knows silver fillings in the mouth are one of the major causes of degenerative disease and so forth. The CDC knows that autism is caused by mercury. They know it. They know that the thimerosal that was used as a preservative, although they took it out. They then put in aluminum, and aluminum causes autism. This country cannot survive until we take back the government from the corporations. It's not Democrat or Republican, and the doctors keep their mouths shut. The media takes ad from the purple pill. They're not going to tell you the truth.

The entire structure is corrupt. There is no way Obamacare will survive with the amount of degenerative disease and autism that's going on. In 1950 autism was unheard of. This is our generation. These are the next generation that is going to preserve this country and bring us forward. In 1950 it was unheard of, in 1970 it was one in 10,000. You know what the rate is today? One in 55 boys. When I did my film "Greed," it was one in 150, that was three years ago, it's now down to one in 55. Something's fishy in Denmark and it is the vaccines and the CDC knows this. They did the Simpsonwood Report. Google it. Because everything I say, Google. Go there, find out you'll see. Read the Simpsonwood Report. There's an abstract of it where you can read it decently quickly. They know it and they lie. They're deceitful and when I say this government is corrupt, it's corrupt down to the core. The CDC knows, that's the Communicative Disease Center in Atlanta, the Simpsonwood was a conference where they sat around and they talk about how mercury in the vaccines were giving the wrong numbers. So they fudged the numbers.

Ty: Let me ask you this, Burton. One of the things that it sounds to me that is causing some of these treatments that you're talking about to be so effective is that they're not cookie cutter treatments. The treatments that you're talking about in Germany and Greece are specific for that person due to a blood analysis and they're able to target those specific cancer cells using a much lower dose of chemo for that person.

Burton: Which brings up, that's actually true. Which brings up the subject of double blind studies. They are as corrupt as can be. One size shoe, one size bra fits all. In integrative and alternative medicine you must use multiple therapies. You can't just do a silver bullet. There is no silver bullet. You need a whole bunch of these bullets. So you have to go to the cause. Find out what caused it and one of the best ways of doing it is using quantum physics a device called electrodermal screening. The ability to tap into the body noninvasively. All my clients go to a medical detective who uses a quantum physics device to tap into the body noninvasively and know what poisons prohibited the organs and systems to function optimally. Which allowed you to come down with cancer.

Ty: Specific to that person?

Burton: Specific to that person because one can have cadmium or lead or mercury or zinc or who knows. You don't know and that's why you have to do individual diagnosis with each patient and there are certain tests for finding out certain metals. Metals have to be pulled out, toxins and poisons.

Look, today it's impossible to avoid cancer. Even if you're a vegetarian, which incidentally I don't believe most Americans can be vegetarians. Most Americans who come from Europe background have been eating meat for century upon century and they need it. But what meat? Our meat supply is corrupt. Mad cow disease is prevalent in the United States today. I did the film called Greed which never did get out. Where I talked about cancer, autism and mad cow disease, 15 percent of Alzheimer patients are Creutzfeldt-Jakob form of mad cow disease. This is a double university study. Yale, and Pittsburgh. The Pittsburgh study was done by a friend. I asked that friend scientist to go on camera. He refused. The other one was done by a female scientist in Yale, refused to go on camera.

But, when you extrapolate all the numbers, a percentage of Alzheimer's have Creutzfeldt-Jakob or mad cow disease. We taught the French and the English how to use it. And the corruption in this country is they're hiding it from the public. The only meat that I eat is grass fed beef, organic chicken. I won't use GMO's because GMO's cause cancer. The study in the Frenchman was cooperated by a man in Bangkok under the government of Thailand. After seven months, tumors arise, where Monsanto only did it for three. I think the Séralini's study and then it was withdrawn from the medical journal but the Thai study did the same study and it turned out to be accurate. In minute concentrations GMO's cause cancer. Nuclear energy, there are higher rates of cancer around every nuclear power plant.

We know this because of the Tooth Fairy Project that was started under the Kennedy administration. He put the testing underground because of the scientist who went to him who told him, you're hurting the population. You're coming down with more cancer. We have in this country for Genobyl we still have thyroid cancer fexo thyroid in just everybody. That's why one of the reasons for obesity. The thyroid malfunctions. The thyroid's a thermostat, it's poisoned. There are higher rates of cancer around every nuclear power plant and what happens is strontium-90 never existed on the globe until nuclear energy. The bomb and nuclear power plants. Goes up in the sky. The wind blows it downwind. It goes on the grasses, the cows eat the grass. Strontium-90 has an affinity for calcium. It goes into the milk. The child drinks the milk, comes down with cancer. You have ice cream comes into you.

There's no way of avoiding it, so if you want your loved ones to survive you must pay attention to integrative medicine. You must vote, you must become politically active. The only ray of hope I see is if you take back your government from the corporation. If you don't we're dead ducks. Autism is now one in 55 boys, in 1970 it was one in 10,000. Have you ever heard a pediatrician yell, "what's causing autism"? "What's causing cancer," from your oncologist? They all play the game. They keep the ball rolling. They keep their mouths shut. But you, to protect yourself and your loved ones, better learn this. By the time we wake up and by the time the public gets the information it will be too late. So, you must vote and you must vote people in who are conscious of your health. Look, they've robbed our banks, not one individual who robbed us for that 2008 bankruptcy of this nation. Not one of them went to jail, not one. They're not only robbing your money, they're robbing your health and the media who takes money from the big purple pill are not going to tell you the truth. Agriculture, the head of the FDA is on the board of the Shrine Company, the largest manufactures of silver fillings which have 50 percent mercury in it.

Ty: Conflict of interest.

Burton: The head of the FDA. She knows that Bisphenol A is one of the major causes. She has the research of the cancer of the breast and prostate. Plastics are one of the major causations of cancer in this nation. She knows it and it's not banned. Every single can that you use has a lining. Here's a can of water that was given to me. Guaranteed Bisphenol A is lining every can. It comes in plastic. Harvard just did a study. They gave a man a can of minestrone soup. It happened to be a brand, it doesn't matter. They're all the same whether it's beer, whether it's water or minestrone. They checked his body burden of bisphenol A. one week later after eating the can of Progresso minestrone his BPA level went up 1,200 percent in one week it was still 1,200 percent. It goes in, does its problem in the prostate, in the breast and because it makes the organ heavier and it turns it into cancer. It's a perfect storm. It's not just one thing, it's a multiple bunch of things. And dentistry we talked about diet, the GMO's the pesticides and herbicides.

Ty: We're surrounded by toxicities that are compromising our immune system. Talk about the lymphatic system.

Burton: We're being poisoned to death. One of the systems, the garbage removal system of our body, is the lymph system and very few cancer physicians pay attention to the lymph system. It is the basis of lymphocytes, these are the good guys. And it also is the garbage removal system of the body and I use a device myself. I have one that I use on myself called the light beam generator. But there's a few of them that fractionalize the molecules. Women who have surgery in the breast and the lymphedema happens. As a matter of fact that's how I earned my doctorate.

A woman in Pennsylvania had a leg that was so swollen she was about to die. Her husband who was a retired Rear Admiral in the Navy buys my book and sees a doctor in Oregon. Takes his wife Muffy Fanning to Oregon and they're looking through the electric thermal screening device in the dark field microscope and they finally put her to sleep and then wake her up. Takes her blood and they see the parasite for Elephantiasis. And they use conventional drug here, see I'm not against medicine, I'm against, in emergency and trauma they're the best in the world. But in degenerative disease there are certain drugs and heroic surgeries. I would have been blind, I'm 87 without these cataracts removed and I have lenses sewn in. I can see close with one eye and it's amazing what wonderful medicine can do. But, don't confuse that with degenerative diseases where they become legalized drug pushers. And pay no attention to the immune system except to cut it out when they find cancer near the breast. So you must fractionalize the molecules and open up. Now, very few cancer clinics use it and need it and do it. But, that's one of the ways you get the immune system functioning optimally.

Ty: They are stimulating the lymph through fractionizing.

Burton: Fractionalizing, the trampoline is also another way of opening up but, and the Vodder method where they did a massage on the lymph system, but the lengthening generators or the youth noble gasses. I saw a study years ago when I was doing my book of a clot in a dog and these clots can kill you. So they put the lightning generator on. It disappeared like a cloud in the sky. They had a camera in the vein of the dog and that's how it works. It fractionalizes molecules and opens it up. So Muffy Fanning ended up living and her husband in payback became chairman of the board of Little Medical School for doctors in Washington D.C. and they honored me with a doctorate back in 1999.

Ty: What a great story. I've heard you say, Burton, before, that we're being starved to death.

Burton: We're not only being starved to death, we're being poisoned to death and that's the purpose. Wake up America. There's things you can do. But the number one thing you need to do in addition to protecting you and your loved ones is vote and make sure you put people in who are not hacks. This president Obama is no different than the two before. Democrat, Republican, Clinton was as bad as Bush, was as bad as Obama. The agencies that were designed to protect us are staffed by people who are protecting in industry and until you take back the government from the corporations you're going to be dead ducks. See, the doctors can't say this. They'll lose their license. I don't practice. I'm an old Jew so there's nothing they can do.

Ty: Nothing they can do to you. So, kind of shifting gears here, Burton. You were featured in Suzanne Somers book *Knockout*. Tell me a little bit about that.

Burton: Well, Suzanne, my first run-in with her, well, see she was on Larry King and many, many years ago, and he said why did you have liposuction on your breast. She said Larry, these scandalous magazines reported her. She said, Larry, I had cancer of the breast and I wanted to level the look of my breasts. He said you had cancer? He said how did you get into, what are you doing for it. She says I'm doing alternative medicine. He said alternative medicine, how did you get into that? She said another nice Jewish boy by the name of Burton Goldberg did a book called *Alternative Medicine Definitive Guide*.

That's the book I put out in 1997. And this was a year or two later. And so CNN called and I came down and they wanted to know about mistletoe which helps the immune system. And so I was seen all over the world on that. So that's how she first came in contact with me. And then other doctors had recommended me for the book. And although I'm not a medical doctor I do have knowledge because I've been traveling the world trying to find the best that will work on cancer. So, she interviewed me. She's very bright. And she has done more for alternative cancer and integrative cancer treatment than anyone else because of her celebrityship and she's a stunning, bright human being. Courageous, caring and has saved a lot of lives.

Ty: And, I'm sure that I'm not going out on a limb here when I say that you have saved a lot of lives as well with your books. With the reach that you had. So that's something to be really proud of, because you have changed the world in no small way. Through your publications, through your research through your books and you're one of my heroes. So I just want you to know that. We've only got a couple of minutes left. Anything that you want to touch that we haven't touched. I was going to ask you as far as who you would recommend, what doctors, what clinics you might recommend so...

Burton: I have several clinics around the United States. Depends on the case, the financing and so forth. So I do consultations. My website is BurtonGoldberg.com. I would highly recommend you see my film Cancer Conquest. You can pay 20 bucks and see an hour and a half. I promise you if you have cancer it will change your life. Cancer Conquest is the film yes. You can see it online.

Ty: Burton, tell us a little bit about your involvement with anti-aging.

Burton: Well, I think I'm a poster boy. At 87 I look, feel, have the energy and I've been on stem cells for many years and I guide people in the art of staying young and healthy and I send them to medical detectives to find out and look for disease before it manifests. Don't wait for diagnosis. One of the biggest problems in medicine today is when your doctor tells you, you have this, or you have that look for trouble. And don't do mammograms. Thermography, ultrasound and electrodermal screening. Tap into the body noninvasively. I can't stress enough. I'm here today because about eight million years ago I had kidney failure. I almost died and I went to Charlotte, North Carolina and I had been sent from Germany with cancer of the stomach and I went to Buttar. I flew back to the United States because I had insurance here and he put me in a hospital. He says you don't have stomach cancer, you have a large prostate and you have kidney failure. So I went to Germany and I tried to shrink it. I couldn't shrink it so I had green laser therapy on my prostate and now I'm living happily ever after.

Ty: That's a great story. Early detection is what we focus on and a lot of times the conventional cancer industry focuses on early detection. That's not necessarily a bad thing, it's just what method are you using to detect it is what I'm hearing from you.

Burton: Yeah. There's too many false positives with mammograms and the mammograms are medical x-rays. When you go to the dentist they cover your sexual organs and they run out of the room. Why are they running? Because the radiation from x-rays mutates cells. And when they replicate, they replicate outwardly. So, it's very important to not use x-rays. There are times when you need it. There are times you need PET scans, so the doctor knows as a base where to go, and what to do, and you're going to be very careful. But using the blood test to see circulating tumor cells are one of the most important things you can do if you have cancer.

Ty: And I've heard the same thing from Dr. Connealy. Really, she's very heavily into the detection of...

Burton: She's one of the best doctors in the United States. She is a master. I've known her for many years. When this test was developed I brought it to her. She went over to Germany and studied it. She's a dear friend and I have the most admiration for her type of medicine.

Ty: Well Burton, I want to thank you for taking the time to share some of your knowledge. I'm sure just a tiny bit of your knowledge with us today. "The voice of alternative medicine." You're passionate and you're rational and you've got a lot of wisdom you've shared with us today. Thank you. **[end transcript]**

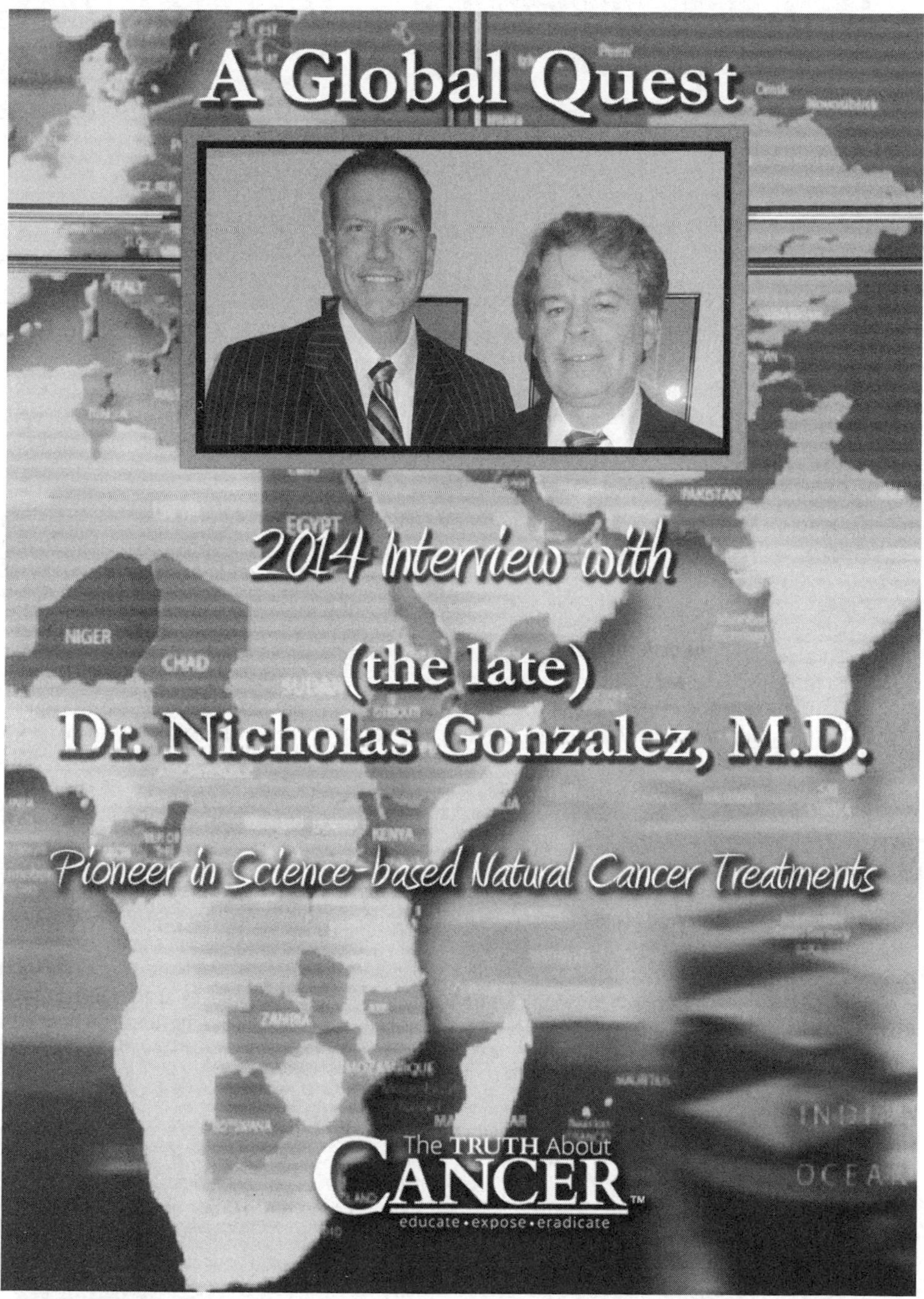
A Global Quest
2014 Interview with
(the late)
Dr. Nicholas Gonzalez, M.D.
Pioneer in Science-based Natural Cancer Treatments
The TRUTH About CANCER
educate • expose • eradicate

Ty: I am here in New York City today at the office of Dr. Nicholas Gonzalez. Dr. Nick, thank you so much for taking the time with us today.

Dr. Gonzalez: Thank you for the opportunity to have the interview. I appreciate it.

Ty: Really excited to have you on the series. If you could to start with just telling us a little about yourself and how you got to become a medical doctor specializing in cancer.

Dr. Gonzalez: When I was in college at Brown University 1,000 years ago, the last thing on earth I ever thought I would be doing would be practicing medicine, working in science and treating cancer patients. I had absolutely no interest in science. I thought science was the most uninteresting subject—any kind of science—you could possibly pursue. My degree was in English Literature. I went to Brown because there were no required courses so I could design my own writing major, and I had very good teachers there. After college my first job was at Time, Inc. That is pre-internet, which will show how old I am—and those were the days when print media reigned supreme and Time, Inc. was considered the Rolls Royce of the publishing industry. Now it is kind of like the forgotten stray dog because the internet has taken over. It was a wonderful place to work and I had wonderful mentors in journalism that really guided me wonderfully.

One of my first editors was Byron Dobell, who was famous in those days and published many, many well-known writers. He really guided my editorial career and well into my career as a journalist one of my editors challenged me and said, "I want you to do some investigative work in medicine." I said, "What is this? A punishment? I haven't been good enough?" And he said, "No, no. I wanted to be in Paris in the spring, not doing something like that." He said, "No, no one wants to do it but this is a fascinating subject." So, against my better judgment, and screaming and hollering, I started to do some investigative work in journalism and did a big piece on cancer research. It was a long piece that got a lot of publicity. As a result of that article I got to meet many well-known researchers like Linus Pauling—researchers doing really avant-garde type work. I first interviewed Linus Pauling in 1972 when he came out with his book on vitamin C and the common cold, and I interviewed him for the book on cancer. What I began to realize, contrary to my earlier misguided prejudices, these creative scientists were as creative as any journalist or writer or artist and they really were doing extraordinary work. They were great thinkers. I befriended a lot of them.

Actually, it was Linus Pauling who challenged me and said, "You know, you're smart enough to go to medical school." The first time he said it I kind of laughed and said, "Sure, right. I want to go to France and do my novel." He said, "No, think about it. Medicine is really fascinating. You should do it." So, with some encouragement like that, I eventually decided to go back and study medicine. Having my degree in English, I had to do my pre-med work, which I did at Columbia. I gave up my apartment in New York and my girlfriend thought I was crazy. My friends bet how long I would last—the longest was about six weeks. I moved home to my parents' house in Queens. They really graciously took me on as I did my pre-med work and really took to it.

I applied to medical school, got in, decided to go to Cornell because it was associated with Memorial Sloan-Kettering Cancer Center and I was interested in doing cancer research. The president of Sloan-Kettering at the time was Robert Good. In fact, he had been on the cover of *Time* when I was at Time in about 1973. He was the most famous immunologist of his generation and the most published author in the history of medicine with over 2,000 articles to his credit. He was known as being very innovative and, in fact, it got him into trouble where he was being criticized by the board of directors. A lot of controversy surrounded him but I wanted to work under him so I chose Cornell as a second-year medical student. Dr. Good adopted me into his research group. I was with a great scientist as a second-year medical student having been a journalist. He, like my journalism mentors, took me under his wing and guided my career. At the end of my second year of medical school back in July 1981, I had the opportunity to meet William Kelley under the strangest series of circumstances. Kelley was the controversial, alternative dentist who developed a very aggressive new approach to cancer and other diseases. He was based in Dallas at the time and he had been involved with the famous Steve McQueen episode. Everyone knows Steve McQueen was the famous actor, kind of daredevil wild guy who was kind of an icon in Hollywood who died of mesothelioma, allegedly under Kelley's care. The press really had started to attack Kelley late in 1980 after McQueen died. He was being harassed, he was being followed by National Enquirer reporters, so he left Dallas, took a train ride across Canada just to get away from the media (this was 6 months after McQueen died), was coming through New York and a journalist friend of mine who knew he was going to be in New York wanted him as a subject for a book. He said, "That guy has been all over the media, attacked because of Steve McQueen, it might make for a good book." She talked to him for a few times. He agreed to meet with her for lunch but she couldn't make any sense out of what he was talking about. She was a journalist—she had no scientific background. She said, "Look, you were a journalist for seven years, you study medicine now and you have two years under your belt, would you meet with him?" I said, "No. I don't want to meet the guy. He sounds like a nut case." She called three times. Usually if people persist three times—kind of a rule I learned in journalism—if someone persists three times they are probably worth meeting with]. It is the three call rule. I said, "Okay, okay!" Just to get her off my back I said I would meet with her so we met in a chiropractor's office in Queens—the strangest story how we met.

I went in there so skeptical, having been an investigative reporter, and I was interested in becoming a straight-line medical researcher at Sloan-Kettering. The reason I went to Cornell is I expected to spend the rest of my academic life at Memorial Sloan-Kettering doing basic science research. I meet Kelley and within five minutes my life was going to change. I realized within five minutes that he was probably the smartest man I was ever going to meet. He was very humble and contrary to what I expected him to say—a lot of bravado and how he was being vilified. He said, "Look, I think I am doing something useful and I need an outside research group to look into it." He already knew from my friend that I was working under Robert Good and he said he knew about Robert Good. He said the only person he knew in academic medicine that could fairly evaluate his work would be Robert Good. After several hours of talking to him the first thing I told him to do was not to do a popular book, which is what my friend wanted to write. I said, "If you want your works taken seriously you have to avoid that right now because you are too involved with Steve McQueen. The last thing you need is a bestselling book attacking you because you were involved with Steve McQueen." I said, forget that. My friend the journalist, who brought us together, was so angry with me that I told him not to get involved with the book that she wouldn't talk to me for 16 years. We finally met at a conference and she gave me a hug and we made up.

That afternoon I went to Robert Good, to the president's office at Sloan-Kettering. It is about 30 blocks north of my office, overlooking Manhattan and I talked with him. Here is a guy who is president of Sloan-Kettering, who meets with Rockefellers and the rich donors and the board of trustees and Nobel Laureates, and he always took the time to talk to his scientists—young science students and medical students that he thought had something interesting to say. He gave me like an hour and a half and we talked about my meeting with Kelley. He said, "Look, this is what I suggest. I have always learned as a teacher that if you pursue a project of your own devising you will learn more medicine than if I assign something to you." I had the summer off and I had some funding to do research. Kelley was leaving for Texas the next day. He said, "You go with Kelley tomorrow and start going through his records." He said, "Will Kelley open his records?" Kelly had already promised he would open his records and he said, "That's a good sign." He said, "A lot of fringe/alternative practitioners won't open their records. They will make a lot of claims but they won't open their records." That impressed me right away that Kelley had no secrets and he was willing to open his records.

The next day I was on a plane to Dallas with Kelley with Dr. Wood's blessing and that is how my life changed. Over the next three weeks I went through hundreds of Kelley's records that he kept in his Dallas office and within a couple of days I found case after case of appropriately diagnosed, biopsy proven, terrible prognosis cancers ... metastatic prostate, metastatic lung cancer, metastatic colon and pancreatic cancer, acute leukemia...the worst of the worst of the worst Kelley had treated, and these people were alive five and 10 years later. Kelley allowed me to call them. He would call them first and say, "This isn't a set-up. I trust this guy Gonzalez." And they would talk to me. They had the most incredible stories. Even though I wasn't a physician—I just finished two years of medical school—I had enough medicine to realize that these were extraordinary cases. After about three weeks I copied a whole batch of Kelley's records, brought them back to New York and met with Dr. Good in his president's office at Sloan-Kettering. We were on our hands and knees on the floor with all of these records opened up. He was very cautious. He had to protect his reputation. He didn't want to jump to conclusions, but he admitted right away—he would never say it in public—but he said, "I've never seen anything like this." Five-year survivors of pancreatic cancer. He encouraged me to develop this into a formal research project, which I did under his guidance while a medical student.

Presidents of Sloan-Kettering are given about 10 years and if they don't find the cure for cancer they are booted out and his tenure was just about up. So in about 1982-1983, when I was still a medical student, he was booted out. He first went to the University of Oklahoma where he set up a cancer research unit and then All Children's Hospital in Florida where he set up a cancer research unit and bone marrow transplant unit. He was famous for bone marrow transplantation and was one of the darlings of the conventional cancer world because he did the first bone marrow transplant in history at the University of Minnesota where he was chief of pathology back in 1969. I followed him down to Florida, finished my fellowship and one of the ironies of ironies—I actually trained under Dr. Good to do bone marrow transplantation so I am conventionally trained by about the most aggressive oncologist you could ever wish to know. But, in addition, for five years he supported my nutritional research under Kelley. I went through over 10,000 of Kelley's records, interviewed over 1,000 of his patients, evaluated 455 of his advanced cancer patients who had done well, evaluated 50 at great length, representing 26 different types of cancer. Some of these patients we actually saw in our own immunology clinic with Dr. Good. It was really amazing. I wish I had film of Dr. Good examining these Kelley patients and writing notes on official hospital records with his white coat and stethoscope.

We put it together in monograph form. I did the writing, I did the research, and he was my mentor. I evaluated 50 patients with 26 different types of cancer—all poor prognosis or terminal or advanced who enjoyed extraordinary responses that could only be attributed to Dr. Kelley's nutritional program. We put this together in monograph form in 1986, finished my immunology fellowship. Now, here I have Dr. Good as my mentor—the most published author in the history of medicine, 50 books to his credit. He was either editor or co-writer of 50 books, over 2,000 papers published. The general responses were one of two. First, a lot of the editors didn't believe it and in fact, I have some of the letters in my office from editors who warned Dr. Good this had to be a scam, fraudulent, and I conned him or something even though we saw the patients at our own clinic and Dr. Good knew they were real. The other thing is, editors would say, "This isn't real but if it is real it is the most extraordinary thing in medicine but it is also the most controversial." A nutritional approach to cancer? This was 1986 where, to mention nutrition and cancer in the same sentence was tantamount to a felony and the editors said this would be the end of my publishing career. The American Cancer Society and the National Institute of Health and National Cancer Institute would make sure that I can't feed my children so they would pass. I tried for two years, couldn't get it published and eventually put it away but finally in 2010 we published an updated, rewritten version with a long introduction about being updated in 2010.

At that point, Dr. Good was not at Sloan-Kettering, I finished my immunology fellowship, and we had a long talk. We went out to dinner, and he said something very interesting. I don't have it on tape so I can't confirm it but he said, "You know, some of these cases are so extraordinary, like a five-year survivor of pancreatic cancer—" which he had never seen. One of his former wives—he was married three times—had died of pancreatic cancer two months into his presidency at Sloan-Kettering. He couldn't save his own wife—she died quickly. He said, "You are showing me these cases," and he said, "I don't know how Kelley is doing this. I have never seen anything like this and I am president of Sloan-Kettering. People come from all over the world for my advice about cancer."

The whole Iranian crisis began because of Dr. Good. The Shah of Iran got sick so he wanted the best physician in the world to come evaluate him so he picked Robert Good, flew Robert Good in the Shah's private jet to Iran, Dr. Good examined him—he was a brilliant clinician as well as researcher—and within 10 minutes made the diagnosis. He said, "You have gallbladder cancer. You have to come to New York," and so he came to New York Hospital and that is when the Iranian Revolution began, so it actually … no one knows this at all. No one knows that the Iranian Revolution began because of Robert Good, president of Sloan- Kettering and my mentor. I lived in his house when I joined his research group. That is an incredible story.

Ty: That's fascinating that the Iran dilemma began because of Dr. Good.

Dr. Gonzalez: Robert Good. He brought the Shah of Iran to New York and then he died here and that led to the Iranian Revolution. It is an interesting story. But, we couldn't get that book published and Dr. Good met with me before, at the end of, when I finished the book and finished my fellowship and I had a choice—stay with Dr. Good or find another place to be. We had dinner and we were talking and he said, "You know, people come from all over the world for my expertise. I don't have the slightest idea what Dr. Kelley is doing and yet I have seen cases in our own immunology clinic that I can't explain and you are telling me that I, one of the leaders of cancer medicine, a former president of Sloan-Kettering…" And he was just listing, not egotistically, just factually, the most published author in the history of medicine—you are telling me that I don't know anything about cancer. He said, "I can't emotionally live with that." So, I knew I had to leave his group and I did. We talked about it. I said, "You know, what I'm going to do is go to New York, open a practice and start seeing patients and try and keep Kelley's work alive." Because, by that point, our failure to publish the monograph really had devastated Kelley. He thought his work would never get accepted and he really went off the deep end. He closed down his practice, stopped seeing patients—which was kind of a tragedy—but he was burned out. The Steve McQueen thing had a devastating effect on him. He couldn't open a newspaper for months without being attacked in every major media outlet. This was pre-internet. All the major TV shows, all the minor TV shows, the news, the major news, the weekly news, the local news, "Kelley Quack" The American Cancer Society held a press conference attacking Kelley and invited all the media to come. Dozens of reporters showed up. All the cancer groups had these press conferences attacking Kelley.

The Steve McQueen story has never been properly told. That is another big thing. There are all kinds of biographies about Steve McQueen and they mention Kelley, the crazy guy. I have talked to some of these authors. They never really investigated it properly. I know the whole story. In fact, in this office about 25 feet from where we are sitting I have Steve McQueen's complete medical records even when he used assumed names. I have all of his records here—I got them from Kelley. They are in this office. I know the whole story. I know it like nobody else has because no one else has ever had his complete medical file. McQueen was kind of a reckless guy. Motorcycle racer, smoker, drinker and lived a hard life as he is famous for. He started getting sick in 1978 and 1979 and went to his fancy Los Angeles doctors and they kind of blew it off. "You live too hard … you've got to cut down the smoking. No one took him seriously." Finally he was so debilitated he went to his doctors and said, "You've got to do something." Finally the genius said, "Hey, let's do a chest x-ray." He had tumors in both lungs. They worked him up and he had metastatic mesothelioma. Mesothelioma is associated with asbestos exposure. Well, he was a motorcycle fanatic and in those days the pipes of motorcycles were lined with asbestos and he would work on his own motorcycles. He was a great mechanic. He was exposed to a huge amount of asbestos and he ended up with mesothelioma. In those days, 35 years ago and today, mesothelioma is completely incurable once it spreads. The only hope is to get it early and do surgery. Well, the doctors had completely missed the diagnosis for a year so by the time it was diagnosed it was metastatic.

Then the geniuses decided to give him immunotherapy. Well, I am trained as a classical immunologist under Robert Good. There has never been a study in the history of the world showing immunotherapy has any effect on mesothelioma. Talk about quackery … but they gave it to him. It didn't work so then they decided to give him radiation. Maybe they gave him the radiation first, I have to pull out my notes. There has never been a study in the history of the world showing radiation works with mesothelioma. Guess what? It didn't work so he ends up with stage IV advanced cancer and weeks from death he goes to see Kelley. Kelley made one fatal mistake in treating Steve McQueen. He took him on as a patient. He was too advanced, and he was a reckless guy. He was still smoking, still drinking but he pleaded and Kelley was a very compassionate guy. He said, "I will treat you but you are too weak. You can't do this at home the way most of my patients do." There was a hospital in Mexico at the time that was administering parts of Kelley's therapy. He said, "Go down to that hospital in Mexico and I'll kind of direct them." And he did. McQueen wasn't 100 percent compliant. He still had the Haagen-Dazs ice cream and cigarettes smuggled in from his friends, but he did enough of the treatment that he started getting better. Then one of the doctors in Mexico gets the brilliant idea, "Let's open him up," because they think that the tumor—he had a tumor in his abdomen as well as in his chest. "Let's take it out—we think it's a dead tumor." They do the surgery and the next day he dies of a pulmonary embolism, which is a blood clot in the lungs. He did not die of mesothelioma and, in fact, the tumor was a dead tumor. Kelley used to have it in his office in formaldehyde—a dead tumor that had shrunk down from a huge tumor down to nothing. It was dead. He didn't die from—the way the media reports read, which I have, is like Kelley took a gun and shot McQueen—his crazy quack doctor.

The true story has never been told. First, his brilliant conventional doctors missed the diagnosis for a year. Then they gave him immunotherapy, which was worthless. Then they gave him radiation, which is worthless. When all that failed then he goes to see Kelley, who keeps him alive and kills the tumor and then he gets blamed for killing Steve McQueen. It is a bizarre story. In none of the media reports did they mention the fact that the diagnosis had been missed and the conventional doctors had done everything they could do and even today in 2014, metastatic mesothelioma is universally 100 percent incurable by standard therapy. Now, we have patients who have done beautifully, but Kelley got blamed for that. He was absolutely devastated by that. It really threw him off. He never really recovered.

So, here it is in 1987 and I know that I can't continue with Dr. Good because emotionally he can't accept the fact that this might work, and he wasn't at Sloan, and he didn't have the power base he had before, and he was getting older. Kelley was going nuts. I never spoke to him after 1987. He accused me of being part of a CIA plot to steal his work or something crazy ... part of a great conspiracy to steal his work. After 1987, I never talked to him.

Dr. Isaacs and I, we worked together in research, came back to New York to set up a practice in late 1987 and started seeing patients, and from the beginning we saw the results. The first good thing is we learned, it was transferable and this wasn't some miracle of magic that only Kelley could do in la-la land or something, and you could teach it to other people and get the same results. One of my first patients was a wonderful lady who lived in New Jersey but she came to me. I'll never forget ... December 3, 1987. She was so memorable I remember the day. I had only been in practice a couple of months. She had stage IV breast cancer. Very interesting story. In 1985, she developed a mass in her right breast. The breast turned red and the doctor thought it was mastitis which is an infected breast, puts her on antibiotics and it doesn't get better. He gives her more antibiotics and it doesn't get better. The breast gets bigger and redder and looks nasty so he sends her to a surgeon who biopsies it and it comes back inflammatory breast cancer. As physicians know, inflammatory breast cancer is the most aggressive type of breast cancer there is. It is virtually incurable by standard approaches. It was huge at that point. So big that when she was sent to the surgeon for surgery he said, "It's too big. I can't operate on you. What you need to do is have radiation first to shrink it down." She goes through five weeks of radiation. The tumor shrinks down enough so the surgeon said, "I'll try to take it out." He takes it out, and it was eight cm which, for breast cancer after radiation, is huge. But, more importantly, 17 of 17 lymph nodes were involved with cancer. All of those that were evaluated had cancer, which is a dire prognosis.

The way it works in cancer medicine, whenever you have more than nine lymph nodes involved it is a death sentence. They did a bone scan but they didn't see anything in the bone. But when you have 17 of 17 lymph nodes positive you are dealing with a deadly disease. Her oncologist decides that they are going to give her aggressive chemotherapy—a triple-agent regimen, very aggressive in those days. It was the standard for metastatic disease: CMF-Cytoxan. Years into it—August 1987, she develops pain in the sternum. They do a bone scan and she has multiple lesions in her ribs consistent with metastatic disease and a huge tumor in the sternum. They do an x-ray and it confirms the tumor. The oncologist—an honest guy—throws his hands in the air and says, "There is nothing else we can do."

I had only been in practice two months. It is not like I had this kind of international reputation. I was as well-known as dog poop. Nobody knew who I was. I happened to be on the Bob Adkins show. Bob Adkins is an old friend from my journalism days I had included in a couple of my articles, so we had been personal friends. He had a very well listened-to national radio show back in those days, and he knew about my Kelley study. I had given him a copy, which I couldn't get published. He had me on his show and this patient's social worker who she was consulting with because of the stress of cancer happened to have an interest in alternative. Actually, ironically, she worked for the American Cancer Society. She kept her interest in alternative medicine secret. It was like pornography—you have to keep it secret. You have to hide it because they might do something and you might lose your job and end up in jail. So she had a secret interest in alternative medicine and heard me on the show and tells the patient, "You have to see Gonzalez," even though I had only been in practice two months. It was something on the radio show—Bob gave me like, an hour—that resonated with the social worker, and the patient believed what the social worker said and came to see me. It's interesting. In 1987, I had been practicing two months—why would anyone trust me dealing with stage IV cancer? But she did.

We have learned that often the difference between success and failure is the attitude of the patient. We treat people biochemically and my goal in life once I adopted science as my new lifestyle was to spend my life at Sloan-Kettering doing basic science research. I never even thought I would see patients, but I learned I had to change that. I learned a lot of this from Kelley. The attitude and the mind of the patient is the single most important that determines. Patients who are at peace with their situation, who have faith in the practitioner always do the best. I always tell patients, when you don't trust your practitioner, whether it is me or Joe Schmo down the street at Sloan-Kettering, leave. Find someone you believe in, because your lack of belief, your lack of faith, and your lack of trust will undermine your treatment, whatever it is—chemo, radiation, or voodoo. She trusted me from the beginning, did the program. I don't know why she did but it was something that resonated. We got along great. She did the program, didn't want scans. She said, "What's the point? They told me I would be dead so why do scans? Why expose myself to the radiation?" Even back in the 1980's she was thinking like that.

Finally in 2001, 14 years later, I said, "Look, I'm trained as an academician. Humor me. Do a bone scan. We won't do CT scans okay? I don't want you getting radiation but let me do a bone scan." She did, and all the tumors were gone. She is alive and well now. It has been 26-and--a-half years since her diagnosis with stage IV metastatic inflammatory breast cancer, who developed metastasis while on aggressive chemotherapy with total regression of disease on my treatment, 26-and-a-half years out. Having been a journalist it is so funny. I have a different personality now. I am obsessed with the conventional medical literature and I study the literature because it helps me with my own work. I know of no case in the history of medicine of a 26-and-a-half year survivor of metastatic inflammatory breast cancer to the bone with development of metastasis while on chemo with total regression on a nutritional program. I don't know of any other case. She is alive and well and doing fine. She is getting older, that's all, but she still takes the enzymes that we use.

From the beginning we saw that this therapy worked and we just plowed ahead and never looked back. Back in the late 80's and early 90's, two of my professors from Cornell who I knew quite well and followed me as I worked under Dr. Good invited me, both times to breakfast, both at Sloan-Kettering. I met with them and they said, "You know, you have such a promising academic career and Dr. Good is your mentor. I want you to join our group." In both cases the provision was, but you've got to give up this crazy alternative thing of yours. It is like some kind of psychological—they didn't say this but—some kind of crazy psychological defect. I was so honored. To be offered a job not once, but twice, at Sloan-Kettering, was very gracious and even though I was already getting to be controversial … As I got better known, controversy follows. They still thought that I had a career in science which, again, I am honored that they even thought that. In each case I turned it down. I have turned down two positions at Sloan, which I don't say proudly. It is just an interesting footnote to the story.

Ty: You may be the only person in history who has.

Dr. Gonzalez: I have been told that I am the only person in history to turn down two jobs at Sloan-Kettering. Most oncologists would not necessarily shoot their mother, but maybe sell her into slavery to get a job there. Yeah, I turned it down twice, but I never looked back because I knew what we were doing was working and Sloan-Kettering in 1989, 1990, 1991 wasn't ready to hear it. I didn't belong there. It would be like taking a wild animal and putting it in a cage. I needed to be free to do what I needed to do with freedom and I just needed that.

Ty: Well, Dr. Gonzalez, talk about the protocol that you are using. If you could, go back and kind of give a few details about what protocol Dr. Kelley was using and then how you have adopted that into your practice now. What are you using?

Dr. Gonzalez: Kelley's program and our program have three basic components. Our therapy today, 25, 27 years later, is really a derivation of Kelley's. We follow his model pretty closely. It involves three basic components: individualized diet, individualized supplement programs, which for cancer patients is large doses of pancreatic enzymes, and detoxification routines like the coffee enemas.

Now, unlike a lot of alternative practitioners who use one diet for everybody, like Atkins thought everyone should be on a meat diet, and there are groups of people who think everyone should be a vegetarian—Kelley realized early on different people need different diets. Some people do well with a plant-based diet and other patients need fatty red meat two to three times a day. He had 10 basic diets and 94 variations. Investigative journalist that I was at heart, when I first met him I challenged him. He showed me on his computer the 10 basic diets and 94 variations. Even then he would individualize the diet so he didn't have, and we don't have, one diet. We follow that tradition. We have 10 diets with dozens of variations.

Secondly, large doses of nutritional supplements. Vitamins, minerals, trace element and glandular extracts from animals like liver, thymus, lung, pancreas and heart. These glandular products are made for us in New Zealand. We don't believe the vitamins and minerals, trace elements and glandular products are going to cure or reverse cancer. What they do provide is nutritional support. Now we are doing two things. We are trying to attack the cancer directly, but we are also trying to rebuild a ravaged body. A lot of the patients who came to Kelley and a lot of the patients that we see not only have advanced cancer, which just wrecks the body, but also have been treated with aggressive chemo, radiation and all kinds of combinations that also ravage the body. We try to rebuild the body and also attack the cancer. You can attack the cancer better if you rebuild the body. So, the vitamins, minerals, trace elements and glandular products help restore the normal equilibrium and homeostasis of the body and even then supplement programs are very individualized. Kelly did, and we do, individualize all of these supplement programs. No two patients are on exactly the same protocol although some of them, of course, are similar.

Now, in addition to the vitamins, minerals, trace elements etc., designed specifically for each patient, and for cancer patients large doses of pancreatic enzymes. This was Kelley's great innovation, which he traditionally followed of course. Pancreatic enzymes have been known since the 1850s or 1860s and they are known as digestive enzymes. They help us break down proteins, fats and carbohydrates. In addition, Dr. John Beard was the great professor at the University of Edinburgh. English by birth, Scottish by profession, and was in Edinburgh all of his professional life. He was a very brilliant embryologist and got his doctorate in 1884 from the University of Freiburg in Germany, and he was one of the great embryologists. His work in embryology is still quoted today in the literature.

His work in embryology led him on a side tangent into pancreatic enzymes and cancer. He was not trained as a cancer researcher but he was a brilliant man and like a lot of brilliant men, like Linus Pauling, he became an expert in a lot of different fields. In 1902, he wrote the first paper on pancreatic enzymes in addition to the digestive capability, which had been well documented by that point, that the body's main defense against cancer would be useful as a cancer treatment. And brilliant man that he was, he did animal studies. When you think about it, 110 years ago, it was a primitive time in science where scientists worked out of caves with candles. Well, actually he was very sophisticated, and by 1902, pathologists and Sloan-Kettering already existed by that point. Brilliant pathologists in the US and Europe had already evaluated and diagnosed and defined 100 different types of cancer. They knew what cancer was, they knew what it looked like, they knew how it behaved and they knew how to examine it and get a biopsy and look under a microscope.

Beard took an animal model, which they had at that time for cancer, and used his enzymes—first study of enzymes in history, and got 100 percent regression of cancer in the animals that he treated, whereas the control group died very quickly. He was not a physician, he was an ScD—he had a doctorate degree—so he was not able to treat patients directly but physicians working under him began using enzymes. The first case was in 1905—a case of head and neck cancer. The person who administered it, Dr. Clarence Rice, had an office about five blocks from this office where we are sitting now right on Madison Avenue, so it is kind of a historic place to be in terms of enzymes. The tumor completely regressed, and it was published in conventional medical literature. I have collected dozens of articles in peer-reviewed conventional literature from the period of 1905-1911, and physicians under Beard's guidance treated advanced cancer: colon cancer, rectal cancer, breast cancer, endometrial cancer, lung cancer, successfully with the enzymes. He wrote a book in 1911: *The Enzyme Treatment of Cancer,* where he actually photographed—sequential photographs—of patients with head and neck cancer where tumors actually disappeared and the skin healed normally 100 years ago! More than 100 years ago. The work then, as it is today, is considered too controversial.

There is another footnote which we don't often talk about in my lectures. At the same time Beard was showing that enzymes could reverse cancer, Madame Curie, the great French—well, she was Polish by birth but she was working in University of Paris—she was investigating radiation. X-rays had been discovered in 1895 and by 1900 they were used diagnostically. They were miraculous. You could do an x-ray and see the inside of the chest and see the lungs. By 1905, Madame Curie was saying that radiation would be a simple, easy and non-toxic way of treating all cancer. She had two Nobel prizes already, one of the few people—Linus Pauling also had two—few people that ever had won one let alone two and she was well loved by the media. She was the first great media star. She knew how to use the media. She knew how to call press conferences and she announced radiation as the cure of cancer to the media.

Beard was this nerdy, ivory tower scientist who thought the media was a bunch of morons and had no use for them, no use for his critics. He wasn't the most diplomatic person, whereas Madame Curie knew how to nurture the media. All over the world, Madame Curie, the greatly beloved. She was the first woman to get a PhD in theoretical physics from the University of Paris. She is extraordinary in history. Movies have been made about her. The press loved her. Who cared about Dr. Beard and pancreatic enzymes? Well, nobody, apparently, so his book went unheeded, radiation came into the forefront of cancer treatment. Of course, Madame Curie was completely wrong on all counts. It isn't non-toxic and in fact she, herself, died as a result of radiation exposure. She died of aplastic anemia caused by radiation. Most tumors that regressed come back very quickly, more deadly, and only a few cancers actually responded to it, so radiation was not the simple, easy, non-toxic way of treating all cancer. She was wrong. By that point, by the time scientists realized it, hundreds of scientists involved in radiation had died because of her cavalier exposure to radiation. It is invisible, the rays are invisible.

By that point, Beard died in 1924. He died in obscurity, his book forgotten. Kelley revived that. Kelley himself had cancer and was trying to fight his own battle. He was an orthodontist by training.

***Ty*:** What type of cancer did he have?

Dr. Gonzalez: He had pancreatic cancer. I spoke to his doctors. When I first did my research 30 years ago they were still alive. They never biopsied it. They said he was too unstable and they didn't want to bring him to surgery. This was before CT scans, in the early 1960s. They did x-rays, and he had tumors in both lungs, fluid in his lungs, and a tumor in his hip. In fact, he always walked with a limp because the tumor ate through his hip bone. He had a tumor in his heart which is rare for pancreatic cancer but it was in his bone and they said there was nothing they could do. He had two months to live, with four young kids, all of them adopted. He had mumps as a teenager so mumps can make you sterile and he couldn't have kids, so he adopted four kids out of the orphanages. He was afraid that if he died they would end up back in the orphanages, so he said, "I can't die." Kelley was a very determined guy. He also had an IQ twice of most of us. He said, "I'm not going to die." He went through the literature and realized the only thing he could do was change his diet, and then he learned about Beard's work from, at that point, 60 years earlier, added in enzymes and got well.

Then the local doctors—Kelley was very well known in the town where he lived. He lived in Grapevine, Texas, which is a suburb of Dallas/Fort Worth. In those days it was a poky, professional suburb, and now Dallas has taken over the world, but it was a poky town—Grapevine. He was in the country club and taught Bible study on Sundays and was at the church and school board and everyone knew him. At the country club the doctors saw him rise from the dead like Lazarus, so they started quietly—this is 1964,1965—sending their cancer patients to Kelley because they knew him and trusted him. He was in the same country club and same church.

Ty: So the medical doctors were sending their patients to a dentist?

Dr. Gonzalez: That's right. Legally he didn't have the right to treat cancer. Dentists can't. But they would send them and they would get well. That was the good news and the bad news. The good news is word-of-mouth network started to spread. Now someone's cousin in Houston heard about how my cousin got well, and they would come to Kelley, and then it was a person in New Mexico, and pretty soon people would come from all over the country to Kelley, to a dental office outside of Dallas, getting well.

Well, guess what? The Medical Board wasn't too happy about it because sooner or later they heard about it. Kelley once told me that at one time 14 government agencies were investigating him. Now investigative reporter that I am, I know people tend to exaggerate, but I looked through the data and indeed, 14 government agencies, from the local county attorney, to the State Medical Board, to the Dental Board. The Dental Board actually took away his license for practicing medicine without a license. He didn't care because he just said he was doing nutrition and kept seeing patients anyway. State Attorney, the State Attorney General, federal attorneys, the IRS—they all colluded like going after the Tea Party groups together to try and get Kelley. Here is a guy giving cancer patients nutrition. This isn't like he committed the Holocaust. He was just giving patients with nothing else to do ... you can't treat them successfully with any conventional therapy and he was giving them nutrition. Lo and behold, the problem was a lot of them were getting well, which started to upset the medical authorities.

It is interesting too, and as far as I know these are stories that have never been told before—at one point he was arrested at gunpoint, kind of like typical equivalent of a SWAT team in those days, and arrested. They always do those things to try and embarrass you. They came at midnight in front of his kids in pajamas, dragging him away. Well, there was a very prominent Washington politician high up in the Justice Department—I mean, really high up in the Justice Department. The next day he called the local sheriff and said, "Let Kelley out, or I am going to have the entire federal government investigating every one of you, audited for income taxes for the last 25 years." He said, "You don't want to mess with me." Kelley was let out of jail within five minutes of that phone call and they never went after him again. He continued to practice. He just had patients sign a form saying, I am not a medical doctor, I am doing nutrition, and they left him alone.

All of these incredible stories. I would interview patients who would confirm all of this and his family. I knew three of his four kids. They didn't have an easy time because they were the kids of this crazy, cancer quack doctor. The Dallas newspapers would carry it and all over radio—again, pre-internet. It was tough. They would go to school and be laughed at—crazy quack doctor—so it was tough. Their relationship was a little rocky for a while.

Ty: What is it about it, Dr. Gonzalez, in the pancreatic enzymes that is so successful at reversing the cancer?

Dr. Gonzalez: No one has ever had the financing to do the work. Now, Beard did animal studies 100 years ago, and we have done animal studies too. We were fortunate that we had funding from two major international corporations. People laugh when I say it, but Proctor & Gamble gave us millions of dollars to help perfect the enzyme, and Nestle—the chief of research at Nestle—Pierre Guesry was the former medical director of the Pasteur Institute. Nestle lured him away to run the research division. Nestle in those days had a $600 million basic science division. They have a campus in Switzerland that rivals the NIH. It is unbelievable. I have lectured there several times. Guesry was a real scientist and physician by training. He was head of Pasteur Institute, one of the preeminent research institutions in the world, and he had heard about my work back in 1992. This was pre-internet. I don't know how people heard about me.

Actually I do know so I kind of exaggerate. Pierre is still alive, he lives in Balta now, retired and has a sailboat and sails around the Mediterranean. He set up a research group to travel the world, looking for alternative therapies that might be useful. These are genius people. They don't tend to have prejudices. They just want to see if it works. They don't care if it is moondust or spooky stuff or radioactive waves—they don't care as long as it works. They actually set up a division very quietly, highly funded, and sent a team around the world from the jungles of New Guinea to New York and to me.

Ty: A division within Nestle?

Dr. Gonzalez: Within Nestle, to look into alternative therapies. Unknown. it never was publicized. They traveled the world. One day I got a phone call—I'm going off on a tangent about enzymes but you can edit this down ...

Ty: No, this is great stuff.

Dr. Gonzalez: I get a call from the research director of Nestle and I said, "What the heck does the research director of Nestle want to do with me?" Then they told me his name—Pierre Guesry, and I said, "That rings a bell." This was before internet so you couldn't Google but I found him and I said, Oh, this is the guy that ran the Pasteur Institute. So, I called him back and he said, "I want to come to New York to meet with you," and I said, "Why? I don't eat chocolate." He said, "No ..."He laughed, "Nothing to do with chocolate." He explained that he had been looking into alternative therapies and my name kept coming up and wanted to meet with me, and the end result was Nestle agreed to fund studies. They funded our first clinical studies very successfully with pancreatic cancer and also animal studies back in 2002-2004. They were done at the University of Nebraska by Parviz Pour, who is one of the preeminent researchers in molecular biology of pancreatic cancer. Dr. Pour developed an animal model for pancreatic cancer that they used in our study. He used the most aggressive animal model at his disposal and Nestle funded him to do this. They were going to really put my enzymes to the test. It was extremely successful. Pour told me that this is the first time in his lifetime that he saw this particular model respond to anything. It didn't respond to chemo or anything. He published in a peer-reviewed journal of the pancreas in 2004—I have copies around.

We know from animal models it worked, and from my first clinical study that it works, but we don't know the molecular biology to answer your question. We don't know how it actually kills cancer. What we think is that proteolytic, which is the protein digestive pancreatic enzymes like trypsin and chymotrypsin, actually tear apart the cell membrane. Cell membranes are a little bit fatty but they also have protein molecules that are receptors, and pores that allow nutrients to get in, and waste products to get out ... that is how cells survive, with the protein pores and membrane. These proteins—I think the enzymes chew them up. They don't affect normal tissue. Beard said in his book more than 100 years ago that there is reason that cancer cells have the opposite electrical charge as the normal cells, and everyone laughed at him at that time but we now know that it is true. Normal cells repulse the pancreatic enzymes in the blood stream, but cancer cells attract them, and the enzymes go right to the cancer cell, and, we believe, chew up the proteins on the cell membrane. We think it is that simple, but we haven't had the trillions of dollars of funding to substantiate that. Pour wanted to do that, and Nestle was willing to fund more, but the key with Nestle is, I would have had to turn over my own intellectual property. It would have been a co-ownership. They had their patent lawyers in the US filing patents but it would have been Nestle and me as co-owners. The problem with that is, Pierre retires, and the next person may think it is all quackery, and then Nestle owns my work and I can't do anything with it so I said, no thank you. We're still friends, Pierre and I. He understood why.

We haven't had any other funding to do that kind of work and figure out why the molecular model enzymes kill cancer, but clearly they do, both clinically and in animal models. People are, "Well, you never did any clinical studies." Well, we did animal studies. They have been published in a peer-reviewed journal. There is no question that they kill cancer both in animals and Kelley's experience proved that and our experience shows that 26-and-a-half years later. We know that they work.

So, to answer your original question. The three components—individualized diet, individualized supplements and larger doses of pancreatic enzymes. The third component is detoxification, which is often the component of therapy that elicits the most mockery from conventional doctors, but it is really very simple. When Kelley was treating himself he was taking the pancreatic enzymes, the tumors were breaking down, and that is when he got really sick—almost life threateningly sick. At first he thought the enzymes weren't working any longer and then he realized the tumors were shrinking and he realized, I am reacting to the tumor waste, and indeed, as conventional oncologists know today in 2014, nothing is more toxic to the human body than dead cancer. In fact, chemotherapy, though it doesn't work for most cancers, does work for some like Hodgkin's and certain leukemias. In a Hodgkin's patient, if you break a tumor down too fast with chemo you kill the patient from the dead tumor. They call it tumor lysis and it is recognized in the textbooks and conventional textbooks talk about it. Well, Kelley recognized that back in 1963 when he was trying to get over his own cancer. He started going into the literature as he always did.

He was a great scholar. He would go into the literature and try and find some technique that would help his liver and kidneys work better. The liver and the kidneys are the body's main detoxification organs and that is where the environmental chemicals and metabolic waste and dead cancer process and neutralize and prepare for excretion. He opens up the Merck Manual, and lo and behold, there are coffee enemas. The interesting thing, or the sad thing, and the ironic thing—Kelley was brutalized in the media for his use of coffee enemas, and we get attacked about it today too, but they come right out of the conventional medical literature. He didn't learn about it from alien space beings who projected it into his brain from some mystic psychic experience. He didn't learn about it through some alternative throw-away journal. He learned about it from conventional medical textbooks. The Merck Manual is a compendium of conventional therapies. They were in the Merck Manual. Coffee enemas were in the Merck Manual right up until the 1970s.

When I was doing my investigation of Kelley, trained investigative reporter that I was, I called up the editor of the Merck Manual then and I had a talk with him. He said the only reason they were taken out is that it was kind of folksy and we had all this high tech stuff to use. He had files on coffee enemas, which he sent me—dozens of studies from the '20's and '30's and '40's at major institutions where they used coffee enemas for a variety of things: arthritis, mental illness ... I have a study from The New England Journal of Medicine, a preeminent medical journal of the US. In 1932, from Harvard Medical School research, psychiatrists successfully treated what we today call bipolar illness and in those days they called it manic depressive ... with enemas. Their hypothesis was that there were toxins through the intestinal tract that were polluting the mind, and that is what was causing the mental illness. They put these people on enemas and colonics, and they got well and they got them off medication and out of the hospital. It was in The New England Journal. I have a copy of 1932. I have a study from Uruguay. Just because it is Uruguay doesn't mean there weren't serious scientists. People downplay anything that is not from Boston. It was a good study. They had patients with septic shock and in those days septic shock occurred because of gram-negative bacteria producing polysaccharide, a kind of carbohydrate that is toxic to you, and people die from that. The death rate today is still at a rate of 40 percent or 50 percent with septic shock and those days it was 90 percent. People in Uruguay in the intensive care unit had learned about coffee enemas from the conventional medical world and started treating the patients with coffee enemas and had great success and published it in a peer- reviewed journal. We have a translation. It was originally published in Spanish. Almost 90 percent reversal of septic shock that should have changed the way hospitalists treat septic shock all over the world was ignored because it was folksy and wasn't high tech even then in 1941-1942.

We have dozens of articles. Kelley collected dozens of articles from the mainstream, peer-reviewed medical literature discussing the use of enemas, coffee enemas and other types of colonics, for successful treatment of all kinds of illnesses. He incorporated them into his practice and it helped, and he added other things like liver flushes, colon cleanses, juice fasts and skin brushing, which was an all-natural homeopathic technique to get the lymphatics to work better, kidney flushes … all kinds of techniques that we still use today.

Ty: What is it about the coffee in the enemas that helps to detoxify the body?

Dr. Gonzalez: Interestingly enough, when you drink coffee it tends to suppress the liver. When you take coffee as an enema, rectally, the caffeine stimulates a bunch of nerves in the lower colon called the sacral parasympathetic nerves. When they are turned on by caffeine, they feed back to the liver through a reflex arc, and within seconds causes the liver to release all the toxins. Nothing helps the liver clean out faster and more efficiently or more effectively than coffee enemas. For cancer patients, when you are breaking down a tumor quickly with the enzyme and you get all this tumor debris that can be deadly and life threatening. It gets the liver to work better so it processes tumor debris very effectively and then you just poop them out with the enemas. Interestingly enough, when you drink coffee, it is really toxic to a cancer patient, but if you take it rectally it opens up the liver so the liver dumps into the small intestine and you get rid of all the dead tumor waste very effectively. I have patients that, when they are breaking down tumor, they have a reaction to the tumor, and get fevers of 103 and 104. Do an enema, and literally within 20 minutes of the enema, the fever is down to normal. I see this routinely. They will feel like they are dying and we will do an enema and they will feel better. Guesry reported this. He had his own alternative therapy in the '40's and '50's. He died in 1959 but he wrote a book of 50 cases in 1959 discussing his approach to cancer and his success, and he used coffee enemas for the same reason. He found that if the program worked too quickly, patients would die from the dead tumor waste, so he incorporated coffee enemas back in the '40's and '50's.

I often get criticized when I lecture, as I don't mention Guesry as the source of coffee enemas. Well, Kelley actually didn't learn about the enemas from Guesry. He knew of Guesry later but when he was fighting his own cancer he learned about it from the conventional medical literature like the Merck Manual. So, when you take coffee rectally it just helps the liver run better and that saves your life.

Ty: So you have got the nutritional approach with all of the scores of supplements. And I have seen the scores because recently I saw an interview with you on Fox with Carol Alt and she pulled out her bag of supplements and it was a big supplement bag that she uses every day and you pulled yours out as well.

Dr. Gonzalez: Did I pull mine out on TV?

Ty: You did.

Dr. Gonzalez: This is my lunch dose which I took dutifully.

Ty: Yeah, you both pulled out the bags of supplements at the same time. That was neat.

Dr. Gonzalez: She takes more than I do, though.

Ty: So you have the massive doses of supplements and you have the coffee enemas and the other detoxification techniques and the individualized diet …

Dr. Gonzalez: That's what it is. It is really simple in its basis. Three components.

Ty: That was the three-pronged approach that Kelley used and you pretty much adopted that.

Dr. Gonzalez: We did. We updated. When Kelley was practicing, for example, no one knew what coenzyme Q10 was, and now it is available as a supplement, so we have incorporated that as we need to in our protocols. As new supplements become available we evaluate them and decide whether or not they will fit into our model and use them accordingly. We are always trying to update our program, but it is basically the same model that Kelley developed, which worked then and works now.

Ty: What was the name of your 2010 book that you finally got published?

Dr. Gonzalez: *One Man Alone: An Investigation of Nutrition, Cancer and William Donald Kelley.* In there, we have the 50 case reports. Now, initially the patients actually gave us permission not only to use their medical records but to use their names, but over the internet … a lot of them are still alive in their 80's and 90's. We didn't want them being harassed and reporters tracking them down, so we blacked out their names with one exception—Arlene, I can use her name because she is a good friend. In fact, she called today, Arlene Van Straten—she was one of Kelley's great patients, and I now follow her. In 1982, Appleton, Wisconsin—typical American success story. She and her husband ran a gas station seven days a week and worked their tail feathers off adding a store to it. They were later bought out by a big chain and they were able to put their kids and grandkids through college. She starts getting gallbladder pain and the doctor said, "You've got a gallbladder problem." This is 1982 before they routinely did CT scans. They took her to surgery to take out her gallbladder and opened her up. She had a tumor in her pancreas, tumor in her liver. They biopsied the liver lesion, and it is adenocarcinoma—metastatic pancreatic. They close her up, she meets with an oncologist, and chemo wasn't going to do nothing in 1982. It still does nothing today in 2014. She goes to the Mayo Clinic, and I have the note from the Mayo Clinic guy who said, "I'm not going to give you chemo. It will just ruin your quality of life. Enjoy your life." She went to the best of the best and they said they can't do anything. She learned about Kelley from this 32-page book, *One Answer to Cancer* in 1969 at a local health food store. She reads it, calls Kelley, and he said, "Well, I've trained this chiropractor locally and he trained some people who do it really well. He is near your town. Why don't you go see him?" And she does.

She never went back to a doctor and never had it scanned. The fact is, here it is 2014, and she is alive and well. Interestingly enough, paradoxically, ironically, today she called and said she wants to chat. Usually it is about her family. She is 32 years out. In August it will be 32 years, stage IV pancreatic cancer, biopsy proven with liver metastases confirmed at the Mayo Clinic. To put it in perspective and to give Kelley his credit, I searched the literature religiously. I know of no patient in the history of medicine with stage IV pancreatic cancer, adenocarcinoma of the worst kind, biopsy-proven liver metastases confirmed at the Mayo Clinic—not some local hospital in Guatemala but by the Mayo Clinic—who is alive 32 years later. Never found a case like that. I have challenged doctors at conferences and lectures to match it and they haven't been able to.

Ty: Thirty-two years.

Dr. Gonzalez: Thirty-two years. In August of 1982 she was diagnosed with stage IV pancreatic cancer and alive 32 years later. Technically I cannot say the tumors went away because she has refused scans for 32 years.

Ty: She is alive.

Dr. Gonzalez: She is alive. You don't need to know anything else. The average survival for stage IV pancreatic cancer in those days, and today, is three, four, five months. Nobody lives beyond about 18 months with that kind of disease.

Ty: Right. And this is 32 years.

Dr. Gonzalez: Thirty-two years later. If she had been a conventional patient and treated in a conventional institution the American Cancer Society would have held a press conference and it would have been on the cover of *Time* Magazine. I remember about 10 years ago there was a new chemo drug that was being touted and Harvard was pushing it and it ended upon "Good Morning America" and ABC, CBS and all the morning shows. One patient who had a regression of disease at six months, and she was like a show horse, being shown around at all the TV shows. Well, that drug was later taken off the market because it did absolutely nothing, but that didn't stop the Harvard team. They are a publicity machine at Harvard Medical School. If they have a chihuahua that lives two months longer they get on national TV. We have a patient with stage IV pancreatic cancer. I challenge anyone who watches this to match the case. Criticize. Criticism is easy. Any critics out there? Match the case. I will be impressed.

Ty: Thirty-two years. What is it do you think about the protocol—this is just your opinion because you have already said that the testing has not been done as far as the exact mechanism—but why would it be that pancreatic enzymes help so much with pancreatic cancer? Would it be the fact that the pancreas is no longer secreting those enzymes?

Dr. Gonzalez: No, it helps with all kinds of cancer from toenail cancer to brain cancer.

Ty: *I mean specifically with pancreatic. I know it helps…*

Dr. Gonzalez: They work for any cancer so I think the ability to kill cancer cells of the pancreas is no different from the ability to kill brain cancer or leukemia or any other cancer. That is why in the book I deliberately chose 26 different types of cancer—50 patients and 26 different types of cancer—to make the point that it works for all different types of cancer. Leukemias, lymphomas, blood cancer, solid tumors, breast, colon, rectal, metastatic prostate and a whole series of them. Five or six patients with metastatic prostate who did beautifully. It isn't just specifically for pancreatic. It is for all cancers. It seems to be a universal cancer killer. As Beard said, it isn't my own ego, I didn't develop this. Beard did 100 years ago.

Ty: I guess that the pancreatic cancer patient just caught my attention because that is unheard of. 30-plus years out.

Dr. Gonzalez: Yeah, in August it will be 32. Appleton, Wisconsin—she still lives in Appleton. If you want to talk to her she is happy to talk to people. She is getting old. Her only problem is she is old but she has seen her kids and grandkids go through college. She is real proud of all of them.

Ty: It is just really amazing to me that nobody knows about this—a 30 year survivor which—you are right. If it had been conventionally treated it would have been all over every magazine and every TV show.

Dr. Gonzalez: The story I told you was about Iressa … I didn't make that up. Iressa was the drug and it was being touted as the new magical cure for metastatic lung cancer. Based on the prestige of certain conventional research, and the FDA actually approved it in the absence of any legitimate data. The idea that conventional science is well-proven medicine is absolutely nonsensical. Most of it is done through friends and phone calls and lobbying. The FDA actually approved it before there was any clinical study done. There was this one patient who was being touted. I assume she is dead now. When they finally did controlled clinical studies they found it didn't work at all and the FDA withdrew its approval for lung cancer. There was a case where it got approved before anybody did research so don't tell me that conventional doctors are sincere and subjective scientists evaluating data and using only proven therapies. They use whatever suits them based on their prejudices, biases and opinions of what should work.

Pancreatic cancer…to answer your question, pancreatic enzymes, nutrients, coffee enemas can't possibly work so they don't work … because we don't believe they work, they can't work, because they can't work, we are not interested in them, and because it can't work there can't be any cases. That is the kind of logic that you see in conventional scientists who claim they have no bias, prejudice, and we objectively evaluate the scientific data when in fact they are driven by their emotions and opinions. What they believe should be true and what they were taught 20 years earlier in school. It is all driven by bias and prejudice of what they believe should be the truth, not what actually is the truth.

Ty: The truth is that we have a patient that is alive with pancreatic cancer 30 years later. That should be enough to pique their interest.

Dr. Gonzalez: Well, if you can't match that one case in all of the thousands of patients with pancreatic cancer that have been treated at Sloan-Kettering, Columbia and the medical schools here in New York, and they see 75 cases a year at Columbia and Harvard Medical School and MDA Anderson and Johns Hopkins has a big pancreatic cancer research center, Jefferson Medical School … 43,000 people died of pancreatic cancer last year according to the data I read and there are supposed to be more this year, like 47,000 or 48,000 this year.

There are a lot of patients out there diagnosed with pancreatic cancer, and 95 percent of them die, so if anyone out there has a stage IV pancreatic cancer with biopsy-proven liver metastases confirmed at a major institution equivalent to that of the Mayo Clinic, match the case. I want to know. I am a scientist.The reason I do what I do is I was very fortunate in that I didn't go to medical school first. I was an investigative journalist and I had some really good mentors. Byron Dobell is still alive now. He was the executive editor of *New York Magazine*—very famous editor, the first that published Mario Puzo, Tom Wolfe, and kept him alive until he did his first book that was a bestseller, Truman Capote ... his Rolodex was unbelievable with writers that he had helped and he said one thing. He said, "If you go into a story as a journalist with a preconceived notion of what the truth is going to be, that's anathema to a journalist." He said, "No matter how weird the story is you have to go in with no prejudices." He just instilled that.

In journalism, he was like my Robert Good. We would have dinner together. I would have dinner at his house and he would say, "You have talent, but any prejudice, you have to get rid of. Approaching a story is completely objective. Otherwise you are going to miss some great truth. Historically you look like a horse's ass. You had the truth and you missed it because you had some biopsy or prejudice that blurred your vision." I really took that seriously. Even with Kelley, I had a prejudice. I didn't want to have lunch with him. My friend had to call me three times. She met the three-call rule. If anyone calls me three times and wants to meet with me they must have some reason. God must have a reason. Once I can blow off, twice is ... eh, so what? Three times? Okay, I'll take it seriously. That is the three-call rule and that is when I met with him. I didn't want to meet with him but he changed my life. My comfortable, scientific career at Sloan-Kettering where my colleagues really liked me and I would have probably won some minor award and proven some mouse gene has an effect with some obscure cancer that is only found in penguins in Madagascar or something. People would have lauded me, I would have been accepted at conferences, and the American Cancer Society would have given me free lunch at one of their conferences but it would have amounted to a hill of beans.

Ty: Well I'm glad you met with him, Dr. Gonzalez, because what you are doing now is amounting to much more than just a hill of beans.

Dr. Gonzalez: It is an interesting constellation of events and I know that you believe, as I do, that God runs the place. It was the oddest constellation of events and Kelley was so hounded by the media that he took a train ride across Canada to get away from the press because he was being followed. At that point he lived in Washington state. There were long-distance lenses on him. His kids wouldn't talk to him because they were being offered money to spill the beans on their crazy quack father. He did it just to get away and be quiet in a train car. Five days to cross through British Columbia and down through Montreal to New York City to meet with this journalist. The only reason he came to New York was to meet with the journalist who wanted to do this book and I said, "Don't do this book because it will just revive all the Steve McQueen stuff which you don't need. The book would have been Steve McQueen this, and Steve McQueen that." I said, "You don't need that." She set up the meeting and I just destroyed the book that she saw as a best-seller. She had million-selling books before. She didn't talk to me for 16 years and then we met at a conference because she came to hear me talk in New York and she gave me a hug and we made up.

Ty: So you're back together now?

Dr. Gonzalez: I haven't spoken to her since that conference. We were quite good friends for a while from my journalism days. I can't say we are best buds but she forgave me for wrecking her book.

Ty: That's good. I'm glad to hear that. Dr. Gonzalez, I really appreciate you spending the time today. I can honestly sit and listen to you all afternoon. This has been fascinating and I think it is going to be really enlightening for the people that are watching the show. I just appreciate you spending the time with us today.

Dr. Gonzalez: That's great. I hope we didn't go too long. It's great that you are here and I really appreciate the opportunity to talk about my work with you. **[end transcript]**

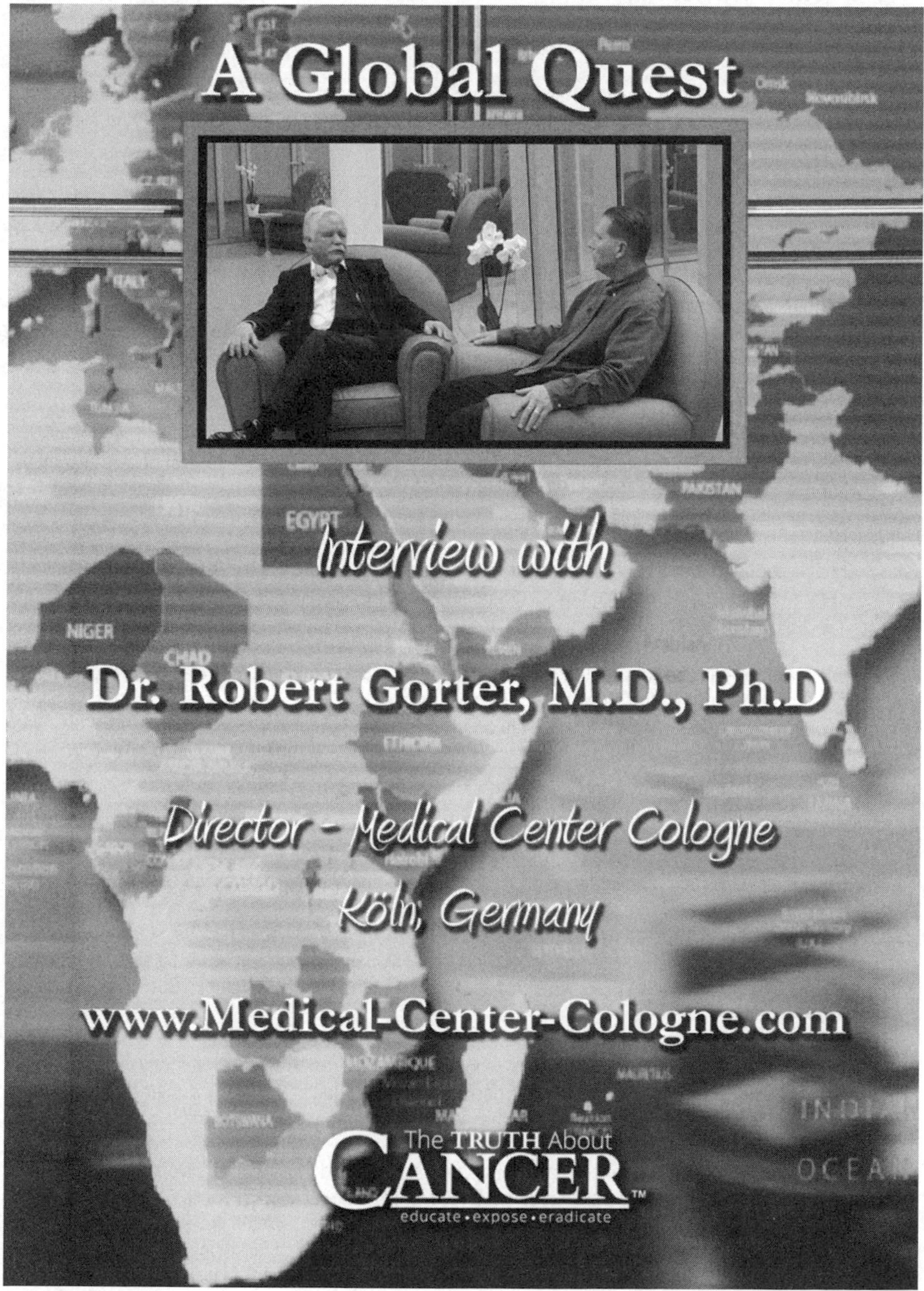
A Global Quest
Interview with
Dr. Robert Gorter, M.D., Ph.D
Director - Medical Center Cologne
Köln, Germany
www.Medical-Center-Cologne.com
The TRUTH About
CANCER
educate • expose • eradicate

Ty: I'm really glad to be here in Cologne, Germany tonight at the Medical Center of Cologne. Dr. Robert Gorter, thank you for the invitation to come and tour your clinic.

Dr. Gorter: Well, thank you for your interest and what you do.

Ty: Absolutely. I'm really interested to see the clinic. We'll go look at in here in a few minutes but before we do that could you share with us a little bit about your background and your education. And your diagnosis of cancer a long time ago.

Dr. Gorter: Well I'm originally from Holland, Amsterdam where I did my medical training. Then I did extra training in oncology in an anthroposophical hospital in Basel, Switzerland. And then I started my own clinic. But almost on day number one I was diagnosed myself with a very far advanced germ cell carcinoma.

So they start in a woman from an ovary and in man from a testicle. And they grow very, very fast. And so when I was diagnosed they said, "three months, with some luck maximum six months." I would do a chemo, do this, do that. And I said, "No, no, no." Because I knew as a doctor what I would go through. So I thought even if it is true that I live six weeks longer but on the blood of others—

I am not afraid of death and I would rather die then, statistically, a few weeks earlier. They always said I was crazy but I said, "No, there are other options." I also had this idea that the root of cancer is in an immune suppression so I should improve immune function. So I did. I treated myself with mistletoe, or *Viscum album*, mistletoe injection.

I get hyperthermia so I went in a hot water bath so the temperature was up to forty degrees. I did a few of those things and now, remarkably, I got better and better. So probably about a year and a half later I was free of cancer.

Of course, I didn't check every day because I thought, "you know, if I have to die, I'll die so I won't change anything." But it was clear that after about a year and a half, when I really checked, nothing could be found. So I was perfectly back in order.

Ty: How many years ago was this? What year was that?

Dr. Gorter: 43 years ago.

Ty: Forty three years ago? Did you ever go back to see the doctors that told you were crazy?

Dr. Gorter: No. Because all had died by now, because there were little or nothing. I had just started as a doctor and these were big professors, they were all in their fifties and in their sixties. And I said, "I don't want chemo." They said, "How stupid." But probably I was right and they were stupid. But anyway, who knows?

But also, I don't feel I should have any revenge or any—I did get better. So I went my way and it worked. Since then, for some reason, as people were told, I had many, many cancer patients always my whole life. Because for some reason they were drawn to me or my team.

And then after 11 years I went to San Francisco, California and I was at the University of California, San Francisco. I right away was very much forced to take care of people with HIV infection and AIDS.

And for many years I was the director of the Department of AIDS Epidemiology and Biostatistics at the University of San Francisco. And much of what is known about the medical history or the natural history of HIV, and also leading to cancer or other problems comes from this group of these 3,000 men in San Francisco.

I was very much interested, from one comes to the other. So when I decided to come back to Germany, or to Europe, I said, "I want to focus my whole life, first of all, to understand cancer better and what would be the best form of therapy." Because a lot of patients, they are very afraid of cancer.

Because it is not a nice disease. But if you don't treat it with chemo or radiation—often patients have so many side effects of the treatment. In the United Kingdom 28 percent of all hospital admissions are due to side effects of the treatment. Not just only for cancer.

Almost a third of all people must be admitted because of the toxicity. I've fared well, or I live shorter but no toxicity. So now it shows. Also the Nobel Prize for medicine in 2011 was awarded for three researchers who discovered the function of dendritic cells. And in a quieter way we jumped on the research and we further developed how to make dendritic cells from patients' simple own white blood cells.

So that's what we do. And you can say that dendritic cells can be seen as the policemen of the immune system. Because these dendritic cells, they migrate through your whole body, everywhere. They can come to tip of your nose, your liver, your prostate. They look for abnormal cells and when they find one, then they quickly in the lymph node form killer, natural killer, cells and they kill. So dendritic cells can only sort of see what is right or wrong but then they inform cells which as have a function to kill. And that's what happens.

And if it functions well, then within 24 hours a cancer cell which has been detected is then also killed. And now when you get cancer you could see in the image these policemen all need reading glasses, they can't see so well anymore. And therefore, cancer cells get a chance. They are unnoticed and then they pass by and they start to grow.

What we do, we can make from one simple blood draw, from monocytes or simple white blood cells, we can make a whole new generation of policemen, dendritic cells. And they are given back. And so it is very safe because it is autologous, our body's own tissue.

So there is nowhere something from a donor—I come from the AIDS epidemic so you're always afraid that you might transport something unknown from blood product. So it's absolutely safe. No side effects, no rejection. And that is what we do. And then suddenly I say to a patient, "You get 20 million young fit policemen from the police academy and they really like to make hell in your body."

Ty: I like that analogy of the policemen.

Dr. Gorter: But it's really true. The policemen, as an image it's really true. Because good policemen will recognize rapists and a bank robber, and the banker or other things like that. So they don't only notice cancer cells but also cells which are one way or another damaged by a virus infection or another way, or from mutation. So therefore these dendritic cells are very important. But really a patient understands right away when you give that image of the policeman. That they see more than just one bad guy.

Ty: So you've got the dendritic cells that you're using here.

Dr. Gorter: Yes. Then we have the hyperthermia, we like to do before we give the dendritic cells. The patients go through a moderate period of fever which we initiate by infrared lamps. And also if people have metastasis, or cancer in the lungs and liver or elsewhere, then we treat that in addition with local hyperthermia. And the principle is that we bring through a region with cancer, cancer tissue, these electromagnetic fields. And very selectively, only cancer cells are quickly increased in the temperature. And cancer cells always make lactic acid and the production of lactic acid is almost tripled. And then the pH goes down so it gets more and more acidity in the cell and then the cell dies during the treatment.

And also no side effects, no toxicity. Except for people that have a pacemaker. That's the only contraindication because the pacemaker can cause strain when you put a strong electromagnetic field on it. So that's the only contraindication.

Ty: Little bit different than the traditional treatments for cancer with the chemo and the radiation and all the side effects. No side effects?

Dr. Gorter: No side effects because we don't have people throwing up, people don't need blood transfusions. We have never had to treat side effects. Because you see that after the treatment with the dendritic cells, two or three hours later patients have for a couple of hours some flu like symptoms. And all the patients who [have] flu like symptoms after the vaccination, they always do well or they go in complete remission.

So patients are happy, "I have a couple of hours that I feel slight (inaudible - 08:56)." And by midnight they are fine again. Then they know that the chances that it really worked for them quickly increase.

Ty: That's a good sign, isn't it.

Dr. Gorter: Yes.

Ty: We typically want to suppress the fever. When we begin to get a fever we take an aspirin or an Advil, or whatever it might be to suppress the fever. You don't want to do that. Fever is good, isn't it?

Dr. Gorter: Yes. Often in medical school it is often portrayed that fever is the cause of illness, but it's the opposite. Your body—the last attempt to activate the immune system is to produce a fever. When your body temperature goes up one degree your immune system is in an absolute state of alert.

Because at normal core body temperature the immune system is on automatic pilot. It doesn't think. But if there is an emergency, the only way to activate the immune system is through fever. There is no other way. So you should really embrace your fever.

There are studies showing that little kids, before they are six—if you suppress fever, when children cannot have at least four and a half times statistically a fever, when people can remember the little child was sick, then they have no way to well develop their immune system. So they get more allergies in puberty and more and at an early age cancer.

When I was a medical student, I will never forget, the surgery professor showed us a woman who was 34 with breast cancer, and he had never seen that in his life before. Because breast cancer, 50 years ago was always the cancer of middle age and elderly women. Now she was 34. Now, 25, 26, you start to see breast cancer.

Ty: Why do you think we're seeing cancer so early now?

Dr. Gorter: Well, because the immune system can never really develop. What you need, and I really believe this, that the childhood diseases are there because, what do all childhood diseases have in common? Fever.

A child has a couple of days of high fever but the immune system can then really—so aerobics for the immune system. The immune system goes through a ripening phase. So if you suppress it, then you take a chance away for the immune system to work well. So that we have allergies, hay fever, and also all these food allergies.

When I went to medical school, a hundred years ago—when I was still in high school, we had one person in the whole high school who had hay fever. So sneezing in the spring, we all made fun of that because we had never seen allergies. Now everybody has a gluten, and this and that, and pollen, and light.

But 30 percent of all teenagers nowadays have some form of allergy that they seek treatment [for], they have symptoms. And, again, 50 years ago, 40-50 years ago, it was really rare. So I think it is because of many theories. But for sure, if you prevent a child from running it will not develop well its muscular system. If you can't play certain qualities are not well developed. And to develop your immune system you need to go few times through fever. I'm absolutely sure.

Ty: That makes a lot of sense. So maybe that's one of the reasons that we're getting childhood cancers. Is we're stopping them from running a fever?

Dr. Gorter: All this happened but it is more common. And also for adults, cancer is on the increase. And it also comes at an early age. Now, there are some statistics also in my book, Statistics from the NIH, the National Institute of Health, that are good reliable data of the cause of death since 1950. So over the last 60 years, good data on why people die in the United States, and it's very similar in Europe.

And you see that western medicine, academic medicine, had made big progress, great progress in treating heart attacks. So less people die of a heart attack or strokes. There is no difference in cancer. The same amount of people die—America's official statistics, the same amount of people die now from cancer as in 1950.

Therefore, we have to say there's something wrong [with how] we look at cancer and what we think is the cause and how to treat it. So we should rethink more now. Acknowledge the immune system and the function of the immune system in early detection and killing of cancer cells.

So it should really be bothersome that all the trillions of dollars which went into cancer treatment and research didn't bring anything. And that must really put people to think, and also public health officials, that there is something wrong [with what] we do and we should really rethink how to treat.

Ty: Yes. You mentioned early detection. What are some good early detection techniques?

Dr. Gorter: Well, of course, a couple of things. First thing is to see your core body temperature. Many patients, and also family members who turned out to be at risk, they have a lower body temperature. So we advise people—also when they come and are treated here they have always too low a body temperature. And they measure it in the morning and then over the month we treat them, we see that the temperature increases to what is normal for a healthy person.

Plus there is viability. So all these cycles—almost anything which is alive goes through cycles, usually a 24-hour cycle. Now, your core body temperature should be lowest early in the morning when you wake up. And during the day also when you don't do much. It should increase at around five or six in the afternoon, it should be at its highest. And it is more than than half a degree difference. And in the evening when you go to bed, it slowly goes down. And then hits in early morning its lowest point again.

Now, if you have that, you can't have cancer, or it is extremely rare. So often people think, "Well, my mother and my aunt, and my father. So maybe I'm at risk." And just a simple detection where you take two or three weeks of temperature in the morning and the evening, it really tells you. If you don't have this nice circadian rhythm you're much more at risk. And people also say, "Oh, cancer patient has cold feet in the evening, or they easily cool off in the nose and hands."

But lots of people don't notice anymore because they have it lifelong. But you're also at risk if you cool off easily or when you don't have this nice 24-hour rhythm, you're also at high risk.

Ty: Very interesting.

Dr. Gorter: There's much more known about chronobiology, as it's called. So how time—we also have a moon month rhythm, four weeks rhythm, and a week rhythm for certain cells. But what is most dominant is the 24-hour rhythm. That's why we go to bed and we wake up. But it is expressed in that your body temperature goes up and down like in a sinus graph. Practically a sinus graph.

Ty: What do you think are some of the main causes of cancer?

Dr. Gorter: Now I think one is that children cannot mount a fever anymore. Which parent, unless they know, will sit there and say, "Okay, my child has the chicken pox, has a couple of days' fever. It's fine?" And the other reason is because of nutrition and all kinds of medications that people take.

I was a family practitioner an Amsterdam, I then moved to the United States, and did all the residency and a specialty training program again. I also spent a month or more in the emergency room. And I was amazed that for any little snot, any little cough in a little child, they got antibiotics. Strong, broadband antibiotics.

So it's that also. One thing is you create a resistance if you use it too much. And finally, I would like to say, if I have a viral infection, a sore throat, I take seven days of antibiotic, and I take a week without. There's no difference.

Ty: No difference.

Dr. Gorter: Because antibiotics only work really on bacterial infections. And patients have little kids that don't get fever. And I think it all is a component. Look at a little child or little kids when they go to school—here in Germany in the streetcar, they all have them, their earphones. And in the meantime they are all chatting and chewing bubble gum.

So they are bombarded with sense perception and that really also is disturbing. (inaudible - 17:35) children one reason, they get taller and taller, but thinner and thinner. And they always have back problems. I think 50 years ago, for teenagers it was rare. Maybe two percent or so had some back problems. Now, about 30 percent. And how tall? Children get taller and taller, but paler and paler.

So you must see that it's a whole complex, a whole syndrome, which is also an expression of our time. I'm not pessimistic, but I saw certain things are taken out of the relation to other things, functions, and then you get this one side of that. Of course, if a child has a very high fever, you want to know why and maybe then intervene.

But it's part of childhood that you have fevers. In the United States, a little infant, the first 12 months, it has on the average seven viral infections. An ear infection, in order to produce a fever. That's the main reason.

And now more and more pediatricians and immunologists, they will say, "Yes, actually we shouldn't right away jump when a child has a little bit of a fever." All these things are a part of that we are actually, we look healthier, but we're actually worse off.

They say, "How can it be that cancer is on the rise?" But almost 50 percent of all Americans and Europeans get somewhere in their life a cancer diagnosis, and more than 70 percent will die. But it's the same in 1950 and now. Therefore, we should see what are all the possible reasons of cancer and how we will treat it.

Ty: What's your message to somebody that might have recently been diagnosed with something that the oncologist says is terminal? "You've got terminal cancer." What would you tell them? Is there hope?

Dr. Gorter: Well, I would say we will all die one day. Some people die from cancer, also, who come to us. But I think—I did a lot of clinical trials, or was the director of the site for where the trial was done, or the principal investigator. And what was always of concern to me, that all these clinical trials to prove that something works, it is in a very selective population.

So we always did inquiries in the inclusion and exclusion criteria. So often we had patients who we thought, "Well, they're a good candidate." But they were then rejected because whatever reason, they didn't fit the ideal profile. So usually, if 20 patients could apply with the diagnosis, only one is accepted.

Therefore, you have very selective sampling of people with a certain cancer, and then you do your study. So these drug companies, they sort of pick out the raisins out of the raisin bread. Or they think, "Well, if it works, this is the best population." But your regular population is very different.

So, of course, the whole concern of the drug companies, that we do all the data. And all the, the research files are then picked up, it goes to the pharmaceutical company. And they do the statistics.

Ty: So it's not independent?

Dr. Gorter: No. It's not independent. It also briefly was a big scandal but nobody really paid attention. The FDA approved, about four years ago, an antibiotic. The data was submitted by a French company but it turned out the study was never done.

Ty: Falsified completely.

Dr. Gorter: It wasn't even done. So therefore it is of concern. If a lot of money is involved, then we get this whole complex human interaction. If a lot of money is somewhere.

And there's also—with our western medicine, drug companies and doctors or hospitals, make money when you're ill. When you're healthy, they make no money. So to tell you how to stay healthier, or stay healthy, what can you ask for? Consultation, do nutrition, don't smoke. You can ask nothing essentially.

Therefore, in the whole western world, anything we do, there is always an economical side to it. It means making money, making money. And even now quicker and quicker. It's also unfortunately in medicine.

So that is of course of concern. But also these studies, people always ask you, "Yes, this is statistically proven." When I lecture for new students, medical students, and must know something about statistics. I tell them to following—this is from a long, long time ago. This image that babies are born, and there's a stork, this big bird, that brings down the babies. It has in its beak, a baby hanging in its diaper.

Since the 60s in Europe, this big bird, this stork, less and less come back from North Africa because they go in the winter to North Africa to survive. In the summer they fly to Northern Europe. That is over 6,000 kilometers. And then they get here, the babies, when they are big enough, they fly back. So they migrate.

But it turns out that less and less of these birds are returning because they are eaten in the Nile delta. But also the number of babies goes down, the birth rate goes down. Now statistically, that is very significant correlation. It's statistically proven, that because there are less of these birds, there are less babies. We know these birds don't bring babies. Other way the babies come.

But statistically it's true. So that's why I give it as an example when people say, "statistically proven." Churchill, I know some people in the United States—and one of my biostatisticians helped me. She had a picture of Churchill, Winston Churchill with this quote, and he said, "The only statistics I really believe are the ones I manipulated myself." And it's really sort of true.

Ty: That's a good way to—

Dr. Gorter: You have to be very careful.

Ty: That's a good way to summarize statistics. You make them prove anything you want.

Dr. Gorter: Or it is too bizarre but if I make this as a bizarre example, of course, then we all know that these big birds don't bring babies to mothers. But statistically, I can prove it. It's true. So they have to be a little more—when people say "evidence-based" and "statistically proven," "No, wait a moment. I would like to see the statistical analysis." But you never get to see that.

Ty: Well let's go take a tour of your clinic. What do you say?

Dr. Gorter: Okay. Good. You're welcome. I'll give you a little tour. Show you a little bit of what we do. And we cannot go too much in detail but I have an impression. I would love to do that.

Ty: Very good.

Dr. Gorter: First, over here is the waiting area. All the patients come when they have an appointment. So they don't have to wait, but sometimes the treatments take several hours and family members come. So they want to hang out here. There is, of course, Wi-Fi. There is a buffet usually with organic apples and juice, and that's available.

So essentially you can walk all around the clinic, but I'll show you the part which we mainly use. But if it's busy, we use also the other side. But what we do here, total body fever range, total body hyperthermia, the local hyperthermia. We do ozone therapy. We do vaccinations for dendritic cells. And all kinds of things for immune restoration, including mistletoe, *Viscum album*, also there's other preparations made from cannabis.

So I'll give you the tour. Let's start from this side.

Ty: You're hitting it from all the different angles, aren't you?

Dr. Gorter: Well, we have a concept. Maybe there are certain patients we feel maybe this is best for them to start. So we don't have a protocol where everybody goes through in the same way. But we have the different components, and what the patient needs, we will adjust them.

So here is one side of the clinic. We wanted the clinic to be not like a typical clinic, where it smells like alcohol or where people feel like they are at a dentist office. So therefore it's a little bit like a hotel-like setting.

Makes you sort of feel comfortable and that we have all the time. So we're never in a hurry. This also supports special patients who have been in university hospitals, where it's often you go in and out, in and out, and here you have all the time. But patients can't stay overnight. Buy six, seven o'clock, we slowly have to get the patients done, back to their apartment or hotel.

So they maybe start on this side of the clinic where we have a couple of rooms with local hyperthermia. But we also have a difference in the beds, so maybe you first start here.

These are the principal—after local hyperthermia. A patient, let's say, with a brain tumor—we have many, many patients with brain tumor every day. And that is like this that we put this. Let's say we have the patient's legs here, and the head is in between the two electrodes. And what is built up straight through the patient and with minimal pressure—there's contact of course, and then there is an electromagnetic field, very similar to an MRI scan. So no radiation, nothing.

Nothing is unsafe. So none of us disappears. And then in a period of an hour, there's an electromagnetic field is built up, a little bit like a microwave, the same principle. And cancer cells always have an increased resistance inside of an electromagnetic field. So if you have more resistance and then you get friction, then you get warmth production.

And this method is almost too nice to be true. But it shows—Siemens, a big German company, is behind us—that I can selectively in cancer cells, quickly increase temperature. So after about 50 minutes, the cancer cell has increased in the cell its temperature 43-44 degrees, to like 110 or so Fahrenheit.

And then a cancer cell also makes a lot of lactic acid, it's really an acid. And so when it's this high up, it will be forced to make three times as much lactic acid as when at normal body temperature. And then there is an accumulation of lactic acid, so the pH goes down. So it gets more and more, and more and more acidity inside the cell, and the cell then collapses and dies during the treatment.

So it causes what's called necrosis. And that is the whole principle. So we can—right away when a patient has a lot of pain because of growing tumors, within a couple sessions often they have no pain anymore because there's so much reduction of tumor tissue that there is less pressure or it doesn't grow anymore. And the patient notices after a couple of times the relief from symptoms, because they have much less tumor tissue.

Ty: So it doesn't affect the other cells, just the tumor cells?

Dr. Gorter: No. Also if I would bring the brain, the normal brain cells to 44 degrees Celsius or 109 or so Fahrenheit, the patient would die. Because that's not longer—you can no longer live with that kind of temperature in the brain. But it's not one point of a degree up because it is not effected normal cells, because they don't have an increased cell membrane resistance.

Ty: Oh, okay. So it's the resistance that causes the heat?

Dr. Gorter: Yes.

Ty: Got it.

Dr. Gorter: That's correct. So therefore, it is very selective, so patients never really feel much. It's very comfortable, often they fall asleep, and there's also no contraindication. The only contraindication is in people that have a pacemaker. Because a pacemaker, it is an electric apparatus under your skin, and if you put a strong electromagnetic field on it, it might go astray. And you don't want that to happen.

So you also see here on the door. Each door where we have the local hyperthermia, it has the sign. Anybody who has a pacemaker knows, "Oh, I should not enter here when the therapy is going."

Ty: I see.

Dr. Gorter: Because then they have or could be—that's what's the only risk. So we have maybe once every four years a patient who couldn't do that because they have a pacemaker.

Ty: Okay. But no other side effects?

Dr. Gorter: No side effects, absolutely none.

Ty: You just don't want to come in here with a pacemaker.

Dr. Gorter: Yeah. Make sure you never need to (inaudible - 31:13).

Now we have here the same, similar, but here's one different. Also a local hyperthermia bed. But here—so on the other batch, you have that you built up very concentrated this electromagnetic field between two electrodes. Here you have one electrode to the one side, the patient lays here, but this is a waterbed. And the whole mattress is the other electrode.

And we have some patients, they're very sick, very cachectic. So very skinny, skin off the bone. So they can't lay long on these other beds, they too hard. But this is a waterbed, so they can comfortably lay here. That's what I use, the only drawback is that we have less concentrated electromagnetic field. So we see when the patients can't handle to lay there for one or two hours, then we have this as an alternative. And this is always fine.

Ty: And you said that this—even patients that are in the cachexia cycle. They're okay?

Dr. Gorter: They're fine here. Because it's never stressful. The total body—when they produce fever that's a whole other issue. But here, patients lay here or sometimes they read a book or they listen to music or something. And there's never, ever distress. We're doing it now for 15 years, on this type of bed, and we have never had a patient who said, "oh [*making raspberry sound*]." Never.

Ty: Great.

Dr. Gorter: Now here is a room where patients come for ozone therapy. Then they lay here in the bed the infusion takes about 45 minutes to an hour. We take like 100 milliliters, 100 ml, of blood, and we saturate it. We let ozone go through it and then it is given back as a drip for about 45 minutes to an hour, it's given back. Why it's so effective—so when you put all these white blood cells in the bloods which took off under stress, because ozone is stress, and then they excrete practically all the interferons and the cytokines they have, they express that.

And then you get, in this 100 milliliter blood, a little bunch of all kinds of cytokines which will then, when it comes back in the body, will really activate many of the immune functions.

Ty: I see.

Dr. Gorter: It's a little bit a-specific, but it works well. Also for viral infections. Before really effective AIDS treatment was there, we treated many, many people, HIV positives, we treated them also with ozone. And for now, like six, seven years, nobody show progression. (inaudible 3402-05) but also in cancer.

Ty: So that, is that the primary way that you use the ozone, is you take the blood out, you infuse it, it causes the cytokine release, and then put it back in?

Dr. Gorter: That's right.

Ty: Got it.

Dr. Gorter: And there never any toxicity, any side effects. One of the family members, or one of the nurses, or I sit here a little bit and we talk.

Ty: Got it. Very cool. Total body hyperthermia.

Dr. Gorter: Yes. We call this fever-range total body hyperthermia to emphasize that we don't do extreme temperatures. As always you can get—when you really have a nice rule, in centigrade is 38.5, maybe to 39, which when you're healthy, you can easily produce, make that. And that's what we do. And it's a computer that's all computer programmed that monitors heart rate, and cardiogram, like in an intensive care unit. But we never, ever have seen any problems.

Ty: This is total body hyperthermia, so it's basically the equivalent of getting a good sweat if you're sick.

Dr. Gorter: Yes. And they get a fever.

Ty: Fever sweat.

Dr. Gorter: The core is also monitored with a thermometer and a little sonar. It is monitored, so we know exactly from minute to minute what the core body temperature is. And the heat, it comes from these lamps. They have infrared.

The principle is so that infrared doesn't go deep but maybe a centimeter through the skin, and the blood flow in the skin works like a central heating system. We have hot water running through the house. So the blood is heated up, so to speak, and then it circulates through the body, and then the whole body is warmed up, slowly but surely.

It's a very elegant way. Usually after about two hours, the patient is at 38.5, 39 degrees Celsius. Then we switch off the lamps and we leave the patient for an hour. Then they are at steady state, and then we slowly cool them off. And when they're cooled off, then we have here a shower, and the patients take a shower. Here patients shower.

Ty: Very nice.

Dr. Gorter: Of course, a nurse is always there. So you cannot slip or so. And then afterwards—that is what we do. Then we give patients the vaccination with dendritic cells.

Ty: Dendritic cell vaccination.

Dr. Gorter: Yes. Dendritic cell vaccination.

Ty: What exactly are dendritic cells?

Dr. Gorter: Well, they are often called the policemen of the immune system. Because usually often cancer patients say, "Well, over the last 30 years I have not missed a day of work." What they mean, "I've never never really had a fever." That's what they mean, "I wasn't sick." Because you feel sore throat, muscle aches and so, but if you don't have a fever—people associate fever with being ill. Where that fever is the cause of an illness.

But it's actually the opposite. Fever is an attempt by the body to overcome an infection or a trauma. So what we do is, we first bring a patient to this fever state, and then the immune system is really activated. Only way to improve immune function or to activate immune system is through fever, to increase body temperature. There's no other way.

It's a very delicate center in the brain stem which regulates very nicely the temperature. And if it has to go quick up because it's hurt, an infection is set, then you can either have the chills and these little muscle contractions, they produce actually more warmth. So within half an hour, an hour, you have a big fever.

But what we do—cancer cells have all kinds of escape mechanisms. They make themselves less visible, also for dendritic cells. As if we're the policemen. So as if they walk through the shopping mall and the street, as if they do this all day. You can't really see them, they're hiding. But it takes energy. If we put on a lot of stress then temperature goes up, they make more and more lactic acid. They will put all that energy only in surviving. That's all. And then they drop their escape mechanisms. Of course, that takes a lot of energy. And then they become more and more visible for dendritic cells.

So what we do? Before we give patients dendritic cell vaccination, we first let them go through a period of moderate fever and then for sure—animal studies show that these cancer cells are in a lot of stress or maybe in the act of dying, so they can easily be seen by these policemen, by these dendritic cells.

And in (inaudible 39:04), like in patients with glioblastoma multiforme, the most aggressive brain cancer. Why it is so aggressive is because they have such a good escape mechanism that the dendritic cells can practically not see them. But we have still—when they come to us and they already have a relapse, we still have 46 percent, almost half, still in complete remission. We have patients now 8-10 years down the road that were dying from glioblastoma, and without any glioblastoma, any cancer. But they come here with breast cancer, almost any cancer—we have actually, in all humbleness, pretty good results, because we combine the hyperthermia with the dendritic cells.

Ty: So that's a good one-two punch. Hyperthermia with dendritic cells.

Dr. Gorter: I think we should—it is our public secret that we say you should, if you vaccinate, if at all possible, you should also activate immune function with moderate fever. And it works, I think also for breast cancer patients. Practically, we only get patients who are on their last phases. They have been told, "There's nothing we can do anymore, this is it. Now you must say goodbye. We'll make you comfortable, and so on."

And often they come to us as a last hope. And still, quite a few turn completely around, and a number of years completely without cancer. The brain, metastases, liver, bone. And there's a lot of also video documentaries on these kind of patients. We see them every two years again. Maybe (inaudible - 40:37-39). But again, it's impressive how people go in complete remission. But you like to know how they do four or eight years later. So every couple of years, there's an update.

Ty: That's great. That's great. You've got some interesting protocols here.

Dr. Gorter: Well, we do our best. But there's always privacy. We never put two people who don't know each other in a room. And upstairs there's a couple of suites, because we also have patients who have a little crown on their head or are public figures. So we can offer safety. But also they don't always want people say, "Oh, is he not so and so?" So we have them upstairs.

Ty: Some private.

Dr. Gorter: Some private suites. In order to have people—also for safety. First of all for safety. Because it speaks around that they—and a dictator of country is here, I don't know, we might have a bombshell going or something.

And here is the apparatus for ozone.

Ty: Ozone, got you.

Dr. Gorter: So this is ozone. And a certain amount—the pressure puts through in 100 millimeter blood, and then given back slowly as a drip. And the principle is that you put all these immune cells on a lot of stress, they excrete the many things they have and then you have a big bomb of these cytokines, which have a significant effect on the immune system.

It's a little bit a-specific, like fever, but it works. But also in cancer, also in chronic viral infections. Especially those two, are very well documented by others and by us, with good efficacy.

Ty: So you really are working on getting the cancer cells weak, and then giving the immune system a bump.

Dr. Gorter: That's right.

Ty: Got it.

Dr. Gorter: Here's another total body hyperthermia. So we have more, but you've seen one or two and that is enough. But it is the same principle. One more.

And then here is the doctors' rooms. During the day when the clinic is up and running usually two doctors sit here to be easily available and so on. And to put in infusions. But this is their office. And then, again, you have here two more local hyperthermia beds. Which in principle have—

Ty: You've got several of those.

Dr. Gorter: Yes. Because treatment takes one, two, or maybe three hours. And somebody can have metastases in lung, liver, and maybe in a knee, they will need three sessions of an hour. And then it wouldn't be good if people have to wait for each other, so we can always do a couple of treatments parallel. Same treatment, parallel.

And over here is something for children. Because the children maybe need some blood draw or this or that, or infusion. So we have a bat, dog or lion.

Ty: Got it.

Dr. Gorter: For children. And also if you're very good you can take it home. So all the time, they take bats and dogs home. But it's special for children. It's in the corner here, so it's not that much if maybe once a child screams or so. We don't watch of course. But children can scream and everybody is not upset and saying, "Oh, what's going on? What's going on?"

Ty: Right. No, this is fascinating. I love it. This is a great clinic.

Dr. Gorter: Well, thank you.

Ty: I like the way that you focused on peacefulness. And also integrated with the physicians. So the doctors aren't somewhere separate, they're accessible.

Dr. Gorter: A lot of times they walk around. And I, of course, am often here, maybe not nonstop, but we do that also. And also the nurses are very well trained, also love what they do. In practically almost 15 years, we've only had one nurse who left us. But she got married so that was a good reason.

But because our staff and nurses see how many people come here, and they are told or they say, "I'm dying." And then 10 years later they still come once a year for their dendritic vaccine. There is also motivation here. If you can help a lot of people, then it motivates them to do better. (inaudible - 0:45:08) something happens.

It's almost 15 years, we had nothing happen. Because what we do, nothing is toxic, so we don't have this whole ordeal. Let's say, like the cancer clinics, with the slowing up the blood transfusion, the side effects, nothing.

Ty: No side effects.

Dr. Gorter: No.

Ty: That's what it's all about, right there.

Dr. Gorter: Because if you improve immune function, it can never have toxicity. Because toxicity means that you suppress, or push, or kill. And in local hyperthermia, that only kills cancer cells, which are not normal cells.

Ty: Selectively toxic.

Dr. Gorter: Yes. So therefore it's not toxic, only for cancer cells. And if lot of cancer cells die, then some lactic acid is excreted, but the bloodstream takes this and your body is extremely well fit to absorb lactic acid. Like if you run to the bus stop, also you make lactic acid in your calves or so.

Ty: Right. Lactic acid. Sure. I love the light in the middle of the clinic here.

Dr. Gorter: Yes. If it wouldn't be here, it would be maybe a little dark. So a lot of lights on the things, and sunlight, there's a lot of light here. But actually we don't really have lights on this one, one in the corner.

And on the other side, we have very similar. Two more rooms where people can just rest for a while. A few less beds for us on this side. But the same thing, you can just walk around. And this is the center, where the light is.

Ty: And you were telling me earlier that you can treat, what, 30-40 patients?

Dr. Gorter: No, 30. We don't really do much more. Because we want everybody to get full attention. And so the patient notice right away, we're never in a hurry. That's often a problem. You go in clinics—there's always, if you talk to a doctor more than 10 minutes, he looks, "umm." Often patients come and they tell a story, I take two hours to talk with them.

Ty: I can attest to that. We're here almost eight o'clock at night, and you're just taking your time, giving us a tour, not in a hurry.

Dr. Gorter: Let's just say I'm married to my work.

Ty: Married to your work.

Dr. Gorter: Because I had cancer myself, so that gives an extra motivation to be available. You know what they go through.

You know, I was for a year, the dean of a medical school in Germany, but I didn't like it. It was too political, so I quit. But I got all the students, medical students, before they went on the floors and they had patient contact, they first had to have one weekend themselves in a hospital bed.

Ty: To know what it feels like.

Dr. Gorter: Yes. Well, they were not sick, but they had to pretend. And they had bed privileges. So if they had to go to the bathroom, they had to do it in the bed. That's very difficult to have a bowel movement in your bed. It's very against all your instincts. But they had to do that. And the nurses were instructed, if they call, they want tea or coffee, wait a little bit, they can wait 20 minutes or so. So we treat them a little bit badly, but they were not sick. Just to feel how it is so easy—when doctors say, "bed rest" but the consequences of that. And when you're sick, what it is.

So I know many of these medical students they hated me. But years later, once I was in Vienna in a meeting, suddenly this guy comes to me and taps me on the shoulder. He said, "I know you can't remember me, but I was one of your students in Herdecke, and I hated you. I had a beautiful weekend and my girlfriend was waiting, but I had to be here in the stupid bed." But he said that now he understood what I wanted to show. I feel that respect is worth something.

Ty: It's probably a really good lesson for them to learn, how it feels to be on the other side.

Dr. Gorter, thanks for the tour. Thanks for the interview today.

Dr. Gorter: You're welcome.

Ty: Great information.

Dr. Gorter: Thank you that you came to have a look at what we do. And I will like to participate in interviews like this because it is important that more people, and also doctors, know there's more to do. And also scientifically based, proven, like the dendritic cells. And that there are other ways to treat cancer patients. When you ask me what do I say to a cancer patient who is at an end stage disease and told, "There's nothing we can do." I say, "Well, possibly we can still do something and give you hope, because we do it very differently."

Ty: Thinking outside the box. I like that. Well thank you for the interview today, and thank you for the tour.

Dr. Gorter: Thank you for coming.

Ty: Alright.

[end of transcript]

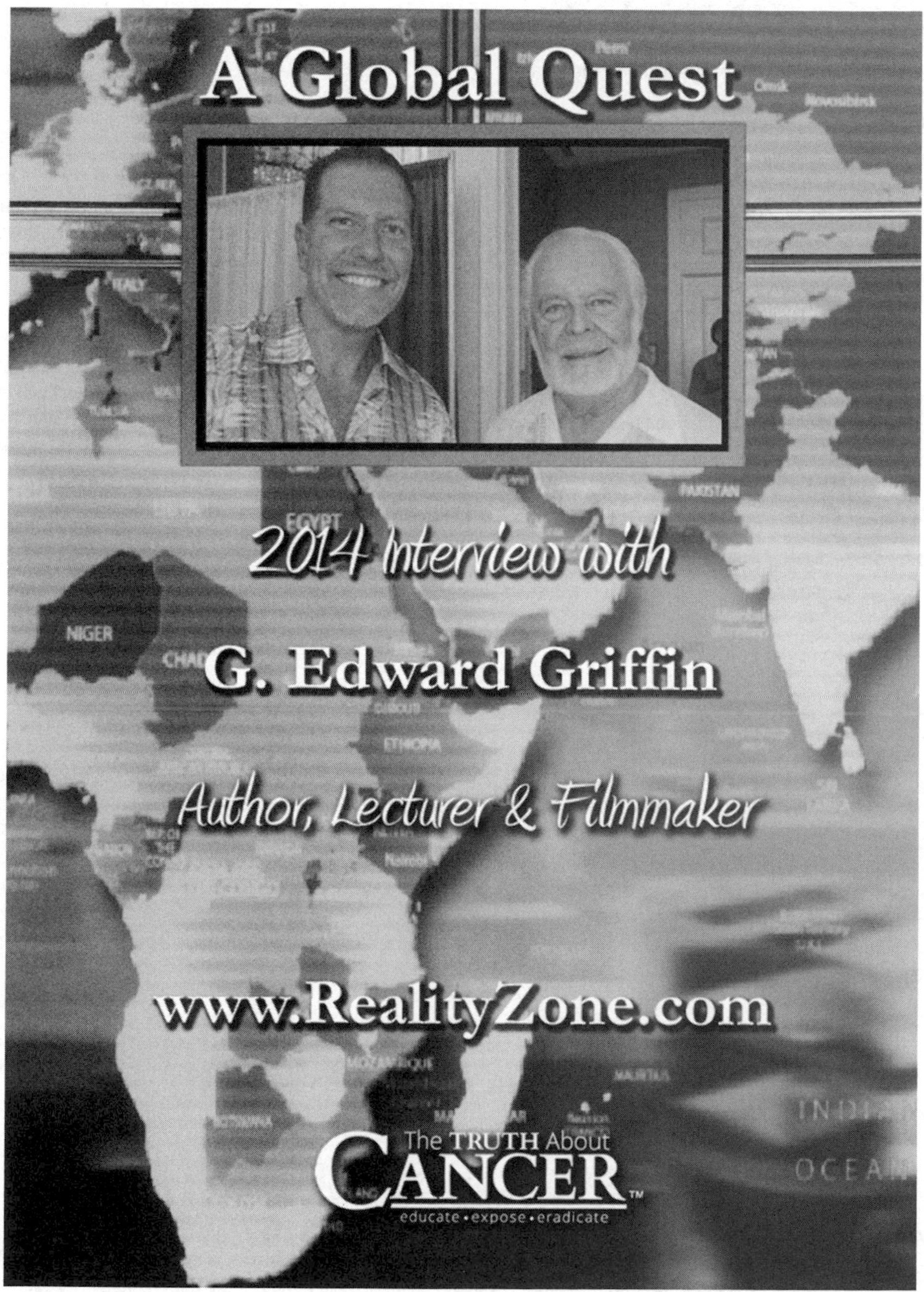
A Global Quest
2014 Interview with
G. Edward Griffin
Author, Lecturer & Filmmaker
www.RealityZone.com
The TRUTH About
CANCER
educate • expose • eradicate

Ty: So I'm here today with G. Edward Griffin. We're here in Southern California and I just want to say thank you for taking the time to spend with us today to share some your knowledge. Thank you for being with us today.

Edward: Well thanks, thanks a lot. My pleasure.

Ty: Tell us, Mr. Griffin, about your experience, your background, what got you to where you are today?

Edward: I have to confess all, I guess. Well, I don't know where I am today, that's the hard part, but I know where I came from. Yeah, I'm just a guy that likes to delve into esoteric subjects and mysterious things and I like to write about them. I'd much rather investigate them than write about them. That's where the fun is. But anyway I've written some books on upstream topics. My favorite areas are alternative health and natural health. I get into geopolitics. I'm very interested in some pre-history geology and things like that nobody else cares about. I really became kind of a crusader at a young age and I take on mostly topics that, as mentioned, are upstream, meaning that I have a point of view that is different than what is the common point of view. Conventional wisdom, and not only that but these are topics that I think are extremely important. Not just to me and my family but to everybody and to the world. So I have that kind of bigger picture that some people find to be strange but I can't help myself. I'm a crusader so naturally I find topics that I think need some support. So that leads me right into the field of geopolitical areas and also alternative health. So I've written books. I produced a couple of documentary films and I've done that ever since, 1962, I think is when I started down that path.

Ty: Since that time you've written multiple books, two of the most popular being *The Creature from Jekyll Island* about the Federal Reserve System ...

Edward: Right.

Ty: ... and *World Without Cancer.*

G. Edward: Right. Those are probably the most important ones and although now they have a little age on them they continue to be very popular. We update both of those books a couple of times year. We go through a couple of printings a year and so we keep them as current as possible. In the case of the Federal Reserve book, it's in it's fifth edition and I think in it's 38th printing right now so ...

Ty: Wow.

Edward: ...it just keeps rolling along.

Ty: And *World Without Cancer,* you'll continually updating that as well?

Edward: Yes, absolutely.

Ty: Tell us about the book World Without Cancer.

Edward: *World Without Cancer* is, on the surface, it's about a specific alternative cancer therapy called Laetrile, that's its common word. Its common title. The substance itself is really called amygdalin, but on the surface it appears to be about that and, in fact, it is but it's also about the bigger picture. The fact that medical establishment, in the Western World at least today, is oriented very strongly toward drug therapy and radiation, of course, and some very expensive procedures, which in my view and the view of the doctors and researchers that I have relied upon for my research, in their view it's not the best treatment at all. So it's about the bigger picture about how the industry, the cancer industry, particularly the pharmaceutical cancer industry has dominated that field and not necessarily conscientiously but as a result of that it has certainly filtered away all of these natural approaches for cancer treatment.

So that's the real picture because it's not just that the Laetrile is necessarily the most effective treatment. I think there are many different types of treatments that are very good but they all have one thing in common, and that is that they come from nature. Now that may not seem like a big deal, but when you understand how the industry works you realize that if anything comes from nature it cannot be patented. It has to be invented before you can patent it, which is why the pharmaceutical industry is not interested in anything that comes from nature. What they are interested in is to find out if something works in nature, take it to the laboratory, pull it apart, look at the molecule, see what the active ingredient is and then see if they can reassemble it and call it ours, you know. Now they can patent it and that's the bigger story. I think once people understand that there's this commercial bias that's built into the industry and that bias is not just about money but it's about their lives and their health. Then it becomes a very, very important story and here comes the crusader galloping on his white house. He's got to tell this story.

Ty: Fascinating. I want to get to Laetrile here in a few minutes. First of all you mentioned the fact that we got the pharmaceutical industry, we've got kind of industry driven by money, and we've got doctors who are really smart people today, brilliant medical doctors. They're using treatments that really don't seem to work as well as some of these natural things. Why is it? Can you go back into the history of the medical association, The American Medical Association, AMA, and maybe take us back 100 years and then to current day and explain why that is, because I've heard you talk about this in the past and your explanation is fascinating and I want the listeners to be able to hear this.

Edward: Well thank you for that. It is a fascinating story. It's an important story. I suppose we don't have time to go into all of it, but maybe the best way here is to kind of back into it to start with where we are and then go back and see how we got there. Where we are today is that, just as you described, these very smart doctors, let's face it, they're very selective process there. You just don't get into med school unless you got a pretty good brain on top of your shoulders there, so yeah, it's the cream of the crop. The best students go into these schools, these medical schools but they're not taught anything about natural cures. They're taught only about drugs, primarily, and drug reactions and the chemistry of this and the chemistry of that and they have to become really pharmacists in a way, they have to become chemists, before they can even make it through pre-med. So that's not necessarily bad, but it is a bias. I have come to know a lot of doctors in the last couple of decades since we've been working in this field, many doctors who came from that lair of education and who gradually, and sometimes very painfully, had to break away from that and go back and re-examine some of these fundamental issues. Many of them have made the transition and they speak quite openly about it now. They say, for instance, they'll say, "When I went to medical school we never learned anything about vitamins except we had maybe two hours of instruction on the structures of vitamins and minerals and so forth." Two hours compared to hundreds and hundreds of hours about pharmaceuticals and chemical reactions and so forth. I remember there was one doctor he said, "My wife knows more about nutrition than I do when I came out of school." That is not surprising when you realize—now we start to go backward in time. How did that happen? The fact that these great medical teaching universities and teaching centers are so great is because they've had a lot of money given to them. Where did the money come from? Now we're on the trail. You know the old saying following the money …

Ty: Yeah, follow the money.

Edward: …and usually that'll take you right to it. Well, if you follow the money you'll find out that most of it came from the pharmaceutical industry. The pharmaceutical industry knows that if they give large grants to these universities they have a double benefit. First of all, they have the appearance of being philanthropists. You know they're doing good things and that's always—that's good for public relations. I'm not saying that they're not doing good things, they probably think they are, but anyway, that's one advantage to giving tax-exempt or tax-free deductible donations to universities. The other advantage is far more important because once you have financed a research project you now have sort of a first right to whatever comes out of that research and consequently you can determine in what areas the research will go. I could assure that if I'm a big pharmaceutical company and I give a $20 million grant to a research group I'm not going to be very happy if they start to research whether or not dandelions can be used in the control of cancer. I want to make sure they're going to research a drug that I am working on in the laboratories right now. That's where I want the research go. So they realize that they can take their own research budget and transfer it to a university or some research laboratory and get a tax deduction for it, knowing full well that if that's what they're researching that's where the data is going to be. So I don't need to go any further.

You can understand when the money is coming from a source, which has a vested interest in the outcome, now what's going to happen is the outcome is going to be what the donor wants it to be, generally. So this is the problem and that goes back even further in time to the turn of the last century when the Rockefeller group and the Carnegie group actually came together and they decided that they would reform medical education in America. At that time the quality of medical education or medical treatment was really quite low because there were no standards. There were no ways to determine who really had an understanding of science and who was a quack. If you had a few bucks in your pocket you could send them through the mail and get a diploma in the mail and now you're doctor. You could put that up on your wall. Needless to say this is not a very good situation.

Ty: There literally were mail order doctors then?

Edward: There literally were, and some of them were good, by the way. Interestingly enough I discovered some of them were pretty good because they were working on the basis of traditional cures. What they learned from their grandmother. What they learned from the medicine man and so forth.

Ty: I want to stop you there. Traditional cures. Now today we hear traditional medicine and we think drug-intensive but traditional cures really are cures that go back hundreds, and even thousands, of years.

Edward: That's right.

Ty: That's interesting that you said traditional cures because today we think of traditional cures as being drug intensive cures that the modern medical industry uses but really the true definition of traditional is cures that have been used for thousands, hundreds of years.

Edward: Yeah, I guess it's just whoever's using the word whatever they have in mind. But anyway, that was the case, and yes, there were diploma mills. The Rockefellers and the Carnegies decided that here was an opportunity to do some apparent good that people would say, "Well, gee they're going to reform and upgrade medical education," and at the same time these groups realized that since they were heavily invested in the pharmaceutical industry that this would be a way of getting some of their money back in a way that could magnify or multiply their investment. They looked at as an investment, not really an act of philanthropy. So they hired a guy by the name of Dr. Abraham Flexner. They wrote the famous Flexner report, I think it was 1910 if I remember correctly, and Flexner did the obvious. He surveyed the state of medical education in America and said it's pretty bad. Then came up with a solution. Well, the solution was to make it better. That means to hire more qualified people, to determine a very high-quality curriculum, to determine what textbooks were to be used to hire top people in these research centers and so forth. All of that required money, and so then the money followed from the Carnegies and the Rockefellers, they donated quite a bit of money to the teaching universities in America. Not all of them accepted the money. Those that accepted the money grew and actually a huge influx of finance and they grew. They were able to build buildings. Hire the best people. Get the best equipment in there and these are the ones that survived to today we consider them to be the great medical centers of America and that's how they got to be there in the beginning. Those that declined the money sort of fell by the wayside, they couldn't compete and most of them are out of business now.

So the result of that little piece of history is, oh by the way, when they donated the money the donors would say, "Well, now we've given you a lot of money and we know you're going to do the right thing with it but would you object if we had someone from our staff appointed to your board of directors just to see how our money is being spent?" That was really a condition of getting the money so you know the university said, "That would be fine. Anybody you would suggest would be, I'm sure, more than adequate." So they began to load up the boards of directors of these teaching centers with people who literally were on the payroll of the donors. So once that was in place, the curriculum of the universities, the teaching centers, swung completely in the direction of pharmaceutical drugs, and it has remained that way ever since.

Now does that mean it's a conspiracy? No, it doesn't mean that at all. It just means if you follow the money this is what motivates people. I think many of us, if we're going to give money to some charity, we don't want to see that money spent on something that would be competitive with our line of work. We wouldn't do it. So it can be too harsh on these people because they're just making good business decisions, at least in their mind. Then you follow it through, and you realize that now this whole medical field has been skewed in the direction of pharmaceutical drugs, which can be patented and produce great profits for the producers. Then the next step is, that means that anything coming from nature is excluded. That's where we think, some of us think, that most of the promise lies in these very complex substances found in herbs and plants and trees and things like that, seeds. Some of us feel like it is was probably meant to be that way. So you come out of all of this analysis and all of this history with the realization that the medical profession is really like a lap dog of the pharmaceutical industry. Most of the doctors have no idea that that's the case. They don't understand this history.

Ty: That is a good way to put it. I have not heard it put that way before. A lap dog of the pharmaceutical industry. That explains my next question. My question was going to be why is that medical doctors today are so heavily biased towards drugs and not nutrition? You just explained it.

Edward: That's it, yeah.

Ty: It's not because they're dumb people. They're brilliant people. Most doctors have a brain much larger than mine. They're very smart people, but they have not been taught the nutritional protocols.

Edward: It's as simple as that, yeah.

Ty: Even a genius can't teach you something that he or she doesn't know.

Edward: That's right.

Ty: Talk about nutritional protocols for cancer. You had mentioned *World Without Cancer* and you've mentioned nutrition. Talk about the Hunza Indians. I remember reading about the Hunza Indians and I remember hearing you talk about cancer being a nutritional deficiency. Could you expound on that?

Edward: Yeah, this is the big question. You have to be careful you don't get too deeply into the details without establishing some big assumptions. So let's back up to the basic assumption, which is the answer to the question. What is cancer? Believe it or not, after all of these years and all these billions of dollars that have been spent on a so-called war against cancer, those in the highest levels of this war, they still do not agree as what cancer is. It's amazing to me. They got these theories about, well it's a gene, or it's maybe it's a deficiency, maybe it's something awry, there's a receptor here and, you know, they get into all these highfalutin', very complex technicalities that the average person cannot understand and, frankly, some of the technicians don't understand.

Ty: How can you declare a war on something that you don't know what it is?

Edward: You don't even know what it is. Yes. I'm not saying that I'm smarter than anybody else, but I am going to say that when I talked to the doctors and the researchers who advocate alternative therapies, there answer is as to what cancer is made a lot of sense to me. Much more sense than anything that you would get from the other side, from the so-called orthodox field. These men and women believe that, well let me start off with the traditional view. Now we have to rephrase that word "traditional." The present orthodox view is that cancer is a lump or a bump. That's the cancer. That's the assumption. Now if that is true then to get rid of cancer all you have to do is get rid of the lump or the bump and hence we have surgery. Well that gets rid of the lump or the bump or we have chemotherapy, which poisons the lump or the bump, or we have radiation, which burns it and got rid of it and you undergo these three therapies and to get rid of the lump or the bump the doctor will say, "It looks like we got it all." That famous line, "We got it all." But did they? No. The statistics show that in most cases it comes back. They didn't get it all because that was never the cancer in the first place.

If you're a farmer and see all these little black spots on your corn leaves and you think, well those are black spots. That's the disease. You get scissors out and you cut all the black spots away, well, you say, "We got it all," right? No, you didn't because that wasn't the disease. What caused those black spots is still present and so the same thing these men believe, the alternative doctors believe. They are more concerned with what caused the lump or the bump. So they start looking at the body as a whole and they believe, therefore, that cancer is not caused by something. It is caused by the lack of something. Whole different perspective. The lack of something, a breakdown in the body's normal ability to remain healthy. They believe that cancer is really a natural process. It's related to the healing process and it's over simplification, you might say, that cancer is nothing but healing gone awry.

If I were to scratch my hand now, just then with that thumbnail I've probably scraped, oh I don't know hundreds of cells. Right now already my body is responding to that and is sending signals out, chemical signals and electrical signals and a lot of electricity in the body and it's triggering the mechanism to start growing new cells. This is natural. This is the healing process. When those cells are finally replaced, they will send signals out and the body says that's enough, stop now, but now if the signals are not working right because of a chemical imbalance or some toxic intervention of some kind, the signals are not working right. Now it doesn't say stop healing. So it just continues to heal and heal and over heal and finally we have that famous lump or bump and ah, it's cancer. No, that's a symptom of the cancer. The cancer is why didn't the signals work? There's something wrong with the signaling mechanism. That's sort of the difference between the orthodox view and the alternative doctors view of what cancer is.

So the orthodox physicians are always looking for ways to reinforce the body's defenses. They know there's something wrong. The body broke down. The body failed. It wasn't because of a bacterium or a virus or something that attacked the body and then it grew the cancer. It's the body itself, which was unable to do it's normal job. So the search then becomes, what is that breakdown? Now we get to the really interesting part of the saga. There are a lot of things that can break down that could result in a cancerous growth. A lot of things. Almost anything as a matter of fact. The cellular maintenance of healing is a very complex substance. I know just a little bit about it, and even what I know is just mind boggling, as to how complex and beautiful it all works. So you don't know really quite where to start. Most of these physicians will start everywhere. They'll say, "Let's do a blood test and see what your panel looks like. If you're deficient in this let's build it up. If you have too much of that, especially if it's something toxic like radioactive particles in your body, let's get rid of that," and so forth to get you back to what they think is a healthy state, and the search then is for something else. Maybe you're missing something from the outside.

Those who follow the Laetrile theory, and it's a theory, very well proven I think, but still it's a theory. They recognize that there are two factors that need to be focused upon. There's the intrinsic factor and the extrinsic factor. Meaning intrinsic from the inside and extrinsic something from the outside. The easiest one to look at, I don't how deeply you want to go into this, but the easiest one to look at is the extrinsic factor. Meaning something you eat. Something you take in from the outside. It doesn't come from inside the body. You have to put it into your body. Food, in other words. Now we're into this thing called nutrition, an extrinsic factor. Well, what is that? They have found that there is a substance in nature, again, can't be patented, it's in nature, it's in about 1,400 edible plants, it's ubiquitous. It's everywhere except on the plates of modern man, because it has a bitter taste to it. If you have choice, you know, if you're not just living in a primitive society and you can chose what foods you want, you normally don't chose bitter.

Ty: We like sweet.

Edward: We like sweet and that is the beginning of the problem or least the answer to the question, why does modern man have cancer and primitive man does not? There's a part of the answer. Well anyway, this substance is called amygdalin. It's well known. It's been in the pharmacopeia for almost a hundred years. I think it was first isolated and described in Germany and it's been used for medicinal purposes for a long, long time. Amygdalin is a substance that is bitter, and it's found in grasses and in seeds primarily. They have found that in those cultures, those places in the world, where the diet, the native diet is rich in amygdalin foods, the cancer rate is very low if not zero. You compare the diet to the same food or you compare that diet to the diet of the people in modern societies where cancer rates are high, and you find there's practically no amygdalin at all. It's just a complete eye opener. What are those cultures? Hunzas I think you mentioned a moment ago are probably the best known, from a little kingdom up in Northwest Pakistan. It's a very idyllic place, I'm told. The story Shangri-La, they say, was actually written based upon Hunza as the model. Everybody knows the story of Shangri-La. Well Hunza's pretty much like that. It's very remote. If you risk your life getting into it, and I always thought I wanted to go visit Hunza after I read about it until some photographs of these deep ravines that you have to walk across on a rope bridge and it's about a mile and a half straight down, go along the cliffs like this, you know, I said no, I think I'll just read about it.

Ty: I'll read about it. Yeah.

Edward: But anyway that is really the way it was. I guess they have a road in now. The people in Hunza never had cancer but afterwards when they come out of Hunza and they go into other countries and they start eating the same foods that those people eat they come down with cancer like everyone else. In Hunza, at least in the beginning when all this research was done, there was no such thing as money. It's kind of a primitive society and a man's wealth was measured by the number of apricot trees he owns. People eat apricot seeds there, a little sweeter than the ones in California but still loaded with amygdalin and they eat them like candy. It was like a delicacy there. Well there's just one example. There are other cultures, the Bilcabamba's, the Navajo and Hopi Indians, the aboriginal Eskimos, all of those cultures have zero or very low cancer rates. If you look at the native diet, in every case their foods are at least 200 times, if not more, rich in amygdalin than anything that you would find in a major city or even in the countryside in our western world. So that's a clue. So then the next question is what is this thing amygdalin? How does it work? It's very simple. Amygdalin is a molecule that has four components in it locked together. There are two components of sugar or glucose. There's one component of cyanide and there's the word that scares people, we'll come back to that in a minute and one component of benzaldehyde. Now people say why cyanide, you want to take cyanide to treat cancer?

Ty: Right.

Edward: The answer is, yes, of course. Well, doesn't cyanide kill you? Well, yes, if it's real pure, gaseous cyanide, if it's pure cyanide, yes. When it's in a molecule with other components it's not cyanide. It's something else. It's like vitamin B12. It's called cyanocobalamin. We would be dead if we didn't have cyanide in our bodies in that form. In cyanocobalamin it's not cyanide it's cyanocobalamin. It's a molecule that's made up of several components, one being cyanide. Well, there's a big difference between free cyanide, which is gaseous or when it's locked with other components or elements …

Ty: Sure.

Edward: …so that's the key to understanding why we're not worried about cyanide being part of the molecule. The real question is, what is it that would release cyanide? By the way, benzaldehyde is toxic too. Most people don't know that and the two together are even more toxic than two times each so it's—if you release the cyanide and the benzaldehyde you've released a very toxic component so you have to be very careful about that. The next question is what releases it? I'm glad you're sitting down for this, I think you already know this but I hope everybody watching this is sitting down because the thing that releases the cyanide and the benzaldehyde is an enzyme called Beta-glucosidase. Beta-glucosidase. It's an enzyme. Where is that found? In cancer cells and only in cancer cells.

Ty: Wow.

Edward: It's a beautiful mechanism of nature that could not have been accidental if the body's natural method of controlling overgrowth, over healing, because once you get one cell that is an over-healing cell, it contains this unlocking enzyme, as we call it. The unlocking enzyme comes in contact with amygdalin, if you are eating food with amygdalin …

Ty: That's the big "if" isn't it…

Edward: That's the big "if" yeah…

Ty: **…you have to eat it.**

Edward: …if you're not eating food with amygdalin in it then it doesn't work but if you are, it doesn't take much, just a little bit, and if you are eating it and it's in your bloodstream, it comes in contact with that overgrowth cell, the overgrowth cell releases the toxic components and commits hara-kiri and you don't even know that anything happened. You come to the conclusion that everybody has cancer all the time but it's continually being controlled and eliminated by a natural mechanism of the body. It's nothing to worry about. It's part of nature. It's part of the healing process. Only time you need to worry about it is if you've messed up your body in some way then you've not given it the fuel. You haven't given it the components it needs to do its job. So that's the big difference between the alternative view of cancer and the orthodox view of cancer.

Ty: Now let me ask you this, Mr. Griffin. So we've got this huge epidemic of cancer, especially here in the United States. It's all over the world. It's a pandemic but here especially. A lot of the reason you're saying is because potentially our diets are deficient in a simple nutrient. This amygdalin. I've also heard it called vitamin B17, and I've also seen a lot of warnings on the Internet, it's funny that you mention the cyanide. If you look for B17 on the Internet you get the warnings, "Watch out it's cyanide, it'll kill you, but you just mentioned vitamin B12 contains a molecule of cyanide as well but it's bound to other molecules so it's not really cyanide."

Edward: With no warnings on B12. Why is that?

Ty: That was my question. Why is there no warnings on B12?

Edward: Because you'd be laughed off the Internet if you did that that's why.

Ty: But we have the warnings against B17.

Edward: Yeah, yeah.

Ty: Why do you think that is?

Edward: I don't know. I have to think about motive. I suppose mostly it's just ignorance. Most people who are putting those warnings up probably don't know about what I just said. They really believe that, oh, yeah there's cyanide in there and so we need to warn people. Maybe some of them are putting it up there for legal protection, just in case somebody wants to sue them. Maybe their attorneys have advised it. I don't know. The third possibility is that maybe somebody from the pharmaceutical industry says, "Look, we need a campaign to discourage people from exploring this nutritional approach so they'll come to us for our expensive chemotherapy drugs." It could be any one of those three.

Ty: Okay. I have a question for you. You said that this enzyme Beta-glucosidase unlocks the molecules. Once it unlocks the molecules and it kills that cancerous site why doesn't it kill the rest of the body?

Edward: Well, it's a good question. I'm not sure I can answer the why. All I know is that the laboratory results show that it does not. In fact, it becomes a nutrient for normal cells. It does not negatively affect them all. It's sort of like vitamin B12 in a way. In fact you mentioned vitamin B17 was another name for it. That was a name given to it by Dr. Ernst T. Krebs, Jr. who was the co-discover of this. He thought it should be named B17 because it has a lot of characteristics of the other B vitamins and there are 16 of them identified and officially recognized, he thought this should be 17. Never has been officially recognized, but the point is that it's similar to other B vitamins. So when this breaks down, it acts like a vitamin in normal tissue.

Ty: I'm friends with a man in Michigan that actually used vitamin B17, Laetrile, amygdalin, whatever you want to call it, for his cancer. He was given a terminal cancer sentence. He used it, and he said not only did it kill his cancer but it got rid of all his pain. So what you said about it being used as a natural painkiller, helping the normal cells, that's a real life experience that I'm familiar with.

Edward: Yes and I'm glad you brought that up because let's face it, Laetrile doesn't work in all cancer patients. Mainly because when people turn to alternative therapy, they usually have been through the mill. They've tried everything else. They've had their chemotherapy, their radiation or surgery, and most of them have been told by their doctors there's nothing more we can do for you. You better go home and get your affairs in order. You may have two or three more weeks to live. At that point somebody says, "Why don't you try Laetrile?" Some family member or well-wisher and so forth and most of them, of course, say, "No, no I just want to die, it's my time to die." But some people say, "Okay, I'll try anything at that stage." Now they go onto Laetrile therapy, I mean the fact that anybody would survive at that point is pretty rare. The truth is that about 15 percent of them do, whereas if they didn't go on Laetrile there's no chance for them. But 15 percent is not a very good rate, but it's only because they're practically dead at that point anyway. There's not much you can do there. Now if you take these patients with cancer and they start taking Laetrile as a first alternative, the first choice, now the numbers switch around and 85 percent will make it. Only 15 percent will lose the battle. So it just depends on how far the cancer has progressed when you start into that mode.

Ty: So really what you're saying is that Laetrile is really good as a preventative. You add it to your diet and then down the road you've got this nutrient that is doing this reaction in your body you don't even know what's happened.

Edward: That's exactly the way you should look at it. Cancer is a breakdown of the natural mechanism. It's not a disease. It's not something to be treated. It's a breakdown of the natural mechanism. You got to find out what that natural mechanism is and support it. Then you never have to worry about treating it. Now it can be treated, of course, but it's much better not to have to deal with clinical cancer in the first place. Now the reason I brought that up before is because you talked about pain. They found that cancer patients, even if they can't be saved because they've gone too far down the road, their pain goes away and they don't need all the morphine and the heavy sedation that is typical. So at least a person can pass in dignity.

Ty: Yeah.

Edward: I think that is of great value too.

Ty: It is. It is. Talk about the California report of 1953. I've heard you—I've read some of your writings about the California report, and it's a very interesting topic.

Edward: It is, and it's a clear example of the degree to which, I guess there's no other word, but fraud. The degree to which fraud, deliberate, conscious fraud can be injected into what we would normally think is a scientific process. Early in the days of development of Laetrile there were stories circulating that people were getting well. They were being treated and coming back from the edge of the grave and so forth. So naturally the pharmaceutical industry wanted to put an end to this, and so they set up a deal where they wanted to have it tested. The idea is okay, none of this discussion about people getting saved, none of these little stories, let's do a scientific test. Not everybody was in favor of that, except they insisted that only those who were opponents of Laetrile do the tests and nobody else could do the tests, you see. It had to be the oncologists and the people on the staff of the pharmaceutical industry and so forth. Well, anyway, to make a long story short, and it is a long story, the California branch of the AMA, California Medical Association was given the task of doing a test on Laetrile, and the people who were in charge of this were all in the cancer industry.

The two men, as I remember the names correctly that wrote the analysis of the report were Drs. McDonald and Garland and McDonald, I think, was a surgeon, and Garland, I think, was a radiologist or maybe it was the other way around, but there was a surgeon and a radiologist and the other members of the panel were all in similar positions. Most of them were radiologists, interestingly enough. So anyway they all had kind of a vested interest in not finding something that would interfere with their businesses, you see. So there was sort of a bias built in. Anyway they did this very fine scientific study using mice and so forth. They spent a lot of money, they produced the report, and McDonald and Garland announced that there was no evidence whatsoever that Laetrile had any effect in the control of cancer. So that was all anybody needed to hear. There was something done by the California Medical Association and two fine upstanding doctors. Well these doctors, just to give you an idea of how fine and scientifically astute they were. These were the guys, both of them said that there was no connection at all between cigarette smoking and lung cancer.

Ty: Same doctors?

Edward: Same doctors, yeah, before they got involved in this report. They had already been bought and paid for by the tobacco industry, of course. In fact I think it was McDonald who even made this fantastic quote: "A pack a day keeps cancer away."

Ty: I've seen the newspapers ads that they used to run.

Edward: Yeah.

Ty: That had that exact quote. That was from him?

Edward: That was from him. He was one of the guys. Incidentally, he died in bed some years later in a fire started by his cigarette in bed.

Ty: Wow.

Edward: Burned him up. I mean I'm sorry to see anybody die, especially from fire, but I thought it was there a certain irony to that.

Ty: Poetic justice.

Edward: Poetic justice or something and the other died of cancer of the lung. They were both heavy smokers. So anyway that gives you a little idea of the scientific expertise of these guys. Well, as far as most doctors are concerned, if they see a report from the California Medical Association and it's accepted by the teaching institutions, there's no question that—that is—that science right there is authentic.

Ty: That's gospel truth.

Edward: That is gospel truth. Well it was accepted as gospel truth for quite a while, and then we got a hold of a copy of the full report. I've forgotten how we did it, but we did. It was a big, thick report. All anybody ever read was that cover page where McDonald and Farland, no McFarland and Garland, I'll get it straight. Sounds like a comedy routine.

Ty: **Who's on first?**

Edward: Who's on first, yeah? Anyway all anybody ever saw was that little summary that they wrote and it turns out that these guys never used Laetrile themselves. They were just sort of analyzing the laboratory results of the study and this was their summary. Well when you go back and read the actual pages of the report the summary was a lie. An absolute lie.

Ty: Kind of like the cliff notes being incorrect.

Edward: The cliff notes were incorrect.

Ty: **Okay.**

Edward: Nobody ever went back to look at—there was plenty of evidence in the laboratory work that it did retard the growth of cancer in spite of the fact that there was a question about the quality of the Laetrile they were using. In fact, it was pretty obvious that they did not have a good quality Laetrile. It was also obvious they were using lower dosage than were being used in the clinics, and in spite of those two handicaps, the laboratory results were reporting case after case after case where these mice were recovering from cancer. Right in the body of the report, and yet the summary was there was absolutely no evidence that, you know, etc,, etc. This was sort of the flagship of what had been repeated many times since then. Sloan-Kettering report did pretty much the same thing. It goes on and on and on, and once people realize that not only is there just ineptitude or bias in the cancer industry, bias against natural therapy but also deliberate fraud. Now we're dealing with a different animal. Because when you consider the number of people who die from cancer this amounts to genocide.

Ty: I would have to agree. If they are lying about the information that is causing people to follow these protocols that end up in their death, that is genocide.

Edward: It's murder.

Ty: Wow. You mentioned in that description there, you mentioned the term "control the cancer" and it stuck with me. Correct me if I'm incorrect but you mentioned the fact that cancer is a normal process in the body. So you really wouldn't cure cancer. You would control it.

Edward: Yeah, you would control it. Yes.

Ty: I like the term. So we're not really looking for a cure for cancer, we're looking for a control of a natural bodily process that has gone out of control.

Edward: Yes. We're looking for prevention, really. If you can maintain a healthy body you're not going to get cancer. Now that's not so easy, to maintain a healthy body, even though you know what you should do, because increasingly we live in an environment where there're all kinds of toxic things that cause the body to go into healing mode. If you remember a moment ago I said we kind of look at cancer as a over-healing process so, therefore, anything that would cause the body to need to heal is the initiation of the cancer process if we don't have these controls in place. So that is why, you take a look at a group of people like the Seventh Day Adventists, who generally don't smoke and they have no lung cancer or very little of it, but their rate of cancer is the same as everyone else. It just happened somewhere else. If they have this deficiency of whatever it is, Laetrile or other things we haven't even talked about, but there are other things too, then the cancer's going to happen somewhere. So it just happens wherever there's a healing process going on, and if you're a smoker that happens to be the lungs. If you live under a high tension wire you might be getting—having your genetic code fried and your chromosomes getting all twisted out of shape…

Ty: Right.

Edward: …electromagnetic stimulation. If you're drinking beverages with all kinds of toxic additives in it maybe you're poisoning your digestive tract and your kidneys and so forth. That all triggers the healing process. Now if you're deficient in what the body needs to fight back you're going to get cancer wherever the healing process is going on.

Ty: I would like to find out from you what you would recommend as far as maybe the top five or six foods that would contain Laetrile because after hearing this I want to make sure we're eating foods that contain Laetrile. Where would we find them in a typical grocery store or can you find them in a grocery store?

Edward: Oh yeah. They're there. In fact we published, our little company published a book some years ago called *The Little Cyanide Cookbook*. Had a lot of fun.

Ty: I like the name.

Edward: Yeah. We were afraid a lot of ladies might want the book for other reasons.

Ty: I would buy the book just because of the ingenious title.

Edward: Yeah. It is all about how to cook delicious meals with foods that contain natural sources of cyanide in this vitamin B17 format or amygdalin format. So if anybody wants to know the complete list we've got the list there in the back of that book called *The Little Cyanide Cookbook*. But getting past that, and if you want to go down to the grocery store today … it's hard to find foods that are really rich in that because people don't buy them. They don't want them. The best source, easiest source is an apple seed. Get apples and if you chew those seeds, your grandmother might have said don't chew those seeds it's poisonous…

Ty: Poison.

Edward: ...yeah, poisonous. Well it's not poisonous. It's got amygdalin in it. That's what makes it so bitter. So if you're eating apple seeds and really chew them up you'll get that bitter taste. Now you know what amygdalin tastes like. That's one good source. Apricot seeds are very good. You can find those in some health food stores or you can go on the Internet. There are companies that sell them on the Internet, apricot seeds. The California seeds are the most bitter, meaning they have the most amygdalin in them. They also import them from Turkey, and they're a little sweeter but you have to eat more of them to get the same amount. So those are two good sources. Peach seeds. Plum seeds. If you can crack these hard shells open and get those little seeds out. Almonds, no. Now it used to be that all almonds were very rich in amygdalin but they are very bitter.

Ty: Right. The bitter almond tree.

Edward: The bitter almond tree was the almond tree that at one time 80 or 90 years ago, that's all there was. Some farmer found a tree in his pasture that, hey, this isn't bitter. This is sweet, and everybody started grafting onto the twigs from that tree and now you can drive through mid-California orchards and you can drive for miles and miles and miles and thousands of these almond trees about this far off the ground you can see where the color and the texture of the bark changes. They've all been grafted. So all almonds today are grafted trees. They're not natural. So that's sort of a symbol of what's been going on in the modern world. We're getting rid of all the bitter stuff. Lima beans. Not my favorite bean even today but I understand that at one time they were very bitter. They had amygdalin in them but they've been hybridized out. Lima beans have a very low amount of amygdalin in them today. So through this process, you know, we've been killing ourselves by getting rid of that natural flavor. So anyway, to answer your question I would say you want to have a steady source or a reliable source would be apricot seeds and apple seeds.

Ty: So eat the seeds.

Edward: Eat the seeds. No, a caution, you can eat too much, because you'll get sick. So I think there's natural law there. How many apricot seeds would you eat if you're also eating the whole apricot? Well, what six, seven, how many apricots can you eat? You know six maybe, that's a lot. Maybe seven. Perfectly safe, but now somebody might say, "Gee, if six or seven are good maybe 20 or 30 are even better." I wouldn't' do that because I know that you can get an overdose and you get nauseous and get dizzy and it's not good for you.

Ty: Good rule of thumb then is don't eat more than you would eat the actual fruit.

Edward: Exactly.

Ty: Mr. Griffin, tell us a little bit about the role that pancreatic enzymes might play in prevention and/or treatment of cancer.

Edward: Very important. Thanks for asking that. A moment ago I said there were two factors, the extrinsic factor and intrinsic factor, and we've talking about the extrinsic factor so far, the food that comes in from outside. But there are certain things that are generated within the body that are very, very important. One of those happens to be the pancreatic enzymes. You've got digestive enzymes that have a special mission of digesting meat protein. Why is that important? It's a fascinating story. They had known for a long time that the, let me back up a little bit by saying one of the questions that puzzled scientists for a long time is, why doesn't the immune system attack cancer cells? If you're working with the assumption that cancer is something that's foreign to the body, which is not our assumption of course, our assumption is that cancer is natural to the body that's gone awry, but the orthodox view of cancer is that it's something foreign to the body. It's not suppose to be there. Why doesn't the immune system attack it and destroy it? The answer is that cancer cells have a protein coating around them. Protein coating. That has a negative electrostatic charge.

It's amazing the more I learn about how much electricity plays a role inside the body. I used to think it was all chemistry. Well, chemistry is basically electricity. Little balances, you see, the pluses and minuses on the chart and so forth. It's all electricity or the chemistry doesn't work. Anyway this protein coating around the cancer cell, one of its unique qualities has a negative electrostatic charge. Well the immune cells, the lymphocytes, leukocytes, monocytes, all these white blood cells that are supposed to attack the foreign invaders, they have a negative electrostatic charge also. Well everyone knows that common polarities repel each other, so the cancer cell is well protected against the white blood cell, and I believe the reason is because the cancer cell is not foreign to the body. It's part of the natural protectants. Hey, I'm a friend not a foe. Even though I'm out of whack I'm still a friend you know. So now if you are eating foods that have a lot of meat protein in them you're probably going to use most, if not all, of that digestive enzyme produced by your pancreas to digest the meat. That's what it's meant to do.

Ty: Yeah, makes sense.

Edward: There's very little left over, if anything left over, to do anything else. If your diet is low in meat protein, and if your pancreas is normally functioning okay, you should have plenty of digestive enzymes to take care of the meat and there still be plenty in the blood stream. Now when these digestive enzymes come to the cancer cell they say, "Ah, protein, meat," and they will actually digest away that coating. Now the underlying cancer cell is exposed and it has a positive electrostatic charge. Now here come the white blood cells, and they do literally attack the cancer cell once it's been stripped of its electrical protection. So all of the physicians who I have ever met that are following this alternative therapy, this concept, one of the things they focus on is making sure that the patient changes the diet to either eliminate meat all together or make sure it's very, very low. A lot of people don't understand that. They think, well, what is it, just some kind of vegetarian nut? We have to eat vegetables too and along with it. Well yeah you do. If you want to have the full mechanism working in your favor you definitely, at least if you have clinical cancer, you definitely want to make sure that whatever your pancreas is producing in the way of these digestive enzymes is completely available to do that job.

Ty: That would explain then why many physicians part of their protocol to treat cancer is, add pancreatic enzymes to the protocol.

Edward: Exactly. That's exactly it.

Ty: Okay. Tell us a little bit about your website Reality Zone and what people might be able to find there.

Edward: Reality Zone is our commercial site where we sell the books and recordings on topics such as this, and you'll find everything that we're talking about there. It's Reality Zone.com and we have a section for health. You'll find my book, plus a lot of other books and audio recordings and video recordings on this topic. So that's Reality Zone.com.

Ty: Well, Mr. Griffin, I really appreciate you taking the time to spend with us today. Sharing just a tad of your knowledge because I can tell you have a lot more but it's been very beneficial to me, and I know that the people that are viewing this show have benefited as well. Thank you so much.

Edward: Well, thank you. My pleasure.

[end transcript]

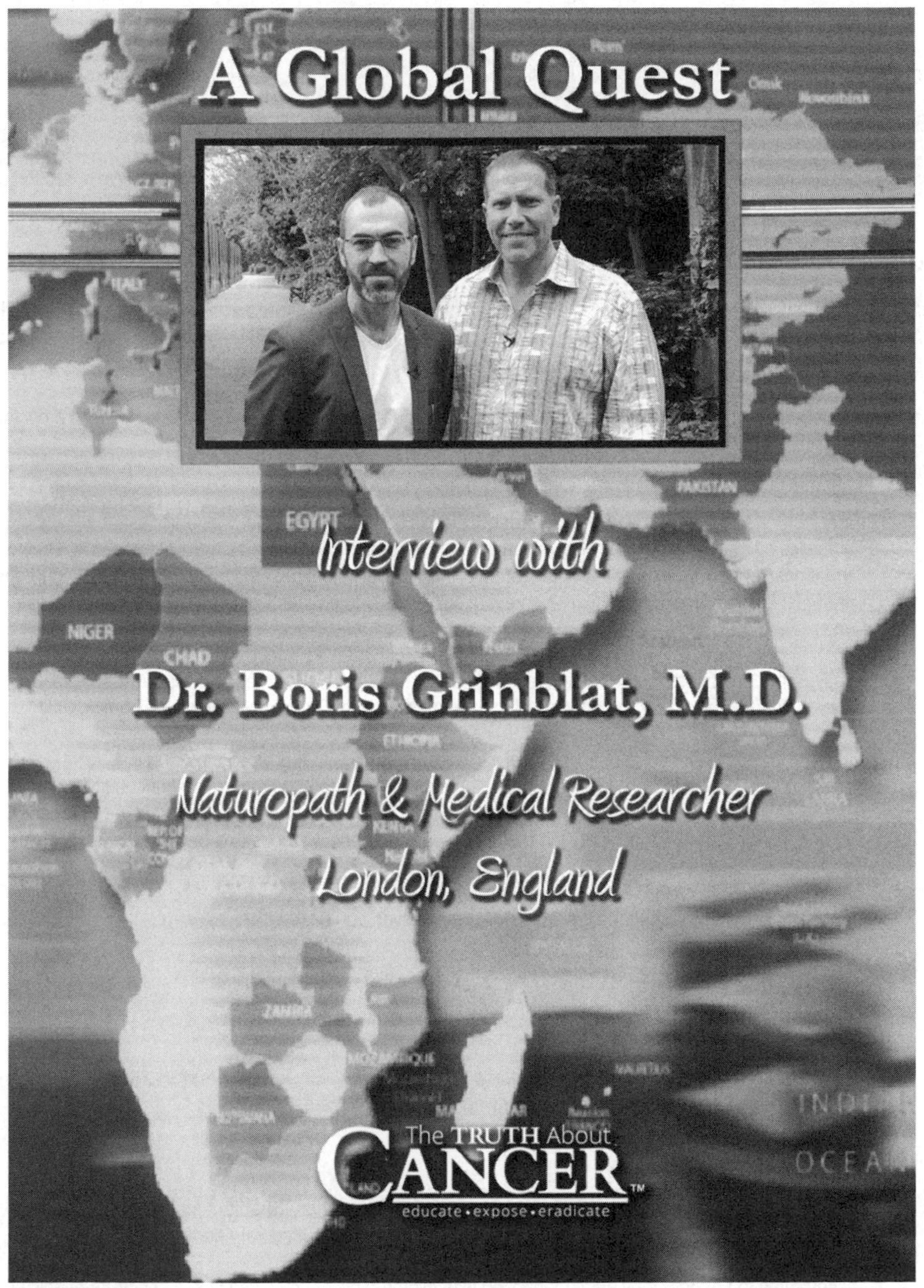
A Global Quest
Interview with
Dr. Boris Grinblat, M.D.
Naturopath & Medical Researcher
London, England
The TRUTH About CANCER
educate • expose • eradicate

Ty: Boris, thank you for joining me here today.

Dr. Grinblat: My pleasure.

Ty: You are originally from Moscow, Russia.

Dr. Grinblat: Yes. Correct, yeah.

Ty: And your last name is Grinblat which appropriately means green leaf in Yiddish, right? We're around all these green leaves today.

Dr. Grinblat: Yes, so I feel home.

Ty: We've been corresponding on email for quite some time and you shared with me a story that I wanted to share with our viewers about working in a children's oncology ward in London. Can you share with us some of the things that happened while you were there?

Dr. Grinblat: Okay. First of all I want to point out that I had an administrative post there. I wasn't a doctor.

Ty: Right.

Dr. Grinblat: But having a medical background, I understood perfectly what was going on and I was appalled by the same picture repeating over and over again. I was working with Russian kids. They were coming from Russia and it was sponsored by a government based charity that was paying for the treatment. Huge money, sounds like on every sick—300,000 pounds for every kid. So story was like this.

In Russia, doctors stopped treating these kids at a certain point because they were not successful and then parents were asking the charity to fund treatment abroad. That's how they were coming.

When they came to the hospital, they were treated basically with the same trio—surgery, chemotherapy, radiotherapy. And after each chemotherapy, the kids were in terrible condition. They were very often in intensive care. It was taking them days or sometimes weeks to recover to repeat chemotherapy again. Unfortunately it was like usually from a few weeks to a few months. Kids were dying.

Ty: Boris, the treatments on these children they rarely if ever worked, right?

Dr. Grinblat: Well, for three years that I've been working there they've never worked.

Ty: Never worked.

Dr. Grinblat: Never worked. It was all the same story. Mind you, very sick kids were coming for treatment, but they were all dying and they were all dying from the treatment.

Ty: Dying from the treatment.

Dr. Grinblat: And I remember one case which was out of the ordinary when the mother came, was (inaudible 00:02:30). The mother was a neurosurgeon so she spotted very early symptoms.

They came to London, they were diagnosed with glioma. This girl received whole spectrum of official treatment and a few months later she died. This was only one case out of ordinary. But again, she died from the treatment and her last few months were terrible.

Ty: I bet.

Dr. Grinblat: No parent wants to see that. No one wants to see that.

Ty: Terrible side effects.

Dr. Grinblat: Absolutely yes. She was on steroids and she had tripled in the weight. It was really terrible. But generally that's what was happening all over again. To my surprise, oncologists were doing the same. I was working there for three years, it was too much for me, but the oncologists worked there for years and they do the same protocols with the same results.

Ty: In that, do you remember a quote by Einstein, "Insanity is doing the same thing over and over and expecting different results."

Dr. Grinblat: Absolutely! But you know what I also noticed? There was one good doctor who was allowing some natural treatments while parents were asking to introduce them. But he could not offer it himself, and when I asked him why, he said, "I couldn't do it. I would lose my job."

So it means oncologists here and in many other countries, I'm sure they are very restricted in protocols. They are not free to offer good treatment. They are very restricted in their protocols.

Ty: The oncologists—or I'm not sure if they're called oncologists in Russia. The cancer doctors.

Dr. Grinblat: Oncologists.

Ty: Okay. In Russia the oncologists apparently they don't go as far on the conventional treatments as in other places.

Dr. Grinblat: Yes, that's true. They have to stick to a certain number of protocols and then they have a kind of a regulation that they couldn't step over the line. That's where people who can afford to, who get funding they go abroad to continue treatments thinking that the Russian doctors are not able to continue because they don't know how to do it further. That's the reason why they go abroad. Basically the result is always the same unfortunately.

Ty: So in actuality, it may be almost a hidden blessing in Russia that you can't get more chemotherapy because you are going to get less poisoned.

Dr. Grinblat: Absolutely. Many patients who I'm trying to help, they are exactly that type of people who went through all official treatments, official treatments stopped, and then they were trying to find some business themselves. So basically yes, it is a blessing in disguise.

Ty: Yeah. What types of treatments have you seen over the years that actually work to mitigate cancer?

Dr. Grinblat: You're talking about official ones?

Ty: Well, are there any official treatments?

Dr. Grinblat: No.

Ty: None.

Dr. Grinblat: None. Not to my knowledge, no.

Ty: Are there any alternative treatments? When I use the quotes for "alternative" they really shouldn't be alternative. They really are the ones that are the most effective.

Dr. Grinblat: Oh, totally, I agree with you. Well, again to my knowledge, and I'm not only a practitioner, I'm also a researcher, only alternative treatments work, or natural treatments.

Ty: You're a naturopath.

Dr. Grinblat: Yes.

Ty: Okay. Talk about the natural treatments that work.

Dr. Grinblat: Well, again, there are about 600 of them. If you do it in competency, it has to be comprehensive to cover all milestones of natural treatments. Once you do that, there is a very big chance of success.

I said there are about 600 things, but you don't have to know the 600. You just have to understand the principles, and if you understand that idea, then you can compile this protocol from a means available to the patient.

Ty: What are the underlying principles that you've seen that make a cancer treatment successful?

Dr. Grinblat: Basically those are the ones that you talk of in your series. That is detoxification, immuno-stimulation, antimicrobial and anti-tumor measures, oxygenation, a psychological work—this very important—physical exercises, diet. It all has to be comprehensive. But what do you put in this comprehensive, what do you use for each aspect? It's up to you or up to the patient conditions.

Ty: It really depends upon what is available to the patient. And what you're saying is it's comprehensive. There is not really a silver bullet of one thing that can defeat cancer, right?

Dr. Grinblat: Well, there is a silver bullet, if you call it comprehensive natural protocol.

Ty: Comprehensive natural protocol. I like that.

Dr. Grinblat: This is a silver bullet.

Ty: Yeah.

Dr. Grinblat: But what you put in it, as I said, depends on where this patient is, it depends on his personality, of finances as well, where this person is because Russia is a huge country. Some people can get stuff, for some it would be very difficult. I have to consider all this when I help them to compile this protocol.

Ty: One thing Boris that caught my attention, one of the protocols that you mentioned to me via email that immediately made me think of Russia was vodka in oil, is that it?

Dr. Grinblat: Yes. Vodka and oil.

Ty: Talk about that protocol.

Dr. Grinblat: Well, that is quite a strange one, but I don't want you to laugh. You have to mix vodka and sunflower oil, unrefined sunflower oil, 30 mils of each. You have to shake it very hard three to five minutes and then you have to drink it like it's vodka three times a day.

It sounds a bit strange, Vodka and oil, but in fact it has quite a good scientific base. In some ways, talking about mechanism, it is similar a little bit to Johanna Budwig.

Ty: The Budwig Protocol.

Dr. Grinblat: Yes.

Ty: I've thought about the Budwig Protocol when you mentioned the oil. Because of the good flax oil and the sunflower oil.

Dr. Grinblat: Sunflower oil is rich with all the unsaturated fats which are very important building blocks of membrane. They carry lots of benefits. They help mitochondria to produce more energy and that's the reason why a cancer cell gets more energy.

When mitochondria start working again, that's when apoptosis surge is on. These cancer cells die, not through necrosis and inflammation. They just die through the biological death or they get back to normal. So that's the plus of this treatment.

Ty: What part does the vodka play in it?

Dr. Grinblat: My understanding is that it helps to get oil into the cell and also it gives a lot of energy. Oil of vodka is ethanol gets into the cell and gives off lots of energy, helps the mitochondria to produce energy. That's the problem with the cancer cells with the mitochondria. First of all there are much less of them in numbers and then they work on a very low capacity.

Ty: Okay. Talk about some other protocols that you had mentioned. You mentioned there was actually a Russian version of the—was it the Gerson Protocol?

Dr. Grinblat: Yes, the Gerson Protocol. There is a girl specialist and she is a physician and biochemist and her name is Martha (inaudible - 00:10:38) and she is a proponent of right diet, juicing. This part is part is very similar to the Gerson Protocol, but also she puts a lot of emphasis on colonics which helps.

Ty: Detoxification then.

Dr. Grinblat: Yes. Well yes, detoxification, but she is using herbs like yarrow, beans, chamomile, plantain, lots of colonics. It is almost like with coffee enemas. They use it initially a few times a day. Say it was your herbal colonics. As I said, she puts lots of emphasis on the diet. Again, it is quite intensive. For the colon, she's quite popular.

Ty: Is it a diet that would be considered to be similar to the Gerson Diet, very high in antioxidants and vegetables?

Dr. Grinblat: Absolutely yes. The only thing is she suggests a vegetarian diet not a vegan diet or a diet like many of your specialists now. She stays with the vegetarian diet.

Ty: I see.

Dr. Grinblat: But generally it is intensive for producing colonics diet.

Ty: Okay. One popular protocol is—it's an antifungal protocol that was developed by Dr. Simoncini out of Italy and it is using sodium bicarbonate, or baking soda. Now in Russia, you've got a different spin on that. Could you share that with us?

Dr. Grinblat: Yes. First of all I think Simoncini Protocol is very popular in Russian, but some patients combine it with the protocol from Professor Neumyvakin who is a proponent of using hydrogen peroxide. I know one survivor who actually combined—to my knowledge he was the first one to combine it—he was using Simoncini Protocol and on top of that he was using Neumyvakin Protocol.

He was using soda bicarbonate and hydrogen peroxide. Also he was using diet and he was supplementing himself. That guy had pancreatic cancer, incurable pancreatic cancer.

Basically, as we were talking about at the beginning of the conversation, he was at home. He wasn't even treated. It was—yes, at this stage. He was a simple guy. He was a truck driver, so he sat a few evenings behind his computer and he chose these protocols for himself.

Ty: Did he combine hydrogen peroxide with the baking soda?

Dr. Grinblat: Yes, that's what he used.

Ty: Was he putting it together? Was it food grade hydrogen peroxide?

Dr. Grinblat: No, it was three percent hydrogen peroxide which you can easily buy in any pharmacy in Russia, and he was drinking it with water, like 15 drops three times a day in half a glass of water, and he was using the full Simoncini Protocol which is drinking soda and also intravenously. Drops like 500 mils of five percent of soda.

Ty: So really a protocol that someone that doesn't have much money could use.

Dr. Grinblat: Absolutely.

Ty: Very inexpensive protocol.

Dr. Grinblat: Absolutely and that was his decision. He didn't have much money. It's very cheap and it's very effective because, as you know, pancreatic cancer is one of the most difficult ones to treat.

Ty: Sure. And this man is still alive?

Dr. Grinblat: Yes, almost two years after that and he is now helping other patients. He is filming himself, he's explained this protocol and it's getting very popular. I think it is a very good protocol.

But Simoncini is a little bit of a reductionist approach. He's got only soda, but what this Vladimir Lazai did, he actually expanded it and now it's basically called a comprehensive protocol.

Ty: Which, again, as you mentioned earlier, that's the key.

Dr. Grinblat: Absolutely.

Ty: A comprehensive protocol.

Dr. Grinblat: Absolutely.

Ty: No silver bullet, but you hit it from different directions, right?

Dr. Grinblat: Absolutely. Yeah.

Ty: Talk about Tesla and energy and frequency.

Dr. Grinblat: I was reading a lot about this subject and then it dawned on me that it should play—well, it plays a very serious role in what we are doing. I think that all this treatment allows a patient to get his body producing high frequencies.

What happens then? Through these high frequencies, a person can get information. A person can communicate with say, with universal wisdom.

There was these great minds like Tesla and the British scientist Rupert Sheldrake. They think that all information about ourselves, about all species, even our collective memory, and the information about our health is all around us. It's not just empty space.

We're surrounded by fields and this information is in these fields. We can extrapolate this information. When we reach these high vibrations, we can get the right information.

Most of the people live in the metropolises and the Western type of life they need low vibrations. They cannot get to this necessary, vital information for them to be healthy and to live happy lives. Tesla's famous words, he said that to understand the universe, you have to think vibrations and energy.

Ty: And the ambulance back here is not emitting a good energy, is it?

Dr. Grinblat: Absolutely not. Yes, so basically what's the end goal of natural treatment? To my view it is to get a patient to this high vibrations. To some patients it's much easier to understand instead of giving them difficulty about, say, difficult metabolical process. To some it's inexorable [inaudible]. I can understand that.

Ty: Right. Right. We know that one of the problems with cancer is the cell's lack of communication. We know also just from recent research over the last couple of decades that even the plants communicate.

Dr. Grinblat: Absolutely.

Ty: So we're in a world that we're not the only ones that are communicating. Other beings or other living forms are communicating.

Dr. Grinblat: And not only that. We don't feel it, but every cell in our body communicates now with this universal wisdom and gets information how to survive or what to do, everything, every organ, every cell.

And we have to allow our body to communicate on the right frequency, and for that, we have to give ourselves, our body, everything it needs for that including positive thoughts, including good food, including good surroundings like the ones that you have now.

Ty: Yeah. Beautiful surroundings here.

Dr. Grinblat: Yes. There are three sources for this high vibrations that a person can get. It is from surroundings like this one, in nature, when they communicate with nature. When you nourish your body with the right food and when you think in the right way, when you project love. Because projecting love and forgiveness, that is what gives you the right frequencies.

When you tap all the three sources, then you have a very good chance of getting well if you are sick, or getting all the information that you basically need for leading a happy life, a healthy life.

Ty: To sum up those three, you have to ingest healthy things, you have to think healthy things, and you have to be in a healthy environment.

Dr. Grinblat: Absolutely. And get rid of all things that prevent you from getting these vibrations.

Ty: \Right. You talked earlier of pediatric cancer. Boris, why do you think that we have this huge rise over the last couple of decades in children with cancer, even infants being born with cancer on day one? The infant born with cancer, why is this happening now?

Dr. Grinblat: Well, I'm convinced that a very important role in this plays vaccination. Interestingly enough, every parent that came to that clinic that I was working in who has a sick kid, I was asking if they had vaccinations. Everyone had vaccinations and almost every parent can recall some complication from this vaccination.

This is a major reason. Another major reason is all these toxins that mother ingests, like BPA, for instance. When the child is born, all of this in his system are lots of these toxins which lead to these problems. Basically it's the modern way of life, vaccination and these toxins which surround us.

Ty: From day one, some of these kids don't even have a chance.

Dr. Grinblat: Absolutely. There was research and umbilical blood was taken from newly born kids and they had over 200 chemical substances which were carcinogens or toxins or bad for the health.

Ty: Yeah. I remember that study.

Dr. Grinblat: Over 200. Yeah.

Ty: Yeah. I think it was close to 300 total chemicals and over 200 and something were known carcinogens, so wow! It's really amazing that we have kids that are born without cancer, isn't it, in light of that fact.

Dr. Grinblat: Yes. I would agree with that. Yeah.

Ty: Boris, talk about the importance of fasting, that fasting might play in overcoming cancer because it is very popular in the United States. And I know in Russia you mentioned that fasting is done as well.

Dr. Grinblat: Yes, it's popular in Russia, it doesn't take much money. Cancer cells they differ from regular cells and we can play on those differences. One of the differences is they don't take heat as well as normal cells and they cannot survive without food for them, which is usually mostly glucose.

In fasting, they suffer more than normal cells. Even for normal cells it is good. They detoxify themselves so nothing is happening to them, but cancer cells they die. That's the reason why it's good. It's a plus for normal cells and it's minus for cancer cells.

Ty: So the fasting eliminates the food for the cancer cells, but you also mentioned they don't respond well to heat, so hyperthermia.

Dr. Grinblat: Absolutely. In Russia, what they do—it's a famous Russian banya or sauna. In the clinics, it's hypothermia. You can do it a double whammy. You can do a fast and then you can do this hypothermia in the Russian banya. So you can use this normal physiological difference of cancer cells and kill them with heat and with fasting.

Ty: Double whammy. I like the way you put that. Now with the fasting, is it water only fast or is it juice fast? What do you mean by fasting that is typical in Russia?

Dr. Grinblat: A different type of fasting. Russians are quite tough people, so usually it's fasting only with water.

Ty: And how many days?

Dr. Grinblat: Up to 40 days. It has to be done with a specialist though because it is a very difficult thing. You have to prepare yourself and then you have to get out of the fasting. But usually it is up to 40 days only water.

Ty: Russians are tough people.

Dr. Grinblat: Absolutely.

Ty: Most Americans have a hard time making it from noon to 6 p.m. for their next meal much less going 40 days without food. Have you done a 40 day fast before?

Dr. Grinblat: No. I find the treatment—well, actually I'm a proponent of a softer approach. I don't like stresses like this and I think it is not for everyone. A 40 day fast is not for everyone. That's why there has to be a choice.

Some people, some patients would like to go on this fasting. For some it would be very difficult. There is always a mild approach. Some specialists say that even when you do a treatment and it causes you stress, then it shouldn't be done.

Ty: Because emotionally it's harmful.

Dr. Grinblat: Absolutely. You can do in this case fasting with juices.

Ty: Okay. I've never done a 40 day water fast, but I've done a 30 day juice fast and just fresh juices. That's difficult, but it's doable because you are still getting in nutrition. You know past the first couple of days you're not really hungry. You pass that hunger stage, but you're still getting some nutrition into your body. You're not in any danger of harming yourself by doing just juices.

As a matter of fact they do 30 days, sometimes 60 days each year of just juice and it's really healthy.

Dr. Grinblat: Absolutely. It's the right way. You have to do it regularly.

Ty: Yeah. Boris, I want you to go into some of the treatments in Russia that are based on what you call "folk remedies," which are the chaga mushroom, red clover, some of the ingredients in essiac tea, hemlock even.

Dr. Grinblat: Yes, yes. Well hemlock is quite popular in Russia. It's called болиголов.

Ty: And it's poison, right?

Dr. Grinblat: Yes, it is poison. There is a special way of doing it. I think it's called [Russian] which is one drop. You have to start with one drop, add one drop every day up to 40 drops and then go back to one drop and then a few days' rest.

There is another protocol when you add drops more like, not three times a day, but first day one drop, one drop a second time, two drops and that way. And for that type of protocol, you add drops even quicker and stop when you are feeling unwell. Then go back.

Another very famous thing in Russia is chaga.

Ty: Chaga mushroom.

Dr. Grinblat: Chaga mushroom. It has so many benefits it is almost like curcumin. You can say it's like a Russian curcumin because it basically does everything. It is anti-cancer. It is a stimulant. It is anti-inflammatory. It's got lots of minerals and 15 percent of chaga is ash. Ash has lots of manganese and manganese is a very important factor in enzymes, activating enzymes.

Ty: Manganese. Okay.

Dr. Grinblat: Yeah. It's unique, but it is taken from a birch tree. So in those places where there are birch trees, I think chaga is very good to use.

Ty: You have medicine growing on the tree and all of the chaga mushrooms...

Dr. Grinblat: Yeah. That's what they do, and it's very easy to prepare it. Lots of them they use it and there's lots of birch trees in Russia.

Ty: Yeah, and you mentioned also burdock root which is one of the components of essiac tea.

Dr. Grinblat: Absolutely. You can find those everywhere. It gets used a lot. The only minus is that some patients use only herbs. They have a kind of reductionist approach and I think this is the greatest minus of some folk remedies. But if you include this into this comprehensive protocol, then I think it is very beneficial.

Ty: The key is, I'm hearing you say over and over, you need a comprehensive protocol to hit it from different directions. You've mentioned the herbs. We've got the hyperthermia, detoxification, the mental and emotional...

Dr. Grinblat: It's extremely important. Diet and also some substances which have direct anti-tumor effect and some substances which have direct anti-microbial effect just to help our immune system. All this complex. It's like eight to ten different aspects. Each one has to be given certain attention.

Ty: You previously worked in an oncology ward so you've seen these scenarios. What would your advice be to someone that has been recently diagnosed with cancer? What kind of questions should they ask their oncologist?

Dr. Grinblat: First of all, I think they should not be afraid. They should take their time and prepare those questions for oncologists. After a certain—when they search, when they prepare those questions, if the oncologist cannot answer those questions, then they have to go somewhere else, find specialists who can answer those questions.

Ty: One of the questions that I've been told from other people, other doctors that you should ask your oncologist is, "What are the side effects of this treatment?" Many times the oncologists don't tell them the side effects.

And then secondly, "What are the success rates for my particular type of cancer?" A lot of times the statistics they give, a generalization of all cancers. You want to know how it works for your cancer.

Dr. Grinblat: And that could be the questions. When they give the answers, you just go somewhere else. Actually, I was present on many consultations where this oncologist was speaking to parents of Russian kids, and they were given those percentages.

You know what was surprising to me? Even when the oncologists were saying that you have two to four percent chance, like with gliomas—and that oncologist, he was a very honest guy—parents still would go for it. You know why? Because they didn't know that there was an alternative.

Ty: They didn't know that there was an option.

Dr. Grinblat: They still think that two or four percent is still a chance.

Ty: It's better than nothing.

Dr. Grinblat: Absolutely. That's what they thought.

Ty: Okay. Really I think that the message that I'm hearing is it is so important to let people know that they have options. Then they have a real choice at that point.

Dr. Grinblat: Absolutely, but it's only half of the problem to get information to people. Unfortunately, from my experience, I found that some people are not able to accept this information. There are quite a lot of people like that. They think if the oncologist is not mentioning it, it's not worth it. If they don't hear it from mass media, it's not worth it. And when they hear it, there is always a conspiracy theory. Some people are simply not able to accept this information.

Ty: Because if their doctor didn't know it, it must not be true.

Dr. Grinblat: Absolutely. They trust their doctors.

Ty: It's the same in Russia as it is in America.

Dr. Grinblat: Yes. Unfortunately, yeah.

Ty: Boris, this has been a fascinating interview. I really have enjoyed getting your perspective on things from the Russian perspective. I see that we're very much alike. We have the same problems. The people have the same misperceptions, misconceptions about cancer and about the treatments. The doctors in both countries are miseducated, under-educated. It's the same worldwide, isn't it?

Dr. Grinblat: Absolutely.

Ty: Same problems.

Dr. Grinblat: That is why what you are doing is extremely important. And now a few of your films are now being translated into Russian and it is getting very popular. People are very interested. As you just mentioned, same problems in Russia. People are very interested what they can hear from your specialists because lots of those things they can use at home. They can use to treat themselves.

Ty: I think that when they see this series, when they see this global quest, they're going to learn that there are a lot of things they can do that don't even have to be wealthy to do and that their fellow Russian comrades are doing as well that you just shared with us, these treatments that are so inexpensive, but very effective.

Thank you for sharing.

Dr. Grinblat: Thank you for inviting me.

Ty: I really appreciate it. How do you say "Thank you" in Russian.

Dr. Grinblat: Spasiba.

Ty: Spasiba.

[end of transcript]

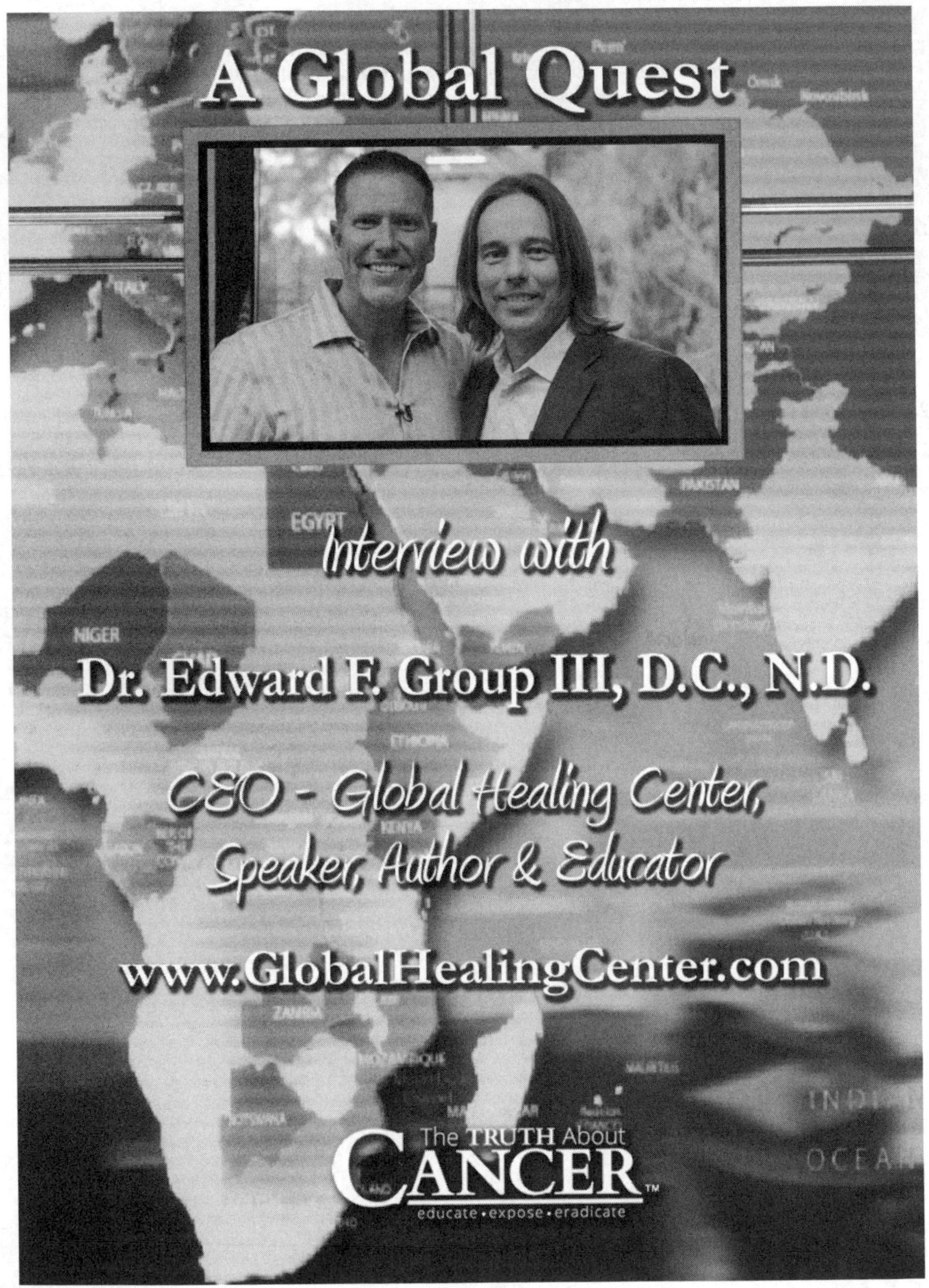
A Global Quest
Interview with
Dr. Edward F. Group III, D.C., N.D.
CEO - Global Healing Center,
Speaker, Author & Educator
www.GlobalHealingCenter.com
The TRUTH About CANCER
educate • expose • eradicate

Ty: I'm really excited to be here in Houston, Texas with Dr. Edward Group at your beautiful office here in the reserve. Thanks for inviting us here.

Dr. Group: Thanks for coming down. I love your stuff and it's always nice to be able to be part of helping people understand the root cause of cancer and degenerative disease and also share some of the technology that we've found and developed over the years that could help people not only prevent, but recover from any type of cancer or disease.

Ty: So Dr. Edward Group, when we were in Detroit speaking earlier this year, you shared some things that really resonated with me. And you have a unique perspective in treating cancer, but we also have a lot in common. So if you could, share with the viewing audience a little bit about your history, what's happened to you to make you interested in overall health, and specifically in treating cancer?

Dr. Group: Well, I originally wanted to go to medical school and be an allopathic doctor, and I lost my dad to cancer in 1990, throat cancer, and then later on lost my mom to cancer. But after my dad died of cancer and I was involved in that whole process with chemo and radiation and standing by his side and seeing him deteriorate, I really wanted to focus on natural, or figuring out why my dad had cancer.

So at that point in time, I really kind of devoted my life to developing or figuring out what could be done for cancer, and not only cancer, for degenerative disease. I wanted to find the root cause. I couldn't find that anywhere. So at that that point in time, I decided to go the natural route and become a chiropractor, a naturopathic doctor, but at the same time focus my research on alternative oncology and figure out exactly how cancer comes about and what can be done to prevent cancer, and not only prevent cancer, but actually reverse cancer.

Ty: Admirable because you lost your father. I can relate, of course. I lost my father and mother and several other family members, but you did as well, right?

Dr. Group: Yeah, I ended up losing all my family members pretty much within a two-year period, but my mom and dad are the ones that died of cancer, and I figured if you can come up with a way to eliminate cancer, then you can pretty much figure out how to work with every single disease. I started a research group back in the late 90s then when I really started getting into it around 1996 and 1998, and we were focused on learning all the different types of alternative cancer therapies, and also tracing back the root cause of cancer.

We traveled to all the cancer clinics in Mexico, interviewed the doctors down there, studied all their protocols, the natural practitioners in Germany, Switzerland—every bit of information we could find from emotional stability to detoxification to different types of herbal compounds, ozone, far infrared, everything you could think of in how it works and how it affects the body considering the body is already damaged to the point of non-repair or too toxic at that point and that's why cancer develops in the first place.

Ty: What were your conclusions after traveling the world? You've done what we're doing now. You've already done that.

Dr. Group: Exactly. What I was doing is what you're doing now and my conclusions were there were a lot of effective natural therapies that could boost the immune system and that could attack cancer cells. But we were still trying to focus on the root cause and we found that talking to all these doctors and looking at all the different exposure to different types of chemicals in the air the people were breathing, the food that people were eating, the beverages they were drinking, the alcohol, the genetically modified foods, all the herbicides, pesticides, the phthalates.

The chemical slough in the water supply, everything that was coming in the body, we could link to every different form of cancer. So the next step was let's trace this back and figure out where these toxins are coming into the body because if we can identify that first exposure point, then we might be able to prevent those toxins from ever getting in and heal the body.

So after years of research, the first exposure point that we found was the intestinal lining. We figured that cancer would not exist in the body if these chemicals and toxins were not coming through the intestines and ultimately getting in the bloodstream. Once they were in the bloodstream, they went through the liver. So our first focus was let's eliminate and we looked at people's dietary habits. We looked at the sedentary lifestyle, we were looking at emotional components to cancer, and we found that everybody with cancer was completely toxic and infested, and the liver was toxic, the intestines weren't working properly, the liver wasn't functioning properly. Usually below 18-20 percent activity.

We found that they were extremely toxic and heavy metals and chemicals in their fat storage. We found that they were emotionally unstable, usually holding on to anger, fear emotions, which we then traced also back to the liver. Then we noticed that when we looked at all the other protocols that the cancer doctors were using out there, we found that there really wasn't anybody that was taking two steps back before taking two steps forward. Another analysis that we did was we looked at a lot of the patients that came in and we looked at the protocols. For example, a cancer patient would come in and the doctor would prescribe ozone or prescribe 30 different supplements for the individual to take. Well, what was happening is their body was already toxic, and anybody with cancer, especially Stage III, Stage IV, their body can't handle—their self-healing mechanism is suppressed.

So we found that what we wanted to do was kind of change that whole philosophy and start with fixing the intestines where, you know, the immune system resides, the neurological system, because we traced back the appendix, which our medical systems still says is useless. We had to translate Russian research to figure out how important the appendix actually is. The appendix actually regulates the lymphatic system, the neurological system, the immune system, regulates everything in the bowel, sends signals to the brain, sends signals to all the endocrine system. Every system in the body is regulated by the appendix. Why wouldn't it be, right?

We traced everything back, all disease-causing agents, and cancer-causing agents to coming in to the intestines. So that's the first exposure point to all your foods, your protein, your fats, carbohydrates, minerals, vitamins, everything. So your microcomputer system is really located at the juncture of your large intestine and your small intestine. Then we started figuring out how little doctors were being taught about the importance of the intestines. And we started interviewing doctors and gastroenterologists, and we found out that it's the closely guarded secret of the medical profession, and it's the closely guarded secret of big pharma as well as the liver as well. So basically, they're not teaching doctors how to properly balance the intestines because they know that if they poison the intestines, it's eventually going to burn holes with the genetically modified foods and all the acid compounds.

All the chemicals and disease-causing toxins are going to leak into the bloodstream, then they're going to poison the liver and they know that if they poison the intestines, and they poison the liver, that you're going to get some degenerative disease or you're going to get cancer fairly rapidly. And also we linked that to all mental illness. There's no such thing as mental illness. There is no depression, anxiety, bipolar, any of that stuff. That was all created for the big pharma to prescribe medications because they knew that when the liver becomes toxic and the intestines become toxic, the intestines can't secrete serotonin, regulate the neurotransmitters, and you're going to get heavy metals, and they're going to alter the neurotransmitters in the brain.

So we traced back all this chemical toxicity really to two organs: the intestines and the liver. And the liver is the only organ in the body that regenerates itself. So when we opened our cancer clinic in 1998, our main focus was how can we keep the intestines clean on a regular basis because we found most people—prescription drugs, over 900 prescription drugs, 90 percent of them cause constipation, they also kill the intestinal flora, chemotherapy ruins the intestinal lining. Chemotherapy also kills liver cells. Radiation does as well.

So we found that the allopathic approach to treating cancer was only putting a band-aid over the problem. Yes, you might kill the cancer for a short period of time, but that's why they set that four-year window because they know after four years, most likely, it's going to come back with a vengeance because you're not focusing on increasing and boosting the body self-healing mechanism, which is another thing that we discovered. That everybody has the most powerful medicine within themselves. So if we know that each person has the most powerful medicine, way more powerful than chemotherapy and radiation, within themself, which is the body's immune system and the self-healing mechanism. And we know the body can heal itself just with thought. There's been proof of that to where people have manifested with and visualized their cancer going away and their cancer went away with no other type of medicine internally or externally.

Ty: Which we would think of as maybe almost the placebo effect, and the mental influence.

Dr. Group: Exactly, but it's not really placebo because that person actually manifested the change and the enhancement of their body's self-healing mechanism. And that's not taught anywhere. I mean, where do you go where they teach you about the self-healing mechanism? Okay. You know you hear a little bit about immune, but the self-healing mechanism is a balance of all your systems in the body working together. And what we found is if part of your body is toxic and chemical ridden, your body's self-healing mechanism is going to go below 50 percent.

When it goes below 50 percent and you're taking in a million toxins on a daily basis and you're only able to eliminate 500,000 toxins on a daily basis, the body has to dump those toxins and chemicals somewhere and it doesn't usually dump them everywhere because your body is smart enough, it doesn't want to destroy every organ. So usually, it picks one specific area to dump all the chemicals and toxins. Usually, it's an area of trauma, genetic area. You might have had some damage to that area or your mom or your dad or something like that. Or you have a spinal injury somewhere, or a bone out of position and that organ is not getting enough neurological impulses.

So, we traced it back, the root cause of disease, then we found out that the body has a self-healing mechanism, so the next step was how do we reactivate the body self-healing mechanism. We used to have 260 something different medications and when we opened our cancer clinic, we wanted to do things different. We wanted to focus on cleansing the intestines and repairing the intestines because we knew that there's so many immune properties in the intestinal tract that we knew that the gut flora by itself can produce strong interferons and strong anti-cancer agents, and anti-disease causing agents, and antivirals because we found that not only were people toxic with chemicals, but when your body is toxic with chemicals and your PH levels fall and you become acidic, you also are a breeding ground for parasites. And parasites are anything that lives off of a host mechanism, which is going to be viruses, bacteria, microplasms, fungus, candida.

You know, all of these things overrun the body and these organisms constantly secrete formaldehyde, isopropyl alcohol, formalin, very acidic substances. So even people that we were seeing that said, "Hey I was on a juice diet for six weeks. What's going on? I'm still acid." Well, what happens with that scenario is nobody had done a parasite cleanse. You haven't addressed getting rid of all the parasites, and just juicing is not going to get rid of the parasites because a lot of parasites can thrive on vitamins, and minerals, and nutrients like that. So we realized that there was more to it. So we realized we had a big problem with cancer and degenerative disease patients, number one with the gut, number two with the liver, and number three with parasites. And even Will Rife determined in his research that the BX virus was associated with cancer. Now we have all different types of viruses and with vaccines and flu shots and everything else coming into the system.

So he found every cancer patient had over a trillion microbes living inside their body. And we found the same thing. There is no cancer patient out there that doesn't have massive amounts of organisms feeding off their body. So at that point in time, not only were we using the high tech cancer treatments that you talk about all the time—and every patient had a specific protocol developed for them whether we were using ozone, 714-X, laetrile, cesium chloride.

I mean, we had the same technology that all natural doctors have right now. But the only thing that made our program different is that we found out that cancer patients, liver function—well, first of all their bowel function was below 25 percent and their liver function was below 18 percent. So we had to find a way to repair the intestines *and* the liver because we knew that even everything that we're going to be giving them that's natural, still has to go and be processed through the intestine and the liver. It has to be absorbed and utilized.

So the next stage was what can we find that can clean and repair the intestines, the small intestines and the large intestines. There was only a little bit of research out there that was done by Nikola Tesla, and Eugene Blass in 1898 about stabilizing a reactive oxygen species onto a magnesium compound. We looked at all the different herbs, but really the herbs are not going to repair your intestinal tract. They're going to increase mucus. You know the psyllium is going to add fiber. But nothing is actually going to work as an oxidation reduction reaction to where it's going to bubble away all of the hard compaction in the small intestine and oxygenate the villae and actually repair the valve.

The only thing that we could find—I mean if you look at cascara sagrada, if you look at marshmallow, if you look at any of the herbs out there, they can actually cause permanent damage to the valve over a period of time. So the only thing that we found that could work was an oxygen-based intestinal cleanser because what we found was—think of how much food, and junk, and garbage people put into their body every single day. Well we take a shower to wash our skin every day, but we don't clean the inside of our body, and our intestines are just our skin turned inside out.

Ty: They're technically outside the body.

Dr. Group: Yeah. Exactly.

Ty: Your whole intestinal tract is technically outside. There should be no leaky, right?

Dr. Group: It's the only linkage to the outside environment. It's exactly, it's epithelial tissue just like the skin is. And that's why when you have problems with your skin, you really have problems with your intestines.

Ty: Right, right because that basically is your internal skin, right. Somebody that's watching now and they're saying, "Okay, I've used these other products for the intestines, for the colon, how do you clean it using this reactive oxygen and magnesium? Do you have a supplement that you developed for it? How do you do that?

Dr. Group: Yes, we actually had to develop a supplement and we called it Oxy-Powder and then we ran it through Phase 1, 2, and 3 FDA clinical trials, and we were using that and seeing amazing results with our—well, first it was a product called Homozon that was out there that was one of the original ones by George Freibott. It was inconsistent with oxygen testing, so we wanted to soup it up and really make it more effective and release more oxygen. So we developed the Oxy-Powder product and started using that as an intestinal cleanser. I still feel that people need to clean their intestines at least once a week, twice a week.

Ty: I agree.

Dr. Group: Because you take a shower every day to rinse your skin, right. What happens if you don't take a shower for a week? I mean, that's just—as a preventative, you need to clean your intestines on a regular basis.

Ty: Still available? Oxy-Powder?

Dr. Group: Still available. It's one of our best-selling products and amazing results. Thousands upon thousands of users. Thousands upon thousands of reviews. 4.8 stars. I highly recommend people go online, look, and read all the reviews

Ty: So that's something you would use once a week or something just to maintain cleansing your internal skin, right?

Dr. Group: Yes. Once a week, once or twice a week just to clean your internal skin. And the second thing we wanted to do was put people on a good probiotic formula. There's a lot of good probiotic formulas out there. We developed one, which has an exclusive 18-strain blend with over 50 billion organisms, kind of the ones that we use that were successful with repairing the bowel pretty rapidly, especially with cancer patients. Then we always used enzymes too because cancer patients have a problem breaking down their foods and absorbing their foods and it helps—it's an energy balance.

You want to conserve as much energy for that self-healing mechanism to reactivate and we were the first ones in the world because of all the cancer research that we were doing, I found a rare enzyme. It's actually the enzyme that keeps honey from never going bad. It's called glucose oxidase, and we're the first company in the world to develop a complete vegan enzyme formula, and the only company in the world to use glucose oxidase. And the reason I put glucose oxidase in there is because glucose oxidase converts glucose to hydrogen peroxide inside the cell.

Now if you think about cancer cells which feed on glucose, and we're doing some preliminary—this is the first time I've actually said this on air, but we're doing some preliminary research on cancer with straight dosage of glucose oxidase because if you—the cancer cells will pull in the glucose oxidase and inside the cell, it'll convert the glucose to hydrogen peroxide, and hydrogen peroxide will then kill the cancer cell. So that's kind of an exclusive right now that we're working on.

So by cleaning the intestinal lining and then repairing that, automatically, that self-healing mechanism goes up five to ten points. The next step was cleaning the liver and purging the liver because we really have to have a functioning liver in order to boost the self-healing mechanism to the point where all of the stuff that you're doing, all the cancer supplements and everything else you're doing work at 75 percent or above. Right now if you don't do that and you go and you start taking all these anti-cancer supplements, those supplements are only going to be working maybe 25 percent. You're just going to get a tiny amount of therapeutic value to that. And that's why sometimes you have cancer patients that take this natural protocol and get better, and sometimes you have cancer patients that take that natural protocol and don't get better.

Ty: Right. Yeah, that was my next question. That's a very frequent question. Why does it work for somebody and not for somebody else?

Dr. Group: So if everybody cleaned and repaired their intestines and their liver, then you would have a more consistent success rate across the board. The problem is those individuals that their liver is only functioning below 18 percent that they're not going to be getting better faster. But I…

Ty: The liver is the key.

Dr. Group: The liver is the key. The gut and the liver is the key. There's no doubt about it.

Ty: So what kind of supplement do you have, or what type of product do you use to detox the liver? Because we've heard of a lot of different detoxification processes for the liver, starting with coffee enemas, and on down the line.

Dr. Group: Right. I mean, coffee enemas are great, but you need something that's going to actually purge the liver. Now, oil pulling is one of the new things. I kind of refer it to this. Just think if you have an oil filter in your car and you've never changed it in ten years, it's going to be so gunked up that you need to take the filter out and put a new one in. There's no way to really clean that, right. You can take it out and rinse it with water, you know, all this stuff, but you're not really going to rinse all that gunk off, unless it was some way where you could just purge it out and push all that stuff out of there.

We've tried to figure out ways that we can clean the liver with just taking different types of herbs, coffee enemas, all these different things. And they work to a certain degree to help the hepatocytes regenerate and maybe stimulate the Phase 1 and Phase 2 detoxifications systems in the liver. Well, what they didn't do was push out all the liver stones and they didn't push out all the congestion in the liver. This goes back years, and years, and years in research is actually drinking oils because oils are the only thing that are going to actually push the congestion out of the liver.

So we developed a program based on ancient philosophies and techniques with modern philosophies and techniques and experimented with different products and different herbs. So we developed an herbal formula, which uses borututu bark, and chanca piedra, which are rare rainforest Brazilian herbs which will actually loosen and dissolve stones in the liver. Then we have them do that for four days and on day five, they drink an extra virgin olive oil with some Epsom salt and they push. So it cause contractions of the liver and it actually pushes all of that congestion out.

What we found with evaluating over 100,000 liver cleanses is liver cleansing is probably the most effective ways of boosting your self-healing mechanism. Each liver cleanse is going to boost the liver production and efficiency by 10-15 percent, which means—another thing we found in research is that most cancer and degenerative disease patients need multiple liver cleanses, usually, three, six, or nine in order to boost their liver above 80 percent, is where you really need the liver functioning, at about 80 percent. If you want your self-healing mechanism to be working at 100 percent.

Ty: So how often can they do this liver cleanse? One a month for nine months?

Dr. Group: What we recommend is doing the five days. It's really like a six day because on Day 6, you're still eating healthy. Take three days off and do another one, then six days, take three days off, then they can do another one. Take three days off, six days on. So you can do this in conjunction—the beauty of cleansing is you can do it in conjunction with any doctor that you're seeing or any cancer doctor. You know, I've been trying to tell the cancer doctors for years that they need to incorporate these cleansing protocols because this is what I've been focusing on for close to 25 years.

Ty: Is this something that they could do on their own then?

Dr. Group: They could do it on their own. [crosstalk] As a matter of fact, we've had IV Stage cancer patients that have just done intestinal cleansing and balancing and multiple liver and gall bladder cleansing without taking any other supplement, fourth stage with two weeks left to live that have been sent home to die, that if continued liver cleansing and intestinal biosis, you know, fixing their intestines and just doing liver cleanse, liver cleanse, liver cleanse.

Ty: Is this something that needs to be done with fasting or just with your normal diet?

Dr. Group: Well, I always recommend changing the diet because that's the root cause of why you got the problem to begin with. You want to change to an organic diet, you want to avoid any of the chemicals, MSG, artificial sweeteners, aspartate, all those chemicals you want to avoid. But at the same time, when the liver function is so low, that's when those chemicals really have an effect on your body because the liver is no longer able to function. As a matter of fact, we're seeing liver problems in children right now. I would say that 100 percent of the population right now in the United States, their liver is only functioning at maybe 60 percent.

That's why we're seeing so many mental issues. That's why we're seeing so much of every type of symptom, whether it's fatigue to skin conditions, to hair loss, to hormone dysfunction to everything. I mean, every single thing can be traced back to the intestines and a congested liver. I was talking about oil pulling in the mouth, well, when you drink the olive oil, the olive oil goes down and it goes inside the liver and it kind of works like oil pulling. So it pulls out all these chemicals, and toxins, and fats that the liver doesn't want, that's congested in there and forms these little oil globules. There are stones in the liver, but most of the things that come out when you do a liver cleanse are just globulates of toxins of oil. And so you pass all these out. You pass all these stones out and what you're doing is you're getting rid of all these chemicals, and toxins and garbage that's inside your liver.

Ty: This is olive oil that you use?

Dr. Group: This is olive oil, yes. I mean, it's by drinking on day—once you prepare the liver for the first five days, on Day 5, actually, is where you drink the Epsom salt, which kind of loosens up the bile duct and everything and gets the intestines ready. And then you drink the olive oil, and the olive oil will actually go into the liver, start sucking out, and pulling out all the chemicals and toxins and then you'll push it out the next day.

Ty: So you said this is after you prepare the liver for the first five days, which is taking a chunk of the piedra and the other herbs, right? And then also is that in conjunction with—let's say you've already changed your diet. You're eating a clean, organic GMO free diet, is this something that you would continue to eat that diet, or do you fast during a liver cleanse?

Dr. Group: No you continue—we have a diet that you can follow, but whatever your natural healthcare practitioner has you on because a diet should really be—there is no one diet that works for everybody. I mean, you should really evaluate that individual, their environment that they live in and see what grows naturally there. And then I also think every cancer patient, their doctor should evaluate their home as well because they'll always tell you that they live in a clean home.

Every single person—one of our procedures that we did with ever cancer patient was to go to their home. And we found memory foam mattresses that they were sleeping on with fire retardants and VOCs. We found usually mold, we found geopathic stress lines, we found toxic paint. We found all kinds of toxic cleaning supplies. We found in their kitchen, all kinds of toxic foods. Even when they tell you, "Oh, yes, I'm eating good and I'm…" The air, we wanted to clean up their air in their house, put some plants in there, you know, create an environment, an outside environment. We've been talking about the inside environment, but we also want to create a pure outside environment for their self-healing mechanism and their skin, what they're exposed to, so we're not having all these chemicals and toxins coming in continually to the intestines and the liver while we're trying to clean the intestines and the liver. Then we would do a parasite cleanse as well after the first liver cleanse because we knew that then the intestines would be ready to expel them, and then the liver would be able to deal with the toxins produced by the parasites once we start killing them off inside the body.

Ty: Okay. Great. What were the ingredients in the parasite cleanse?

Dr. Group: Well, we looked at a lot of different ingredients and we decided that we would use the black walnut hull from the green hull, we would use American worm seed, epazote. We would use worm wood, we would use clove, kamala, and that combination with a couple of other ones, with romaleon. We would be able to—also using diatomaceous earth as a flow agent—we would be able to get rid of and purge the majority of the parasites inside the body.

Ty: How long does the parasite cleanse portion take, how many days?

Dr. Group: Parasite cleanse takes six weeks because that's the cycle of most parasites from the time that they lay eggs until the time that they're an adult. So if you do a parasite cleanse for shorter period than six weeks, then there might be eggs still left in there that might hatch. Now the good news is this can all be done in conjunction with whatever doctor supplements that you're currently taking whether you're doing ozone or anything. There's not any contraindications of doing an oxygen intestinal cleansing, doing liver and gall bladder cleansing, doing parasite cleansing. And then the last thing we would do would be chemical and heavy metal cleansing, which is also another factor that needs to be considered in conjunction with your cancer care.

Ty: Sure. The parasite cleansing, those different ingredients, you formulated into a product?

Dr. Group: Yes, I formulated it into a product called Paratrex. A lot of doctors use it all across the nation. I, personally, think everybody should do a parasite cleanse at least once or twice a year because there's just no way around it. I mean, even if you're a raw foodist, you're still going to have an overgrowth of parasites in your body.

Ty: Yeah. Yeah.

Dr. Group: I mean, one square inch of sushi has up to 10,000 parasite larva in it. So I mean, it's something that—we're living in a world, we're all living in a toxic world. The world is sick, and the world has cancer right now. Trees are dying, the chemtrails, the soil is sick. The water is contaminated. The air in the world is contaminated. The only thing that we can do is to keep our self-healing mechanism strong. And in order to keep our self-healing mechanism strong, we have to keep our bodies clean. It all comes back to simplicity.

I mean after years of looking out here for the answer, I finally realized that the answer was right here and realized that no disease can exist inside of a clean body. If you put clean, pure water inside your system, if you put clean, pure food inside your system, if you detoxify your body on a regular basis and keep your self-healing mechanism strong, you never have to worry about getting any type of disease.

And the same thing goes for if you have cancer, if you have a degenerative disease, what your body's telling you is it's dirty, it's toxic and it needs to be clean. So it's begging you and giving you those signs. Because your self-healing mechanism will start giving you signs and symptoms to try to tell you something is wrong.

Ty: What you just said is profound. It really was. I felt like you just went Bam! Because you just nailed it. The world's sick, but if we can keep ourselves clean, we can be healthy. When you said that a cancer patient is begging for this clean environment, the cancer can't live in this clean environment, the cancer patient is not begging, or the cancerous body is not begging for more chemicals, right. It's begging for purity.

And so the way—I think the reason that the whole conventional paradigm is skewed is that we take a sick body and we treat it with something that'll make it sicker, right. You have a sick body that's overburdened with chemicals, so what do we do? We inject it with more chemicals, and it just can't ever have a good long-term result because the whole philosophy is backwards isn't it?

Dr. Group: It's the difference of addressing the root cause of cancer and disease or addressing the symptoms of cancer and disease. That's the way the medical system is and the way that they want to stay because there's no money in addressing the root cause. We would ask every single cancer patient that came in our clinic—and by the way, they had usually been seen by 15 different doctors and we were the last resort, and they would come in with bags full of supplements. And we would say, "Tell us how or why you have cancer?" And they would look and say, "I don't know." We would say, "Well, didn't any doctor explain to you why you have cancer?" And they would say, "No." "Well, don't you need to understand why you have cancer first before you understand how to get rid of your cancer?"

I mean, you're not going—you have to understand how to be an electrician before you rewire a house or any job. And the body's the same way. I mean, your body is really a job. You need to pay attention, you need to learn about your body, but that's another subject. They keep that information from you. They don't want you to learn about your body because then they want you to be dependent on the medical system.

So that's what we would do. "Let me explain to you why you have cancer." And the first step in our cancer program, our treatment program was explaining to the patient and teaching them. Education. Educating them as to why they have cancer, which is exactly what we're talking about. You have a self-healing mechanism. Your self-healing mechanism is suppressed, blah, blah, blah, and we would talk about that.

The second question that we would ask them is what they know about their body and their self-healing mechanism and how that works, and if they're motivated enough to start doing some sort of a cancer program. We would say, "What do you do for fun?" or, "What makes you happy in life?" And I can tell you probably every cancer patient started crying at that point in time, because you know how it is. They've been through so much and they don't really have anything that they're doing for fun or anything that they love to do.

So we would explain to them how simple it is to clean the body and reactivate the body self-healing mechanism. I would say, "It took you 40 years to get cancer and disease. What if I was to sit here and say it's going to take another 40 years to get rid of it?" But the good news is, you get a new liver every three months. You get new intestinal cells every 24 hours. So, what if I told you, you could reactivate your self-healing mechanism and you could start your journey towards health within 90 days.

Ty: Yeah, well, you got the intestines today, you got the liver every three months. You got about 60 days to kill the parasites, so you're right, within three months you could be completely regenerated.

Dr. Group: So even though the people came in and we would start them on whatever we were using. We would evaluate their condition, go to their house, start eliminating all the chemicals and toxins coming in, start on the intestines, then move to the liver, then move to parasites.

At the same time, you could still be doing those things like ozone and laetrile, or whatever those patients want to be doing and your success rates are going to go through the roof because it all boils down to the self-healing mechanism and how active it is, and how good the liver and how good the intestines are functioning.

Ty: Got it. Dr. Group, when we were in Detroit, you shared a story that I want to get you to share about being kidnapped and put in the back of a van and taken to a restaurant in Houston.

Dr. Group: Yeah, that was—well, first of all what happened is when the word start getting out—and by the way I didn't mention a couple of things that we found that pretty much every cancer patient and every person in the world needs, and it was vital, was iodine. Iodine is one thing that I would highly recommend every single person look at, at detoxified iodine because we found that it's crucial in the oxidation. Like I was talking to you about glucose oxidase, a new project we're kind of secretly working on. Well, we're finding is that every single person—and Dr. Brownstein is also verified this with testing of over 9,000 patients. Every single person is deficient in iodine and when you're deficient in iodine, cancer can be one of the consequences, but also every single cancer patient should be on, probably a minimum of 10-20,000 micrograms of a detoxified iodine a day. Two other things is Vitamin D3 also that everybody is deficient in, and then also B12, like a methyl- or adenosylcobalamin.

But yes, what happened was, with our cancer clinic we were so successful, that we were having all the other cancer doctors send us their hardest patients. It didn't get—we were right down the road from Burzynski, which is also a fantastic clinic, but also M.D. Anderson. And word got out at M.D. Anderson, and all of a sudden we had people leaving M.D. Anderson and coming to our clinic.

We actually had the chief oncologist from M.D. Anderson come in, bring a patient into our clinic one time. I sat down for two hours and gave a class on the cause of cancer because I asked a patient, "Did they explain at M.D. Anderson what caused your cancer?" She looked at me and the doctors looked at me with this angry look, and then I said, "Well, let me explain to you the cause of cancer." And I took the chief oncologist, his main oncologist that worked underneath him, and their patient that they tried to trick me with, wheeling in in a wheelchair that had an IV hooked up in their arm, and for two hours I—he tried to interrupt me a couple of times and I just said, "Well, let me just finish and I'll take any of your questions after."

So I went through the whole self-healing mechanism, the root cause of all disease and after the whole thing was over with, I looked at him and I said, "Do you have any questions?" And he said, "No," and they got the patient and wheeled him out of my office. About a month after that, I got raided by the FDA, all my good files were stolen and everything. Then, what you're talking about, the story I told you, was they thought they would follow me around. They basically told me I had death threats, don't do anything in this country, they don't want cures in this country, and a black car pulled up and asked me to get in before they would throw me in. So I got in, they took me to a location here in Houston where it's a secret meeting place for people high up in the illuminati. Went into the restaurant, I noticed on the restaurant walls, I saw the President, all these pictures of all these dignitaries and famous people, and this was just a tiny little Chinese restaurant. I'm thinking to myself, "What in the world are all these people coming to this Chinese restaurant for?"

Ty: Must be great food.

Dr. Group: Yeah, must be great food, right. Well, then the wall opened up in the back and there was a secret meeting room and then the wall closed. And they basically said, "Hey we want…" The government and these secret organizations have remote viewers and the military's been using remote viewers.

Ty: I had General Major Al Stubblebine, who—the guy that they did the movie, *The Men Who Stare at Goats*. He's the guy, he was a remote viewer. He had a whole team of remote viewers.

Dr. Group: So, I found this out later because I was like well, why did they just try to shut me down and then why are they pulling me in here. So they said, "Listen, we want you to come join with us." And I think part of it was that they wanted me to help all the other people because I mean, these guys, even though they do have high technology, they still want somebody to oversee them when they get cancer, when the get sick and stuff like that. But then I found out it had to do with my lineage also because my great-great-great-great-great-great grandfather was the one, [Palatial] Webster that actually wrote the US Constitution, and Webster's Dictionary. They wrote the Masonic Code in Webster's Dictionary. He was like my great-great-great-great-great grandfather. My dad was also involved with the government, which I think he was killed off. He was working with Reagan and them, and one of the developers of PVC Plastics and Saran Wrap.

So anyway, they bring me in there and they say, "We want you to join us. We're going to make you a senator." I was like "Make me a senator? I mean, how you going to make me a senator?" They said, "Well, don't worry about it. We put everybody in office." I said, "Well, okay." They were like "You have 24 hours to get back with us. Here's a number to call. Call this number and just say 'yes' or 'no' and we'll take care of the rest. But if you don't call in 24 hours, then you'll never hear from us again, and you'll never have this opportunity again."

Another thing they said is, "You'll never have to worry about money. You'll have so much money, you'll never know what to do with it all. You'll have bank accounts and you'll just have as much money as you'll ever need." So then they took me, put me in the car, dropped me off, gave me the little number, and that was it. After that, of course, I didn't call. But after that it was—I never heard from them again, and then the FDA comes in my office still and harasses me probably once or twice a year. But also believe that I have a lot of good power and protection, and it's all about getting this information out.

I can get out information on the importance of cleansing and repairing your liver and your intestines. Those aren't diseases. That's just going back to the basics. What everybody needs to be doing. And I know now the power of detoxification and cleansing. There's not one case of any disease to where they haven't cleansed their body and their environment to where their disease has gone away.

Ty: Very important, isn't it.

Dr. Group: Unless it's just your time. I mean you can't—there's nothing you can do about that. If it's your time to go, it's your time to go.

Ty: But even that, you recently, you just told me a story about somebody that was literally minutes away from dying that was revived. You don't have to share the details, but it may seem like your time…

Dr. Group: There's always hope. There's always hope. The body is amazing. The self-healing mechanism is amazing within the body. Just like you, that's what we do. Our mission is to help heal the world, help heal the planet, get rid of the Monsanto's, get rid of the fluoride in the water, get rid of all the toxic chemicals everywhere that are causing all the diseases and educate people as to the root cause of all disease, and educate people on how they can reactivate their body's own self-healing mechanisms and the importance of cleansing. I mean, think of all the junk people put in their body on a daily basis. I mean, I can talk to 100 people on the streets right now, and 100 out of those 100 probably have not done an intestinal cleanse, have not done a liver cleanse, have not done a parasite cleanse.

Ty: Sure. I think that's a pretty safe bet. So Dr. Group, it sounds like we're on the same mission. We're searching for the opportunities to share truth. We want to educate and we want people to be healthy. We want to heal the world, we want to heal people. We want to get everybody the education that they need to make informed decisions, right. I mean, I think really, when I look at what we're doing, it's almost more of a freedom-fighting mission than anything for people to be educated and then just have the freedom to make choices, right.

At least right now, we're in a relatively free country, right. So we can choose to do what we think we need to do except in certain states like California, where now they're going to force jab you, or forced vaccines. But what can we do to maintain this freedom, and what can we do to continue to spread this message to reach the masses and give the world hope?

Dr. Group: Well, the good news is we've come a long way. I mean, we've woken people up about GMOs, we've woken people up about fluoride. I think that right now, compared to ten years ago, compared to even five years ago, we're at critical mass, or almost critical point right now because with Obamacare and people not getting the medical care that they need, people looking at their—watching their parents die with the standard medical system, this new generation is waking up. They're online, they're researching things more.

There's more information that's available through your videos, through our information about what people need to do and what they can avoid. It all starts with education. It really starts with the root cause of why we're dealing with all these things today, which are just chemical toxicity. And how you change things is the more people that are talking about it the more people that you put this information in front of their face. Those people are sharing through social media and even the people five years ago that were saying "Fluoride's good for you."

Now you're starting to see a shift and they're saying "Well, wait a second. Maybe it's not." Fluoride calcifies the pineal gland. They knew that back in Nazi Germany when they put fluoride in there for one reason: to reduce our consciousness, to make us non-aggressive, to make us controllable, to make us like zombies literally to where we walk around unmotivated and uncontrollable. So the answer is to detoxify the fluoride from the body, reactivate the body self-healing mechanism because what does that do? It opens up your consciousness.

If you decalcify the pineal gland of fluoride, which iodine does by the way. It's the only thing that does. That's another reason they took iodine out of everything and they wanted to suppress iodine because they knew that if people had iodine in their bodies it would raise the conscious level and the thinking of all humanity. So it's all through detoxification and the cleaner you are the more your self-healing mechanism is active, the more conscious you are, the more people see that, the more educated you become, and it's all about changing the planet and your body one step at a time

Ty: I think we've taken a big step today. I thank you for what you're doing. We're all on the same mission. So keep up what you're doing and we'll keep up what we're doing, and together we will change the world.

Dr. Group: Thanks. Appreciate it.

Ty: Appreciate it, Dr. Group. ***[end of transcript]***

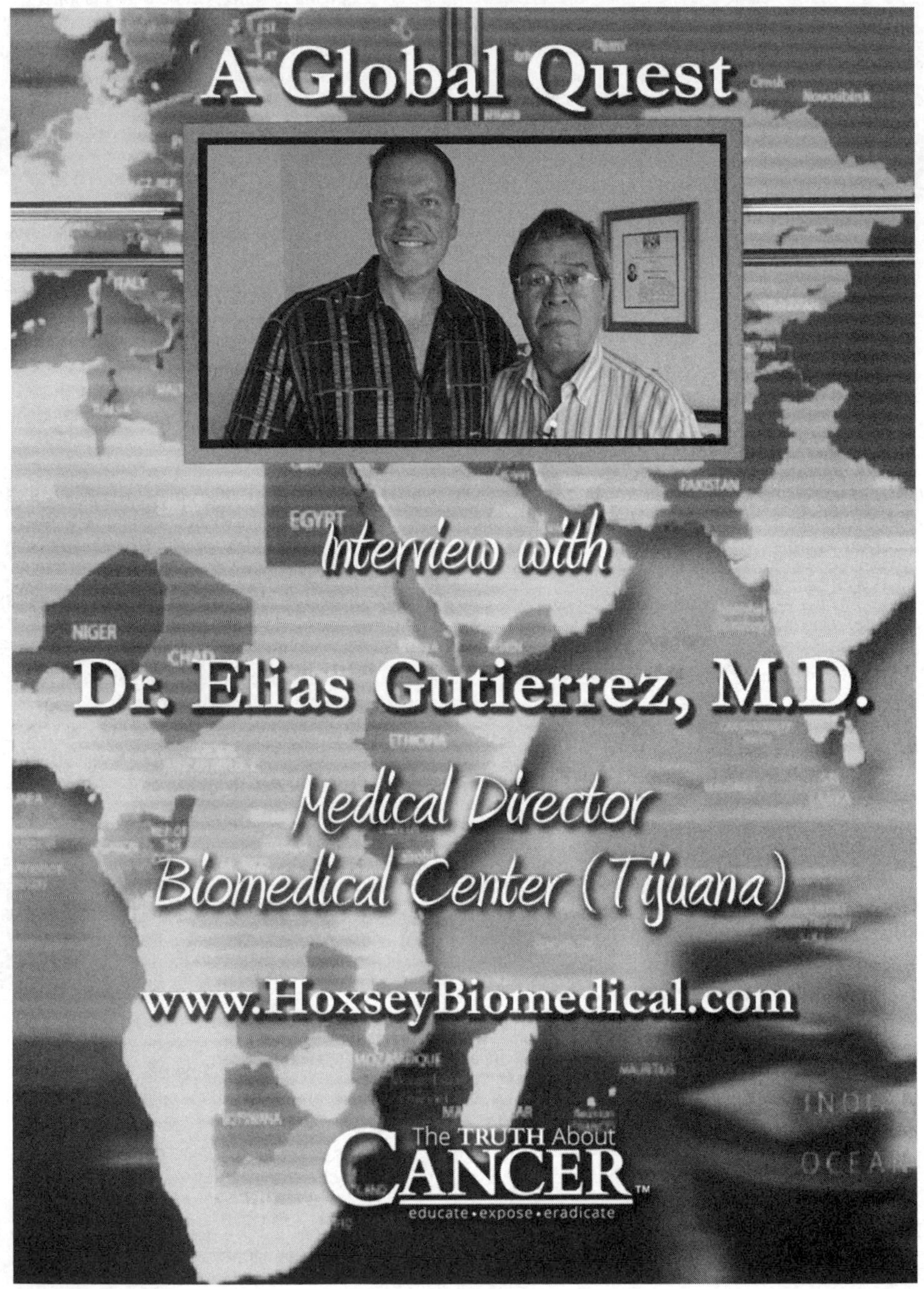
A Global Quest
Interview with
Dr. Elias Gutierrez, M.D.
Medical Director
Biomedical Center (Tijuana)
www.HoxseyBiomedical.com
The TRUTH About
CANCER
educate • expose • eradicate

Ty: I'm here at the Bio-Medical Center which was formerly known as the Hoxsey Clinic in Tijuana, Mexico with Dr. Elias Gutierrez.

Thank you for joining me today.

Dr. Gutierrez: Nice to meet you.

Ty: I'm really excited to get your perspective on the Hoxsey treatment; what I called the Hoxsey treatment. As I was sharing with you earlier, when my dad was diagnosed with cancer in 1996, we wanted to get him here to the clinic but he died in 25 days.

One of the things that really impressed me about the clinic was the success that you'd had with a lot of different types of cancers as I began to research back in the mid-90s. So, if you could Dr. Gutierrez, share with me and with the viewers, what exactly is the—I call it the Hoxsey treatment. I don't know if you even call it that anymore.

What treatments do you use here at the Bio-Medical Center and how long have you been here?

Dr. Gutierrez: Well, I've been here for about a little bit more than 30 years, maybe 34. Basically, what everything spins around is what is known as the Hoxsey formula. It's a liquid made with a combination of several herbs and minerals. Because of the way that it is put together it selectively targets only the malignant cells. Any cell with the bad DNA or a bad metabolism, those are the ones that are going to be destroyed.

Of course there are a few vitamins, there's a diet which is not a difficult one to follow, and we also use a lot of both occidental and Chinese herbal formulas.

Ty: What exactly is in the Hoxsey formula? What are the herbs that are in it now?

Dr. Gutierrez: There are several herbs like licorice, potassium iodine, and there are a couple of more things. There are about eight or nine ingredients in it.

Ty: Do they all have different mechanisms by which they are selectively toxic to the cancer?

Dr. Gutierrez: Yes, definitely, each one. Besides, you have to remember that there is a mechanism called potentialization, or when you combine several ingredients together. You can take one herb and it is just going to have a simple effect, but if you put them together, each one will potentialize each other and you will get a combined effect.

Ty: It's kind of a synergistic effect.

Dr. Gutierrez: Synergistic effect. Yes, yes.

Ty: The formula that you're using, is this pretty much the same formula that Harry Hoxsey used 80, 100 years ago?

Dr. Gutierrez: Exactly the same.

It was first passed down from Hoxsey over to Mildred. Then Mildred brought it into the clinic and then she passed it on to Liz, she's the owner now, Mildred's sister. We still use basically exactly the same formula that was being used in Texas.

Ty: Share a little bit with the viewers about the history of Harry Hoxsey before the clinic moved here and what happened with him. Why did he have to leave the United States?

Dr. Gutierrez: I think essentially it was because the treatment was getting pretty famous. There was a time when there were about 14 Hoxsey clinics scattered across the United States and I think it was a big threat to the medical profession. It was threatening the pharmaceutical companies, the big hospitals, everybody that makes a lot of money out of medical treatments. So they definitely had to get rid of him because this was an effective and cheap treatment. So they had to get rid of it.

Ty: And one of the things that I read about Harry is that he wanted to make sure that if people didn't have the money that they would be treated for free.

Dr. Gutierrez: That's correct.

Ty: And at that time, if I remember correctly, the AMA wanted to buy the formula but he was afraid.

Dr. Gutierrez: Definitely, he didn't sell it to them. That's correct.

Ty: Are there certain types of cancer that the Hoxsey formula works better with? Or is it just cancer in general?

Dr. Gutierrez: No, there are a few types. In general, it works really well for most of the malignancies we treat. But there are a few that we know we only get like a 50-50 response. With cancers like sarcomas and multiple myeloma, we only get about a 50-50 response.

Ty: If somebody comes in to the Hoxsey clinic and they want treatment, how long does a treatment typically last?

Dr. Gutierrez: This is a clinic that does something in a different way than most of the regular clinics. We try to do everything in a single day. People come in in the morning, they register, they go through the laboratory, they go through the x-rays, they get their consultations, and they go through a very thorough physical examination. Then we have to wait until we get the reports from the laboratory and x-rays, which takes a couple of hours. Then we call people up for a second visit in the afternoon and we explain all the findings to them. We give them their instructions, their treatments. They just pick up their supplies and make their payments and they go home.

Ty: Wow. And so you're about to start seeing patients today. So it's just before nine o'clock in the morning and by this afternoon they'll have their treatments and they'll be able to go back?

Dr. Gutierrez: Exactly. They will be able to go back home.

Ty: So it's a home treatment then really that is supervised by you here?

Dr. Gutierrez: Yes.

Ty: So you're in touch with the patients once they leave?

Dr. Gutierrez: Yes. They take their supplements. Most of the medications are taken by mouth so there are hardly any medications that are going to be injected. So they take their supplements and they do the diet. This is something that you can do at home. You don't have to be necessarily hospitalized to do it.

They stay on the diet and they come back for a checkup every three, six months, every year. Eventually they just come back every two to three years.

Ty: Okay. So the Hoxsey tonic then, is this something that they would take back bottles of or do they brew it themselves?

Dr. Gutierrez: No, they take bottles of concentrate so that makes it easy for them to take at home, but they get instructed on how to dilute it and how much to take. The amount is different for each particular patient.

Ty: I see. Generally, how long would someone take the Hoxsey tonic after they've been in the clinic? They go home, three months, six months, a year? How long?

Dr. Gutierrez: You mean the length of the whole treatment?

Ty: Yes, how long will they take the Hoxsey treatment?

Dr. Gutierrez: I'd say on average four to five years.

Ty: So you take it several years afterwards. Okay.

Dr. Gutierrez: Yes, yes. Then on the fourth or the fifth year, if you cannot find any detectable traces of any malignancy in their bodies through PET scans, CT scans, laboratories, and physicals, if there's no sign of any more trouble, then we tell them, "Hey, you can stop the treatment." Some of them say, "Yeah, I'd like to get rid of it" and then start eating regular things. But some people say, "Hey, I don't want to stop it. I just want to continue taking it the rest of my life."

Ty: So they take the tonic and then they—What does the diet look like?

Dr. Gutierrez: We asked them to stay away from things that are normally not so good for you like alcohol, carbonated beverages, refined sugar, artificial sweets, and that kind of stuff. There are six or seven things.

Ty: Other than that, not really all that restrictive?

Dr. Gutierrez: Oh no, no. Except for the things that we specifically recommend people not to take, they can eat whatever they want. Being conscientious of what they eat.

Ty: Right. So staying away from the refined sugars, carbonated beverages, and alcohol. What else?

Dr. Gutierrez: Pork, tomatoes, vinegar, regular table salt, refined sweets, and artificial sweeteners.

Ty: Why tomatoes?

Dr. Gutierrez: One of the mechanisms of action of the formula is to change the PH of your blood to make it more alkaline. So if you eat anything with acidity in it, that's going to reverse the alkalinity for the treatment and that's going to ruin the whole thing.

Ty: So tomatoes will do that. What about grapefruit?

Dr. Gutierrez: No, because the citrus has a completely different mechanism of action. They mix with the acids in your stomach and become a very strong alkaline.

You see, cancer cells cannot tolerate alkalinity but they thrive in acidity. So if you put acidic food into your system, your PH becomes really acidic and that's wonderful for cancer cells. So we ask people to avoid acidic fruit.

Ty: So, the Hoxsey tonic really works on the alkalinity of the blood?

Dr. Gutierrez: That's only one of the four or five mechanisms of action. That's only one of them.

Ty: What are the others?

Dr. Gutierrez: It stimulates the bone marrow so you can produce more of the specific cells that fight cancer cells. Somehow your immune cells get used to the malignant tissue in your body and don't do enough to stop it. With the effect of the medicine, I mean the Hoxsey formula, you're going to produce a new generation of more aggressive immune cells that are going to specifically destroy the malignant tissue.

Then you break the fibrotic tissue, which normally surrounds cancer cells, to break it open and allow the immune cells to go in there and destroy them. It works on the DNA of the cancer cells, several things.

Ty: Okay. So back to the ingredients of the Hoxsey tonic. You said it has licorice? What is it about licorice that is beneficial against cancer?

Dr. Gutierrez: You have to go to into the literature. There is tons and tons of information about licorice and rhubarb and—

Ty: Is rhubarb one of the ingredients as well?

Dr. Gutierrez: In some of the formulas, yes. Not in ours.

Ty: Not in yours.

Dr. Gutierrez: No. I have a collection of books which say that they have the Hoxsey formula and there are all kinds of different variations of the formula. But that's not the real one.

Ty: So what are the specific ingredients in the one that you use or is that proprietary?

Dr. Gutierrez: I think it's proprietary, but you can get the official copy of the list of ingredients from the girls at the front desk and they will give it to you. That's not a big deal.

Ty: Very good. So as far as terminal patients, let say somebody comes in here and they have undergone chemo and radiation. And their body is really in bad shape. Do you have success with people that are terminal?

Dr. Gutierrez: No, no. It depends. If you have somebody that is really just grasping for breath and really on the last minutes of their life, there is nothing you can do about it. People have to still have a certain degree of capacity to respond to the medication. If they don't, you won't be able to do anything about it. They still need to be able to swallow their food, to be able to stick to the diet, and do a number of things. You have to use your clinical, your common sense to be able to tell some people, "Hey, unfortunately, there is nothing we can do about it."

Ty: It's too late.

Dr. Gutierrez: Yes.

Ty: Do you recommend that people, if they call and ask, do you recommend that they stay away from chemo and radiation?

Dr. Gutierrez: No. In most cases, we can help them without necessarily having to go to chemo and radiation or surgery. But there are some cases in which you feel, according to the opinion of the team here that the best thing for them to do is to get surgery, to get chemo. And we're the first one to tell them, "Hey, go ahead and get this operated on because you're going to get obstructed..."

Ty: Brain Tumor.

Dr. Gutierrez: Exactly. "Your arteries are going to burst. You need to get chemo, you need to get radiation." Whatever they need we tell them. But in most cases, like I said, we can manage to help them without having to go through those conventional means.

Ty: Very good. So what would you recommend to someone that is looking at different clinics to go to to treat cancer? What's the most important question that a cancer patient should ask so they can figure out if they're going to the right place?

Dr. Gutierrez: I don't know. There are so many options and so many therapies out there. That's a really difficult question to answer. I guess they just have to inquire into every single one of them and then there's the economical issue. They have to inquire into every single one on what they will use and do their own research. And then maybe talk to people that have been going to different places to see which one seems to be getting better results and then go for that one.

Ty: Well, those are good questions.

Dr. Gutierrez: Yes.

Ty: Being a one day treatment, is the Hoxsey treatment really affordable?

Dr. Gutierrez: I think so. We're the cheapest clinic in town.

Ty: Are you really?

Dr. Gutierrez: Oh, yes. At some of these other places you have to sell your house to be able to be treated. Crazy.

Ty: Well, Dr. Gutierrez thank you for sharing with us today. I wish that my Dad had been able to get down here before he died.

Dr. Gutierrez: Well, what can we do?

Ty: Sometimes you're just too late.

Dr. Gutierrez: Yes, yes. That's correct.

Ty: Well, keep up the good work.

Dr. Gutierrez: Thank you. Appreciate it.

Ty: Thank you.

[end of transcript]

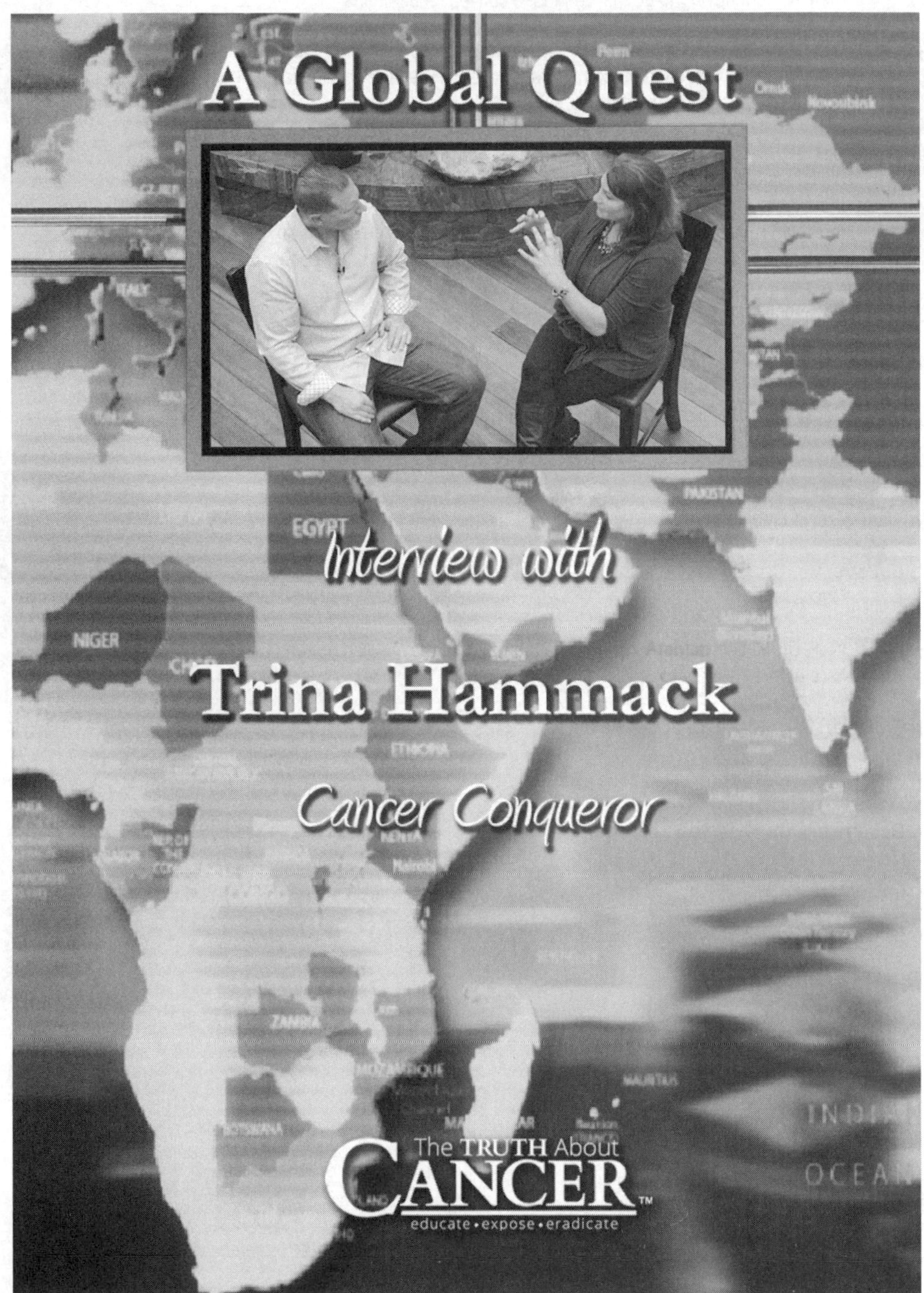
A Global Quest
Interview with
Trina Hammack
Cancer Conqueror
The TRUTH About
CANCER™
educate • expose • eradicate

Ty: I'm here with Trina at the Hope for Cancer Institute in Tijuana, Mexico. Thank you for joining us today.

Trina: Thank you for having me.

Ty: We were at dinner last night, not you and I, but Dr. Tony and I were at dinner, and he was telling me a little bit about your story. And he said you were going to be here today so I'm really excited to hear your story of being diagnosed with cancer. You are a wellness practitioner, yourself.

Trina: I am.

Ty: Walk us back. How many years was it that you were diagnosed? And tell us about your story.

Trina: Sure. It was back in 2008. My nine-year-old son said, "Mom, mom, you're getting fat." And I'm like, "Yeah, my belly is getting kind of big." I would kind of palpate my belly a little bit and feel in there and it felt like there was a bubble inside my belly. And it was rather large, and so I went to the doctor and he did an ultrasound and on the spot he diagnosed me with stage IV ovarian cancer. And so I about passed out with that kind of a diagnosis, and it was unbelievably scary.

Ty: I'll bet. You had one son at the time. Any other children?

Trina: One child. And I was not going to leave this world and leave him without a mom.

Ty: Was that your first thought?

Trina: Oh yeah. Five years before I had healed myself from Lyme disease in my brain, and he, again, was my motivation for doing whatever it took to get well. And I knew I had to do something different. I lost my mom to breast cancer when she was 48 and my grandmother died of ovarian cancer at 36.

Ty: Wow.

Trina: So when I got this diagnosis at 46 I knew that I had to do something differently than what they did. So I called up Tony.

Ty: You already knew him.

Trina: I knew him because I had been sending my clients to the clinic for cancer situations and I said if it ever happened to me he would be my first call. And it was. I called him at home and I said, "What do I do?" And he said, "You get that thing taken out and you get me the pathology report." So that's what I did. They took out a melon-sized tumor.

Ty: Huge.

Trina: Huge tumor.

Ty: Huge tumor.

Trina: Huge. And then I sent him my pathology report and I came down and he actually created a home program for me so I didn't actually have to come down here and stay down here.

Ty: What was involved in the home program? What did you do that you had not been doing before?

Trina: The main part of my home program was the Sono Photo Dynamic therapy. I would do my light treatments for an hour and then I would go into the bathtub and do an ultrasound treatment. So the first thing you do is you ingest a chlorophyll type agent, in the dark, and you let that go and seed itself inside any cancer cells in your body. And then I think it was 24 or 48 hours later you start your treatment.

So when I went under the lights for the first time I remember feeling this interesting sensation. So with this chlorophyll type agent in my cells, if it is inside the cell, and you get exposed to the full spectrum light, then the chlorophyll will bloom and it will create more oxygen and kill any cancer from the inside out. So when I got under my lights for the first time it was just this bubbly feeling throughout my whole body. It was really interesting.

Ty: It was killing the cancer cells.

Trina: Yeah, it was killing cancer. I think it also helps go deeper for Lyme and helps kill Lyme even deeper. So I would do that. And then, I lived in Big Sur, California so I was out in the country and my tub was outdoors, and I would have to go into the bathtub and use ultrasound to do the same thing, so the sound waves would do the same thing and activate and kill cancer cells.

So I was so dedicated, I would be out there in my outdoor bathtub, in storms, and there are sticks flying, and wind blowing, and rain coming down, and I was out there shivering and doing my treatment. I never passed up on my treatment. And so that was the main thing, the Sono Photo Dynamic Therapy that I did. Tony had also done a urine therapy where he took my urine and he made injections, and so I would give myself a series of injections from my urine. That was another piece to it that I did, as well.

Ty: So the diagnosis was what year?

Trina: 2008.

Ty: 2008. Okay, so how many months or years did it take before you conversed with Tony, or talked to him on the phone, or whatever, and he said, "Hey, your cancer is in complete remission now?"

Trina: You know, I think it was about a six-month program, and then I decided to go for a full year, and I just did it for a year because I just felt so good on it. So, it's been seven years. It will be seven years next week.

Ty: Seven years. So what was the diagnosis when they found this tumor? What was the conditional prognosis?

Trina: When they tell you that you have Stage IV ovarian cancer, blah-blah-blah, they wanted me to do chemo, and I said no. I knew in every cell of my being not to touch chemo with a ten-foot pole—for me. I watched what it did to my grandmother and my mother and I wasn't going to be that statistic either. And I knew I had to be here for my son. I was not leaving this earth. I was not. And so it was my will and I just knew what to do.

Ty: Did they try to steer you toward chemo? Did they try to scare you about it or anything?

Trina: Oh my gosh, absolutely. They absolutely tried to scare me. An interesting story was, the day after my surgery—we took it out, and then the largest wildfire in California history started a mile from my home. And so we couldn't go home for five weeks. So I was healing elsewhere and when I got home I was able to check my messages, and I got a message from an oncologist saying, "You're scheduled for chemo tomorrow."

They went ahead and scheduled me even though I had declined it. I sat across the desk from one of my surgeons and he called me a fool three times for declining chemo. And then I finally said, "You know, I'm not just sitting down in Big Sur rubbing crystals and rocks and feathers together, wishing this away. I'm working with a doctor who knows alternative protocols. And then he finally was quiet about it.

But they went ahead and they scheduled the chemo anyway. So I get home after being away five weeks and I get this message and I called the oncologist and I said, "I respectfully decline this therapy, I'm doing something else." And they were actually really kind about it but they went ahead and they scheduled me anyway even though I said no.

Ty: Wow, that's kind of strange. It's also strange that within one sit-down you were called a fool three times.

Trina: Oh yeah, and I had to finally say, "Can I talk now?" And I'm glad I took the route I took.

Ty: Yeah, because Stage IV ovarian cancer—the statistics are not good. You're seven years out. You would not be alive today if you had gone with traditional chemo.

Trina: No way. Not a chance. And like I said, my "why" I had to do something different was for my son. I didn't want to leave. I wasn't leaving him without a mom.

Ty: Right.

Trina: I looked deep inside myself and I knew what I had to do, and this was what I had to do.

Ty: Yeah.

Trina: That's what I did.

Ty: So your son, I'm sure now he is just completely on board with what you're doing.

Trina: Oh yeah.

Ty: He's seen you live it.

Trina: Oh, absolutely. He is 16 going on 17.

Ty: Have you ever—since you've been treated here, or treated with this protocol at home, have you ever gone back to those oncologists or doctors that you met with initially?

Trina: Not yet. I kind of have this little fantasy in my mind that someday I will walk into his office, but I haven't yet. One of my surgeons, though—I had two—she was my gynecologist for a while, and she was actually open to some of the things that I was doing, and she has since opened up her referrals to naturopaths and other practitioners. But that one gynecological oncologist—he was something else.

Ty: And he was the one that called you a fool?

Trina: He called me a fool three times. And that wasn't good for me.

Ty: Right. That would be the one I'd want to visit.

Trina: Yeah, and I actually was thinking about that.

Ty: I'd like to visit back with a T-shirt that has "Fool" written three times.

Trina: That's a great idea. That's exactly what I'll do.

Ty: Do you remember you told me this seven years ago?

Trina: Yes. And I'm here today. And so I educate even more about getting to the source, getting to the roots, on an emotional level, on a physical level, you have to heal the cell to get well, and you have to do…

Ty: That's what you're doing now in your clinic, as well, teaching people how to do that.

Trina: Yes, we have programs that are amazing, right in alignment with this natural approach. And it works.

Ty: But for those that do get a diagnosis of cancer this is something you would recommend, Hope for Cancer?

Trina: Oh, absolutely, Hope for Cancer is the best. The people are so nice and they're knowledgeable. You know, I think we've been indoctrinated for so many years that cancer is a death sentence. When I got my first diagnosis the first thing I saw was a coffin, one of those old-fashioned coffins with nails, from the Westerns. That was the image I saw in my brain. And cancer equals death in our society, but if you know what to do and where to go then it's not true.

Ty: It's not true. Cancer is not necessarily a death sentence.

Trina: No, it's not. But it's a message that you need to clean up what's going on inside in order to be healthy.

Ty: What would your message be to someone that is watching this that has been recently diagnosed with cancer, and maybe they've got a really "sensitive" oncologist, like you had, that says, "Hey, you're dead in X number of months," or "You're a fool if you don't do these treatments that I have prescribed?"

Trina: I'd say, "Look outside the box, absolutely. Call around and see what feels right for you, because it's not a death sentence. It doesn't have to be a death sentence." I knew chemo would have killed, not only me, but if it didn't kill me it would have killed my spirit. So look outside the box. There is a lot out there.

Ty: And maybe be educated and be prepared ahead of time, like you were, right? You were diagnosed but you knew, "If I'm diagnosed, I'm calling you, Dr. Jimenez."

Trina: Oh, absolutely.

Ty: And so maybe that is good advice, as well, to prepare ahead of time instead of just being scared to death when you get that diagnosis if you don't know what you're going to do.

Trina: Exactly. And start looking at your lifestyle now before you end up getting that diagnosis or it's too late. Start cleaning up your diet. Start living a healthy lifestyle, because that's all part of it.

Ty: Yes. And you're here today to be a testimony to that.

Trina: And I will continue to be. I continue to teach and share and inspire, because there is hope, there really is hope. We are taught to be afraid—taught to be afraid of this, and forced to go into chemo, and radiation, and cutting and chopping us up. And it doesn't have to be that way.

Ty: Yes.

Trina: Most of the people that I have sent down to Hope for Cancer, they always said, "We wish we would have come here first."

Ty: That's good advice.

Trina: Yes.

Ty: Trina, thanks for giving everyone out there hope today, and for teaching them and inspiring them. You've inspired me, and I appreciate you.

Trina: Oh, thank you so much.

[end of transcript]

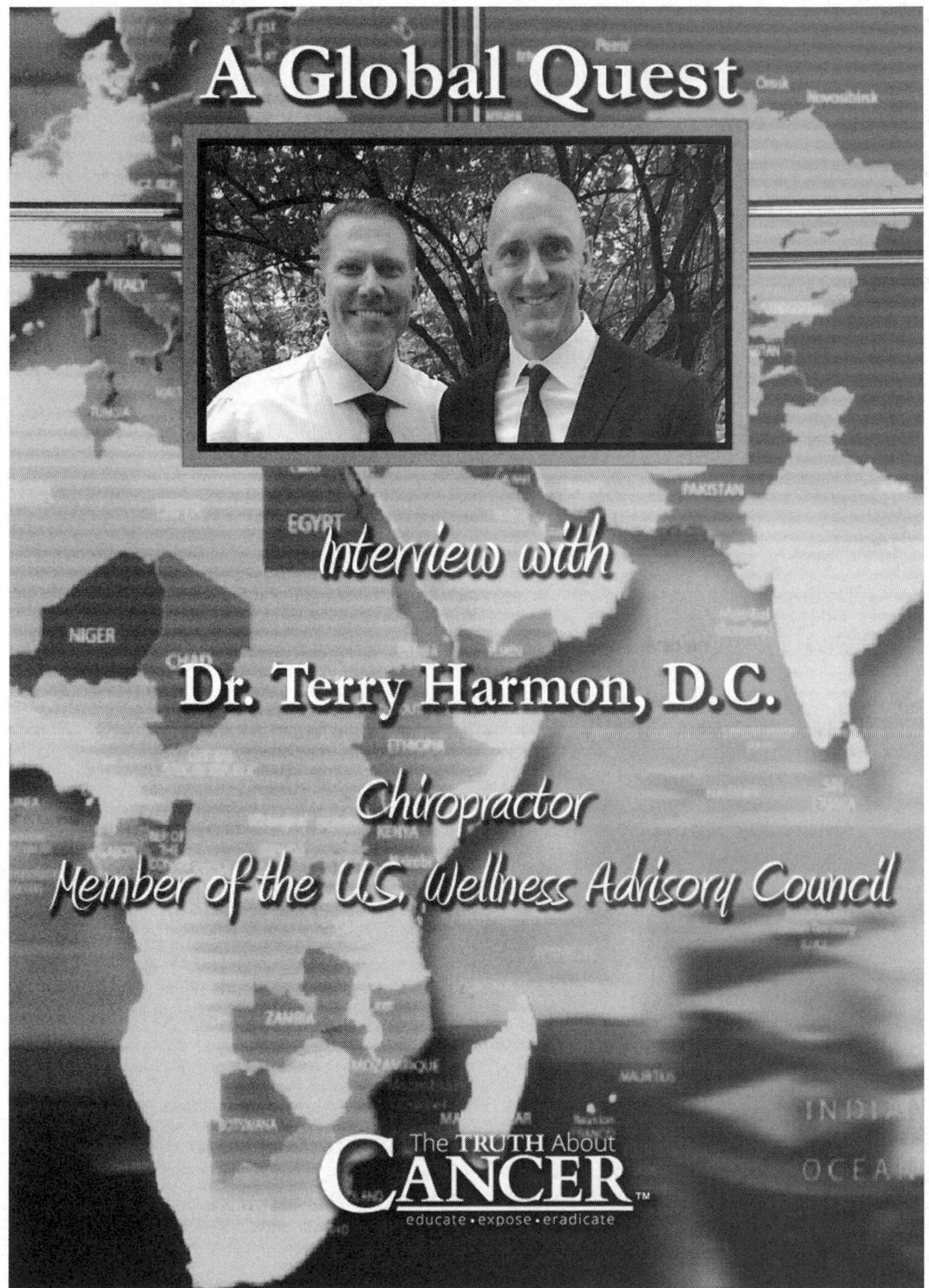
A Global Quest
Interview with
Dr. Terry Harmon, D.C.
Chiropractor
Member of the U.S. Wellness Advisory Council
The TRUTH About CANCER
educate • expose • eradicate

Ty: Well, Dr. Terry, thanks for being here with me today.

Dr. Harmon: Thanks for having me.

Ty: I appreciate you making the long drive down to Nashville from up in, where in Kentucky?

Dr. Harmon: We're in northwest Kentucky. Morganfield, Kentucky.

Ty: Okay. I appreciate you being here and really looking forward to getting your input on the importance of the spine in overall health, which was kind of a little bit of the piece of the puzzle that we missed in the last documentary.

Dr. Harmon: Right.

Ty: And also some other issues. I've heard some really amazing testimonials from people that you have helped that are now cancer-free thanks to some of the things that you've implemented. I'm really looking forward to the interview today.

Dr. Harmon: I'm excited to be here. Honored to be here as well, and excited to share, also.

Ty: Yeah.

Dr. Harmon: For sure.

Ty: Dr. Harmon, what I want to do today is really pick your brain about the importance of the spine. As I mentioned, that's an area that is often overlooked in overall health and even cancer. Share with us, initially, how did you get into becoming a doctor of chiropractics?

Dr. Harmon: I had a great experience growing up with my chiropractor and just thought this will be a great thing to do. So, that's why I pursued chiropractic and after getting into chiropractic and loving it and having a great time with it, that's when I began to see patients in my practice who had cancer and I loved working with them, but had no clue that really—I could really help them.

And then there was one day in practice, I had a patient, I'll never forget it. He had cancer that was eating away at his face and he came in with a bag of commercial food. We'll call it commercial food. I said, "What are you doing?" I knew enough about the body, obviously, and the spine and the nerve system and nutrition to say, "These two things don't add up. You have cancer, it's not looking good, why are you doing that?" He said this specifically, I'll never forget it. He said, "My doctors told me to get as many calories as possible and this type of food was the best thing I could put in my body during this treatment. It was literally at that moment I said, "I'm not going to stand around anymore and act like I can't contribute something." I began to study even more and then I began to hold workshops on boosting the immune system and that's how it all started.

Ty: That was your "aha" moment.

Dr. Harmon: It all really started when I was young. My mother had cancer, lymphoma, when I was really young and I got to witness that my whole life growing up. I got to witness the ups and downs of cancer, the ups and downs of cancer treatment, the ravages of conventional treatment. Yet, even at that, I didn't feel as if I had the knowledge to help that until that fellow came in and I had been in practice a couple years and I said, "I know I can do more than I'm doing," and then I said, "I'm going to commit myself the rest of my life to learning and studying and figuring out to help this thing."

Ty: Okay. So it was really more of an "aha" period of time to where you saw the failure of conventional medicine with your mother and then you saw this man coming in with an aggressive cancer eating things that you knew couldn't be good for his body and you said, enough's enough.

Dr. Harmon: Up until that point, I believed the lie, if you will, so to speak, that the cancer experts are the cancer experts, and even though I knew things that could help people, I felt like they knew more—if you would. There was something that happened there, I said, "No, I will do more from this point on," and this was probably 15 years ago. The studying really, really commenced and over the last probably five years especially, the things that we've been able to see and do with people has been quite amazing.

Ty: So, Dr. Harmon, talk about being a doctor of chiropractic, you deal with the spine.

Dr. Harmon: Correct.

Ty: Why is the spine so important?

Dr. Harmon: That's a big thing, because oftentimes even when patients come to see me, they're thinking nutrition if they're coming with a cancer diagnosis, but when we start to study the body, and you're looking at the "Quest for Cures" and other things out there, we look at what system is the most important system for fending off cancer and most people will say the immune system. Right?

Ty: Right.

Dr. Harmon: Most people say, absolutely the immune system. I would agree with them. But then, we look at the immune system is comprised of a series of glands and organs that make this immune response, and those glands and organs are controlled by the nerve system.

Ty: Okay. First of all, what are the glands and the organs of the immune system?

Dr. Harmon: Right. So we're going to look at the thymus, we're going to look at the spleen, we're going to look at the bone marrow, and then the gut.

Ty: Okay.

Dr. Harmon: So when we look at the gut, a majority of our immune response comes from the gut tissue

Ty: Right.

Dr. Harmon: Yet all of that hinders upon or rests upon the vitality of the nerve system. So when we look at the spine, the spine is the tissue that surrounds and protects the spinal cord, so the brain communicates to the body via the spinal cord.

Ty: Right.

Dr. Harmon: When we look at that, oftentimes as we work with patients, a lot of people don't understand that our spine is designed to have a certain structure, a very specific structure. And any deviation off that structure directly interferes with the nerve system's ability to adapt and respond to stress. What are we doing more of now than ever before?

Ty: Stressing about everything.

Dr. Harmon: Stressing about everything, we're sitting now more than ever, we're looking at our technology more than ever...

Ty: Right.

Dr. Harmon: Even if we go to the gym, we're kind of thinking fitness; we're not thinking structure. When we look at all the research, some of the most research on the planet is coming out right nowadays, and it says that the nerve system controls the immune system and then I tell people, what impacts your nerve system and they say, "Everything." Everything we do impacts the nerve system. The only question is, are we doing the things that make it healthier, or are we doing the things that break it down?

Ty: Okay.

Dr. Harmon: So absolutely important to understand.

Ty: That's fascinating to look at because we do hear about the immune system and the importance of the immune system and for any cancer or other diseases, but what you're saying is that really the controller, the quarterback for the immune system, maybe a football analogy, might be the nervous system.

Dr. Harmon: Absolutely. It absolutely is. The immune system is absolutely paramount and vital, but it really is regulated by the nerve system. We want to work with patients and teach people all of the things they can do nurture their nerve system, to understand the nerve system, and also to nurture and understand their immune system as well.

Ty: Okay. So, how can they do that? Let's look at the nervous system as the quarterback, right?

Dr. Harmon: Yes.

Ty: Not Tom Brady quarterback, not the deflate—

Dr. Harmon: Not that kind.

Ty: But a quarterback, right?

Dr. Harmon: Absolutely.

Ty: So controlling the immune system so how do they nurture that quarterback—the nervous system?

Dr. Harmon: There's three things that I like people to become aware of. Number one is their actual spinal structure. If we had a chart in front of us and we looked at the spine from the side, it's designed to have these amazing curves in it. When we look at the spine from the front, it's supposed to be straight. I tell people, on a scale of one to 10, we're shooting for a 10, as far as moving people towards optimal structure. You can actually work on correcting your spine, just like you would correct your teeth with an orthodontist.

Ty: Okay.

Dr. Harmon: Everybody knows that if you want to make your teeth line up better, there's a profession that deals with that. That's an orthodontist. Awesome! Absolutely amazing. It's the same way that goes with the spine. Number one is becoming aware of your structure. Number two is becoming aware of your mobility. Are you mobile where you're supposed to be mobile or are you not? If you're not, if you score subpar there, then that's hindering or impacting your nerve system. And then the third thing, which is amazing, Ty, is the fact that there's technology today, where you can monitor your nerve system in real time. And that's called heart rate variability. So, literally, there's technology we have in the office, but then there's technology with your smartphone and a heart rate monitor that will tell you exactly, literally to the tenth of a percentage point, how your nerve system is doing.

Ty: Wow! So technology is amazing when it comes to this area of science, right?

Dr. Harmon: Yeah. It wasn't available even five years ago in relation to utilizing on your smartphone. Now anybody watching this or listening to this, within 10 minutes can find out exactly how their nerve system is doing, if it's swung one way or another, and then how to address that.

Ty: Speaking of which, I interviewed a man recently that is a patient of yours—

Dr. Harmon: Yes.

Ty: Right?

Dr. Harmon: Yes.

Ty: And he said that he went to you—he had been diagnosed with terminal cancer—

Dr. Harmon: Correct.

Ty: Kidney cancer—

Dr. Harmon: Yes.

Ty: And he comes to you and you found out there was [sic] some issues in his spine. Could you talk about that and then tell us how he's doing today?

Dr. Harmon: Foundationally, when we analyze a patient, when I look at him, we're going to look at the spine, we're going to look at structure, and right off the bat you could see and it was amazing that his structure was not good, just visually. Then we took films and saw over a 200 percent shifting in the wrong direction and then obviously we began a program to work on correcting that. Along with that, we did functional lab work. We're going to look at deficiencies, toxicities, inflammation. Same thing—write up a plan to address deficiencies, toxicities, and inflammation, and this began in August of 2014. We're filming this May of 2015, and he's completely cancer-free, was Stage IV, told he wasn't going to live beyond Christmas, and the most amazing thing with working with that fellow is he said, "I feel better now, than I felt in my entire life." Why is that? Well, it's because possibly for his entire life that nerve system never really clicked optimally, and now it's actually starting to do what it's supposed to do.

Ty: He's a great guy.

Dr. Harmon: Yes.

Ty: And he's going to be in the "Quest" here, "The Global Quest"; we're going to put his testimony somewhere, but you can tell he's just vibrant. When you talk to him and you can tell that he's so thankful for you and for what you've done for him. But I wonder how many people are out there that have been diagnosed with the same type of cancer or another similar cancer that that is the problem—that their spine is the problem and they never find that out.

Dr. Harmon: I tell people—it's such a huge component and it's a piece of the puzzle that oftentimes has been missed and really because chiropractic as a whole, that's my primary degree is chiropractic, really hasn't put as much of an emphasis on it as it could. So, on some level, it's our own fault as a profession and it's really my passion and the colleagues that I associate with and work with and teach with that we're going to reestablish that is what chiropractic is. We're going to work on structure and we're going to establish healthy nerve systems. It's powerful.

There's a scripture, and all the talks I give, I share all of the time, Psalm 139:14, King David says, "*I praise you Lord, for I am fearfully and wonderfully made, he says that my soul knows well.*" It's just a powerful, short scripture and the reason is it's so powerful is because so many people have lost belief or hope that they're fearfully and wonderfully made. Because of what we've been led to believe culturally that we're made defective, that we don't stand a chance—that cancer is going to get all of us—that causes fear in so many, especially if you've seen loved ones, like you've seen, like I've seen. Even patients—when I first started I saw—it's just horrible to see people suffer.

We begin to potentially believe that we're not fearfully and wonderfully made. The reality is we are. We're fearfully and wonderfully made; however, things happen that alter, if you will, the way we work. We just have to restore ourselves back to the way we're made to begin with.

Ty: That kind of goes into your deficiency, right? Talk about some deficiencies that could be causing us to not be as healthy as we were made to be.

Dr. Harmon: Three primary deficiencies on lab work that we see. We look at Vitamin D, a huge one. We see that most people's Vitamin D levels are around 20, and we want around 60 to 80. That's huge because Vitamin D is huge for the immune system. B-12—really, really huge. We see that being low a lot of the times and that ties into with methylation, and then the third thing we may see is ferritin. We may see that low or we may actually see that really high.

Ty: What is ferritin?

Dr. Harmon: Ferritin—iron. Iron to the blood. Iron to your tissues.

Ty: Got it.

Dr. Harmon: So that's major as well, and we can see that really low or we can see that really high and usually with inflammation we'll see it really high. There's a number of other toxicities and deficiencies as well. Heavy metals, right?

Ty: Yeah.

Dr. Harmon: Major. If we have a patient who is loaded with heavy metals, it's going to be hard for their nerve system to work well and their immune system and their endocrine system. We're going to look at deficiencies, we're going to look at toxicities, and then we're going to look at inflammation.

Ty: Speaking of the heavy metals. You've got your deficiencies you analyze through the lab work if they're deficient and then you true those levels up.

Dr. Harmon: Absolutely.

Ty: The heavy metals, though, the toxicities. How do you get rid of heavy metals? For somebody who comes in and they're high on mercury.

Dr. Harmon: Absolutely.

Ty: What happens? How do you get rid of that?

Dr. Harmon: You're going to do specific chelation protocols.

Ty: Right.

Dr. Harmon: So, chelation means, "to draw or to pull or to claw," and you've got to do very specific protocols to pull those out. Because if you go, for example, online and you say I want to get rid of heavy metals and you're going to find five pages of Google talking about how to get that out. There's safe ways and there's not safe ways to do that. We use very specific protocols in the office to pull the different metals out.

Ty: Okay. So how might these deficiencies and these toxicities combine to result in the inflammation?

Dr. Harmon: Absolutely huge. Because foundationally, again, if you look at the research as well, you almost jump from one thing to another, but inflammation is the root cause, if you will—the root cause of all 21st century diseases. All kinds of research on that.

So we want to address that and then we want to work with the nerve system as well, but if we're deficient in something or we're toxic in something, it stresses the body and when the body is stressed, it's going to inflame in an attempt to heal. Too much inflammation—bad, it's going to clog down nutrients to the cells, toxins out of the cells. It's major, major issues. Like with our friend, Bill, that we worked with, you interviewed Bill as well, is you start to put three or four of these things together and, unfortunately, in most cases, if you only address one or two, sometimes people don't heal and they die. But when you start to put all of the pieces together and you address them, "fearfully and wonderfully made," manifests itself.

Ty: Wow! Then there's not really a magic bullet. You're talking about there's so many different components. There's like moving pieces to the puzzle to this cancer equation.

Dr. Harmon: Absolutely.

Ty: There's not a magic bullet.

Dr. Harmon: Correct. People will ask me all of the time—I live in Kentucky, it's awesome, I love it there so they'll say, so what's causing all of this cancer? Thinking about that one thing. It's the water; it's the air; it's this, that, and the other. The reality is multi-factorial, but I'll say really, we assess all of that, the nerve system, inflammation, deficiencies, toxicities, and the other component that can play a major positive role in this is exercise. We want people exercising to flood the body with oxygen because oxygen is great for cells and bad for cancer cells, but, ultimately, again, we've got to make sure, again, we're addressing nerve system and inflammation.

Ty: What's a good exercise that you would recommend to somebody that may have been diagnosed with cancer that not only gets the oxygen to the cells, but also might help with the nerve system and the inflammation?

Dr. Harmon: That's a great question. That's where we start to get more specific in relation to the nerve system. Are they parasympathetic dominant, or are they sympathetic dominant.

Ty: What's the difference?

Dr. Harmon: Two branches of the autonomic nerve system, the nerve system that controls and coordinates every cell tissue and organ in the body and the part of the nerve system that we don't directly control. We indirectly control it. So parasympathetic is rest, recovery, healing, repair, and sympathetic is fight or flight, which is what most people actually are overstimulated with, it's wake up, tackle the day, go until midnight, do it again—groundhog day. So when we test—when we do heart rate variability, it will tell us. It will tell us whether you're sympathetic dominant, parasympathetic dominant, and then we'll teach you how to use the technology on a daily basis to really monitor what your nerve system is doing. So if you were parasympathetic dominant, then we'd want you to get more active. To the best of your ability, we want you to do more high-intensity workouts. If you're sympathetic dominant, overstimulated, stressed, fight or flight, then we move you towards walking. We may move you towards yoga. Those type of things.

Ty: To calm you almost.

Dr. Harmon: Absolutely. Because your nerve system is already overstimulated, it's already stressed. We need to bring it back. Ideally, the autonomic nerve system is supposed to work as a pendulum. If you go really, really hard today and your nerve system automatically swings over into sympathetic dominance, it's doing what it's supposed to do. Then tonight it's designed to go back hard the other way with parasympathetic to heal and then as you wake up, you're rebalanced and able to do the day again. But most people, they've lost the ability to ascertain that and so over a period of time Dr. Nick Gonzalez, in one of his books—it's absolutely amazing I'll never forget reading it and he says that people who are sympathetic dominant, they are prone to solid tumors of the organs. He says, conversely, people who are parasympathetic dominant, are prone to cancers—immunological cancers, like leukemia, lymphoma, myeloma, and sarcoma.

Ty: Really?

Dr. Harmon: Yes.

Ty: That's pretty amazing.

Dr. Harmon: Then the question I ask people is, "What are you?" and then let's work on what we need to do to be able to get that thing balanced and able to pendulum the way it's supposed to. Swing back and forth because sometimes for a day, a week, or whatever, we're going to go hard.

Ty: Yeah.

Dr. Harmon: We're going to push hard, life is going to be busy, fine. Then the idea is, is that nerve system is able to come back just as hard in the parasympathetic, and then ultimately to balance out.

Ty: Right. The equilibrium. The homeostasis. That's what you're after.

Dr. Harmon: Absolutely. The problem is most people have lost that and they don't realize it. Then the other thing is we know about cancers is because it takes years and years and years to really fully manifest because this didn't start yesterday.

Ty: Right.

Dr. Harmon: This started years ago and if and when, hopefully nobody ever gets a diagnosis again, but if people get the diagnosis, that's the thing that I encourage them to know is, okay, from this moment forward, just understand that this took years to develop, and now you get the opportunity to live differently.

Ty: Right.

Dr. Harmon: For the rest of your life you get to live differently.

Ty: Right. I've heard people say that cancer is not a death sentence is actually a life sentence.

Dr. Harmon: Absolutely. I've seen that many times. People, so to speak, get their eyes opened and say, okay, from this moment forward, we're going to do life differently.

Ty: Right.

Dr. Harmon: It's awesome.

Ty: Yeah. I've heard people say it was the biggest blessing. Not to minimize the diagnosis, and the importance of after you're diagnosed there's a lot of things that you must do. But a lot of people are living healthier lives now because of that diagnosis. But Bill's not an isolated incident.

Dr. Harmon: No.

Ty: You've been telling me about other people. Share with me some more of the stories of people that have shared with you recently about their success with cancer.

Dr. Harmon: Absolutely. Many, many, many cases now. It's really the norm if you will, in our practice through the Grace of God, just that when a patient comes in, typically, I tell patients in our practice and again, we don't treat or cure cancer, we boost the immune system, boost the nerve system, but when they come into our practice, we're going to look at these foundational components.

My other doctor in the practice as well, when we sit down and look at the cases, it's, okay, how bad is structure, we're going to address structure, and then we get the functional labs in and we look at those, and then we go to work at correcting. Just on Saturday when we're in the office looking and just to give you an example, of another fellow with Stage IV cancer, started in his liver and already spread throughout his body. We're looking at his spine, it had improved by 75 percent in eight weeks, and then we looked at his inflammation and there's a lab marker we look at called CRP—C-reactive protein. His first C-reactive protein was 33. We like it below 3, his was 33—massively high, very scary. It went from 33 to 1.9 in eight weeks.

Ty: Would it have been that—the reduction—the drastic reduction because of the fact that you aligned his spine and there's no more inflammation?

Dr. Harmon: It's both.

Ty: So the CRP went down?

Dr. Harmon: It's both. So there's specific nutrition protocols that we're going to recommend for people with high inflammatory markers, so very specific diet, and then also very specific supplements to support that. It's very powerful.

Ty: So talk about that specifically. What is the diet, what are the supplements?

Dr. Harmon: So the diet. Depending on the patient, a high amount of good fats. Healthy fats, avocados, coconut oil, olive oil, good fish oil.

Ty: In line with ketogenic.

Dr. Harmon: Absolutely, ketogenic. Absolutely, that's exactly what it is. It's ketogenic, lots of spices, lots of herbs, lots of vegetables, low to no sugar essentially, clean protein sources, berries, etc.

Ty: And sugar, although we love sugar, and as Casey said, sugar should be a fun food occasionally. We tend to glom it on with everything. Sugar not only feeds cancer cells, but recent studies have come out showing that sugar is actually oncogenic.

Dr. Harmon: Absolutely oncogenic. Massively inflammatory. There's a new book that just came out called "The Sugar Crush," which is awesome, again, written by a neurologist, and so everybody is really starting to see this. It's not just about weight; it's about inflammation and the fact that it is oncogenic.

Ty: What does that mean?

Dr. Harmon: Sure, cancer-causing.

Ty: Even though I brought up the word.

Dr. Harmon: Cancer-causing.

Ty: Cancer-causing.

Dr. Harmon: It's turning on genes or stimulating genes that actually trigger cancer in the body.

Ty: That's a good reason to stay away from sugar.

Dr. Harmon: Right.

Ty: And also the studies have shown that it's four, five, seven times as addictive as cocaine?

Dr. Harmon: As addictive as cocaine and opium. When we work with patients—I teach classes on this—we say, look, plan on three days to maybe two weeks of maybe not feeling very great. If you have loved ones around you, know to be prepared, this may be a tough three days to two weeks, but you can get through this and you can get over this. It's a ketogenic-type diet, and then from a supplement standpoint, we're going to supplement based upon deficiencies, toxicities, and inflammation.

Ty: Very specific.

Dr. Harmon: One of my favorite supplements for inflammation, one of them, is turmeric. Highly concentrated turmeric but absolutely incredible. We haven't seen anything come close to turmeric in relation to knocking out inflammation. It's just that powerful and we're looking at it from a standpoint of labs. We can see labs, CRP drop, 33 points, 32 points in a matter of eight weeks, along with everything else we're doing is awesome.

Ty: That's huge.

Dr. Harmon: Absolutely awesome.

Ty: Okay, and so, other than turmeric—people think of that is maybe curry, turmeric. Are they the same?

Dr. Harmon: Turmeric is an extract of curcumin, right. When we look at that though, we need to look at amounts, because sometimes people will say I'll start to put that in my smoothies, good idea. Real good idea. They'll incorporate it into their food.

Ty: I love to cook with it.

Dr. Harmon: It's a good idea. A teaspoon is equal to about 150 milligrams of turmeric, and we're looking at more of 3,000 to maybe 4,000 or 5,000 milligrams—

Ty: You need the extract.

Dr. Harmon: You need the extract to really address that. Now, just from a, hey, if everything is good standpoint, you might be able to get by just on your cooking. Once you become aware of it, using it more. It really is a targeted approach to reducing that inflammation. Another supplement that I really like is kind of new on the scene is berberine.

Ty: Berberine.

Dr. Harmon: Berberine is a very powerful and been shown to stimulate apoptosis in cancer cells. Cancer-cell suicide. We love that. We don't like suicide unless it's cancer, right? Berberine is awesome and that also is for blood sugar regulation. So when people get started usually their blood sugar is up and down, we monitor hemoglobin A1C, so that's blood sugar over time, and if we see a high reading, then we want to address that. One of the ways to do that in addition to the ketogenic diet, is also going to be through a supplement called berberine.

Ty: Berberine.

Dr. Harmon: Yes. It's all lab-based.

Ty: A good friend of mine, Dr. Michael Farley, said berberine coupled with dong quai, *Angelica sinensis*, will wipe out the bubonic plague.

Dr. Harmon: It's absolutely amazing when you start to put these pieces of the puzzle. Remember, don't forget about Vitamin D. It really became popular five years ago, so a lot of people like you and I really caught on to it, but it does play a major role. We definitely want to get that Vitamin D where it needs to be and everybody, but especially people who are battling cancer.

Ty: But isn't the sun our enemy?

Dr. Harmon: Right. Isn't that the big thing that we heard if you're going to go outside, you better lather up with toxic sunscreen? That's where a lot of people as well are getting sicker and sicker and sicker because they're not optimizing Vitamin D levels. As well, even if you are getting sun exposure, if you don't have a healthy liver and healthy kidneys your body won't be able to make it.

Ty: Because it has to make the Vitamin D3 from the ultraviolet B coupled with—

Dr. Harmon: Cholesterol.

Ty: In your skin.

Dr. Harmon: Through the liver and kidneys in order to manufacture Vitamin D in the body.

Ty: That's why detox is so important.

Dr. Harmon: Back in the day, I used to—way back I'd tell patients in the summer if they were in the sun a lot, "Hey, don't worry about supplementing." They looked like they were getting a lot of sun, but then we would test levels and they would have low levels. That's why I say for $10.00 or $20.00, get your levels checked and then just work towards optimization.

Ty: So even if you're out in the sun getting enough sun exposure, if your liver and your kidneys aren't working properly, you're not going to convert that to Vitamin D3.

Dr. Harmon: Correct, so a $20.00 test we'll call it, you can get your baseline. Over time, test it periodically, so you know that what you need to do throughout the year. For example, a person may need to supplement with 1,000 IUs in the summer and 3,000 in the winter, and that's just an example, but you can really start to figure out what you need.

Ty: Right.

Dr. Harmon: Over time. Then as your liver and kidney get healthier, it can go down. Very powerful.

Ty: A question that's a little bit not in the same genre here, but it's regarding children.

Dr. Harmon: Yes.

Ty: We're getting a lot of kids with cancer now.

Dr. Harmon: Yes.

Ty: Literally, it's an explosion. All of the cases of these kids, these babies, even newborns, with cancer. Any ideas as to why that be happening?

Dr. Harmon: We know that we live in a society that's exposed to more chemicals now than ever before. EWG, ***environmentalworkinggroup.org*** did a study where they tested umbilical cord blood in babies and they found that the average baby born in that study had about 287 known toxins in their body, 180 approximately of which are cancer-causing. So, again, that's terrible and it's sad that by the time these babies are handed to mom or dad, they have these chemicals flowing through their body, then we add in vaccines, typically a lot of antibiotics, potentially the baby is not nursed so now they may have toxic formula. The next thing you know, these kids, they're so compromised today, it's terrible.

Ty: What do you mean "toxic formula"?

Dr. Harmon: Toxic formula, so baby formula. Ideally, babies were born to ingest something called breast milk. That's what they're designed to do. Studies have shown it boosts IQ, boosts immune system. Now when we have a synthetic baby formula that can come from soy, toxic soy, which is known to be cancer-causing, or it could be even a rice formula or a dairy formula, it's still going to have all kinds of additives and preservatives, bad fats, sugars, etc. It's not what the body is designed for. That "fearfully and wonderfully made" baby, their nerve system and immune system is going to be stressed. Terrible.

Ty: I guess the question is not why do so many kids have cancer, is how do any kids not have cancer when they're born?

Dr. Harmon: Psalm 139:14. "We are fearfully and wonderfully made"—that a baby could be born—think about it, with 287 chemicals in its body—and still look and smell amazing like babies do, that's a testament to the God that created us. Right? It really is—versus the other way around.

Ty: Right.

Dr. Harmon: Childhood cancer is a horrific. I've seen it several times now. It's horrible, but it's not so much that cancer is the thing that's overwhelming us. It's the toxins and the stress on our bodies.

Ty: So, really, I guess it would be safe to say, if you kind of go out on a limb, that there's not any cures for cancer.

Dr. Harmon: Right.

Ty: There are—are substances that make our bodies work better or substances that we can eliminate that we're impeding our bodies from working the way that they were supposed to.

Dr. Harmon: Yeah.

Ty: It's really a matter of giving the body what it needs, removing what it doesn't need, so that it works the way that it was made to.

Dr. Harmon: Absolutely. We're "fearfully and wonderfully made"—and if we take care of it, it will work the way that it's designed to work and it will flourish. And it will flourish in incredible health. That's the big deal. I tell people our job is to—in our office, is to remove the interference, and teach how to take care of the body. Thomas Edison, so the doctor of the future, "Will give no medicine, but will interest his patients in the cause and prevention of disease and the care of the human frame." Hopefully, that's where we're at now. At least we're moving towards there rapidly.

Ty: We're moving very rapidly towards there I believe. Quick question, last question.

Dr. Harmon: Yeah.

Ty: As a DC, did you take the Hippocratic Oath?

Dr. Harmon: Absolutely.

Ty: So the Hippocratic Oath says, in essence, to sum it up for us—

Dr. Harmon: "Do no harm."

Ty: "First, do no harm."

Dr. Harmon: "First, do no harm." Absolutely. That's what we're called to do. We're called to help and certainly, absolutely, do no harm. Hippocrates said, "Let thy food be thy medicine and let thy medicine be thy food." He also said this; you ready? "Look well to the spine, for the cause of disease."

Ty: Hippocrates?

Dr. Harmon: Yeah.

Ty: He knew what he was talking about.

Dr. Harmon: He did know what he was talking about, absolutely. He would have been a great guy to interview.

Ty: He would have. Since he's not here, I'm glad you're here to share that with us.

Dr. Harmon: I'm glad I'm here.

Ty: I think the addition of this information about the spine, the importance of the spine in health and cancer, is invaluable for the people that are watching. I really thank you for coming today.

Dr. Harmon: It's my pleasure. Thank you for having us.

Ty: God bless.

Dr. Harmon: God bless.

[end of transcript]

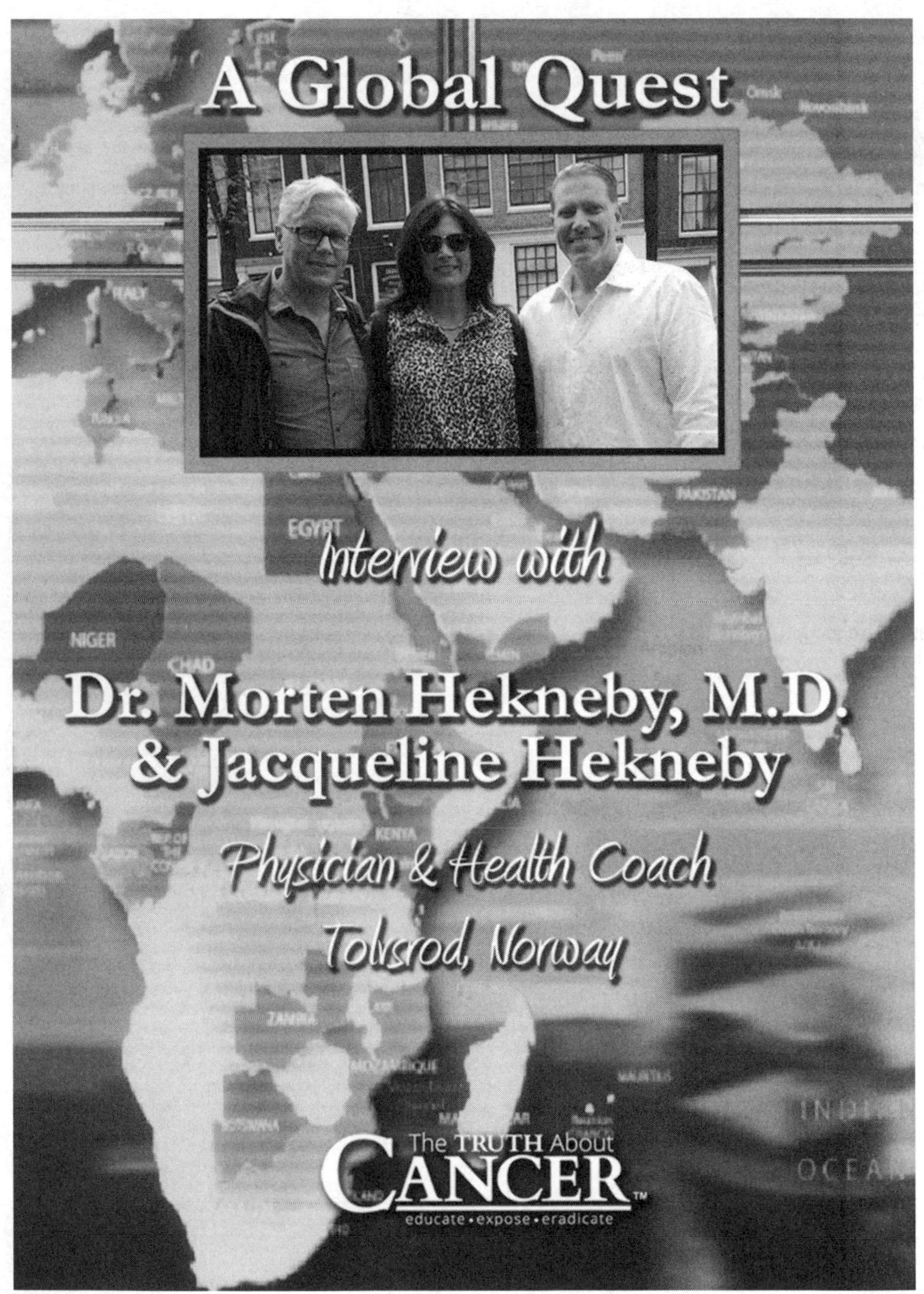
A Global Quest
Interview with
Dr. Morten Hekneby, M.D.
& Jacqueline Hekneby
Physician & Health Coach
Tolvsrod, Norway
The TRUTH About
CANCER
educate • expose • eradicate
EGYPT
NIGER
CHAD
PAKISTAN
KENYA
ZAMBIA
INDI
OCEAN

THE TRUTH ABOUT CANCER

Ty: Well, I'm really excited to be here in Amsterdam, Netherlands with Jackie and Morten Hekneby. Nice to see you and meet you finally. We have been in touch for many years. And finally we're able to meet in person. So thank you for joining us here in Amsterdam. But you're not from here. And tell us your name because I'm sure I butchered it. How do you pronounce your last name? And tell us a little bit about where you're from.

Dr. Hekneby: Hekneby is our last name. And that's Jacqueline and I'm Morten. I'm from Oslo. Jacqueline is from London. We've been married for 32 years and we have seven children.

Ty: You've always been into sports?

Dr. Hekneby: Yes. For many years. For 30 years. I have had my own club for 12 years and been an internationally accredited athlete.

Ty: Okay. International athlete. Swimmer?

Dr. Hekneby: No. Kickboxing.

Ty: Kickboxing?

Dr. Hekneby: Yes.

Ty: Wow. You look tall and lanky like a swimmer, but kickboxing? Okay. So I don't want to mess with you. I'll be sure to be really nice to you during the interview. And then you're also a doctor?

Dr. Hekneby: A medical doctor. For many years we lived a right life when it came to food and training and lifestyle generally. But I became suddenly very ill four years ago and that was a shock for us all because I got something called sepsis. Blood poisoning. And we didn't know where it came from. Because we had just been on two weeks holiday in Spain and I think you must...

Jackie: I think I'll just tell you because Morten didn't really remember much of it, what happened.

Dr. Hekneby: I was quite ill.

Ty: So Morten was very ill. And you being his wife wanted to help him. You took over at at that point, right? And give us a little bit of your background too, Jackie.

Jackie: I grew up in London, England. I was a top model in the UK for seven years and worked internationally in 12 different countries. I married Morten at the age of 22. And didn't go skiing, didn't know what to do in Norway. So we ended up having a big family. What else do you say? I didn't like studying Norwegian. Studying Norwegian was hard enough than English. So I just enjoyed my family and had no idea what the future would bring for me.

Ty: And you do have a lovely family. I've seen pictures. Incredible family.

Jackie: We have a fantastic family. Thank you. We're very close and have a lot of fun. Totally crazy.

Ty: So, once you began to do some research on Morten's condition, what did you find and where did you go?

Jackie: I was always interested in natural health like most people. I was taking vitamin pills from the age of 15. And going to take the best ones. We had organic food for many years. We had vegetarian for many years. We thought we were better than others, but then again I was still addicted to chocolate and Pepsi Max.

We know things but we don't always how to do it. Or we want to do it but we can't. And so it was a kind of fight in me to do the right thing. The flesh is weak, right? It started really in 2009 when I got a call. My mum called me and said my aunt had called her and said that she had cancer.

And that it was a family thing. That I was the next one to get it. And that everybody in father's family had died of cancer. And I didn't know that. I just never had met any of the family. I hadn't seen my dad for 10 years.

So I didn't know about this. So both the men and the women had all died of breast cancer. And then she got it and she died of it. So I was the next one. I was 48 years old and they had all died in their early 50s. So it was like being given a death sentence. So I started to do a search.

I really didn't know where to turn. So I just started researching and what I found out was that people removed their breasts to avoid getting this, the ones with the genes. It was a horrifying thought. I thought, you know what? I would do it if I have to.

I started contacting people who had done it. And it was like a little bit of a family feeling and getting to know people who have done it and that was the thing to do.

Ty: So really you were seriously considering prophylactic surgery just in case you might be diagnosed in the future?

Jackie: If I had that gene. So I took a gene test at the Norwegian Cancer Hospital.

Ty: When you say that gene, you're talking about the BRCA?

Jackie: Yes. And they said it would take almost a year to get the results. It was like having a death sentence over me that year. So I started to look into things. And my father – I call him once a year on his birthday.

And I called him and I just mentioned, your sister had called up and said that she had cancer and I was the next one out. And he said, "Oh, you don't have to die of cancer. There's loads of things you can do."

But my dad is an eccentric. He's an inventor and he's a bit crazy. But I have to be careful what I say because my family is a lot more like him. So he did recommend your book, *Cancer: Step Outside the Box*. He'd recommended stuff to me for 30 years. I never listened to him.

But for some reason I actually ordered that book and I had it next to me for a few months. We went on holiday to Spain where I had the time to read it. So I read it on the beach, in peace. And when I first read it Ty, I wasn't sure if you were a bit of a nutter yourself. Really.

Ty: Well, actually I am.

Jackie: Some of what you'd written made sense. Some of it was completely new. And I thought, is it really true that there's power in food to cure? I mean if it's new when you read it the first time you think it can help a little bit, but that much? Can it really cure cancer? I really didn't know if I believed it. I didn't know if it was fact or fancy.

So when I closed the book I didn't tell anybody what I read. I just kept it in my heart and I thought if I ever hit any of the serious problems with health in my family I would go that way.

That was in 2009. It turned I didn't have the gene. I have never been back since to have any test or anything. It's just now that I know what I do. I just don't go near that.

But in 2011 we came back from Spain as Morten said. And Morten fell suddenly very ill. We were busy. We'd been on holiday. We had first our daughter's wedding and then the holiday. You come back home, you got massive to do. So I didn't notice actually how fast Morten was going downhill. We were just so busy.

So suddenly I saw that you were looking a bit thin. And then you said you've lost five kilos in one week. And you said "I've got a really busy day." You just had a shower and you laid on the bed, you looked really tired.

And you said, "I've got so much to do today, I just got to get on with it." And I said, you know what? You've got to go the doctor. And you said, "I haven't got time." I said, you've got to go to the doctor. But getting a doctor to a doctor is really tough. I don't know if you know that.

Dr. Hekneby: Well my, she always has the—if I've been a little bit tired, I just do it a little bit harder.

Jackie: Typical athlete.

Dr. Hekneby: It was not every wise in this situation. But luckily I had Jacqueline that took me to the doctor.

Jackie: I got a hold of the doctor and got an appointment. Emergency appointment at 11am. We went in the waiting room. But during the waiting time of 20 minutes, Morten got a lot worse. And he had to lay down.

And when we did get the doctor, the doctor was asking questions and he was struggling to sit. And the doctor's hand started shaking as he was on the computer.

Obviously as he asked the questions he was starting to realize that the situation was serious. And I really didn't know what was going on. But he went to call an ambulance. So I said, I have a car outside.

Ty: He wanted to call an ambulance?

Jackie: But I regret that because I should have called an ambulance. Because Morten got so bad in the car and we got to hospital and I had to go and park the car. And I found him just sitting on the chair. They hadn't taken it seriously. Then you were having trouble breathing.

So then they suddenly rushed him into the room enclosed with wires. Oh my gosh, they were all coming in, all the doctors and nurses. Basically started a six months in that hospital. Many weeks at a time in hospital. And then he nearly died three times.

He was resuscitated one time. Just seem to get worse and worse and worse. They didn't know what it was. Well, Morten went downhill really fast and they didn't know what it was. They took some tests. They thought it was Legionella, because we came from Spain. And they took all the tests but it didn't turn out to be that.

So they thought it was atypical. But nothing seemed to work. The antibiotics wasn't working. So they were pumping with so much his one arm went on green and I was really worried. And they did the other arm. And they did that until it went green.

And I thought what happens if it doesn't work? Then they thought it was lung cancer that had spread to the rest of the body. Then I thought it was lymphoma spread to the rest of the body.

Ty: So they didn't really know what was going on?

Jackie: No. They didn't.

Dr. Hekneby: They didn't know. My symptom was I got very high inflammation. CRP.

Ty: C-reactive protein. Sure.

Dr. Hekneby: And it was really high. And my blood pressure went down and I was resuscitated one time in the hospital, just one week after they let me go from the hospital.

Ty: So they thought you were gone a few times. Did you ever get the family together and say, "Hey, Dad's not going to make it?"

Jackie: We were not aware. We never thought about death. I don't know why. But in the six months—Morten only 55 and had never been ill before. We actually didn't think about him dying. It wasn't until two days before Christmas, they called Morten in for a meeting when they said that this could be literally only three months to live.

It's so complicated. It's been in the body for many years because it really came up in the PET scan all over the body. They literally said, "We'll call you in a week's time and see the results; tell you the results of the PET scan." They called 8am the next morning and said, "Get to your doctor before 9."

Dr. Hekneby: And it was lighting up all over my body, except the brain. So they thought I had metastasis all over – in the bone marrow, limb system, lungs, all over. And then I had to go very fast into hospital and took biopsies from the lung. Biopsy from the bone marrow, and from the lymph. They took out a huge lymph node and they found inflammatory that proved that it was sarcoidosis.

Ty: Wow, sarcoidosis?

Dr. Hekneby: Sarcoidosis.

Jackie: Which no one seems to have heard of. And there's not much research done on it. But there's actually, in fact, a very high death rate on sarcoidosis that people aren't aware of.

Dr. Hekneby: You don't really die of sarcoidosis. You die of other disorders. You die of pneumonia and infections, because sarcoidosis suppresses the immune system. And that happened to me. And if sarcoidosis goes into different organs, you have to transplant. I have a colleague that had to have new lungs and get a new heart. It's very serious.

Ty: So how is it that you're standing here with us in Amsterdam today? Why are you alive? What happened?

Dr. Hekneby: You can tell that story because you're the reason for it. And you [Ty] are actually a reason for it too. You're the main reason, actually.

Jackie: It's quite crazy really because, well, the doctors basically gave up. Morten was just getting worse and worse over that period he was in their care. After the last visit to the hospital, the biopsy just was really bad. You weren't producing enough white blood cells. You didn't produce any hormones. Your heart was beating irregularly.

Dr. Hekneby: I got chronic obstructive lung disorder. Of course I have that now. I got jumping heart arrhythmia. And it's a lot of diagnosis.

Jackie: You had no energy at all. Absolutely no energy. Couldn't take a single conversation. Couldn't walk down the stairs. Nothing. You said walking down the stairs on Christmas day was like running several kilometers.

Dr. Hekneby: Yes.

Jackie: That's when it hit us that Morten was dying. It hit so hard that I had no idea. I wasn't prepared. So the first day I just screamed like a pig that's being stabbed with a dagger. And the kids were just clinging to me.

But the second day I went out in the garden and I just prayed because I've done it before when I had a crisis with the family before. I said "Lord, I just need you. You're just going to have to guide me." I felt the Lord say, put Morten in a chair and get the family to pray.

So I gathered the family. And we're quite a big family. So everyone laid their hands on Morten and we prayed. Then we all felt peace which was very strange in that situation. When you have peace you're able to think straight.

And then I remembered your book. And I hadn't thought about that for the whole six months when Morten was ill. Because the doctors were taking care of him. But when they were out the picture, I picked up the book.

And you can tell me if I'm wrong but I picked it up and I opened it up and I read, if you've been given a diagnosis of terminal cancer you've still got a 90% chance of survival. I've never found that again since. But when I read that to you, they thought the blood came back into your veins. It gave hope.

Dr. Hekneby: And I was yellow in my skin. I was yellow in my eyes. I had a wax look in my skin and I was shining. I was really, really—I had three, four percent, I think, of life in me.

Ty: You were very jaundiced.

Jackie: It was really, really bad. Morten's colleagues started to phone up and say they wanted to come and say goodbye to him. And I wasn't ready to say goodbye myself. And it was like the phone was going. I'd turn everyone away.

I'd say, "You can't come and say goodbye because we're not saying goodbye. You can come and join the party like someone who's celebrating survival." And they got really cross with me. They thought I was in denial. I ended up taking the phone off the hook, and I put a notice down on the gate saying, no one is to come in. No exceptions.

And I updated Facebook once a day and told people to not disturb us. That was fantastic because then we were able to think straight. Since it was Christmas, I remembered in your book how to start, so I just started by saying to Morten, "Okay. I want to give it a go. Give it a shot. We'll start with no sugar today and no alcohol and keep off the white flour."

That was over the two days of Christmas. Then the shops opened and I literally took everything out of the cupboards. All the food, all the skin products, hair products, and I put them on the front door. And I put it on Facebook that if anybody wanted, they could come and get them.

And I went down to the health shop and I restocked with everything organic. And our second daughter, Rosanne, she just dropped everything to be my right hand. And I really think it took two people a full-time job to do this. People need to know that it's a lot of work. And then I remembered what you had to do with the food.

So I literally made a list for my daughter of the food that's supposed to be cancer fighting like garlic and ginger. Rosanne made a plate of lovely food. We started off with the Budwig Diet in the morning. Then this plate of raw food that you had to chew.

She made it look beautiful, but it was pretty awful some of it. And then in the evening she made an Indian curry out of all these ingredients that were cancer-fighting.

But on Christmas day I wrote to you. And that was a lesson for me because I've always been annoyed of people calling Morten Sundays in the middle of dinner. Their crisis you know. I kind of got really annoyed. Then I would beat everybody by writing to you Christmas day.

So there was a lesson to learn there. But you answered me two days later and we started to communicate. And I asked you for the world's best doctor and you recommended a doctor. This is kind of weird for many people to understand.

But he wanted 150,000 kroner. I don't know what that is in dollars. Twenty thousand for six months follow-up. And I wasn't so worried about the money as I was, was this the right direction? So I just said, "Lord, if it's the right direction please give me that money within the week to give it this doctor. Doctor Farley."

And a lady I didn't even know came and gave me 100,000 kroner. She said the Lord told her to give it to me. And an aunt I hadn't seen in 30 years called my mum and gave me 30,000 kroner.

And some youths that were in and of our house when they were younger, we always had an open home. They had made a Facebook group and had gathered money. And they delivered that. So I got 150,000 kroner six days later without putting it on Facebook, without asking anybody.

Ty: That's amazing.

Jackie: It is. It's crazy. So I knew then that I was going the right way. So I decided to talk to this doctor, Mike Farley. I don't know if he likes his name mentioned or not.

Ty: That's okay.

Jackie: And I learned a lot from him and he just gave everything to help me with Morten. He made a herbal mixture.

Ty: Yes. Doctor Farley developed LifeOne.

Jackie: LifeOne was—well, he had cured 3,000 terminal cancer and AIDS patients in eight years with that. And he thought he was going to get a medical prize for it. But he wasn't very popular when he made it. It took about a month to get it into Norway because of the toll system is really, really strict to Norway.

Dr. Hekneby: But it worked.

Ty: It worked, didn't it?

Dr. Hekneby: And he was a fantastic support.

Jackie: Yeah, he was amazing.

Dr. Hekneby: We were talking sometimes and he was an amazing person.

Jackie: We're still in contact with him. Basically, really, honestly four days after I changed the products out, you started to feel stronger – less pain, breathing easier.

Ty: Four days is all it took to see a difference.

Dr. Hekneby: More power. Strength.

Jackie: We all saw it and you felt it. But your eyes were still really yellow. At the time Morten said, "are my eyes yellow?" And I said no. Because I knew that if he knew his eyes were yellow he would have understand the seriousness of the situation. So I didn't tell him, but I didn't know if I had the time. I could see it was working.

I really didn't know if I had the time. So, every night when we went to bed I wasn't sure Morten would be awake in the morning. It was that bad. We didn't get any LifeOne for a month. But basically, this process, Morten went back to work in two months.

Dr. Hekneby: And the core in it was the information from your book. And that strengthened you up and you strengthened me up. And we changed the diet totally. And that made me go from three, four percent energy to 20 percent. But that was a huge difference in four days. And I knew I would live.

Jackie: By two months you were about 60 percent I think, if I remember correctly.

Ty: And within two months he was back to work.

Jackie: Yes, it wasn't 100 percent at all, but probably up to about 60 percent. And I was thinking there must be more to this, we can do more than this. And that's when you called me in May 2013 and told me about the Moringa product. It takes time to understand that product, even if you know a lot.

Ty: Well, I mean it's a product that has just amazing amounts of nutrition.

Jackie: That's why the body can take it out 90-99 percent. I got it in the country and I saw the difference it made in Morten. And I start taking it myself and it completely changed my life as well. Morten has never had any medication since I took over. And he's now gone how long? Two and a half years?

Dr. Hekneby: If I had taken chemotherapy or cortisone, I think I wouldn't live today.

Jackie: That's what they recommended.

Ty: They recommended chemotherapy and cortisone?

Jackie: For sarcoidosis, yes.

Ty: So Morten, what do your colleagues think now that you're four years later and you're doing so well? Do they ever ask you what you did to get better?

Jackie: They don't ask, do they?

Dr. Hekneby: They don't understand it really. And they don't ask. They don't—they think that it maybe was not so serious as it was. I think that is the general thing they're thinking.

Ty: That seems odd to me. That seems odd to me that you're at one point apparently they thought that you might not live through the day and then you're alive four years later and your colleagues don't ask. That seems odd.

Dr. Hekneby: It's not so strange really because the traditional medicine, we think we know everything. And what we don't know it's not so necessary to know because we know everything. So when someone gets ill, it's probably a part of what they're doing. I mean it's crazy.

Ty: It is.

Dr. Hekneby: The way a traditional doctors thinks, like myself.

Ty: Well, you know what's interesting, we interviewed a lady in Riga, Latvia a few days ago. And she was late stage, stage 4 cancer undergoing chemotherapy. She got so bad that she could not walk.

And her family literally carried her out on a stretcher, put her in the car, and drove her to Latvia to begin another treatment. She's recovered now, doing great. And she went back to see her oncologist. And he said that she probably recovered from a delayed reaction to chemotherapy.

Dr. Hekneby: Yes, that's the same reaction I got. The same thinking.

Jackie: There's been no interest at all in what happened. But among friends, a lot of interest. So we had several friends come and knock on the door. It was very strange. They would pass Morten as a doctor and come to me and say can you help us? And I said, "I don't know." But they say, "Please, please help us."

And I end up doing the same thing with them. And I saw people recovering up to three diseases in one body. And I've also seen cancer go back. I found that very frightening. I was very frightened the first time I saw it.

Dr. Hekneby: I read on the net that 70 percent of the people with sarcoidosis get spontaneously healed. But the 30 percent that is left, there is about 1/3 of those that die of sarcoidosis. But this huge group, as I said that don't die of sarcoidosis but the effect of it, because it suppresses the immune system. So they die of infections. So sarcoidosis, you don't know any sort of medications or anything that can take it, because we don't know the origin. What causes it except this inflammatory big groups of like tumors in the body?

Jackie: In the bones as well.

Dr. Hekneby: In the bones.

Ty: So what does a typical day look like in the Hekneby household as far as nutrition? What do you typically eat?

Jackie: Well, when I changed I didn't change immediately because I was so busy helping Morten that I didn't think about myself. And I looked a pretty big mess actually. I was overweight, my hair was falling out, and I had sleep problems. For 17 years I've been on medication for not being able to sleep. There's a whole lot of stuff.

So when I started doing the same thing for myself, I couldn't believe how I came back to life. And I've counted 10 things that have gone after three months. I've slept naturally ever since, after 23 years of problems with sleep. I've gone down 20 kilos and I've started running again after 24 years. So I run every second day.

My hair got thick and grew out again. I had a great big stomach. I thought it was because I had six children. I'd say to Morten, "I've had six children." And he'd say, "And lots of lovely food." No mercy. But you know what? It was toxic. I just didn't know that it was toxic because of the cola drinks and the lite products and the aspartame.

Ty: Aspartame. A lot of aspartame.

Jackie: It toxifies the liver. And you're never going to go down in weight. So I went cold turkey on those drinks. And I had a migraine for three days. And a lot of that—just uphill really. I never thought I could feel so good. I'm now 54 this summer and I haven't felt this good since I was 30.

So I'm so grateful for the knowledge I have. I'm not sure they'll all take the knowledge with them. We eat organic food. We eat mainly vegan. We cut back on meat. We eat meat, but we don't eat as much as we ate before. We'd rather eat quality and not so often. So we exercise. Morten exercises every morning. I exercise every second day. We go for a long walk together every day.

Dr. Hekneby: I have health care 70 percent now; 50 percent as a consultant and 20 percent as a psychotherapist in my own private practice.

Jackie: And I started working. I started my own company called Natural Health Hope two years ago. And I've started to travel around with a doctor you introduced me to called Doctor Howard Fischer.

And we work daily together for two years. And we've actually toured Europe together. Spreading the word about natural health and the product that you recommended us. Changing lives. So it's duplicating.

Ty: So what would your message be to someone that's recently been diagnosed with a terminal prognosis of cancer or any other disease? What would your message be to them?

Jackie: I would say think outside the box. A lot people don't dare because they really—we're brought up in our society to respect our parents and our teachers and the police and then the doctors, and people are not used to thinking for themselves. But you need to think for yourself and do your own research. The best research is in Ty's book *Step Outside the Box*. That is all done for us. I would say just go organic food, organic products for hair and skin products. And boost your immune system with the best possible plant in the world: moringa oleifera, I would recommend. And detoxification is also done naturally by moringa oleifera. Drink only purified water, and exercise or go for gentle walks, don't use up all your energy. If you have naught to ten and you're eight. Then only use six. Never use more than you have of energy. So keep it low and see what happens.

Ty: Give it a shot.

Jackie: Yeah, if it doesn't work, you can go in other directions and within a month you'll know. What I've seen with the people that come to me is it works really quickly. It's shockingly fast.

Ty: So is there always hope?

Jackie: Definitely.

Ty: There's always hope.

Jackie: Definitely. And even if someone has done all the traditional therapies and the body is destroyed with the chemotherapy, I think you can have less pain and longer time if you change things around.

Ty: Higher quality of life. That's important.

Jackie: Hope is important.

Ty: It is.

Jackie: Just hope itself is amazing what it does to people.

Ty: Well, you know what? Jackie, Morten, this interview, this testimony is going to give hope to a lot of people that watch it. So thank you for travelling all the way from Norway here to Amsterdam to do this interview. And I really look forward to the impact this is going to have on everyone's lives.

Dr. Hekneby: And thank you, Ty.

Ty: Thank you.

Jackie: Thank you again, Ty.

Ty: Thank you and God bless both of you.

Jackie: God bless you too.

[end of transcript]

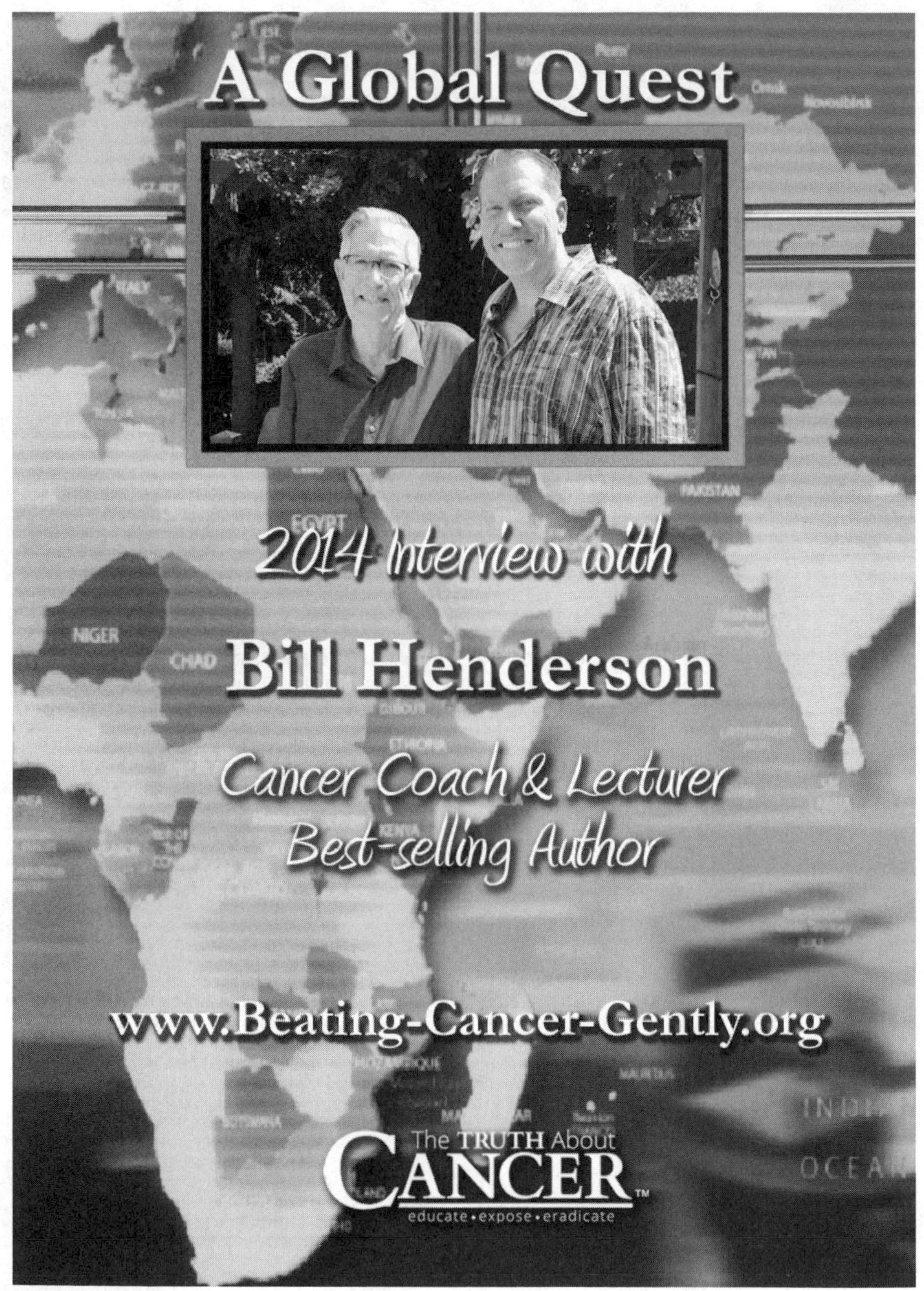
A Global Quest
2014 Interview with
Bill Henderson
Cancer Coach & Lecturer
Best-selling Author
www.Beating-Cancer-Gently.org
The TRUTH About
CANCER
educate • expose • eradicate

Ty: Well, this afternoon we have the privilege of having Bill Henderson with us. Bill is the author of several books on cancer and actually coaches people to help to treat their cancer. So, Bill, first of all, I just want to thank you for spending the time with us this afternoon.

Bill: Thank you, Ty, for inviting me, and really I am delighted to be here.

Ty: Can you give us a little bit of your background? What got you into this field?

Bill: Yeah, well, it started about 23 or 4 years ago, my late wife developed ovarian cancer and she went through, really, four years straight of conventional treatment. And, during that time, this was the early 90s, I looked all over the place for alternatives, for things that might be options that she could try, and I could not find anything. I went to the library and there were books on cancer, but there was nothing really that I could find that would help her. And, she just wasted away at the chemotherapy and the several surgeries, and it was horrible. She died in 94.

Ty: Sorry to hear that.

Bill: And, the doctors put on her death certificate heart failure as the cause of her death, and she had had cancer for four years at the time. So, it led me to believe that the cancer statistics are not very believable, frankly. But, what it inspired me to do later, in 98 or so, when I started discovering the Internet and how much information even then—this was 16 years ago—was there on the Internet about natural cancer healing. And, I said, "Wow, if I can help people avoid her fate, maybe I should try that." And, I said, "Okay." And, I started a process, published the first book in 2000.

Ty: What was the name of your first book?

Bill: The name, the first book was called Cure Your Cancer. I discovered somewhat later that that is really not a very good concept, simply because you cannot cure cancer, there is no way. We will talk about that later if you like, but the cancer cure is never going to happen. Cancer is us. Every day we have cancer cells in our bodies, all of us that have no cancer diagnosis. And, I finally learned that and I decided, well, what you want to help people do is get cancer under control. That is the concept. Get this cancer under control. It has gotten out of control in your body, temporarily. And, it is not that difficult as it turns out.

Ty: So, control the cancer is a better term.

Bill: Absolutely, yeah, absolutely. It is much better.

Ty: Because, you mentioned just now that we all produce cancer cells every day.

Bill: Every single day, yeah, probably hundreds of thousands. Nobody know the count, millions it could be. But, think about it. We have 75 trillion cells in our body, and about 300 billion of those divide every single day. The cancer cells are a very, very small portion of that, and if it is like 3/10,000 of 1 percent of cancer cells, of those dividing cells, that is a million cells every day. Well, it could easily be that many, and the body takes care of these. The immune system, with 130 different types of immune cells, and about 14 trillion of them approximately, is about 20 percent of our cells, it is taking care of these things that are non-self cells. Cancer cells just basically get controlled by the immune system until it cannot do it anymore, and then we get a cancer diagnosis, because the cells have exceeded our immune system's ability to handle them and they form something, usually a tumor. Ninety percent of the time, it is some kind of swelling in an organ somewhere. The other 10 percent, it is not a tumor, it is melanoma on the skin or it is lymphoma, leukemia. But, it is all the same thing in my experience, and I think you agree, cancer is cancer. It is all the same thing, it is an imbalance in our bodies where the immune system has been overwhelmed temporarily. We can restore that almost entirely with almost any kind of cancer. But, we have to be aware of what this is in order to deal with it. And, unfortunately, the medical system does not teach us that. It teaches us that this is some kind of enemy that has invaded our body. It is the medical model of cancer the doctors are trained in, as you know. It is simply that this enemy has to be attacked with all of the armament at their disposal, poison it with chemotherapy, burn it with radiation, cu it out of your body and dispose of parts of your body to get rid of this enemy. Well, that is completely ridiculous, okay. And, the entire medical treatment system of cancer is based on that model of what cancer is. What is it? Well, I will tell you what I believe, see if you agree. I think cancer is simply a symptom of an imbalance. It is sort of like diabetes, fibromyalgia, arthritis. It is a chronic, degenerative condition in our body caused by an imbalance. And, that imbalance, once you understand that that is what it is, you realize that this is not random, something randomly that happened to you. It has happened for a reason. Something has gone wrong in your body that has caused this cancer tumor to appear, or in whatever other form. And, once you correct that reason, the cause of the imbalance, it goes away. The body is very capable of shrinking cancer tumors.

There has been an interesting study done. I read about where thousands of people who died of something other than cancer had autopsies done, and what they found was, in the thyroid gland of every single person, were microscopic cancer tumors. They died of something else, heart disease or something. And, cancer is us. It occurs every day in our bodies, and we probably, you and I, have had microscopic cancer tumors in our bodies that the body has taken care of. Once it grows out of control, where the body cannot handle it, the body gets pretty smart. It has a backup system, okay. It says, "My immune system didn't handle it. I need to control these malignant cells that are creating in excess." And, it creates a tumor. Well, a tumor is just tissue surrounding malignant cancer cells to keep them from spreading elsewhere. That is what the body is doing. It is a very smart mechanism.

Ty: So, the tumor may be a protective type mechanism.

Bill: It, yeah, I feel it is, and of course, it is not perfectly protective against the rest of the cancer spreading throughout your body, and it will eventually metastasize elsewhere. But, the body is attempting to control it. The medical system, among other things, looks at the tumor as the enemy, and in order to identify this enemy and cover the behinds, if you will pardon the expression, of the doctors involved, they poke holes in the tumor. It is called a biopsy, and they take with a needle some example of what is inside the tumor and have it analyzed in the lab. And, if it comes out malignant, well, certainly our diagnosis was correct. You have cancer, and on Monday, three days from now, we need to start chemotherapy on your body if you are ever going to survive this. And, most people are so emotionally upset and in fear with this diagnosis called cancer that they accept what the doctors say and they have no real time or effort to explore their own options at that point. So, if the person has not studied this before they get the cancer, in most cases they are going to submit to the doctors' treatment. And, in my opinion, 95 percent of deaths attributed to cancer, approximately, are caused by the treatment of the cancer. And, once people understand this, it may be too late. It is possible to pass a point of no return in the treatment of cancer, as you know. I mean, most cases we can help people recover, but if they go on too long with this kind of damaging treatment to their body's immune system. What makes no sense at all to me, is that they are trying to treat something, which is caused by an immune system that was too weak to handle it, they are treating it with something that further damages the immune system. Every single thing doctors do...

Ty: That is a common thread.

Bill: ...chemotherapy, all types...damages the immune system. Radiation damages cells beyond those that are cancerous, weakens your immune system, causes other cancers, it is carcinogenic. Even surgery is very, very stressing on our immune system, and it causes a very difficult recovery in a body that is already weak, with an immune system that has been overwhelmed.

Ty: Let me ask you this. Could a biopsy spread the cancer?

Bill: Absolutely, yeah. They estimate, well, surgery and biopsy both involve, of course, disturbing this tumor that has been formed by the body to try and seal off the cancer cells from the rest of the body. Well, you are damaging the integrity of this thing with the biopsy. You are poking holes in it, and you get what is called needle tracking. Needle tracking just simply means the malignant cells inside the tumor have been released and they travel elsewhere where they might not have otherwise. So, I try to encourage people to avoid biopsies if they can. But, by the time I get to them, usually, they have already had it done and/or the surgery. And, even the statistics gathered by the American Cancer Society and some of the surgeons involved, the surgical organizations, admit that about 50 percent of the time surgery causes the cancer to spread elsewhere.

Ty: Bill, you mentioned fear. So, can you talk about the role that fear plays in the cancer equation?

Bill: Oh, yeah. Well, what is important for people to understand about cancer is that it is a response to something that has happened to our bodies. One of the things, of course, is emotional upset, as you know. Emotions of all kinds affect our bodies in a way that is quite harmful, simply because one of the things it produces physically in our body is something called cortisol. Cortisol is a hormone. The brain signals the endocrine system to produce it when we are under stress. When it is produced, it causes acidity in our body. So, in any kind of emotional upset, stress, whatever, it is producing acidity, which is conducive to cancer. Cancer loves an acid state in our body's fluid. The other thing it does, of course, is weaken our immune system. So, any reaction like that, panic or fear, is causing an emotion that is harmful to our health.

Ty: So, Bill, if you have an oncologist that tells his or her patient that you have got terminal cancer, you are going to be dead in six months. That creates, I can see that creating a response that would be then more detrimental. The patient would be in worse shape than before they had heard that diagnosis, because of the emotional reaction.

Bill: Yeah, it is very well proven that not only does this program the brain literally to listen to this god, this doctor that we all worship from toddlerhood on as the person that has the answers when we are sick. And, he has just given you a death sentence. Well, this programs your mind, this guy must be correct, and your mind controls your body in major ways. The other thing, of course, that those kind of things cause is a continuing emotional problem, where the person literally is trying to live out the six months they have been given to live in, but they are living in an atmosphere of fear. And, it is extremely damaging to have those kind of death notices, I call them, the terminal notice that somehow you are not going to survive. This is very, very vicious. It should be criminal, but it is not, unfortunately. The doctors, basically, as I understand it, with those kind of prognoses, are trying to cover their behinds, basically, that is all. I mean, if the person dies within two or three months and they have not anticipated it, they could be sued by the family. So, they give you a death notice. If you do not die, well, they are okay. If you do, they have covered themselves.

Ty: And, you mentioned the immune system, Bill. What role does the immune system play in preventing cancer, and/or treating cancer, and can you go into certain ways that you have uncovered in your research that you can make the immune system work the way it is supposed to?

Bill: Oh, absolutely. The immune system is a function in our body that is responsive to almost everything we do to our bodies, what we eat, drink, the kind of exercise we get, what we think, our thoughts, our beliefs, etc. All of these affect our immune system, and we can make this as strong as possible by doing, among other things, what we recommend in our book. There are about seven items in our regimen that we recommend. One of them is directly related to strengthening the immune system and taking something called beta-glucan, and that is quite effective for that. But, it is, the whole idea is to re-energize the system that has been overwhelmed by the cancer, that there is no person who has cancer who does not have a weak immune system. My friend, Mike Adams, you probably know Mike and Natural News. He wrote an article and said, "You know, doctors use a term that was more descriptive to describe cancer and not as emotional, we'd probably be more likely to do sensible things about it." And, he said, "Cancer should be called SISD." What the heck is that? Well, he said, "Sluggish immune system disease is what they call it, SISD."

Ty: I like that.

Bill: Yeah, well, I do, too, because, obviously, you are not going to think that putting poison in your veins is going to help a sluggish immune system disease. I do not even like the term disease, Ty. I like the term reaction. Cancer is really a reaction of your body to whatever has happened to it. And, whatever those things are, they have challenged your immune system. And, one of them is stress that you mentioned. There are two others. One is fairly obvious, which is what we put in our mouth. Obviously, that affects our whole immune system. Smoking, drinking to excess, which most of us do not do, but just diet, just eating and drinking. What we normally do as part of the standard American diet, the old SAD, is pretty bad. I mean, it really challenges our immune system. But, the thing that most people do not even think about that I found is so common is dental toxins, okay. What is coming out of our jaw for most people, from the dental work we have had done, generally, root canals, cavitation sites, they are called, where you have had wisdom teeth or other teeth removed, mercury amalgam fillings, metal that the dentists put in our mouth. All of this stuff affects our system dramatically, because our jaw is intimately connected, and every tooth in our mouth intimately connected to organs in our body through the old Chinese meridian system, if you will.For example, on each side of the jaw, there are two molars, upper and lower, that are directly connected to the mammary glands in both men and women. I mean, men get breast cancer, too. But, these are probably the most common cause of all breast cancers, simply because they are directly connected to a gland that brings on the breas cancer.

And, when they are dealt with, what I have found, literally thousands of my clients, once that type of thing is cleared up, the cancer disappears, it goes away. And, these are mostly people, again, they are coming to me, Ty, so kind of as a last resort in many cases. They have been through chemo and surgery and whatever and it has not worked, and the cancer has recurred. And, they start doing something more sensible, generally, they do a diet change, they talk supplements, and what have you that we recommend. That does not seem to work either in most cases. This cancer is still there. They feel better, they get more energy, they lose some weight, but they do not get over the cancer. They finally get their jaw cleaned up by some competent dentist, and the cancer goes away. Six, eight weeks later it is gone, and this is hundreds of people I have worked with now, Ty, hundreds all over the world, literally.

Ty: So, that is a fundamental part of the protocol that you put people on once they have been diagnosed, is to clean up their mouth, get...

Bill: Absolutely.

Ty: ...the mercury out of their mouth. Because, the silver amalgams are not really silver, they are mercury.

Bill: That is right.

Ty: And, also, what do you recommend if somebody has had a root canal?

Bill: Well, again, it is the most deadly thing you can have in your body, practically. One of the dentists I work with calls them, calls it taxidermy of the jaw. What it is, is taking a tooth that cannot be filled with a cavity, because the cavity would invade the center portion, the nerve of the tooth and make it incredibly painful.

Ty: Okay, so you take a tooth that cannot be filled.

Bill: Right. Instead, they take the center portion out, which is the nerve and the pulp surrounding the nerve, and in the process they have a dead piece of bone in your jaw, basically. There is no circulation through it. The bacteria in it cannot be eliminated, and the doctor tries to do this, the dentist tries to sterilize the tooth. It is impossible to do, because there are millions of what they call little tubules inside the dentin. The dentin is inside the enamel of the tooth, and it has these tubules in it that are all connected with little connecting tunnels. And, it is impossible to sterilize it completely, and so the bacteria in the tooth remain there, and they mutate, because of the lack of oxygen, into anaerobic bacteria, which are extremely toxic. I have heard they are a thousand times more toxic than any other bacteria. They put out toxins that are more toxic than botulism, literally.

Ty: And, these are sealed into a tooth that has been root canaled.

Bill: Yeah, and the root canal, the idea, the name is a little misleading, because the root canal is what goes down through the tooth into the roots of the tooth. So, what you get is a filling put into that area where they have taken out the nerve and the pulp. And, it is kind of a rubbery substance called gutta percha in most cases. But, it does not seal off this millions of little tubules, unfortunately, like it is supposed to. And, this was discovered over a hundred years ago, and very well-documented that the anaerobic bacteria that accumulate there cause all kinds of chronic degenerative stuff, heart disease, cancer, rheumatoid arthritis, proven beyond any doubt. But, this study which was completed in 1923, believe it or not, after 60 prominent dentists tried to figure out how to do a safe root canal, and they threw up their hands and published this 1174 pages of their study of root canals. And, found that they could not be done safely. And, now, almost 100 years later, they are still done the same way.

Ty: Isn't that the definition of insanity?

Bill: Well, it is, yes, indeed it is. And, why would it be done? Well, if you calculate the income of the endodontist, this is the specialist in root canal, it comes to several billion dollars a year, doing approximately 30 million root canals each year in the United States. This is a very big money-making exercise, and believe it or not, the dentists are in denial about this. Their union, which is the American Dental Association, is in denial about it, as they are about mercury. And, so people listen to their dentist down the street. "Don't worry about those root canals, Alice, they're okay. You must have some problem originating somewhere else." When in almost every case, 95 percent of the time, the primary cause of the cancer in my experience is coming out of their jaw.

Ty: I have heard that statistic from other people that upwards of 90 percent of cancers are related to some issue in the mouth. So, what would you recommend, Bill, if somebody is listening to this, they have a root canal tooth. What do you recommend for that person that is now, it is too late to not get the root canal.

Bill: Yeah. Well, it is an interesting question, because so few tent to fix this problem. The reason, of course, is that not only is this an extraction, it is a surgical procedure to clean up the infected bone. The ligament surrounding the tooth is always 400 percent more infected apparently than the root canal tooth itself? So, the average dentist will, if you insist, will pull the tooth out with the root canal fill space in it, but they will not clean up the socket correctly. And, this is the major problem with root canals. They have to be removed by a competent dentist who has trained himself or herself after dental school to do this correctly. And, these are the people that I try to refer people to every day. Very few of them in the United States. Out of 160,000 dentists in the American Dental Association, there are less than 50 that I would trust to clean up my jaw.

Ty: Wow.

Bill: And, that is in 50 states. There are 30 states where I do not any dentist that I would refer people to. Some states like California and Texas have several.

Ty: So, the cleanup, who does the cleanup is as important as getting the cleanup done.

Bill: Absolutely. And, you have to get a competent dentist. And, these are the dentists who have learned this from other dentists, or doctors, or somebody. The physiological interrelationship that is intimate between your teeth and your organs in your body. And, I try to educate people about, you need to look at a diagram of this, because there are lots of them. There are some on the Internet that are kind of interesting. They're an interactive chart that comes up on the computer, and it shows you all of your 32 teeth, and you just click on one of them with the mouse and you can see which organs that tooth is connected to. It is a very educational process, because all of our organs are directly connected to teeth. It can actually be a two-way street, they have found. You can have an infected organ, affected tooth, but in almost every case, it is the other way around. It is the tooth that is affecting the organ. And, if you do not fix the jaw, you do not get over the cancer, unfortunately.

Ty: So, that is a primary ingredient in the protocol that you put people on, because in your book—now this is the second book that you wrote, is called what?

Bill: Well, it was called Cancer Free, and it came out first in 2004 and ten years later we are on the fourth edition.

Ty: Great book, by the way. I have read it. Fantastic book.

Bill: Well, thank you. I appreciate it. Yeah, I have got a co-author now, Dr. Carlos Garcia, who is a formally trained M.D., and he and I are soul brothers. We believe the same things about cancer and what causes it and how people get over it. And, he has a clinic in Florida that he helps people heal cancer. But, he says they heal themselves, and I believe that. Doctors can kick start your healing process for cancer, they cannot heal it for you. You have to heal it yourself, and he is well aware of that. So, yeah, we both help people in different ways. I have found that most people can heal themselves without going to a clinic. You may agree, but, in most cases, the cancer can be reversed if you understand the causes and how to reverse those, you can usually get it under control. And, you usually have plenty of time, and this is why the doctors' death sentences are so misleading. Because, most cases, you have at least six months to two years minimum to treat cancer. And, it does not matter how advanced it is. I have had people, stage four, given up on completely by their doctors, people in hospice, and they recover.

Ty: Oh, I, yeah, I have seen on your website, I have seen the dozens and dozens and hundreds of people that you have worked with, that you have helped to control their cancer.

Bill: Yeah, it is amazing how almost anyone can recover, if they get the information. I feel cancer deaths, and what are there, eight million a year in the world, something like that, they are all caused by lack of information, Ty, lack of information. And, now days, no real excuse for that, because it is there.

Ty: Well, that is what you are doing, you are providing information for people with, through your books...

Bill: I try to do the best...

Ty: ...through your website and your newsletters. I firmly believe that my mother and father may still be alive if they had had the information that you share on your website. So, I admire what you are doing. Let me ask you this. If somebody came to you, and they probably have, because you do coach cancer patients. If somebody came to you and said, "Bill, I have terminal pancreatic cancer. My doctor just told me I have terminal pancreatic cancer and that there is no treatment, because conventional treatments don't work for pancreatic cancer. What should I do, Bill?" What would you tell them? And, based on your responses thus far, I do not mean to cut you off, I know it would be clean up your mouth.

Bill: Well, sure.

Ty: And, then, what would you tell them from there?

Bill: Yeah, it would obviously be focusing on the cause, but at the same time, radically changing their dietary, daily regimen, taking supplements that are necessary and desirable.

Ty: You would put them on the Bill Henderson protocol, I am guessing.

Bill: Yeah, initially, and with pancreatic cancer, it is pretty aggressive. It is pretty difficult to reverse. They may want to try even more than our regular regimen, if they feel that they are that far along.

Ty: What is your regular regimen that you could put somebody on?

Bill: Well, it consists basically of about five supplements. The immune boosting product I mentioned, the beta-glucan, Vitamin D3, something that stops the spread of cancer, which is called Heart Plus, and green tea extract, a vitamin mineral substance, which is very effective, and something called Barley Power, which is a barley product, which is very, very helpful as well.

Ty: You put it in a smoothie?

Bill: Like eating a bunch of vegetables. Well, it comes in a capsule. Veggie cap, you can take it that way, or you can take the powder out if you like. But, then, of course, the diet, which we recommend, on cottage cheese/flax seed oil mixture, which is extremely helpful for rebuilding your health cells...

Ty: And, that was, the cottage cheese and flax seed is called the...

Bill: Well, the Budwig, Budwig diet. It is a major part of that. It is the only part that we feel is essential of her diet. It was a more complex diet, but there has been a lot of research done since Dr. Budwig discovered this wonderful mixture of cottage cheese and flax seed oil, which is still unique as far as I know.

Ty: What is the science behind the flax oil with the cottage cheese?

Bill: Yeah, the flax seed oil, of course, contains a high proportion of Omega 3 essential fatty acid, which is, our cells are very deficient in it, because we do not eat anything that has Omega 3 in it. We eat a lot of Omega 6 and so on, and we get this imbalance in our cell membranes, which need essential fatty acids to operate efficiently. Well, what she found was that this sulphurated protein, which is the cottage cheese, when mixed with the oil, it loses its dairy properties, the casein, the lactose go away, but what it results in is a carrier, which takes the oil directly to the cell membrane and the cell nucleus really. And, reforms your healthy cells, it gets them communicating more efficiently. Well, the whole process of cancer, in my opinion, is a breakdown of communication among your cells. It is cellular malfunction, basically, if you want to look at it that way. And, this is restoring your normal cells, but then at the same time, it is attracting oxygen to the cancer cells, which they cannot stand. Oxygen is like murder to cancer cells. They need glucose really to survive. It is a fermenting cell, as you know. So, the oxygen attracted to the cancer cells kills them off. Well, I do not know anything in the world that does those two things.

Ty: Because cancer cells are anaerobic, they do not, they produce energy without oxygen, is what I have been getting from doctor after doctor, researcher after researcher, throughout this series.

Bill: Absolutely. So, if you get something that attracts oxygen to them, and they say, "Oops, we can't survive in this environment. We're out of here." I do not know anything in the world, I would certainly recommend it that does those two functions. It is a unique substance, and everyone can mix it their own kitchen. There are even things you can take on a tour, where you are travelling, that are in a powder form or a capsule form now that emulate this mixture. So, there is no excuse for not doing it every day, and believe me, it has helped thousands of people I have worked with, about 5,000 who I have coached personally, approximately, to heal themselves. Nobody can claim 100 percent, I certainly do not. I do not even have statistics on how many of these people complied and got over it and so on.

About all I have is what you mentioned, lots of stories from people, of healing themselves this way from virtually every kind of cancer. And, it becomes very, very convincing. The statistics are pretty difficult to accumulate, as you can imagine. It is hard, because, how do you determine the compliance of someone with a regimen that you recommend, that you are, are they taking the pills every day? Are they being very disciplined about their diet, about everything that goes in their mouth? Are they really paying enough attention to the causes? Are they getting, can they afford to have their dental work taken care of, cleaned up? It tends to be pretty expensive for most people. They do not have dental insurance, so that is a difficult process for many, many people with cancer. And, they may get education they need, but they may not be able to afford to do what they have to do. So, it is hard. But, a high proportion of people seem to recover if they follow this regimen and particularly paying attention to the causes.

Ty: Yeah, that is what I have read. I have read testimony after testimony from your website, and people just, they love you, and they rave about your protocol, because it works. And, we, the cottage cheese and flax oil, that is, it is actually yummy. We, it tastes good. We put it, we will put blueberries in it, and maybe a little bit of stevia to sweeten it, and it almost tastes like a homemade cheesecake, if you mix it right. So, it is really a good tasting food.

Bill: Yeah, you need to probably experiment around a little bit first, but most people say, "Yuck, you know, I don't want to eat that stuff."

Ty: Right.

Bill: But, once they experiment enough to make it palatable, it is the healthiest you can put in your mouth, honestly, really. I have eaten it every day for 13 years and I am only going to be 83 here shortly.

Ty: 83? You are doing great.

Bill: I attribute a lot of it to cottage cheese and flaxseed oil.

Ty: And, so you practice what you preach.

Bill: Yeah, absolutely.

Ty: Right. And, I know that you are consistent with what you tell people, and there is something to be said for that. I know people in the health industry that are somewhat hypocrites. They will practice something different than they tell, and I know you are not that way. And, that is one of the many things I appreciate about you. It is your consistency.

Bill: Thank you. I am delighted to meet the people, as we are doing during this conference here, who have really come from far away. A lady from Dubai in the Middle East is here, and a lady from Vietnam, and another gentleman from Chile.

Ty: Yeah, I think I met the man from Chile.

Bill: Yeah, interesting...

Ty: Encouraging.

Bill: These are, they are just wonderful people who have healed themselves and they are caring enough that they want to pass on this information to other people. And, believe me, I tell them it is the most fulfilling thing you can do with your life, as you know.

Ty: It is, it is.

Bill: There is nothing better that I know of.

Ty: Yeah, and that is the real purpose of this investigative mini-series that we are doing as well. It is just to help more people learn that they do have options that the cancer does not have to be a death sentence, that there are options to the big three.

Bill: Yeah, if we can just satisfy this information shortage that people have, and the opposite extreme, which of course, is information overload. There is way too much information available now, try and sift through all of that and, that is why we have tried to simplify it as much as we can.

Ty: That is why your books are so valuable, because you have taken that information that is out there, that is overwhelming, quite honestly, with somebody that is, that faces a cancer diagnosis. And, you have simplified it and put it all into one book.

Bill: Yeah, and it is not really that difficult. Cancer is frightening simply because of the media and all of the doctors and so on who pass on this terrible vision of cancer as something that is incredibly difficult to overcome. It is not, as you know. It is relatively simple, if and when you capture it in time and do the right things and concentrate on the causes.

Ty: And, if you correct. You mentioned earlier that it is a result of an underlying imbalance.

Bill: Absolutely.

Ty: So, if you correct that imbalance, then the symptom, which is the cancer, goes away.

Bill: Yeah, the body is very capable of handling cancer, and if you give it the support it needs, it is going to take care of it, really, no matter where it is. The metastasized cancer, the doctors tend to give up on, because none of the treatments they use will spread throughout the body and kill the cancer wherever it is. It kind of concentrates on a particular shrinking of a particular tumor or something. But, the body is capable of handling cancer, and once you understand that, you say, "Okay, I'm going to give it all the help it needs," you are on the way to healing yourself, really. The attitude, you have discovered this, I am sure. The attitude that people have, to me, is quite evident when I talk to them. It involves understanding that they are in charge of their own healthcare. Once they reach that point, they are halfway home. And, the other part, of course, is a commitment to a regimen that they believe in 100 percent, because they have studied it enough, they have done the research themselves. And, part of that regimen, of course, is pursuing the cause. Why did this happen to me, and what can I do about that to reverse the thing. It is about that simple, really.

Ty: Tell us about the four A's for conquering cancer.

Bill: Yeah, we say there are four A's. Well, the first one, of course, is your essentials. The first one is attitude that I mentioned. It has to be very, very well-defined. And, you got to basically say, "I'm in charge here." The second one is an advocate. We recommend you get somebody to help you, if you have cancer. It may or not be a spouse. A spouse may not agree with you, but if not, it needs to be somebody that you are really close to, and you can have humorous episodes with, who can accompany you to the doctor, who can help you jot down things you need to recall. If you have cancer, you tend to get pretty emotional and you may not understand what the doctors are saying, or the naturopathic doctor, whoever you are talking to. So, an advocate is a very helpful person and they should provide you or help you with the proper questions to ask any doctor that you are seeing, a naturopathic doctor or a chiropractor or even a conventional doctor. The third, and we call it assistance, which is basically seeking out the right medical professional. Unfortunately, your normal family doctor and, of course, the cancer doctors are not going to help you with the cancer healing. They are going to do pretty much the opposite. They are going to, whatever they do is going to cause you to get worse. So, you need to seek out assistance from someone. It may be someone like me or you, Ty that can coach people, so that they can heal themselves. If it is a medical professional and you need to look around, okay. And, we give you, in this book we give you some online directories, about ten of them, of holistic physicians that can help you heal yourself, basically. And, they deal with the person, not the disease. These are not cancer doctors, they are holistic physicians, we call them, and their purpose is to help you heal yourself.

Ty: Heal the whole body.

Bill: Sure. And, number four of the A's, is action. Cancer is not stabilized normally. It is a process that is going on in your body. And, the cancer cells are going to continue to divide and to become more prolific, and to spread and cause metastasis, which is the only thing that kills cancer patients generally, is spreading to more vital organs. So, action, you need to do something. You do not have to be concerned about acting too quickly, but you need to lay out a good game plan, we call it. Something that says, "Okay, I'm going to do the research for the next few weeks. I'm going to get smart enough to where I can develop a procedure for myself that I believe in. And, then I'm going to set up some kind of a fork in the road date, okay. I'm going to use something, some test like we recommend in the book, to determine my progress. And, at some point, I'm going to set up a calendar date that I'm comfortable with, three, four, five months, whatever it is in the future." I might select five months, but if you are not as confident as I am, maybe three months. And, you say, "At this point, I am going to decide. Is what I'm doing working?" which is the only question you need answered. You need to answer that question with tests of some kind. Is what I am doing working, and if not, try something else, okay. Do not give up on any options, and keep open in your mind the fact that there are at least 400 different ways I know of that people have healed themselves, that do not involve invasive chemo, radiation, surgery, that are natural healing, that are non-toxic and very gentle in most cases. They are not all where you can do them coincident with each other. Some of them you have to avoid if you are doing the other one. So, there are certain complexities like that. But, in most cases, there are many, many things beyond what we recommend in here, if it does not work. It does work for most people, and we encourage people to at least try it, three months, four months, whatever you are comfortable with. And, then, let's decide, and if, and I do coaching for people, as you know. And, one of the things I try to do with them is monitor their recovery enough to where if it is not working, we try some other things. There are lots of others, as you know.

Ty: Well, Bill, your books are a wealth of information. Your website is a wealth of information and you are a wealth of information. And, I really appreciate you spending the time with us today, for us to pick your brain, and to share this vital information with our audience. So, thank you so much, Bill.

Bill: Thank you, Ty, and God bless you for doing this kind of work, because this word needs to get out as much as possible to people. They need to understand that they can heal themselves, and we will help them. If they give us a chance, we will help them.

Ty: Thank you, Bill.

[end transcript]

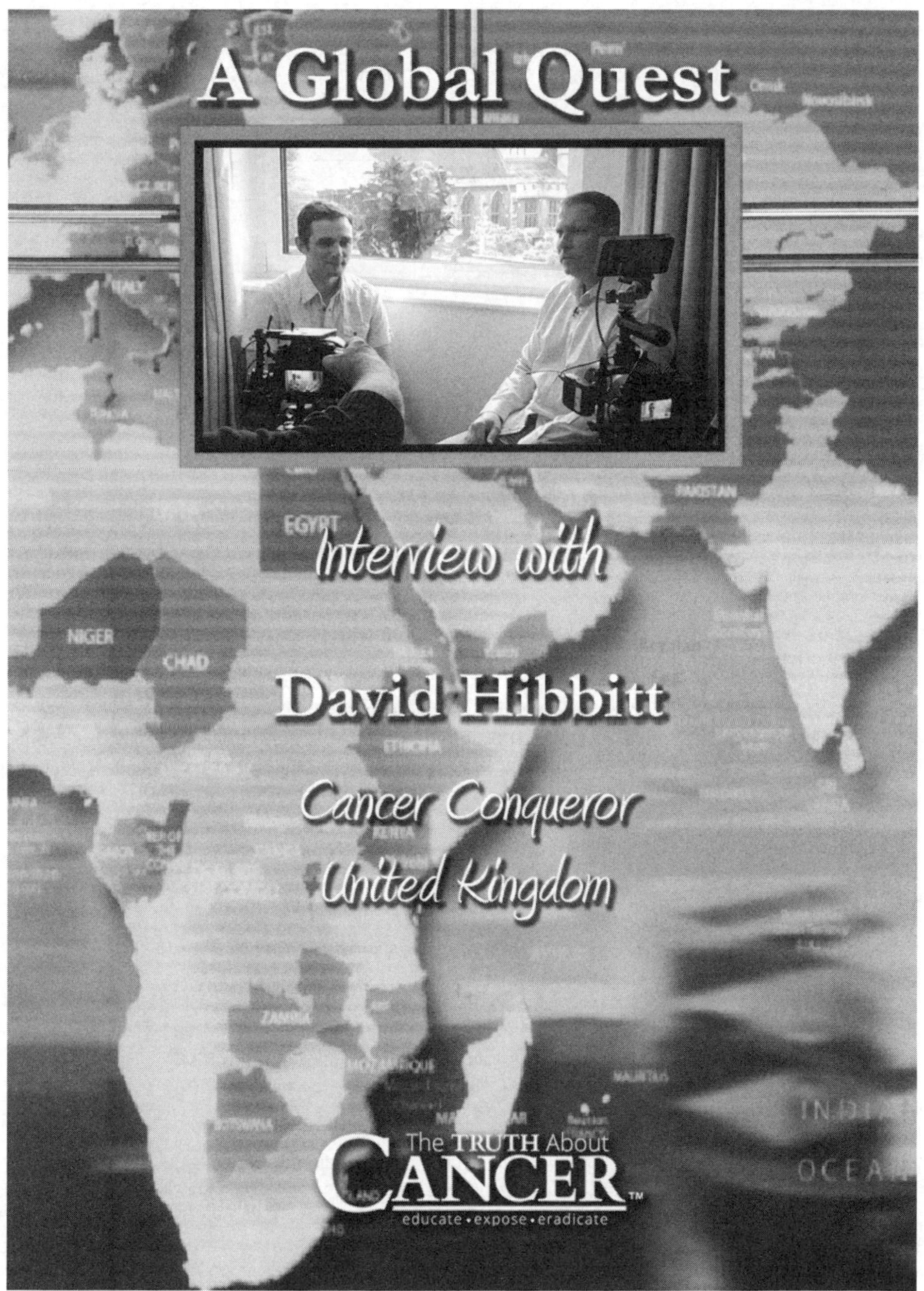
A Global Quest
Interview with
David Hibbitt
Cancer Conqueror
United Kingdom
The TRUTH About
CANCER
educate • expose • eradicate

Ty: So here we are in partly sunny, partly foggy, rainy, London, England. David Hibbitt, thank you for joining me today.

David: Nice to be here.

Ty: I really appreciate you coming down. You came down from where?

David: Stoke-on-Trent, Staffordshire.

Ty: So we're talking a few hour drive, huh?

David: Yeah, it's been three hours. Just over.

Ty: Okay. Not a bad drive?

David: It's been okay. A bit of traffic when you get into London.

Ty: Yeah, we noticed the traffic when we came down Sunday from the US. Pretty bad traffic.

David: Yeah. It does.

Ty: So you look really healthy right now, but that hadn't always been the case.

David: No, no it's true. My cancer, two and a half years—up until only recently got the all clear in January of last year.

Ty: Okay. Talk about—walk us backwards to the day. When were you diagnosed? You got diagnosed with cancer a few years ago, right?

David: Yeah. It was July 2012, and I was diagnosed with ball cancer, and it was actually stage 3. It was already in my lymph nodes. And at the time, I went to radiotherapy, alongside chemotherapy tablets. And after this, they had my large ball removed. And then I was going to be all clear then. And that was in March 2013.

Ty: So you did about six months of treatment?

David: Yeah.

Ty: Okay. How many cycles of chemo, and how many cycles of radiotherapy?

David: Radiotherapy was actually five days a week for six weeks, and then the chemotherapy tablets was—I think it was eight tablets a day I had to have, and that for right about three months. Then I had to have a little bit of a break, because I had to have an operation to remove my ball shortly after.

Ty: Okay. What kind of side effects did you experience from the treatments?

David: At that time it wasn't too bad. I had a bit of mild irritated skin where the radiotherapy was and appetite suffered a little bit. But it wasn't too bad at the time. But shortly after getting the all-clear in March, when it returned—and I went on chemotherapy again.

Ty: Okay. Well, just so we get the story straight. So you were given the all-clear. What exactly did your oncologist say? You're cancer-free? Or it's in remission? What was the terminology?

David: I honestly can't remember what the actual terminology was.

Ty: But you thought you were okay.

David: Yeah, he expected that there'd be no cancer to return.

Ty: And then how many months until you found out that it had returned?

David: It was three more months. And then it returned again in my lymph nodes of the groin and that was immediately removed. And then I had chemotherapy after, from July up until I think it was the end of October, early November 2014.

Ty: So another six months of chemo?

David: Yeah. That one was pretty bad. And side effects from upset-ness, and nausea, weakness basically—I was very tired, but couldn't sleep. It was quite hard to explain. And I had numbing in my fingers and toes and I was very sensitive to the cold. Even eating something out of the fridge made my mouth go all pins and needles, actually, in my mouth.

And I was told that a lot of that would actually never go away. And that led on—like I say, finished at the end of October, early November. And again, I can't remember terminology right off the top, but I was led to believe I'd be okay.

Ty: Yeah, the first time you were told that you were okay, you probably believed it. Second time, were you a little bit more skeptical in light of the fact that it had already returned once?

David: Yeah. I obviously had that in the back of my mind, but I wanted to believe that I would be okay I suppose. At the time I tried not to think about that too much. And especially just coming out of chemotherapy as well, and how bad it made me feel—I just wanted to get better. Christmas was coming up as well, so…

Ty: Right. And you're a young man, so how old were you when you were diagnosed?

David: Thirty. I'm 33 now. But actually, soon after Christmas, when it came back again for the third time—again in the lymph nodes. And this time—this is when they told me, you know, to be honest, there's very little they could do.

Ty: What kind of an emotional blow was that? To hear that after the first two—you go through the two rounds of treatments, you're told you're cancer-free twice, and now they say, "Well, actually it's terminal."

David: Can't put it into words. Devastated, completely devastated. I've got a little boy who was three or four at the time, and now—I just couldn't accept it from him. And I couldn't believe it, but I struggled to see how I was going to get through it after them telling me that.

I was with my family. You know, my mom's passed away. It's devastating for everyone, it really was.

Ty: I'll bet it was. I've got children, too. I know the feeling I could assume that I would feel if I were faced with potentially leaving them without a father. I know that had to have been hard for you.

David: It really was. It was actually the hardest thing to think about. It really was. You know, because he is one of the reasons why I had that positive attitude all the way through and I believe positivity has helped me as well. I really do. And I've always said that I'll be okay and I'll get through it. But that little thing in the back of my mind—obviously knowing it might not happen. The best part—I've always said I'll get through it, and so far I have.

Ty: Well, you know, I can kind of tell that. We just met—we corresponded via email—met for the first time in person, and when you meet somebody, you can kind of get a sense about them initially, and I could tell that about you, that you're a very positive type person. Just the smile on your face when I greeted you for the first time. So tell me about after the terminal diagnosis. You're devastated emotionally, you're thinking, "I can't leave my son." Where did you go from there?

David: Well, initially I went with the treatments they offered me, and I went onto chemotherapy. I did about four, three months.

Ty: Even though they said it was terminal?

David: Yeah. They told me that this would possibly extend my life. If I didn't start the treatments they were saying I've got about six months to live. And with the treatments, depending on the success, I could have 18 months. And so, to me, at the time, I thought, "An extra 12 months with my little boy. I'll do it."

And three months into the chemo, I had another scan. It had been reasonably successful, the tumors had shrunk a bit. But they were still giving me the same prognosis. And then—it was then—because I'd started getting a lot more sick, three months into it—it was then I was thinking, you know, I'm not going to last 18 months anyway. My body's telling me it can't go on no more. And then I'd been told about alternative treatments by people, even up to this point, but to be honest with you, I didn't actually believe them back then.

And it just came to a point where I knew I had to try something, whether I believed it or not. And I looked on the Internet and there was one particular thing that kept coming up more than anything, and there seemed to be certain amounts of research done. Maybe not on humans as such, but in a lot of laboratories. And so I went ahead with this treatment and it's done really well for me.

Ty: What did you decide to do?

David: It's cannabis oil. And it's extracted from a cannabis plant. It has high THC content. And it's something that I take orally. I just put a little bit in my mouth, let it absorb. And I took that alongside chemotherapy initially and for a couple of months. And then it made me feel hell of a lot better just on the chemotherapy. My hair stopped falling out.

The pins and needles that I got from the last chemotherapy, which I was told that I'd have for the rest of my life, actually have disappeared. They started to disappear when I started taking this oil. And I actually started missing chemotherapy sessions then. I only went once a month for the next couple of months and then eventually stopped it at the beginning of August.

I then went on to have scans, and the fear of it growing or spreading that the doctors thought was going to happen never happened. And they've gone on to remove my lymph nodes. Now the measurement when they took the lymph node out is actually a little bit smaller than it was after I stopped the chemo.

And after the operation, I just changed my diet, was very healthy. They couldn't give me radiotherapy because I'd had the legal amounts already, and I didn't want the regular chemotherapy, so I just carried on with the oil and good diet. This time, three months on, the scan was clear.

That's the first time it's happened for me. And I've got another scan due in a month, so we're going to touch forward, that one is going to be clear, too. And so yeah, like you say, I don't know what else to say about that.

Ty: I mean it's awesome. So you just recently received the first clear scan?

David: Yeah, January that was. And I've the next one June, next month.

Ty: Maybe five, six months ago. That's awesome. So you said you took the hemp oil. Now, here in the UK, how do you get hemp oil? Do you have to go to the doctor to get it prescribed?

David: It's actually illegal in the UK.

Ty: Is it?

David: Yeah. And it's illegal medically. It's illegal recreationally. It's not seen as having any medical use in the UK at the moment.

Ty: I see.

David: And—

Ty: It's illegal in many states in the United States, too.

David: Yes, I believe it is.

Ty: It depends on the state, but many states it's illegal as well.

David: Yeah, and—it's a lot of the countries. It's still illegal as well. And so I had to—I made some myself, by purchasing the cannabis illegally. And I also purchased some oil from I suppose what you'd call a local drug dealer.

Ty: Isn't it absurd, David that you have to go to an underground drug dealer to buy a plant that can heal your cancer?

David: It's crazy, absolutely crazy. I just don't understand it. I really don't. And now I've gone back to the doctors, I've looked at my records, and they're actually telling me to continue doing what I'm doing.

Ty: They're telling you to continue?

David: Yeah.

Ty: That's great.

David: But I've not got it in writing, unfortunately. But if the doctors are willing to say that to me, then I can't understand why it's classed as an illegal drug, if, you know, it's being used for medicinal use. It just does not make sense.

Ty: Right. It doesn't. It does not make sense.

David: No.

Ty: And did you learn about it through Rick Simpson initially?

David: Yes, that was one of the videos I kept getting shown by my friends. It was obviously one of the friends who was devastated about the news, and they were saying, "Try this. Try that." And Rick Simpson was the main one, and we pretty much followed his protocol when I made the oil for the first time.

Ty: Okay. Yeah, he's got a great video series out there on how to make the hemp oil.

David: Yes. I've seen it many times.

Ty: So how did you feel after you go through your first scan, it's completely clear, you go home and see your boy? Emotionally contrast that with how you felt before, when you had the diagnosis?

David: Oh man, I don't know.

Ty: You can't even describe it?

David: It makes me emotional now thinking about it. Honestly, after being told that—and then such a short time as well to get told that it's pretty much the exact opposite. It's unreal, the journey I've gone through, as well as taking the oil. And my friends and family didn't want me to do the oil and stop chemotherapy.

Ty: Right.

David: Nobody wanted me to, because even if we thought it might work—we hoped it might work—nobody knew. So it's been an emotional roller coaster and to get that news…

Ty: I'll bet it was fantastic.

David: It's amazing, yeah. It's surreal.

Ty: Now your friends and family now—how are they now?

David: Yes they're all for it now.

Ty: Right.

David: They're backing me to try and get this available to cancer patients in this country. I've started off my own little petition. And to have it illegal for a cancer patient, it's just absolutely crazy. And if you want to try it, you should be allowed to.

Ty: Sure. And here's the thing, it's not like it's snake oil.

David: No.

Ty: Okay? That has no benefit. There have been literally dozens and dozens of studies over the last 40 years that prove that THC, hemp oil, cures up to 12 types of cancer. All over the world. So in the United States, it's considered a Class 1 drug, a Class 1 narcotic. It is right in the same category with heroin and cocaine. And, in order to be considered Class 1—in the United States at least—it has to have no medicinal benefit.

Well, it's still considered a Class 1, even though we've got dozens of studies that show that there is medicinal benefit. So it's a complete contradiction for it to still be considered in the same class of drug with heroin and with cocaine. And it's basically a plant.

David: Yeah, it just does not make sense does it?

Ty: No. I did not know that it was illegal here as well.

David: Yeah. It's how it's been as far I've been a child. It's not classed the same as heroin and cocaine, but it's on line with amphetamines as a Class B drug. And I just can't see how it is. It's just—like you say, it's a plant. It doesn't make sense.

Ty: Right.

David: You know, you're told to believe in God, and believe in faiths, and embrace other people's faiths. So if it's a plant, if it's been put on the earth, I don't understand why the governments are telling us we're not allowed to have it.

Ty: It doesn't make any sense at all.

David: No, no it doesn't.

Ty: So you started the hemp oil. You said you changed your diet. Can you kind of describe what you did from an eating perspective?

David: Yeah. Before I had the operation, I didn't change it too much, because I was pretty weak after chemotherapy. And I was advised to do an alkalizing diet, which I was going to start, but when I was told I was going to have the operation, I thought I'd wait until then, because I was a little bit weak anyway from the chemo and I lost a bit of weight.

But as soon—from day one, as soon as the cancer was removed, I basically did an alkalizing diet. Cut out carbs, eating a lot of vegetables, organic foods. I would actually eat meat, but I'd make sure it was organic meat. And my shopping bill must have increased by 300 percent. And I eat a lot of seeds as well, and nuts.

Ty: Do you have pretty good access to organic food where you live?

David: Not really, no. It's very limited, what we can get organic in. It's basically supermarket, local (inaudible - 00:14:55), what other good organic foods they stock. We do have local farm shops, which are locally produced products, but when I went in and asked them if they were organic, they actually said no. And a lot of people do actually believe them to be, but then the shop owner said that they're not. So organic food is pretty hard to come by and it's a lot more expensive as well.

Ty: Right.

David: The supermarket's a lot more expensive.

Ty: Do you grow any of your own up there?

David: No. I did have an allotment, but because of how poorly I was from the chemotherapy, I couldn't keep it going, so I ended up giving it to someone else.

Ty: I see. So other than hemp oil and the change of the diet, anything else that you—the people are watching might be in the situation you're in—that you could recommend to them that they could try?

David: Yeah, definitely. Before the operation, after stopping the chemo, I took vitamin D tablets, and—a biochemist actually recommended me to take 10,000 IU of vitamin D a day, which is 10 times the recommended daily allowance.

Ty: Right.

David: Didn't actually take that many. I only took three times the amount. And don't know how much benefit that did have for me, but it seemed to (inaudible 0:16:02).

Ty: No, there's a mountain of research behind vitamin D to prevent cancer.

David: That was really the main other thing that I did. And those graviola capsules. I mustn't forget them. I bought them off Amazon, those capsules with the graviola leaf. And it was them, vitamin D, the cannabis oil, and I improved my diet pre-op. I took out processed food completely. And like I say, after op I went 90 percent organic.

Ty: And you're still here today?

David: I'm still here today. Talk to you, still cancer free. Next scan will hopefully show that again. And the more I go on being cancer-free—I think it shows you don't necessarily have to have some of these chemotherapy treatments, or radiotherapy, like if you're offering me, you know… I haven't had it, and I'm doing okay, so…

Ty: Yeah. You seem to be doing great. Well, you know, one of the—the cannabis oil not only helps to target the cancer cells and kill cancer, but it also really gives your immune system a boost.

David: Yeah, well definitely, because I mean—if you looked at me, three months before taking cannabis oil, and then looked at me now, the difference—I look 10 years younger. It's truly amazing. My family have commented on it a lot. I personally didn't realize. And then I looked back at photographs, and I saw it for myself. You know, I was shocked. I really was. It was crazy. I looked like an old man.

Ty: You've got some of those pictures on Facebook.

David: Yes.

Ty: Because I've seen some and you do look younger. Because when I first saw you down there in the lobby, I didn't recognize you, because you actually do look younger than some of the pictures I saw.

David: Yeah, I mean, I suppose as the months go by, I'm gradually starting to look better and better, and I put that down to the diet and the oil. I'm doing nothing else, so that's all I think it can be.

Ty: What would you recommend, David, to somebody that's watching the documentary here that may have been recently diagnosed with cancer—what would your advice to them be, coming from someone that was diagnosed as having terminal cancer?

David: I suppose you need to take advice from your doctors, and listen to the doctors, but don't necessarily believe 100 percent what they're saying. There are other things out there. Cannabis oil can't definitely work for every single cancer, but if you can find your actual type of cancer and type it into Google with the cannabis oil, you might be able to find certain studies that have been done with that particular cancer—because there are hundreds of different cancers. And the laboratory stories will actually tell you if the THC has been effective for it or not. Most of them have been done in a petri dish. At least it gives you an idea that there is a chance.

And if you're terminal, the doctor's saying there's no chance at least that gives you some sort of hope. Your diet as well. If you're strong enough, look into the alkalizing diet. Things like back off soda, if you do have to eat carbs. And if you are weak, obviously you need to eat what you can to build yourself back up. But once you get yourself at a good strength, look at the alkalizing diet. It's true that your body needs an acidic environment for cancer to grow, so if you can bring the pH of your body up, that can at least slow down the growth, if not do more.

Ty: So your message to somebody that might have recently received a terminal diagnosis is—not necessarily terminal, don't necessarily believe that. You've always got hope, right?

David: Yeah. Well, I was told I was terminal, and now I'm told I'm not, so, you know, there is hope there. It's not just me as well, there's plenty of other people that have gone through it.

Ty: Yeah, most definitely.

David: And if I can, well, they can, too.

Ty: If you can, they can too, right? You're living proof.

David: Yes. I am. You say it's all betting margins, you know. Everything's gone so quickly. It's just crazy, and it's really frustrating as well that I've been able to do this, but using something illegal. And the fact that it's still illegal is, you know—it can't go on. Something needs to change, really.

Ty: To me that's criminal, to withhold a potential treatment from someone.

David: If it's someone for medicine—I've even spoke to the police—and I don't want to say the police person's name—but they said to me, if it's for a medicinal reason, they don't want to arrest anyone for it.

Ty: Right.

David: Why would they? The high is a side effect. So if you're not taking it to get high, you're taking it to make you feel a little bit better—all I can say is how can you arrest someone for it?

Ty: Right. One of the additional benefits for people that are late-stage cancer is—a lot of them are kind of wasting away. They're losing weight, have a hard time putting weight on, don't have an appetite, a lot of times from the chemotherapy. And what the THC will do is it will give you an appetite.

It will make you hungry, eat more, stop that cycle, which is called cachexia, the wasting syndrome. That's another reason to allow it—just because it makes cancer patients have an appetite and feel better.

David: Yes. Definitely. And since I've been in the local paper recently, I've had a lot of contact with other cancer patients, and a lot of them are actually taking cannabis oil. And the ones that do, have been saying to me, the appetite, since they've been taking it, has been a hundred times better.

And also, sleeping pattern, you know—if you can actually sleep now. Because when you're on chemo, you do feel tired and weak, but sleeping's actually really difficult. It messes with appetite and with the sleep. So that alone, even if it doesn't slow down the tumor growth, that alone is helping them get through the chemotherapy, making them feel better in them final days and weeks.

That's all some people want. Some people, they're trying it and not expecting it to cure them. They just want to feel a little bit better and maybe have an extra few days or a few weeks with their family.

Ty: And not feel so sick the last days.

David: Exactly. The drugs that they do give you, and the painkillers that they give you, their side effects stop you from eating, and you need to eat. When you're that poorly, you need to eat. To give someone something that can actually make the appetite suffer, it's—again, it just doesn't make sense to me. It really doesn't.

Ty: No, it doesn't. And you know, even if somebody takes it with just the intent to feel better, get better sleep, have more of an appetite, they might realize pretty soon they're getting healed and didn't even expect it.

David: Exactly, yeah. Anyway, that's just amazing. It's a double bonus for them. It really is.

Ty: Yeah it is. It's amazing stuff. You're a living testimonial to the power of hemp oil.

David: Yes, and like I said, I just want more people to come forward as well, because I know there are others out there, and I think people are just a little bit scared because of the legality around it. But imagine what would happen in the UK if a policeman arrested you for treating a terminal diagnosis with cannabis oil and it got in the papers. It would just be crazy. So it's not going to happen. People shouldn't be scared if you want to come forward. Come tell your story. Get it out there so that we can help others.

Ty: Yeah. That's not the kind of PR that they want.

David: No.

Ty: Right?

David: Exactly. No, it's not. They're supposed to be helping people. The government's supposed to look after us, so to do the exact opposite to someone who's helped himself—they wouldn't do it.

Ty: So David, I've got a question for you. In light of the fact you're a father, you've got a son you don't want to leave behind without a father, and you're two cycles of chemo, then the terminal diagnosis. At that point, you begin to use the hemp oil, and you've got the mental state, you can't leave your son, you believe this is going to work, and you talk about the importance of belief and this positive attitude that you have—that you have now and you had to have had then. How important was that in your cancer recovery?

David: I think it was vital. I really do. Because in myself I completely believed that I was going to do this. I had to focus on seeing my son growing up, being there for him when he grew up. And I suppose it's hard for me to put into words, but I think if you feel too negative about something, you can end up making yourself feel quite bad.

And I think if you feel positive about something, you generally stay in a good mood, and things tend to work out better, if you just have a positive outlook, just in general. I think that is extremely important in any walk of life, not just through illness, to be positive.

A smile makes other people smile. You can walk down the street with a smile and someone will smile back. You walk down the street with a sad face, you just don't see all the positivity around you. Positivity creates positivity. And like I say, any walk of life, not just through illness.

You need to be positive. Because if you're not, your body knows that, and your body can release certain chemicals through the brain. I'm no scientist. I don't know exactly how it works, but I do know mood can control certain things in your body. So 100 percent, be positive, and just keep that positive outlook.

Ty: And I'm sure that your positive outlook is a part of your recovery. Not to exclude the efficacy of the hemp oil, because I know that was a big part of it, but I know that your positive belief that you were going to be healed—that was a big part of it as well.

David: Yeah, definitely. The positivity, the oil, the diet, it's all had a—it's all had an effect, I think, and it's all helped me to get me to where I am today.

Ty: Well, David, thank you for your courage. Thank you for stepping out and sharing your story with us. I've been touched, just from your story—perspective of a father who wants to stay alive for his son, and I'm so thankful you're doing well. And I know that you're going to continue to stay well.

David: Thank you. Cheers.

Ty: Cheers.

David: Safe traveling.

Ty: You bet.

[end of transcript]

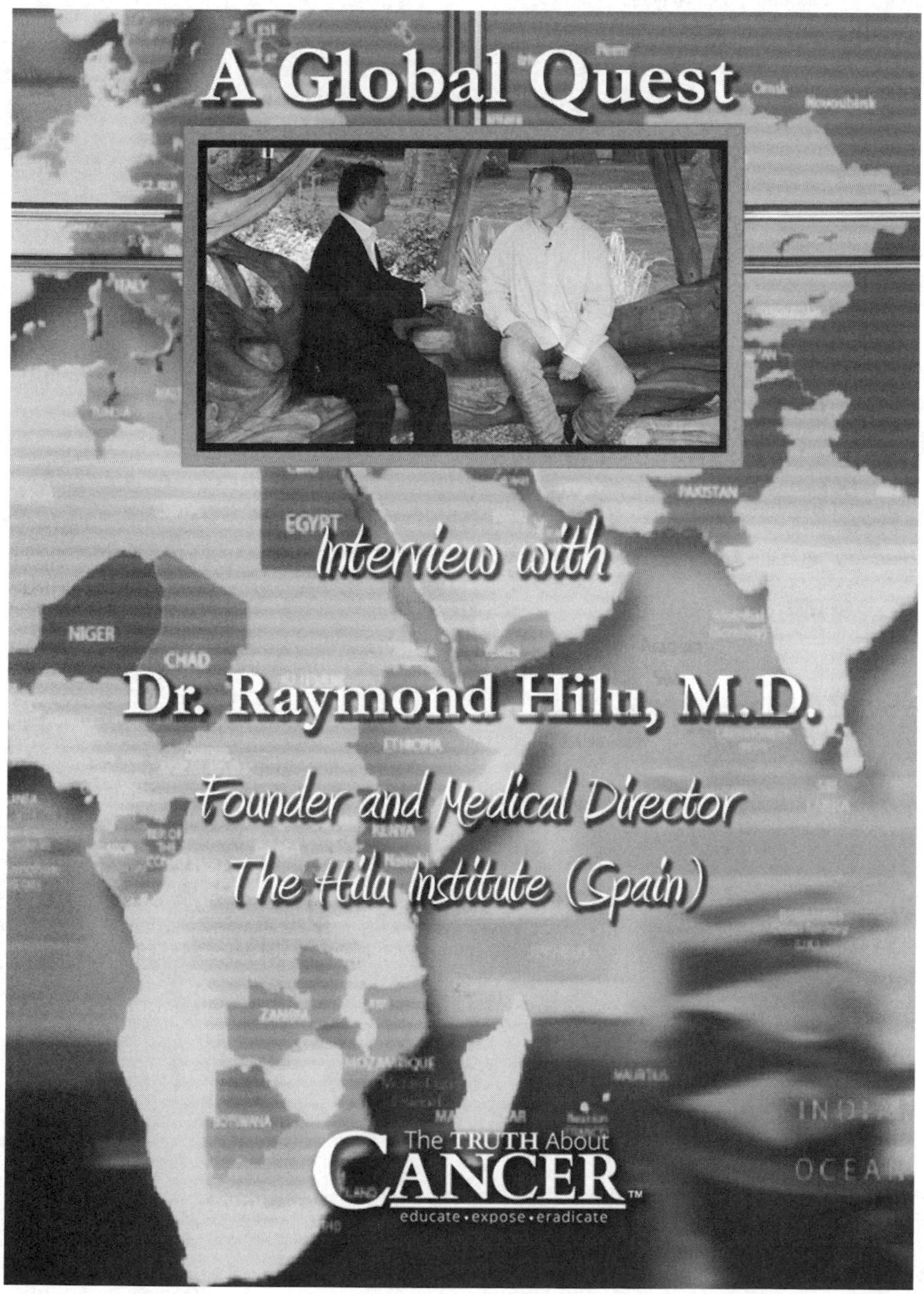
A Global Quest
Interview with
Dr. Raymond Hilu, M.D.
Founder and Medical Director
The Hilu Institute (Spain)
The TRUTH About
CANCER
educate • expose • eradicate

Ty: So Dr. Raymond Hilu. I really appreciate you joining us today.

Dr. Hilu: Thank you for the invitation.

Ty: Yeah. So your practice is in what areas of Spain?

Dr. Hilu: I have a practice, the main practice is in Marbella, that's South Spain. My second most important, or largest, practice is in Barcelona. And I have a third practice in Madrid, in the capital.

Ty: Okay. So that's three?

Dr. Hilu: Three, four years ago.

Ty: Okay. Three different practices then.

Dr. Hilu: Yeah.

Ty: Okay. And your training is as a conventional medical doctor?

Dr. Hilu: Yes, a general surgeon and conventional medical doctor.

Ty: Okay. Where did you go to school?

Dr. Hilu: I went to the American University of Beirut.

Ty: Okay.

Dr. Hilu: That was in Lebanon when I was very, very young.

Ty: Okay. So one of the things that I've read about you is that—in your writings—is about what you call—is it HRB analysis? Could you talk about HRB analysis to begin with?

Dr. Hilu: Yeah. This is a high resolution cellular study of the blood. You just need a couple of drops from the finger. And of course there are different ways of doing that, but the method I'm using nowadays is a special microscope built specifically for me.

We magnify the sample up to 65,000 times, so I'm able to see what's happening even inside the cells. It gives me a very good idea of the imbalances, deficiencies, irregular morphologies, and the contents of the blood serum. So whatever is wrong, I take note of it, and try to put it right. As simple as that.

Ty: 65,000 times?

Dr. Hilu: Yes. Not many. The thing is—

Ty: Wow. Just from a couple drops of blood?

Dr. Hilu: Yes.

Ty: That's amazing.

Dr. Hilu: It's quite common in the states.

Ty: How many physicians are using this type of analysis?

Dr. Hilu: I think are 3,000 in the states that use this method. In Holland, are a couple of them. In England, there's one. In Spain there are two or three. But in Russia there are quite a few. I did some training in Russia as well, which was really good.

But the thing is, that the morphologies, or the things they see under the microscope, some see up to 20, others see 30, Dr. Bradford, from the states, who was one of my professors, managed to discover 58 different morphologies.

Ty: Now when you say morphologies, what does that mean?

Dr. Hilu: Shapes. Shapes you see and are able to identify after examining them. So what I've done—I've trained with everybody who knew something about it. I've been doing that for the last 30 years. And I ended up managing 840 morphologies. So the way I do it, to my knowledge, nobody else is doing, because the maximum that one physician does is less than 60.

Ty: And so, is this particular—and that's amazing that you're, what 15 times more than anyone else? You're able to determine more morphologies than anyone else. Are you able to determine if someone has cancer from just a few drops of blood in this HRB analysis?

Dr. Hilu: Yeah, although this is not a diagnostic tool, it does help us to even prevent cancer, because cancer or any other disease—call it fibromyalgia, call it chronic fatigue syndrome, call it whatever you want to call it—any disease starts up with cellular imbalances.

That's the beginning of any disease. Things start to go wrong on a cellular level—and this is where the microscope becomes a very useful tool. Because we start seeing these irregularities before the disease appears, even cancer, years in advance. So we can prevent diseases from happening.

Of course, if the patient is already suffering from cancer, we will see the imbalances that the patient is suffering and the things that are making cancer grow worse and we try to correct them as well. So it's useful to treat, but mainly I love to use this tool to prevent the disease from happening.

Ty: Okay. So seeing these morphologies allows you to catch it early, before it manifests?

Dr. Hilu: That's the idea. Some cancers we can detect five years in advance, which is great.

Ty: That's awesome. Because most of what we think of as diagnostics are really not diagnostics at all. I mean, it's not early detection I mean.

Dr. Hilu: It's too late.

Ty: Right. It's too late. So we hear about early detection is your best protection with mammograms. By the time you see it on a mammogram, it's too late, typically. You want to catch it early and that's what this allows you to do.

Dr. Hilu: We want to catch it even before it becomes a tumor. But when there's a cellular imbalance that is precancerous, that's when we want to catch it.

Ty: And then you've got a much higher cure rate.

Dr. Hilu: Yeah. It can be even—more than 95 percent we can save.

Ty: Right. Dr. Hilu, why is there this huge explosion in childhood cancer? We were talking about this on the walk over. Could you elaborate for our audience?

Dr. Hilu: This is a very difficult question because to begin with, cancer is a very complex disease. It's multi-factorial. It's not caused by just one thing, not even two, not even three. A minimum, in my experience—it's four. It's four issues.

Ty: And what would they be?

Dr. Hilu: Mostly it's—but it doesn't apply to children, that's why it's not so easy. Mostly it's radiation, contamination—be it chemical or any other one—genetics, and nutrition. These are the four main causes. We cannot refer to nutrition as a cause—or maybe yes—when we talk about babies, because they have not started to eat on their own yet. But in a way, they have been receiving nutrition from Mom.

And who knows what nutrition has been received if they ended up with cancer. We don't really know. And also about contamination, they're still inside, so how could contamination bother them? Well, also from Mom, in a way, especially when it comes to metallic contamination.

Ty: Metallic?

Dr. Hilu: Like mercury from amalgam fillings. Such fillings contain a mix of different metals, one of them being carcinogenic, which is mercury. It's banned by the WHO.

Ty: Is it banned in Spain?

Dr. Hilu: It's banned all over the world in fact, but they still find a way to use it. The year they banned it was the year the thermometers, the glass thermometers with the mercury inside, they disappeared all of a sudden.

Ty: I remember that, when I was a kid.

Dr. Hilu: Yeah. Some kids used to play with them. They used to play even with the mercury thing, with the drops.

Ty: Right.

Dr. Hilu: Because are very funny the way they move. They're quite heavy for little amounts. But the thing is, just one contact with mercury can be fatal. But it's cancerous, that's the thing. It can provoke cancer. And from Mom, it always gets to the fetus, without exception.

Ty: And so—

Dr. Hilu: The metals end up there.

Ty: So a mom has mercury fillings, they're out gassing mercury, and you're saying it gets into the fetus through the umbilical cord?

Dr. Hilu: Yeah. So that can be another cause in a way. Also electromagnetic fields that surround us. We know that there are more and more electromagnetic fields. There are no good enough studies, technical studies, about which is the bad ones, and which ones can be tolerable by the human body.

But we know that mobile phones, microwaves, GPSs, and similar do alter body chemistry. And also, when there are a mix of things, like if you have amalgam fillings, and you use the mobile phone a lot, the filling, which is metallic, acts as an aerial, as an antenna. It amplifies the signal and pulls more radiation into your body and it also affects the fetus.

Ty: So they see a correlation between mothers with amalgam fillings and then babies with cancer?

Dr. Hilu: I do see it in the practice. I do see it. Emotions can affect as well and, of course, there's the genetics. I mean, you have this altered gene.

Ty: Sure.

Dr. Hilu: If the other factors exist as well—so the co-factor of genetics is there, it becomes easier for the baby to develop some sort of tumor or some sort of cancer.

Ty: I see. Can you describe the fact that—I've heard you mention cancer being an imbalance in the body?

Dr. Hilu: Yes. Yes it does, because cancer normally is a very slow-growing disease. It doesn't happen in 24 hours. It's not like an accident. Things have to go wrong for some time. And these things that go wrong for some time, go wrong on a cellular level. Cells start to behave wrongly.

And this is why I'm so much in love with cellular medicine, looking at the blood under the microscope, because we start seeing those imbalances before the disease shows. And we're able to correct them once we are able to identify them. The hardest thing in medicine is to treat things by just treating the symptoms, not treating the cause.

If we see the cause, we see the real imbalances, it's much easier to deal with such things. So if we see that the size of a certain cell is not the right one, we can make it bigger. If we see that the shape of a certain cell is not the right one, we can correct its shape.

If we see that the amount of taurine inside the white cell is not enough, we can get the person to take more taurine and fix it. So it's—to certain degree it's easy, if you know what you're dealing with.

Ty: Right. And you mentioned symptoms versus causes, right?

Dr. Hilu: Yes.

Ty: Treating symptoms versus causes. One of the things that conventional medicine does, specifically with cancer, is really to treat the symptom, the tumor, rather than the cause.

Dr. Hilu: Yeah.

Ty: Can you talk about being conventionally trained as a medical doctor—what was your aha moment, where you really woke up and you realized that, specifically for treating cancer, that conventional medicine really wasn't doing all that great of a job?

Dr. Hilu: Well, sadly I didn't have experience of this aha moment whilst practicing conventional medicine, because this aha moment came to me as soon as I finished medical school. I discovered that the tools I had were not good enough for me. I was not happy with the treatment tools.

I was very happy with the knowledge about the human body. I was very happy knowing the names of the diseases and of the microbes and how things happen inside the human body. But the treatment tools, the therapeutical tools, I was not happy with.

And that's when I started to train all over the world, trying to discover, or get hold of, or acquire specific knowledge that can help me be minimally invasive and maximally effective when treating diseases.

Ty: So it gave you the foundation that you needed?

Dr. Hilu: Yes, absolutely.

Ty: Right?

Dr. Hilu: Good. What I needed.

Ty: A good, working knowledge of the body and the way it works and then you built on that. Let me ask you this. Last year, in *The Quest for the Cures*, I interviewed dozens of medical doctors in the states. I asked them, how much training did you get while you were in medical school on nutrition? Now the typical answer in the states is nothing, maybe an hour or two. What about you?

Dr. Hilu: Thirty hours.

Ty: Thirty hours?

Dr. Hilu: Which is nothing.

Ty: So you got more outside of the United States than they do in the United States. You got 30 hours?

Dr. Hilu: Thirty hours. That was it.

Ty: Okay. And in comparison to—what was the total workload over the course of your medical education? 1,000 hours?

Dr. Hilu: Yes. 1,500 maybe.

Ty: 1,500 hours?

Dr. Hilu: Yep.

Ty: Okay, so 30 out of 1,500. A little bit more than in the states.

Dr. Hilu: It's nothing.

Ty: But small in comparison to the total.

Dr. Hilu: Because bear in mind—if we get back to one of your questions before, nutrition probably is 25 percent of health or of disease. So you need a 25 percent training hours to be fair with a patient. If not, you are not qualified, shouldn't treat the patient.

Ty: Right. So how can a doctor teach you about how to be healthy when nutrition's such a big part, when they don't know?

Dr. Hilu: They use TV adverts. I've seen it so many times. There's a very famous TV advert in Spain. It's about margarine.

Ty: Margarine?

Dr. Hilu: Yeah. And you see a helicopter coming down with margarine and spreading the margarine on the toast of the children, saying, "It's very healthy, very good for you." And then doctors end up prescribing or recommending margarine as good for you.

They haven't read a word about margarine in their life, because there is not one decent publication that talks well about margarine. In fact, Dr. Budwig—you know of her don't you?

Ty: Yes.

Dr. Hilu: She tried, through the German government, to ban margarine worldwide. I have some of the letters that they interchanged between the Ministry of Health and Dr. Budwig personally.

And it's amazing how—not amazing, that's not the right word—but worrying, how dangerous margarine is for health. Because if you refine margarine, just one more time, it will become plastic.

Ty: Yeah. You know, my father died of cancer in the 90s. And before he died, three or four years before that, I remember him talking to us about margarine, telling us that it was close to plastic. Now, at that time, I thought, "Ah, Dad's off his rocker. He doesn't know what he's talking about." Because I'd never heard that. They didn't tell us that on TV. But that's the truth.

Dr. Hilu: Dr. Budwig said so in 1953. So…

Ty: It's been a long time.

Dr. Hilu: A long time.

Ty: Talk about the Budwig diet.

Dr. Hilu: Oh yes. This was maybe a big—what did you call before, aha?

Ty: Aha moment.

Dr. Hilu: Aha moment—

Ty: Yeah, aha moment.

Dr. Hilu: —in my medical life. Because up til then, I was critical with naturopath and people who spoke about diet and nutrition, because I am a good gourmet. I love my food. So I used to be critical with whoever was vegetarian or macrobiotic. I thought that they were a bit out of balance and I used to use myself as an example.

I could eat anything and I was alright and I was healthy. And I still am in fact. I'm lucky in that regards. Until I met Dr. Budwig. I was trying hard for many years to get to convince her to train me. And she was refusing. She always refuse. She never trained anyone in fact.

Until one day, I just went there along with a friend and an interpreter, a German interpreter. Because back then, my German was not good enough. And I didn't even have an appointment with her. I just popped into her house in South Germany. It was in the year 1996 I think and I had a little chat with her. And she considered that she liked me.

Her English was very good. She took a stick and kicked out the German translator. She was like that, very aggressive. So Barbara went away, a good friend of mine. And she also refused to train my partner, the gentleman that came with me, a Canadian man who's also into medical things.

And she allowed me to participate with her, you know, experiments and to help her out with redefining certain medical expressions and conclusions of some of her work. So I was going—coming and going to Freudenstadt, the city where she used to live, and got the full training. And realized how nutrition—how important nutrition is.

I even went to do some of your work, in Freudenstadt, because she treated 2,200 people only with diet. And they were cancer patients. And almost all of them were cured. Of course, I wouldn't believe that just by listening to her.

So I went personally to different ones and I interviewed them, to make sure that what she was saying was true, and it was. And this was my aha moment. I decided to use her diet, to incorporate this discovery into my clinical work.

Ty: So over 2,000 patients?

Dr. Hilu: 2,200, yes.

Ty: How many of them did you talk to personally?

Dr. Hilu: I talked to about—maybe 300.

Ty: 300?

Dr. Hilu: Yes. Over the years.

Ty: And that was your aha moment?

Dr. Hilu: Yes, of course. Because there was an intersection, a clear intersection with all their, let's say, confessions.

Ty: What is the principle behind the Budwig diet? First of all, describe it real quickly for somebody that's watching that may not know what it is, and then why does it work?

Dr. Hilu: Yes. It's very simple in fact, very clever and very simple. It consists of mixing cottage cheese, preferably low fat, with flaxseed oil. That's it. Banning the bad foods, the sugars and the red meat and so on.

But the main ingredient is this buttercream mix, which is cottage cheese, flaxseed oil—two tablespoons of flaxseed oil. The amount of cottage cheese is not important, just enough to mix it well so that you can't see the oil anymore. And that's it. And you can add to the mix whatever you like, use your imagination and make it nicer, or—

Ty: Add fruit and bulgur.

Dr. Hilu: You can make it go sweet and make it like a dessert or go more salty and put herbs and add it to your salad, whatever. So it's a matter of choice, of whatever your flavors tell you to do.

Ty: Right.

Dr. Hilu: Now, the scientific basic behind it, in fact, is the same scientific basics behind work of Dr. Otto Warburg, the Nobel Prize winner, who discovered—and that's why he had his Nobel Prize—that cancer cells would not normally grow in oxygen rich atmosphere. They need hypoxia to grow. And presence of oxygen—it's difficult for them to grow. And the basics of Dr. Budwig's diet is the providing of oxygen to the tissues and organs of the body.

How is that? Well, flaxseed oil, even the industrial flaxseed oil, the one that is used in paint, you use it to make quick paints, quick drying paints. So if you mix flaxseed oil with paint and you paint a façade, you paint a wall, it will dry quickly.

Ty: The flaxseed brings the oxygen quicker?

Dr. Hilu: That's the basics. As simple as that.

Ty: Ah!

Dr. Hilu: So she does the same thing inside the human body. She managed to do it better than others, because the difficulty with flaxseed oil, and poly-unsaturated fat in general, is that it's not easily absorbed in the intestinal tract. It's difficult to absorb.

The intestinal lining has a negative charge to it, and flaxseed oil—just to put it simple—has a negative charge to it. So negative and negative, they repel each other, and it's not absorbed. Her discovery as a biochemist was that if you mix well this flaxseed oil with a positively charged protein—sulfur based in this case—like cottage cheese then it's readily absorbed. In a few minutes, it's in your bloodstream and it gets to the cells, oxygenates them, and makes life difficult for cancer cells. Easy.

Ty: It seems so simple, the way you explained it.

Dr. Hilu: It is.

Ty: Okay. So it's really a deal of electricity.

Dr. Hilu: Yeah.

Ty: Like charges repel, opposites attract.

Dr. Hilu: Yeah.

Ty: So you're changing the actual charge of that mixture from negative to positive.

Dr. Hilu: Yeah. In fact, Dr. Budwig talks a lot about electricity and positive and negative charges. Part of her treatments have to do with that directly. She asks people to go barefooted and walk on grass, or on sand—wet sand, while sunbathing, so that electricity in the body gets corrected.

Ty: Earthing.

Dr. Hilu: Earthing.

Ty: Right.

Dr. Hilu: Earthing is very good, very good. And different tricks to earth yourself, apart from the psychological things—but it's good for the body. We need it because we are surrounded by things that contaminate us, electrically speaking.

Ty: So there's something to be said—I remember growing up, I used to see people that thought it was good to go out and walk in nature barefooted, and—being raised in the United States—we thought that was kooky. But there was a lot to it. We were just mis-educated growing up. We didn't know that there was something to that.

Dr. Hilu: Yes. Probably, cancer is the outcome of mis-education, in general.

Ty: Talk about detoxification as part of your protocol, because I know that's a big part of what you do to treat cancer patients.

Dr. Hilu: Yes. But again, the basic principle will still be oxygenation. The cells of the body are interconnected by interstitial tissue, or by matrix. This area in between the cells is where things happen. This is where the nutrients are, and they enter into the cell. The dirt inside the cell go out into this area and then the lymphatic system drains them away.

So this interstitial tissue, this matrix, has to be clean. If it is contaminated, then oxygen won't be able to go through and the cell can become cancerous. The proper nutrients cannot go through, and the cell can become cancerous. Potassium and magnesium cannot go through, so the cell becomes acidic in this case, and they can turn cancerous. That's why detoxification is very, very important. Because it allows for this homeostasis to happen, and for the cells to behave naturally.

Ty: That's a fascinating explanation of detoxification. I've heard detox explained as the fact that it's compromising the immune system, these toxins in your body. But on the flip side of the coin, you're talking about detoxifying in order to improve the uptake of oxygen and energy, and nutrients into the cells.

Dr. Hilu: I'm not against the series of the importance of the immune system. In fact, I do believe that they have a very, very important role. But over the years of treating many, many patients, many cancer patients, who were concentrating very hard on their immune system, taking lots of stuff to improve their immune system—and under the microscope they had a fantastic immune system.

But cancer was still growing. Because if you don't access the area that is contaminated and clean it up, even if you have the best immune system in the world—useless. Again, cancer does not depend on just one issue.

So immune system, on its own, is not enough. Food on its own is not enough. Good emotions on their own are not enough. You have to do everything simultaneously. That's another difficulty, because if you just correct the immune system and don't correct the rest, the rest will end up ruining the immune system again.

Ty: Right.

Dr. Hilu: If you detoxify, but you don't do the nutritional part, and other things, then toxicity will accumulate again. So you will end up falling into the same mistakes once, and again, and again. That's why it's so important—that's the secret of our work, in our clinics, that we do everything simultaneously.

The four, five, six approaches that are needed, ten, no matter how many it was, we discover what's needed and do it—always to fit of course—but we do it simultaneously.

Ty: So there's really a synergism with the concurrent approaches—all at the same time.

Dr. Hilu: Yes.

Ty: Right? They work together to make each other more powerful, I guess.

Dr. Hilu: Exactly. That's a very good way of putting it.

Ty: Dr. Hilu, talk about the importance of electricity when it comes to our bodies, the way they function, and even regarding cancer.

Dr. Hilu: Yes. Again, it's the same basics that happen inside the intestinal tract, when we spoke earlier about flaxseed oil and its absorption. Everything in the body is electric, yeah? The heart is an electric engine, automatic electric engine that doesn't even depend on the brain. It can work on its own—fantastic piece of design.

But every single bit of the body is also like that. For instance, the red blood cells, they have a membrane, and the membrane has got an electric charge, which is a negative charge, and for this cell, this globule, to function properly, it needs to trap the oxygen, which is an o+, positively charged, and distribute oxygen in the body, then collect the carbon dioxide in the lungs, interchange of gases again, pick up the oxygen and distribute it again.

This is only possible because the electric charge of the cell membrane is negative, and the electric charge of the oxygen is positive. If we don't have the right charge, the oxygen does not pick up and cancer and other diseases would occur, even just tiredness because there's not enough fuel.

Because oxygen is the fuel of the body. It's so basic to be electrically balanced. And the balance of the cell membranes, when it comes to electric charge, is thanks to the composition of the cell membrane, which is amino acids and phospholipids. And guess what? Phospholipids are made from the same ingredient that we find in flaxseed oil.

Ty: Okay. So you know, any child that's played with magnets recognizes the fact that, you know, opposites attract, like charges repel. So talk about medical biomagnetism. I've read some of your papers on medical biomagnetism. Fascinating subject. Could you explain a little bit about that?

Dr. Hilu: Yes. This is a discovery of Dr. Isaac Goiz from Mexico. He's the father of this technology. And it started—the first observation occurred when the first astronaut, Neil Armstrong, who—when he came back from space, they observed that there was a shortening in one of the legs. And when they did a treatment, a magnetic treatment on him, it came back to its initial measure.

Ty: His leg lengthened?

Dr. Hilu: Yes. Lengthened or shortened. I can't remember if they treated the longer one to become shorter, or the shorter one to become longer. I can't remember. In fact, that was in 1967, 1968. From then, they discovered that magnetic imbalances do affect limbs. In fact, this is one of the basics of a science called kinesiology.

Kinesiology, they measure the contraction of muscle as a response to accepting or rejecting some product, or some idea, or some—it's a complex science, in fact. And after that, Dr. Goiz mixed the two things together, plus his own discoveries as he worked for many years in a hospital in Mexico that was specialized in asthma and breathing diseases, breathing-related diseases.

And he started his first experiments there by using this magnetic field treatment to balance the pH, which seems to be the reason why muscles shorten. If the area that is to be impacted is out of balance, then there's a shortening of the muscle, there's a contraction. Once you balance it, it goes back to its place.

And it seems also—that's what was discovered at the same time—that once you do that, you also eliminate, by this impact, the microorganisms that are in this area that cause disease. And that's how this science started to grow.

And nowadays you can relate different points of the body, shortening or elongating, with pH balances and different microbes that find the, like niche, in this specific place of the body, and could provoke a disease. So it gets rid of them by just using powerful magnets, of 3,000 gauss potency.

Ty: That's fascinating. So I'm assuming it's a completely nontoxic type approach. It doesn't have any negative side effects.

Dr. Hilu: No, only if you have a pacemaker. You shouldn't put it on top of a pacemaker.

Ty: Right.

Dr. Hilu: But besides that, no, nothing.

Ty: Okay. Once you had your aha moment, what was the reaction of your colleagues, at that point, that you worked with? Now that you began to go more of a natural, holistic type approach, as opposed to conventional medicine.

Dr. Hilu: Well, most of them thought—and that's how they expressed their thoughts to me—that I was nuts. Probably they were right, but I don't care. So I was not very social back then and I'm still not very social anyway. I'm half autistic in a sense. I don't care.

Ty: Okay.

Dr. Hilu: It doesn't bother me. No, most of them did not see a good point in what I was doing. They thought that I was losing my time, I was risking my future, that I was risking the life of my patients, no matter how hard I tried to convince them to look what I'm doing, has got no side effects.

What you are doing, what you are prescribing on this paper, any paper you write out to your patients, is loaded with side effects. I never write out on a prescription anything that may have any side effects. I don't agree and I don't care.

Ty: That's a good approach. Many people think I'm nuts, too. So we have that in common.

Dr. Hilu: Okay, welcome to the club.

Ty: Welcome to the kookoo club, right? Now one of the things you mentioned really struck a nerve, because—you're right, doctors regularly write out prescriptions for drugs that actually can kill. One of the alarming statistics that I've quoted many times, is—in the Unites States we have the FDA. On their own website, they admit that each year, 100,000 people die in the United States alone from properly prescribed drugs.

Dr. Hilu: There you go.

Ty: Properly prescribed drugs, not illegal drugs. From drugs that a doctor wrote properly for a certain symptom and it kills the person.

Dr. Hilu: You mean that's—these are prescriptions written by doctors, and those prescriptions are killing the patients, and the patients cannot sue the doctors for that, because everything was legal and proper, and ethically correct.

Ty: It was approved. It was approved. Budwig diet has never killed anyone, has it?

Dr. Hilu: No. But many doctors who've used Budwig diet have been taken to court.

Ty: I've heard about them in the United States. So they've been globally as well?

Dr. Hilu: Yeah.

Ty: Wow. Because it's not an approved procedure, I guess, an approved standard of care treatment. You mentioned earlier about conventional medicine versus natural medicine. We look at symptoms versus causes. Can you talk briefly about a tumor? We look at that as the cancer, but isn't it really just a symptom of the cancer?

Dr. Hilu: It is a symptom. Of course it is. Some—I can't remember the name of the doctor—but some scientist and a few doctors, in fact, refer to the tumor as the, like the head of the iceberg, like the showing bit of the iceberg, but all the cause is under the water. Tumors are just a little symptom.

It's like a little grain that grows because there's something going wrong. Of course, if this grain, or this tumor, is bothering you, you can get rid of it, and it stops bothering you. And this is what conventional medicine does. When it comes to cancer, they do so normally using four methods.

One is cut it off—surgery. Two, chemotherapy, which is a cytotoxic poisonous product that goes into your blood and destroys the weakest cells first. The weakest cells include cancer cells. Cancer cells are very weak. The same as hair follicles and intestinal mucosa. These are very weak cells, so they get destroyed by chemotherapy.

So that's a second method to get rid of the grain of the tumor. Radiation also destroys cancer cells before destroying healthy cells. And in specific tumors that are hormone related, they use hormones to destroy the tumor.

Ty: Okay.

Dr. Hilu: But nobody in traditional oncology looks for the cause. Nobody looks under the water. They get rid of this tumor. That's it. It comes up again, we'll get rid of it again. But they don't treat the cause behind it. The reason they don't treat the cause behind it, is because they don't know the cause behind it. I don't know the cause behind it.

Probably nobody knows the cause behind it, because every cancer, every tumor, every grain, is different. It's individual. It's like personalized bit of tumor. But we need to work hard to discover what's the cause in the case of this particular patient—is very hard work. We need to look into too many issues, and doctors don't bother to do that.

Ty: So there are many causes potentially, and the treatment needs to be individualized, not just a, you know—you have x-y-z cancer so you get this drug and that drug and that drug, it needs to be more individual, person specific.

Dr. Hilu: Yeah. That's why it's very, very important, at least for me, to utilize the 840 parameters that I look for when I'm studying a cell.

Ty: So then again, we go back to the HRB analysis. That's why that's so important to you?

Dr. Hilu: Yeah.

Ty: I like the analogy that you just used of a tumor being just the tip of the iceberg. You know, I've heard it referred to as like there's something wrong in your car. It's the check engine light, and we just smash the light. But I like the iceberg.

Dr. Hilu: This is nice also.

Ty: That's good, too. But the iceberg's good, too, because let's say you get rid of the tip of that iceberg sticking out of the water. That wouldn't have done much good for the Titanic.

Dr. Hilu: No.

Ty: It still hit. The majority of that iceberg—you have a tip here, and you've got this much under the water. That's what the real problem is. It's not the tip. And so you still have that underlying problem in your body.

Dr. Hilu: Yeah.

Ty: What would your advice, Dr. Hilu, be to a person that's been recently diagnosed with cancer, and they're talking to their oncologist? What questions should they ask to determine if they're going to receive adequate treatment?

Dr. Hilu: You know, there's one very, very important question that some patients don't dare to ask. But oncologists are very dedicated doctors. They work really hard. So knowing that, they could—patients could have use of that, in a sense, of this knowledge I'm mentioning now, that they are dedicated doctors and they want the best for their patients.

Their intentions are always good. They don't want to kill the patients. They are trained to save lives. All doctors are trained to save lives, that's—because it's a sort of work, if you don't love people, you can't do it. So there are always good intentions behind what an oncologist suggests, explains. But of course, there's a limit to their knowledge.

Ty: Right.

Dr. Hilu: Your knowledge, my knowledge, and everybody else's knowledge, oncologists included. So a very good question would be, "Doctor, in your opinion, what are the chances of survival if I did this, if I did that, if I didn't do any of what you are saying and I went that way? Please tell me your opinion."

And then it could be much easier for the patient to make up his or her mind. Because if a doctor says, "Well, look, in your case, if we employ chemotherapy, your chances of getting cured are going to be 2 percent more." I don't want that.

Or if the oncologist says, "Well, in your case, for this specific type of leukemia—,"that's one of the diseases where chemotherapy can be very effective, in some cases can be the only way to deal with the problem,"—it's 95 percent chances that you get cured." Much easier for the patient to make up his mind.

Ty: Right.

Dr. Hilu: This would be number one. Number two would be side effects. And again, the patient needs to evaluate if they want to go through such side effects or not. They have to be questions directly related to the treatments regarding benefits and side effects.

Ty: So it's really a risk/benefit analysis, right? Is it worth it?

Dr. Hilu: Yeah. And what the patient should never do is ask the doctor, or naturopath, or his father, or his son-in-law, whether he has to go this way, that way, or the other. Once the patient's got all this information in mind, the patient has to make up his or her mind. "That's it. I'm going that way and I'll get all the help I'm able to collect in order to heal myself."

Ty: Right. And we just hope and pray that we continue to live in a society, a global society, where those choices are available to the patient and not forced on us.

Dr. Hilu: Yes. We should never allow any treatment to be forced on us, in fact. We don't have to view the oncologist or any doctor as somebody who can obligate us to do something. They are tools that we pay with our own taxes to get help from. So we need to use such tools wisely. So just use them.

Ty: Use them and use your own brain to make your own decision to keep up with your own health or to regain your own health. I think that's what—a common thread that I see, is that we need to remain to have the choices to treat our own health the way that we see fit.

And that's one of our goals with *The Truth About Cancer* here and I just want to thank you for spending the time with us today to share your knowledge. It's been very valuable, and you shared with us some things that no one else has shared with us thus far. And so it's going to be very beneficial for our audience. So thank you again.

Dr. Hilu: I'm glad to hear this. Thank you. It's been an opportunity for me as well. I do thank you for it.

Ty: You betcha.

Dr. Hilu: Okay. ***[end of transcript]***

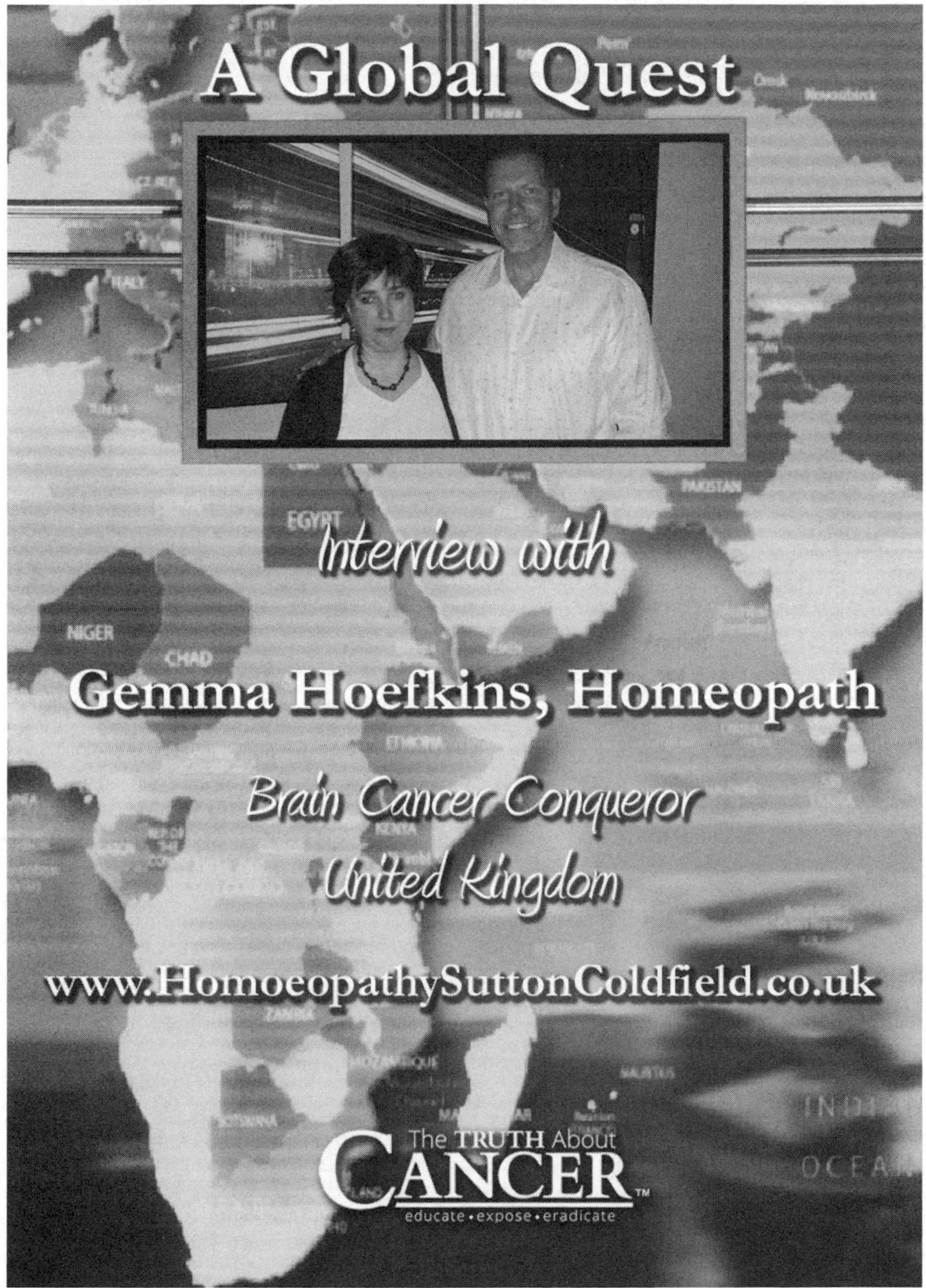
A Global Quest
Interview with
Gemma Hoefkins, Homeopath
Brain Cancer Conqueror
United Kingdom
www.HomoeopathySuttonColdfield.co.uk
The TRUTH About
CANCER
educate • expose • eradicate

Ty: I am really excited to be here in London, England today with Gemma Hoefkens. I've known you, Gemma, via email and the Internet, for several years now. It's a pleasure to finally meet you.

Gemma: Yes, and you. Very good to see you. Very good to be here.

Ty: Thank you. Where did you travel from here?

Gemma: From Birmingham.

Ty: From Birmingham. So, north of London?

Gemma: North of London, yes.

Ty: Thank you for joining us today.

Gemma: Pleasure.

Ty: I'm really excited to get your story because you are a homeopath, but you also have a cancer story—a cancer survival story. So let's rewind back about 20 years and if you could, begin to share with us your story of overcoming a cancer diagnosis back in the mid-90s, if I remember correctly.

Gemma: It was 1996. I was sent home to die, really. Previous to that, when I was 23 years old, I had hydrocephalus and they said that was a really successful operation. Hydrocephalus is water on the brain which is a tube going from your head, going down to your abdomen, draining fluid. Everybody has got synovial fluid that goes down. And then, a couple of years later on I started getting problems, many problems—dizziness, headaches—and they kept doing scans. I was worried about the shunt coming down, whether that was damaged or not working properly. And they gave me MRI scans and checking and checking, nothing wrong. And then they finally found there was a tumor in my pineal gland, which is right in the middle of your head. So they couldn't do—well, they didn't want to do anything with it anyway because it was so tiny. They said, just see what happens, really.

And basically, what happened was it grew a little bit bigger, and then it spread to my pituitary gland in the head. But because it was so delicate, and the pineal, the initial tumor, was in the middle of your head, you couldn't have surgery because it could be too damaging to the body. You would die if you had surgery. So they said, "It's not causing you too much problems." But gradually it was getting worse and worse. I was getting little stars—you know in cartoons you get little stars going around you, or lots of memory problems, especially I would bump into things. And gradually, they said, "It has grown." And they said, "We're going to do a biopsy." So I did a biopsy and they found that I needed radiology, which was pretty horrific.

Ty: So, did you undergo the radiation treatments?

Gemma: Oh yes. I had that and I was fitted with a mask and you lie there as still as you can and it's really quite frightening. You have all these rays at you and you can't move because if you do the rays are going to go in the wrong place. I didn't get it, really. I'm not a scientist, I didn't understand, but there are rays going into you and nobody is to come in the room, they are all outside the room. Nobody will come in because it was so damaging. But it was supposed to help me anyway.

Ty: Didn't make sense to you?

Gemma: Didn't make sense to me. If it is going through your head, why isn't it damaging everything? Why is it just damaging your tumor? So I was frightened. What if I sneezed? They're going to do it the wrong place, aren't they? So I was really worried. And then on the first radiology session they leapt into the room and said, "Stop it," because they had found another tumor. This was one on my pituitary gland. This one had spread so they had to mark up the mask and so it was aimed at that, as well.

Ty: So did they hit them both at the same time? Did they try to get both tumors with the first treatment? Or did you do that after that?

Gemma: I don't know.

Ty: Not sure.

Gemma: I don't know, I'm not sure.

Ty: Was this considered to be brain cancer?

Gemma: They weren't sure, to be honest. There were tumors, and they were acting irregularly, well, they began acting irregularly. Then it went down my spine. And they did some more radiology down my spine. And then they did some boosters, so that wasn't enough. They did the radiology and said, "That's not enough, we need—there hasn't been enough improvement and we need to do boosters." So I had the boosters.

Ty: So that's more radiation.

Gemma: More radiation. And then I got the results and they were looking through them and they said, "Oh, actually, this is quite good," because the ones in my back had actually gone. So they thought that was great, but then they said, "It's not improvement enough. We need to do chemotherapy." Which was, again, confusing. I was thinking, "Well, why don't you carry on with what's working?" But the doctors said no. So I thought, "Okay, good news." But I was a bit confused because I was going on to chemotherapy. So I had the chemotherapy. I was supposed to have three sessions of it, and I think I had two. I didn't have the third. They said to me, basically, "Our treatment is making you worse." I was getting worse.

Ty: The chemo was making you worse.

Gemma: "Our treatment is making you worse." I don't know if it was the chemo or the drugs. I had steroids and lots of different drugs and the radiology. All my hair fell out with the radiology in two weeks, and I was nauseous and vomiting.

Ty: Two weeks to lose all your hair.

Gemma: Yes.

Ty: Is that what you said? It took two weeks?

Gemma: No, no, no. My hair fell out in one weekend.

Ty: One weekend?

Gemma: Yes. It was devastating for me.

Ty: I've never heard of that quick of a reaction to the…

Gemma: I don't know how long. I can't remember how long it was, but when I was having radiology, I can't remember what number session it was, but it all fell out in one weekend.

Ty: At that point, what were you feeling when you see all of your hair falling out?

Gemma: Can you imagine, particularly a young woman? I'm 26, my hair was shoulder-length hair, I always had long hair. I was actually staying at my friend's house and it was all coming out as I was in the shower. It was all coming out and I just put it in a bin and forgot to tell her it was in the bin, and she looked later and she saw all this hair in the bin.

Ty: So what was the protocol after your doctors told you, "Our treatments are making you worse?" Where did you go from there?

Gemma: So that was after my chemotherapy. They came in and basically they said, "Would you like to stay in hospital? Would you like to go home? Or would you like to go to a hospice?"

Ty: To hospice?

Gemma: Yes.

Ty: So it was a grim prognosis, then?

Gemma: Oh yes. Oh yes. So I thought, "Well, I don't want to go to a hospice." As far as I was concerned, you go to hospice because you die. And I thought, "I don't want to stay in this hospital, everybody's dying." Remember, I was in the oncology ward and I could hear people having their last rites in the middle of the night and things like that, and I couldn't wait to get out of there. So I thought, I'll go to my mom's. You want your mom to look after you, mom and dad. I went back to their place.

But just before then—I used to go back and forth to my mom and dad to be looked after now and again. I lived in London, they lived in Worcestershire. And my sister-in-law phoned me up and she said, "Look, I've heard about this woman. She's helped with my eczema, and my daughter's eczema has gone completely away. Do you want to speak to her? She is a homeopath." I thought, "What's that? I don't know what that is."

Ty: You didn't know what homeopathy was at that point?

Gemma: No, I didn't know what homeopathy was. I didn't know. But I thought, "I'm really, really, poor I might as well give it a go, I'm not getting anywhere." And so I started having some treatment from her and so I had a bit of faith in her, I didn't have a lot of faith, and I was very skeptical. But I didn't have any alternative, to be honest.

And I thought all these things that were happening to me were a bit of a coincidence, but they kept happening, again, and again, and again. So I thought, "Okay, okay." So I kept them in there. And then when I was sent home to die I just did homeopathy ever since then. And now, this is 18 years later on and I've never needed to go to a doctor again. Yes. In fact, anything wrong I go to my homeopath.

Ty: So homeopathy is what you attribute to saving your life because you were sent home to die?

Gemma: Yes.

Ty: What particular homeopathic remedies did you use at that time?

Gemma: Oh, there were lots. I did lots. There were lots of detoxing ones. And then, for instance, I got to the point where I could barely get out of bed. Well, I couldn't get out of bed on my own, I needed to have help. And I couldn't even open up my eyelid, I would have to lift it with my finger. And then, I had to have a stick to walk with just to go to the toilet. I had to have a stick on there, and the balance was really, really bad.

Ty: And you were in your late 20s.

Gemma: I was 26.

Ty: So what did you—did you use your particular homeopathic to help those symptoms?

Gemma: Yes, she was doing great. And I said, "Look, If you could just to get my eyelids to work." And she gave me a particular remedy that really helped. And it went on and on and on.

Ty: Did you change anything about the way that you were eating at that point? Did you change your nutrition?

Gemma: Oh yes, a strict diet.

Ty: What does that mean?

Gemma: No dairy, no sugar. Sugar feeds cancer. Dairy can produce mucus. Mucus produces tumors, I was told. No E numbers. Eat organic food. Luckily, my dad had an organic garden, which was absolutely perfect. I didn't realize. I (inaudible - 10:52) things, snails. But it was absolutely perfect for me at that point.

Ty: That's really amazing that your dad had an organic garden, just for you.

Gemma: It wasn't for me.

Ty: It was for you, you just didn't know it, right?

Gemma: I know.

Ty: It was for you. That's awesome. So you changed your diet, eating organic. Did you eliminate anything that you had been previously eating, and did you change anything else about your daily routine?

Gemma: My daily routine—meant I was literally in bed. I couldn't do anything much. I mean, I could see about that far, and it was all fuzzy, and double vision, and so I couldn't read. I couldn't read a book, I couldn't watch TV. I was just lying there waiting to die.

Ty: So the brain tumors really affected your vision, as well.

Gemma: Yes.

Ty: In the 18 years since you began the homeopathic treatments have you had any contact with the doctors that told you there was nothing that they could do, that their treatments were making you worse?

Gemma: I called back two years later, I think. I had gone back to live in London. And I was furious, really, with them. Why hadn't they gotten back to me? They just said that was it, I think. Actually, my sister ran after them after they said, "Did I want to go to a hospice, etc.?" She ran after them and said, "Look, the family needs to know. How long have we got? What's the prognosis?" And basically, he said to me at the time, "Have a good Christmas." This was in October, and I was thinking—I realize now he was probably saying, "Because this is going to be your last one." He basically gave me about three months to live.

Ty: And have you seen him since then?

Gemma: I went back two years later. I was very proud about doing this because I could walk down the road on my own, get a bus, and get to the hospital on my own. And I told him to put it down to homeopathy. And it's in my notes, he puts it down to homeopathy. But he said it was remarkable recovery and he couldn't understand it. And then he turned round and he went to shuffle some papers and said, "Well, maybe it's a delayed effect from the chemotherapy."

Ty: Really?

Gemma: Really.

Ty: A delayed effect of the chemotherapy.

Gemma: This is two years since they said it was making me worse, and there is nothing more we can do. It's on my notes, his registrar said, "Gemma knows there are no other viable options for her." No other viable options. And I want to tell people, this is one of my missions, that there are other options to health.

Ty: Talk about some of the things that you incorporated in your treatment protocol in addition to the homeopathy and the changing of the diet. Was there anything else that you could share with people that you included as far as supplements or anything like that, specifically, that might help somebody that is watching that has been diagnosed?

Gemma: Well, I think organic food. I think, good water. I think you've done enough work on that, I'm not going to repeat all that. Getting out your issue, finding out your issue. If you go to a homeopathic practitioner, getting out your issues and sorting them out. If you're on your deathbed, whether you live or die—I thought, "Well, it's not fair, I want to go and do it." Maybe you could get your future, write it down, do a mind map, sort it out. I thought, "I haven't told people that I love them. I haven't told my dad I love him."

Because that was my way. I was very closed and I was embarrassed about saying things like that. So start telling people how you feel. Here's your dad, tell him you love him if you love him. So I always go for a big hug now and so it's not a problem now. Think about what you want to do. What's the thing? You don't want to die regretting you haven't done this, this or that. Make your plans now and get a future.

Ty: Live your life.

Gemma: Live your life.

Ty: Right? And you have, because now you're a homeopath, right?

Gemma: I didn't know about it, and of course, that's what I wanted to do. I wasn't happy with the job I was doing. I was doing admin work, and it was not really what I wanted to do. It's all waiting for something to happen, for some job to come up, or this to happen. And you've got to make your luck and go out there and do it.

Ty: So when did you go to school to become a homeopath? When did you decide to do that?

Gemma: It was about three years after that, and then I graduated in 2000.

Ty: So you've been a homeopath for 15 years?

Gemma: Yes.

Ty: That's awesome. Are you helping any cancer patients at this point?

Gemma: I am, yes.

Ty: I'm sure you are, with the testimony that you have.

Gemma: Well, I can't even say that, we're not allowed to say that. I'm helping people and they might have different ailments, and some people have this ailment or that one, and some people have cancer.

Ty: But you're not treating cancer, right?

Gemma: No, no, no, no. I treat the individual.

Ty: You treat the person.

Gemma: Because, say somebody has an illness—if there are three people here, right? You all have the same illness. I might give you all a different remedy, depending on your medical history, what you like to do, how you react to things.

Ty: So it's an individualized approach.

Gemma: Really holistic and individualized.

Ty: So that's very different than what you get with the conventional treatments for cancer. Because you get this kind of cancer, you're going to get X, Y, Z drug, just like everybody else. It has no individual protocol. I think that's part of the power of homeopathy.

Gemma: Yes, I think so.

Ty: What would be your message to a cancer patient that has been recently diagnosed that has gone to the oncologist who has said, "Hey, you're a dead man walking, you have three months"—what's your message to a cancer patient that might be watching?

Gemma: Well, for me, I can only say that I know what helped me and that was homeopathy. So I would recommend homeopathy and there are lots of other things that can help. And watch Ty's episodes to find out other things. I can talk more authoritatively about homeopathy.

Ty: Sure. Is there hope for a cancer patient that has been told they are going to die?

Gemma: Of course there is. They say, "Oh, you are giving false hope." Well, actually, I'd rather die with hope than without it. I'm not saying it's just hope, because it isn't. I would much rather die with hope than without hope.

Ty: And a lot of what the conventional treatments for cancer, or the conventional prognosis does is create despair, doesn't it?

Gemma: It certainly did with me, yes. Absolutely. People often don't call it cancer, they call it "the C" or "the big C."

Ty: They don't even want to say the word.

Gemma: No.

Ty: Talk about the effect that the belief and emotions might play in that, in light of the fact that we know that fear, stress, anger, all suppress the immune system.

Gemma: Exactly. So it is much better to be positive.

Ty: Do you think that has a big—

Gemma: A positive effect, of course.

Ty: Do you think that has something to do with somebody recovering? The positive mental attitude?

Gemma: Absolutely. Yes, it's one part. But then people will say, "Oh, it's just placebo." It's not placebo. Homeopathy can work on animals and children, and they don't know what…

Ty: There is no placebo effect with animals.

Gemma: No.

Ty: Or children.

Gemma: No.

Ty: Talk about that real quickly, because I wasn't even thinking about this direction, but with the epidemic that we have of children's cancer lately, why do you think that we have this huge increase in the numbers of children, even infants, that are diagnosed with cancer?

Gemma: Health can be for all sorts of reasons—bad health, it could be geopathic stress. You could be living under an electric pylon for the last ten days, or two years. It might affect you or it might not. Some people can have a bottle of whiskey a week and smoke 80 fags and it won't affect them, and they live to 110, or whatever. But some people, it will affect them. And so, it could be a geopathic thing, it could be a really bad diet. It could be a combination of things. It could be some awful emotional state of grief, or people they have loved and have died.

Ty: What do you mean when you say geopathic stress?

Gemma: Okay, things like mobile phones, computers, might affect some people rather than other people. It will affect some people and stay in the body, along with other things, as well—bad diet, bad water, all these horrible emotional things that might have happened to you.

Ty: So, once you free yourself of that baggage, whether it be emotional baggage or the toxic load, or the baggage that…

Gemma: All of it. You deal with all of it.

Ty: So there isn't a single magic bullet, then, to treat cancer.

Gemma: I don't know of it. If it was, I'd be a very rich lady.

Ty: Yes. A lot of different factors that you need to change, aren't there?

Gemma: Yes, that's why I think homeopathy is good because it looks at all aspects of it.

Ty: Well, Gemma, it has been a pleasure to interview you today. I'm really honored to be able to meet you after all these years. And I know that some of the things that you have said today are going to impact people that are watching, so really grateful to you for all that you are doing.

Gemma: Thank you, and I was very pleased to be here. And I don't mean just here, I mean living—to be here in this world.

Ty: I am glad you are living, as well, too, and I attribute it to the homeopathy and the other things that you did. And to getting out from underneath the umbrella of those conventional treatments that were killing you.

Gemma: Yes, thank you. ***[end of transcript]***

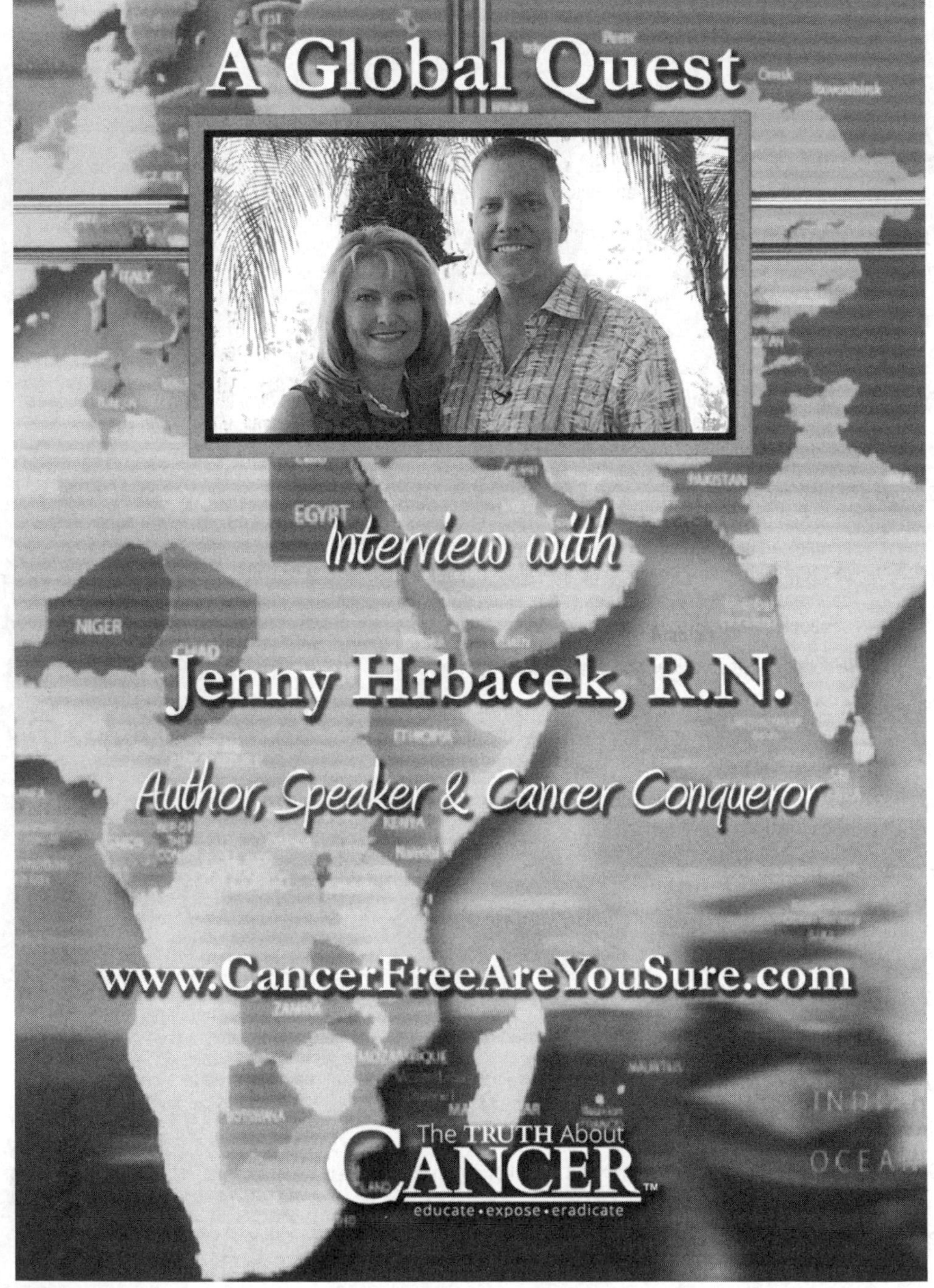
A Global Quest
Interview with
Jenny Hrbacek, R.N.
Author, Speaker & Cancer Conqueror
www.CancerFreeAreYouSure.com
The TRUTH About
CANCER
educate • expose • eradicate

THE TRUTH ABOUT CANCER

Ty: So Jenny, thank you for hanging out with me today.

Jenny: What a pleasure.

Ty: You're going to share your story with us, and last night you came up to me and you began to share the story. You're a breast cancer survivor. You've written a book on breast cancer. I'm going to just plug it here, this is amazing, *Cancer Free! Are You Sure?* Foreword by Dr. Gordon, Garry Gordon. A guide to early detection tests. Get tested and validate your "cancer free" status. Do not be a victim of cancer or experience recurrence. Stop cancer before it's unstoppable.

I love this title. I love the contents of this book. Thank you again. You gave me a copy of the book, but this is something that I want to get you to share because we've done these, *The Quest for the Cures*, last year and this is for the *Global Quest for the Cures* that this is a part of now. One of the most frequent questions that we got after last year's series is, "How can I detect cancer?" You know we preach against mammograms because they are ionizing radiation. We preach against a lot of these invasive testing methods, but we didn't really last year give people a lot of options of what they can do.

***Jenny*:** Right.

Ty: So tell us about your breast cancer diagnosis. You told me you were cured and then in remission when you weren't, and then the foundation of this book.

Jenny: Okay, I'll try and give you the short version, but the title of the book is called *Cancer Free! Are You Sure?* And the reason that I have that title is because people say to me, "Oh my wife or my loved one is cancer-free. They had clean surgical margins. The PET scan is clear. Everything's great." I look at them and I say, "Are you sure?" They look back at me. And I say, "Well, does your doctor want to see you in six months?" And they say, "Yes." I'm like, "Well are you sure that your doctor is sure?" So all of the sudden they're thinking, "Well, wait a minute. I thought I was cancer-free, but why does my doctor want to keep seeing me and checking me?"

Anyway I had received a diagnosis of breast cancer in 2009. I was a registered nurse, and I wanted it out as fast as possible. I went ahead quickly, did surgery, did lots of reconstruction, did everything. Then I decided I'm going to be involved with a breast cancer support group. Well, in the middle of that, at the first meeting we had about 60 ladies show up. I asked everyone to introduce themselves and tell a little bit of their history. In doing that I found that half the women in the room had had a recurrence.

I thought, "Okay, they had the same kind of cancer that I had, the same treatment I had and they're going through cancer now two and three times." I thought. "Do I have a target on my back? Something is not right." So, anyway, I thought, "Not me I'm going to figure this out. I've got to get out of these shoes." It's terrible to walk the halls of an oncology hospital. It's something that I don't want anyone to ever have to do.

Ty: There's no hope there is there?

Jenny: I would sit and watch people doing chemotherapy. I only did four rounds. There was a young man across the little—they call them a chemo suite and they have all these big lounge chairs like you're going to the movie. This kid across from me has a recurrent brain tumor. He's eating Nutter Butters. The lady across from me on the other side has on a nasal cannula with oxygen. I'm talking with her and that's because the Adriamycin has damaged her heart. She's having a hamburger and fries.

I look over at the snack machine, and it's full. It's not even what I would consider food. We need to change our thinking in America. We think food is one thing, and it's not really food. It's just that the package says it's, you know, food. Anyway so I was very upset so I decided I'm going to fix my immune system. That's when I went to Dallas because I think I had exhausted all my resources in Houston. I had fired two oncologists. One of them because I told him about his snack machine, he told me he was not in charge of the snack machine. So I said, "Well, you know what, I don't think you're going to be in charge of me either." I got up and walked out.

Ty: I love it.

Jenny: I was done, there's more to this story that you have to read in the book.

Ty: You know what? Doctors work for us and so if a doctor's doing that, just like you did, fire him and find somebody who knows what they're doing.

Jenny: Yes. So anyway, so I went to Dallas and I thought, "I'm going to go to this naturopathic guy. I'm going to build up my immune system, because if that's what faltered and somehow it let cancer grow and my body didn't recognize it, I don't ever want to go through this again." So when I went to see Ray Hammond. I don't know if anyone knows him. He's out of Rowlett, Texas.

Ty: I used to live in Rockwell so I know him. I know about Ray.

Jenny: Okay, it's a beautiful area there. He said, "Before we built up your immune system, let's make sure you don't have any cancer. I told him immediately, "Oh no, I'm cancer free. My PET scan is clear, I had clean margins, everything's good." "Well," he said. "Just humor me."

So he took some blood and he sent it to Research Genetic Cancer Center over in Greece to do what was called a CTC count, which is a circulating tumor cell count, which is what I now know why all those women had breast cancer and their breasts were cut off, in the trash can, that tissue was gone, because would have breast cancer come back in their liver, in their lungs or in their bones because any tumor over two millimeters has blood profusion. Those cells were circulating, and they took up shop in another place. I didn't know that and I was a registered nurse, I was trained.

Ty: But the surgery did nothing for the circulating tumor cells.

Jenny: All it did was make sure these women did not get cancer in the tissue that was thrown in the trash can. Ty, I said to all my doctors, "The only reason I'm doing this surgery is because I don't ever want to deal with breast cancer again." And no one ever corrected that misconception. I had to figure it out on my own.

Anyway at the same time my tumor markers had gone up a little bit. I had just finished chemotherapy, my hair was about this long. I was really attractive, if you can picture that. Anyway, my tumor markers went up so, with my second oncologist after I'd already fired oncologist number one, in Houston. She said, "Let's check a circulating tumor cell count test," and that one's through Cell Surge, which is a company subsidiary of Johnson & Johnson.

At the same time Dr. Hammond sent my blood for another CTC test to Greece and I really expected them all to be fine. Well, the tests came back from Research Genetic Cancer Center saying I had 14.2 cancer cells per 7.5 ccs of my blood. For a visual on that, If you took a little insulin syringe that's one cc and you put all my blood in insulin syringes, I would have over two cancer cells in every syringe.

All of a sudden my thought went back to that day in that breast cancer support group, and I thought, "I am just like those women. If I don't do something, I'm going to have these cells circulating. They're going to take up residence somewhere, and I'm going to have a metastasis and when that happens, it's stage four and it's dramatic, it's life threatening." Anyway so when that came back so he immediately starting me doing intravenous vitamin C and some poly MVA and curcumin and just all the great things that we know work.

Ty: All the things that have affected the immune system.

Jenny: I stayed in Dallas for a couple of weeks. I did that and I thought, "Oh gee, I've got this lab slip. I need to go back to Houston and get this other test because insurance was going to pay for that one." They will only pay for the Cell Surge test if you have an indicator that you have a metastatic lesion, a breast, colon, or prostate cancer. They will not pay for it if—you can't just go to your doctor and say, "I want a CTC."

Ty: So they'll only pay for it if it's too late.

Jenny: Exactly. I had asked oncologist number two, "What are we going to do if this comes back positive?" She said ,"We'll do a PET scan. We'll see where the cancer's at and we'll start more chemotherapy." I thought, "Oh my gosh." That's why I stayed in Dallas when my tests came back positive and got right on it. Her tests came back and the count was zero.

So she left room, you know how you have the little cubbies, they're so much fun to wait in and when she went out the room, I got on the phone and I called Dr. Hammond. I said, "Get Dr. Hammon on the phone. I'm in the oncologist office. They're giving me a zero here and I have a 14.2 from him. I need to know what's going on." He got on the phone before she came back in and he says, "Jenny, you've had five or six IV vitamin C's. You had a 65% apoptosis which is cancer death with IV vitamin C and we probably knocked it down below five. Their tests won't pick it up unless it's above five or it has metastasized to another organ."

So I thought, "Oh well." I was happy that we had gotten it down. She came back in. I showed her my RGC paperwork, and she didn't want to hear it. She says, "You do not have cancer." She says, "You are fine." She insisted I did not have cancer even though my tumor markers were elevated. So I said, "Okay, let me just make sure I understand you." I said, "What was my CTC when I came in and I had the original breast cancer that we can see on the PET scan?" She said, "We don't check that." I said, "What do you mean you don't check it? I had all kinds of tests. I mean you all were sticking me with needles and heart scans and nuclear scans and MRIs and blood tests, you didn't check this?"

She said, "No, we don't check it because it will not show cancer until it has metastasized to another organ." So I said, "So you're telling me it was zero when I was diagnosed and that I did have cancer and that you're telling me it's zero now and you're sure I don't have cancer." and her face was a little bit blank and she just said, "Well just go take a multivitamin, eat cupcakes and exercise. You're fine."

Ty: Eat cupcakes?

Jenny: Yes.

Ty: That's good advice, okay.

Jenny: So that was the end of oncologist number two. Through this whole journey I thought there's got to be more. So I found out about Best Answer for Cancer and I signed up to go to the conference. I did not know this was a conference mainly for physicians. And I showed up there and I'm sitting in a room with 200, 300 doctors and I see all these MDs, I'm like, "Where are the normal people?" There were not very many normal people, just people off the street.

I am a registered nurse, but I was there for my own personal benefit to try and learn. In the exhibit hall, I walked up to one of the tables and aid, "Hi." I said, "So what do you do?" They said, "We're Oncoblot and we have a test and we can find cancer years before it will show up on a PET scan." I'm like, "Really? Why isn't there a line here?" Why are people out here on the street with cancer and they should be in here. Go to the next booth, it's Red Drop and I said, "Tell me what you do." And they said, "Well we have a test and we can test for thymidine kinase. It's an enzyme that's put out when cancer cells replicate, and we can find cancer growing in you long before a tumor would ever show up on a PET scan." I'm like, "You're kidding me."

Ty: So there are two tests you know a bit about.

Jenny: Yes. So I go around the room and I run into Dr. Emil Schandl with American Metabolic Laboratories and I say, "Hi, what do you do?" and he says, "I have a CA profile and I can find cancer before you have to—you know before eight to 10 years because—" and Ty, I'm blown away. I'm thinking, "Why are people not in here? Why do people not know about this?"

At this point I had picked up your book, which is amazing, and I had picked up every cancer book I could find, and there was nothing that had a compilation. I ended up with nine tests in my book and I tell you how to get it, how much they cost. A lot of them you can get without a doctor's help. I tell you what to do when the kit comes, where to go to get the blood drawn.

Ty: Go through them real quickly, Jenny. Go through the nine tests.

Jenny: Okay.

Ty: You already mentioned Oncoblot and the Red Drop.

Jenny: Hand me my book here so I don't miss one. I have them all lined out here.

Ty: Yeah, let's go through them because I want to get all of these tests for the people that are watching.

Jenny: And I'm going to put on my glasses.

Ty: Sure.

Jenny: And then I want to tell you all about my ball because this is so critical. So critical to how we diagnose cancer today, in 2015. And I think it's a little bit archaic because we can find it early. People tell me, "You know, Jenny, I don't know that I would want to know that I had cancer early." I'm like, "Are you kidding me? Then do you go for a mammogram? Do you go for a PSA count? Obviously you do want to know."

Ty, the first thing that people ask their doctor when they're told they have cancer is, "Well how bad is it?" They want to know. Wouldn't it be a blessing to find out that you had cancer when it won't even show up on the PET scan? We're finding here today these doctors are saying it could take 10 to 20 years before the cancer will be bad enough to show up. We know from epigenetics that cancer is lifestyle-related. You can make some choices and changes and potentially never get that diagnosis.

Anyway, let me go over this. The CA profile plus is one. I even tell people who don't have a lot of money just a simple occult colon blood test you order on the internet, you drop it in the toilet with your stool and if changes colors, it shows that you have an invisible blot in your stool. A lot of times you can't see it, but that's just a sign of colon cancer. A lot of times people do a colonoscopy, but cancer is up in the small intestine. It's a simple test, $20 that you can order on the internet.

Ty: Okay.

Jenny: There's a test that I go over called the early CDT. It's a test for lung cancer. You do have to meet the criteria where you've had to smoke so many packs of cigarettes for so many years, but that one they will bill your insurance company for. There is coverage, or they'll bill Medicare Part B or I think. It's $150 just self-pay, but for people, who have been smoking, they're at high risk for lung cancer and you can't live without your lungs. So you know —

Ty: Can't cut it off.

Jenny: No and then I have—have you heard of Dr. Navarro?

Ty: Sure, the urine test.

Jenny: Right. You know, $55 for just his HCG test, which you know is a little controversial, but it's certainly a great indicator. You can buy the stuff that you need for it at the art supply, some acetone, coffee filters, alcohol and a spoon. You can get you a stamp to go to the Philippines at the post office. It does require a little effort, but I did it.

Another one I have is the nagalase test and that one's about $85. I tell you a lab where you can get that because nagalase is important. It shuts down the immune system and without that the cancer can go undetected. I talk about Oncoblot, which is the enox2 protein that's present. Cancer cells produce that and that test can tell you even what type of cancer it would be. I'm following a couple people now that have had a positive result and they're trying to convert that back to negative because their PET scans don't show anything.

Ty: Right, the Oncoblot is a great test. Several people have mentioned Oncoblot.

Jenny: Yes, but also I mean it's—so you get a positive Oncoblot and then you go down to MD Anderson, or I was at Texas Oncology, and your scan is negative, you can't dismiss this result because it might take 10 years for that cancer to get big enough. I'll explain why in a minute for it to show up on that PET scan. It doesn't just appear there that one day.

I tell people—this lady came by and talked to me today and she had a positive Oncoblot. She goes, "I'm so concerned." And I said, "Oh, my gosh you should be blessed because you're finding it way earlier than anybody else who goes the traditional route. The odds are that you can take some interactive measures and can stop the process or at least can significantly slow it down." Then I talk about getting a PAP and a HPV test, which those are usually covered by insurance and they do find cancer.

The Red Drop, which is your thymidine kinase and then I go into Research Genetic Cancer Center because they have the Oncocount and they do also the big Oncostat, which will tell you kind of like doing sensitivity testing or a culture if you have a bacterial infection. It'll tell you which chemo would work best for you, which you need to know. Chemo never kills all the cancer, but if you're going to take it, it will at least tell you ones that at that point in time worked better and which supplements your cancer responded to.

I did the RGCC sensitivity test for nutrients, and I got my count down from 14.2 to 5.5 in three months. Then in another three months down to 2.9. I did the things that my test showed and with cancer, as you know, not everything works for everyone. Everybody's a little bit different. But I give you a whole tool and then I have another 15 or 16 tests in this book that you can do or ask your doctor about that will indicate that there might be something happening in the body that could lead to cancer that you might want to correct like your hemoglobin A1C, keeping that low, your C Reactive protein, getting an energy meridian test and getting a spinal analysis.

You got to have good energy to those organs. That's pretty much what it is. I know I'm coming up against a huge industry and I really don't care because that—it's your option. You can wait for the cancer to be on the PET scan to show up or you can find it really early.

Ty: This is a great resource for people and this is great information that you've shared with us because now people are going to have a good, long laundry list of tests that they can use to diagnose cancer way earlier than the tests that we use.

Jenny: And Ty, if they've had it they can confirm they're really cancer-free and don't let a recurrence come back up because that's deadly. Ninety percent of circulating tumor cells that are left behind can, you get them...

Ty: And chemotherapy doesn't kill circulating tumor cells anyway.

Jenny: No, no it doesn't.

Ty: So tell me about pinhead here. This is scary. This is pinhead.

Jenny: These are my tennis balls. When I started on this journey my phone would ring and people would call me. I would never not answer the phone for a cancer patient, and I would end up spending two, three, four hours with people trying to explain. I thought, I have got to get through to them because they're like, "But my doctor wants me to have a PET scan." I'm like, "Do you understand what a PET scan is? Do you understand why the sugar is an issue?"

So I made these little tennis balls. These little—this is a cell, we're just going to pretend these are both cells. The little pins that I've stuck in, and I have 10 pins in this ball. These represent insulin receptors. We know that when we eat even a piece of whole wheat bread that it has as much glycemic rise as a little snickers bar, but we don't think about the bread as being sugar. That's a lot of us, me included, how we got into this situation, but you eat that, your blood sugar rises and the pancreas spits out some insulin, which opens these little doors so the sugar can get in the cell for energy. So the doctors use these—what happens is we run high blood sugars systemically as Americans, because of the standard American diet.

Ty: Because we eat a bad diet.

Jenny: Yes, and so the body, it doesn't like that. It doesn't like that high blood sugar because it burns your neurons, it messes with your vision, people get numb feet, their wounds won't heal. So the body's going to put more and more of these little receptors in to try and get the sugar out of the blood into the cell and so eventually you end up with this.

This is what a cancer cell looks like. A cancer cell, from my research, has 15 to 16 times the number of insulin receptors as a regular cell. So when you go for your PET scan, which in the United States, right now in 2015, the way that they diagnose cancer is with a positive PET scan or a biopsy. It takes years for the tumor to get to be at least half a centimeter so it will show up. So you go in for the test, they start an IV and they inject you with radioactive glucose.

Ty: Sugar.

Jenny: Yes, it goes around the body. You wait for about an hour in a little room by yourself because nobody else wants to be around you because you're radioactive. The radioactive glucose, the glucose will go to these insulin receptors and it goes into the cell and so then when they take your picture these cells light up.

Ty: It shows up.

Jenny: So you have to wait long enough for enough of these cells to grow, to absorb enough of that radioactive glucose to light up on the screen or you can do some other things and find cancer much, much earlier, but this is my little visual.

Ty: This is a great visual demonstration and this is a great visual demonstration as well for the fact that we've talked on and on during this miniseries about the fact that cancer cells love sugar. Look at all the receptors. Of course they're going to love sugar. They have all the receptors for it.

Jenny: Yeah and I—Jenny loves sugar too, but you know.

Ty: We all love sugar, and as Casey Gray she said last year, "We all love sugar, but it should be part of our fun foods that we eat occasionally and not a staple that we eat every meal." And unfortunately with our diet the way it is, we eat it every meal whether we know we're eating it or not because as you mentioned, these whole grains, the pasta meals, they convert to sugar.

Jenny: Oatmeal and cereal for breakfast, it's like starting your day with a bowl of sugar and I thought I was doing good, Ty. I would spend 20 minutes looking at the cereal boxes at the grocery store because I would want to pick the best whole grain cereal, you know, and I had no idea what I was doing.

Ty: Right.

Jenny: I hope to share that information with people because I don't want anyone, anyone to have to walk through the shoes that I've walked through and it's a journey.

Ty: You've shared it very concisely with us tonight, very clearly and I'm sure that this information's going to be very powerful to people who are watching it. It's going to empower them to know, you don't have to go for a mammogram, you don't have to go for a PSA test, you don't have to have a biopsy, you don't have to have a PET scan. There're a lot of other tests that are non-invasive that detect cancer a lot earlier.

Jenny: Right, when it's still curable and manageable. It doesn't have to be life changing.

Ty: Yeah, well, Jenny, this is great information, thank you so much.

Jenny: Thank you.

Ty: All right.

Jenny: Thank you. God bless.

Ty: God bless you too.

[end of transcript]

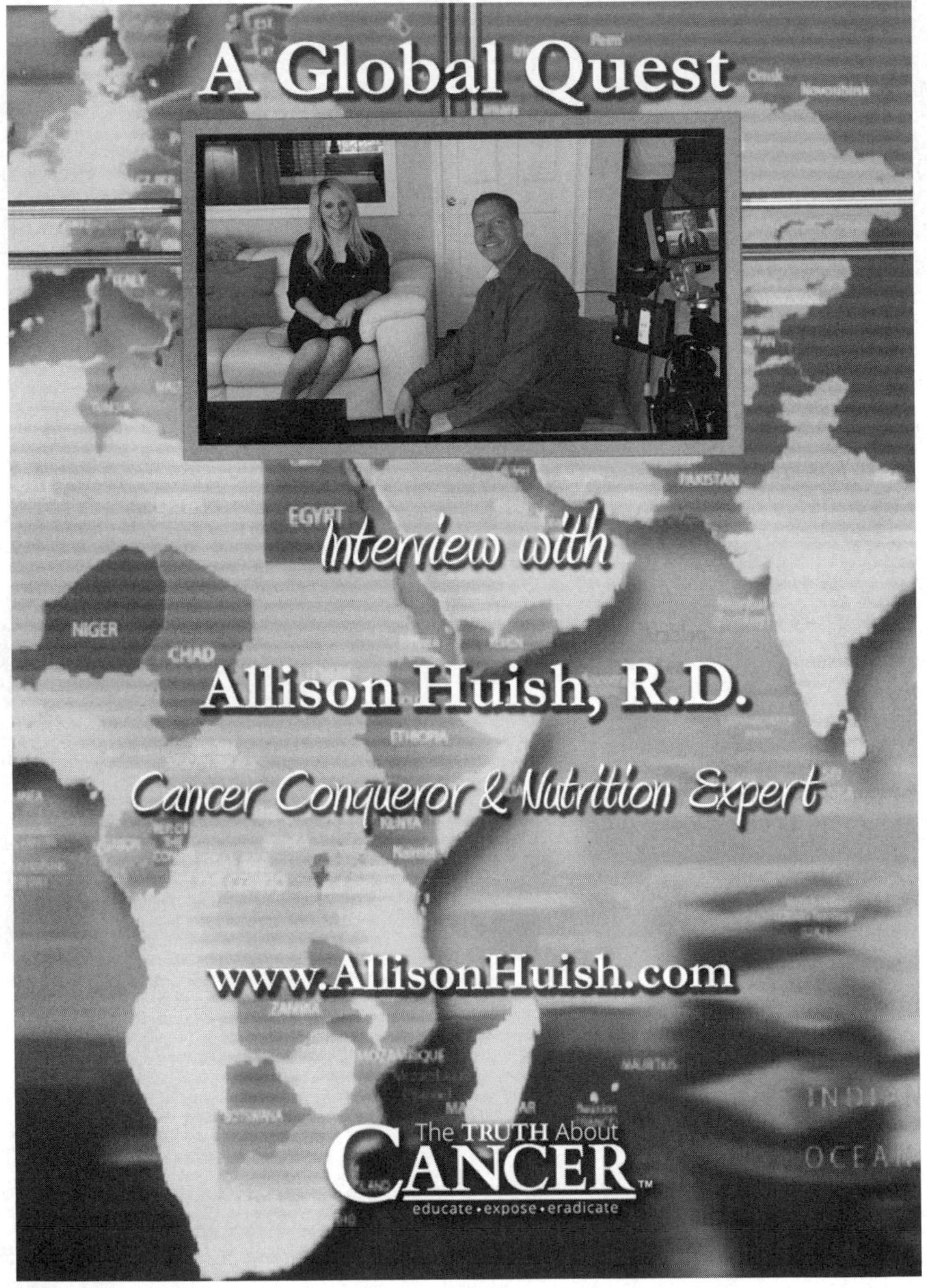
A Global Quest
Interview with
Allison Huish, R.D.
Cancer Conqueror & Nutrition Expert
www.AllisonHuish.com
The TRUTH About
CANCER
educate • expose • eradicate

Ty: I'm here just outside of Atlanta, Georgia today, with Allison Huish. She flew in from Arizona?

Allison: Yeah, Mesa, Arizona.

Ty: Thank you so much for being with us today.

Allison: Thank you.

Ty: So I really want to get your story today, of being healed from cancer. So let's go back several years ago to when you were a little girl. And if you could just share your story about the beginning of your health problems.

Allison: So my health issues are a little bit different than most people. Starting at age six, I started to have some noticeable health issues. From a young age, my head started to tilt just a little bit to the right. No one knew quite why that was going on. And then also, my hearing in my left ear just started to get progressively worse.

Then that kept going on for a few years. I also had stomach issues that started. So we couldn't figure out what was going on. It was very interesting. We went to a lot of different doctors. I was diagnosed with, you know, high acidic level, anorexia, bulimia, all of these things that were just very different.

Ty: And this is at what age?

Allison: This was about age seven to ten.

Ty: Okay.

Allison: Went to numerous doctors, and just nothing worked. We couldn't find answers. We were just frustrated. My health started to just go down. I got very, very skinny. Junior High I was probably about 70-80 pounds, just very, very skinny, very emaciated, eyes were bulging out.

But we couldn't figure out what was going on, and was very frustrated. So one of my appointments, at age 13, I went to go see a pediatric GI specialist, because I had all these stomach issues. I would wake up every morning and just want to almost throw up. It just was not comfortable.

So I went to go see a pediatric GI specialist, and she did the initial tests. She did the test follow my finger with your eye. And she went side to side, and then she went up and down. And she went up and down, and then she kept going up and down. And she did that many times, and I'm like, "Why? Why is she doing this? This is frustrating."

Well, what happened was, she noticed when I looked up, that my eyes were shaking a little bit. And she's like, "You need to go get an MRI, like right now." So she cleared her schedule. I went and got an immediate MRI that afternoon. Well, after my MRI, they made me sit in the waiting room for a long time. I couldn't figure out why. They wouldn't let me see my mom, they just made me sit there.

Ty: By yourself?

Allison: Yeah, by myself. They just said, "You have to wait here. We'll let you know when you can come out." And I was kind of worried to sit on that cold table, like what's going on here? Well, I walked out of the waiting room about an hour later to see my mom, who had just hung up the phone with tears in her eyes.

And she told me, she said, "Allison, you have a brain stem tumor." And I didn't know quite what that meant, at 13 years old, I just started Junior High School a couple weeks prior. But I knew at that moment that my life would be different from there on out.

So we immediately went to go see my doctor, to my pediatric neurologist, and he showed my parents what the tumor was. Basically it was a brain stem tumor, pilocytic astrocytoma is what it was, about the size of an egg, and it rested on my brain stem.

So that next day, I was scheduled for emergency surgery, and they were able to get rid of about half my tumor. Now the thing with tumors is, why mine was so serious, was because it's all about location.

It was right there with the brain stem, and you're toying with all the nerves, which explained why I had the head tilt, why I had the hearing loss, and why I had the stomach issues. Most people, when they have tumors, they have headaches and blackouts, and seizures. Mine were very different.

Ty: And the reason it was different was because it was a brain stem, and it was mixed in there with the nerve tissue?

Allison: Mm-hmm. It's just very different. It was all about the location, which was, you know, the gradual hearing loss. Because as my tumor was getting bigger, was pressing on that nerve, so I had the gradual hearing loss in that ear. So I had surgery, and they were able to get rid of about half of it.

But a large part of it was still inoperable due to the location. And so grateful for an amazing neurologist. He closed me up and said, "You know what? We'll take care of this later." So closed me up, sent me on my way, and I had an amazing recovery.

I went home about a week later, after being in the ICU at the hospital, and we began going home, and started looking for answers. You know, we had heard stories about people who had beat cancers naturally, beat tumors naturally, and we knew there was something out there.

Ty: Yeah.

Allison: So we began searching. We said, "What is it? What do those people do, that are doing these incredible things?" And I would say at the time we were an average healthy family, but we learned what nutrition does, and it was very interesting. My doctor told me, you know, "The calories count. If you'll eat pizza, if you'll eat ice cream," because I was very skinny, "Just get calories in you, whatever you'll take."

But in our research we learned how nutrition was so important. I needed to give my body good calories to help support good healthy weight gain, support the cells so I would function better.

Ty: And this was at the age of 13?

Allison: Yeah, at the age of 13.

Ty: What was the emotion of your family like at that point? What was the mental state?

Allison: Yeah, you know what? It was very interesting. It was hard because a lot of my family, they cared about me, but they didn't know what was going on. And so they were frustrated. So there was a lot of contention with the family, honestly. There was some because we couldn't figure out what was going on. So it was tiring.

It was very hard to be this young girl, and I see many people just fighting over what to do next for me. That was very hard to see at a young age. And then we started doing research on what to do.

And of course, many people were pushing us to go see our radiologist and go that direction. My mom and I, we did go meet with our radiologist. And I still to this day remember sitting in that room, the feelings that I felt in there.

Ty: What were they?

Allison: It was very cold. It was very cold. It was not what I wanted to do. And I actually left that appointment, and I grabbed my mom's hand, and I told my mom, "Mom, this isn't the process for me." And so she said she also felt the same way. But we left that radiologist's appointment knowing we needed something else. There has to be something else out there. Thirteen years old, just started Junior High School, radiation to the brain stem 15 years ago just didn't sound like a good thing for us.

Ty: Right.

Allison: So we started doing a lot of research on what to do, and that's where it came a lot with nutrition. We learned about giving the body a lot of greens, a lot of good calories, a lot of nutrition to help heal myself. Because I needed to gain weight, I needed to gain probably about 30-40 healthy pounds.

I needed to get rid of stomach issues. I wanted hair to grow back. All these things. And then we also kept doing research on what else can we do? And that's where we were really drawn to these essential oils. They kept coming across in a lot of our research. We noticed how essential oils did incredible things.

There's medical studies out there showing what essential oils can do. And in particular, with the essential oils, we were really drawn towards frankincense essential oil. I love frankincense oil. It's a very powerful oil. I think there's a reason why it's called liquid gold, or why it's one of the oils that the Christ child was given.

It's a very, very precious oil. So we did our research, and we came across the oils, and frankincense oil, and all of these studies pointed towards what these oils could do, how they could boost white blood cell count, how they could help bring oxygen into the cell, how they helped balance the cell.

I'm a very science-based person. I loved reading about that, and I found that all my research about either nutrition or essential oils pointed towards healing the cell. And so that became my goal. My goal became giving the body lots of oxygen. It became getting the body to an alkaline state.

So I used a lot of oils. I used a lot of frankincense oil. I also used clove oil, because clove oil's a very oxygenating oil. I also used a lot of digestive enzymes, things to support the cell. But primarily, as far as oils, I did the frankincense oil and the clove oil.

Ty: And how did you take it? Did you ingest it, or did you rub it on your skin? Or did you do the aromatherapy? How did you do that?

Allison: You know, it was really interesting how we did it. So I did do it back here where my scar is, but I don't know how effective that was, because you do have a very thick skull. But one way that I did, and this was probably the way that I was most consistent is, I would put a drop of frankincense oil on my tongue, and raise the tongue to the roof of my mouth.

And I did that probably about every two hours. Because I figured, hey, that's probably the closest way I can get to my brain stem without interfering with bones, or things like that.

Ty: And a lot of blood vessels there too, to absorb.

Allison: Mm-hmm.

Ty: Right.

Allison: A lot of blood vessels, so just a lot internally. I did some on the reflexology points, bottoms of my feet. But the primary way was on internal through my tongue. So I did that about every couple of hours. And what happened was actually quite incredible. So I started to gain health pretty quickly. Like I said, I started Junior High School and I was diagnosed three weeks later. So I came home and started to regain health after my surgery. I was able to start school again with my peers the next semester.

Ty: Great.

Allison: And that was pretty incredible.

Ty: That's quick for a brain tumor.

Allison: You know what? It was interesting. I was only in the hospital for about a week and a half. Most people are in there for about six weeks. But once I had my tumor, we started on good nutrition, we started on oils. And I just had an amazing recovery. So I was able to graduate with my peers on time. And that was huge. I was able to regain strength, regain health. So what happened with my tumor is that my tumor basically started to do what tumors aren't supposed to do. Tumors are supposed to get fuzzy, supposed to spread, and get bigger.

My tumor started to do the opposite of that. My tumor started to encapsulate, that's what my doctor told me. He's like, "It looks like it's encapsulating." It started to come together and like whole, you know pull apart, where it had little fingers before, started to pull together. And then, over time, it would just start to slowly shrink. And it was really interesting. I would go see my neurologist every six months, and I'd have MRIs done. And he would have to look at the dates very closely, because he thought he had them backwards.

Ty: Because it was shrinking instead of growing?

Allison: Because it was shrinking. He's like, "Wait. Do we have these backwards?" He wasn't quite sure what was going on. And so he always told me, "Allison, you're doing awesome. Keep doing what you're doing, and we'll see you in six months." And so I would go see him for about every six months.

Ty: For how long?

Allison: That took about three years.

Ty: Okay.

Allison: It took about three years. I would go see him. But every time I would go see him, it just slowly was improving. It wasn't dramatic, overnight. It was a slow, gradual process. But it took about three years. Then I remember the point where I went to go see my neurologist and he told me, "You have no more tumor."

Ty: Really?

Allison: "It's completely disintegrated."

Ty: What did you feel like at that point?

Allison: You know what? Words can't describe it. It was just like such an emotional relief. You know, I had been praying, and I wanted my tumor to go away. I was like, I need another chance at life.

Ty: Yeah.

Allison: And so, when those words were said, it was invigorating. It was like I had a new life again.

Ty: Alright.

Allison: You know, I wanted to go to college. I wanted to become a registered dietician. I wanted to tell people my story. And when I was told those words, it was like, "This happened."

Ty: And that was at the age of 16 then?

Allison: That was about, yeah, the age of 16, 17.

Ty: Okay.

Allison: That's when that happened.

Ty: Great.

Allison: So, ever since then, my health has just been improving with what happened. But I'm just so grateful for essential oils, for what we learned as far as diet, as far as just taking care of your body, to know that you can heal it.

Ty: How many years ago was this?

Allison: So, I'm 28 right now. I was diagnosed 15 years ago. So about 12 years ago. I remember the point where I also hit my five year mark of being completely tumor free, because that five year mark is where it's kind of written off your record. And I remember hitting the five year mark, knowing that the tumor's not coming back.

I got personal confirmation, but I have the medical tests to show that this is something that's done. So to this day I still take my essential oils daily. I'm a very big believer in frankincense oil every day. But I'm grateful for what they did, and I credit them for being the reason why I'm here. You know, I didn't do anything consistent throughout my tumor process except for essential oils.

So I will never know, you know, did oils cure it 80 percent, 90 percent, 20 percent? I'll never know that guarantee. But I know that was the only thing I was consistent in. So that is why I love them, why I'm a very big fan of them.

Ty: That's awesome. What an inspiring story. So what would your message be to people that are watching today that are cancer patients? What would your message be to them?

Allison: You know, my big message I try and let people know, is that realize there are options out there. I get almost frustrated or sad when someone goes to their doctor and gets a prognosis, and they accept it. And they say that this is just what's going to happen. I'm going to pass away, or this disease is going to progress.

And I want to tell them no. There are answers out there. There are many people online like yourself, my story, that have had experiences that are willing to help. So my message to people is, don't accept one answer to be the answer. If it's not an answer you like. If you want to live and live an awesome life, there are answers, there are solutions out there.

Ty: And you're living proof of that.

Allison: Well, thank you.

Ty: Yeah, well what an inspiration, Allison. Thank you so much for sharing with us today.

Allison: Thank you for letting me come here.

Ty: May God bless you.

[end of transcript]

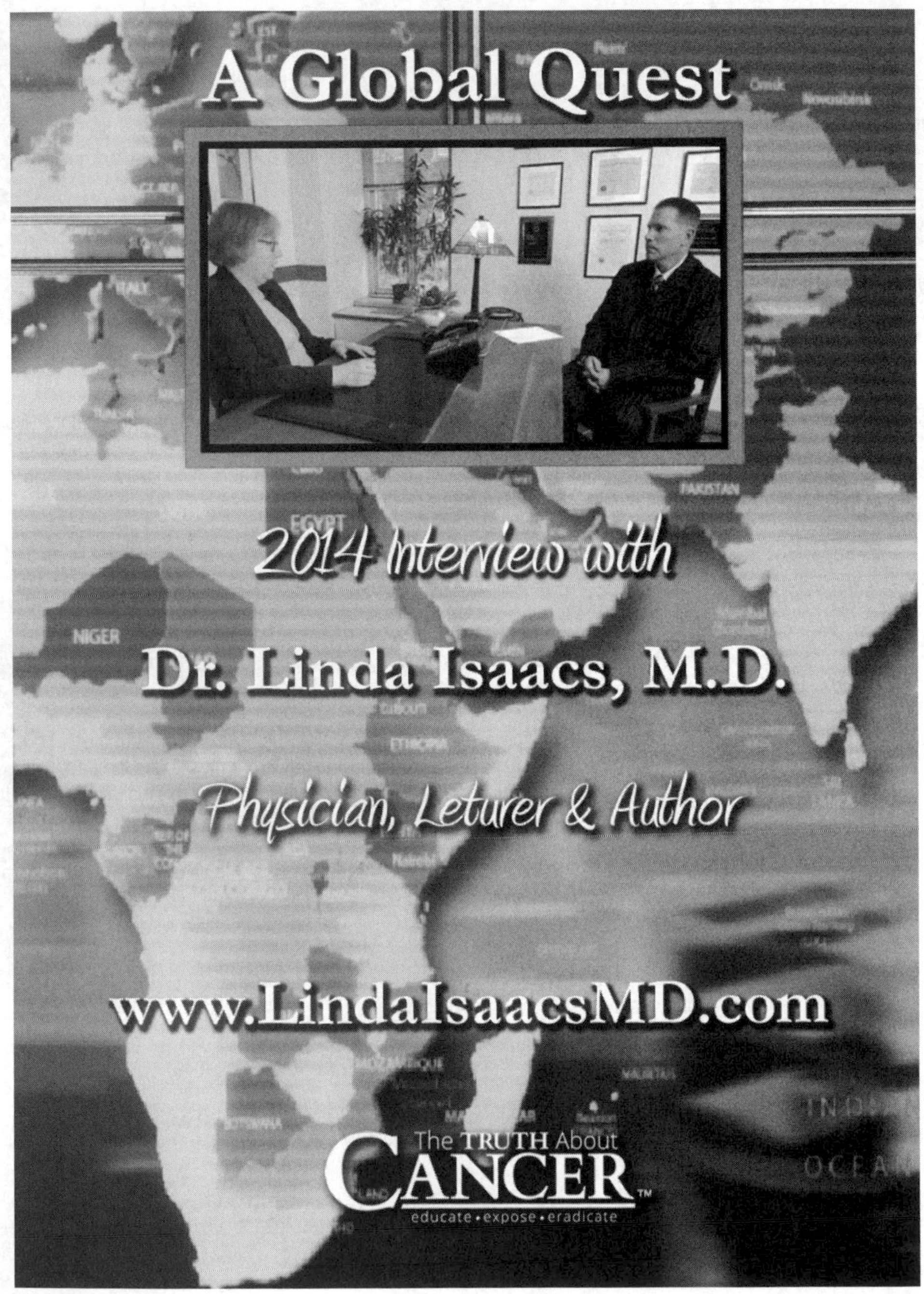
A Global Quest
2014 Interview with
Dr. Linda Isaacs, M.D.
Physician, Leturer & Author
www.LindaIsaacsMD.com
The TRUTH About
CANCER
educate • expose • eradicate

Ty: I am here today in New York City. And it is my privilege to interview Dr. Linda Isaacs. Thank you so much for being with us, doctor.

Dr. Isaacs: It is a real pleasure being here. Thank you.

Ty: So tell our listeners, our viewers, a little bit about yourself; how you got into the medical field.

Dr. Isaacs: Well, I started off mainly interested in science and math. And I went to college thinking I was going to be an engineer. But what I found was that engineering was not as interesting as I thought it would be. Meanwhile, my older sister is a physician. And I worked in a lab where she was working for a couple of summers in my early years in college. I found that much more interesting. So I took a college level biology class and from there I got interested in biochemistry and eventually applied to medical school. So that is how I got into the medical field. Now I would have thought, I was expecting to be just a general internist more or less mainstream physician so to speak. And I actually have the training. I am board certified in internal medicine. But I had always had some openness to the concept of alternatives that are out there. And partly because of my mother, she had always been interested in nutrition. And it turns out in talking to her and just in the last few years that her grandmother was the local herbal medicine person in her corner of West Virginia.

Ty: Oh really?

Dr. Isaacs: Yes. So perhaps an interest in alternative and less mainstream approaches goes way back in my family, who knows? But when I was in medical school, when I was doing my internal medicine rotation, was when I met Nick Gonzales, who is one of the other folks you are interviewing for your series, and who is a doctor that I work with now. So I learned about the research he was doing and that got me interested in pursuing this line of work myself.

Ty: Now how long have you been working with Dr. Gonzalez here?

Dr. Isaacs: Well, one way or another we have been working together since nineteen eighty five. In terms of this particular office space we have been in here for a little over twenty years.

Ty: Wow. Now this documentary miniseries that we are doing is really focused on cancer, of course.

Dr. Isaacs: Yes.

Ty: So just go back—let me go back to a basic question: what is cancer?

Dr. Isaacs: Cancer is a condition where some cells in the body are no longer responding to the signals that tell them when to quit. In other words, most cells that have a purpose for developing, they develop to a certain point and then they stop. Cancer cells keep reproducing. So they keep growing and they can spread to other places. That is what is called a metastasis. So cancer cells have escaped the normal controls for regulation and how big a bunch of cells is supposed to become.

Ty: So what might be some of the reasons that these cells have lost their regulatory mechanism, I guess for lack of a better way to put it?

Dr. Isaacs: Well hmm, that is a huge question, actually. That is the sort of thing that molecular biologists could give you an answer that could go on for hours. And I am not—most people, including myself, probably could not understand more words than—than one word in ten out of it. But what we believe is that cancer cells actually originate from cells that are there for a reason, to provide replacement cells for the body, stem cells as they are called. And that some of those stem cells come—they are no longer regulated because the body is not making enough of the thing that keeps them regulated, which is pancreatic enzymes. The underpinnings, the background, of what we are—the approach that we take and that theory actually is more than a hundred years old. It comes from the work of a Dr. John Beard who noticed the similarities between what is called the trophoblast, the early stages of the placenta, and cancer cells. Now trophoblast cells have a purpose in the body. They are part of the embryo that creates a new human being.

And cells similar to that trophoblast have a purpose in our body that create the replacement cells for instance, our skin, our intestinal tract replaces itself quite rapidly and we need that to happen. But if those cells are no longer under the regulatory control then they can turn into a cancer like a skin cancer or a colon cancer. What we think is that the regulation is really pancreatic enzymes. So if for whatever reason a person is not making enough of those enzymes to keep the stem cells under control you can wind up with a cancer.

Ty: Now here—here is a question that I am not sure if you are prepared to answer or not. And if you are not we will just cut it. But it deals with HCG. That is something I read about HCG, the pancreatic enzymes, and something that happens in the placenta at eight weeks.

Dr. Isaacs: Yes.

Ty: So Dr. Isaacs, I have ready something in the literature about the relationship between HCG and the placenta and then something that happens around two months or eight weeks in the pregnancy. Can you—do you know what I am talking about? Can you expand on that?

Dr. Isaacs: Well, HCG is something that is made by the trophoblast, the early stage of a placenta. And the reason it is made is that it stimulates progesterone to be made by the body to help maintain the pregnancy. So HCG, though, is very specific to trophoblast types of cells. And what happens at around eight weeks with the trophoblast is that there comes a point that, the early stages of the trophoblast, the goal is to invade into the uterus, to create that solid attachment. But if it kept going like that indefinitely it would eat through the uterus and kill the mother. And that is no good for either the mother or the baby. So there is a point at which the trophoblast stops working its way in and becomes a more mature organ but not penetrating more deeply into the uterus, just kind of maturing, so to speak. That happens at around fifty-seven days which, if my math has not deserted me here in the moment, is roughly the eight week period you are talking about.

Now so HCG is something that is specifically made by the trophoblast and it picks up so that progesterone can continue to be made. So some people have looked to see whether HCG is present in various cancer cells, and actually it is in a wide variety of different cancer cells. It is not something that you would predict if you are not taking into account the trophoblast as the origin of cancer.

Ty: Now is it also at about that same time—doesn't—isn't it at that time that the trophoblast, the placenta, begins to produce its own pancreatic enzymes? Does that happen about the same time?

Dr. Isaacs: It is when the baby starts making pancreatic enzymes. In other words, the growing fetus, which is by this time differentiated from the placenta. The placenta is eventually going to be sloughed off and not part of the finished product, so to speak. So when the baby starts making pancreatic enzymes is when the trophoblast changes its character.

Ty: I see.

Dr. Isaacs: And one of the big questions, of course, is why does a baby need to make pancreatic enzymes. And this happens very early in development. Nature tends to be pretty conservative. In other words, the lungs are not ready to go until the last month or two because the baby is not breathing. But here the baby is making pancreatic enzymes and yet in classic physiology we are taught that pancreatic enzymes are only good for digesting food. But here the baby is making them really two months into the development. But it would make all kinds of sense if the purpose for those pancreatic enzymes was to control the growth of the trophoblast. Because again, uncontrolled growth is no good for the baby and no good for the mother because it would kill the mother.

Ty: So then based on that presupposition or that deduction from the given facts, it seems only logical that the treatment that you and Dr. Gonzales are currently using, the pancreatic enzymes, which was based on the work of Dr. Beard and then Dr. Kelly, that is why it might work. That might be the mechanism by which it works.

Dr. Isaacs: That is what we think, yes.

Ty: Talk about the work of Dr. Kelly. We have already interviewed Dr. Gonzales a little bit about it, but talk about the work of Dr. Kelly and how that has impacted your career.

Dr. Isaacs: Well, when I met Nick Gonzales he was investigating Dr. Kelly's work. And so much of what I would have to say is in effect taken second hand. I mean, I met Dr. Kelly myself. But much of Nick's work was done before I actually came on the scene, so to speak. But on the other hand I could say that the data that Nick was collecting was part of what got me convinced that this is the direction I needed to go because it was compelling data and there was nobody else but Nick and me to follow up on this. Dr. Kelly was an orthodontist by training. And he got into cancer treatment because he himself got very, very ill with what was almost certainly pancreatic cancer.

Now this was in the early sixties so there were no CAT scans and the only way to make a biopsy was to do an operation. And so many times pancreatic cancer was diagnosed by autopsy in that day and age because there was no reason to take somebody to the operating room to prove an academic point when everyone could tell that they were sick and on their way to death. So Dr. Kelly had lost enormous amounts of weight. His report had a mass sticking out of his abdomen. And his doctor said looks like pancreatic cancer. And he had four young children. He had a lot of reasons to live. He was actually in his late thirties, early forties, something like that. So he was very motivated to try to figure something out. Apparently the first thing that happened was, his mother came to visit, and threw out all his junk food because he had—he was a dentist, an orthodontist. He knew all about nutrition he just was not doing it.

She threw out all his junk food and he stabilized but still was not doing too well. Then he added on pancreatic enzymes in an effort to help his digestive problems, because like many patients with pancreatic cancer, he was having enormous difficulty just digesting his food, a lot of gas, et cetera. So he took large amounts of pancreatic enzymes. And then he started taking them in between his meals and found that the character of the tumor seemed to be changing. So based on that he did a little investigating and found out about the work of Dr. Beard. But he noticed a change in the tumor sticking out of his abdomen when he himself started taking large doses of pancreatic enzymes. So the pieces of his treatment program came together bit by bit. He found that as he took more and more enzymes he started to feel bad. And he discovered that coffee enemas could help him feel better. So the idea there is that the enzymes as they do their work create waste materials, the coffee enemas help get rid of those.

And what happened was that bit by bit, with good quality food, with the pancreatic enzymes, and with the coffee enemas, he got better. Because he got better, that meant that people, word of mouth being what it is, there was no internet back then but people still heard, and people started coming to him. So bit by bit his practice changed from people who wanted their teeth straightened to people who wanted their cancer straightened out. And he collected more and more cases of people that should have been dead that were still alive and doing well after many, many years. That is when Nick came on the scene and started doing the research to collect the data to try to move forward in terms of documenting this particular approach.

Ty: Now the numbers that I have read, and we interviewed Dr. Gonzalez, he said he personally looked through I think ten thousand cases.

Dr. Isaacs: Right.

Ty: But the numbers I read is that, in total, Dr. Kelly had in excess of thirty thousand documented cases of different types of cancers. And it was an excess of a ninety percent, I think, five year survival rate with those thirty thousand plus cases. That—that is pretty amazing.

Dr. Isaacs: That is. I cannot really comment on the accuracy of those statistics. But he certainly had enormous numbers of patients who were doing well when they should have been gone.

Ty: Right. One of the stories that Dr. Gonzalez told us was about a woman with pancreatic cancer that is now alive thirty-two years out from diagnosis.

Dr. Isaacs: That is correct, yes.

Ty: Now that is something that, if it had happened with conventional medicine, it would have been on every newspaper, every TV show, but nobody has heard about it. So that leads me to this next question. In nineteen seventy one President declared a war on cancer.

Dr. Isaacs: Yes.

Ty: Are we winning the war on cancer?

Dr. Isaacs: I think cancer is definitely holding its own in this war. I mean, I am an orthodox trained physician, so I do not want to totally discount what progress has been made. And what I would say, though, is that people smoke less is a huge blow in the war against cancer, but it has got nothing to do with its treatment. It has to do with people changing their habits. And I think that colonoscopy, for example, I would definitely encourage everyone to get that, because it can find early stage colon cancer and it can remove polyps that can turn into colon cancer. There has been progress made in childhood leukemia, for example, or testicular cancer. There are a number of cancers that the war has had some effect. But for the major killers of adults, which would be lung cancer, colon cancer once it is metastatic, breast cancer once it is metastatic, prostate cancer once it is metastatic, pancreatic cancer, really have not gotten much of anywhere I am afraid.

Ty: One of the staples in your protocol to treat cancer is nutrition.

Dr. Isaacs: Correct, yes.

Ty: Can you talk about the importance of nutrition in treating cancer? Why does it play such a big role?

Dr. Isaacs: Well, part of the issue with the work that we do is that as patients take the pancreatic enzymes, and the enzymes work on the body, you need the body to be as strong as possible to handle that whole process, because a lot of waste materials are formed. And if you are eating, in effect, a lot of things that need to be processed and gotten rid of, like pesticide residues, or sprays or waxes or chemicals, those sorts of things, we think that that just puts an extra load on the body to process and deal with that kind of thing. So you need good quality food to be able to have the energy to fight the cancer and to get rid of the waste materials as the enzymes work on cancer. And certainly I think that nutritional issues can have a big part of why people get cancer in the first place. So it does not make sense to think that an illness created by a lifestyle can be managed without modifying that lifestyle. In other words why would you want to go back to the same lifestyle that got you to where you did not want to be? You need to make some changes and diet has a big part to do with it.

Ty: I love that. I love the quote about why would you want to go back to that lifestyle. If you have got a disease that is caused by these lifestyle issues, do not go back to where you came from. It reminds me of a recent communication that I had from a cancer patient that had changed the diet, had done all these things, and then went back and ended up—this was an email from a relative that the cancer patient had died. And it was—it is really sad to see that they had successfully reverted the cancer, cured the cancer, whatever you want to call it, the cancer, they were not being affected in a negative way from the cancer. And then they went back to their old eating habits, went back to their old lifestyle habits, and the cancer came back.

And that is a common thread that I have seen over my years of research and I am guessing that that is a common thread that you have seen as well.

Dr. Isaacs: Unfortunately, yes, but as much as I can, I try to focus on the patients that do follow through because those are—that is how you can see what is possible. All I can do is give people the tools; they have to choose to pick them up and keep using them.

Ty: Kind of like the difference in—biblically speaking, between knowledge and wisdom. Knowledge is knowing it, but not necessarily applying it. Wisdom is when you apply it.

Dr. Isaacs: Right, right.

Ty: So we want to be wise with this knowledge that we are obtaining on cancer and apply it to our lives.

Dr. Isaacs: Exactly.

Ty: Yes. So Dr. Isaacs in, I guess, September this last year, we both had the privilege of speaking at a conference in Atlanta. And I was able to speak to a patient of yours that is a pancreatic cancer survivor of thirteen years.

Dr. Isaacs: That is right.

Ty: Can you talk a little bit about her? I will mention her name, Sarah Cooper, and talk about the treatment protocol that you have used with Sarah to be out thirteen years with pancreatic cancer which is supposed to be a death sentence.

Dr. Isaacs: Right. Well, she was originally diagnosed in the fall of two thousand. She had been having some digestive issues, and then she started losing a lot of weight. And she was not trying to lose weight. So she lost the weight. She was having these digestive issues. And she went to see her primary care physician, whom I have to give a lot of credit to for instantly doing a CAT scan. Now the symptoms for pancreatic cancer can be kind of vague, in other words, digestive problems. A lot of people have digestive problems and most of them do not have pancreatic cancer. But when you add in weight loss, that becomes the signal that it is time to do a scan. And her doctor jumped on it. And she was found to have a mass in the pancreas.

So a few months later, it took a little time, I think people were telling her she should get surgery and that is what they were advocating, but she was not too keen on that idea. So eventually she did, though, get a needle biopsy which showed that she had a poorly differentiated adenocarcinoma which is another way of saying it was really bad news. And there are different types of pancreatic cancer, so just to be absolutely sure, the hospital sent the slides on to an expert at the Mayo Clinic, who also looked at them and said, yes, this is pancreatic cancer. It is the adenocarcinoma, the nasty kind. So they once again suggested that she really should have surgery. But she had done her research. She is a very smart woman. And she had checked into how well surgery works for pancreatic cancer.

Now surgery can be curative. But even when they think they can cure it, in other words when they do all the scans there is no evidence of spread in terms of CAT scans and the like, and they go in and they do the surgery, it is a big procedure. Some people die from the procedure itself. And only twenty-five percent of the people that have that operation are in fact cured by it. The other seventy-five percent wind up having a recurrence. So Sarah's gut feeling was, this is not a good idea. She did not want to have the surgery. And so she wound up actually applying for a clinical trial that we were engaged in at that time. She was told that she was ineligible for it because, oddly enough, she could have surgery. And so they felt very strongly that she could have the surgery so therefore she could not be in the trial which was only for people who could not have surgery.

Ty: I think I follow that illogic...

Dr. Isaacs: Now her feeling on that was, that she was choosing not to get the surgery, so why then was she different than other people that could not have it for whatever technical reason. But regardless, that was their decision, a strange decision, but that was done. So she wound up going on our program off the protocol, so to speak. And what she was advised to do then, the nuts and bolts of the program for her, large doses of pancreatic enzymes, some other supplements that are designed to help support the body as she fought against the cancer, and a diet. In her case it was predominantly vegetarian, although it does include eggs and fish, some dairy products. And the coffee enemas, other detoxification routines. So that is the program that she was on which she has implemented over the last thirteen years now.

Ty: Quite an impressive lady, too, by the way.

Dr. Isaacs: Yes she really is.

Ty: Let me ask you this, Dr. Isaacs, what would you recommend to people that are watching this that do not have cancer that are wondering what can I do to lessen my chances, to prevent cancer? What are good basic steps that a medical doctor like yourself would give to try to prevent cancer? Because if I were diagnosed, let me tell you, I would be calling you and Dr. Gonzalez.

Dr. Isaacs: Yes.

Ty: But I do not want to be diagnosed. And people that are watching this, if they do not have cancer they do not want to be diagnosed. How can we prevent it?

Dr. Isaacs: Well, a few very basic things would be do not smoke. One would like to think that would be obvious but there are still people out there that are smoking. So if you smoke, stop, no matter what it is that you are smoking, whether it be tobacco or something else, stop smoking it. Secondly I do recommend colonoscopy like I said earlier. It can get rid of the polyps that are early stage. The thirdly, eat a healthy diet. What do I mean by healthy? I mean whole grains, organic food, unprocessed food, freshly prepared food, raw food as much as you can. Beyond that I really cannot be too specific because we believe that different people need different things. So there are some people that thrive on a more vegetarian diet and there are other people we think actually do need some red meat in their diet. Most people, with the exception of sugar, which we all like and none of us should eat, most people are pretty much attracted to the foods that are good for them, I believe.

And so usually when I see someone who would fit into our meat eater model, the people with things like melanoma, leukemia, those types of illnesses, when I tell them that they can eat red meat they are so happy. If I had to eat the diet that I was giving them I would probably feel sick because I cannot eat that much red meat and feel well. But that is not my metabolism. I need something different. So I think, vegetable juice I think is good for everyone. I they think that having that on a daily basis is very helpful. And beyond that it would start to be different for different people so that is about as extensive as I can get.

Ty: No, I appreciate that. But what I am hearing you say is that it is an individualized approach but there are some basic guidelines. Like one thing I did not hear you mention is eating processed foods. So you are not recommending anybody go out and increase their uptake of processed foods that have a shelf life of eight billion years, whatever it is.

Dr. Isaacs: That is correct. And I would certainly say to avoid the unpronounceable ingredients.

Ty: Yes, I cannot remember who it was that I was interviewing, but he said that if there are more than five ingredients that you cannot pronounce in this list of ingredients, do not buy it.

Dr. Isaacs: Right.

Ty: Because he said, even he as a medical doctor, he understands what they mean, some of them he still does not know what they mean. So a layperson, you do not want to buy things that you do not know what you are eating.

Dr. Isaacs: Exactly, yes.

Ty: Now concerning Sarah Cooper, one of your patients, pancreatic cancer patient that is thirteen years out, conventionally speaking, though, pancreatic cancer is not curable.

Dr. Isaacs: That is correct.

Ty: Why in your opinion is it so difficult to treat pancreatic cancer conventionally? Not with your protocol because you have had a great success, but conventionally.

Dr. Isaacs: Well, what I would say there, is that most of the solid tumors as they are called, the adenocarcinomas, once they become metastatic, if surgery is not going to be curative, then perhaps a little progress has been made, but they are not curable. Again, lung cancer, colon cancer, breast cancer, once it is metastatic, prostate cancer, all of the adenocarcinomas, once they have spread you cannot cure them. So what I would say is that standard medicine has not figured out what the trick is for that. We think, again, it's pancreatic enzymes, but that is a different discussion. Pancreatic cancer can also be difficult, because the cells in that can tend to create a lot of scar tissue around themselves sometimes which can make it hard for any kind of treatment to get into the cells. They kind of wall themselves up in scar tissue. So that can create some challenges potentially.

Ty: Here is something that I have heard, you tell me what you think of this. This is just a theory that I have heard about pancreatic cancer, is that one of the reasons that it is harder to treat is because since the pancreas is affected, the production of the proteolytic enzymes, the quantity has been decreased. And so then with other cancers, let us say you have lung cancer, the pancreas is still secreting those enzymes. Maybe not to the level that it should but it is still secreting. But when that organ of itself is affected then you have got even less secretion of the pancreatic enzymes. Have you heard that? Is that—?

Dr. Isaacs: That would make some sense. But what I would say just abstractly, lung cancer can be just as aggressive and just as deadly. Lung cancer, pancreatic cancer, either one of those do not really get as much attention as they deserve in many ways in the mainstream world, because people pass away from them, as opposed to breast cancer, where many people are surgically cured but they are still a force out there going on the walks for raising research dollars and et cetera. So lung cancer can be just as aggressive.

Ty: What do you think about the effect of environmental toxins on the cancer equation? When I say environmental toxins, you mentioned pesticides earlier, so we have got these toxins that are on our food. We have toxins that we are breathing in the air. We have electromagnetic frequencies that are, according to some, toxic to the energy of our body, the frequencies of our body. What is your opinion on the impact of environmental toxins on cancer?

Dr. Isaacs: Well, I think all of those things certainly—environmental chemicals, for example, farmers have been shown to have higher incidence of lymphoma, a type of cancer. I believe the same thing is true for dry cleaners or people that live in a building where a dry cleaning establishment is. Bladder cancer has been associated with different types of industrial chemicals. I think for all of us, though, and we live in a world that is kind of a low grade soup of a lot of different chemicals. And I think all of that can add up. I think pancreatic enzymes are part of the body's way of keeping things clean and keeping things managed, so to speak. And when we are creating an environment where there is a lot of extra chemicals, well, those enzymes have more to do and you can in effect run out of them. We think that that is when you would start to develop a cancer.

Ty: And you also have the inability to excrete the toxins which is why you have implemented the coffee enemas.

Dr. Isaacs: Correct.

Ty: It helps you get rid of that toxic load especially when the enzymes are digesting the cancerous tumors and you are trying to get rid of those. What is that called, herxheimer reaction? When you have too much toxins in your system.

Dr. Isaacs: Yes.

Ty: Now this, Dr. Isaacs, is a loaded question but feel free to answer it appropriately. Does modern medicine play—play—let us do this again. Dr. Isaacs this is a loaded question but you feel free to answer it appropriately. Does modern medicine pay too much attention to drugs and not enough attention to natural types of treatments?

Dr. Isaacs: Yes. That is the short answer. Yes, that is correct. And I think a lot of that is how is research funded. And much of research is funded by the pharmaceutical industry. And they, for better or worse, are—their goal is to make money for their stockholders. And so their goal is to develop drugs that can be patented, that can be sold to treat illness. So they are funding the research and, not unexpectedly, then the medical world is looking for research to know how to treat patients, and what is available is drugs. One of the problems I think that doctors feel is that if they—even if they prescribe some sort of nutritional approach or nutritional modification, that the patient is not going to follow through on it.

You think about it, what is easier? To talk to a patient about the dietary influences on cholesterol, for example, or the benefit of exercise. They feel like the patient probably is not going to do it. It is much easier to write a prescription for a pill. And many times when a patient comes in complaining about some issue or problem, the doctor feels like what is wanted is a prescription. In many cases they are correct. So I think that if you want to get nutritional input or guidance from a physician you either have to ask for it very bluntly or go to a doctor who is oriented that way in the first place. Many doctors' own diets are not that impressive. So that is another consideration, is that it is hard, if you are a doctor, working eighty hour weeks, eating on the run, mostly eating junk, they are not going to talk about nutrition too much, because they know they are not doing it themselves. And they would rather not think about it. So they just keep writing prescriptions.

Ty: I appreciate your candor in that answer. One of the things that is interesting to me is that you are a medical doctor, and I have heard from other medical doctors that I am good friends with, several, that going through medical school did not really receive much training in nutrition. It was more of a drug based program that you went through in college. Talk about your own medical school. Did you receive much nutritional training through medical school?

Dr. Isaacs: We did not receive much medical—nutritional training in medical school. And I think part of it is that much of the training that you get in medical school is really crisis intervention. It is not really about dealing with people that are well and how to keep them well. It is really about dealing with people that are in a crisis either because of trauma or because of some disease process that is well on its way, quite advanced. And so nutrition really is not discussed because pharmaceuticals is what helps you deal with somebody who has got pneumonia or somebody who is in heart failure and has fluid up to their eyeballs so to speak. Pharmaceuticals is what is going to help turn that situation around fast, but what, as a patient, one wants is help in staying healthy as long as possible. But that is not really what doctors are trained in.

Ty: And I am glad you made the distinction, lest anything think that I am being down on medical doctors. I think that the state of trauma medicine in the United States today is second to none. If you have—like I have often used the analogy, if I am shot with a shotgun blast to the chest, I am not going to go rub aloe vera juice on it or something natural. I am going to go to the hospital and the emergency room doctors are going to have the best knowledge of anybody to save me. If I have a limb amputated, they may be able to reattach it and still function. So I think that our state of medicine concerning trauma is just amazing today.

Dr. Isaacs: Yes.

Ty: So lest anybody think I am being overly critical just asking the questions here.

Dr. Isaacs: Right.

Ty: Do you think that sometimes doctors might fear backlash if they use a nutritional or a natural approach as opposed to the standard of care for treating cancer? Because at least if they use the standard of care, and the patient does not make it, they did what was protocol. And if they kind of step outside the box and use some kind of nutritional advice or a natural approach and the patient does not make it then they are in legal trouble.

Dr. Isaacs: Yes, that is correct. There is a standard of care, as it is called. And when you are operating within that standard of care, you have, in effect, a safety net. If you are not operating in that, then you lose that safety net. There can also be an issue of, a doctor works in a community of other doctors. So if they are doing something that is outside the norm, that can create repercussions in terms of working with other doctors, in terms of hospital privileges, or a lot of different factors that can tie into that. So it is certainly something that I think a patient should be aware of, that a doctor is in effect stepping outside of some of the safety net, like I said.

Ty: Last question, and I am not trying to get you here, but if you were diagnosed with cancer, I am not going to say any particular kind, just if you had cancer, what would your approach be to treating?

Dr. Isaacs: Well, what I would say there, I think surgery has a place in the treatment of cancer. And I know that there are some alternative minded people that would disagree with me on that. But I think that there is something to be said for surgical intervention if that can cure somebody. Now, I use the word "cure" perhaps a little differently, in that I would say there is still something going on with the body that made a person develop cancer in the first place. But having said that, if I had—like for instance, my mother had a melanoma taken off her shoulder. And I had actually been bugging her for months to get that looked at, even before she did. So she finally went in and it was a fairly deep melanoma, and she got it out, and she finally got compliant with the program that I told them to do. And she has done fine. Now in her particular case it was fairly deep. She had a thirty percent chance of not having a recurrence. So is she good enough to write up? No. But she did beat the odds and she is going to be ninety-two in June and she is still doing quite a bit of the program that I prescribed for her.

Ty: Great, and I am assuming the program you prescribed is what you are using with the three pronged approach that you and Dr. Gonzalez use?

Dr. Isaacs: But I also told her to get the surgery. My feeling is, that is a good way to approach it. Beyond that, what would I personally do? I would do my own program. I already do my own program for health maintenance.

I do not take a lot of enzymes. If I developed a cancer I would start taking a lot of enzymes. But I take pills with my meals. I watch my diet. I do coffee enemas and other detox type protocols. So I would intensify what I do already, which is my own treatment.

Ty: Sorry, I lied, that was not the last; one more question.

Dr. Isaacs: That is quite all right.

Ty: Concerning coffee enemas, is that something you think would be appropriate, that may not have been diagnosed with cancer but just in light of the toxic overload that we have today? That is something that could stimulate the liver to help secrete all of the toxins. Is that something that is good for people that do not have cancer?

Dr. Isaacs: I believe so. Now, I have to put in a disclaimer when I say something like that, since we live in a litigious world. So I will say that I am not telling any of your audience—I am not advising them to do it. They need to get instruction on how to do it properly. But having said that, yes, I do think that they are beneficial for anybody. And I think most people find they feel better with them. So they tend to sell themselves. None of our patients coming in for the first time ever believe this. But I tell them it is going to be your favorite part of the program. And they come back and say you are absolutely right, I never miss the coffee enemas, because they made me feel so much better.

Ty: Because the enemas help them to get the toxins out of their body?

Dr. Isaacs: Well, that is what I think is happening, but I can tell you they feel better and they swear by them.

Ty: And that does matter; feeling better does matter.

Dr. Isaacs: Feeling better does matter, and that can replace a whole bunch of those things that people must be buying based on those advertisements for headaches and tension and ibuprofen, all the different ads for all the different ailments that people are having. Our patients really do not use over the counter medications. They use things like coffee enemas which seem to keep them going pretty well without any Tylenol at all.

Ty: Without the side effects.

Dr. Isaacs: Exactly.

Ty: Well Dr. Isaacs, I think that based upon what you have shared with me today a lot of people are out there feeling better because of what you and Dr. Gonzalez are doing here so I really appreciate you spending the time with us today. And I know that our audience has benefitted from the information you have shared.

Dr. Isaacs: Well thank you, it was a pleasure to be here with you.

[end transcript]

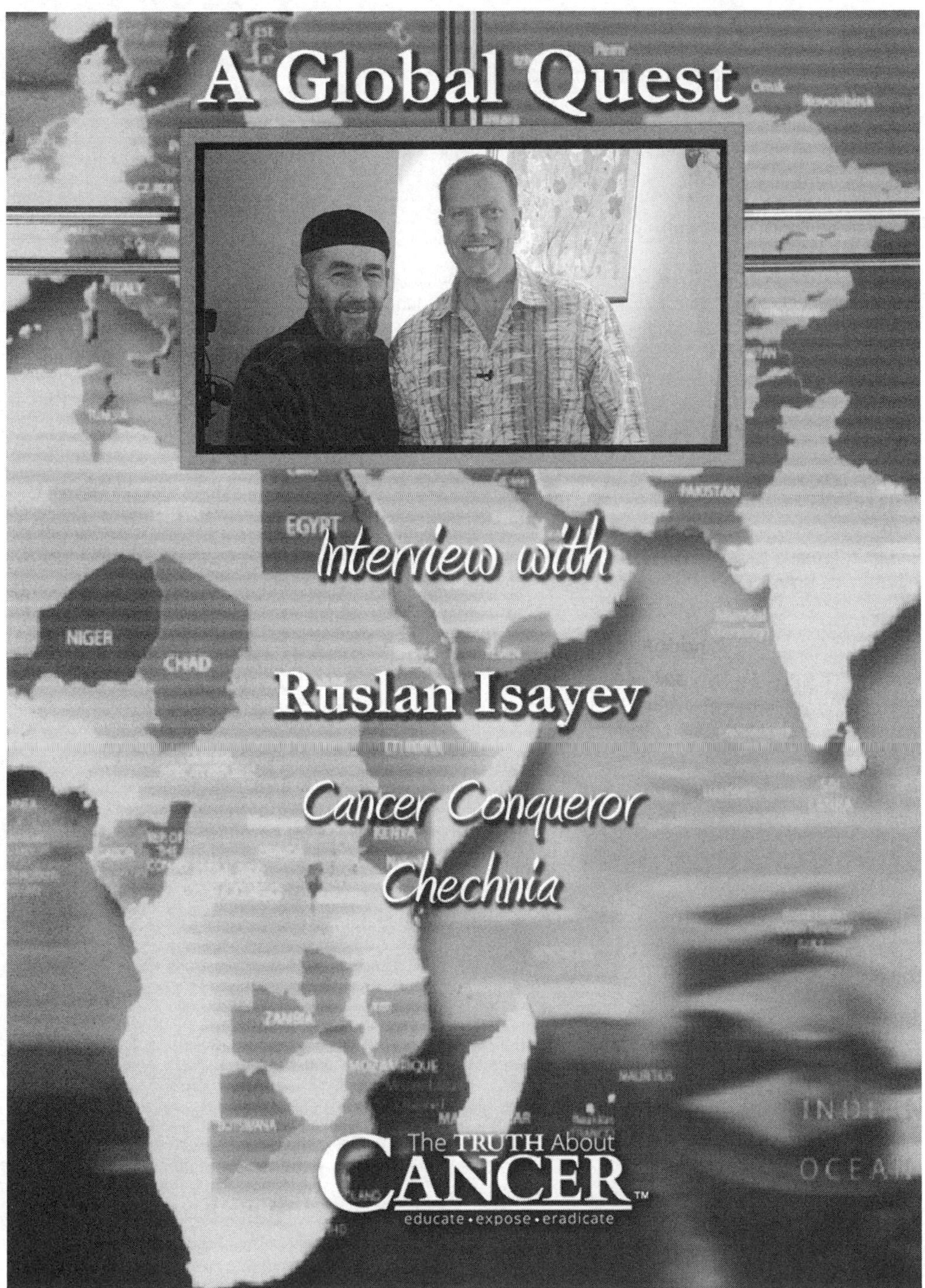
A Global Quest
EGYPT
Interview with
NIGER
CHAD
Ruslan Isayev
Cancer Conqueror
Chechnia
ZAMBIA
The TRUTH About
CANCER
educate • expose • eradicate

Ty: Ruslan, thank you for joining us today. I'm looking forward to getting your story.

Tell us about your cancer diagnosis several years ago.

Ruslan: [Translated 00:00:17 to 00:00:22] I was diagnosed at the end of 2009. [Translated 00:00:26 to 00:00:38] It was extremely sudden, and I got really afraid. So I said, "Please cut it off immediately from my body."

Ty: What type of cancer did you have?

Ruslan: [Translated 00:00:50 to 00:01:12] It was a melanoma, a skin melanoma and it was localized in the general localizations and in the back bone. And the tumor of the back bone was 37 centimeters, and I had surgery. They had to cut it off.

Ty: What stage cancer was it?

Ruslan: [Translated 00:01:34 to 00:01:40] It was third-stage malignant and progressing.

Ty: Okay, so it's third stage, it was spreading. What after you got it cut out, what was the treatment recommendation in Russia?

Ruslan: [Translated 00:01:59 to 00:02:11] The only recommendation we have in Russia, in our country, after surgery, is chemotherapy, and doctors sent me home with seven months to live.

Ty: So seven months to live. There was really no hope that they offered you.

Ruslan: [Translated 00:02:31 to 00:02:44] They said, "No, you've no hope. You can make ready for the last periods of your life." And when I got home, they prescribed chemotherapy.

Ty: To me that just not make any sense that you are given no hope, seven months to live but they still prescribed chemotherapy. Why would they prescribe chemotherapy if it's not going to help?

Ruslan: [Translated 00:03:16 to 00:03:25] They said that there's a little possibility that it could just prolong this period slightly, but the possibility was really, really small.

Ty: So you did chemotherapy at that point?

Ruslan: [Translated 00:03:40 to 00:03:51] Yes, I did receive chemotherapy, but I was feeling really bad after that. But I wanted to live. I had my family and the will for life was very strong.

Ty: So what choice of treatment did you pursue after the chemotherapy? Because obviously you are sitting here with us so you're alive today. You must have done something that worked.

Ruslan: [Translated 00:04:22 to 00:04:42] After the very first course of chemotherapy I was feeling really bad and my condition was really, really weak. I rejected continuing the chemotherapy even though I had a very serious disease. And somehow I survived one year more without the chemotherapy. And after that I decided to find another treatment method. Yes, this is the one, this is the one.

[Translated 00:05:09] This is the one that saved me. [Translated 00:05:14 to 00:05:24] I think, I know that it is the best medicine for patients who have cancer. I was too weak to walk on my own, I had to have support to walk. But after that I was able to walk.

Ty: Tell us about your son who is a miracle because of Rigvir. I've heard the story but go ahead and share it with us please.

Ruslan: [Translated 00:05:57 to 00:06:05] This is a very hard topic, okay? I become very emotional.

Ty: Tell him to take his time.

Ruslan: [Translated 00:06:20 to 00:06:29] We were sitting at home having dinner, ordinary evening and my wife said that she's pregnant. [Translated 00:06:36 to 00:06:44] Before that her doctor said due to my disease it would be very hard to have kids so everyone said it would be impossible to have kids.

[Translated 00:06:57 to 00:07:23] And the day when my wife told me we were having a baby, after this very serious and difficult time, I thanked God and give my word that if there will be a girl, a daughter, I will name her after Aina Muceniece, the professor who was to discover the great person, so Aina. [Translated 00:07:43] And if there will be a boy, then I will name him after the Chairman of Philanthropy, St. Urgis, who is at the same time who is the grandson of Professor Aina Muceniece.

Ty: So Ruslan, you named your son Urgis after the grandson of the inventor of Rigvir. Do you have a picture of your son that you could show us?

Ruslan: [Translated 00:08:04 to 00:08:15] Sure I have; I will show it. [Translated 00:08:24 to 00:08:25] See what Rigvir does.

Ty: Is Urgis a common name in Chechnya?

Ruslan: [Translated 00:08:33 to 00:08:40] No. They are laughing at me that this is a Chechnyan legend.

Ty: Okay. But you don't care. You are so happy about Rigvir that they can laugh all they want and it doesn't matter to you.

Ruslan: [Translated 00:08:57 to 00:09:04] They aren't making fun in a negative way though, and they are also happy for me. They're supporting me.

Ty: It's a happy laughter.

Ruslan: [Translated 00:09:12 to 00:09:27] Before taking Rigvir, it was difficult for me to walk. I had to take the support of a staff to walk. But after taking Rigvir when I got this cream from Riga for treatment, I started to feel much better.

[Translated 00:09:43 to 00:09:54] And in two months after following this scheme, this protocol from Virotherapy Center, I didn't need the support of things. I simply started to walk by myself.

Ty: Were you able to – once you began to recover – were you able to connect with the people back home or did you share with them about Rigvir® to either your other cancer patients or the doctors and tell them about this treatment?

Ruslan: [Translated 00:10:34 to 00:10:37] I wanted exactly to say this, what the doctor told me. [Translated 00:10:41 to 00:10:46] And after that, I just completely one year I didn't go to the clinic. I simply visited the lab to take the blood test analysis to send them to Riga.

[Translated 00:10:57 to 00:11:04] And after a year when I came, I had to come to the hospital for recommendations. I had another doctor.

[Translated 00:11:16 to 00:11:22] And the doctor looked at my history of my disease, at these papers and documents and he said, "Please invite the patient. I want to see him." [Translated 00:11:32 to 00:11:33] Because he didn't know me. He was a new doctor for me. He didn't know me. He didn't know the story.

[Translated 00:11:38 to 00:11:42] And I said, "It's me. I'm the patient." He said, "No, it cannot be you because the history's so…" [Translated 00:11:49 to 00:11:59] "It's impossible. It can't be you because through all my practice I had not such a case when the person had such serious disease and such a negative condition and now he's completely healthy, he's walking without any support.

Ty: At that point, he had never seen a case of recovery like that, that was that amazing. Did he want to learn more about what you had done?

Ruslan: Yes. I started to introduce Rigvir because this doctor is a new one in our district. He is a young person and very passionate. He's very interested in new treatments and methods.

Ty: Good. So maybe because of your input to your doctor back in Russia, maybe one day Rigvir will be available there.

Ruslan: [Translated 00:13:29 to 00:13:32] I hope for it. I hope for it. I pray to God for it.

[Translated 00:13:39 to 00:13:47] Then he made the consilium of other specialists about my case in our country. [Translated 00:13:53 to 00:14:06] And I told my story about the treatment, about the way I feel now that I'm healthy, and there were many patients when I was receiving chemotherapy. There were many patients also receiving chemotherapy and they knew these people.

[Translated 00:14:24 to 00:14:30] And people when they started to speak, people want a miracle, one injection and immediately the disease fades. Well, it can be so from the very first injection.

[Translated 00:14:42 to 00:14:57] And they explained then that it can't be so from the very first time. You need to follow strictly these indications and protocols in the Virotherapy Center and you have to listen to these doctors and follow their indications from the Virotherapy Center again but not the ones in our country who don't actually know much about this method.

[Translated 00:15:21 to 00:15:39] When I was receiving chemotherapy, I made friends with nine of the patients and as I started to receive Rigvir I recommended to one of them, "Please try because there is a chance that you can survive and you can have a long life." But this chemotherapy will definitely kill you.

Ty: Are any of those chemotherapy patients still alive that you stay in contact with?

Ruslan: [Translated 00:16:06 to 00:16:18] And also this was three years ago I forgot to say, and after when I was going today, recently, to Riga there was only one left but he was in the hospital. He was feeling really weak. He was looking very bad and I think that his condition got even worse and the rest, eight, they passed away. They're gone.

[Translated 00:16:46 to 00:16:58] I've attended the funerals for all of these people and the family, the relatives they were crying. They were begging, saying, "Oh, why they didn't try the treatment you tried?" And I said, "I recommended it but it's their choice. They had to make the choice."

Ty: Why do you think it was, Ruslan, that they did not try Rigvir when you recommended it?

Ruslan: [Translated 00:17:29 to 00:17:59] Our people are like soldiers. It's very hard for them to believe and they didn't trust. Maybe they think that it's an advertisement or it will not work or something. They were not sure. Usually people who have enough money, they, for example, go visit such countries as Israel which have a reputation. I had a friend who brought his mother to Israel and he was paying $8,000 per week. But she passed away anyway, and he brought her back to the funeral in the homeland.

[Translated 00:18:33 to 00:18:55] But if you compare the cost for this treatment it's incomparable. When I needed it I simply communicated with my family and friends, and they supported me also financially and well, it worked, and it was really worth it.

[Translated 00:19:12 to 00:19:33] It would be great if the people who have money would be kind enough to for other people who don't have enough money simply to support them financially to buy this course of Rigvir and to give them not telling what it is, but to give them and tell them, "Try it. I want to help you." And I'm sure that these patients would survive and they would feel great and have it.

Ty: I think that, Ruslan, as a result of this interview today that there are going to be potentially millions of people around the world that see your success story, that see your miracle son that are the result of Rigvir. So I think that many people are going to know about Rigvir because of this interview, so thank you for spending the time with us today.

Ruslan: Thank you.

Ty: Thank you.

Interpreter: Thank you.

Ty: So Ruslan, are you able to work now?

Ruslan: [Translated 00:21:29 to 00:21:39] During the winter while I'm taking my blood tests I have work. I'm driving a car that delivers bread in this district.

Ty: So you went from being diagnosed that there was no hope back to work again.

Ruslan: [Translated 00:22:00 to 00:22:04] Yes, it's all thanks to Rigvir. [Translated 00:22:09 to 00:22:14] This is the thing that saved me. I want to show it like this. [Translated 00:22:17 to 00:22:19] This is life.

Ty: Very good. Okay, so I'll redo the intro. Intro. I'm going to leave the same outro. I just didn't do a full intro at first. You're fine. I think we're not going to move.

Rolling there Therese.

Technician: Hold on one second. Okay.

Ty: I'm really excited to be here with Ruslan from Chechnya Republic in Russia and he is going to share with us a story—

Oh yeah, I'm looking at this – yeah.

I'm here in Riga, Latvia. I'm really excited to share with you the story of Ruslan, who is going to share with us a miracle story of recovery from cancer today. He came all the way from Chechnya Republic in Russia. Thank you so much for joining us today.

Ruslan: [needs to translate/language 00:23:13]

Ty: Okay. Awesome.

Technician: Got it.

Ty: Good?

Technician: Yep.

[end of transcript]

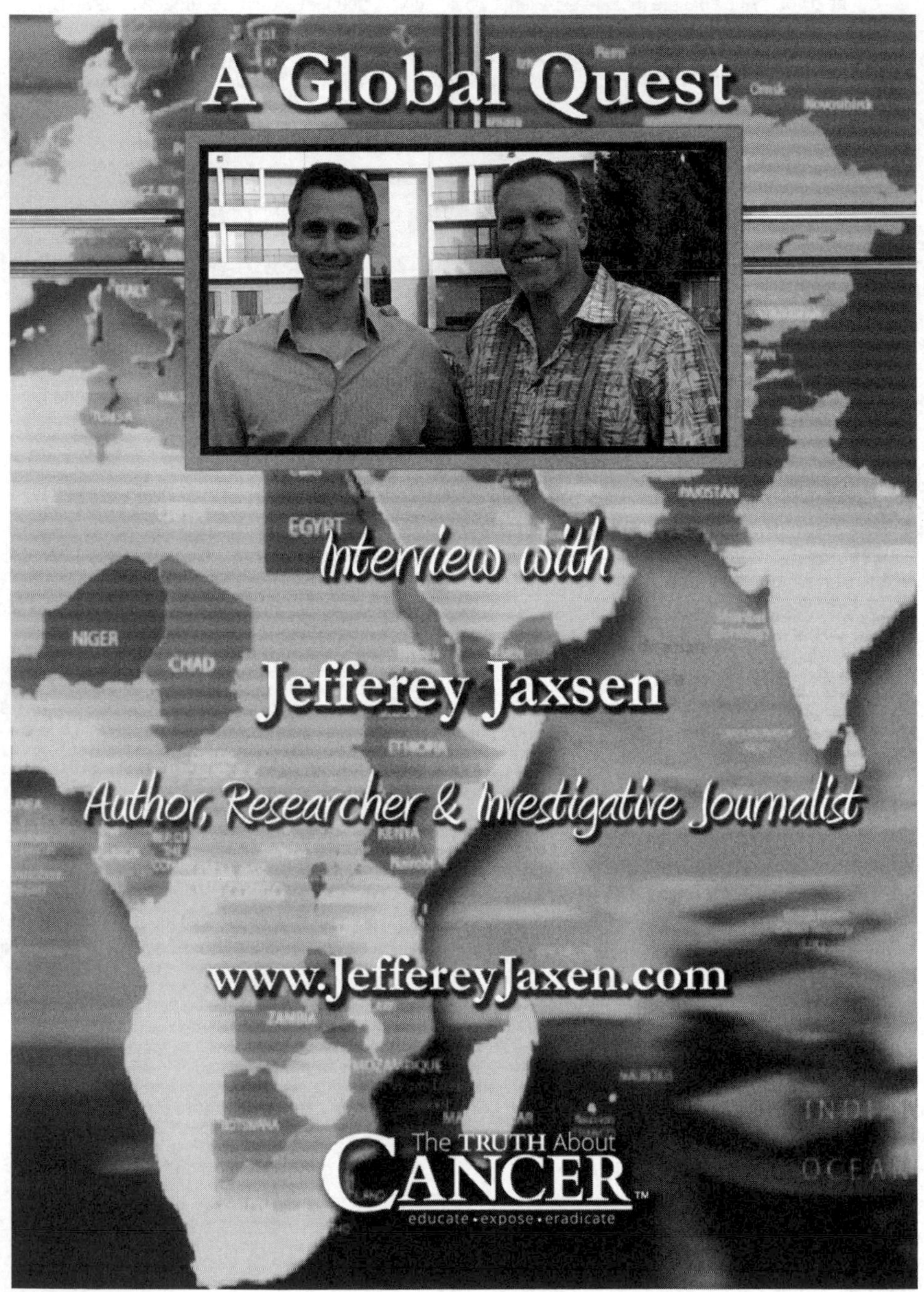
A Global Quest
Interview with
Jefferey Jaxsen
Author, Researcher & Investigative Journalist
www.JeffereyJaxen.com
The TRUTH About
CANCER™
educate • expose • eradicate

Ty: Jefferey, how are you doing today, brother?

Jefferey: How you doing Ty?

Ty: Good, good to be here. I'm looking up at the skies and I see these trails of chemicals. So what can we do in today's toxic world to avoid all these traps and detoxify our bodies?

Jefferey: It doesn't matter where the chemicals are coming from. It all goes back to the solution is nature, comes back to nature, so that's where you're going to be looking for the solutions, doesn't matter where the chemicals are.

Ty: Back to nature. So Jefferey, I agree with you that nature has the answer for a lot of our problems, but here's something that really stumps me. Why is it that we have so many children now that are being born with cancer? Because it seems like a child being born, that's the most close to nature state you can be right? You've been exposed to less toxins than you will be later in life.

I don't understand why we have this epidemic of childhood cancer. Can you help me understand that?

Jefferey: That's true, but in a perfect world, and unfortunately we're in a toxic world, what happens is children's cells are developing so rapidly, they're splitting very rapidly, so if they get introduced to a toxin, which studies have shown there's toxins in the breast milk of women as they give that to their child. There's toxins in—the child's experiencing toxins when it's in the womb. When it's getting hit with these toxins at that point these cells are dividing rapidly and they're mutating. So they don't have the correct information to develop correctly and quickly like they should. So you get these cancers, and they're getting hit from so many different angles now.

We have vaccines, we have GMOs; I mean the list is as long as my arm and it really goes back to nutrition. The mother has to start before she even conceives the child, she has to clean her body and detoxify her body, and then when that baby's in there, when that baby's developing, that is nine months of the best pure lifestyle you could possibly have. The mother and the father have to take it upon themselves to learn all there is to know about toxins and detoxification before they decide to have a child at this point, and unfortunately that's where we've come.

Ty: So, it's important before the mother even gets pregnant to detoxify.

Jefferey: Correct.

Ty: Because then those toxins are going to get into the bloodstream of the baby. You mentioned two things that I want to hit on. You mentioned GMOs and vaccines. You've written a lot of articles about both of these topics. Let's talk about the vaccines initially. We know that there are known carcinogens in many vaccines.

Jefferey: Yes.

Ty: So what—let's go to California. Okay, over the summer we had this big hubbub in California about mandatory vaccines. Give us your perspective on that.

Jefferey: Well, mandatory vaccines are—it's a medical device. This is a medical product from a private company, with risks. The safe and effective line is not true, that's a paid line for people to say that get paid by the companies that make the vaccines.

So what's happening here is you're getting vaccines, which is a medical product, pushed on children against their parents' wishes. So essentially this state is saying we don't trust your parent's judgment. We don't trust the judgment what you want to do with your kid and your child's health. So we're going to step in and give them a risky medical product that has, basically funds associated with it, that doctors are getting kickbacks with, lobbyists are getting kickbacks with.

It's unfortunately very dirty right now, but I believe it'll clean up and I believe it won't stand, because mothers and fathers aren't going to stand for having the state come in and take away their choice when it comes to medicine. Certainly in America, freedom has to start with what you allow or what you get to do with your body especially, if it's sick and then it goes into the chemotherapy as well, with children being taken away from their families.

Ty: So—and I agree with you completely. It is a freedom issue. Without a doubt, it's a freedom issue. Unfortunately, it seems that our freedoms are being trampled, and one of the ways I believe that they're being trampled, not just with vaccines, is with GMOs because genetically modified organisms are not being labeled, and so we don't even know what's in our food.

Jefferey: Right.

Ty: Right, and one of the things that you've written a lot about is GMOs, so could you address GMOs and are they really as bad as people say they are?

Jefferey: Well, that's a big topic and I'm going to step back and say, Dr. Oz was attacked a while back for that. And he came out and he pushed back against his attackers who turned out to be people from the biotech industry that were getting money, the doctors that attacked him were, and he had Joel Fuhrman on. Dr. Joel Fuhrman said this attack was anti-human, anti-freedom, and anti-American.

In my opinion, I believe that's what GMOs are and that's what forced vaccinations are. These are things that go against medical consent. So essentially, we're fighting simply for the right to know, we're not even fighting to keep this stuff away from our body, we just want to know. So you have companies now that— I wrote an article, "GMO food is the best product, according to the manufacturers of GMO food, that no one knows where to buy, and no one knows how to find, and it flies in the face of basic finance." If you're a company that has a product, you want people to know where it is.

But they're spending millions fighting legally in the courts to keep people from knowing this. But, it doesn't matter anymore, because the tide has turned and the backlash—I call it the end of the American GMO experiment, it's over and people want to know and the more they push back and try to keep it secret, the more people are going to wake up to the fact that it's dangerous stuff.

Ty: I think that's a good point, Jefferey. If they were so good for us, then the manufacturers would want us to know that they're in the products, right?

Jefferey: Absolutely.

Ty: If they're so good for us, yes this product has GMOs, it's got tons of GMOs and they're good for you. They don't want us to know, so that should tell us something about the fact that it's really not that good for you.

Jefferey: Right, and that goes with the vaccines too, since we're on the topic, in 1986 Ronald Reagan passed a Vaccine Protection Act. Basically, what was happening is manufacturers were making these products and it was for profit with the vaccines, and there was so much damage that was happening. They were getting sued, their pants were getting sued off in court and they went to the government and said, "Hey, look we need protection otherwise our companies are not going to thrive, they're going to go under."

So Ronald Reagan passed this act in 1986, a lot of people don't know about, that you do not get to sue the manufacturers or the doctor if you have any damages and in fact, you have a very limited time if your child is damaged after the vaccine to seek representation to sue. To date, as I stand here today over $3 billion have been paid out to damaged children and families in the United States, and just recently in the UK, $63 million GlaxoSmithKline paid out for damage from swine flu vaccine that they forced on the population. So the safe and effective, I always say the safe and effective route is it's only safe and effective until it's not safe and effective, and then it's time to do legal battles.

Ty: Well I mean apparently it's not all—the vaccines aren't all that safe if they've paid out over $3 billion with a 'B'.

Jefferey: Correct.

Ty: In settlements.

Jefferey: Yes.

Ty: And I would think that with those kind of dollars they wouldn't be paying them out if they weren't owed.

Jefferey: Correct.

Ty: Right, I mean if they had—if there's any way where they could have gotten off, they would have and probably most of them out of court settlements?

Jefferey: Yes, and also to keep in mind too, one of the things I brought up all the time. I always try to make this point, vaccines are not tested. On the insert it says, not tested for carcinogenic and mutagenic properties. It also says it's not safe for pregnant women, and it's not tested in children for those same properties. So what that is, is that's your consent form that the doctor doesn't give to you.

When a doctor's pushing or a nurse is pushing a vaccine, this is uninformed consent at the highest level and this goes against the Nuremberg principles, Nuremberg principle number four, actually five, that were in 1940s after World War II. They did this so there was no more human experimentation on people, and this is medical experimentation because we are the last phase of the experimentation process.

So as they're manufacturing these we are—it depends on the lawsuits that come back to the company to tell the company if this product is actually safe. There have not been studies for the vaccines, but now there's not been studies for two and three and four vaccines stacked on each other and up to 60s and 70 and however many they're going to push. There's no studies for all of those on top of it, so you're looking at uninformed consent at the highest level.

Ty: That really blows my mind because what you just said Jefferey, and I know this to be true, is that the vaccine manufacturers tell us that vaccines are safe and effective, but they have not been tested to see if they cause cancer or if they cause mutations, which can then result in cancer and other diseases.

Jefferey: Correct.

Ty: So we're told they're safe and effective, but they've never been tested. We're just told that, and we're supposed to believe it so that's why you say it's the highest level uninformed consent.

Jefferey: That's right.

Ty: Wow. Okay, because my next question was to talk about uninformed consent, that's exactly what uninformed consent is.

Jefferey: There's not only the Nuremberg principles, but the Law of Helsinki. There are about three levels of international laws that they break by doing this. A lot of countries, Japan recalled, not recalled but stopped, the MMR vaccine because it was—there were issues with autism. The children were coming down with autism very quickly.

And even Dr. Wakefield, very controversial character in my opinion, I think he has high integrity and he's out in front of this whole issue by years, but he said, "I'm not against vaccines necessarily. I want to take the MMR vaccine and split it up into three shots." Because when you hit these kids with all three of them at once, you're tripling the androgens, you're tripling the aluminum, you're tripling the mercury, and no one seems to talk about that. Why we keep compounding and adding more shots to these children. They would seem to think that, unless you have a shot, you can't get protected against a germ. And with that theory, the germ theory, you're going to be racing around because there are millions of germs out there. So are we going to possibly see in the future millions of vaccines? I hope not.

Ty: I hope not too. And talking about the germ theory, okay, explain real quickly, what is the germ theory and how does that relate to what I've heard you talk about as our internal terrain? And contrast those two positions.

Jefferey: Yeah, so the germ theory won out over the law of the terrain and the germ theory supports basically—to make it as simple as possible—the germ theory supports products and business. So with the germ theory, you can take a germ and you get a product and you can sell that product to fight that germ.

Now the law of the terrain has to do with your body and keeping the terrain of your body healthy. For example, the soil we're standing on is also terrain and nothing will grow on this soil if this soil's not healthy. So if the soil in your body is unhealthy, you're going to get germs that are already circulating through your system, germs on the outside, you'll be more susceptible to it.

This is what happens with people with chemotherapy, their immune systems get suppressed, they get secondary infections. This is law of the terrain, their terrain has now become not protected anymore, somewhat toxic. So the law of the terrain is really what it's about, keeping yourself healthy and the best way to keep yourself healthy, going right back to nature.

If it comes from the ground and it's organic and non-GMO and all that stuff, that's the best way to do it, and there's certain strategies to do with this that you don't need to take pharmaceutical drugs. You don't need to take these things to fight these germs because if you're going to be fighting germs—I mean Nixon started a war against cancer in the 70s and we've been fighting that ever since and we're at one in three men and one in two women, I believe it is, maybe that's reversed, are going to get cancer in their lifetime and that's right now.

I mean, at some point, I hope it doesn't come to this; it might be one in one the way the toxicity is going. So the law of terrain is where it all starts, people need to take responsibility for their own terrain and not rely on being a patient because, I like to say too, "The best way to become educated is not to be someone's patient. It's to educate yourself to become healthy."

Ty: That's a great contrast with our current medical paradigm, because our current medical paradigm is, wait till you get sick and then go have a doctor treat you. There's no prevention, that's not taught, that's not even focused on. What's focused on is what am I going to do specifically in terms of cancer, what am I going to do after I get cancer? That's the attitude that a lot of people, as opposed to what can I do now, how can I change my diet, how can I change my exposure to these toxins, whatever it might be, so that I don't become one of that one in two men, one in three women that you just mentioned.

Jefferey: Right, exactly.

Ty: And that's where we're lacking, I think.

Jefferey: Yeah. We have a medical system—the Commonwealth Fund in 2014 did a study, a very prestigious study, the US ranked 11th out of all the developed nations they studied. They studied 11 nations, US was 11th. They ranked dead last. When we get the spiel that we are the best and the brightest out there, it's just not true.

Barbara Starfield in the *Journal of American Medicine Association*, JAMA, she did an article and she compiled the research. And this is something you'll never hear a doctor talk about, you'll never hear on the news, she said that 225,000 people per year die from the American medical system, 106,000 of those people are directly from pharmaceutical drugs. Now you times that by any given ten years, you're looking at over two million people that have died. That's more than a lot of wars and these are—this is our medical system. This is what we're looking at; you contrast that with a toxic environment and a medical system that is somewhat inept at this point, it's very dangerous. It's a bad combination.

Ty: And that number you quoted, the 100 plus thousand, that's on the FDA's own website.

Jefferey: Absolutely.

Ty: They admit that 100,000 are due to prescription drugs that are properly prescribed, that's what gets me.

Jefferey: Yes.

Ty: Properly prescribed prescription drugs kill 100,000 people a year that blows my mind.

Jefferey: What people also need to understand is prescription drugs are nothing less than an isolated part of a plant. All prescription drugs, all the constituents are from a plant and they isolate it, they amplify it, and they make it synthetic in a lab and you can grow that same thing in your backyard.

The Chinese have been doing this for years; traditional Chinese medicine has 5,000 years of research backed up to it. The American Indians have been doing it. The literature's out there. You can do something called a backyard pharmacy, and you don't need these pharmaceutical drugs anymore. I'm not a doctor so I can say that and not have to worry about losing my license.

Ty: You mentioned the fact that Chinese medicine, 5,000 years of research, American Indians, they've been using plants for a millennium. Talk about what is real evidence based medicine, because often times you'll hear people that will characterize folks that only go natural, as far as treating cancer naturally and they'll say, "We won't eat—" you should be using evidence based medicine.

Jefferey: Unfortunately, the evidence based medicine is corrupted. It's been shown that the FDA's own reports are—high percentage of them are corrupted, from either conflicts of interest or simply just research fraud, and we're finding that out now. It's coming out on a regular basis.

The USDA just had a scandal where its scientists came forward and said, "We need protection from Bio Tech, from Monsanto, from these companies, because we trying to do studies and tell how bad this stuff is and tell people what it's doing to your health, but our research is being changed before it's published or we're getting threats to our careers and these people are having a hard time coming out."

This is where the controversial CDC whistleblower comes in, he released a statement through his attorney that said, "Look, the autism research we did for the CDC." Now he was one of the CDC's top researchers and he said, "The research I did with two other co-authors was fabricated and the MMR—there was a high correlation of autism in African American boys, young boys and this has been quieted." He has not had any approval to have any testimony with this. It's probably going to go down in the memory banks as a conspiracy theory, but I'm here to say this man released a statement through a lawyer. So evidence-based is not quite evidence-based.

Eating healthy is the best way to do it. Going back to plants, going back to the ground and the earth, it's got to come from there otherwise processed food is dead food. You can't find it there anymore. Not only is it dead, it's toxic and there are a lot of things in processed food, the heavy metals that—I know Mike Adams was doing his own independent lab testing. That was unknown until now, and people are starting to decentralize the testing.

So what's going to happen now is you're going to get—I hope to see at some point an individual testing unit for everybody at the store as they walk through, and they can just test their own food for glyphosate, for metals, for anything, and I hope it comes down to that because that decentralizes this power that we have to trust evidence-based medicine. I'm not going to attack evidence-based medicine anymore because it has gotten to us to a point with a lot of great research and there is valid points to it, but when companies get involved and when products get involved, the integrity is damaged.

Ty: I think a lot of the natural treatments that we would espouse are evidence-based. By definition, they're evidence-based.

Jefferey: Yeah.

Ty: You mentioned glyphosate. So let's talk about glyphosate, it's the primary ingredient in Roundup and we think of Roundup, we think of—go hand in hand with GMO foods, the Roundup-ready corn and soy. You mentioned testing. Aren't the GMO foods tested? I mean haven't they been shown to be safe by, who?

Jefferey: No, no they haven't and I'm not a researcher, as far as for the Biotech company, but they haven't been shown to be safe on people. They've been shown, theoretically, to be safe. They've been shown to be safe for short trials.

I know Jeffrey Smith on one of the episodes of *Quest for the Cure* that you did, he referenced the French study where they took the study past term where they normally are forced to end the study, all the rats had cancerous tumors, or most of them I should say, and this is what we're finding. Glyphosate was just recently labeled a possible human carcinogen by the World Health Organization's Cancer Department, or Cancer Division. And this is in the same category as HPV, as HIV. And you have to ask yourself why is something—I mean could we imagine if HIV was being sprayed on our food? Would that make some people kind of worried?

The other thing that no one really talks about is glyphosate was patented in 1964 by a company called the Stauffer Chemical Company and it was meant to be a chelator of minerals, trace minerals, magnesium especially. So what's happening is, every person tested has some glyphosate typically running through them depending on how they eat. But a majority of people do, including mothers, including newborn babies.

What you're looking at is you're looking at going through your body as a sponge that pulls your minerals out of your body, it pulls your magnesium out of your body and this is coming from also soil that has glyphosate in it that takes up the magnesium. There is a huge push for magnesium deficiency and people to supplement magnesium and that's one of the reasons this is happening right now.

That also affects circulation and it's been shown that magnesium—I'll go on that subject for a second, it's been shown that low magnesium levels are also a probable carcinogen, just having low magnesium levels. Supplementing magnesium with tumors shows tumor shrinkage. This is a huge thing when it comes to cancer, no one does this. If you're going to take magnesium, magnesium chloride is the transdermal, you can put it on your body and magnesium citrate is the type you can take orally. But you can't patent magnesium, so that's why no one's talking about it. The doctors won't talk about it. There's nothing in the journals about it because it's not a product, you can't patent it. It's just out there.

Ty: That's really fascinating that magnesium shrinks tumors and that might be one of the correlations with glyphosate the fact that it absorbs the magnesium.

Jeferey: Right.

Ty: So people that have glyphosate in their systems are magnesium deficient. One of the things that really blew my mind is that you just said that they just declared, I'm not sure what body it was, they just declared glyphosate is a possible carcinogen.

Jefferey: Yes.

Ty: So this kills me, I was just in one of the big box stores recently and was buying some plants and there were literally shelf after shelf of Roundup and I was seeing people in Tennessee, where I live, they were grabbing the Roundup to go spray and it's a possible carcinogen, which means it's a carcinogen.

Jefferey: Most likely.

Ty: If they say it's a possible, there has to be some reason that they—they've got to have some studies that are showing its cause in cancer.

Jefferey: My hypothesis is this is to cover their butt legally. Because now, at this point, we're seeing an influx. I do a lot of research on the influx in independent labs, doctors, small food companies, they're all having their patients tested and their products tested because this is a legal case now.

What happened in California is a class action lawsuit by the people of California has just been filed. And what happened is that they're filing it against glyphosate saying that they misrepresented their studies and this is a possible human carcinogen and you're poisoning us and you knew this all along. This is gaining speed in California. But this can go in every state, in every county, this can go forward and individual food manufacturers need to now watch their butts because they're selling a product that's a cancer causing product, probably. So this is a legal thing that—it's going to really come back to bite them in the butt, if there's not a backlash.

Ty: So you think that was more of a legal maneuver.

Jefferey: I think so, I really do.

Ty: That's a great connection you made with the glyphosate and the magnesium. So what are the best ways to boost your magnesium? What are some natural foods that you can take?

Jefferey: Hemp, hemp seeds, hemp hearts they're called, organic of course. You want to go organic; yeah, you have to do that.

Ty: Eat those all the time.

Jefferey: Pumpkin seeds, leafy greens, now most of these minus the hemp unfortunately in this country, you can grow in your backyard. Leafy greens are the best thing. Pumpkin seeds, save them, come Halloween, cashews, almonds, the list is this long. You can do avocadoes, that's the natural way.

But a lot of the supplements now, the magnesium supplements are pretty good because they come from deep earth sources which have not been touched by toxicity, so they're pretty trustworthy, but the list—if you look up magnesium deficiency online, besides cancer, the list of things that it's associated with, magnesium is part of 300 plus functions in the body and one of the biggest functions it's part of is ATP and energy generation. It's like pulling the plug on you when you get the low magnesium, you get chronic fatigue and a lot of stuff associated with that, adrenal fatigue, but the cancer thing as well, it's a big part of that. The literature is out there. This is not a theory. The literature is out there between cancer and low magnesium.

Ty: So Jefferey, talk about chemotherapy and radiation. A lot of times people, they don't know about natural treatments so they've undergone them. I think we're going to have hundreds of thousands of people that are watching the show now that might have already undergone it or may be in the middle of it. What are some good strategies that you can mitigate the negative effects of these two treatments?

Jefferey: What you're looking at at that point is antioxidants and you want to boost your immunity because chemotherapy destroys immunity, and it just hurts part of your body. I mean, that's what it is, but hopefully it hurts the cancer more than it hurts the rest of you, but when you get out of it, your body went through a war and there's some damages from that war.

I am a big proponent of saying that your body can heal no matter what happens to it and someone may—watching may say something crazy like well what if I lose an arm? There's been studies in other countries where they show limb growth with certain modality. So really anything that happens, you can recover from.

When it comes to people that have taken the chemotherapy or the toxic drugs associated with that, you're going to look at immune boosting, I like to say mushrooms. Reishi and cordyceps, they have to happen, in fact everybody—in my opinion, minus any toxicity or any contradictions, which at this point there are none for cordyceps, should be taking cordyceps in this environment. What the cordyceps mushroom does is it ups your immunity and it ups available oxygen in your body.

Cancer, as you know and everyone watching probably knows, thrives in a non-oxygen based environment or an anaerobic. So when you take these cordyceps, studies have shown that it ups your body's oxygen, internal oxygen by 40 percent, ATP by 28 percent and then it also increases your natural killer cell activity by 400 percent, and that was in people that had cancer for the last one, the natural killer cells.

So athletes in China—it's been Chinese medicine for a long time, and in 1993 it became like right on the radar because the women's' marathon team started shattering all these records. And they were shattering them by not one or two seconds, but 30, 40 seconds. Just huge amounts, and people were trying to figure out what was going on. They were taking cordyceps, they had a supplemented with cordyceps.

Ty: More oxygen.

Jefferey: More oxygen, exactly, more available oxygen for the muscles. So what happened at that point is, the sports commissions and the sports regulation body said, "Look we got to regulate this stuff, because it's very prominent in China and they know how to develop it and they have the best sources. It's not fair for other countries that don't have these sources because, now this is an unfair advantage." So now it's disseminated everywhere. You can buy it everywhere, but cordyceps is the way to go.

Ty: Can you buy it at a health food store?

Jefferey: Yep, health food store.

Ty: Do you take a supplement or the fresh mushroom?

Jefferey: That's a great question. You can take a tincture, which is the drops with water or you can take a pill, either way. Some companies are actually infusing it into coffee to go a step further.

Ty: I've seen that.

Jefferey: There you go. I mean people that don't like to take supplements, if they're coffee drinkers, you do that, but to go a step further, nanotechnology has taken this cordyceps, this is kind of the new wave. Nanotechnology can be good or bad, but in this case, they've taken the cordyceps mushroom and they make it a nanoparticle. In that case, usually only about 30 to 40 percent of the herb or the mushroom gets taken into your body and used. When it's a nanoparticle, smaller, it gets about 98 percent into your body.

Ty: Wow, so it's much more bioavailable to your system.

Jefferey: Bioavailable to your system and you don't have to take as much and it's very powerful. Now the other part of the mushroom I want to talk about is the Rishi mushroom. The biodefense and bioshield department of the United States did studies on the Rishi mushroom before for the big dogs, for swine flu, bird flu, some of the really nasty viruses and at one to 100 dilution, it was showing huge, huge virus killing abilities with this stuff. It ups your microphages; it ups your immune system. There's no toxicity to these things and you can also—there's no contradictions really. So you can take them almost all the time, unless you're immune suppressed.

Ty: So you get the Rishi the same place as the cordyceps?

Jefferey: Yes.

Ty: At a health store? You can buy the tincture or the powder or the pill.

Jefferey: Yes, I don't like to talk about other people's supplements, but in the case this was the researcher, Paul Stamets. When it comes to mushrooms, the word Paul Stamets is basically the same word. He's been around for a long time and he's done the greatest work. In fact, I think he should win a Nobel Prize, but he has a line and his line is pretty high integrity.

So on the cordyceps mushrooms as well, I had the pleasure of working with a guy, his name is Dr. Richard Alan Miller. Dr. Richard Alan Miller, he was responsible for creating the physical parameters or making basically the first Seal team into Super Soldiers, and he was developing that and he used cordyceps with them, way back when, to amplify them and to give more oxygen in their bodies so they can continue to function better.

Ty: Wow. You know I don't take cordyceps regularly now, but I'm going to after hearing you talk about it here. That's pretty amazing. So talk about—like we were talking about the gut earlier. Is the gut full of good bacteria or bad bacteria?

What makes somebody that's exposed to a virus gets sick where another person exposed to the same virus to the same bacteria, doesn't get sick, what is that? They're not exposed to different viruses. So what is it that's the defining difference between the two?

Jefferey: Well, when it comes to the gut, the gut is just now the tip of the iceberg being studied. There are so many levels of what this does in your body. It's called the second brain, but we'll get into that, I'll get into that in a second. When it comes to the immune system, it's an integral part of your immune system and we go back to GMOs, when it comes to GMOs we basically—it's replacing your gut bacteria.

Jeffery Smith talked about this, with GMO and other nasties down there. So what happens is it eliminates your good gut bacteria and changes the flora of your body. When your flora is changed, that leads the way to fungal infections, to all types of stuff and that's lack of oxygen and cancer. That goes hand in hand with that. So we go back to the GMOs, everyone should be taking a probiotic when it comes to—even if you don't eat GMOs, they're going to be snuck in there somewhere.

The glyphosate has a lot of food with the drift going on, so it's an integral part of your immune system, you have to do it. Now the gut as well is part of your intuition. So back to the Navy Seals for a second, they were taught to think with their gut. Your gut has—now this is proven, I was deciding if I wanted to talk about this here because it goes a little outside of *Quest for the Cures*, which you normally talk about, but when it comes to making decisions, your gut has access to information outside of space and time.

Your mind is working on parameters that are—they can see calculable parameters. Your gut has access beyond that. The Institute of Heartmath in California has done studies, and this is documentable and this is what the Navy Seals were doing, they would develop that to make decisions at key junctures and they wouldn't use their head, they would use their gut.

So I go back to when I talk to people that are having cancer that come to me, I say, "Hey use your gut, don't use your heads, don't use your fear; use your gut for that. It has the answers and it's influenced."

And one way it was described to me, and I use this all the time, your gut checks it out to see if it's right, your heart brings it and you resonate it out with your heart and that's where you put your passion into it and maybe at the last minute. If you need to use your brain for last minute calculations that's what that's there for.

Most people, the mainstream medical community, the first thing they do with cancer patients is give them fear. They hit them with fear and out of all the instincts we have, fear is the only one that causes no motion. Fear is the only one that paralyzes us. So when you get into a fear based mindset, which cancer—the word cancer already invokes fear. I tell people to think of it this way, thank your body for giving you the warning in time so you can make a decision to change it, instead of worrying about fear and listening to a doctor that says we got to get you in tomorrow. There's time, listen to your gut, take a breath.

Ty: That's where the term, "that's what my gut instinct says".

Jefferey: Exactly.

Ty: It's there for a reason.

Jefferey: That's right.

Ty: Right, and that phrase is a century old.

Jefferey: And it's scientifically proven now. So people can't say this is mumbo, jumbo. This is scientifically proven stuff.

Ty: That's interesting. So what would you say to a cancer patient that's been diagnosed with cancer and their oncologist has, as you just said, instilled fear into them, what would your message be to that patient?

Jefferey: I would say take a day or two and think about it, without the fear. Do your best to think about that mindset I just talked about. Instead of thinking about why me, it's fear hating your body, flip it around and say, "Thanks. Now, you're giving me this opportunity to make a change otherwise you would've killed me and you wouldn't have given me the opportunity. I wouldn't have seen it coming. Help me work, help me do this, lead me to the right things." Start doing some research, get some education.

There's so much info online right now with people with high integrity, they can find this info, they can go to the right people. The cancer documentary, your cancer documentary, that's 11 hours. If they wanted to have a marathon cancer documentary and do a matrix download, there's a good place to start. There's a laundry list of doctors now because of your work and other people's work, that aren't afraid to come out and talk about other ways to deal with cancer. There's a lot of choices out there. That's why I say don't have fear, don't settle into that fear mindset.

Ty: I think that's good advice and too, and fear has also been shown, they can empirically measure your immune response to fear, to anger, to stress, and it shows that it suppresses your immune system.

Jefferey: Exactly.

Ty: That's another reason to not buy into all the fear.

Jefferey: Think of this way, I used to do stress research with Henry Ford Hospital and one of the things that we always said was, stress speaks cancer's language, stress is cancer's food. And stress has been shown to in some cases, 50 percent of the immune system gets knocked out right away in levels of stress. When you knock out the immune system, anytime you knock out your body's ability to defend itself, you're opening up to cancer. That's a big part of it.

One of the real big things I wanted to talk about was the way people hold stress. The reason you'll never hear doctors talk about stress much, because they can't measure it, and they're physical, so you tell doctor, show me some stress. Show me a tincture of a stress, they can't show you it because stress is bunch of symptoms and what these symptoms are—if you control these symptoms you control the stress response in your body and you can control that immune system drop.

What happens is, I always say picture a child's balloon and when a clown blows up that balloon, that's your body. When you have stress, squeeze one side of that balloon real hard and the other side pops up, the side that you're squeezing is parts of your body that's not getting oxygen. That's your stress in there and it's a pressurized container and when there's no oxygen, once again, no oxygen, anaerobic, stress, or I'm sorry, cancer, feeds off anaerobic conditions so if you already have a predetermined spots in your body or organs that aren't getting the correct oxygen and you go under heavy stress, there's a bad situation right there, still brewing.

Ty: You mentioned something about the lack of oxygen - a recent story, somebody told me that had seen the *Quest for the Cures* a year ago. He was told he had terminal cancer. There were parts in his spine that were dead, they were not getting oxygen. The chiropractor went in and realigned it and got the energy to flow and he's healed. He was told he would be dead in six months, he had terminal renal carcinoma, right kidney cancer and he's completely well a year later and he's in the *Quest for the Cures*. This global quest, I got an interview with him.

Jefferey: Good.

Ty: We will see that here either later in this episode, or whenever you've seen it, but that's really fascinating. So, the energy, the oxygen energy I've heard you talk about, you're a very renowned writer and you've written about energy and frequency, and you call it the new health paradigm.

Jefferey: Yes.

Ty: Talk about that.

Jefferey: Well, let me go back to that example right there, I can tie it right in. So we have something in our body called micro-circulation. This is something along with magnesium and mushrooms, you don't hear about very much because it's powerful, potent information.

Ty: Triple M—microcirculation, magnesium and mushrooms.

Jefferey: There it is. And microcirculation can't be measured because it's micro, microns, some of its micron level. Some of it's so small that a blood cell has to squeeze down to one blood cell to get through there, and these are like roots through your whole body. There are parts of your body when that microcirculation gets cut off for whatever reason, dies. And for the chiropractor—for that example you gave me perhaps it was the way that his body had contorted had cut off that certain circulation to those certain areas, but I'm no chiropractor.

My point with microcirculation is, microcirculation, oxygen, blood, and energy all are pretty much levels of the same thing. So those are four roads that all merge into one road. So when people hear about this it's kind of confusing, well what are we talking about? Energy or blood cells, it's all the same thing. So when you take, for example, the glyphosate that's in your body and it's taking the magnesium away, or even a better example the aluminum, or the aluminum in the soil or the aluminum in vaccines or in deodorant, aluminum, when that gets in your bloodstream it piggy backs onto a blood cell and it takes away the blood's ability to carry oxygen.

Blood cells also carry a charge. So when that happens your oxygen, the charge and the blood flow all do something, they slow down at each of their respective levels and on the physical level, they do something called flocculate and flocculation is, if you go online and search flocculation, what that is, is basically when water treatment plants get the dirty water, there are all kinds of dirty stuff suspended in this water. They use aluminum in there to flocculate or congeal this and combine it and it drops to the bottom of the container so they can remove it. That's what aluminum does in your blood. So it hits your bloodstream, these positive charges in your blood drop out so your blood is a coital substance and when they drop out, that's when they start clumping, that's when oxygen is less and it can be measured in millivolts.

So we go back to the energy now, millivolts is 20 to 30 millivolts the human system operates at. At 10 millivolts you become open to chronic disease, at plus 30 you have to get cancer. So people that have this—now this is just another way of saying you have less oxygen in your body because the voltage is correlated with the oxygen, but another way to say it is voltage is correlated with PH. So an acidic body is a body with low voltage and low acid. It's all the same thing and these metals, these toxic metals that we talk about, all work on - they're taking away oxygen, they're taking away voltage and they're also taking away the mitochondria's ability to make energy.

Ty: So you're talking about low voltage, low oxygen, low pH.

Jefferey: Correct.

Ty: Okay.

Jefferey: It's all the same thing. It's just different levels of how you want to talk about that. Doctors talk about mitochondria, blood cells, erythrocytes. People in the energy paradigm will talk about voltage, frequency, energy, but also too, let us not forget in 1940 and 30, this was talked about in your other episode, Royal Rife, this was, in my opinion, this was the golden goose that laid the egg that no one saw. This was swept under the carpet very quickly.

Royal Rife basically hit a cancer cell with a frequency and it exploded. He described a glass, a crystal glass because he noticed that the cell, the outside of the cancer cell was kind of like crystalline structure. He found the frequency, and it exploded it. The biggest problem his patient's had was after the cancer cell exploded, instantly there was too much of a toxic dump of the internal constituents of this cancer cell. So the detox is usually what hit them pretty hard and they went into a major detox. So he found if he hit the frequency a lot slower, now this is a whole different viewpoint of cancer that we're starting to get into now, but it's going to take a big paradigm shift. It's coming, but it's a way from the physical into the energetic.

Ty: Royal Raymond Rife was very successful with his frequency machine. He was a brilliant scientist. There were dozens of articles that were run about him on the West Coast and he was really attacked and he was—by what I call the Medical Mafia.

Jefferey: Absolutely, unfortunately that was before the Internet, because if that was during the time of the Internet it would have changed and they can't stop the information now. The fact that we're sitting here talking is the fact that back then they controlled the papers and the only reason that he—it was like whack-a-mole. He popped up because the paper made, the paper ran an ad or not an ad, but a headline that said, "Man cures cancer." And everyone went, "Wait a minute, what?" and it attracted the wrong type of attention at that point by the medical mafia, the Rockefeller Medical Mafia.

Ty: Well, Hippocrates is the father of medicine. He's been quoted as saying, "Let food be thy medicine and medicine be thy food." So give us a list, for you Jefferey Jaxen, what are your top foods for keeping your voltage at the proper level, the alkalinity at the proper level, the oxygen level in your body, all these things that we've just discussed. What are your top foods, because you're obviously very healthy? So people are watching, wondering, how do I get that healthy, what do you eat? What would you recommend?

Jefferey: Leafy greens, number one, and I know this is been something that's been beaten home by everybody, leafy greens, kale. Leafy greens not only have high voltage, but they are also highly oxygenating so it's a double whammy for your body. The third part is it also pulls out toxins. So it's detoxifying at the same time. It has antioxidants, so we're now up to four things, it's a functional food, four things for one.

Ty: When you say leafy greens, give me a few examples of leafy greens.

Jefferey: Kale, spinach, chard, I like to grow those here, because in Michigan we have some hard winters and I know that the kale winters very well. I can grow that with snow on the ground. Also cilantro, that's a big one too, because cilantro is one of the best metal chelators. So you're taking it out, cilantro gets rid of that aluminum that's in your body slowing down your blood stream. It gets rid of the mercury; it gets rid of all that stuff, the lead.

Ty: Parsley?

Jefferey: Parsley as well, now a side note, parsley and there's something called lovage. Lovage isn't talked about very much. These are the two foods with the highest antioxidant flavonoid called quercetin. Quercetin is another functional food, it's probably one of the most, perhaps the highest, anti-cancer flavonoid and it's also a metals detoxifier. Again, it's like a three in one hit there.

You can grow this stuff in your garden, you don't need to spend money on supplements, and in fact, I would argue it's better coming from your garden because the food we get takes a while to get here and in that time of travel, it loses voltage, it loses energy, it loses it's effectiveness—it's minerals and it's vitamins, which is probably all the same thing we're talking about here. So when you pick it directly out of your garden, you're getting stuff that your body's never seen before. This is supercharge time.

Ty: Same reasons why if you're juicing, you want to juice fresh greens, fresh vegetables, fresh fruits at your house, drink it immediately instead of going to the market and buying juice that was fresh juice two days ago. Because, by the time you get it to your house you just, you don't get the same effect, right.

Jefferey: Yes, the other stuff I do, I go gluten free and in my opinion from the research I've done, everyone has gluten intolerance. Gluten is a neurotoxin, a very potent neurotoxin, so even though the outward signs you may not see gluten sensitivities, the inward stuff's going on, and you can better believe that.

Ty: Do you think that's potentially because of the way that they've changed the wheat to where it's not ancient grains any longer?

Jefferey: Correct, yeah, 100 percent.

Ty: Because one of the things that we eat at our house is Einkorn Ancient Grains Wheats, so it's the old stuff. I mean it cost a fortune to buy, but it's different than the wheat that we eat today in almost any bakery.

Jefferey: Yeah, unfortunately the wheat today, and then you're also talking about the wheat today, the flour has metals in it, so you have to watch out for that.

The other thing I'm a big proponent of is hemp. Hemp for hemp protein and hemp hearts, one of the highest magnesium leveled proteins and on top of that too, you want to make sure you're getting it from Canada until these laws change. There are two sources, Canada and China. China, you got the heavy metal problem again, because of the toxicity that's going through the air and it drops into the crops. So China, I'm sorry, Canada organic hemp, that's another thing I live off that stuff.

Ty: And it's a superfood right?

Jefferey: It's a superfood, absolutely. A couple other things I do sometimes, I do the detoxification, spirulina, chlorella, I have to make sure those are also from sources that are sources. I know there's a source in Hawaii and I actually wrote the company and I asked them if Fukushima was a problem because they're growing basically a superfood that takes out radiation from your body, in an area that you know arguably has radiation.

Ty: It's full of radiation.

Jefferey: It's full of radiation, and they said they independently test it, they grow it indoors, the letter they wrote me back was—it satisfied all my answers and actually I posted it online about a year ago. So people can go read that.

Ty: Yea,h that was interesting, I saw a news report just a few days ago about an area very close to Fukushima that, they're measuring people's radioactivity and they're all radioactive.

Jefferey: Fukushima, I believe we'll be talking about this—I'll start over. I believe that what we're talking about right now, people may look back in 10 or 20 years and say, "Look at that, they had it. Someone should have listened to them." Because Fukushima is probably one of the largest disasters of our time, totally unreported. Reporters, mainstream reporters that talk about it get canned immediately. There's a gag order on it, and one of the things though, I like to always balance out bad news with good news.

There are two things that I've—we have the natural products. We have the spirulina and the chlorella, the cilantro, those are all great radioprotectors and also to detoxify your body from radiation, but there's also things. This is kind of futuristic stuff, but it's called a fullerene and a fullerene is a structured water. They call them the—the nicknames called the buckyball and that was Buckminster Foley. He designed these and it's been known for a long time and they've done this research in Japan and in China.

This is repeated, they fed rats lethal doses of radiation and in the control group, obviously nothing, and they gave them these fullerene, it's a structured water. What the structured water does is it surrounds the radiation and eliminates it from your body immediately and there's a 95 percent recovery rate on the rats. It's huge and at this point, I mean as I'm standing today, not much reporting on it, but this is the kind of research that's happening.

So when people, again when it comes to that fear, when people read a headline and say we're all doomed, or whatever the case may be, you don't know what's going to be coming out next year. You don't know the research that's happening right now or in 10 years from now and people—amazing minds are on this research. So there's hope, there's always hope, your body can always recover.

Ty: So Jefferey, amazing information you shared with us today. I really appreciate it and I love your positive perspective because there is always hope, cancer doesn't need to be a death sentence, and so give us a couple of rays of light and a couple of words of hope for those that are watching here in the interview.

Jefferey: Okay, well, it's not about fear, doesn't matter what your doctor says, this is your time now and you have a path to walk and you've been chosen. You have cancer for a reason and it's probably because to educate yourself, to change something about you.

There are a lot of people watching you that you don't know, walking this path that you have with cancer, and trying to rebalance it and you don't know how many people you're going to inspire by curing your own cancer. So I can say, do it for yourself, but also the world's watching you and when you change, you're changing the world.

Ty: Great words man. You're awesome, Jefferey, I really appreciate the interview today.

Jefferey: Thank you.

Ty: All right.

[end of transcript]

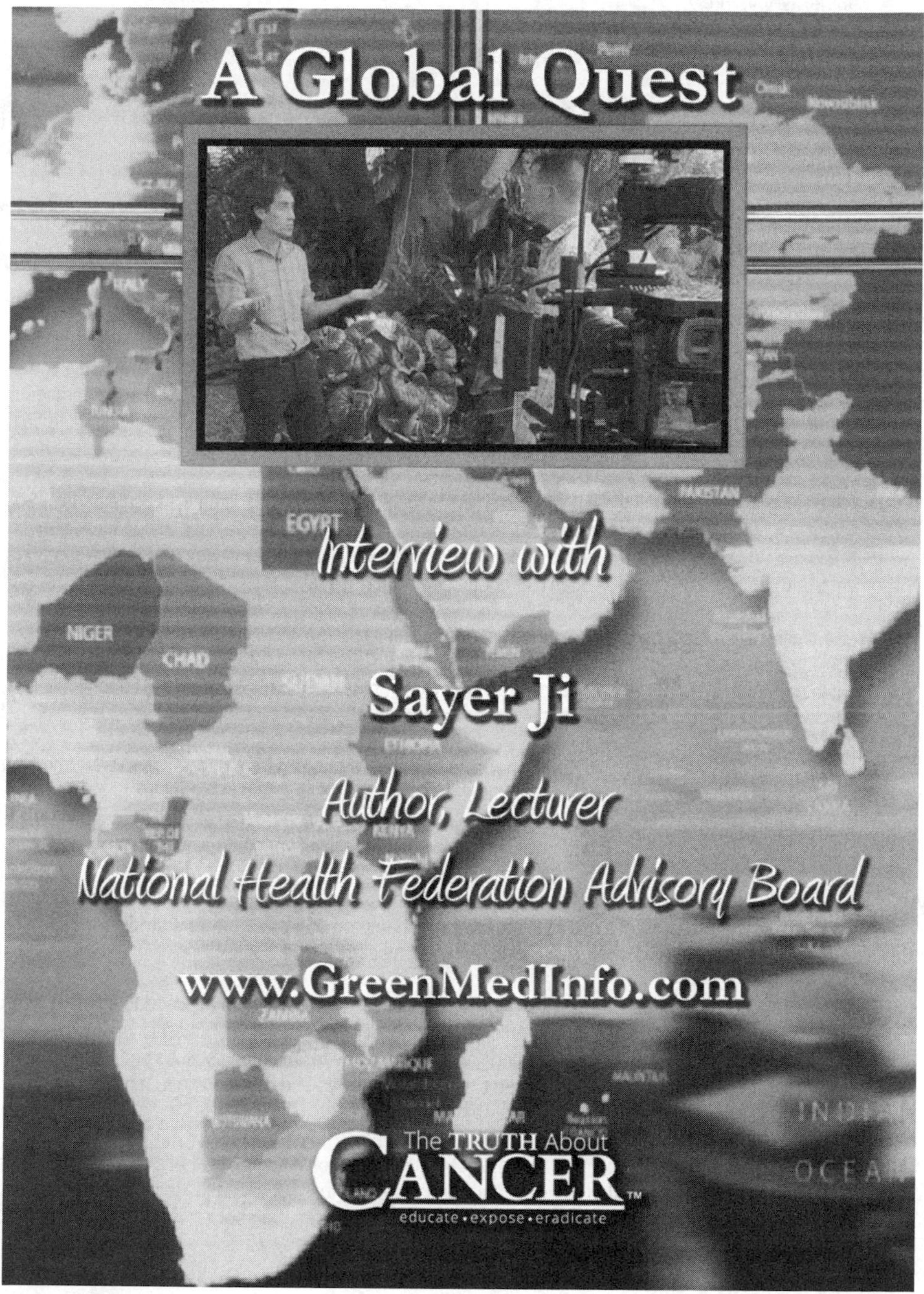
A Global Quest
Interview with
Sayer Ji
Author, Lecturer
National Health Federation Advisory Board
www.GreenMedInfo.com
The TRUTH About
CANCER
educate • expose • eradicate

THE TRUTH ABOUT CANCER

Ty: So, I'm here in Naples, Florida at the Shangri-la Resort and I'm with Sayer Ji. What a pleasure to interview you today.

Sayer: Hey, it's great to be here and see you in person.

Ty: I've been following your work for long time and it's great to finally meet you face-to-face.

Sayer: Same here.

Ty: I'm really looking forward to getting your take on a lot of these serious issues surrounding cancer today.

Sayer: Absolutely.

Ty: So let's start off. I want to talk to you about chemo and radiation resistance.

Sayer: Yes. I feel the word itself is almost euphemism for something really terrible which is that when you are exposed to radiation that is based on gamma radiation, it is basically ionizing, it will cause damage to whatever basic tissue it is being exposed to. In the same way chemotherapy is also designed to be genotoxic.

You are trying to target fast replicating cells and by doing so, it is by definition also carcinogenic. So when we talk about resistance to chemo and radiation, it is really just a way of blaming the victim. Because we are all—when exposed to conventional chemo and radiation—going to be harmed and it is actually going to have a carcinogenic effect and it will often cause secondary cancer.

So technically, I think people need to be aware that this isn't truly a cancer therapy. At best, it's palliative in the sense that it might shrink a tumor but really the main thing that I would like to get across is that it is going to cause an enrichment of the actual mother cell that's beneath the tumor, which is known as the cancer stem cell.

So technically, you are shrinking the tumor size but you are enriching the population of the tumorigenic cells at the very same moment. So again, the idea that some people are resistant to chemo and radiation is really a false concept. Everyone exposed to radiation and chemo will have secondary adverse effects, some of which are worse than the original condition that they're being treated for.

Ty: So Sayer, talk to us about different cells in the body that are also fast-dividing. We know that cancer cells are fast-dividing. That's one of the theories of chemotherapy that it hits fast-dividing cells, which are cancer. But are there other cells in the body that also are fast-dividing?

Sayer: It's a great question. See, basically, our condition in modern times is we're exposed to so many sources of inflammation. And there's a very compelling theory that cancer essentially starts in many cases with unregulated inflammation. So, if we're constantly being hit by toxins and infectious agents, chemicals, what will happen is the cells will be forced to repair themselves and that's going to require inflammation to occur which actually involves proliferative natural chemicals.

So if there's constant frustrated inflammation, the healing is not taking place. Let's say we're smoking daily or we're doing things that are constantly causing injury that will cause those cells to replicate more rapidly. And so over time in many ways, the cancer is a frustrated, unresolved inflammatory response that will eventually emerge into a cancerous phenotype. So in many ways. . .

Ty: What is a phenotype?

Sayer: A phenotype is just a cell changing from its intended purpose. So if I'm a hair or a heart or a skin cell, after being beaten down by all these unnatural modern exposures, I'm trying to adapt so I'm actually becoming a different type of cell to adjust to those conditions. And that type of cells is going to look a lot like a cancer cell.

Ty: Now, are you talking about stem cells? Because those are the ones that can become anything, right?

Sayer: Yes.

Ty: Stem cells.

Sayer: Yes, cancer stem cells are actually a dis-regulated or misinformed normal stem cell that is basically now proliferating wildly, not aware of its role in the whole of the multi-cellular organism. It's gone rogue basically, but again, not for reasons that aren't logical because it's trying to adjust to a very toxic environment.

So those cells will start to try to invade other tissues and they do their own thing. Yes, the cancer stem cell ultimately does come from a normal cell that its job is to keep repairing the daughter cells that had been damaged and keeping on healing the body.

Ty: And so really, when we're talking about chemotherapy, we're talking about a substance that targets cancer cells but not the stem cells, if I understand correctly.

Sayer: Yes, the idea behind a lot of the least genotoxic chemotherapies, which are really poisons—in fact, some of them actually originated, as you know, from the war theatre as sort of chemical weapons. And so, even today, there are forms that are derived from that lineage. So they just destroy any fast replicating cells because when a cell is replicating in mitosis its DNA is exposed, perfect time for it to be genotoxic and, in theory, kill the cell.

Unfortunately though, the cancer stem cells are resistant to chemo-toxic agents. So technically, those cells survive when all of the daughter cells that are in the tumor—again, tumors are not cancer. They're different and they don't themselves have the ability to go out and invade and kill the patient. They do cause problems over time because they can obstruct normal biological processes but the idea is that the cancer stem cell will basically be enriched when you use chemotherapy. And that ultimately puts the clinician, the oncologists to say, "Oh my gosh, we're winning. We've just beat back the tumor. It's smaller."

In fact, you might even beat it back below the threshold of surveillance but ultimately, if you look at what's happened, there's been enrichment in the cancer stem cell. And the cancer stem cell might be one in every 10,000 cells within a tumor and it's erected like a hierarchy. The apex is the cancer stem cell. The mother produces all the daughter cells, all the differentiated roles, but unless you target the cancer stem cell, it will just keep coming back.

And the thing about it is because of the way that the cancer practice and industry really looks at the five-year survival rate, they may "treat" somebody, give them chemo, radiation, see the tumor regress, go into remission. And then five years and two months later when they get another cancer, they can just define it as a new cancer and not look at the root of it which is that it was just those remaining sub-population of cancer stem cells that were not only resistant to chemo and radiation but were enriched and then grew back slowly over time. Because, as you know, a tumor or a cancer can take decades before you actually can get it to be surveilled so sort of just like an antibiotic resistant bacteria.

You have an infection, you take this chemical—which is in the category actually of a chemotherapy, antibiotics generally. And you whacked back 99.9 percent of the infection, of course, with all the good bacteria. And then, that 0.1 percent is now building up this bio-film, it's sitting there in dormancy and is resistant now to that chemical. So you have to come back with even more toxic chemicals when it comes back. Before you know it, obviously, the host immune system is dead, you've poisoned the body and now you have this highly resistant, antibiotic resistant, chemical resistant bacteria.

It's the same with cancer.

Ty: Name a few cells in the body that are also fast-dividing as well as the cancer cells.

Sayer: Fast-dividing tissue in the body, when you look at it, things like hair follicles cells are very fast dividing which is one reason why chemo often causes hair loss. There are intestinal cells that will divide so rapidly that every three days you have a new intestinal lining.

So a lot of the tissues that are susceptible to adverse effects from chemo and radiation are going to be those are constantly having to regenerate. Because when you really look at cancer, it is really a regenerative process in our body that is thwarted and misguided. Ultimately, when you think about cancer, I mean, it is possible to kill it. It's like a metaphor for eternal life and indestructibility and resilience of life versus chemicals.

The problem, of course, is that it's about the micro-environment of the "cancer cell." We have to adjust and change things back, detoxify, we need to supplement with the right nutrition and information from the right foods, hydrate, oxygenate. Those are all the factors that will then re-educate that cell to say, "Wait a second, I'm supposed to do this particular job as a hair cell, this job as a heart cell. I'm not going to go become a cancer and try to take over the whole body."

Ty: Right. Are there certain herbs and supplements that you can take that will target those stem cells that are the real boogers?

Sayer: Yes, absolutely. In fact, there's a term that is used in the research community and this arena called selective cytotoxicity which means that—you know, you could take bleach, obviously, and expose a cancer cell to it, it's going to die. So, when you use herbs sometimes in the cell or petri dish model, it makes everything look pretty good. But the difference is that, when you take an herb like turmeric and you take a compound out of it like polyphenol-rich curcumin, it will actually kill the cancer cell but then you have healthy normal cells there, it'll leave them intact.

In fact, in some cases it'll have a cytoprotective, or cell protective effect. So it's intelligent in the sense that it can target the cancer stem cell and leave other cells that are either tumorous and will never cause harm or are natural healthy cells and totally protect them from damage.

Ty: So turmeric is one?

Sayer: Turmeric is probably the most heavily researched anti-cancer agent which has the ability to selectively target the root of the cancer, which again cancer stem cells, and then leave intact the healthy tissue. But you have other substances such as resveratrol, green tea, quercetin—found in onions and other herbs—sulforaphane from cruciferous vegetables, especially broccoli sprouts. These are the heavy hitters that I'm sure you know a lot about.

Ty: The reason I'm smiling and chuckling a little bit is that we did a recent interview with Dr. David Jockers and he mentioned those same exact herbs but not for this reason, but for other reasons. But they're just different ways that they all hit cancer cells.

Sayer: It's remarkable because really this category is often polyphenol category. And so things like catechins and green tea, resveratrol from red grapes, even peanuts, and curcumin from turmeric—actually, that category of compounds is produced by plants when they are under stress. And it turns out organic plants are the main ones that produced these in any significant amount because they are not basically having pesticides to take care of their pests and petroleum-derived fertilizer to boost their growth. They have to survive the elements like us so they've developed these strong chemistry to protect them.

When we consume those compounds, they activate longevity pathways within our body, similar to what caloric restriction does in fasting. As well as activate things like anti-cancer mechanisms within the cell.

So it is almost like this poetry of positive co-dependency between the plants we've evolved to consume and, of course, our body's needs. We sort of depend on each other and help each other.

Ty: It's really fascinating. One of the things you mentioned that I've never thought about it is the fact that plants, vegetables, fruits that are being sprayed with pesticides, since they are being sprayed with pesticides, they don't have that reaction to pests which protects them. So we don't have that compound or those compounds that we ingest.

I was interviewing Dr. Patrick Quillin—he has written a book, *Beating Cancer with Nutrition.* It was last year, and he was talking about several compounds that plants produce to protect themselves from pests that then benefit us. I had never put that together, that the plants that are sprayed with pesticides, they don't have those.

Sayer: In some cases, organically produced produce will have a hundred times higher polyphenols. So when you look at the ultimate price you're paying—maybe it's 50 percent more for organic but you're getting a hundred times more value as an anti-cancer nutrient. It is clearly a better value. Especially since when you price cancer, then you're talking about a million dollars and financial bankruptcy. Not to mention all of the suffering that it causes.

Ty: One of the things you mentioned earlier, Sayer, was about if you live five years and two days or two months or whatever, and then they may call it another cancer. Talk a little bit about the way statistics are skewed.

Because let's say you have somebody that's diagnosed that they have breast cancer and they douse it with chemotherapy. The tumor shrinks, it's not detectable. They live five years and a month and then they diagnose them with another type of cancer. That's considered to be a cured person now.

Sayer: Exactly. I mean, in terms of the way that there's been a manipulation of this science—and there's been a very dangerous thing called over-diagnosis that has really afflicted millions of women over the past 30 years, especially for breast cancer. Because what they've done is that they convinced women that if they were to basically subscribe to an X-ray mammography screening, even though they have no symptoms, that ultimately, that would help them in the long run. They'd have a lower risk of cancer because they'd find it early.

Ty: Early detection is your best protection.

Sayer: Exactly. They even equated this meme with prevention when in fact you're exposing your breast to a type of radiation that is actually known to have a higher risk of causing cancer in the breast. Especially if you have the BRCA1 and 2 gene mutations that everyone is so concerned about. Because they make it harder for you to damage, to radiate, to protect yourself from radiation-induced damage.

Over-diagnosis, according to a recent study done in *The New England Journal of Medicine*, over the past 30 years in United States resulted in 1.3 million women being diagnosed with early stage breast cancer that technically never had any type of cancer that would cause harm. This is called ductal carcinoma in situ or stage zero cancer, which they equated with actual cancer which now we know is not. So what that basically meant is that they would give them the standard mastectomy or lumpectomy with radiation with chemotherapy. Things like tamoxifen, and then follow up hormone-suppressing therapies like Arimidex.

So basically, what we're dealing with here is kind of a medical holocaust of sorts. Because those women now had to deal with being diagnosed with a cancer they didn't have, being treated for it, having the stigma, and all the psycho-spiritual emotional stress that's caused by that. And then, statistically, the industry told them that they saved their lives when in fact, quite the opposite had happened. So they identify with the aggressor like a Stockholm syndrome.

And millions of people march in these breast cancer awareness marches not realizing that it's funded by the very corporations that make money off the drugs used to treat breast cancer. We're talking about AstraZeneca which actually is a derivative of Imperial Chemical Industries who started breast cancer awareness month in the 80s and has the patent or had the patent for tamoxifen and Arimidex.

So it's a vicious circle of brainwashing and it's used to cover up, really, what has cost the lives, I think, of hundreds of thousands of women ultimately.

Ty: That's really fascinating information. It's really shocking. It's really sad that we've had so many women that potentially have been diagnosed with cancer and have gone through all of these toxic treatments. Potentially even died from the treatments, that never even had cancer to start with.

Sayer: Absolutely. Over-diagnosis is basically causing inflation of the success in terms of what the industry says they're doing. Because of what's called lead time bias. Which is, if you diagnosed something early that would never progress to cause harm in the patient—and surely not take their life—it appears as if, according to statistics, you've saved their life because you have this [additional] time when you diagnosed the cancer from when it would have caused the symptom later.

Ultimately, the mortality statistics remain the same, meaning they don't live longer because you've done that. Lead-time bias is also related to length-time bias which is that when you do these sorts of screenings, you're going to actually detect the slow-growing cancers before you are the fast-growing. It's a statistical fact that fast-growing cancers which are the ones that are malignant are not going to be picked up as fast or as accurately as the slow-growing non-malignant ones.

These two factors lead to ultimately higher mortality than those who subject themselves to breast cancer screening. That's actually the reality. You look at all the trials and it now says that women who do this preventatively to detect it early are actually probably going to end up dying of breast cancer sooner than those who do not.

Ty: You know I've read that. I've also read that you mentioned the fact that mammography actually increases breast cancer risk.

Sayer: Yes.

Ty: That's amazing because the fact that women are urged—this documentary will be airing on October, breast cancer awareness month—and when they are urged to get the mammogram and it's actually an ionizing radiation. And studies have shown over and over, it actually increases the risk of cancer.

Sayer: Yes. Not only that, what they found is exact type of wavelength that is used. It is actually five to six times more carcinogenic than high energy radiation which is how they look at radiological risk today as compared radiation in mammography to the kind released during the Hiroshima event which was based on external exposure of a different wavelength.

And because wavelengths are technically of lower energy but higher carcinogenicity, higher toxicity, it actually causes more radiation-induced breast cancer than letting people know. So the risk of screening is five to six higher than what women are being told.

Ty: I can't remember the study, it was released in 2009. It was by a big independent conglomeration of researchers that determined that from the age of 40 to 50 breast cancer screening through mammography, it does zero good.

Sayer: Right.

Ty: But we're still told that you should start screening at the age 40 even when this independent study said that it doesn't do any good.

Sayer: Well, here's another thing. If we look at it logically, we know that the problem with the breast cancer susceptibility genes, the BRCA-1 and 2, is that it confers greater risk for DNA damaged in the breast tissue because the BRCA protein actually protects you from radiation damage. So if you are not being screened for BRCA-1 and 2, before getting exposed to these X-rays through mammography, then technically, you're not being given informed consent and you're being put in harms way in a way that is unethical.

Ty: And you look at the situation like Angelina Jolie. That had these genes and did a preventive mastectomy.

Sayer: Yes.

Ty: Because of this, talk about—that is probably something they didn't tell her.

Sayer: Well, there's a problem because in the mainstream culture and, of course, the media, they talked about BRCA 1 and 2 variations as if they are, quote, "mutations." We think back to comic book era stuff where someone was exposed to nuclear reactor waste and it just turned him into like some Incredible Hulk or something.

Ty: I used to wish I could be exposed and I could be the Hulk.

Sayer: Right. And that's not what is happening because this single nucleotide polymorphism called snips are variations from a norm. So generally, maybe, one percent or less of the population might have a variation. There have already been a thousand different snips identified for the BRCA genes. Whereas we talked about it as if it's one thing and it just conferred us with certainty of increased risk for breast cancer, it's not like that. Some of the variations have shown to conferred to survival advantage from breast cancer.

So technically, if you really look at the literature, you'll find no unequivocal proof that if you have the co-mutation—and again, there are literally hundreds of them—it doesn't give you a death sentence. It doesn't require you to take any kind of dramatic intervention like prophylactic mastectomy.

Ty: That's something Angelina should have known and probably didn't.

Sayer: Right. I think she was profoundly misinformed about what risk is because when we're doing prognosis, we are doing what is basically taking a crystal ball and reading the future based on truly the failures of what the conventional system has already created. So if they think that, for example, you have some really bad pancreatic cancer and you have a six-month likelihood you're going to be alive, then they are just talking about their failures using chemo-radiation.

You talk to someone like Nicholas Gonzales in New York City and he is healing people that are in their deathbed using things like vegetable juicing enzymes. Those cases will never be recorded in their statistics. So that's when they come to you and they say, "Well, you're going to die, you know, in six months." That's when the power of belief really starts affecting the outcome.

Ty: Talk about that belief and emotions and cancer—and after that, you mentioned Dr. Gonzales and enzymes. I want you to go into that but let's talk about belief and emotions first.

Sayer: Absolutely. This is one of the most powerful studies of our time published in *The New England Journal of Medicine* just three years ago which showed based on a huge group of Swedes —we're talking about 500,000 of these in the study. When they were given the results for their cancer test—we're looking at different types of cancers—they were told positive. What happens is that within one week of that diagnosis, they had up to 26.9 fold increase risk of death from heart related events.

Ty: Just from the diagnosis. Just from the emotional and mental effect.

Sayer: Exactly. There's no way of knowing whether it was an accurate diagnosis, because again, we're getting a lot of over-diagnosis of lesions that are benign being basically identified as being cancer when they're not.

What happens is like it is a shaman in an old culture pointing to a bone in a member and saying, "You're going to die tomorrow." That person is so convinced that that authority is so valid that they go walk off into the woods and the next day, they die. Exactly proven by this new study, the power of belief in what they call the nocebo effect, which is if your physician whom you trust more than your own self-healing ability, comes in and says, "You're going to die. Look at this results-you have six months." Guess what? You're probably end up dying.

What this study showed was that the belief is so powerful, your heart fails on you within one week. It crashes. You die because of your belief. It is not based on evidence. It is based on the belief that someone else knows your fate better than yourself. And that is why we have to be extremely careful about conventional medicine in this type of diagnosis.

Ty: You mentioned nocebo effect. What is nocebo effect?

Sayer: The placebo effect is really, "I will help," basically because if you believe your physician like your mother who is taking care of you who is going to heal you with her—

Ty: With her sugar pill.

Sayer: Exactly. The thing is true is that if you believe, or your doctor comes to you and you feel negative vibe or you think they don't like you and they think you are going to die, it means it will harm and it means you believe that and you incorporate it in your life, in your belief-system, feeds it into your physiology and then you end up having adverse effect or dying.

Ty: So the nocebo effect. So it's like the flip side of that coin.

Sayer: It's the exact opposite.

Ty: Placebo is positive, nocebo is negative.

Sayer: It's true and it's also tells us that physicians have an ethical and medical responsibility to be aware of their effect, to be aware of their belief system and realize if they are quoting from some statistical data set of four outcomes based on really outdated cancer therapies, let say, radiation and chemo, which is just absurd ultimately. It's on them.

They have to educate themselves and they should be inculcating into the patient a belief in the healing power that they have. If they don't know, I understand, they weren't trained on this, but they should probably be doing something else than treating people with cancer if they don't know that.

Ty: Right. I agree. I mean, to me that's almost the equivalent to a crime to have a cancer patient be diagnosed and tell them that they are going to die because you just sentenced them to death.

Sayer: Exactly. And it's no longer just a bunch of people on the periphery like us saying, "You know, you've got to do better." In *The New England Journal of Medicine*, one of the highest impact journals, stating this is a lethal force. Nocebo effect is as real as the placebo. They are responsible for what they say, what they know. They should never pronounce someone dead based on statistics of an outdated way of treating people with cancer.

Ty: Our emotions have a huge impact on cancer diagnosis and treatment, don't they?

Sayer: And belief. Because ultimately when we liberate ourselves believing in the priest of the body, and realized the placebo effect is the basis of evidence-based on medicine, they have to control for it for even to have a sort of hierarchy of power structure saying that they have the evidence and the truth, right?

Double-blind randomized placebo controlled trials. That's the absolute truth in their model. And why are they controlling for the placebo? It's so powerful. It's even more powerful than most medication that you are using. And so what the placebo is is basically the self-healing ability that I've now outsourced to you because you're the doctor and I believe in you.

When you tell someone that their body is constantly self-healing to overcome cancer in the same way that they may have a scratch on their knee and they can watch it heal and they believe that, they do the right things. Then they will heal cancer and that is really the power that we have that the medical profession really doesn't either, they don't either know it, or they don't want you to know about it.

Ty: So Sayer, let's take a step back here real quickly and just get in to the basics. What exactly is cancer?

Sayer: It's a great question because until we, obviously, answer that correctly we can treat it. And so understanding cancer is has been an on-going pursuit. For at least 50 years, the dominant view is called the mutational theory which is through happenstance, something goes wrong in the nucleus of the cell that causes it to get deranged, go rogue, and just want to replicate clonally into this tissue that invades everything.

But that view has been completely disproven because they identified that cancer is actually rather intelligent. It's capable of invading the immune system by changing the structures on its surface like something out of the Matrix. It can go and produce its own enzyme supply that dissolve through tissues, produce its own blood supply.

It has a hierarchical arrangement of cells which have their own little duties and little village, so to speak. There's a root cell, a cancer cell called the cancer stem cell, which we talked about—the mother behind it all. And so the view that cancer is just rogue terrorists in our body has justified using literally "weapons of mass destruction." Things like chemotherapy which came from the war theatre, actual chemical weapons-grade material being administered to patients as well as radiation which is called from nuclear reactors might as well be culled from nuclear munitions to try to just destroy the terrorist within the body and not think about what it does to all the civilian population. It's the same basic models, pretty much insane.

So what we now know is that view is not correct and that cancer is a survival mechanism that's unmasked. In fact, it's quite amazing if you think about it that these cells can survive things that even in a chemical weapons war or atomic blast a normal human shouldn't survive but these cells were able to.

So it speaks to how cancer truly is. It's an amazing life-force, a regenerative energy that is able to survive the modern apocalypse of chemicals and inappropriate nutrients and pseudo foods and electromagnetic energy and viruses—vaccines for example—and be able to still live.

So when we look at cancer through that lens, we start understanding that the real answer is to adjust back to what is a more natural, healthy state of living, get the cells again to be healed, detoxification, proper nutrition. Things like that and not, obviously, blasting it with poisons and radiation.

Ty: Two things you just said I want to expound on. You were talking about chemotherapy coming from the war theatre. What do you mean?

Sayer: Well, what they did was that they did a number of studies on mustard gas and how that is able to destroy fast-replicating blood cells, the white blood cells in sort of what they called hemotological malignancies. And because it was able to kill those fast replicating cells they, of course, used it to try to treat that cancer because they saw some effect that seemed to put it into remission.

Of course, we know now that that type of chemical is able to cause damage to all the cells in our body and then ultimately, once you've taken that route and ultimately seen it fail because you don't get a very long survival advantage, you blame the victim. You say the cancer is resistant to the chemotherapy. Wen in fact we know you shouldn't use that approach. You should have used the natural approach.

Ty: I see. And so some of the roots of chemotherapy go back to the mustard gases from previous war.

Sayer: Absolutely, yeah. The origin of that category which is still being used today. In fact, in pediatric cancers, they use it sometimes, is really from the war.

Ty: Wow. I bet many people don't know that.

Sayer: No, in fact, if they did know it, I'm sure they would think about alternatives with much more interest.

Ty: Right, right. You also mentioned a few minutes ago viruses and vaccines. Talk about vaccines containing known carcinogens, many of them being used on our infants and could that be contributing to some of these cancers today?

Sayer: That's a really good question. In fact, I believe that the canary in the coal mine, so to speak, in our children when it comes to cancers. In fact, the fastest growing population for cancers today is the pediatric community. And there's a number of reasons for this one and that their results are replicating so fast anyway. We know that is a target for cancer because if you're replicating cells a lot of damage is occurring in that process, you know, electromagnetic radiation, there are poisons, it can cause, quote, "mutation" changes in the sequences and it can lead to cancer.

But the other side of it is that, right now in history we have vaccinated our children to the point where there is no precedent. There's no evidence to in any way vet whether it is safe, for one, to give our children, for example, 60 different vaccines. Any one of which has over 40 different ingredients in its manufacture, or present as excipients within the vaccines.

So we're talking about potentially thousand if not tens of thousands of antigens, ultimately being introduced into their immature immune system. At times when none of these were even studied. The vaccine schedule, of course, is based on very minimal clinical research on one vaccine at a time. There's no true placebo ever used. They don't use saline.

Ty: They never do double-blind placebo tests with vaccines, do they?

Sayer: Exactly. If they were to do that, they would find invariably—and this is why they don't do that—that the harms done by the vaccine far out-weigh any perceived benefit because the placebo group would end up being much healthier. They do have in a way a placebo group called the Amish. They have very low levels of autism.

In New Jersey, one in every 25 boys has autism. I mean, it has grown from the 70s to one in 10,000 to right now to about one in 50 perhaps, one in 75 children today have autism. So this is part of the question. The real problem with vaccines when it comes to cancer is that since the polio campaigns originally, they extracted the material for the vaccines which were oral and live from green kidney cells from these monkeys. The green monkey kidney cells.

Now, they discovered after they administered it to actually 98 million different Americans. They received it—according to the CDC's web page before it was scrubbed recently and it's gone, but it's in the historical record—is that it contains onco virus.

It's oncogenic virus, meaning it causes cancer. It's called simian virus 40, because it is the 40th virus identified in this cell. If you could just imagine what a plague of potential vectors of infection we've unleashed by taking other tissues from animals, torturing them, poisoning them, extracting serums and tissues from them and injecting them live into our children. It turns out that simian virus 40 is trans-generationally transmitted.

So if our parents received that vaccine—and of course, it was cancelled in this country in favor of the inactivated form, because of the fact that oral vaccine was causing the only cases of paralytic polio in this country. And so people don't know that, but it is transmitted from the vaccinated parents through the child. So even though we haven't received that oral vaccine, it's still in our bodies and it's associated with a wide range of very hard to treat cancers.

Ty: Yeah, as a matter fact if I remember it right, it was a study, a 2002 study in *The Lancet* that indicated that non-Hodgkins lymphoma, I think it was, or maybe leukemia, I can't remember but something like 50 percent of the cases were attributable to SV40. I can't remember the exact statistics.

Sayer: No problem. In fact, we at Green Med Info, one of the things we do is catalogue all the research on SV40 and then reference to different cancers and studies on different cancers. Like mesothelioma, for example, has been linked to SV40 as well as, obviously, to environmental exposures. There are a number of very hard to treat cancers that basically are related to the presence of what are known as surreptitious or secret viruses they didn't know were in there that were then transmitted to the body unknowingly.

And because of the vaccine schedule today—like the MMR vaccine for example, still contains living tissues from not only animals but from aborted fetuses. They're called diploid cells, and they intentionally harvested those fetuses to produce the master stock for the vaccine schedule and they have to be replenished. So there's a huge ethical issue because we're using those tissue types and they are full of viruses because the human genome is up to eight percent viral in origin. It has actual onco retro-viruses which are known to cause cancer.

HIV is an example of a retro-virus. That's the material we're using to quote, "improve the immunity" of our children. It doesn't make any sense at all.

Ty: It doesn't. Perhaps that's one of the reasons we've seen this explosion in childhood cancers.

Sayer: I believe it is. In fact, Judy Mikovits who is the author of the *Plague* along with Kent Heckenlively from *Age of Autism,* have written a whole book exposing the reality that there is a plague-like phenomena of non-HIV retro-viral infections which likely were caused by the original vaccines and the production of other biologicals like monoclonal antibodies, which were produced through tumors grown through splicing of human cells with mice cells. This is how they are producing the material to improve our immunity today.

And that cause infections of literally millions of Americans with these retro-viruses that still the CDC and all the associated health organizations are covering up.

Ty: That is not something you're going to hear on the nightly news, is it?

Sayer: No, it is not. But *The Plague*, the book about it, is really worth looking up because it documents the facts of the matter. And it is well known that no one would engage the vaccine schedule if they knew the true risk and the lack of safety.

The government has paid out since 1986 through the national vaccine injury compensation fund over three billion dollars.

Ty: Three billion?

Sayer: Three billion dollars for literally thousands and thousands of cases of children that received the vaccines and they were injured and their families have suffered profoundly. And they are just a fraction of those who were compensated. It's been declared by the government that vaccines are unavoidably unsafe and yet they claimed that they are safe and they claimed they are effective. If you look at the research on the effectiveness—Cochrane database reviews which is one of the most authoritative sources—you will find, no evidence unequivocally proves that the vaccines on schedule today are safe. It doesn't exist. It's completely a lie.

Ty: And one of the things that Dr. Sherri Tenpenny told me last year is that no vaccines are ever evaluated for carcinogenicity. They are not tested to see if they cause cancer.

Sayer: And that's probably intentional. In fact, that was a huge debate before they started to use the animal cells for vaccine production early on in the 50s because they were afraid if they use cancer cells which are much better because they are constantly living and producing antigen that it had an oncogenic factor that can be transmitted to humans.

So what did they do? They decided to not use cancer cells from humans. They used animals cells instead which then they later found had cancer-causing viruses in them. So the history is so well written. They don't do the carcinogenicity study because they know they do cause cancer.

Ty: And you also got other additives to the vaccines, whether it be the mercury in the thimerosal, the aluminium, the formaldehyde, right?

Sayer: Exactly.

Ty: Known carcinogen.

Sayer: It's a known carcinogen, it's not a mystery, it's not a conspiracy theory. It's a fact. The only problem is that we have this sort of blind faith in health authorities, it's called evidence-based medicine. It's not evidence-based medicine, it's science by proclamation. The CDC says, that's not science. Double-blind peer review published research, placebo controlled trials on vaccines , that's not even been done. There has never been a study, ever, in existence on the present vaccine schedule, much less two vaccines simultaneously in the schedule. That isn't evidence. That is completely religious-based faith and it's absolutely destroying the health of our children.

Ty: That's sickening to me because one of my cousin's children is autistic and it happened within a couple of days of the vaccines.

Sayer: Yes, it's one of the main causes. Of course, it's multi-factorial, as you know, C-sections, Tylenol for fevers early on, say after a vaccine. All types of issues with nutrition. There are many factors contributing and that's why they can always say, "Of course it's not vaccines causing autism." Well, of course, logically, but we know the exponential increase, there is no such thing as genetic epidemic. What they are basically implying that's the cause.

That's absurd when you look at the scientifically. So they have to acknowledge the 800 pound gorilla in the room staring at the problem and it is the vaccine schedule.

Ty: You mentioned nutrition. Talk about cancer as being a deficiency disease.

Sayer: You know, one of the most profound discoveries for me over the past few years is the discovery that food isn't just a source of calories and material building blocks for the cell—carbohydrates, proteins, things like that—but has information which is essential to regulate the DNA in our body and make sure the cells know what to do. So when you pull the rug out under our bodies—and for literally hundreds of thousands of years, our diets have consisted of certain types of foods, of certain type of quality—you put a GMO, Roundup-saturated corn, you take oxidized fats from vegetable oils and all these things have never existed before. They carry information that promote cancer.

So if we take those sources of information out of the diet and put back those that are from what our bodies involved with or if you're more biblically oriented, the Garden of Eden approach, you know. Get rid of all these GMO grains and let's add in some of the high quality fruits. Things that were designed by nature, by the Creator, to be taken directly from the tree, eaten. That is really what we need to do. It's to go back to the ancestral diet. And then all the practices of permaculture bio-dynamic farming and intention and getting our soil to be based again on healthy microbes. That's really what is going to be the root of healing cancer.

Of course, you have supplements that are very effective. The research is clear. On Green Man Info, we have 18,000 studies on over 600 compounds that have been shown to kill cancer, at least in the cell model, all the way up to human. So there's no lack of evidence to say that nutrition is the key.

Ty: Right. And your website is fantastic as far as the scientific evidence for these different substances because one of the things that it claims is that we don't have any proof for natural treatments working for these supplements. It's just all quackery.

That's completely false, isn't it?

Sayer: Absolutely. In fact, the real interesting thing, Ty, is what they do. Drug companies literally pour a billion dollars into the research needed to get FDA drug approval. So that starts by finding lead compounds to produce a synthetic chemical and then they go to phase one, two, three, human trials. But when they do this, they pour inadvertently a billion dollars or more. All of these drug companies are into looking at turmeric, resveratrol, green tea, and literally thousands of compounds and they find all this research showing it's superior to chemotherapy.

And so those studies are there and people don't know about them. But they also can't expect those studies on things that grow in your backyard that cure cancer, to receive a billion dollars of capital. Because the whole game is based on producing a synthetic analog to get a patent, to get FDA drug approval. And then of course, more than 50 percent of FDA approved drugs before the patent life expires, get pulled off the market because of the devastation and the death that they caused.

So the whole system is rigged. So you have to read between the lines, look at the research. It is there. You can use grandma's recipes. You can go find an herb in your backyard. You can use your food and that's the way we truly prevent and treat cancer.

Ty: We probably got a couple dozen herbs within a stone's throw of us right here that will treat cancer, don't we?

Sayer: Absolutely. In fact, that knowledge has been passed down since the origin of life, you know, of our species. We're just now re-capturing it. People should know that science is now coming back and confirming that the old wisdom is absolutely scientifically validated.

Ty: Last question, Sayer. Talk about wheatgrass.

Sayer: Oh, wheatgrass.

Ty: Wheatgrass, with a lot of green around here.

Sayer: Oh, I love it because for me, wheatgrass was always a double-edged sword. Because it's from wheat, and yes, gluten-reduced, I used to actually go get it, use it, work with people that would take it. So when someone got sick, someone would feel the great healing effects. Have you seen research on how, for example, on the old-dog-model, it will completely reverse cataracts in some cases by just giving wheatgrass powder.

So when I started looking at the research—and there's more to this—it turns out chlorophyll is an alternative source of energy for the human body. And actually, all animals have this ability because it goes into the mitochondria as metabulae. It enables the mitochondria to capture sunlight energy which photo-energizes the Krebs cycle in such a way that produces significantly more ATP which is sort of the energy currency of the body without increasing oxidative stress.

This is a new study that came out last year which completely undermines our classical understanding of our bodies as only being able to eat other things to live. Basically, we can, if we have adequate chlorophyll in our diet—wheatgrass being one of the best sources—directly capture the sunlight. And not only it does increase the production and efficiency of ATP in our body, it increases the longevity, at least in the earthworm model which they used it for. We will see animal studies and probably human studies soon because basically, this reclassifies as from heterotrophs which depend on other things to photo-heterotrophs, which means we can actually take sunlight directly into our body.

Keep in mind it doesn't just mean the wavelengths, like you know, obviously the sunlight we see. Red, for example, is a wavelength that goes deep into our tissue as well, and it can even penetrate the skull and go into our brain and energize our brain. So this research reveals how—because cancer loves glucose, right? It loves to ferment it, produces all these biomass and it's the ATP-based model of energy is more about bio-mass and less about how we can actually capture energy to fuel our body.

Ty: I want you to talk about sugar because recently I interviewed Dr. Russell Blaylock. He mentioned that sugar and glutamate, actually, are two fuels for cancer cells which was new information. Sugar feeds cancer, we all know about that, but talk about new studies about sugar.

Sayer: A new study came out that showed for the first time that cancer doesn't just only feed on sugar but that sugar can induce a cancerous phenotype in cells, which means it basically changed it from a cell that just likes glucose to one that exhibits invasive activity. Where it's basically becoming an independent cell that wants to go out and invade their tissue.

So it was the first time that we saw that sugar is a cancer risk, much like smoking is. It's not just that it feeds cancer, that it can actually cause cancer.

Ty: Wow, that's amazing information that I was not familiar with.

Sayer: Yeah, absolutely. The thing about cancer that we know so much about, thanks to Otto Warburg's work from the 20's which is—he's a scientist which identified that cancer generally has a particular metabolic type—which is that it loves to ferment glucose. And it does this even when adequate oxygen is available for it to flip in to the normal oxygen dependent oxidative phosphorylation which is far more efficient in producing ATP. Cancer cells are like, "No way. I want to do a less-efficient fermentation of sugar." And then it produces all this biomass which it needs to grow and produce more tumor.

So that concept helped us to realize that sugar is a big risk. And when we're talking about sugar, we're not just talking about table sugar or fructose. We're talking about hidden sugar which is processed grains contain often high glycemic index rating than actual sugar itself.

So if you have puffed rice, that could be almost double as effective at making your blood sweet and feeding the cancer cells than something that actually tastes sweet like actual sugar.

Ty: Wow.

Sayer: Yeah, so, it helps us to understand that our body needs more good fats, obviously. Higher quality sources of plant material, not grains which are really starches and hidden sugar. And then of course, a lot of the protein sources that are high quality as well.

Ty: So name a few high quality protein sources.

Sayer: Well, it's interesting because now that I understand the cell metabolism differently—not so much depending on glucose—protein is important but maybe not as important as I used to think. Now, of course, protein can be turned into glucose, too, that's why we talked about the glucose-centric model of cell metabolism.

So some high quality protein sources—whey for example. I like one that is completely divorced from casein which is what you make cheese from. Whey is usually thrown away when you make casein which is liquid protein but it is also very good for immunity and you can get goat-based sources, too, if you wanted to just eliminate the whole cow factor.

But interestingly enough, protein is prevalent throughout the plant kingdom. And I do believe that our bodies, with the help of the gut bacteria—which contributes 99 times more genetic material than our own body so they have their all this incredible capabilities in terms of degrading anti-nutrients in plants helping to convert amino acids into important things like neurotransmitters. So we can get a lot of our protein actually from whole plant foods as well.

Ty: So that is what you recommend then?

Sayer: I'm actually open. I think there's a lot of research that supports the use of high quality animal products. I think there are some cases where the ethical problem with that is more of an issue where some people might not want to go there. So it's always a matter of balance. They do feel the high quality meats and in some cases, are very therapeutic.

Ty: Great. We're going to go over to Food & Thought later tonight.

Sayer: Yeah.

Ty: And they may have some quality meats.

Sayer: They will and you're going to indulge. I know that they do.

Ty: Well, Sayer, the information that you shared with us today is just fascinating. It's cutting-edge and it's well documented. I really want to say thank you for your time today.

Sayer: It's my pleasure. Thanks for what you do, Ty.

Ty: Thank you.

[end of transcript]

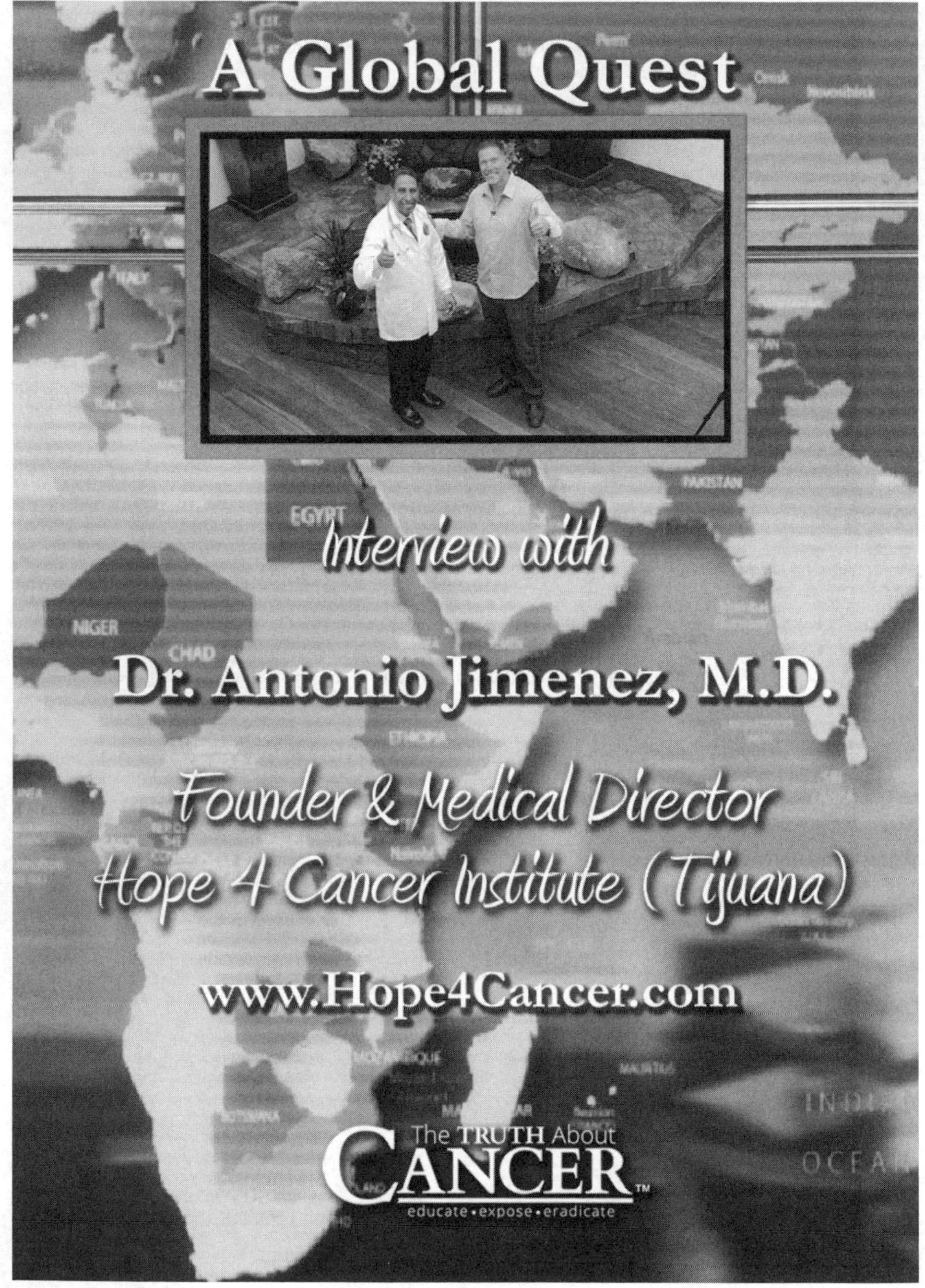
A Global Quest
Interview with
Dr. Antonio Jimenez, M.D.
Founder & Medical Director
Hope 4 Cancer Institute (Tijuana)
www.Hope4Cancer.com
The TRUTH About
CANCER
educate • expose • eradicate

Ty: Well, Dr. Tony Jimenez—good to be with you again, brother.

Dr. Jimenez: Nice to see you, brother.

Ty: Yeah.

Dr. Jimenez: Nice to see you again.

Ty: So, this is the first time we've been together in your clinic.

Dr. Jimenez: That's right.

Ty: We're here at the Hope4Cancer Clinic, Tijuana.

Dr. Jimenez: Yes.

Ty: You know, we've done many interviews before. I mean, we did one on the boat in Latvia together.

Dr. Jimenez: That's right. Yes.

Ty: And then last year—interview in San Diego, but your clinic—first time I visited it. So what I'd like to do today is to see if you can kind of walk me through the clinic and show us what you have here as far as the different machines.

But before we do that, I want to address something that I saw—a video that I saw about this clinic and I saw it and it made me so angry that I wanted to address it. Apparently, someone from England—she shaved her head—

Dr. Jimenez: Shaved her head.

Ty: —and she came to the clinic and without permission, secretly filmed you and basically painted you to be a snake oil salesman, huckster, scam-artist, whatever.

Dr. Jimenez: Exactly.

Ty: Several things were just blatant lies in the video and they bothered me. One of the biggest things that bothered me was at the point where she was filming you, you know—illegally, it was illegal filming by the way, because you were—

Dr. Jimenez: It was falsified medical records

Ty: —with falsified medical records and she's in your clinic, illegally filming you—claiming you're the criminal—

Dr. Jimenez: That's right.

Ty: —while she's committing crimes.

Dr. Jimenez: Exactly.

Ty: Regardless. You're up there at the—you had a chalkboard at this point.

Dr. Jimenez: That's right.

Ty: And one of the things she said was that, "As Dr. Tony begun to spew all of these unscientifically proven lies," or whatever she said—you were talking about cancer, how chemotherapy makes cancer stem cells resistant.

Dr. Jimenez: More resistant, more aggressive. As you know, this is documented information. You know, this is not, "Dr. Tony said."

Ty: Right.

Dr. Jimenez: These are major universities.

Ty: That was the thing that got me so mad because she says, at that exact point, how you were spewing rubbish and lies. And what are there, like, three dozen studies over the last two years that prove that's the truth?

Dr. Jimenez: It's likely.

Ty: I mean, on reputable medical—in reputable medical literature, Pub Med. It's everywhere.

Dr. Jimenez: Everywhere. You know, the Pittsburgh Medical Center is one of them. Extensive study in this area.

Ty: Yeah. So that was one of the things. There were so many things about that video. There were just blatant lies and it really bothered me because I know from knowing you, from interviewing you, the protocols that you are using—you are using things that work.

Dr. Jimenez: We've been here at Hope4Cancer, Ty, for 15 years, you know. 15 years of hard work. I've been in the alternative, integrated fields for 25 years. We've published. We have a lot of science.

Oftentimes, in the medical community, they think because you're doing integrated medicine or alternative medicine, it's quackery or there's no science behind it. On the contrary, there's a lot of science behind it.

Ty: There is. There is. And a lot of these treatments that you're using, you've described to us before, but I want you to walk us through the clinic and show us. I want to see the Far Infrared, the Sono-Photo Dynamic Therapy, the PEMF. I said Far Infrared. There's one other machine I wanted you to show us. I'll think of it.

Dr. Jimenez: The Hyperbaric?

Ty: The Hyperbaric. I want to see the Hyperbaric.

Dr. Jimenez: Indiba Hyperthermia.

Ty: Right. So these are all protocols that have mountains of literature—

Dr. Jimenez: Exactly.

Ty: —that show that they are toxic to cancer cells or that they stimulate the immune system or that they do one thing or another that helps cancer patients. So this is not a center for snake oil salesmen. This is a center for science. So I would like to see some of the scientifically proven treatments.

Dr. Jimenez: Let's take a walk.

Ty: Sounds good.

So Dr. Tony, what's the first room that we're going to go to in to here?

Dr. Jimenez: The first room that we're going into is the Sono-Photo Dynamic Therapy room.

Ty: Okay. Sono-Photo Dynamic Therapy. Say that six-times fast. Okay, so what do we have here?

Dr. Jimenez: At the core of Hope4Cancer for cancer is energy medicine. And we know we use energy medicines for diagnosis, right? Like PET-scan, positive emission tomography, that's energy. We use MRI, CT-scan, ultrasound. For our heart, we check EKG. Those are all energy diagnostic tools, but when we are using energy to help patients with cancer, then that is not conventionally accepted.

And we know that in 1954, Richard Gerber, MD, wrote a book called *Vibrational Medicine*, which at that time—it was far ahead of its time. And now here at Hope4Cancer, we have the Sono, part of Sono-Photo Dynamic Therapy and this therapy is available at Hope4Cancer. We've been doing this for nine years now. We're using sound to affect cancer cells. So we provide a—what's called a sensitizer and the patient takes this under the tongue, based on their body weight, okay? This is absorbed by cancer cells 70 to one. So, for every 70 cancer cells, one normal cell absorbs this molecule.

Ty: What's is the sensitizer?

Dr. Jimenez: The sensitizer is a derivative of chlorophyll or seaweed. It's a naturally-occurring product. It has no toxicity and it's absorbed by cancer cells 70 to one. We wait 24-36 hours after administration. This way, most of the cancer cells have now all absorbed it and normal cells release it. We don't know the mechanism why normal cell release it. I think it's a God thing, but, you know, it's another story.

Ty: But it works.

Dr. Jimenez: But it works. So, cancer cells retain it, but this substance by itself does nothing until we wake it up.

Ty: Okay.

Dr. Jimenez: Or activate it. That is done using sound therapy—a specific frequency, amplitude, intensity—and this is something that patients can do, not only while they're at Hope4Cancer, but for an extended period of time at home as a home program because this is totally nontoxic.

Ty: Right. And then we get the photo part.

Dr. Jimenez: And then, we have the photo therapy and this is a—as you see, it has red lights, blue lights and a row of lights that are not on because when they are on, it is just invisible light in the near infrared spectrum.

So, photodynamic therapy will also wake up the sensitizer and allow it to activate itself within cancer cells and that forms oxygen radicals—O minus. O minus, as you know, are toxic to cancer cells and they set off the apoptosis or programmed cell death.

In addition to that, it provides local inflammatory response. Thereby, the immune system could come and target that area.

Ty: Wow! Very cool. So what does this have to do with it here?

Dr. Jimenez: Yes, this is another type of Photo Dynamic Therapy. We are using full spectrum lights. The patient lies on the bed, this comes down, and they lie here for 30 minutes on the back and 30 minutes on the stomach and they're getting full-body photodynamic therapy.

Ty: Okay, and that same substance that they ingested for the Sono part, that chlorophyll-type substance reacts to the light as well?

Dr. Jimenez: Reacts to the light.

Ty: So you are hitting with—from two different directions on the cancer cells.

Dr. Jimenez: Right. Exactly.

Ty: Fascinating.

Dr. Jimenez: Nontoxic, very effective, and this is proven science how Sono-Photo Dynamic Therapy works.

Ty: So this is not the spectrum that would actually give them a tan or anything.

Dr. Jimenez: Exactly.

Ty: It's a different type of light because—it looks like tanning bed lights to me, but it's different.

Dr. Jimenez: Yes, yes. This is full spectrum. There is no mercury being released from here. This is not fluorescent light. This is full spectrum light. The closest we can come to mimicking the light of the sun. And you know, from historical records, we know that the sun has healed many diseases.

Ty: Right. Cool. Let see what we have in here the clinic.

Dr. Jimenez: Excellent.

Ty: Great.

Dr. Jimenez: Now, we're going to the Hyperbaric Oxygen Chamber room and here, we have hyperbaric oxygen. What this does is the patient comes in here. It's lying down very comfortable. We're increasing the pressure of oxygen to about 4 to 4.5 pounds per square inch. We know oxygen and cancer don't combine. And so, the one hour that the patient is in here, you're saturating the cells with oxygen.

Ty: What's the normal pressure? You said, 4.5 pounds per square—what's the normal pressure?

Dr. Jimenez: About 1.3.

Ty: So, this is like four times as strong?

Dr. Jimenez: Exactly.

Ty: So that pressure is then forcing oxygen into the cells?

Dr. Jimenez: Yes, and patients love this therapy because you feel that oxygen load. And some patients tell me, "Can I stay in here two hours or three hours?" Literally, you can—you can, right, because you can't get too much oxygen in this sense, but one hour is the duration of the treatment. This is one of the preferred treatments of the cancer, not only for its efficacy, but because it allows the patient to relax there for an hour. You know, you kind of are in the bubble, and you forget of what—the fears, the conflicts that you have. It's just a good therapy in that sense as well.

Ty: Very cool. So everybody that's in the treatment protocol here is going to lay in the hyperbaric once a day?

Dr. Jimenez: Once a day. We do it daily for an hour.

Ty: For an hour. Okay.

Dr. Jimenez: Oftentimes, I'd like to do it before bedtime because it kind of relaxes them. Even though they're getting a lot of oxygen which stimulates, but it also mentally relaxes them and they sleep better.

Ty: Because the brain's getting the oxygen it needs.

Dr. Jimenez: Exactly, exactly. They sleep better. Pain is controlled better. Even their stresses, you know, their—it does something that maybe is not described yet to the emotion, but oxygen is the main field for the human body.

Ty: I bet this would be big with athletes.

Dr. Jimenez: It is. It is. Yes. Many sports teams have hyperbaric oxygen chambers.

Ty: Something like this—like a chamber like this—if somebody wanted to buy it themselves—is this affordable for someone or is it pretty expensive?

Dr. Jimenez: This is the higher model ones. And this is about 12, 13 thousand US dollars. It starts out at about $8,000 and I have one at home.

Ty: One of the higher end or the lower end?

Dr. Jimenez:Well, I got this one also because my wife sometimes likes to go in there with myself. So we both go in and the lower end ones are smaller. And my kids—I have 5-year-old twins, so of course, you know, we're educating and teaching them now about how to wear these so they go in here with myself or with my wife and it's excellent.

Ty: Great. What else do we got across the hall here, Dr. Tony?

Dr. Jimenez: Okay, let's go to the—more energy medicine.

Ty: Okay. So, what do we have here?

Dr. Jimenez: Well, this is more energy medicine, the best from across the world. Because we are in Mexico, this doesn't mean we're only using technology in Mexico. Here at Hope4Cancer, we have technology—the best of the best from all over the world.

This device comes from Germany and it's called the Ondamed. *Onda* meaning wave, *Med*—medicine. So like the medical wave, right? Healing wave. This is subtle, pulsating, electromagnetic energy. With this technology, you can scan an individual and also you could treat them.

So, what are we treating? We're treating any energetic aberrations or energetic deficiencies or excesses to balance. Remember those...

Ty: Are those, like, headphones? It looks like you put on your head. What is this?

Dr. Jimenez: Actually, this is placed right here. Right there.

Ty: Okay.

Dr. Jimenez: And then, there's another apparatus that goes in the abdomen, wherever the cancer is. Remember that cells resonate at different frequencies. Cancer cells are about minus 20 to minus 30 milibles, whereas normal human cells are about minus 70 to minus 90 milibles. So, as people age or disease sets in, the cells are losing that electrical conductivity. So with this technology, we're able to up-regulate that electrical conductivity. What happens here is everything works better. Food is absorbed better, water is absorbed better, supplements are absorbed better, the cell is more able to detoxify.

So at the core level, remember cells make up tissues, tissues make up organs, organs make up the system like the digestive system, respiratory system and all the system make up the body. So with this technology, we're able to affect at the basic unit of life which is the cell.

Ty: The cell. The organs—

Dr. Jimenez: Disease starts and ends—

Ty: At the cellular level.

Dr. Jimenez: —at the cellular level.

Ty: Okay. So what is this, Dr. Tony?

Dr. Jimenez: This is Pulsating Electromagnetic Field Therapy. Again, to affect the cell, we can pulsate water, we can pulsate the cells. We can help reduce the tumor size by energy. Can I try it on you, Ty?

Ty: Absolutely. Sure.

Dr. Jimenez: Okay.

Ty: Can I sit down here?

Dr. Jimenez: Yeah. Have a sit please. Make yourself comfortable. I know you had a long day.

Ty: I'll take any relaxation I can get at this point.

Dr. Jimenez: Let's put this around your neck.

Ty: You're not tying this to a truck or anything are you?

Dr. Jimenez: Oh no. We'll start with a 3-minute session and I'm going to increase the intensity. You're going to feel maybe your muscles jumping a little bit.

Ty: Okay.

Dr. Jimenez: And here, we're affecting—you begin to feel that?

Ty: Yeah, I feel it twitching. Yeah.

Dr. Jimenez: You feel it twitching. So now, we're sending electromagnetic fields.

Ty: That's interesting.

Dr. Jimenez: This goes back to the Papimi in Greece. When this was developed back many years ago, it was like a washing machine. Now, technology has consolidated it and we have it this small.

Ty: Wow! This is really interesting.

Dr. Jimenez: It's very good for pain, very good for inflammation.

Ty: I've been having pain in the back of my neck. Should this help?

Dr. Jimenez: Yeah, that should help. Sometimes with one treatment

Ty: So I guess you could—if you'll turn it up too high, I would be like—zzzzttt!

Dr. Jimenez: You know, the intensity is regulated here and whether it is high or low, you're still getting the same amount of energy. It is whether it's here like this—or here. But at the end it's the same amount of intensity. So if that's comfortable, that's what where we're leaving it.

Ty: Yeah, this is great.

Dr. Jimenez: Exactly.

Ty: It feels funny. It's not uncomfortable, but it does kind of feel funny that your muscle is twitching like this.

Dr. Jimenez: Especially when it's your first one.

Ty: Yeah, but it's kind of like when you—almost when you get a Charlie horse, kind of, in your calf or something and you're trying to work it out.

Dr. Jimenez: And there's different adapt—ways to provide this if you want to do the shoulder for example, you put it like this. For knee problems—and athletes or anyone you could do the knee—we would do the four different ways. And then from the back. We give this...

Ty: You can hit different areas of the body right? Localizing it.

Dr. Jimenez: Different areas of the body.

Ty: So if this is around my neck, is this is really focusing on the upper torso?

Dr. Jimenez: It is focusing on the upper torso, but the energy is going all the way to your back. Remember here, we have the thymus gland.

Ty: Right.

Dr. Jimenez: One of the very important immune glands. So, we are stimulating the thymus gland. You know, people that work in energy medicine, you could be affecting the chakras as well. Right balance to the energetic meridians—very powerful.

Ty: One thing I found here while sitting, when I flex my muscle, it twitches harder.

Dr. Jimenez: It twitches harder.

Ty: And when I relax, it doesn't twitch as much.

Dr. Jimenez: Because of the contraction, huh?

Ty: Yeah, just take it easy.

Dr. Jimenez: This is one of the favourite therapies of the patients. And oftentimes, we want them to start the day with this because anything that they could do after a PEMF treatment will be absorbed and work better.

Ty: Better. What does a machine like this run?

Dr. Jimenez: This is 22,000 US dollars.

Ty: Oh, this is—

Dr. Jimenez: This, I don't have one at home.

Ty: Wow! 22,000 is— I guess you want to make sure that these are accurate or that they are good.

Dr. Jimenez: Right.

Ty: I mean you don't want the cheap ones that people can fry themselves on.

Dr. Jimenez: Exactly. Yes. We're waiting for the 3-minute cycle to finish.

Ty: I like this. It actually feels good.

Dr. Jimenez: Yeah, it does. It does.

Ty: Yeah. At the very first it was kind of odd, but now it feels good.

Dr. Jimenez: So Ty, is it done? If you want to see what kind of energy we gave you?

Ty: Yeah.

Dr. Jimenez: Alright. Could you stand up for a second, please?

Ty: Sure.

Dr. Jimenez: And hold this like this. Alright, this is a chain, as you see.

Ty: Wow!

Dr. Jimenez: So, it closes the loop.

Ty: Some serious energy.

Dr. Jimenez: Serious energy. But if I crank it up more, maybe we could take it this way so they can see it. Hold the bottom. Keep it that way. It forms a loop. It stops.

Ty: Right.

Dr. Jimenez: We'll take it away and it's stabilizing the energy pattern.

Ty: Wow. That's interesting. Yeah. So this is the favorite treatment of many patients, the PEMF.

Dr. Jimenez: Yes, absolutely sure. Very simple to use, very effective and one of the staple treatments at Hope4Cancer.

Ty: Very cool. Thanks for showing me.

Dr. Jimenez: Surely. I'm glad you enjoyed it.

Ty: I appreciate you letting me be your guinea pig. It was enjoyable actually.

Dr. Jimenez: Okay, excellent.

Ty: So, Dr. Tony, this is a sauna. What kind of a sauna is it?

Dr. Jimenez: This is a Near Infrared Sauna as opposed to a Far Infrared Sauna.

Ty: So Dr. Tony, what is the difference between Far Infrared Sauna and Near Infrared? I got a little personal Far Infrared at the house, but I think one of your patients today that I talked to said, "No, it's not a Far Infrared. It's Near Infrared." What's the difference?

Dr. Jimenez: Near Infrared light has a greater depth of penetration than Far Infrared. Near Infrared light is more detoxing. You know that saunas and infrared light pulls out toxic and heavy metals. Also, most Far Infrared Saunas in the market have too much EMF—electromagnetic fields—that are toxic, like a cellphone, right?

There's a book called *Sauna and Detoxification* by Dr. Lawrence Wilson, MD, in Arizona. And there, he is considered the guru of Sauna Therapy and he talks about what I have just mentioned to you about the importance of using the Near Infrared as opposed to Far Infrared.

Ty: So, Near Infrared has less EMF and penetrates further. But why are so many people pushing Far Infrared? Is it just more affordable?

Dr. Jimenez: I don't know because this is not that expensive.

Ty: It's not? Okay.

Dr. Jimenez: Actually, you can even build one of these yourself. As you see, it has a light bulb like the ones that I use to heat a bathroom, you know, generating the infrared heat and light. Also, with respect to the Sono-Photo Dynamic Therapy, it's been shown that Near Infrared light also activates the sensitizer in Photo Dynamic Therapy. So it has that added benefit.

Ty: That same chlorophyll molecule that you're taking.

Dr. Jimenez: Yes. Yes.

Ty: Interesting. Dr. Tony, this is the hyperthermia room? So, what's going on here? What kind of machine is thic?

Dr. Jimenez: Here we have a local, direct, hyperthermia. What is hyperthermia? High heat. We know, science knows, that cancer cells are heat sensitive. Normal human cells are heat resistant. That's why when we have a flu or virus and infection, we get a fever to kill the bugs, but it doesn't kill our healthy cells.

So now, even in the US, they're using hyperthermia with radiation and they're saying, "Wow! The results are better." Well, of course, because most of the damage selectively to the cancer cells are being done by the local hyperthermia.

Ty: And so that is what it is, it's a local hyperthermia machine.

Dr. Jimenez: It's a very easy, non-invasive therapy. This is the one. Of course if—let's say the patient has a tumor in the breast, we put a conductive gel—natural non-toxic—we crank up the device and then the treatment is done externally. This is using both capacitance and resistance—diffent types of energy to get to superficial as well as to deep tumors.

This is another favorite, Ty. I know I told you several of them are our favorites, but this is not only a feel-good therapy, but a very effective therapy. With the combination of Sono-Photo Dynamic Therapy and local hyperthermia, we're getting at least a 52 percent decrease in blood supply to the cancer tumors or masses during the stay of the patient here. We know that angiogenesis, right? It's one of the characteristics—hallmarks of cancer, so if we could decrease the blood flow to the tumor, we are well on our way to having an effective therapy.

Ty: Yeah.

Dr. Jimenez: And you know, maybe you saw some patients today who had an 80 or 90 percent blood flow.

Ty: Yeah, we did, as a matter of fact. Now, as opposed to what we have already seen with the Near Infrared Sauna—that's also hyperthermia, isn't it?

Dr. Jimenez: That's correct.

Ty: This is a different machine that does the same thing?

Dr. Jimenez: Not exactly. It doesn't do the same thing because that's more for pulling out toxins, that's more for superficial opening up of the pores for cleansing the toxins. This local hyperthermia—and we also have full body hyperthermia here—is a therapeutic treatment for cancer, meaning it is going after the cancer cells, it's going after the bugs—

Ty: Got it.

Dr. Jimenez: —the viruses, the bacteria, the fungus.

Ty: So it's good doing both?

Dr. Jimenez: It's good doing both.

Ty: Great. Dr. Tony, here we are, Hope4Cancer Center in Tijuana.

You gave me an outstanding tour and I really appreciate it. I feel like now, I've got a better understanding what you do here. I knew the therapies before, but it really helps to be able see it.

I'm hopeful that this has been helpful to the viewing audience to be able to see these treatments that you've been doing so successfully here. They got a good taste of your—the survivors here, your staff is fantastic. Your clinic is really doing good work.

So thank you for spending the time with us today to do that.

Dr. Jimenez: Thank you. Thank you for your work, Ty. It's been marvellous.

Ty: Keep up the good work. We'll keep up the good work and together, we're going to eradicate cancer once and for all.

Dr. Jimenez: No doubt.

Ty: No doubt. God bless you, brother.

Dr. Jimenez: God bless you.

[end of transcript]

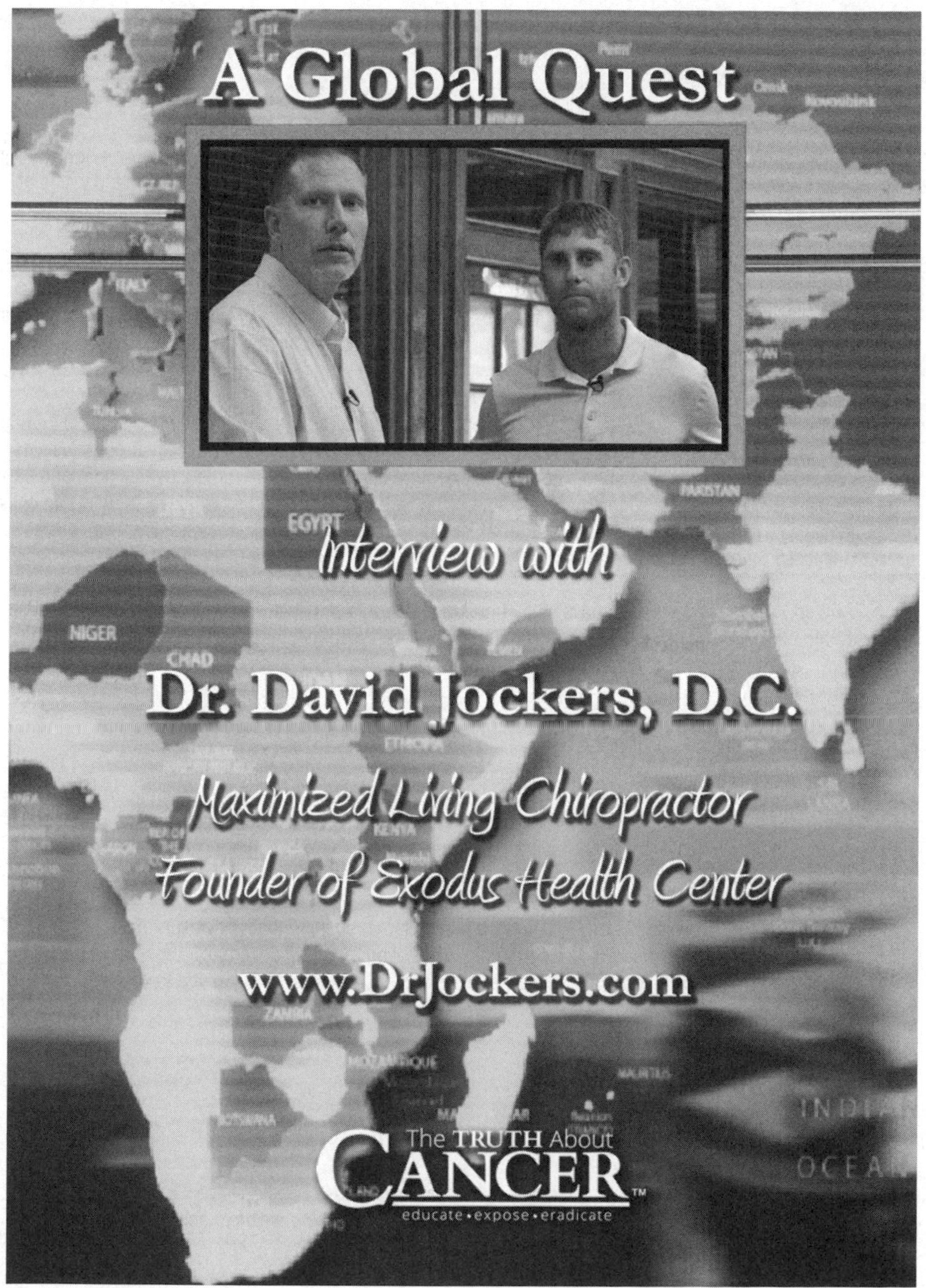
A Global Quest
Interview with
Dr. David Jockers, D.C.
Maximized Living Chiropractor
Founder of Exodus Health Center
www.DrJockers.com
The TRUTH About
CANCER
educate • expose • eradicate

Ty: I'm here today with Dr. David Jockers. If you remember Dr. Jockers from last year with *The Quest for the Cures*, we interviewed you before, but I wanted to go a little bit further today and go into more details than what you shared last year.

So my first question, after I thank you for being with us, Dr. Jockersis concerning sugar. We talked a lot about sugar in "The Quest for the Cures," but can you elaborate more as to how sugar plays into this cancer equation?

Dr. Jockers: Yes, sugar really impairs the immune system. In fact, in the 1970s there was a scientist named John Ely. What Dr. Ely actually did—he actually looked in detail at what happens—how do white blood cells run? What is different about white blood cells and normal cells? What he found was that white blood cells actually need 20 times more vitamin C than normal cells.

Now, he also looked at what the pathway is for white blood cells to get the vitamin C that they need because we know vitamin C is an anti-oxidant, it protects the white blood cells from oxidative stress, and of course, most of your listeners, most people should know, white cells are kind of like your military, right? So they're going out and they're fighting wars every single day, and so they need a lot of protection.

So how does vitamin C actually get into the white blood cell? That's the question. And what he found was that it goes through the same pathway that sugar, or glucose, gets into the cell, through insulin. And so what that means is when blood sugar elevates, our body naturally produces this hormone called insulin. Insulin takes the sugar, puts it into the cell where it belongs. And so what we know is that cells, including white blood cells, have a greater affinity for glucose—the insulin receptor itself has a greater affinity for glucose than it does vitamin C.

And so what that actually means is that when blood sugar is elevated, we are unable to get the vitamin C into the cell. And so there is something that Dr. Ely came up with that was called the Phagocytic Index and it was really just this measurement of how good a white blood cell is at destroying either abnormal cells like cancer or a bacteria or a virus, something along those lines.

Ty: How many bad guys can it kill?

Dr. Jockers: Yes, exactly. That is exactly what he was looking at. And so, here's what he found. A blood sugar of 120 actually reduces your Phagocytic Index by 75 percent. So when we look at our blood sugar of 120, we know that if you have a fasting blood sugar of 120, you are considered basically pre-diabetic—125, 126 is diabetic.

So most people are like, "Well, I don't have a fasting blood sugar of that," however, most people in society, let's say you eat cereal in the morning, just eating that bowl of cereal in the morning, for the next three to four hours you are going to have a blood sugar above 120—most people are.

Ty: Just from cereal.

Dr. Jockers: Just from cereal, right?

Ty: Not even sugared cereal, just because of the grains?

Dr. Jockers: Exactly. Just eating Cheerios, right? Having a glass of orange juice with that, right? Your blood sugar is going to be pumped up and what is happening there is you're actually reducing your white blood cell's ability to break down cancer cells. Then if you go in at lunch, you have a sandwich, you have these high-carb meals—all throughout the day you're actually reducing your Phagocytic Index. Most people are spending 16 hours a day with reduced immune function.

Ty: Or more.

Dr. Jockers: And they are people we think are healthy because they haven't been diagnosed with a disease.

Ty: And how many people get up in the middle of the night and have a glass of juice? And they may have even killed it further—I mean, for more hours.

Dr. Jockers: For the next 24 hours.

Ty: Wow, that's really amazing.

Dr. Jockers: Huge.

Ty: So in that same context, let's expand a little further about the role that oxygen plays in cancer.

Dr. Jockers: Absolutely.

Ty: We mentioned it last year, but let's take it up a little bit.

Dr. Jockers: Yes, absolutely. We look at oxygen therapy. For example, in my clinic we use a hyperbaric oxygen chamber to help people who have chronic disease. Now, we know with cancer, as cancer is developing, these are mutated abnormal cells, so they are no longer running off of what normal cells run off of, which is oxygen. They become hypoxic. And so, what happens is the core of the cancer is highly hypoxic.

Ty: What does hypoxic mean?

Dr. Jockers: That means low-oxygen environment. And that actually provides a protective mechanism against things like chemotherapy and our immune system. And because it is hypoxic in the core that actually signals—it sends out something called VEGF, which is "Vascular Endothelial Growth Factor," which then signals the body to actually start producing blood vessels—abnormal blood vessels—that feed into the whole cancer tumor as it is forming. So it develops its own blood supply that is going to bring more nutrition to the core, and keep it alive.

Ty: And that's what it is called, angiogenesis?

Dr. Jockers: Angiogenesis is the term—forming new blood vessels. That is what that means. So we pump the body with more oxygen. Oxygen therapy, for example, gets more oxygen diffusing into the plasma and into all the cells of the body. That shuts down the production of this VEGF, this "Vascular Endothelial Growth Factor," therefore the cancer, the core, will have a reduced blood supply, which will weaken it and make it more exposed.

Ty: No nourishment.

Dr. Jockers: That's right—make it more exposed to our body's own immune system, which is the greatest defense, that's the greatest military against cancer formation, and it would make it actually more vulnerable to chemotherapy and radiation if that person chose to go that route.

Ty: Wow, so it is really apparent how big of a role oxygen plays in this equation.

Dr. Jockers: Absolutely key.

Ty: That's why the bio-oxidative therapies, those therapies that deal with oxygen, are so important, right?

Dr. Jockers: You've got that right.

Ty: So let's look at another word that has the same prefix—O-X-Y, but oxidative stress. People have heard of oxidative stress. What is it, how can you minimize it, and what kind of a role does it play in cancer?

Dr. Jockers: Absolutely. Oxidative stress is kind of this chemical reaction. The best example for anybody to understand would be when metal rusts. It has all these environmental factors that are coming against it and it ends up rusting. We've all seen that happen. Well, within our body there is this war—this war against rusting ourselves versus our cells actually protecting themselves alone. Our cells—God put this power within us to protect us from oxidation, from environmental stresses.

And what our body does is, every single cell has little signaling mechanism. It is called the KEAP1 pathway. Think about it—keep us healthy. So that KEAP1 is this little receptor and he has just kind of got his hand out there and he is just checking the water. And as the water gets hot—let's say as the water gets hotter—that's more of this environmental oxidative stress that is coming. The water gets hot, it sends a signal, it tags its partner, which is called Nrf2 gene pathway, and this Nrf2 enzyme...

Ty: Nrf2?

Dr. Jockers: Nrf2. You'll hear about that—Nrf2. That, then, goes and it signals our Anti-Oxidant Response Element, A-R-E. The Anti-Oxidant Response Element is a very powerful pathway. What it actually does, is it amplifies our body's entire oxidative stress defense system—all the anti-oxidants are going. So instead of just one anti-oxidant to quench one free radical, a 1 to 1 ratio, it sends out hundreds of thousands of signals to protect the whole cell, the whole genome, from oxidative stress—a very powerful pathway.

Ty: So it's like it opens the floodgates.

Dr. Jockers: That's right—opens the floodgates, like full military defense. We're fully ready, stocked, and on guard.

Ty: So how can you release—how can you open the floodgates? What substances might do this?

Dr. Jockers: Yes, this is huge, because if we want to prevent cancer, we've got to activate this response. We want it to be very sensitive. We want our system to be so good with this pathway. There are four key compounds—many different lifestyle activities, like exercise that help enhance that, but compounds that we can take in from nature that are going to really dramatically improve that antioxidant response are four things, and your listeners may have heard of some of these.

Resveratrol—we find that in berries, so consuming blueberries. Consume grape skins--that is the number one source. We've heard about it in red wine. Resveratrol—very powerful for ramping up that Nrf2, KEAP1, ARE pathway.

You also have it in something called sulforaphane. Sulforaphane is found in cruciferous vegetables—broccoli, cabbage, collard greens, brussels sprouts. The number one source from nature is going to be broccoli sprouts, which you can find at any health—most health food stores nowadays, you can find broccoli sprouts. Put them on your salad every single day—ramp up that pathway.

Also curcumin, which is the active ingredient in turmeric. Curcuminoids help ramp up that pathway, especially if you combine them with a little bit of black pepper, and also good oils, making them fat-soluble—ramps up that pathway.

And the last thing is going to be catechins, which are like ECGC, which is what we find in green tea, chocolate—most people like chocolate—dark chocolate, no sugar in it—loaded with catechins that ramp up this Nrf2 Anti-Oxidant Response Element in our system to protect our genome.

Ty: Wow, that's fascinating. So, four substances that we probably have access to on a daily basis. You have the Resveratrol in the grapes and other berries.

Dr. Jockers: That's right.

Ty: You have the catechins, as you call them, with green tea. You have the curcumin, which is the active ingredient in turmeric, right?

Dr. Jockers: Yes.

Ty: Do you get curcumin if you just sprinkle curry powder on your food?

Dr. Jockers: You will get some.

Ty: Or does have to be more concentrated?

Dr. Jockers: You definitely will get some. Curry, itself, is going to have some Curcuminoid, however, with our modern technology we have been able to isolate curcuminoids, make them much more powerful, so taking a supplement is extremely powerful. I try to do it from both mechanisms. I put turmeric on my foods, put on a little black pepper, and make sure I'm consuming it with some good oils, good fats in there. But at the same time I also like to supplement with specific curcuminoid—extract of curcuminoid—to really ramp up that pathway.

Ty: Okay. And then the last one is sulforaphanes. So we have access to all of these things.

Dr. Jockers: That's right, yes. Very powerful nutrients that are going to really help protect our body from oxidative stress and development of cancer.

Ty: Awesome. And then you said it was the sulforaphanes in broccoli that helps if you add pepper to it? Or was that the…

Dr. Jockers: That's actually the curcuminoids.

Ty: Curcuminoids and good fats.

Dr. Jockers: Yes, the curcuminoids—ten times better absorption when you add that in. And if somebody is supplementing with turmeric extract or curcuminoids, you want to take that with food—very key to take it with food. And if it didn't have black pepper in the supplement, because a lot of supplements don't have that in there—make sure when you are having food, maybe eggs or something like that—put a little black pepper on there to enhance the absorption.

Ty: Wow, sounds great. I think when we leave here, let's go have some broccoli, with some healthy oils, some curcumin, some black pepper, and some…

Dr. Jockers: Some berries. There you go.

Ty: Some berries for the Resveratrol.

Dr. Jockers: Exactly.

Ty: We'll have it all nailed down.

Dr. Jockers: Yes, let's do it.

Ty: Awesome, Dr. J. Thank you so much for joining us today, brother.

Dr. Jockers: Yes, absolutely. My pleasure.

[end of transcript]

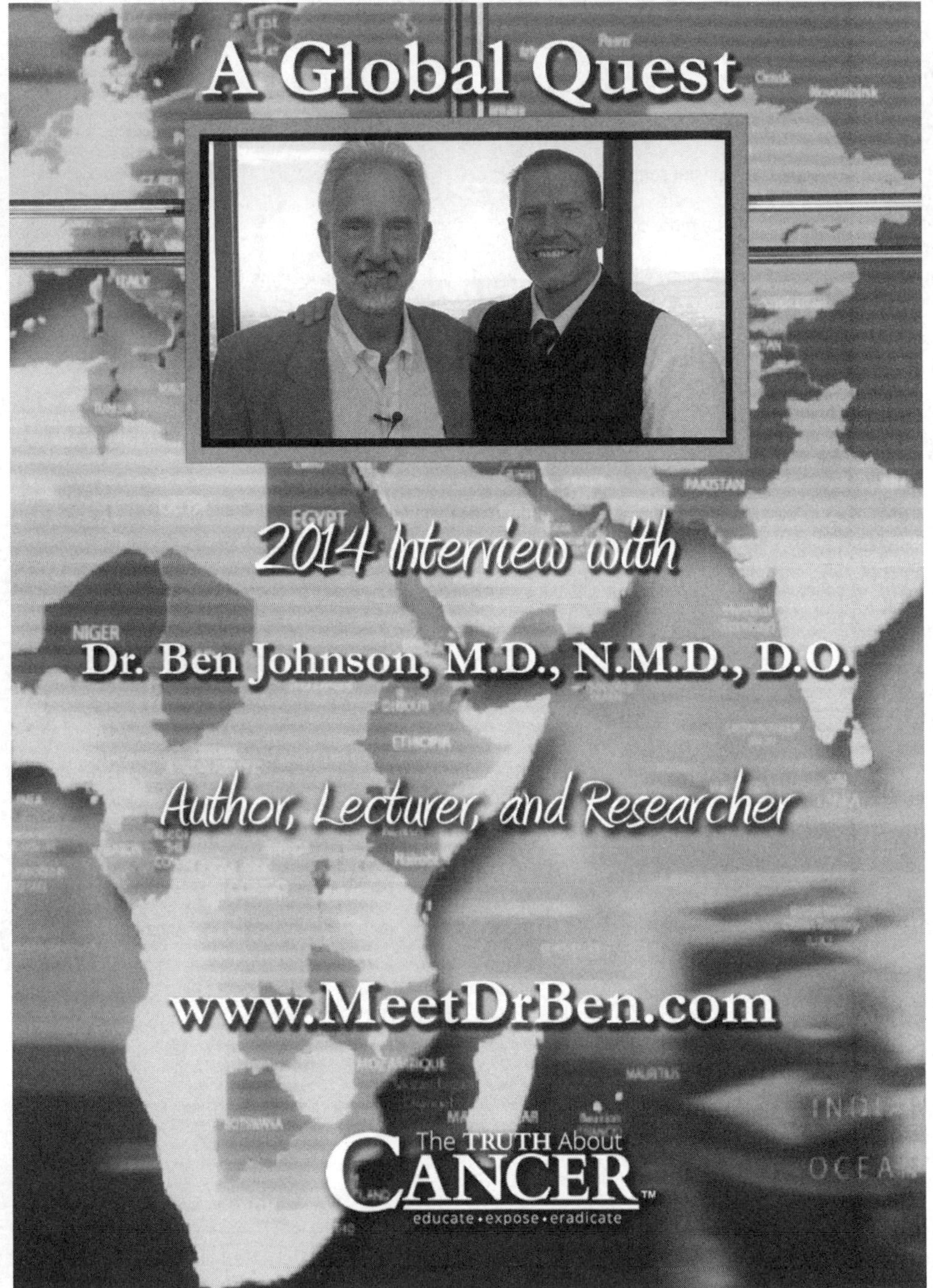
A Global Quest
2014 Interview with
Dr. Ben Johnson, M.D., N.M.D., D.O.
Author, Lecturer, and Researcher
www.MeetDrBen.com
The TRUTH About
CANCER
educate • expose • eradicate

THE TRUTH ABOUT CANCER

Ty: I am honored to be here in Los Angeles, California today with Dr. Ben Johnson. Dr. Ben, thank you so much much for being with us today.

Dr. Johnson: It's a pleasure to be here.

Ty: And Dr. Ben, as I understand it, you are the only medical doctor that was affiliated with "*The Secret*" or in "*The Secret*".

Dr. Johnson: I was, Ty [Laughs].

Ty: Yeah, yeah. That's one of your claims to fame. But tell us a little bit about other things that you've been involved with, in your education. And how did you get involved with, treating cancer?

Dr. Johnson: Well I actually have three medical degrees. My first was D.O., osteopathic, and then my naturopathic medical degree. And then I got my M.D. last fall. But I practiced general practice for many, many years in Colorado Springs and other places, and then kind of backed into alternative medicine. I had an injury and some physical problems myself, and just helping a friend out, with his alternative clinic. And all the patients kept asking about these herbs and these nutritions, these homeopathics. And I would go and read. And I'd go like, oh there's so many ways to get people well besides drugs [laughter]. And so actually, I went back and got my naturopathic medical degree because I realized the field was so broad. There was so much to know and learn, and I wanted to be able to offer that to my patients.

Ty: And so then, once you got your naturopathic medical degree, then you went back and got your M.D.

Dr. Johnson: That's correct.

Ty: Right, and so you started using the herbs and these other natural substances. And so what was the impetus for you going back to get your M.D.?

Dr. Johnson: Well as an osteopathic physician, I had all the privileges of an M.D. The only reason to go back and get the M.D. was because I wanted to speak and write, and unfortunately, nobody knows what a D.O. is.

Ty: You're right. Many people don't.

Dr. Johnson: Yes.

Ty: So now, you are able to start speaking and writing. Talk about some of the things that you've written.

Dr. Johnson: You know, being in "*The Secret*" was a pretty big affair. It really changed so many people's lives. There are much greater secrets in "*The Secret*," okay. Love, joy, peace, patience, so many greater laws than the law of attraction I'm getting. But nevertheless, it really helped a lot of people think about what they were thinking. So, paying attention to what they were thinking, I think, was the real take home message from "*The Secret*."

But, I wrote a book for women, "*The Secret of Health Breast Wisdom*" because, we, as a medical society, are giving women breast cancer with our demanding that they get mammograms. Mammograms cause breast cancer, period. So mammograms are not healthy for women. Women should not be getting routine mammograms.

That's crystal clear, published in the peer review literature. And yet today, if a woman went to her gynecologist or family doc, she would have this shoved down her throat, extreme coercion to go get this mammogram that is causing breast cancer. It's not saving lives. You have a four percent increased risk of dying, if you get mammograms, period.

Ty: So the detection technique that we're using, the primary technique we're using—that we use to detect breast cancer, is causing breast cancer.

Dr. Johnson: Absolutely, it's a terrible test; you know smashing women's breasts and then irradiating with cancer-causing radiation. And then it's so insensitive. For women under 50, it's only like 52 percent effective, sensitive. That means 52 is pretty close to 50, right.

Ty: Yeah.

Dr. Johnson: So about half—that means that half the women that have breast cancer, it would not detect their cancer. That's a terrible test. And so there are much better tests. And yet this is what's still being crammed down women's throats today. Terrible test, causes breast cancer.

Ty: And it doesn't detect, it detects 50 percent and causes cancer. You said there were better options. What, what better options are there for detecting breast cancer?

Dr. Johnson: Well there's two better options. If you've got a lump, if you think you've got something, ultrasound is great. It's a test of anatomy. Mammograms are tests of anatomy. Ultrasounds are tests of anatomy. MRIs are tests of anatomy. So if you've already got a lump, you want a test of anatomy. So that would be like an ultrasound because they see the lump, they can see its consistency. They can see where there's calcium in it. And they can look at blood flow because tumors are going to have increased blood flow. So, for instance, a sensitivity of ultrasound is—is up around 80 percent. It's much higher than mammograms. And the sensitivity is higher too.

But if you're looking about prevention, if you're talking about screening, there's really only one device out there. And that is thermography, an infrared thermal camera. Nothing touches the lady. Nothing smashes her breasts. There's no cancer causing radiation. As we sit here, we are omitting heat in the spectrum called infrared. There's infrared visual and ultraviolet. So this is the infrared spectrum of light, which our eyes don't see, but which is very detectable by the camera. The military developed this so they could see people sneaking at that them at nighttime and so that they could, shoot down missiles and things because they're producing heat.

Ty: Sure, like a night vision goggles.

Dr. Johnson: There you go. Night vision goggles are infrared goggles. So we use it as a medical application to detect hotspots in the breast. Well long before there was a tumor there, there were cancer cells, probably 8 to 10 years before there was a tumor there were cancer cells starting to grow, two cells, four cells, sixteen cells, one hundred forty-four cells, etc., etc.

And it takes about eight years until you get to about a sonometer in size for a mammogram or an ultrasound to detect it. Well that's too late. Because that one-centimeter tumor, about five-sixteenths of an inch, less than half an inch, is about one billion cells. When you get to one billion cells, the cancer has already eroded into the lymphatic system and the venous system and its shedding cancer cells all through the body.

So that's why mammograms—one of the many reasons mammograms don't save lives, it is not early detection. And that's one of the little lies they've propagated along. Early detection saves lives. Get your mammogram today.

Ty: Right.

Dr. Johnson: Well that statement's true. Early detection does save lives. It's just that mammography is not early detection, it's too late, and then the cancer causing radiation. So the long and the short is you're causing much more breast cancer with mammograms that you are detecting.

Ty: Okay, so you mentioned early detection, the phrase that you're going to hear all month this month, October 2014.

Dr. Johnson: Yeah.

Ty: Early detection is your best protection.

Dr. Johnson: Thermography is the only early detection because as—years before that became a tumor, those cells were growing, growing, and growing. They were increasing their blood supply. Some of them were dying off creating nitrous oxide and other debris that dilates the blood vessels and the skin above it. So that reflex has a heat pattern on the thermogram. So thermograms are the only early detection out there. That's because thermography is a test of physiology. It's looking at what's happening in the breast as opposed to the other tests are anatomy. Something already has to be big enough to see.

Ty: I see.

Dr. Johnson: And when it's big enough to see, it's virtually too late.

Ty: It's already beginning to spread. So you hear all month this month, it's breast cancer awareness month about early detection. You're saying they should be using thermography instead of mammography. It's a better early detection technique. Why, in your opinion, are they not using it if it works so much better?

Dr. Johnson: You know there are things that you just want to shoot yourself over that the medical standard medicine, does not do. I'm not much of a conspiracy theory type person. But I've come to believe that American medicine is not about, helping people get well. It's about managing disease and selling drugs and, creating money through the paradigm of patient treatment.

So you can't talk about cure. You can't look at getting people well from cancer. They just want to treat them, and then watch them die. It's really a pretty pathetic state of affairs. So we are not interested in standard medicine and getting people well, just managing their disease until they die. For instance, all of the drugs that you see, if you pick up the label, all of the chemo drugs says causes cancer [laughs]. Think about it.

Ty: Yeah.

Dr. Johnson: We're using a drug to treat cancer that causes cancer, a known carcinogen. How crazy is that? But that's what we do every day in every institution across America. We use radiation. What do x-rays cause, hello, cancer. And we are using that supposedly to treat it. So you know, Stage 4 cancer in America, survival rate is about two percent. You know, that is horrific.

It can't get any worse than two percent. So two percent success rate, for Stage 4 cancers is beyond comprehension. Patients would live much longer and healthier if they did nothing, if they didn't take the drugs, because the drugs are hastening their death.

Ty: Wow! And I've read studies.

Dr. Johnson: Don't get me started [laughs].

Ty: I think you're already started. I think you're already going, which I'm enjoying because it's good information. I've read studies, people saying the same thing. Doctors and scientists saying that you would live longer by doing nothing, than by doing the treatment. And, I can't remember the medical doctor that I was just talking to recently said that in all his years of treating cancer patients that he's never actually seen one that died from the cancer that they always die from the treatment.

Dr. Johnson: Yeah, you know, primary tumors almost never kill anyone unless they're in the brain. The primary tumor can kill you there. But, if you give it long enough, the metastasis can eventually, get you. But almost no one in America today dies of their cancer. They die of the side effects of the chemo. And I shouldn't call those side effects, the direct effects of chemo. Because we call them side effects because they are unwanted. But they are direct effects of the chemo agent.

Ty: Well you know we've talked about breast cancer and mammograms. Tamoxifen, that's a known carcinogen.

Dr. Johnson: Absolutely, it is a known carcinogen. Women should not be taking it. And there are great ways to naturally—what is Tamoxifen? So, on a cancer cell, especially a breast cancer cell; it has receptor sites, tens of thousands, maybe hundreds of thousands of receptor sites. And some of these receptor sites are for estrogen. And so Tamoxifen is a drug that hooks to the estrogen receptor site and occupies it. Now you want that site occupied.

There are three natural female estrogens: estrone, estriol, and estradiol. Estradiol being the more potent, naturally cancer causing one. So you want to occupy that receptor site to keep estradiol from docking there. But you could be giving that patient, and I do give my breast cancer patients, estriol, a normal hormone that their body makes and is used to. I just give it in abundance to block those receptor sites. You can block those receptor sites with soy. You can block those receptor sites with many non-stimulating things. You want those estrogen receptor sites blocked, but not with Tamoxifen.

Ty: Well I know you are not a conspiracy theorist. But nothing better to create repeat business than to perpetuate the disease that you are supposedly trying to treat.

Dr. Johnson: Mammograms, Tamoxifen, you've got a built-in clientele. You're gonna get that patient back. They're going to get, you know, if they don't have breast cancer, you take enough mammograms and they will have breast cancer. You give them Tamoxifen; you know you are going to get that patient back, good repeat business. It's a good business model.

Ty: It's a good business model if you don't have very many morals or—

Dr. Johnson: Yes.

Ty: —or a conscience. Let me ask you this. We've talked about good screening techniques, better screening techniques than mammograms for breast cancer. You've talked about Estriol. Is that the way you pronounce it?

Dr. Johnson: Estriol.

Ty: Estriol as opposed to Estradiol. What other treatments would you recommend for cancer patients that may be a non-toxic treatment that don't create cancer, that don't cause cancer, but that would be able to get cancer under control that wouldn't have the side—the direct effects that the chemo might?

Dr. Johnson: You know I'm actually currently working on the most phenomenal herbal nutritional natural agent that I've seen to date. It's beyond my, belief system right now that it is that good. But I'm under strict confidentiality that I can't share that. But there are good herbals and nutritionals out there.

Salvestrol is a great, nutritional that anyone can get. You can mail order it. Get it—go online and get it. You have to take it with biotin to help it work. Artemisinin, it's the number one anti-malaria drug in the world, great anti-parasitic. But it's a good anti-cancer, natural anti-cancer agent. You have to take it with iron. So you have to know the nuances of a lot of these natural agents to get them to work. And you know you want a coach, someone knowledgeable and understanding, because like Artemisinin, you can't take Risperdal with it because it—or actually that is Salvestrol because it neutralizes it. So you don't want to just—oh, this is good, this is good, this good, and do the….

Ty: You don't want to throw Jell-O at the wall and see if it sticks.

Dr. Johnson: There you go.

Ty: Okay.

Dr. Johnson: You don't want to stir in the pot. You want someone who knows how these things go together.

Ty: Sure.

Dr. Johnson: What's working here, what's working here, what's working so that I am an orchestra director? You know, I tell the oboes when to play and the flutes and the drums. And that's my job, is to orchestrate a patient's treatment back to health. And so that's what I have, is knowledge. And knowledge is very empowering. So you know what fits together. You know when to give what and where and how these things work together so that the patient becomes healthy again because there's such a cascade of events, so many things you have to deal with. So many things cause cancer from spiritual issues. Yes, I said it, spiritual issues, emotional issues, environmental toxins, to mammograms, to x-rays. You know doctors pass out CT scans like they were candy.

Ty: Yeah.

Dr. Johnson: It's estimated by 2020 that 50 percent of all cancer in America will be medical x-ray induced or drug induced. So we will be responsible in a very few short years for 50 percent of all cancer in America.

Ty: Wow!

Dr. Johnson: And that's staggering.

Ty Bollinger Yes.

Dr. Johnson: That's staggering. And the medical society is doing this to us. We are doing it to the people.

Ty: Mm, that's mind blowing that by 2020 we will be responsible for 50 percent of the cancers.

Dr. Johnson: It's staggering.

Ty: Wow!

Dr. Johnson: Yeah.

Ty: And especially in light of the fact that the recent statistics from the WHO and the ACS are indicating that one in two men and one in three women alive today will face cancer. And they're saying that half of that is caused by the medical system.

Dr. Johnson: Absolutely.

Ty: I'm blown away and I don't get blown away easily.

Dr. Johnson: [Laughs]

Ty: Wow! Okay, so talk about this Dr. Ben. You talked about this herbal product that you can't mention. I appreciate that. But what are the characteristics, the methods of action of a good herbal product, a good natural product? How do they control the cancer? And what kind of effect do they have on the immune system, the detoxification process? Share with us the typical methods of action.

Dr. Johnson: There are so many good non-toxic ways to treat cancer that it's laughable what standard medicine is doing. But they all work in different ways. For instance, the Salvestrol works on an enzyme system because cancer cells have an enzyme, IP1B1, I think it is. That's—boy, I'm having a little, escape moment there. But, it's an enzyme, 1B1, which YP -- if I can get it.

Ty: The CYP enzyme.

Dr. Johnson: CYP.

Ty: Yeah.

Dr. Johnson: There you go. Thank you.

Ty: Sure, you bet.

Dr. Johnson: CYP1B1 is the enzyme system that it works on. Well this is a natural product found in fruits and vegetables that CYP1B1 enzymes converts into a toxic product. So this fruit extract, vegetable extract acts as a pro drug. It's not a drug. Your normal cells don't have that enzyme system. So it can't convert it. So it doesn't hurt normal cells. But the cancer cells have the CYP1B1. So it converts it into a toxic substance killing the cancer cells. So that's just an instance of how a particular natural therapy might work. It was found because—and why don't we have Salvestrol today in our body? Well, natural fruits and vegetables produce it just in the last day or two, right, as they become ripe, because that's when they're higher in sugars and that's when fungi tend to attack the fruits and vegetables. So that's when they make Salvestrol. Who eats vine-ripened fruit today?

Ty: Unless you have your own garden, you don't.

Dr. Johnson: That's it, nobody. Because it's all picked green.

Ty: Yeah.

Dr. Johnson: I don't care if you're eating it in a natural food store, an organic food store. It was still picked green to ship to you because that's the only way they can get it there and not lose half their produce to spoilage. So we are eating all this food that's Salvestrol depleted, one of the very agents that mother nature uses to kill cancer cells, which ma and pa got back on the farm. But in the city, buying it from the store, we don't get.

Ty: You mean the fruits and vegetables don't grow at Wal-Mart.

Dr. Johnson: [Laughs]

Ty: There was a survey of school kids a couple years ago. And they surveyed them before Thanksgiving. They said where do turkeys come from?

Dr. Johnson: Yes.

Ty: And close to half of them said Wal-Mart.

Dr. Johnson: Yeah.

Ty: So we don't even understand about the basics of producing our own food anymore so....

Dr. Johnson: Where does from milk come from, the jug?

Ty: The, yeah. Yeah, or used to be they you know, delivered fresh milk every day, fresh raw milk. And now....

Dr. Johnson: Yeah, and it had enzymes....

Ty: Yeah.

Dr. Johnson: ...and bacteria, all kinds of healthy things in it. But they couldn't have that.

Ty: Yeah.

Dr. Johnson: So you know you try to sell natural milk, and....

Ty: You'll get raided like—well by a SWAT team nowadays.

Dr. Johnson: Yes, yes. They will come in with guns drawn, cart everything off, and it's illegal. But that doesn't mean that they won't do it, because what they're trying to do is just crush you. And drag you into court until you have no more financial resources. And they have all the financial resources. They have your wallet behind them.

Ty: They do, they do. And you know one of the worst things you can do today, in my opinion, is to sell natural healthy foods, because the powers that be, the alphabet agencies will—will target those people much more than they will drug manufacturers. I mean you look at Vioxx. It's been implicated in the deaths of tens of thousands of people. That was a legal, FDA approved drug. But you better not sell raw milk.

Dr. Johnson: But you see, they knew there were going to be tens of thousands of deaths from bleeding ulcers. They just didn't know that there would be deaths from heart. So that surprised them.

Ty: Yeah.

Dr. Johnson: But it was acceptable that there were gonna be all these gastrointestinal bleeds and people bleeding to death.

Ty: Yep.

Dr. Johnson: That was acceptable. But you have one herbal or nutritional product, somebody gets sick on that and they're gonna come in and crush that part of the industry.

Ty: Yeah.

Dr. Johnson: Take it all off the market, and just crush it. So there's an extreme double standard. I'm not sure you can even call that a double standard. That's, uh—they just try to crush any alternative that's beneficial, find a way. I'm not sure that they don't even put bad stuff in there and ship it in so that they can crush it. That's not above them.

Ty: No, I would agree with that. You know, I know someone that's a statistician that used to work for the pharmaceutical companies. And he told me that one of the things that they do is they factor in the number of deaths they anticipate from the drugs. How much is that gonna cost them in legal settlements? And then they compare that to how much money they're gonna make off the sales of the drugs.

Dr. Johnson: Sure.

Ty: And if the sales outweigh the risks, the financial risks of letting these people die because they know they're gonna have X number of people that die, that they go ahead and put it to market.

Dr. Johnson: It's just on the spreadsheet. Does it make money?

Ty: Yeah.

Dr. Johnson: It doesn't matter how many people it makes sick, how many it debilitates, how many it kills. Will it make money? That's the only question.

Ty: Wow! Let me ask you this Dr. Ben. So you talked about Salvestrol being one of the chemical constituents of fresh fruits that is produced in the last couple days that we're not getting because we're not growing our own fruits, a lot of us. Name some other foods that you would say are essential in an order to maintain health. What is your typical diet? What does your diet look like?

Dr. Johnson: My diet that I want my patients eating looks green, very green. Vegetables, lots of vegetables, all kinds of vegetables in all forms, but key to that is the fresher the better. So, cutting to you, the less time the better. If you have your own garden, that's awesome. And then secondly is organic, because you don't want those pesticides and chemicals and artificial fertilizers and things working against you.

Ty: Okay.

Dr. Johnson: So fresh, raw, organic are the keys, vegetables and then nuts and fruits. And I do allow my patients to eat small portions of meat. I want it to be organic, free range, or wild caught, harvested.

Ty: Okay. So the way that the animals are raised affects the meat.

Dr. Johnson: You know we have all these studies showing that two eggs a week causes increase in prostate cancer and red meat causes colon cancer in all of these studies. But you don't see anybody comparing organic free range eggs against pen fed, chickens.

Ty: Right.

Dr. Johnson: You don't see the free-range meat. Again, so I would love to see those studies done. Of course, no drug company is going to fund those. And no independent farmer has the money to do that. I don't think the meat, the eggs, the things are the problem. I think it's what we do to them. We put a chicken or a cow in a pen or a hog. And we feed them genetically modified corn.

That's not their diet. I mean they're out there eating grass, including the chickens, and crickets. So they're out there eating things that we, when we raise them commercially, that's not what we're feeding them. So now they have concentrated, genetically modified corn and other chemicals in their body. And then we eat that and concentrate it in ours.

Ty: Wow!

Dr. Johnson: So I don't think it's the—I'm not a vegetarian. I have no problem with vegetarians as long as they get adequate amounts of protein, which is sometimes difficult to do unless they're educated as to how to get those. And there are certain amino acids you just don't find in vegetables at all. But we have nice supplements these days. So you go to a supplement store and get those. So I don't have a problem with a patient being a vegetarian. But I certainly don't have a problem with them being, omnivorian because, we need protein, especially our immune systems need protein. I just want it to be healthy protein.

Ty: Okay. So that leads me to a couple more questions. You mentioned that we need protein for the immune system to function properly. We'll talk about the immune system in a second. But one of the things that you just said, genetically modified grains are being eaten by these cows, these chickens, and these animals that are then concentrated in the animals, and we eat their meat.

I interviewed Jeffrey Smith, the man that's probably the most well-known anti GMO researcher about the GMOs. And that's one of the things he mentioned. The animals are eating these. So we not only have to watch out for the genetically modified corn, and soy, and cottonseed, and all these other crops. We have to watch out for the cows and the chickens that ate them.

Dr. Johnson: Absolutely.

Ty: Because we might be eating an organic produce diet. But if you eat meats that are not fed organic grains or grass, then you could be getting GMO secretly—the back door. And not even know about it.

Dr. Johnson: We are all getting GMOs. And it's like, when I go to get some corn chips. I go and buy the one that says non-GMO and organic. Marketing is so deceptive. You know, it'll say organic. Well, but it's GMO. Or it'll say non-GMO, but it was not organic so....

Ty: You want the non-GMO project verified and organic together.

Dr. Johnson: Yeah, you want them both.

Ty: Right.

Dr. Johnson: Because both are required for a healthy food.

Ty: Right, it is amazing the deception that they're allowed to—

Dr. Johnson: Everything is, this society is so deceptive. And it's just about money, and profit, and sales. And, we've lost the integrity....

Ty: And it reminds me. We're here in California. So and one of the popular arguments that I heard a couple years ago when they were trying to pass Prop 37 to label GMO's was that we can't force companies to label because it would be deceptive labeling. I remember hearing that. I am like, how is that deceptive, to tell us what's genetically modified or not. But the argument against labeling was that that would be deceptive.

Dr. Johnson: As part of the—people that are orchestrating all this are brilliant masterminds of deception. So they did that double-speak. And what it did was immediately confuse people. And they go—it is kind of staggering mentally to hear that phrase.

Ty: Yeah.

Dr. Johnson: And you go like what? And it creates confusion. And so, these pharmaceutical corporations, Monsanto—all these big groups, they actually have disinformation centers where they have writers creating disinformation to create doubt in people's minds about health foods and nutrition, vitamins and things so that it just creates confusion. And people just kinda go like oh, you know. And they just kind of can't make a decision paralysis.

Ty: Yeah, cognitive dizziness as well. And I guess they turn off. And then they say okay, well let's go to the expert.

Dr. Johnson: Yeah.

Ty: And then the experts, what do they always say?

Dr. Johnson: The "gods" in the white coat.

Ty: Exactly, with the stethoscopes.

Dr. Johnson: Go get your chemo and die.

Ty: Exactly! Unfortunately, it was one of the interviewees here. I think it was Dr. Buttar out of North Carolina said when he was going through residency that he remembered oncologists saying, I've got to go, I've got to go poison another cancer patient, when they would do the chemo. Sad! Last question for you Dr. Ben, the immune system. You mentioned that we need to get adequate protein for the immune system. So if you could, just talk about the importance of a healthy immune system in preventing cancer and, staying healthy.

Dr. Johnson: Oh, when I take on—by the way, what I do is concierge cancer. I only take on a few patients. And I go to their homes and take care of them there. But the first thing I do when I get a new patient is—one of the things that I do is, I begin to unimpede their immune system. Because every cancer patient, their immune system has missed the cancer. So it has missed it. And so you have to unimpede their immune system. And then you have to stimulate it back into action because at the end of the day, they will not survive if their immune system is not really stimulated. One of the many fallacies of standard cancer care is they just want to kill cancer cells. Well that's nice. But why did you get cancer?

Ty: Yeah, what was the cause?

Dr. Johnson: They never ask that question. I tell my patients, I encourage them to consider to see their oncologist to give them feedback so as they get well, they will have a witness born to them, that other things work, whereas they know good and well that what they're doing is not working. But I say, two things that you'll be amazed at. They'll never ask what caused this, and deal with that, or try to deal with it in any way. It's just, let's kill cancer cells. And then number two, as you get well, they will never ask you what did you do because they don't want that knowledge, because then they're responsible. So that's two things that the doctors will never ask the patient who is getting well from taking herbals and nutritionals or alternative medical treatment.

But you have to unimpede the immune system. And then you have to stimulate it back in action, because at the end of the day, without your immune system working, you will not live. Because, let's take AIDS patients for a second. They don't die from the AIDS virus. They die because their immune system is no longer able to work. And let's say you have a bacterial infection. We do not have an antibiotic that is good enough to kill one hundred percent of the bacteria, any bacteria. This is one of the many fallacies that we have about medicine and in our worship of medicine. We think oh, antibiotic, it's gonna kill all these—no. It might kill 50 percent of the bacteria or maybe even 60 or 70 percent if it's a great antibiotic.

But at the end of the day, your immune system has to step up and finish off that other 30 or 40 percent or you will not live. That's why AIDS patients die because we don't have an antibiotic good enough to kill any bacteria. We don't have an antifungal good enough to kill one hundred percent of any fungi. We don't have an antiviral good enough to kill one hundred percent of any virus. So at the end of the day, your immune system has to step up. So that's one of the very first things that I do is start working on the immune system. Because at the end of the day, it's gotta work if my patient is going to live.

Ty: And so without that immune system functioning, you're a goner.

Dr. Johnson: Yeah, and standard medicine doesn't even think of it, doesn't even address it. Your immune system what?

Ty: Yeah, well obviously....

Dr. Johnson: Why does that have anything to do with it?

Ty: Right, obviously, they don't because....

Dr. Johnson: That's why you got cancer.

Ty: And that's why when they prescribe chemo or radiation, it's so absurd because they both devastate the immune system.

Dr. Johnson: Well and that is the extreme Achilles heel of chemo is it—and radiation. It damages, severely, the only thing that can possibly save your life, your immune system.

Ty: Unbelievable that those are still the standard of care. But I tell….

Dr. Johnson: Today as we speak.

Ty: With, folks like yourself sharing the knowledge that you've shared with us today, I think we still have a chance.

Dr. Johnson: It is. It will have to stay at a grass roots level until there's probably revolt in the streets from economic, or medical, or a combination of both. Because the echelons that are in power will not be moved. And they have the power to continue to stamp out alternative medicine at will at this point in time.

Ty: Well, we'll just have to keep giving it our best, won't we?

Dr. Johnson: Absolutely.

Ty: Well Dr. Ben, I can see why you were the only medical doctor that was in "*The Secret.*" You've been fascinating today. I really appreciate the knowledge that you've shared with our listening audience. And I know that many of them are going to benefit from what they've heard. So thank you so much Dr. Ben.

Dr. Johnson: Thank you for what you do Ty, in bringing this to the public.

Ty: Thank you. God bless you.

[end transcript]

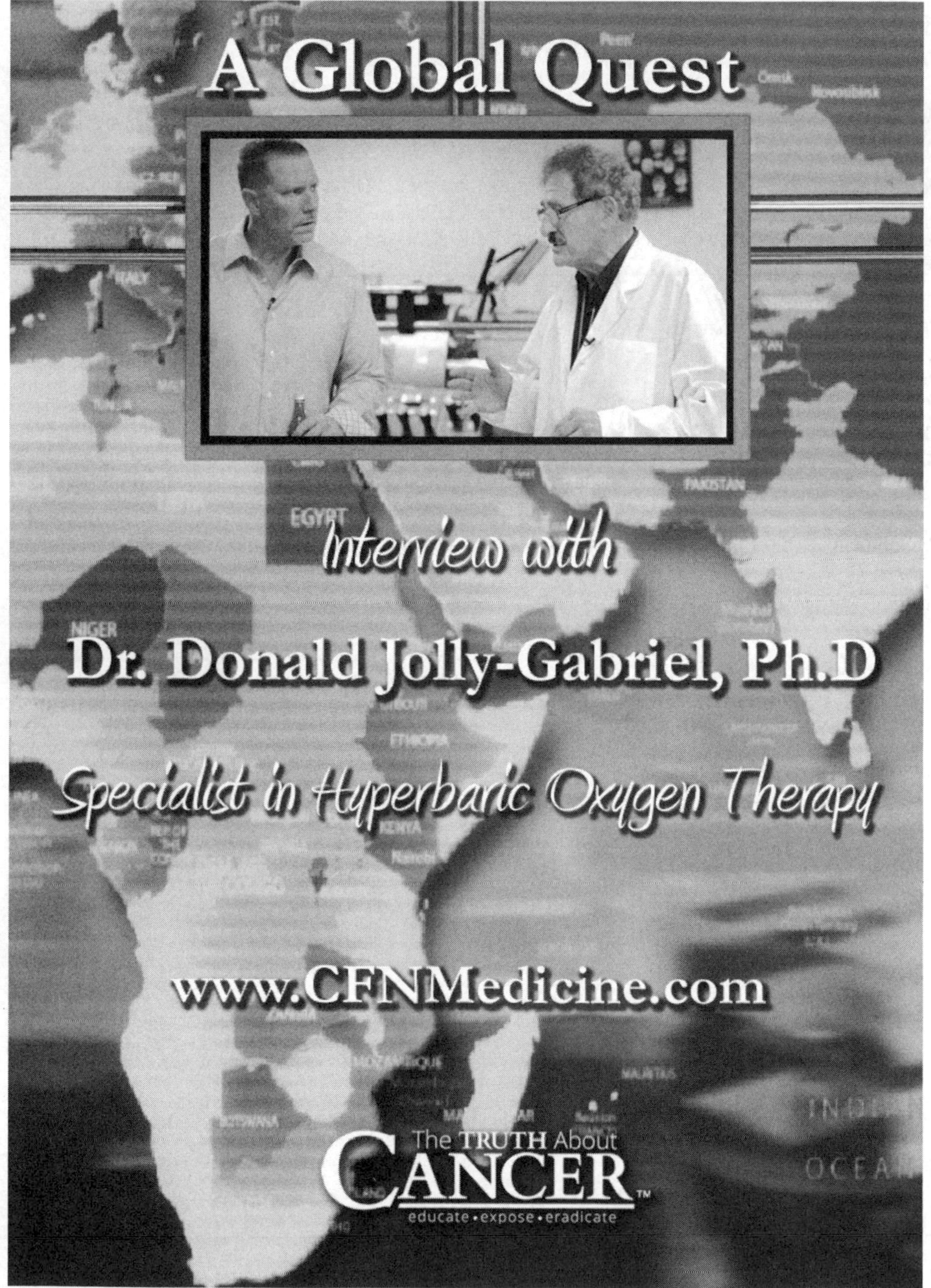
A Global Quest
Interview with
Dr. Donald Jolly-Gabriel, Ph.D
Specialist in Hyperbaric Oxygen Therapy
www.CFNMedicine.com
The TRUTH About CANCER
educate • expose • eradicate

Ty: Well, I'm here with Dr. Jolly. We're about to get a tour of the hyperbaric oxygen lab right?

Dr. Jolly: You are.

Ty: Let's check it out.

Dr. Jolly: You can even have a treatment if you want.

Ty: Alright.

Dr. Jolly: This is the hyperbaric chamber room. And Justin is putting a patient in the chamber, and he will eventually put a mask on him. He will go in the chamber, and he will be in our beautiful glass chamber. We will be watching him constantly and he will communicate with us if he has any problem.

Ty: Okay. So that's going to go to the mask and that's where he's going to be receiving the oxygen?

Dr. Jolly: Yes, hundred percent pure oxygen.

Ty: And what's the purpose then, of the chamber? As opposed to just getting pure oxygen through a mask?

Dr. Jolly: It is necessary to put the patient under pressure so that the pressure causes the gas—any gas in a pressurized environment—to dissolve into all the liquids. And the prime liquid we're trying to get the oxygen to dissolve in is his blood. So we will raise the atmospheric pressure. Oftentimes up to two and a half times. And this will create massive amounts of oxygen going into the blood, which creates a healing mechanism.

Ty: I see. So that's the purpose of the chamber?

Dr. Jolly: Yes. And you know, it's much the same as Coca-Cola. When you manufacture Coca-Cola they mix all the stuff together, they put it under pressure, they infuse a gas called carbon dioxide into the Coke, cap it, and it stays in there until you open it and it sprays out. Except that blood doesn't bubble with oxygen, so you don't have that problem of bubbling, or gaseous extensions occurring at all.

Ty: Okay. How long have you been using hyperbaric chambers, Dr. Jolly?

Dr. Jolly: I've been involved about thirty-five years.

Ty: Really?

Dr. Jolly: Yes. I was very lucky to have some of the world's greatest hyperbaric physicians mentor me and teach me, and I am grateful for that.

Ty: Now, name some of the people that mentored you.

Dr. Jolly: Well, Dr. Bruce Halstead was one of them, he was a pioneer in treating cancer with hyperbarics. Dr. Richard Neubauer, Dr. K. K. Jain was the author of the worldwide textbook on hyperbaric medicine. And these are the kinds of people— much older than I—I was much younger of course—and they're all gone now. Except Dr. Jain is still living, but I am eternally grateful because I got it from the world's greats. And in those days hyperbarics was just emerging.

Ty: You learned from the best didn't you?

Dr. Jolly: I hope so.

Ty: So to recap what we've learned so far, they're in a chamber. The pressurized chamber causes the oxygen to diffuse into the blood.

Dr. Jolly: Absolutely dissolves one hundred percent oxygen into their blood. And there are many benefits from that. It accelerates healing dramatically, any kind of healing. For an athletic injury, for a surgical procedure, any kind of malfunction in the body that has the capacity to heal. The healing mechanism will be accelerated by the hyperbaric chamber.

And then it has some specific effects on things like bacteria and cancer cells and the situation with cancer cells and chemotherapy and also radiation therapy. It accelerates and helps both of them. As a matter of fact, hyperbaric oxygen therapy is one of the only real, efficient treatments for radiation poisoning. And some patients come after they've literally been poisoned with radiation poisoning—they come to hyperbarics for healing. We can heal the tissue, new blood vessels grow, new nerve endings can develop. It's pretty magic.

Ty: It is, it sounds magical. So let's say somebody's watching today and they are going to go on chemo or radiation. Is this something they can use to heal the damage that's been done?

Dr. Jolly: Absolutely. Yes.

Ty: What about during chemo and radiation?

Dr. Jolly: Yes. It can accelerate the effectiveness. We have to take a look at the drugs that are being used. And take a look at the radiation process, where they are in it, and then apply hyperbarics periodically during the process to minimize the production of any negative side effects.

Ty: Dr. Jolly, what is the mechanism by which—when we get oxygen into the blood by one of the hyperbaric chambers—how does that cause healing in the body? I mean, we've heard oxygen is great for the blood, we breathe oxygen, you have to have it to live, but how exactly does that work to heal?

Dr. Jolly: Well, first of all, oxygen is the absolute, essential element to sustain life. If we don't have it for a few minutes, we're gone. We can go without food for days, we can go without water for days—we cannot go without oxygen for more than a few minutes. Number one, it is a sustainer of life. It is also the absolute, necessary product to begin the healing process. Without oxygen, no healing will take place.

We'll develop necrosis, which is a Greek derivative for death. So cellular death can occur in a little part of the body if it's deprived of oxygen. The more oxygen given to it, it will heal faster—and you can completely heal someone who has drastic wounds from diabetes or other causes—putting them in the hyperbaric chamber.

Ninety percent of the time, when I get them at what's called the grade two—which is pretty bad—we're looking at it and saying we may have to amputate. Ninety percent of the time we've been able to save the limb.

Ty: By giving it oxygen?

Dr. Jolly: Absolutely. Put them in the chamber.

Ty: You know, you mentioned that nothing can heal without oxygen. Just a funny story. I live in Tennessee, we have horses—one of our horses got wounded a few weeks ago and just a huge gaping wound on the back of his leg. So we put the hydrogen peroxide and the ointment and everything and we bandaged it, forgot to take the bandage off and the wound started getting worse.

And I had forgotten that we forgot. And I realized, why is the horse limping? And I told my daughter Brianna, "We got to take the bandage off. It's not getting any oxygen." We take if off, within three days the horse is fine.

Dr Jolly: Well, you know something? We have a picture of a horse in the lobby that was treated—that was dying of necrotizing fasciitis. A multimillion dollar horse. And they discussed putting it down. And instead I made a suggestion to the vet and he ordered a hyperbaric chamber delivered and I treated the horse. Twenty treatments later, the horse is back in business.

Ty: Really?

Dr. Jolly: Yes.

Ty: There's no placebo effect for the horse is there?

Dr. Jolly: No, not at all.

Ty: It either works or it doesn't.

Dr. Jolly: Absolutely.

Ty: Great. Anything else you want to share with us while we have this treatment going on about the importance of the hyperbaric chamber that I haven't asked you?

Dr. Jolly: Well, there is so much that I could write another textbook. But I think the most important thing to remember is that oxygen is what we need to stay alive, it's what we need to heal. And when we are in a healing crisis the application of oxygen can be wondrous. Even breathing a little bit more efficiently, raising your oxygen level up to ninety nine, is a good thing.

Standing on a vibratory platform—Dr. Connealy has one in the other part of the medical center—breathing oxygen, elevate your metabolism, and elevate your oxygen level. This elevates it to a degree that nothing else can. And anytime anybody is looking for any kind of acceleration of healing, they should be here.

Ty: Right.

Dr. Jolly: They should be here. I wish we could get every cancer patient to do hyperbarics, because Dr. Otto Warburg—who won the great Nobel prize in medicine—discovered that—and published and won the prize for it—that oxygen is absolutely essential for healing in cancer because cancer cells don't like oxygen.

And many of them cluster and develop an environment where there is no oxygen present and then you have incredible tumor development and that can be helped remarkably with hyperbarics.

Ty: Lends a lot of credibility to the old phrase, somebody is nervous, about to give a speech, "just breathe." Just breathe, right?

Dr. Jolly: Amen. Absolutely.

Ty: Well, Dr. Jolly, thanks for sharing. This is great.

Dr. Jolly: It's been a pleasure.

Ty: Really appreciate it.

Dr. Jolly: Total pleasure. Thank you very much.

Ty: Alright. ***[end of transcript]***

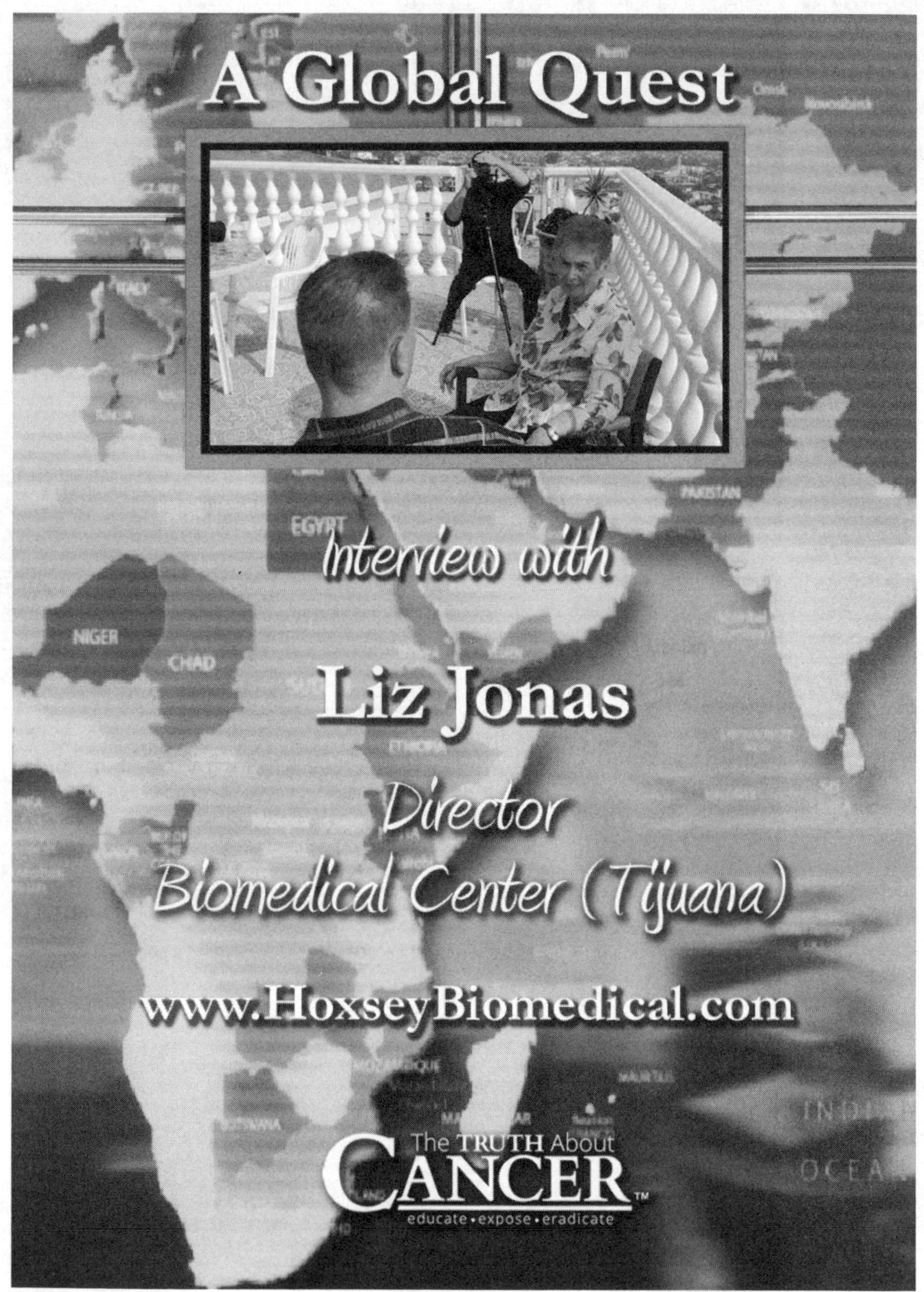
A Global Quest
EGYPT
NIGER
CHAD
ETHIOPIA
PAKISTAN
Interview with
Liz Jonas
Director
Biomedical Center (Tijuana)
www.HoxseyBiomedical.com
The TRUTH About
CANCER
educate • expose • eradicate

Ty: Well, Liz Jonas I'm so happy to be sitting here talking to you.

Liz: Nice to be with you, Ty.

Ty: I've followed the Hoxsey Clinic for a long time, and I know the story of Harry Hoxsey. One thing that you may not know is my father was diagnosed with cancer in 1996, on July 1st· He died the 25th, twenty-five days. But we wanted to get him here. We were trying to get him to the Biomedical Center.

Unfortunately, he didn't live long enough to get him down here. But this is really exciting for me to be able to be here and to interview you about the Hoxsey treatment, I really want to get the history of this clinic all the way back to Harry Hoxsey in the 30s and 40s.

So I'm going to get you to be a historian for us today, Liz, if you could. And first of all, tell the viewers who you are and how you're related to the clinic.

Liz: I'm Liz Jonas and my sister was Mildred Nelson. I have no medical background, mine is business. Mildred was the medical one in our family. My mom had cancer, ovarian and uterus. And they had planted radiation in her body, and burned her very bad, and then told her to go home and die.

My dad heard about Harry Hoxsey who was in Dallas, Texas. We lived in Jacksboro, which is about 90 miles. So my dad called my sister. She was the oldest in our family. There were seven of us, and asked her to come drive for him. He was an old-timey rancher. And she said, "What are you going to Dallas for?" She said, "To get parts for the tractor?" And he said, "I'm taking your mother to the doctor." So she came and drove. And through the day Hoxsey found out she was a nurse and offered her a job. And my dad told them, "No. She doesn't want to work for you. She thinks you're a quack."

He offered for her to go look at all his files but she didn't. And she couldn't talk my mother and daddy out of this. So she decided to go to work for him to prove he was a quack and to save her mom. Our mom lived to be 99 years old.

Ty: So it is true. The things that I've read was that Mildred thought Harry was a quack, and she went to work for him to prove that he was a quack. And ended up being his chief nurse. That's true.

Liz: That is true. She's said that people would come in so sick and she'd think, "We'll never see them again." And in three months, they came back much better. And in six months, better. She said just case after case. So then Harry would tell her some big story and she'd laugh and he'd say, "Go look at the records." But she wouldn't but then it would prove out that it was true.

Ty: And Harry had a big heart, didn't he? He wanted everyone to get treatment if they couldn't afford it.

Liz: Yes. He would buy—if someone didn't have the money to come, he would send them a train ticket or a bus ticket, and then he would put them up in a rooming house close to the clinic, and treat them.

Ty: At no cost to them?

Liz: At no cost, you know.

Ty: Now, one of the things that I've read, and I'm not sure if this is true or not, was that the AMA with Morris Fishbein came and tried to buy the formula.

Liz: True.

Ty: But Harry found out that they weren't going to—either they weren't going to use it properly, or they were not going to give it for free to people that needed it. And refused to sell it to them.

Liz: They got to the point of signing the papers and he said, "You have to make this available to everybody." And they said, "We may not make it available to anybody. We may not use it even." And he said, "No, then I won't sell it."

Ty: So they basically wanted to buy it and bury it.

Liz: Bury it, yes.

Ty: Because it was too effective.

Liz: That's right. In my opinion.

Ty: Mine too. Well, I think anybody that has any kind of a brain capacity would come to that conclusion, right? They wanted to keep it off of the market. Harry was arrested numerous times for, what were the charges?

Liz: All different kinds, just whatever they came up with, you know. But the patients—he always carried a roll of bills in his pocket with him, a big roll of bills. He made his money, in my understanding, in penny stock, all penny stock. But he carried a big roll of bills with him. And sometimes he'd bail himself out, sometimes he'd just stay in jail. The patients would come and bring food and they would circle the whole block. So they would just let him out to get rid of the patients.

Ty: If that's not a testimony to Harry and the treatment, then nothing is. So the patients would surround the jail?

Liz: Yes. Surround the jail. Can you imagine?

Ty: No. I can't, I mean, not today. But this was back when, 40s, 50s?

Liz: In the 40s. But his patients were very loyal to him. Because the AMA and FDA, they would find out they were going to mail medicine to a patient and they would be standing at the patients' door and take the medicine so the patients couldn't have it.

Ty: And it's not like this was something dangerous for them. It's herbs.

Liz: It's herbs. What the Lord meant for us to treat with.

Ty: Exactly. It's natural medicine. And now the story of the Hoxsey tonic and how it came about, from what I've read, was it Harry's granddad?

Liz: Yes.

Ty: Was—could you tell us the story?

Liz: The way I understand it, because that was way before my time too, was that the granddad was a veterinarian and he had a horse that had cancer. He turned him out to die, you know, in a pasture, to let him run free. And he noticed he was getting better and better. So he started watching what he was eating and it was herbs in the field that he was eating. That made him well.

Ty: And then he used those herbs?

Liz: He started gathering some of these herbs and playing around with it. And as he had success on the horses, then people started coming, you know, wanting. They had been giving up. There wasn't anything that could be done. So he started playing around with it a little bit and it was kept very secret. And then Harry's father had it and on his deathbed he gave Harry the formulas for this. And made him promise that he would use it for the benefit of the people.

Ty: And that's one of the reasons he wouldn't sell it, to keep the promise to his father.

Liz: Yes. On a deathbed.

Ty: I imagine even if he hadn't promised, he still wouldn't have because Harry had integrity.

Liz: He did.

Ty: So you've got these herbs that are being used to treat cancer successfully, and, as the story goes, Harry's persecuted heavily in Dallas. And he had many other clinics as well eventually, right?

Liz: He did. And the Dallas clinic was the last clinic that they closed. He had clinics in Ohio, Indiana, all up in the East. There were 11 of them. But they closed each one of them one at a time and then Dallas was the last one. And at that time when they closed Dallas he told Mildred, "If you're going to keep it going, you have to move it." So she moved to Utah. She was not a doctor so she always had to have a medical doctor work for her.

Ty: But she was a nurse?

Liz: She was a registered nurse.

Ty: What was the time period that your mother was treated by Harry and the Hoxsey clinic?

Liz: That was in the 40s and 50s.

Ty: So it was in Dallas?

Liz: It was in Dallas.

Ty: And then as you said, your mother, who had been really badly damaged by the radiation, lived to be 99?

Liz: Ninety nine.

Ty: Now, if that's not a testimony for the Hoxsey clinic, nothing is.

Liz: Yes.

Ty: So after your mom dies, was Mildred still alive?

Liz: Oh yes, Mildred had moved it to Mexico by then. She had moved it several times in the States and they came in and raided her office.

Ty: So was Harry dead by the time that you moved down to Mexico?

Liz: No. He came one time. He was not in good health. Harry had a heart condition. Always had. And really, it was my understanding that's what he died from. Because the [American] Medical Association was after him. His doctor was out of town when he died. So they said he died from prostate cancer.

Ty: I'm glad to know that because you always hear Harry Hoxsey invented this great Hoxsey formula and he died of cancer. That's not true.

Liz: But my understanding was that's the way the [American] Medical Association got back at Harry. When Mildred moved the clinic to Mexico, he told her, he said, "You have to drop the Hoxsey name."

Ty: So that's why you got rid of the Hoxsey name, right?

Liz: That's right. That's why we went Biomedical.

Ty: Because they tried to discredit him. And I've read that from other sources, that he actually did not die of prostate cancer.

Liz: That's not what is on his death certificate.

Ty: Prostate cancer?

Liz: Because his doctor was out of town. So they had a medical examination, another doctor, and they put prostate cancer.

Ty: I see. Well, you know it's too bad that they did that but it's not surprising.

Liz: No, it isn't.

Ty: In light of the fact that he was thrown in jail for curing people with herbs. In light of the fact that they'd stand at the patients' door and snag their formula so they couldn't take them. That's not surprising, is it?

Liz: No it isn't.

Ty: So after your mother dies, Mildred moves the clinic to Mexico.

Liz: No. Mildred moved it before. My mother came out here many times and visited. I have patients today that come and say, "Oh, I met your mother years ago."

Ty: Now, what was the year that your mom died then?

Liz: My mom died in '97.

Ty: I was thinking it a longer—

Liz: No, only two years before Mildred died.

Ty: So then when Mildred died, she had moved the clinic to Mexico. Was this your big ambition to take over the clinic?

Liz: Absolutely not. I was not going to do the clinic. I had helped her with her business in the States but I wasn't going to do the clinic because I had no medical background. I didn't think I could.

Ty: But, what was it that led you to—

Liz: Well, the Lord decided this was what I'd do. And he put obstacles in my way. Like one time when I flew in to San Diego and got off the plane and was walking up when you get—there's a bend you go around to go down on the escalators or you can go out straight and go in front of the airline ticket windows. And there's an elevator there.

And I had had to use the wheelchair a lot so I knew this. And I started out that way and a young lady said, "Ma'am, ma'am. You're going the wrong way." And I said, "No, this is the way I go, but thank you." And I went and got down, was waiting for my luggage, and she comes up a few minutes later.

And she said, "How'd you beat me down?" And I said, "Well, I come every month." And she said, "You come every month? Do you have family out here?" And I said, "No. I run an alternative cancer clinic." She said, "No, no you don't." And I said, "Ma'am, do you have a problem?"

And she said, "I have breast cancer, and I'm trying to cure it myself. And I'm not doing very well." I said, "What are you out here for?" She was out here for a convention. I said, "If you get any time, come over and sit in the waiting room. Come check us out. I'm not saying come do treatment."

And I gave her my card and she came. And she tells the same story today in the waiting room. So is that not God putting people in your way?

Ty: It is. And you know one of the things that I'm really impressed about here is that you're carrying over Harry and his father, and his grandfather, their vision to be able to treat people that can't afford much. Because according to Dr. Gutierrez this is the cheapest treatment in Tijuana.

Liz: It is. And we can't treat for free. Mildred did and Harry did. But times have changed. I have employees to pay, I have the upkeep, we have to buy the medicine, you know.

Ty: But you don't have to mortgage your house to come here.

Liz: No. No they don't.

Ty: Well, that's good to know because a lot of people are looking for natural treatments for cancer. They're looking for clinics. But then, most insurances are not going to pay so they've got to come out of pocket for it. This is a very affordable alternative and very successful. Tell us about some of the patients that have had success here.

Liz: Well, when I first came, or maybe the first five years I was here, the ambulance drove in our driveway. "What's that?" Anyway, they carried this man in and put him in bed. And I had just had both my knees replaced. It was my first week back so I wasn't staying all day.

But I went in and stood and asked this man, "So what are you doing here in an ambulance?" And he said, "Well, I have bone cancers in my spine. I can't sit up." And I said, "Why did you come by yourself? Why didn't you send somebody with your records, and we would have sent you the medicine until you got better."

He said, "I don't have anybody." And I said, "Nobody to come with you?" And he said, "No, I took an ambulance to the motel in the States then the ambulance picked me up this morning, took me to the border, changed me from the US ambulance over to the Mexico border and they brought me up here."

So I stood and visited with this man most of the morning and told him, I said, "You're going to get better if you do what our doctors say. Take your medicines, stay on your diet. And you're going to feel so much better. You're going to get up and you'll break a bone because you have holes in your bones."

I said, "So have somebody put a potty chair right by your bed and be very careful how you turn." Three months later this man walked in, hugs me. I told him, "Don't lift anything. Don't do anything really strenuous." And he said, "You saved my life." And I said, "No, the doctors and you saved your life. I had nothing to do with it."

He said, "Little lady, don't you let me hear you say that. You stood by my bed most of the day and talked to me and I listened." And I didn't even recognize him because when somebody is lying in the bed in a gown they don't look the same as when they're up.

Ty: Right. And how many years ago was that?

Liz: That was five or six years now. But you know, there are many, many cases like that.

Ty: There's a man that I talked to out there that I think we're about to interview. And I think he was told that he was—by the Mayo Clinic I think it was.

Liz: Yes, David Olson.

Ty: David Olson. He was told that he would be dead within a couple weeks.

Liz: He told me he was given a diagnosis by 17 doctors, one day to a year. And then he came here and that was eight years ago.

Ty: Eight years ago?

Liz: Eight years ago.

Ty: And so he's a big Hoxsey success story, isn't he?

Liz: He is.

Ty: Is he still taking the tonic? Do you take it after eight years?

Liz: He may be on three months and off three months, or he might not be taking it at all. I don't know. I haven't asked David. But he comes once a year for a checkup. He always comes for a checkup.

That's where a lot of the patients get in trouble. They don't keep doing their checkups. Unless something shows up, you know. If something does come back, you can get on it right away. Because a lot of patients have maybe even three different kinds of cancer in their life.

Ty: So it's good to keep it monitored.

Liz: Oh yes. You have to keep monitoring.

Ty: So Liz, what would you say to somebody that's been recently diagnosed with cancer, in light of the fact that your mother was being killed by the radiation until she used the Hoxsey.

We talked about David, given a day to a year to live. And so somebody that's been diagnosed with cancer and their doctor says, "You're terminal, you're going to die." What's your message to them?

Liz: My message to them is, "get to the clinic as soon as you can." I own the clinic so maybe you're not going to believe me. But we have miracles there. We can help you. Even the patients that die, they have an easier death. We've been told this by many, many families. We don't save everybody. Nobody can. But we save a lot. We have about an 80 percent cure rate.

Ty: That's amazing.

Liz: And you're not supposed to say cure, but—like Pam Kelsey today, you're going to interview her. She had pancreatic cancer in the 70s. Mildred cured her.

Ty: So 30, 40 years ago?

Liz: She now has liver cancer. You're going to talk to her later, she'll give you her story.

Ty: Yes, but she's still alive.

Liz: She's still alive and well and looks well.

Ty: So Liz, is there always hope?

Liz: There's always hope. There's always hope. We don't want our patients to come if they're not able to travel. We want some family member to bring their records and the doctors will look at it, do the best they can, and diagnose them what they need. Get them started and at a later date they'll be able to come.

We had one patient, I remember, from England. His father-in-law and wife flew over. He had three or four children, little kids. He was in the bed and couldn't get out of the bed. He was bedridden. They came over and got the tonic and six months or a year later he was able to come and they brought one of their children. He played in the yard with him. You know, that's wonderful to see.

Ty: It is. You're influencing the lives of the next generation. Kids are going to have their parents because of these treatments.

Liz: Absolutely.

Ty: Well, I think your mother would be proud. I think she is proud, and I think you're doing God's work here, Liz. Thank you.

Liz: I think I am too, Ty.

Ty: I appreciate the time today. You keep up the good work.

Liz: Of course, I believe in it. You can tell I believe in it.

Ty: I know you do.

Liz: And I think you're doing a wonderful job in all that you're doing. You're doing a great job. By putting the tapes out. Michael has 11 tapes.

Ty: Well thank you, I appreciate that. We're all on the same mission to help people, aren't we?

Liz: That's right. And that's what we're put on this earth for. Really. If you really stop and think about it, we're supposed to help each other.

Ty: That's right. Well, you keep it up, we'll keep it up. Together we'll change the world.

Liz: Great, that's wonderful.

Ty: Thanks Liz.

Liz: Okay, thank you.

[end of transcript]

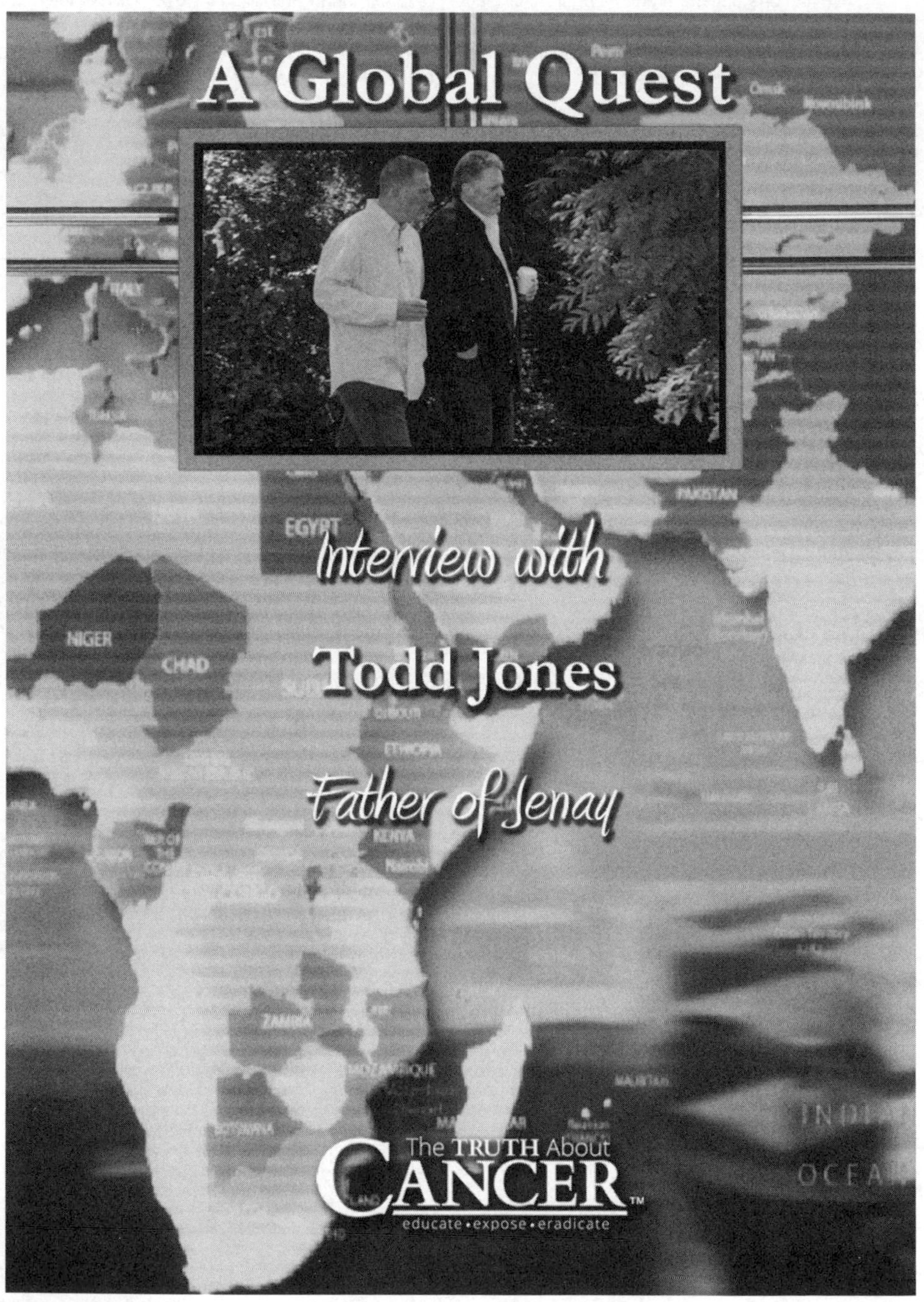
A Global Quest
Interview with
Todd Jones
Father of Jenay
The TRUTH About
CANCER
educate • expose • eradicate

Ty: Really happy to be standing here today with Todd Jones. A man that I've been in contact with over the last six or seven years, and we finally get a chance to meet in person. So thank you for joining us, Todd.

Todd: My pleasure, Ty. It's about time.

Ty: It is about time. I guess what was it, 2008 or 2009 that we first hooked up?

Todd: That's right.

Ty: And the circumstances that we initially met via, you know, online, emails and phone calls was not all that fortunate, was it?

Todd: No. Unfortunately, we had something happen to us that should never happen to any parents. And too many parents are getting the negative news that their child is diagnosed with some form of cancer. In our case it was leukemia. It was the ALL Leukemia which is more common than most but it doesn't really matter as you know.

Cancer is ugly no matter where, when, and how. But with children it just seems to take a different dynamic and it's devastating. And if I hadn't had Living Fuel as part of our family regimen and known about KC Craichy's interview with you—I think it was on his website and I pulled it up that one fine day and I remember the things you were talking about in eating right and everything.

And it just stuck with me. And then when we got the diagnosis that our little Jenay had cancer and we had to do something, I just remember calling up there because I felt like that's a safe place. KC Craichy's building with those people and that product is—you know, you got to get some good word out of there, what do we do? Who's got some information for us at least?

Ty: And so this was what, two thousand—when was she diagnosed?

Todd: That was in 2011. It was in November.

Ty: And how old was Jenay at the time?

Todd: She just turned two. She was two months into two years old. She was born on September 2nd, 2009. She was a great—and still is, thank God—but healthy, energetic little girl. And then about maybe late summer, August, September into her birthday, in October she just started slowing down and her legs were hurting.

She couldn't walk very well and otherwise she's jumping and running with her big sister. And we knew something was wrong. So that's when we started to go take her to the doctors to get some blood work done and get some things checked out and find out why. And she had kind of dark circles going on and there was just—we were going, "Okay, something is different here. We got to find out what."

Ty: So you get the diagnosis and then you contacted me about the Living Fuel, right? I guess you called Living Fuel at KC Craichy's company and they referred you to me?

Todd: Yes. They gave me your name and number, freely. So apparently you don't have anybody guarding your cell number there.

Ty: No.

Todd: I called you up and said, "Hey man, I heard you know about some options here in these kinds of situations."

Ty: And so this was shortly after the diagnosis? Jenay's diagnosis?

Todd: Yes. It was the time where we already knew that there was going to be a medical regimen put together because they told us at the hospital. Actually, they wanted to fly us away down to Oregon's children's hospital down there and immediately begin treatment. And I sort of felt like it was a little too rushed. Even though it was obvious that she needed treatment.

So I asked the hematologist, "Well, do you guys treat here?" And she says, "Yeah, we do." I said, "So we don't have to do that study research treatment down there if you can treat her here?" Because that way I could stay and work and we wouldn't have the stress of breaking the family apart and everything.

So we stayed and opted for that. And then we listened to the doctor but then we wanted to get some other input and not just that rushed kind of almost—it felt like we were rushed into it. We didn't feel like we had a chance to even inform ourselves, really.

So at that point I went into information mode, research mode. Kind of like yourself. I started peeling off everything I knew. And I had already found out a lot of stuff about just health in general. I'd always been fascinated with how things function. Maybe not the perfect picture of health personally but still very interested in what makes a person healthy and stay healthy.

Ty: What was it like for you and your wife to have a two-year-old and then—just from an emotional perspective, I can't imagine.

Todd: Yes. It's something where everything just blurs, your energy just leaves your body, you're in shock, it's traumatic. And you just look at each other and you don't know what to say. And it happens to so many parents now, it's horrible. I guess it's one of the fastest growing segments in the hospital.

Ty: Childhood cancer, yes.

Todd: - Child oncology, it's growing out of control. So, you're speechless and I called my boss, I was supposed to be at a trade show and I was bawling. I said, "Man, we just got some bad news."

So anyway, being the guy I am though, I went into, "Okay, hold on now. We're going to work this through. We're going to pull our boots up by the straps and work this thing out and find out what the best choices are and stuff." My wife was glad about that because she was just as shocked as anybody. But for some reason I just felt confident we were going to just get it done right, whatever we had to do.

And that's why you came into the picture. Because I looked around and I knew that there was somebody out there that I needed to make a phone call to. And just get some alternative options in my mind that I can check into. And is it, mentioning product names here is—

Ty: That's fine.

Todd: It's okay?

Ty: Yes.

Todd: So one of the first things we grabbed on to was the LifeOne product for enhanced immune system support. Because that has such an amazing track record. And I think it was Dr. Michael—

Ty: Farley.

Todd: Yes, Farley and his oncology surgeon partner from Florida.

Ty: Dr. La Rochelle,

Todd: La Rochelle, yes. Those guys put it together, I think. And they just had their ten years of use and just amazing results.

Ty: That product—which nobody has mentioned it thus far, so just briefly for those people who are watching—LifeOne has resveratrol, quercetin, diindolylmethane, green tea extracts, selenium, chrysin. All these things that you've heard about, that you know are all good for cancer, they're all wrapped up in one.

Todd: That's right.

Ty: All these immune stimulants as well as anti-cancer herbs.

Todd: Apparently they got the recipe that's very effective. It's synergy and it just does the job. And so, that with Living Fuel together we said, "Okay, we're going to help little Jenay's immune system right away." Because what happened was that we were told she had to get into treatment. We knew she had to get something done. And we also had no track record or experience like any parent. Nobody knows.

So we said, "Okay let's get her on the treatment." The treatment, it's an intensified treatment for thirty days where they use vincristine chemotherapy and steroids. And that little child just got loaded up with that stuff daily.

Ty: So you were looking to do something while they were doing the chemo?

Todd: I was and I wasn't even sure if that was going to be [during the] chemo or if it was going to be like right after that period was over. Because they told us if everything goes good she should go into remission which is technically, I guess, under one percent of cancer in the blood to be measured. That would verify that.

And as I shared earlier she was at 96 percent. She was full of leukemia in her blood and that's why her legs weren't working very well. And after that initial intense treatment for thirty days it knocked all the way down to under one percent so we were very grateful for that because that's that's remission. I mean, that was an instant response in so many words, right?

Ty: Which, by the way, the chemotherapy will do. It'll kill that cancer but the problem is, that you realized quickly, you got to do something to help the rest of the body that it's killing as well.

Todd: Absolutely. So the collateral damage is very obvious when you bring home a little child every day that's just limp and it's red circles, and pale, and it's no fun at all. So after that initial period we felt like, "Okay, we got the cancer pretty much out of the picture as far as—"

Ty: For now.

Todd: For now. And we started to counsel with Dr. Farley too. Got some blood tests over to the East Coast and we wanted to find out if we could use his LifeOne product and with some Living Fuel which is all-organic, non GMO—

Ty: Super food.

Todd: Nutrient dense super food. I mean the whole palate is in there. Everything from herbs, vitamins, minerals and—you know it, you know it better. So we thought, "okay, if we can get these things to work on her body"—because it's selective and it doesn't kill everything like the chemo did.

We wanted to raise up her immune system and this is stuff that I had to inform myself about. It wasn't like, "Oh, I know what to do now. Now that they've got the cancer down I'll just do this." It was through a lot of counselling and talking about other cases and things like that so that it would be an informed decision.

Ty: Right. And if I recall, we had several phone conversations back then as well.

Todd: Absolutely. You were part of that counselling circle that we were just going through stuff. And I was trying to get information about other children that had done it. They had some kids that were outside of the States because it's critical when you try to treat somebody in the States, as we all know.

Because sometimes you get stopped. And we didn't want to—no parent will ever want to endanger their child. Every parent, though, must stand up and inform themselves and not just give over to, "Here's the regimen." It's one size fits all. It's almost like vaccines. It doesn't matter where you come from, it doesn't matter your disposition, you get vaccinated but some kids don't make it.

Well, it's the same with chemo. Those kids come in there and some kids just can't take that regimen. The growth hormones and... is it the T cells? In the children are very powerful. The stem cells, they reproduce and they can—when you burn down the forest, the greens, grasses, and stuff comes right back up. Children are very resilient but some of them don't make it because it just knocks them down too far.

Ty: Talk about that. You had mentioned earlier about the difference between Jenay when she was going through treatment and then the other kids in the ward.

Todd: Right. That was, for us, it was a tell-all right there because we were watching the other children, and we could see what was going on in the hospital. For example, the food. Right away. If you're a parent you need to pay attention to this because most hospitals just have hospital food and that stuff is french fries and hamburgers. It's corn dogs, and chips, and chicken strips, and canned green beans, and homogenized, pasteurized milk.

Ty: With ice-cream for dessert.

Todd: With ice-cream for dessert, or Jell-O, or canned fruit chunks with corn syrup and GMO everything. So you really want to pay attention to not just letting those children that are being treated just have that stuff with the—as you know, we talked about the steroids that create a desire for salty food.

Parents just want to keep the child happy or satisfied during this horrible treatment period. So they get that salty stuff and all that denatured junk food. And even the hospital staff, doctors, the hematologists, "Oh, they need that because they need something. They're going through all that. Just let them have it." I'm like, "This is not the kind of advice I really feel good about."

So that's why we got these big syringes and we filled them with Living Fuel and we put Stevia in it to sweeten it up. I mean, we stayed clean.

Ty: So you were putting Living Fuel in syringes and giving it to Jenay orally?

Todd: Yes. And she was just sucking it up and she loved it. I mean, we prayed about it too, by the way. When you're in a situation like that there's so many moments when you don't know what to do and if you know the power of prayer you got to use it in these times.

You have to just say, "Lord, we need your help. Guide us on this." Because this is how you help other people when you're conviction and your faith is involved. And then you get—I mean, we were blessed because in this very challenging moment we were demonstrating that we could make a difference too. We didn't have to just listen to the white coat tell us, "This is how it is, this is what you do, this is what you don't."

We looked at everything and, of course, my background is I research stuff happily. I'm a little bit like you. We are just two brothers from another mother but I love to understand why and how things work. And that there's more than just the status quo, or the template solution. We're so amazing in our human beings. We can produce things in our own body.

Ty: The body heals.

Todd: The healing code, for crying out loud.

Ty: That's what we say at the end of our radio show, "The power to heal is yours."

Todd: Yes. Exactly.

Ty: Getting us that in our own bodies.

Todd: So when you're treating a human life let's be careful not to destroy it too much in the process, right? So that's why for us augmentation made a lot of sense. It's was very reasonable.

Ty: So you said you were using Living Fuel in syringes. Did you us LifeOne as well?

Todd: Same deal, you bet. Yes. And we kept that going on alternating and—

Ty: During her treatment? During the chemo?

Todd: Absolutely. During the chemo. And I have to recall here, she did get it during the chemo for sure. She got it throughout the whole three year treatment. But after the first month, and I've shared this with you too, we made a decision that we wanted to—since the cancer was so far down and in remission, as they say, and they told us themselves. We were just like, "Okay, you know what? Thank you for your business. We're good now. We're going to go ahead and build her up naturally. Now that the cancer and half of her system has been 'chemo-ed,' chemically cleansed, we're going to go in and put in the natural good stuff now. And see how we can get her to respond there."

Well, the hospital didn't like that. When I took my daughter and my wife I said, "Okay, let's go and work on this other program." I'm taking responsibility as a parent and I'm doing it with the counsel of people that have been treating people, a lot of people, thousands of patients. And one of them is an oncology surgeon. I felt pretty confident, especially with Ty telling me, "Hey, these are the guys you want to be talking to."

So, when that happened it wasn't three days later and there was that very, very, very, loud, aggressive knock at our door. I'm thinking, "That doesn't sound like anybody I know. Nobody knocks like that." It almost sounded like a boot. So I went to the door and it was the Office of Children's Services and they came and they said, "Look the hospital called. You have taken your child out of treatment and you need to bring your child right back to treatment." I'm like, "Well, we're finished with that treatment. We're just going to continue on with another treatment. I'm the parent."

I even looked up the Alaska statutes. Parents have a legal right to decide how their children get treated. What I didn't know is it doesn't matter what the statutes say. It's the administrative rule that the child is a ward of the state and so you don't have that decision to make. And it got kind of dicey at that point as well because I certainly wasn't into causing more stress than my wife and I had already had.

We were really still in trauma with our little one here. But we were very hopeful because the cancer was down and we were getting things going up in the right direction as far as we were certainly concerned and convicted about. But the Office of Children's Services told us right up front, "We will take both your children and they will both go in foster care if you do not get that child right back into the hospital."

Ty: Take both of your children?

Todd: Both of them. So I'm thinking, "Wow, these guys are making a statement pretty hard right in my face, right up front." And I remember calling you that night saying, "Dude, this is what's happening." And I know, I remember you weren't impressed either. But I made a decision there to not rock the boat and cause more dismay.

I could never imagine my two young girls in the care of other people. I went to two lawyers and got very well informed about this and they said, "Yes, we can get your daughters back. Eight hundred grand and two years later is pretty much what you can count on." Because of all the BS that that—

Ty: And who has that kind of money?

Todd: That's right. I mean it's already bad enough when you're stuck in this treatment program for three years. But we just said, "Okay, let's give this back to God." Let's just say, "Hey, we had faith. We stepped out in faith and we will continue in faith. And we will just do the right thing and we'll just inform ourselves and we'll keep going in the direction that we are shown to go. And do this."

In those three days I remember driving with our daughter over to another hospital to get the stint out of her arm and telling my wife, "Honey, we're doing everything right. Don't worry. God's got us on this. We're just going to pray through things and do what we need to do." So we got her back into treatment and we continued with the regimen and we continued to replace a lot of hospital food with stuff that we would bring from home.

Ty: So you continued on chemo?

Todd: Yes. We're continuing on it because it's a three-year regimen. Well, actually, two and a half and then it sort of fades into three. It seems like forever. But during that time we would observe the children and we could see that our daughter was very resilient. Because there were episodes where she would get heavy dosages and then the steroids on top and you could see how it really wipes out the whole—the natural state of the child was very low energy and just depleted.

But she would bounce back quick. And there also comes a point where, because of the cancer and the chemo, the child, or any patient, has no more desire to eat. Or the taste changes so much that they only go in one direction. We were so amazed that she was still taking the Living Fuel in the syringe. And I think pushing it into the back of the mouth and kind of just swallowing it as you go, helped a little bit. But the point was that we were very grateful because it was working and we knew she was getting all that good stuff in there to clean up the mess that was being made.

Ty: This is something that I think is really important that you're sharing. For people that are watching that may have children that are undergoing chemo now or even themselves currently under chemo. There are things that you can do while you are taking chemotherapy that help your body to rebuild.

Todd: That's right. Especially with children when you're in a forced treatment, if I might say that.

Ty: Well, that's what it was. I mean, if that's not forced, what is? They say they're going to take your other child as well if you don't do it. That is forced.

Todd: Yes. And we watched another little guy in there with brain cancer. Same thing that the parents didn't want him to get a certain radiation and all the other stuff that they were doing because they'd informed themselves that they should be able to get by without the damage that that does. And it is damaging. Maybe not in this episode but in another one, radiation is a topic for itself. Because it's almost irreversible as far as I understand what that stuff does.

But the state took the little guy and brought him into some foster family and he started getting really worse. But then the state saw that he was getting worse and gave him back to the family and the kid started to get better again. But under their authority. So the whole thing was a rough, tough deal. But he made it, by the way, for the sake of this interview. Just to know.

So, as this evolved in the treatment time and we noticed that the other children weren't eating at all anymore, they had to get feeding tubes. I mean, you could just count them. It was like all of a sudden in that month there are three or four more kids who are getting the feeding tube. Well, guess who didn't have to get the feeding tube? Because she was still doing it and she didn't need it.

She was doing LifeOne and Living Fuel and whatever else we'd get in there. It wasn't the perfect diet. She had a couple of little niche areas that we let her have a little bit here and there. But for the most part she got the best stuff we could put in her. Because we're the parents and we love her more than anybody so we're going to do the best thing that you could possibly do.

Ty: Did you have to sneak it in?

Todd: No. This is a great question because they sent the pharmacist up to us to find out what we were doing to her. The other one was—and this, to give the credit to KC Craichy, the omegas.

Ty: Omegas, okay.

Todd: His super omegas. We watched the video where his kids are eating them and popping them in their mouths. My kids both still do that.

Ty: Really?

Todd: I don't anymore.

Ty: Get the good fats.

Todd: And both of them still take them and pop them, make that loud pop. And they just swallow all that stuff, all the amazing omega-3s and the vitamin D and the—you say the word so well, the long chain fatty acids and stuff that are in there. The DHAs and the GHLs. Don't tell me I know more than you on this one.

Ty: I can do the GLA but that's the only one. DH—I can't say those.

Todd: And they're ugly words.

Ty: They are too long

Todd: But the stuff is amazing. And so she did that as well. So no feeding tube and symptoms were minimal even though she was on the double—they ended up putting her on a double intense delayed treatment because it didn't go down to 0.0. You remember I was telling you about that?

Ty: Yes.

Todd: It went under one percent which is remission but it is not 0.0 so they put her on a double dosage. In other words, instead of three months in this particular intense treatment time, it was six months. We were devastated because when we found out about that, my wife, she immediately asked the hematologist, "So what does that do with her survival chances?" And the hematologist just looked at her and said, "Well, that goes down. That's just the way it is. Three make it two don't, out of five."

You don't know. Nobody knows but it's no fun when your numbers get shrunk on you.

Ty: But you continued to give her the Living Fuel and the LifeOne?

Todd: Oh yes. She was so resilient and then—back to the pharmacist, though, who came up and said, "What are you guys giving her?" And I'm like, "Let me think. How much am I going to say today?" But we were pretty cool. We shared. And because it is all natural and it's all food. You can't really say much.

We weren't doing isolated synthetic vitamins and minerals and stuff like that. That's junk anyway. We were doing the full-fledged flavonoid phenol spectrum, if you will. So she stayed on that and did great and they didn't say much. I think I did leave out the LifeOne though. The Living Fuel I brought, but the LifeOne—

Ty: I was wondering about that.

Todd: I left that out.

Ty: So Todd, did you have to push to the pharmacist to get him or her to allow you to continue the Living Fuel given the scenario?

Todd: Great question, Ty, because as I mentioned in our discussion earlier, especially me, I really paid attention to everything. I paid attention when they put the little bag of chemo on that it was exactly what they said. I matched it up, I took pictures, I documented stuff. I read about everything that they were using.

Ty: Did you ever catch them in mistakes?

Todd: Yes. That's what I'm getting at. You got to watch out. You know they're humans just like everybody and they've got a bunch of people they're taking care of and they're changing shifts all day. There are people getting the notes of other people, there are emergencies, there's stuff going on. You have to be on top of this.

Ty: It's like a madhouse.

Todd: That's right. I mean, it's confusion in there, let's be honest. And as a parent it's your obligation to pay attention and to look at stuff. We found one day she was on a bag of antibiotics and I looked at it and I looked at the chart and I said, "That's not even what's on there." Well, I called to the nurses' station and they're like, "what?"

And then all of a sudden, down the hall comes the head infection doctor, ripping down the hall. Runs into our room, unhooks the bag, grabs the bag, runs down to the nurse station and says—you could hear him yelling—"Who put (inaudible - 00:26:56)." And I'm like, "Wow, here we go." Just another example. Got to stay on it. As a parent you just can't let everybody—just because somebody has a white coat on you can't just lay back and let it go.

You got to watch it. So that pharmacist was all good and well but I had to utilize a little authority in my sharing because I really wasn't interested in what they were going to say, yay or nay or nothing. That's what I'm giving my kid. You guys are doing your stuff, I'm doing my stuff.

I've heard people say you shouldn't give a patient antioxidants and things that might keep the chemo from killing things. But if we get real serious about it, nature is so perfect in its ability to be selective, it doesn't mess with the wrong cells. It joins up with the chemo to kill the bad cells.

Ty: KC Craichy, it's funny that you mentioned his Living Fuel, because he shared with us last year that all the recent studies show that if you couple antioxidants with the chemo it actually works better.

Todd: There you go. And it's reasonable and you have to think. And just because the status quo, or the template, was designed 20 years ago—because you know as well as all of us that this cancer thing is still barbaric from fifty years ago. They haven't changed anything.

Just the name of a drug, a little tweak here, a little tweak there. Still the same chemical compounds with still the same bases, and still the same radiation and chemo. War on Cancer 1973, we're going to have it eradicated in five years under Nixon, nothing. Now it's a multi-billion dollar industry, 95 million bucks. Who's going to want to stop that cash flow? But we have to now. Because people are dying.

Ty: And kids are dying.

Todd: Kids are dying. And praise God, our kid made it and we saw a couple that didn't and that just makes your heart break. And that's why I was happy when you shared with me that you're doing another docu-series and I was more than happy to show up and say, "Hey, Ty, man. This is just what we did and hopefully we can help some other parents."

Be assertive, stand your ground, be responsible, love your child. It's hard for anybody to push a parent back who's in love with that child and does the right thing. And I'd just said, "This is what we're giving her. This is food and this is what she's going to take."

Ty: Good for you. You had mentioned earlier that there were some potential for growth impairments, learning disabilities, long-term, anything like that—

Todd: Yes. One of the nurses came to say we have a special department where after the treatment we'll get your kid plugged in for after-treatment treatment for therapy and all that kind of stuff.

Ty: Isn't that something that they have to have a therapy to treat you from the treatment?

Todd: Yes. How about that? And it's all in place too. It's a big old system in there.

Ty: So Todd, did you guys have to go through any of the after-treatment therapy with Jenay?

Todd: Well Ty, no. Not one time.

Ty: Good.

Todd: Jenay, she just perked up after we finished up. The good news was that she was doing so good that she was able to come home and finish out the last six months of her treatment without going to the hospital and staying in there. She did so good but there are times also where because of the treatment, and this happens to almost all parents, the kid will get a massive fever. With leukemia it's common that it goes right up there, 103, 104, 105 and it gets ugly.

One night we up between 105 and 106 and we were praying. We actually also had the nurse in emergency and the hematologist both on one cellphone each. My wife and I were trying to explain it because they tell you once it's over 101 the child needs to come into emergency because they are afraid of infection. When we did that once she got a catheter and my wife vowed never to go in and do that again to our little two-year-old. That just ain't happening.

But my point is there are times when stuff like that happens and you get really nervous. Because you're like, "Whoa, this thing is going up. Where is this going to end?" And I got nervous a couple times and I said, "Okay Lord, we're taking her in because she's at 103 and this is ugly but I need you to do something for me. I need you to give her temperature a 97.3." I just pulled it out of my head. I said, "You give that to them." And when we get there that doctor puts that digital thing on there and writes the report before we go downstairs—"I want to see 97.3 so I know you're there." Guess what?

Ty: You got 97.3.

Todd: My wife just looked at me. The doctor—we didn't even see it, he was doing all this stuff. He came back with the paperwork filled out. He said, "Okay, there is the temperature. It went down." He said, "There you go. It's 97.3." Thank you. We'll go downstairs now and get her done.

How's that for—sometimes you got to call out, you bet. But, like I said, you just keep doing that and keep the faith and you keep doing the right things. And you take care of your child as much as you can.

Ty: We are what? Four years later now?

Todd: Four years? Yes. Let's see, 11 and we are 16, we are 15. Elections aren't yet, darn it. Twenty fifteen, so that's right.

Ty: She's six now?

Todd: She'll be six this September. We're a whole year since treatment. Last spring was the last part of the treatment. So we're a whole year now and a couple of months out of treatment. And she's playing tee-ball and she jumps on the trampoline with her big sister.

Ty: She's doing well.

Todd: And she runs all over the place, and she's at school and she's doing great, yes.

Ty: That's awesome. I'm so glad that she's doing well. I want a picture.

Todd: Yes, you're going to get a picture. I'll give you one of her sport pictures with an autograph.

Ty: I want her to sign it for me.

Todd: That's right. Because she'll know someday that you were part of that support network and that would be a beautiful thing.

Ty: That's great. Well, I'm just so glad to have been a part. And so glad that Jenay is doing well.

Thank you, Todd for coming down here and sharing this. Because I know this is going to encourage parents or maybe people that are going through chemo themselves, parents that have kids going through chemo right now. They know that there's always hope, right?

Todd: Absolutely.

Ty: There's always hope. And there are things that you can do if you undergo the standard treatments—that you can do to build your body while it's being torn down. And that's what you did.

So, kudos to you and your wife for making it through this. I know it's got to be a tremendously tough time as a family. But I'm glad that four years later you're doing well and little Jenay has her tee-ball uniform on playing and—

Todd: She does, man. There is no cognitive dysfunction or learning disability whatsoever. She's sharp as a tack. She's bright as a star. She's full of energy and she's beautiful.

Ty: That's awesome. So tell me in German that you love your little girl.

Todd: [Speaks German 33:58]

Ty: Awesome brother. Enjoyed it. Thanks for sharing that.

[end of transcript]

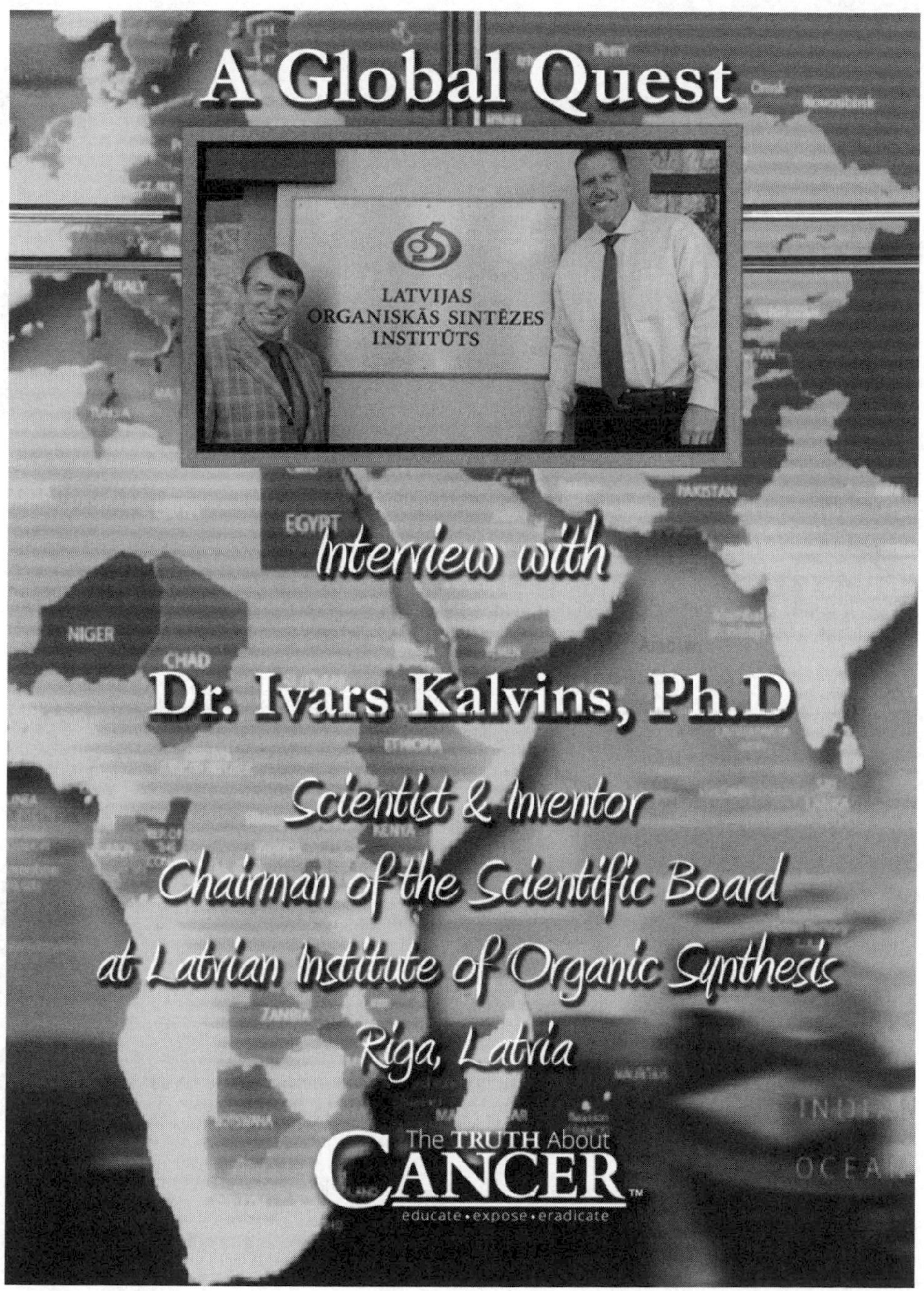
A Global Quest
LATVIJAS
ORGANISKĀS SINTĒZES
INSTITŪTS
Interview with
Dr. Ivars Kalvins, Ph.D
Scientist & Inventor
Chairman of the Scientific Board
at Latvian Institute of Organic Synthesis
Riga, Latvia
The TRUTH About
CANCER
educate • expose • eradicate

Ty: I'm really honored to be sitting here today with Dr. Ivars Kalvins in Riga, Latvia.

Dr. Kalvins: Thank you very much for coming.

Ty: Thank you for joining me here today. Thank you for the invitation. Where are we sitting? In what building are we sitting?

Dr. Kalvins: We are sitting in the Latvian Institute of Organic Synthesis. The leading institution in the drug discovery field in the Baltic.

Ty: You just gave me a brief tour. Really impressive, some of the equipment that you have here.

Dr. Kalvins: Not only the equipment. Equipment is very important, bu the people, the educated and skilled people. This is our passion.

Ty: It is. We met a few of them in passing. You just showed me something in the cabinet here. That you are one of the final three nominees for a very prestigious award. Tell us a little bit about the award.

Dr. Kalvins: Yes. This is very prestigious for scientists in the whole world. This is the European Inventor Award which is given to people who bring something very, very special and new to the market. Everything from science and technology, CD-ROM disks, or discovering computers, and also drugs.

I am among three finalists nominated for this competition for Lifetime Achievement in science. For drug discovery, cardiovascular, anti-cancer, CNS drugs, etc. I'm very proud of that.

Ty: Very nice. Tell us a little bit about the current state of affairs with pharmaceutical companies, cancer treatment specifically. Then I want to get into Rigvir. Specifically Rigvir, because I'm very interested in that.

Dr. Kalvins: The problem for cancer treatment depends on the complexity of this illness, because there are so many types of cancers, as there are many patients with this disease. And the sad knowledge about the movement of this illness in the population.

It is calculated that the new generation, the generation of today, from this generation one in two men and one in three women will have this illness, cancer. And all these achievements in the field of treatment of cancer, even if we are using very, very targeted small molecules, or antibodies, very big molecules against cancer cells, or radiation, or whatever, all of them have a lot of side effects.

The specificity of selectivity is not good enough. That means the drugs are also killing healthy cells, not only the cancer cells.

Ty: So that's what we call selective toxicity.

Dr. Kalvins: Exactly that. The only way to overcome this is to use living species, like viruses. If you can find a virus which specializes in finding cancer cells and penetrating into these cells using the machinery, the factory, these cells use to reproduce themselves, this exhausts their resources and the cells die out.

This is a new approach. There is only one medicine in the world on the market. A little live virus, Rigvir, Riga virus. This was discovered by Professor Muceniece. It's approved by the Latvian FDA, this European country. It's been very successfully used to treat melanoma. And not only melanoma, because this virus is a human virus. It's native, not a modified virus, which has adapted to use as its living space only cancer cells.

Ty: That's a lot of information to get our hands around at one time. So let me summarize to make sure I understand it correctly. Rigvir, which it seems so obvious, Riga virus, Rigvir. I was thinking, "How did they think of the name?" Riga virus, okay. Discovered here.

And it's a human virus, non-genetically modified. So in other words, most people that are watching this documentary know that there's good bacteria and there's bad bacteria. It's the same with viruses.

So this is a good virus that we produce normally. Non-genetically modified. And it's selectively toxic to cancer cells. And it's approved by the Latvian version of the FDA.

Dr. Kalvins: This was found because Professor Muceniece searched for viruses that are present in the stomach and intestine of small children. And she isolated many viruses, and tried to adapt them, to train them to use as cancer cells as their living space.

First of all, cell lines and cancer cell lines are different, and they are in the tissues of cancer, and then adapt to humans. As a result, this virus was selected, and this is fortunately, a virus which is stable. Because the approach they used to stabilize them was not known but they discovered it, and this is used for keeping this stable.

The main problem for all viruses is mutation. This is non-mutating virus. Therefore it is safe, non-pathogenic, but is destroying the cancer cells.

Ty: So it's safe, nonmutagenic, and selectively toxic to cancer cells. I think that's one of the things that really is an eye opener to me about this whole line of treatment with Rigvir. As you mentioned before, you have radiotherapy, the chemo-therapies that are used for cancer, they don't target just the cancer cells, they destroy indiscriminately.

This is a unique product in that it is safe, nonmutagenic, non-GMO, and selectively targets cancer cells. That's fascinating. Can you name the different lines of cancer? You mentioned melanoma, other types of cancer.

Dr. Kalvins: There are at least 10 different cancers, locations of cancer, like renal cancer, breast cancer, stomach, lung, and many others. Also prostate cancer, which is very, very common in men.

But it has only been officially approved for melanoma for now. But this is a very, very big success because we see that the people who use this virus for other types of cancers can also be healed.

Ty: One of the things that is interesting about these type of treatments is that most of the time they're not approved. This one is selectively toxic to cancer cells, it is approved here. How did you go about getting this approved by the Latvian version of the FDA?

Dr. Kalvins: Because all the pre-clinical trials and all the clinical trials were performed. The only problem was that we were able to approve this in the early 80s but there were also doubts about safety.

There were some attempts to use viruses to treat cancer but they were pathogenic viruses and modified. You never know what happens if you apply a modified virus to humans. Because these are living species. They will do what they want, not what you want.

Then the Soviet Union collapsed and there were different problems, political and others. The legislation from the Soviet time could not be used in Latvia or countries that were independent. We had to apply again for approval.

Ty: Something that I'm noticing that differentiates this from many other treatments that may actually be effective is that you've done clinical trials. You've got scientific evidence that this works on melanoma and we've seen the facility here. It's quite impressive.

So you're doing the testing and that's why this got approved. You've done all the tests that are required which takes a lot of money, a lot of time, a lot of effort, a lot of know-how.

Let me ask you a question. What would it be in some one's body that might cause cancer to manifest in the prostate as opposed to in the breast? Or as opposed to in the uterus in a woman? Or as opposed to in the stomach? Why do certain cancers manifest in different places?

Dr. Kalvins: It depends on the origin of the mutations. There are also cancer-causing viruses that induce these mutations in the RNA or DNA of humans. Then these cells mutate during the process of development of cancer. It is not so that the starting cell will be kept during the whole life of the cancer in the body.

No, they are steady state mutating. Only some cancers stop changing their genome. For example, in stomach cancer, or others, thousands of mutations are occurring. Not one point, not two points, thousands, and different. And therefore, it's very, very difficult to find one medicine.

It will never be one medicine if we use chemotherapy because you have to treat different consequences of mutations. And this means that if they are changing during the treatment, it is much more difficult.

But these viruses don't look for mutations in the genes, they are looking for surface properties. They find a channel, the port which they can use to penetrate into the cell, and then they use all the very adaptive mechanisms that the cancer cells are using.

They use all the possibilities of genes that we have but that we will never use. Ninety five percent of genes have never been read in our life. But cancers do, cancers use every gene they want in our genome. Then these viruses are also doing the same.

Ty: It sounds like Rigvir operates on an epigenetic level.

Dr. Kalvins: This is so.

Ty: You mentioned some viruses cause cancer, right? We know that back in the 50s, the Simian Virus 40 that was published 10 years ago, that it caused many cases of cancer.

Dr. Kalvins: Oncovirus also.

Ty: Oncovirus , sure. That virus caused cancer. Why do you think, you mentioned the statistic earlier, one in two men, one in three women, will be facing cancer? Why do we have this explosion of cancer over the past several decades?

Dr. Kalvins: I think there are, from my point of view, but I have not enough evidence to say this is 100 percent true.

Ty: What is your opinion?

Dr. Kalvins: My opinion is that one of the cause is aluminum. Aluminum is an ion which replaces iron in the body in all enzyme systems which defend free radicals. These enzymes are destroying free radicals. Aluminum ion is substituting iron in these enzymes, and that's the reason they don't do this process more.

The second one I think is because of mutagenic influences from outside of the environment. That means all these food additives, preservatives, colorants, pesticides, everything that we use, or even these from my point of view, not dangerous, but still genetically modified food.

Because what we are doing if we are modifying the genes in plants to make them more resistant against bacteria, but what is digesting the food in our stomach and intestine? Bacteria.

Two kilograms of bacteria are in our stomach and intestine. And now you're serving them the food which they can't use normally because these are protected by a genetic approach, to avoid this destruction. And now new combinations of peptides are left in our stomach and our intestine and absorbed by our blood.

And then, we don't know their interaction with the systems in our body. Second, these bacterias try to adapt to the new substance of food. The normal bacteria don't attack our cells from intestine surfaces, etc. because they are normal. But now, you train not normal cells to use food that they don't use. They irritate all of our cells and destroy the membranes. This is another cause for stomach and intestine cancer. Colon and rectal cancer also.

Ty: It's almost like we're the guinea pigs. We don't know how it's going to affect, we're the guinea pigs.

One of the interesting things you just mentioned is your theory about the explosion of cancer with aluminum. Back in the 40s there was aluminum canning. And since that time we've seen a rise in cancer. We've seen all the additives to the foods.

Now we've got the genetically modified organisms and so forth. But aluminum is also used in many vaccines, right? So I want to get clarity on Rigvir because one of the problems with the vaccines is all of the additives and the preservatives, like the thimerosal, which is mercury. This is not a vaccine that has these additives, is it?

Dr. Kalvins: Nothing.

Ty: This is an injection but it's not a vaccine?

Dr. Kalvins: No.

Ty: Talk about how you can contrast Rigvir from the typical vaccine, which is toxic.

Dr. Kalvins: A normal vaccine is used to activate the immune system against the protein applied. This can be a dead virus, dead bacteria or live bacteria or live virus. It can also be the proteins themselves from the cell surfaces, but only the immune system is reacting to these proteins.

But Rigvir, even it would not evoke the immune response. It is going to find, or search for, cancer cells to penetrate into these cells. And then will replicate inside of the cells by using all the factory mechanisms of these cells. The vaccine causes an immune reaction against the protein you apply.

And this can make cross-reactions. That means these proteins are similar to other proteins in the body. This is why there was a problem with the vaccination against hepatitis for very long period of time. Because if you use proteins of these viruses, you immediately beat your own liver.

Because in this cross-reaction, the immune system attacks your liver because they're similar and they can't select between the virus proteins and the liver proteins. This is the main thing. A second issue is that if you apply big molecules the immune system starts forming antibodies against these proteins.

Then by the second injection, this reaction can be very, very active. The third reaction will be that antibodies against antibodies will be formed, and the next application will cause antibodies against antibodies against antibodies. And so a chain reaction of different antibodies is formed by the body.

And as the end, you know a lot of side effects from vaccination.

Ty: That's fascinating. So you've got a selectively toxic virus to cancer cells, that doesn't cause the reaction in the immune system to basically create an autoimmune response against itself, does not—

Dr. Kalvins: It causes, you see, it causes it also, but this virus is very, very small. It has only four proteins on the surface. And the second issue is that this virus uses as the channel the proteins that normally the cancer cells use as (inaudible 21:38) against the immune system.

And how the virus penetrates the cell is that they find, or search for the cells, and then find the pore where the protein is located. It makes a channel, dressing out, leaving the protein outside of the cancer cell receptor, this channel, and only the RNA can penetrate inside.

Now what happens from one side, these proteins are covering the armament of the cancer cell against the immune system. The second, the false protein is bound to the cell. The immune system is activating not against this protein, but against the cell's protein. And this is why the immune system in this case is attacking not the virus themselves, but the cell's virus.

Ty: Okay, so that's why it's selectively toxic. So in other words, the Rigvir virus causes that cancer cell, which is basically invisible to the immune system, it makes it visible. And that's why you have selective toxicity.

Dr. Kalvins: And also, this is destroying the defense system of the cancer cell against the immune system.

Ty: Okay, and that's a big thing because the cancer cells are invisible to the immune system. They have, like you've mentioned, an armament against the immune system. Rigvir targets them, makes them vulnerable. That's why it works so well.

Dr. Kalvins: Exactly so.

Ty: Okay. And that's why it's selectively toxic to just the cancer cells.

Dr. Kalvins: Correct.

Ty: Now the research has been done on the treatment of cancer but, this is my opinion, I think that this would be something that I should take, or anybody should take, maybe even as a preventative. Just my opinion.

Dr. Kalvins: You see, some of our coworkers are using it as a prophylactic. Because what you are doing is that you are simply infecting yourself with a non-pathogenic virus which is watching for cancer cells appearing. That's a very fine defense.

Ty: Where can I get a shot?

Dr. Kalvins: You have to come visit the Rigvir Company, which is Latvia, or this Virotherapy Center of Latvia, or you can ask by Internet to have the vaccine sent to you.

Ty: Or maybe they've got an extra one lying around here somewhere. Well Dr. Ivars, thank you so much for spending time.

Dr. Kalvins: Thank you very much for coming.

[end of transcript]

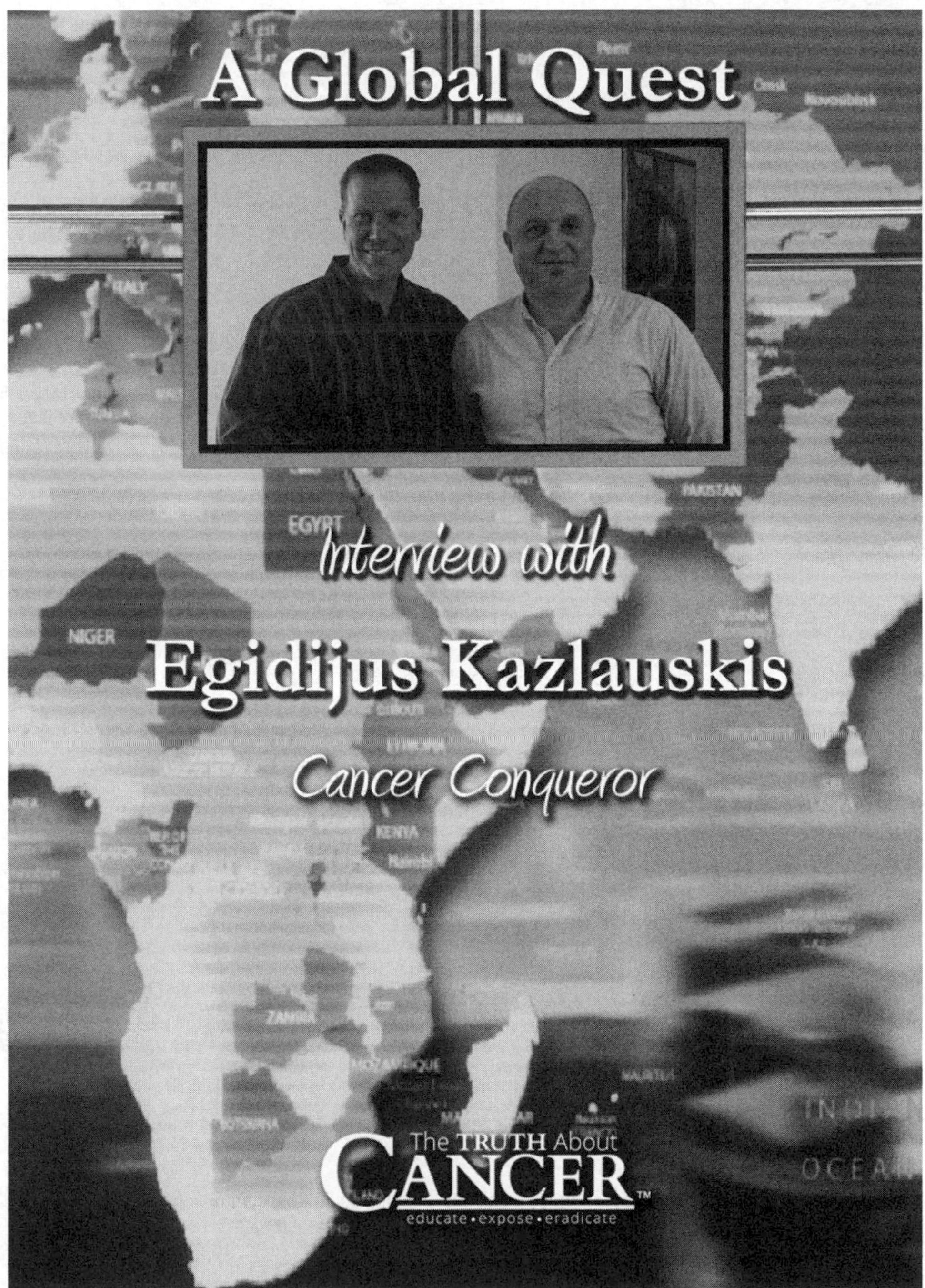
A Global Quest
Interview with
Egidijus Kazlauskis
Cancer Conqueror
The TRUTH About
CANCER
educate • expose • eradicate

Ty: I'm really happy to be sitting here today at the Latvian Biotherapy Center with Egidijus from Lithuania. Thank you for joining me.

So I'm really looking forward to getting your story of success after being diagnosed with a late-stage cancer. Can you walk us back a few years and tell us your story?

Egidijus: [Translated 0:16 to 0:36] Of course, I'm ready to speak about it especially if it will help other people.

Ty: How many years ago were you diagnosed with cancer and what type of cancer did you have?

Egidijus: [Translated 0:48 to 1:27] It was about 2009. It's hard for me to remember because that's the time past—and it was after I went to Alps, to the mountains. I had my vacation there in the mountains and I accidently injured my left hand and when I came back I came here and they sent me to doctor—to see a doctor.

[Translated 1:51 to 2:27] And I went to the doctor to see what's wrong with my left hand but my doctor is very good person, very good doctor. It's a very attentive doctor and he decided also to simply take a look at me, how I am because I'm a rare patient. I don't go to doctors often, and she started to observe me and noticed a small formation, small spot on my back, on the left side of my back. It was not bigger than a tip of a pencil—very small.

Ty: So you had a spot on your back; they did an analysis and what was discovered at that point?

Egidijus: [Translated 3:07 to 3:36] The doctor that I went to, she was just a family doctor and she sent me already to—the same day, the same time—to another department—the skin diseases department, and I received my diagnosis on the very same day, and they said, they concluded that, well, it's a kind of malignant formation.

Ty: So it was a very rushed ordeal, very serious at that point?

Egidijus: [Translated 4:03 to 4:24] Yes it was very serious and, according to my specialist, I understood that I had to contact a surgeon in surgery as soon as possible.

Ty: So did you undergo surgery after that as recommended?

Egidijus: [Translated 4:40 to 4:55] Yes, I had because it was the method. There was a traditional method; first you had to cut off the malignant formation I had and then to do the rest of it.

Ty: So after the surgery did your condition improve?

Egidijus: [Translated 5:11 to 5:38] I wasn't feeling bad. I can't say that I was feeling bad even before operation, surgery, because I think that if my doctor didn't notice it, I would spend many time [sic] because it was not bothering me. I was not feeling weak, I was sleeping well, I was working. I was feeling like a normal person, so everything was okay even before operation.

Ty: So then take us from the period of time that you had your operation until the time that you began to treat your—the cancer with Rigvir.

Egidijus: [Translated 6:10 to 6:32] To be honest I can't say that I felt bad after the surgery before starting Rigvir but only the places that were cut were hurting, but all the rest was normal.

Ty: So it was not a serious form of cancer that you were diagnosed with?

Egidijus: [Translated 0:06:50 to 7:02] Here is when the story begins. That diagnosis was serious. [Translated 0:07:07 to 7:19] The disease was serious and all the research showed that the situation—it continues, it appears again, but not outside on the skin, but inside in the body.

Ty: At the point that you realized that the cancer was internal and not just external, what were the recommendations of the doctors there in Lithuania?

Egidijus: [Translated 7:41 to 8:12] All I was offered—I had a course of chemotherapy and a course of interferon; this was all.

Ty: Why was that the only treatments that were offered? Was that the only treatments that they had available and what was the success rate of those treatments for your cancer?

Egidijus: [Translated 8:31 to 9:14] It was all they offered, I think. Yes, it was the only one that they could prescribe me and I was trying to find out about something else but there wasn't, even in other countries I couldn't find and I simply—well, I followed them. I somehow trust them.

Ty: So, after the course of chemotherapy and interferon, did your condition improve to the point where you did not need any more treatment?

Egidijus: [Translated 9:36 to 10:13] Well, I'd say that I felt the same because only the bruises after the surgery were hurting—were causing pain. After interferon, I had a fever, which was really rather intense, but it was not for a long time and actually after chemotherapy I didn't feel anything.

Ty: So what was it that made you choose to use Rigvir to treat cancer?

Egidijus: [Translated 10:39 to 10:52] Sorry, I'm being maybe too dramatic—too politic [sic]; I simply wanted to live.

Ty: Okay, so I guess maybe I wasn't clear in question. So the prognosis in Lithuania was that it was terminal cancer?

Egidijus: [Translated 11:05 to 11:20] Yes, it was the question of time.

Ty: Okay. So you felt like the treatments that you had available there were not going to save your life and that this was the best option and that's why you chose it?

Egidijus: [Translated 11:31 to 11:52] It was only that I was feeling it, like guessing. I was also feeling it myself and in my body, inside my body, because after the first surgery I had five more and so this situation, occasion, it reappeared every time.

Ty: I see. So how many years ago was it that you began Rigvir treatment?

Egidijus: [Translated 12:17 to 12:30] First time I came to Rigvir in 2010 after the last surgery.

Ty: So five years.

Egidijus: [Inaudible - 00:12:38] Yeah.

Ty: What is your experience been these past five years doing the Rigvir treatment and how has your condition changed?

Egidijus: [Translated 12:48 to 0:13:05] Well, it didn't change. I feel great. I feel okay. [Translated 0:13:08 to 0:13:12] Simply I live and I have a normal life—100 percent life.

Ty: Is the prognosis still that it will be terminal?

Egidijus: [Translated 13:21 to 13:32] You ask it from God; God knows.

Ty: I like that answer.

Egidijus: [Translated 13:38 to 13:43] I don't know why I got this disease. [Translated 13:45 to 13:48] I don't know; will it reappear again? [Translated 13:50 to 13:54] But I really trust and I believe that this medicine help [sic] me, [Translated 13:58 to 14:08] because it's five years, that I don't go to hospital, as I don't have a close, tight relationship with surgeons.

Ty: So the way that you feel really may not have changed much, but despite the fact that five years ago you were told that it would take your life, you're still alive today.

Egidijus: [Translated 14:28 to 15:14] Well, as doctor's ethics, it considers not to say this directly, this negative outcome, so the disease, it's not considered—but, well, I realize that it's not just a bruise that they can put medicine, for example, brilliant green, on and it will simply heal. It was serious, really serious.

Ty: You think this is part of the reason that you're still alive today?

Egidijus: [Translated 15:43 to 15:58] It's not monitored; it's not monitored. [Translated 15:59 to 16:01] I accidently had the same bottle yesterday. [Translated 16:03 to 16:05] Yes, yours is closed, mine's open.

Ty: So you've been taking your Rigvir.

Egidijus: [Translated 16:10 to 16:13] And I'm taking it still today.

Ty: I'll tell you what, your positive mental attitude is infectious and I know that emotions and belief and positivity have a lot to do with success and cancer treatment and if it has—if your emotional state and your positivity has any effect on your lifespan, I think you'll probably live until you're about 200.

Egidijus: [Translated 16:39 to 16:59] I also think so. [Translated 17:00 to 17:08] I agree, totally agree, and this is the reason why I'm here, and I hope and I know that my words will help other people.

Ty: Well thank you for spending the time with us today and I'm completely agreeing with you. If your oncologist has told you that you're terminal, only God knows. Thank you.

[end of transcript]

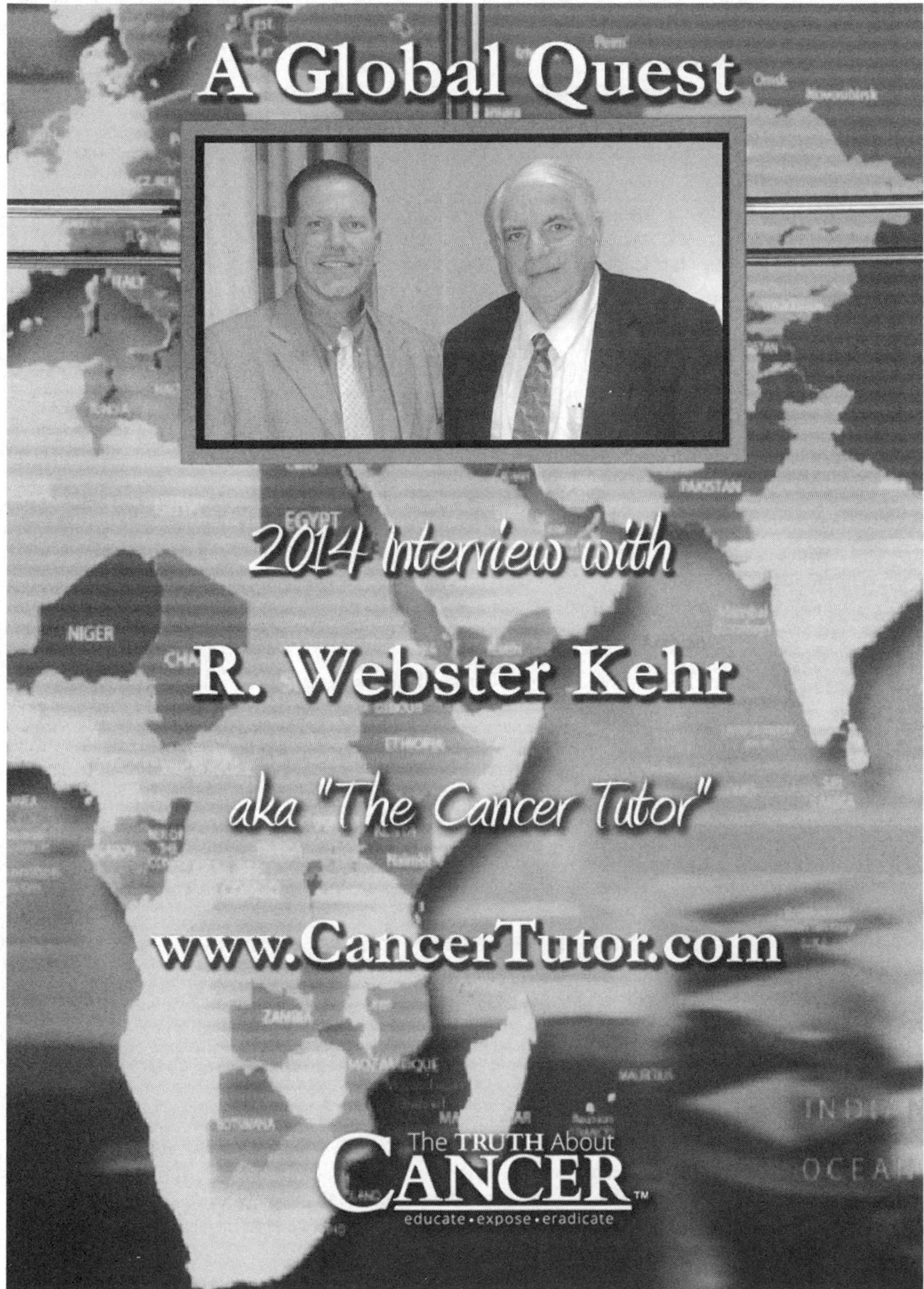
A Global Quest
2014 Interview with
R. Webster Kehr
aka "The Cancer Tutor"
www.CancerTutor.com
The TRUTH About
CANCER™
educate • expose • eradicate

Ty: I'm here today with Webster, the Cancer Tutor, in Kansas City. Webster, I want to thank you for spending the time with us today to share some of your knowledge.

Webster: Thank you, Ty. It's always good to see you.

Ty: Yes. So give us a little bit about your background, your education, and how you got to be who you are today?

Webster: My first college degree was in mathematics, and my second college degree was in accounting. I was over in Europe on assignment by the U.S. Army. I was working for Northrop Grumman at the time. Before I went to Germany I had to take a physical. When I was done with the physical the doctor handed me a prescription for pre-hypertension medication. Now the way I was raised, I'm a little bit skeptical about the pharmaceutical industry. I didn't say this out loud, but I said to myself, "Oh boy, here's another drug they've invented, another disease they've invented." So I took the prescription and I got it filled and I took it over to Germany. I did not like the side effects. I had some time, so I went online to look for natural treatments for hypertension. I found a website of a Doctor Lamb. It was very good. I used his protocol and it worked very fine. But as I was researching natural treatments for hypertension, I accidently came across natural treatments for cancer, particularly carrot juice. I also saw the quackwatch.com website so I thought, "Okay, who's telling the truth here?" Some sites say this cures cancer, and then you have quackwatch.com, which said that all of this natural medicine stuff is quackery. When I got back to the United States I said that I'm going to find out the truth. I started digging and actually talked to somebody face-to-face who had cured their cancer with carrot juice. So I eventually knew what was going on, and I knew that natural cancer treatments were for real. I already had a website and I put a few articles on natural cancer treatments on an existing website. Then I decided I had enough articles and that I should start my own cancer website. So I got the Cancer Tutor name and started the cancertutor.com website, and, as they say, the rest is history. Eventually there were a lot of articles. I work with a lot of people by e-mail. It's very time consuming just to read some of their e-mails, but it's very helpful to the patient.

Ty: I want to personally thank you for cancertutor.com. I know that that was the first Natural Cancer website that I knew about, and it was the website that I went to for years before I published my first book. And then you were kind enough to write the Foreword to it. So you are instrumental in waking me up, helping me to realize about the efficacy of natural cancer treatments.

Webster: That's good. You've added a lot yourself so that's great.

Ty: Let me ask you this. What kind of resistance have you encountered as a result of the www.cancertutor.com website?

Webster: Are you talking about from the authorities?

Ty: Any kind of backlash.

Webster: Occasionally I'll get an email that says what I'm doing is quackery and things like that. That's pretty rare. Most of the e-mails I get are from cancer patients who just want some advice, which direction should they turn. The FDA has never bothered me, and I think the reason is that I don't sell anything. The FDA really is geared to shut down selling products. They've never bothered me and they've never contacted me, because there's nothing sold from the cancertutor.com website. And that will continue. I don't want to sell anything from the website.

Ty: Right. That's where the FDA steps in is if you make claims about natural products.

Webster: Yeah, it's the connection of the natural product and the claim.

Ty: Sure.

Webster: There are three vendors that have told me they don't want their product even mentioned on my website. I can't tell you what they are. But I have a password- protected website from people asking about those products. If they're a password-protected website the search engines cannot find them. So I have to drag people to those websites. With three of the products they have told me, "We'll sue you if you mention our product on your website," because they are afraid of the FDA, and my website makes medical claims. So even though it's not the vendor making the medical claims, I make medical claims and they don't like that.

Ty: With cancertutor.com it's really amazing with just the sheer volume of articles. Anytime that you do a web search for alternative cancer treatments, you're right there at the top.

Webster: Yeah, that's true. I get a lot of hits on the website and I get a lot of emails. That's good. That's why it's there.

Ty: Yeah, that's why you're there to help.

Webster: Yeah.

Ty: So, Webster, we are constantly trying to beat cancer, to cure cancer, to kill cancer, to control cancer. But what exactly is cancer?

Webster: It depends on who you ask. The orthodox charities will say that cancer is caused by DNA damage. The truth of the matter is cancer is caused by microbes. The microbes are inside of the cancer cells. Let me explain briefly why the cell is cancerous and then we'll get back to the microbes. In a normal cell, glucose will enter into the cell. There will be about a 10-step chemical chain reaction to convert glucose to pyruvate. The pyruvate will go inside the mitochondria, and once the pyruvate is inside the mitochondria two chemical chain reactions start. This is a gross simplification, but it's pretty good. The first one is the citric acid cycle, also known as the Krebs cycle. And that starts with pyruvate. That's the complete cycle to create ATP energy. ATP energy is what drives the energy of the cells with adenosine triphosphate. Then about halfway through the Krebs cycle, the electron transport chain spins off. Now the electron transport chain actually creates more ATP than the Krebs cycle, or the citric acid cycle. But together they create more of the ATP energy than anything else. The Nobel Prize was given to Otto Warburg in 1931 for stating that the definition of a cancer cell is low ATP energy. So in a normal cell, glucose is converted to pyruvate, the pyruvate goes through these two chemical chain reactions, and that's where the ATP chemical comes from.

So now the question is, "Why is there low ATP energy?" And the answer is microbes. Helicobacter pylori is the main culprit. This microbe intercepts glucose. That's what microbes do, they eat glucose. So if you're losing a part of that glucose to the helicobacter pylori there's less pyruvate, because if you have less glucose you're going to have less pyruvate. If you have less pyruvate you're going to have less pyruvate going inside of the mitochondria, and you're going to have ATP energy. That is the definition of a cancer cell. A lot of the treatments I have designed were specifically to kill those microbes. And typically, not always, the way to do that is to have a combination of a Trojan horse and something that kills microbes. The Trojan horse is designed to get the thing that kills microbes inside of the cancer cells. I'll give you a good example, honey and curcumin, honey and ginger, honey and cinnamon. Those are three good examples. Honey is the Trojan horse. Cancer cells love sweets and so you mix up the honey with the curcumin/turmeric, or the ginger, and the honey gets the other things in there. What's interesting about this is that down in South America there was a Catholic priest, I think his last name was Romano. He was in a very poor section of Brazil and he had cancer patients. He experimented with his patients with trial and error. He didn't know how to cure cancer. He came up with a formula of honey and aloe arborescens. Aloe arborescens a cousin of aloe vera. He added a little bit of whiskey so that the honey and the aloe arborescens would get a little bit deeper into the tissue to get to where the cancer was.

The formula is in the book, and there's actually a product now called Aloe Arborescens, which has a combination of guess what? Honey, the Trojan horse, and Aloe Arborescens, which kills microbes. He developed it by trial and error. So it's the combination of a Trojan horse and something that kills microbes. DMSO is commonly used as a Trojan horse on my website, MSM and honey. Those are the three main Trojan horses that are used with something that kills microbes. Chlorine Dioxide, which is normally a gas, but it's a liquid for a half an hour or so, or Chlorine Silver. LipH, which is pronounced "life", is commonly used with MSM. That's really what I use for cancer prevention, is MSM and LipH. The formula has worked well. Cancer patients have done well with treatments that use a combination of those two things, a Trojan horse and something that kills microbes. Of course there are also the treatments that actually kill the cancer cells like carrot juice and organic purple grape juice. I mention "organic" because normal grape juice has a lot of chemicals in it. Organic purple grape juice has at least 12 chemicals in it that kill cancer cells. Wheatgrass use. There are multiple ways to deal with cancer.

Ty: Sure. You mention the Trojan horse. You mentioned mixing honey with something else. Why do some of these Trojan horses contain honey or something sweet? You said that cancer likes sugar or sweets?

Webster: Cancer cells have a high number of glucose receptors. That's one of the reasons you don't use processed sugar in a cancer patient, because the cancer cells will gobble up the processed sugar and it will feed the microbes rather than kill them. So you're feeding the microbes with the processed sugar. Cancer patients should not take processed sugar at all. Cancer cells have a high number of glucose receptors and honey is the classic example of a Trojan horse. Maple syrup is used with baking soda. Molasses is also used with baking soda. You can go onto YouTube and find the Kellen protocol, or just look for "molasses" on YouTube. You'll find a lot of testimonies on baking soda also.

Ty: Webster, you mentioned honey in a couple of these Trojan horses. Why honey? You mentioned that the cancer likes sweets, I think you said exactly. Insulin potentiated low-dose chemo is a treatment that I've become familiar with. People have mentioned this in this interview series, this docu-series that we're doing, that they use the insulin as a potentiator to kind of trick the cancer cells into opening up and then the chemo kills them. So it's the same basic principle.

Webster: I'm glad you brought that up, because when I first got started into cancer research, there was a clinic down in the southeast, I can't remember exactly which state it was in. And one of the cancer patients I was working with was going to that clinic. It used DMSO and low-dose chemotherapy. I call it the DMSO potentiation therapy. It doesn't really have a name. That's just my name. But DMSO and the MSM are not glucose products, but they have a propensity to target cancer cells by themselves. They open the ports to the cancer cells. There are four different types of chemotherapy that actually bind to DMSO. And so DMSO and the right kind of low-dose chemotherapy was being used in one of the clinics down there. I never got around to contacting them because they were shut down by the FDA. But that would be even better than insulin potentiation therapy. DMSO is used for example with Vitamin C in clinics, and the FDA had shut down a clinic twice that was using DMSO and vitamin C. The vitamin C kills microbes and DMSO is the ultimate targeting cancer cells. It's just like radar going after those cancer cells. Sugar is bad. Honey, DMSO, MSM, these are three of the more commonly used products to get microbe-killing things inside the cancer cells.

Ty: So you're basically fooling the cancer cells into becoming more vulnerable, and then they're attacked by the substances that kill the microbes?

Webster: Right. It's not so much that the cancer cells are vulnerable. It's the microbes that are vulnerable. You kill those microbes and the cancer cells revert into normal cells. This is a very important concept to understand. There are several ways to deal with cancer. One is you can kill the cancer cells. This is the most common way to do it. The problem with chemotherapy is that it doesn't target cancer cells. Orthodox medicine is not going to use DMSO or MSM to help it target the cancer cells.

Ty: So as a result since it doesn't target cancer cells, it kills indiscriminately?

Webster: That is true, but it has to be used in very, very low doses.

Ty: But the way conventional medicine uses it is in high doses?

Webster: Actually it's very low doses, but because it would kill the patient if they use very high doses. The patient thinks it's high doses.

Ty: Right. I guess what I was saying is relative to the insulin potentiation, which is very, very low dose, correct?

Webster: Yes, very low dose, because it's very, very good at killing the cancer cells.

Ty: Now you mentioned though at high doses chemotherapy would kill the cancer patient.

Webster: Right.

Ty: So in your opinion, talk about the wisdom of using chemotherapy to treat cancer. Is there a place for chemotherapy?

Webster: Let me put it this way. I worked with a lot of cancer patients who are still using chemotherapy. What I will tell them is before you go in there take some MSM, Methylsulfonylmethane, and some of that MSM will turn into DMSO. MSM by itself will open the ports of the cancer cells, and DMSO opens the ports of cancer cells even better. So a little bit of that chemotherapy will target the cancer cells. It's kind of to make chemotherapy a little bit more effective. But the damage is done because they use doses that are very high, so it kills a lot of good cells and it doesn't target the cancer cells. As you may know, the five-year cure rate for chemotherapy, radiation and surgery is about 2.1 percent. If you took non-Hodgkin's lymphoma out it would be less than that. NHL and Hodgkin's disease are really the only two kinds of cancers that do respond fairly well to chemotherapy. But most of the major types of cancer do not respond well to chemotherapy at all. The interesting thing is that all orthodox medicine has to do is use DMSO with chemotherapy. But the problem is if they did that they would use less chemotherapy.

Ty: So then you're implying here that the root of these decision-making processes is what?

Webster: What's best for the medical doctors' pockets and the pharmaceutical industry as well?

Ty: This is a recurring theme that I'm getting is, "Follow the money."

Webster: That's always the case. Yes.

Ty: Let's go back to 1971. President Nixon declared a war on cancer. Are we winning the war on cancer?

Webster: No. I think the cure rate is probably still the same as it was, a 2.1 percent cure rate. I want to say something. This is important because medical doctors will tell a patient that there's a 50 percent response rate that you're going to be alive. What's going through the minds of the medical doctor is probably something like a six-month cure rate. Behind the scenes they're saying, "There's a 50 percent chance you're going to be alive in six months." When they talk about a cure rate and if they don't mention 2.1 percent or three percent, they're not talking about a five-year period. They're talking about a six-month cure rate or a one-year cure rate. I don't know what they're talking about. You have to understand how to interpret what medical doctors, oncologists, are telling you.

Ty: You're a mathematician. You're a smart guy. You know numbers, statistics. I've read on cancertutor.com about the way that the modern medicine manipulates statistics. Talk about some of the ways that chemotherapy statistics may be even manipulated.

Webster: Like I just said, they will typically if they're talking to a patient, they'll use the word "response." There's a 50 percent chance you're going to get a response to this treatment. What does response mean? I don't know. It may mean a three-month cure rate. It may mean a six-month cure rate. What does response mean? It doesn't mean a five-year cure rate, which is what patients want. So they will use these tricky definitions, and I think that's what you're asking. How will they deceive cancer patients? I say "deceive," but it depends on what their expectations are. To a medical doctor that's not deceit, because that's the terminology they're used to using. They're used to thinking in terms of a six-month cure rate or a one-year cure rate. I'm not really sure what their expectations are. But they use terminology like "response" to make it appear like this is a really good cancer treatment. When in fact, it's no better than what they were using in the 1940's. Chemotherapy came out after World War II, but before that they were still using drugs.

Everybody has cancer cells. Everybody watching this has cancer cells. Every one of them, but they also have an immune system. The immune system under normal circumstances keeps the number of cancer cells in check. I have cancer cells. You have cancer cells. What happens is that our immune system gets weak and the cancer cells grow out of control. Why does the immune system get weak? It gets weak primarily because of microbes and parasites as your book talks about. Microbes and parasites in the organs, the liver, pancreas, gall bladder, are weakening the organs. And when the organs get weak the immune system gets weak. One of the ways to treat cancer as you well know is to kill the microbes and parasites in the organs. That's done like Hulda Clark. Which one was your book, the *31-Day Home Cancer Cure?* Is that the name of your book?

Ty: Yeah.

Webster: You use these herbs to kill the microbes and parasites in the organs like garlic. I just got an e-mail a few days ago from somebody who took an entire garlic clove and about a six-foot parasite came out. I was impressed.

Ty: Wow. That would be shocking.

Webster: I got an email from a cancer patient recently who took an entire garlic bulb, not a clove, but a bulb and he had about a six-foot tapeworm come out in their stool. So that was cleaning up some parasites in the organs. That's one of the ways to treat cancer. In fact, it's really important for people that have tumors, otherwise the tumor will come back. There are a lot of things that will shrink tumors, but if you don't fix that root cause of the cancer, the tumors are very likely to come back, whether it's a brain tumor or whatever it is.

Ty: Right. And I think that's one of the themes that I've seen in the difference between conventional and alternative medicine, is that no matter what technique you might use with alternative medicines to take care of the cancer, alternative practitioners look for the cause and treat the cause, whereas conventional treats more symptoms to cut out the tumor, but doesn't do anything to deal with the real cause. That's why you just said that the tumor comes back, because of the underlying imbalance in the body whatever it might be, has not been corrected.

Webster: Yeah. It can even come back with natural medicine if you don't deal with the root cause. I deal with patients and when they describe their situation, the first thing that comes to my mind is, "Your immune system is shot. There is nothing left in your immune system." I could tell you right now that their organs are full of microbes and parasites. Their bloodstream is full of microbes, and right on down the list. They're just full of parasites. Their immune system is shot. They're probably on a processed sugar diet to feed these things.

Ty: So they're feeding the cancer with the diet most likely. And then you said their immune system is shot. So then to me the folly of using chemotherapy is even more then, because chemotherapy is a set of immunocompromising drugs.

Webster: That's correct. Chemotherapy obviously kills microbes, but not in the way that it would really help your cancer. I have an article on the website, which is really critical. It's called, "*ICR Reference Manual.*" Everybody with cancer should really spend several hours studying this article. For example, Step 1 is a list of more than 20 treatments that target and kill cancer cells. Section number two is a list of more than 25 treatments that target and kill the microbes inside of the cancer cells. These revert cancer cells and normal cells as we've talked about. The next one is to kill the microbes and parasites in the organs. Your book is listed in that list. And it goes on and on. There are many different categories. There are more than 15 different categories. There are many different options in most of the categories. It gives you an idea of what you're looking for in terms of what you have to deal with, and what you need to do to deal with that. Now somebody doesn't have to use every one of these. Their dirt cheap protocol is very popular because by the time someone is done with chemotherapy, they cannot afford something like Cellect-Budwig or the cesium chloride protocol or the photon protocol. Cellect is spelled C – E – L – L – E – C – T.

Ty: So this protocol is literally called the "dirt cheap protocol?"

Webster: It's called the dirt cheap protocol. It is the most commonly used protocol on my website that I know about, because the emails I get, the people are poor. I just recently added two more articles. The perfect storm has been around for a while, but it's basically the high dose DMSO and chlorine oxide, a very high dose. And then I just added one a couple of days ago called, "The log cabin protocol." Why would I call a protocol the log cabin?

Ty: I've got a guess. Is it because you use some kind of syrup?

Webster: That's a good guess, but it's actually because when you're in a log cabin you're sequestered from the outside world. It's basically saying, "You're going to sequester yourself from eating bad foods. You're basically eating nothing but foods that kill cancer cells, or revert cancer cells to normal cells." So what can you eat? Carrot juice, purple grape juice, maybe not on the same day, but you can go back and forth on those. And then there's a whole bunch of things from the dirt cheap protocol. I could have called it the sequester protocol. This sequesters you so that everything you eat is treating the cancer. You're not allowed to eat anything that is not a cancer treatment. You can come up with some other things that are also cancer treatments, but the whole concept is the cancer patient eats nothing but treatments for cancer.

Ty: So you're either going to fight your cancer or you're going to fuel it, in other words?

Webster: Well certainly some things fuel it. Yes. And you want to avoid those no matter what. But there are a lot of good foods, broccoli or asparagus. These are actual cancer treatments. You don't want to have too many greens. An orange is really not a cancer treatment, but it's not going to hurt a cancer patient, not like a candy bar would. The typical cancer patient will eat things that are not treating the cancer like oranges and things like that. So this one basically says, "Don't even eat those." Just eat things that are treating the cancer.

Ty: Because of the photon nutrients or whatever chemicals those natural foods might contain that are anticarcinogenic, correct?

Webster: Exactly.

Ty: I've mentioned this many times on this docu-series that Dr. Rashid Buttar in North Carolina, he mentioned in his interview that, "If God made it, it's good. If man made it it's madness." So stay away from the processed foods and eat the natural foods.

Webster: That's a good rule of thumb, but you can take that one step further and only eat the natural foods that are cancer treatments. That's the log cabin protocol. That's the name of it today.

Ty: I like the name. Why is it, Webster, that not more medical doctors today push nutrition? Why don't medical doctors teach patients how to be healthy through eating?

Webster: It's a subject I think all of them at least tell them to use a healthy diet. They could get into a lot of trouble if they actually started using natural cancer treatments. They could lose their license. They can be thrown in jail. There are medical doctors in the United States who are using exclusively natural cancer treatments. They lie low, and some of them don't want me to mention their clinic on my website and I respect that. But I think the average doctor will tell their patient to eat a healthy diet. They just really probably don't even know which foods are cancer treatments and which are not. So they do the best they can. They're just not trained properly.

Ty: They're not trained in nutrition in other words?

Webster: No. They're not trained in cancer nutrition. They may be trained in general nutrition, but not cancer nutrition. It's a different ballgame.

Ty: Yeah, interesting story. One of my good friends is a medical doctor in San Antonio. In 12 years of schooling he told me he had two hours of nutrition.

Webster: Yeah, and I've heard that kind of thing before.

Ty: So while they may be very intelligent people, I'm not debating that, you get through 12 years of schooling in medical school you're a smart guy or a smart gal, you can't teach somebody something that you don't know yourself.

Webster: And they're trained to sell drugs basically. This is not an exaggeration, but I've heard stories of people dropping out of medical school when they were told or they figured out that orthodox medicine had no desire to cure any disease. That's not the direction that orthodox medicine was headed in. I know that's a strong statement. Every doctor is different. I don't want to make a general statement about medical doctors, because every doctor is different. Some of them just don't know any better, and they do the best they can with what they've been taught. I don't want to make too broad of a stroke here, but you're right. In medical school they are not trained to use natural medicine. They are trained to sell drugs.

Ty: Webster, talk about the effects of environmental toxicity on cancer. On the American Cancer Society website they've got a PDF document called "Cancer Facts and Figures, 2013." They state that about 95 percent of cancers are a result of an environmental toxicity or radiation or pollution, some kind of environmental toxin. Talk about that.

Webster: I think that is connected with their theory that cancer is caused by DNA damage. And they're probably saying that these toxins are causing DNA damage and that's what causes cancer. The whole approach is false. It's wrong. DNA damage does not cause cancer. The Virginia Livingston team of cancer researchers discovered that what causes the DNA damage are the microbes that are inside the cancer cells. And basically what they discovered was that these microbes get inside the cell nucleus. And it's well-known that if you have a microbe inside a cell nucleus, the DNA of a cell is going to change, because the DNA of the microbe, the DNA of the cancer cell, or whatever kind of a cell it is, they're going to interact. It's going to change the DNA of the cell. So cancer cells do have DNA damage in a lot of cases, but that's not what causes the cancer. What causes the cancer is the microbes, which not only cause the cancer by eating the glucose, but also as I said, the Virginia Livingston Team showed they get up into the cell nucleus.

This is the whole basis of gene therapy. People with genetic diseases say they try to get a microbe and fit that microbe with a section of DNA, and then they try to get that inside the cell nucleus. So that microbe and that false temporary DNA that they've put in it can change the DNA of the cell. That's the gene therapy right there. So they know that microbes that get inside the cancer cells, the cell nucleus, are going to change the DNA. But they continue to say, "We're going to cure cancer by fixing the DNA"? How is fixing that DNA going to cure cancer? That's what everybody's looking for, "We need billions of dollars more so we can fix this DNA." Well fixing DNA isn't going to cure cancer. Having said that, there may be some rare cases where DNA damage, which is natural DNA damage, does cause cancer like BRCA, BRCA2 genes. These are breast cancer genes. They may create genes that somehow block the production of ATP energy. I do not know that for sure. But it is possible that certain types of DNA damage does cause cancer cells by blocking the ATP energy via some gene that isn't functioning properly. We don't know that. But in general DNA damage has absolutely nothing to do with the cause of cancer. It's a symptom of the microbe that is inside the cancer cells.

Ty: What about the cases of, let's say, nuclear radiation like with the Fukushima meltdown? We've seen an explosion of cancers in Japan from that. Is that one of those instances that you're talking about where maybe it's the exception to the rule?

Webster: I don't know the answer to that question. It could be that radiation could damage the DNA in such a way so it was not able to create the correct proteins. The chemical reactions that are going on inside of the cell are just mind-boggling. There are videos online about the inner life of a cell. One of them was made by the BBC. What goes on inside of a cell is beyond comprehension. You have the DNA, which is constantly pumping proteins into the cell from the genes. It's like a small factory. There are a lot of different ways that something like radiation could cause cancer, because there are so many different ways you can damage the mechanisms inside the cell. If the cell is not creating enough ATP energy, that's the definition of a cancer cell. Radiation can very easily do a lot of damage inside of the cell to the DNA or whatever. It's such that the ATP energy would drop. It's so complex what goes on in there.

Ty: It's going well so far with what you're doing. Are we going? Okay. Talk about Antoine Bechamp and pleomorphism, and how that relates to cancer? First of all who was Bechamp?

Webster: He was talking about the cancer microbe, Helicobacter pylori. Depending upon the alkalinity inside of a cell determines the size and shape to some degree of the microbe. The microbe can be fairly large. This is relatively speaking. I'll just number them from one to 16. At the higher numbers they can be fairly large. At the lower number they get smaller. Again it depends on the alkalinity of the cell. It depends on the acidity of the cell. A cancer cell is very acidic, it's going to have very active and large microbes. When you make the cells alkaline the microbes will slow down and they will get smaller. You would think that that's always good, isn't it? Not necessarily. When down to the smallest size, and different researchers have called this different things, microzymas, and other terms, it goes into hibernation. When it's in hibernation you can't kill it. All along I've been saying, "Let's kill these microbes." Let's not kill the cancer cells. You can't kill the cancer cells. Let's kill the microbes. As the microbes get smaller then particularly when they get to the smallest size like microzyma, you cannot kill them because they're in hibernation. They literally cannot be killed. They will stay in that state for about six months and then they'll come out of that state. I'll give you an example. Let's say somebody is on the cesium chloride protocol and the patient builds up the cesium chloride protocol too slowly, and some of these microbes went into hibernation before enough cesium chloride gets in there to kill them. They will stay in hibernation for six months and then they will come out of hibernation and the cancer will come back because the microbe is now inside of the cancer cell. It was there all along, but for six months it was in hibernation. So basically when this microbe is in hibernation you cannot kill it. It'll stay in hibernation about six months, so cesium chloride for example, if the cesium chloride does not go inside the cancer cells at the right rate, some of these microbes may go into hibernation. And then the cesium chloride will kill the rest of the microbes. The patient will think, "I'm cured of my cancer," and then six months later almost to the day the cancer will come back because these microbes that were in hibernation came out of hibernation. You have cancer again and you have to go through the treatment again. I don't know how often that happens, but it does happen. He wasn't the only one that was familiar with the pleomorphic nature. There are others.

Ty: Talk about the war. I read an article on your website on cancertutor.com. I think it's called, "*The War Against Alternative Cancer Treatments.*" Talk about the war on alternative cancer treatments.

Webster: The war is largely against vendors, and to some degree, researchers. The theory behind it is if the FDA, in other countries it's other organizations, can shut down the vendors, then they can shut down natural cancer treatments. They've thrown people in jail to set an example. There was one person who was using electromedicine. I believe his jail term is that he was sent to jail for 120 years. That's sending a message to everybody else who is doing research. He was selling a product, but he was also a researcher. That sends a message to everyone else that you risk going to jail for the rest of your life. I think he has been let out by now; his sentence was later reduced.

Ty: What was his alleged crime to be sentenced to 120 years?

Webster: I'm not exactly sure what it was, whether it was making a medical device or making medical claims. Usually it's a combination of the claims with the device.

Ty: Or the product maybe.

Webster: Yeah. For example if you go onto the cancertutor.com website, the GB-4000 M.O.P.A. is not always called the GB-4000 M.O.P.A. In some cases it is and in some cases it's called the high RF frequency protocol plasma. And the reason for that is that the vendor did not want, even though I don't get a dime from the vendor and even though he really technically has no control over my website, but he doesn't want that name to show up too many times on my website. So there's a pseudonym a part of the time. As I said before three of the vendors said, "Don't even mention it. We'll sue you if you mention our product on your website."

Ty: Talk about the GB-4000. What is it? What is M.O.P.A.?

Webster: This goes back to the 1930's. It was known in the 1890's; William Russell knew that there were microbes inside the cancer cells. It was rediscovered in the early 1900's. It was rediscovered again and again and again, because back then you didn't have the communication that we have today. In the 1930's, Dr. Royal Rife, who was a microbiologist, knew that there were microbes inside the cancer cells. He came up with an electromedicine device, a couple of them actually, which was designed to do nothing but kill the microbes inside the cancer cells. When he did that, of course the cancer cells reverted into normal cells. One of his major contributions, aside from finding the right frequencies, was that he also determined that you needed a carrier wave to get the microbe killing frequency all the way through the body so that it would kill all of the microbes in the cancer cells. It would not harm natural cells, because healthy cells don't have these microbes in them. It would only affect the microbes in the bloodstream, which are good to kill. There are very few microbes that are good. There are a few that are good, but it's not going to bother them. Even if you kill them it's not really going to have a lot of effect. He developed this technology. The American Medical Association tried to buy him out, and he refused because he did not trust them. Good for him. So the Food and Drug Administration went down and destroyed his laboratory, his equipment, and destroyed all of his inventory. The good news is that 11 of his devices had already been sold before his lab was destroyed. I have to be careful; I'm not going to tell you where they are. I only know where one of them is and it is used for research. Four of them have been found. The other seven have not been found. The GB-4000 devices were based upon that technology, only it uses much better technology in terms of automation. You can't even compare it because of the automation technology of the GB-4000. There's also a GB-4000 SR4.

Ty: What does M.O.P.A. stand for?

Webster: Multi-wave oscillating something. I don't really know. It's a long name, but it has to do with oscillating frequencies.

Ty: Okay. So you mentioned Royal Rife. He's one example of countless numbers of doctors and researchers that have been persecuted for doing something that's not conventional.

Webster: That's right. They were perceived to be cutting into profits. I'm being sarcastic. I've been in this business so long that I've seen too many things to not be sarcastic. I'm sure there are a lot of very good people in the pharmaceutical industry. It's a top-down organization.

Ty: Webster, let me ask you a question. Let's say you went to the doctor and he diagnosed you with pancreatic cancer. What would you do personally?

Webster: The first thing I would think about was, "*Yes, now I can experiment on myself.*" I would probably experiment on myself and if it didn't work then I would use something that's proven to work. I have absolutely no fear of cancer, and I doubt you have a fear of cancer either. So if I was diagnosed with pancreatic cancer I would say, "This is a good opportunity to experiment on myself."

Ty: Do you have any treatments that you would currently recommend that you have on your website that might be effective with that type of cancer? Because I know according to orthodox medicine pancreatic cancer is a death sentence. They don't even claim to try to cure pancreatic cancer. If somebody is out there watching today that has pancreatic cancer, what direction would you send them?

Webster: Let's go back to our house fire example. The faster a house is burning, the more water you need to pour on. Pancreatic cancer is dangerous because it spreads so fast. So this is a case where you need a lot of fire hoses, to use the symbolism. It's true of all advanced cancer patients. Most of the cancer patients I get emails from are very advanced. They've already had the chemotherapy, radiation, surgery. Their body is full of microbes and their immune system is shot for multiple reasons. Pancreatic cancer, even newly diagnosed, would fit into that category. It's a very dangerous cancer even when it's newly diagnosed, because it spreads so fast. So basically I would use pretty much the same treatment I would use on somebody who's already been through the chemotherapy, radiation and surgery. It's a multi-pronged approach. The dirt cheap protocol has 20 different items on it. I have ways, for example the Cellect-Budwig protocol, which we talked about. I literally will say, "Okay. Here's what you need. You need a combination of the Cellect-Budwig and the dirt cheap protocols. That's what you need, because they work in completely different ways." We're not exactly sure how Cellect works because there are ingredients in there that are not mentioned because according to labeling laws they don't need to be mentioned. So we don't really know what's in it.

The things that we do know are in it are things that will slow down the spreading of the cancer and some of them will kill microbes inside the cancer cells. But we kind of categorize it as something that kills the cancer cells, although it may be killing the microbes inside the cancer cells. We're not exactly sure, because we don't know the ingredients. But you're going to use multiple treatments that are killing the microbes inside the cancer cells from the dirt cheap protocol. I may say 10, 12, 15 items from the dirt cheap protocol even on the case. And then with the Cellect-Budwig, which has expert telephone support. When you combine two protocols you can assume that both of these protocols have something in there that's highly alkaline, because that's what slows down the spreading of the cancer. You will have to drop one of those. You will have to decide which one to drop. In this case you would drop the baking soda and maybe even you would drop the asparagus from the dirt cheap protocol. But you would keep everything in the Cellect-Budwig. You would probably have lime juice, which is an option. You would have the GB-4000 which is an option if they can afford it. And then you would add the dirt cheap protocol to it, taking into account you would have to drop one or two items from the Dirt Cheap Protocol. I do that all the time. I recommend that all the time, because of some of the conditions that the patients are in. Maybe they have a really fast spreading cancer. I just kind of lump pancreatic cancer in the same situation as somebody as somebody that's very advanced, so it's deadly.

Ty: I'm hearing your advice would be that you hit it from different directions. In other words, there's not a magic bullet for cancer? You hear people say, "If I had cancer I would do x, y, z." Or, "If I had cancer I would take this one supplement." So what I'm hearing you say is that you hit it from different angles, a multi-pronged approach?

Webster: Right. There's not one treatment I would use in every situation. That's correct. The doctors will create what they call a chemotherapy cocktail. They might combine three or four different types of chemo together into one cocktail. I don't know their reasoning for doing that. But the bottom line is yes. Its chemotherapy, radiation and surgery.

Ty: Webster, when we say chemotherapy, what is chemotherapy? That's kind of a basic question, but I imagine there are some viewers that are wondering, "What is chemotherapy?"

Webster: It's a very powerful drug that kills cancer cells. The problem is it's indiscriminate. The problem is not that it kills cancer cells. The problem is that it's indiscriminate and kills a lot of healthy cells, so that's when it had to be used in very low doses. But basically it's a drug. I have heard, and I do not know the history of this, but chemotherapy came along after World War II and supposedly was basically a use of mustard gas. You've probably heard that too. I don't know whether today's chemotherapy is still based on mustard gas or whatever. But the important thing is that it's very strong. It's a chemical. It's very strong at killing cells. It's very strong at killing cancer cells. Like I said there are four kinds of chemotherapy that actually target and kill, that bind to the DMSO. So if you could combine DMSO with the right kind of chemotherapy—you could use low doses of chemotherapy and target the cancer cells with the DMSO.

Ty: Without the side effects?

Webster: Correct, because you're using low-dose chemotherapy and most of the chemotherapy is targeting the cancer cells. So there would not be the side effects.

Ty: Yeah. And that is one of the biggest complaints about traditional chemo is that, "I feel like I'm about to die when I'm going through the treatments."

Webster: They use insulin because insulin targets cancer cells. And that helps the chemotherapy target the cancer cells better.

Ty: Webster, it's been a fascinating and enlightening for me. And I know that the millions of people that are watching this it's been enlightening for them as well. I just want to thank you for taking the time to share your knowledge with us today.

Webster: Thank you Ty, and you're in this book too as you well know. It's always good to see you Ty.

Ty: Thank you, Webster.

[end transcript]

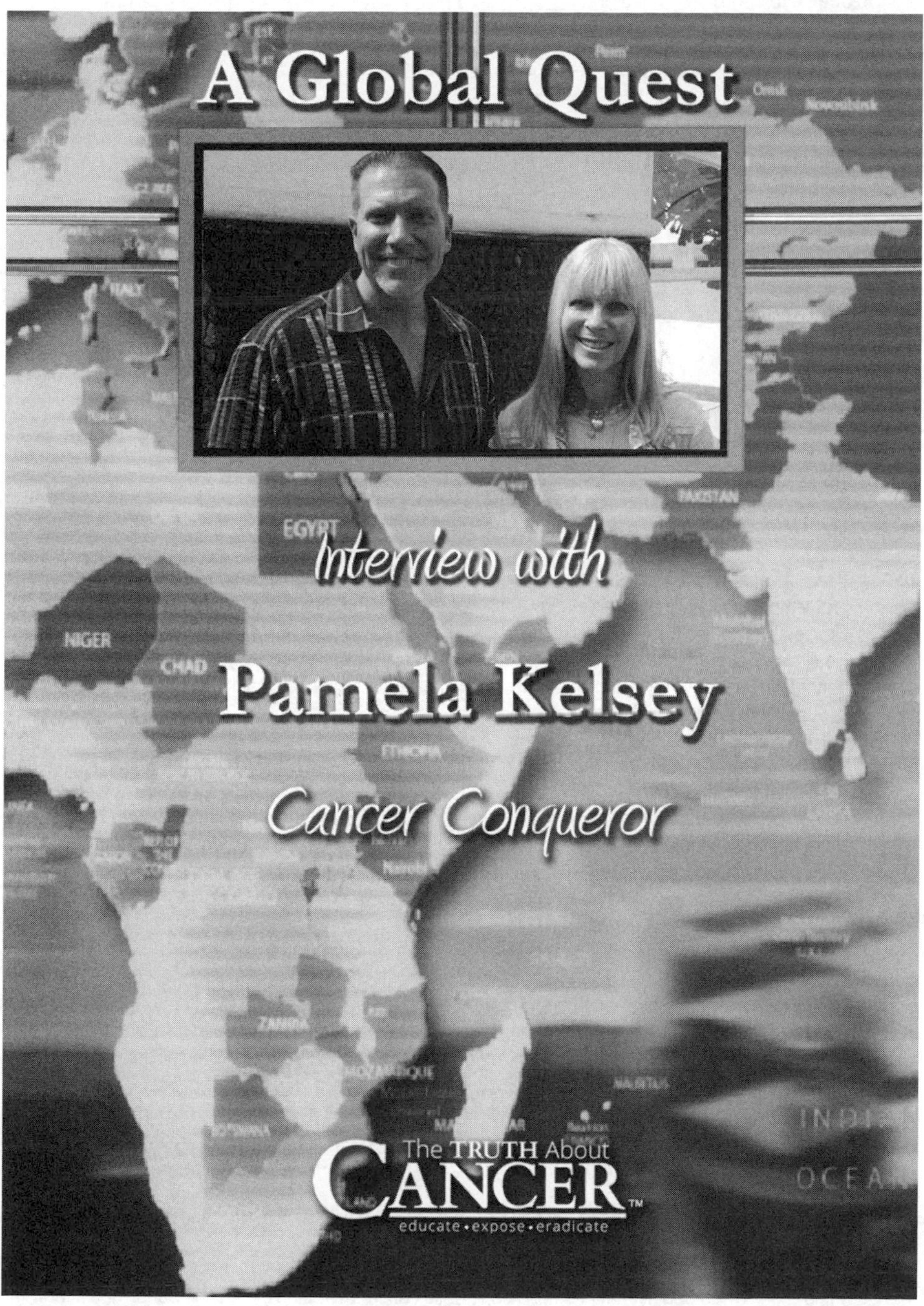
A Global Quest
Interview with
Pamela Kelsey
Cancer Conqueror
The TRUTH About
CANCER
educate • expose • eradicate

Ty: I'm here at the BioMedical Center, the Hoxsey clinic, with Pam Kelsey. I so thank you for joining us today. I'm so grateful to be able to get your story because you had a very difficult type of cancer to treat, didn't you?

Pam: I did.

Ty: Tell us your story, Pam.

Pam: I actually had two. I started with cancer of the pancreas.

Ty: Pancreatic cancer.

Pam: Pancreatic cancer.

Ty: Very difficult cancer to treat.

Pam: Very horrible.

Ty: What year was this?

Pam: This was 1975. Way back. I was 34.

Ty: Forty years ago.

Pam: Yes, 40 years ago. I first was diagnosed with some hypoglycemia. I started having low blood sugar problems and finally it got worse and worse, terrible pain through my abdomen. A friend had been to Hoxsey, as it was called in those days, and she had a friend who was cured of inoperable colon cancer. So she recommended that I see the clinic. So we came down immediately and I was diagnosed with pancreatic cancer. They said I was fortunate because it was just beginning, just starting to go into the intestinal area. It was really good to know.

I felt like I was in good hands because they showed me the x-rays of exactly what was going on. And it was just a day, just like now. They still have the same regimen. You'll get your tonic, they gave me supplements. At that time they giving yeast, vitamin C, calcium, and digestive enzymes. They said in three months I should start to feel better. I was just in intense pain, it was really right through my middle, which I understand is a symptom of pancreatic cancer, just like having a knife go through to your back.

Ty: So you had stomach pain and back pain?

Pam: Yes. It was just like right through the center. And it came out in the back, like literally going through the middle of my chest. And so I went home, started the treatment. I was very religious about what I did. I checked with Mildred Nelson, who was very good to me. If I had questions, I'd call her up, she'd immediately tell me what to do. So within about three months, it was actually almost three months to the day, I noticed a change. I didn't have to take as much pain medication for my headaches. My abdomen started to feel better. I started being able to digest food better. And gradually, from that period of time, I just felt better and better.

Ty: That's really fascinating. I mean, that's fast. Three months with pancreatic cancer. Which many people are dead in three months from pancreatic cancer.

Pam: I know. I followed people that have had pancreatic cancer over the years. Jack Benny had it, and with all the doctors and money he had, he didn't know he had it until it was too late. Michael Landon had it, Steve Jobs, different people that—it's very hard to treat and very low success for recovery.

Ty: I don't know anyone that has had pancreatic cancer that has treated it conventionally that's still alive.

Pam: I don't either. Over all the years.

Ty: And you're alive 40 years later. That's amazing.

Pam: I know, it is, truly. And to have those symptoms, like I said, the pain. And to know that it was just so deadly. And so then I was clear all the years, until 2011. In 2011, I'd had a good physical in January, but I noticed that my abdomen started feeling tighter and tighter. I felt like maybe it was back pain, or just something muscular. But it got tighter and tighter. And I started to have pain on my right side, right in the middle of my right side. So I got more concerned about it. The pain started getting gradually worse and on a Friday afternoon I thought, "This is to the point where it isn't my imagination, I better find out about this." So I called a nurse that was a friend and she suggested that I get to the hospital because it could be appendicitis, it could be a number of things.

So I knew it was too late to come down to BioMedical. So my husband and I got in the car and drove to St. John's hospital, which I had also for medical reasons, I had checked with some of the doctors there. It was a renowned hospital. Elizabeth Taylor went there, Michael Jackson. It was a very well-known hospital, and very reputable. It was a Friday afternoon. I had more symptoms, called a nurse, she said I should get to the hospital to find out what was going on. So my husband and I got in the car, drove to St. John's Hospital in Santa Monica, and told them what was going on. They gave me a CT scan and sent me home because it was the weekend and said to follow up with the doctor on Monday.

So the pain got worse and worse. I called on Monday. I told him what was going on. He said, "Let me call you right back." He read the report and he said, "You need to get to the hospital right away." I said, "Do you think I have cancer?" And then he said, "I think you have what you said." So I knew that I wasn't going to go for further treatment. I said, "Let me think about it." And my husband and I immediately came down to the clinic, got the CT scan here. And Dr. Gutierrez, my old family friend, he informed me that 50 percent of the liver was affected by 22 lesions. And they were up to—St. John's hospital had done the CT scan and they found a number of lesions.

They said they were up to 3.9 centimeters, and they were hypoechoic which means that there was a low echo when they did the CT scan. There was a low echo which indicated a very dense tissue. And they said liver neoplasm could not be excluded. So that's what their diagnosis was. The CT scan here said that there were 22 focal lesions. And the same thing, that they were up from one to five centimeters in size. So I decided to go on the tonic, of course, again. And they put me this time on an organic vegan diet which was more strict. No animal products. I couldn't wait for the three months. I was supposed to come back in three months but I couldn't wait. I was nervous but I was also wanting to find out. Because I know 50 percent, you don't want to wait too long. So I came back in two and a half months and they found that only three of the lesions were remaining in that short of a time.

Ty: Twenty two down to three?

Pam: Twenty two down to three. And I just, home free. I felt really secure and I came down a few weeks later and they were all gone. So it's just been an amazing experience, truly.

Ty: That is amazing. And that was four years ago?

Pam: Yes. Four years ago. And I've done ultrasounds since then. I had one more CT scan and it was clear. And now when Dr. Rodriguez gives me the ultrasounds, he said not only—he checks my whole body, and the abdomen, the pancreas is clear. He said, "It looks like you never—you would never know that you had anything wrong with your pancreas or your liver." Even the scar tissue has healed on my liver.

Ty: That is just amazing.

Pam: Yes. It's incredible.

Ty: I think you're the longest living pancreatic cancer survivor that I've ever heard of.

Pam: I know. And the sad thing, Ty, was that the doctor in the hospital emergency when I went in—I called. I wanted St. John's to know what happened because they have that CT scan. And so I wanted them to know what happened. That I got the treatment and to see what Hoxsey did, what BioMedical did for me. And he said, "that's a very interesting story," but he never followed up to want to see it or anything. Which was just shocking, you know? To have them do that CT and to know that there it was. And he said that it was very interesting.

Ty: I say it's shocking, but it's not shocking anymore. It used to be shocking to me but throughout these interviews, everyone that I talk to that has been diagnosed with some kind of an advanced cancer, they go back to the oncologist and they don't want to know. It's not really shocking. It's a shame. That they don't want to know.

Pam: It's a tragedy really, and I'm so glad you're doing this. Because for a long time—we have a business where we publish a magazine and have a website, and it's kind of known all over the world. And I always wanted the clinic to do more publicity. Of course, they kept a fairly low profile with referrals. But it's really nice to have more publicity and to have more people be able to know that this is such an amazing, simple treatment. That we've known people all over the world, over the years, have been treated for colon cancer, breast cancer, two particular ones were prostate cancer. Given up to die and they're doing well.

Ty: That's really amazing and people need to know this. They need to know that they have options.

Pam: Absolutely. This is so simple, and there's no pain, there's no deterioration of your body, there's no harmful treatment. But it works.

Ty: And it's affordable for most people.

Pam: I know, and it's so fast. The thing that I would really like to always recommend to people is that they come down first. Because for a lot of the patients it's a last resort. And that's the only reason why some people do die. One of two things I've found over the years is that either they're not following their diet and their instructions carefully. Because people think, "well you can cheat here, you can cheat there on your diet." But the tonic is very sensitive to different chemicals like in tomatoes and things like that.

Ty: We heard that from Dr. Gutierrez.

Pam: Yes. So you have to follow it completely and then also they're too weak. We knew one man from Germany who didn't make it but he was absolutely given up to die. He was a skeleton when he walked in here. And it was just too late. So that's the only reason that we've seen anyone not do well.

Ty: What's your message to somebody that's been diagnosed with cancer and they're told that they're terminal? Because you had pancreatic cancer. What would you like to tell them?

Pam: I would just like to tell them, no matter what they're doing, and this is what I tell people whenever I'm contacted or whenever I find out about anyone, to just come here. Even if it's for a second opinion. Send your records down here. Come and see and talk to the doctors. And decide, make an informed decision. Because once you get here and you feel that you just can talk to people, it's so faith-building. Don't give in to just a treatment that's promised. My own mother died of lymphoma and it was just so sad that she completely trusted the doctors. They thought she would do well. She didn't. And so it's a matter of trust. And the medical situation, like with pancreatic cancer, they don't have good records of success rates.

Ty: Is there always hope?

Pam: Absolutely. I mean, here, there really is.

Ty: Pam, you're living proof. Forty years out from pancreatic cancer.

Pam: I feel like a poster child. And they've helped me through different things too over the years. Mildred knew so much. And Dr. Gutierrez—I will say one more thing that might be interesting to people. The doctor that is head of the clinic, Dr. Rodriguez, had his own clinic. He was a radiologist. He had his own clinic in Tijuana. So Mildred used to have him come up at lunchtime to read the x-rays and all the radiology and do the radiology for all the doctors. They'd get together and meet at lunch. He'd come up, help read the x-rays, and then he'd go back.

And he found that when he—because he treated multiple people all over the city—he found that the people that he treated that came here, he would see results on the X-rays. He'd be doing the follow up. And he said, "You're curing cancer. I can see all these results." It was so astounding. So Mildred gradually had him come more and more and now he's head of the clinic. So I think that's very faith-inspiring.

Ty: That really is. He said, "You're curing cancer." Harry Hoxsey was always the quack that cured cancer. He's no quack.

Pam: Reading his story was very interesting too, how it originated. He treated Barnum & Bailey Circus animals and then people wanted to go to him.And it wasn't, well you probably have that story, but anyway. He was a very famous. He was a horseman who raised thoroughbreds. So he had a horse that he put out to pasture. The horse had cancer and he put him out to pasture and the horse healed up. And he thought, "What is this horse doing?"

And so he came up with the formula and then he began treating the Barnum & Bailey Circus animals and they had success. So one man in town had found out he had cancer and he was, I think he was a doctor I'm not sure of that, but anyway, he begged him to treat him. Hoxsey said, "Well this is just for animals." He said, "I don't care. I've got cancer. I don't want to die."

So he gave him the treatment and he did well. And in the beginning days, then the American Medical Association, the AMA, was just starting. There was a political thing. They wanted to go into partnership with Hoxsey and charge $10,000 a patient. And Hoxsey said, "I can't do that, because my father promised I would never refuse to treat patients if they couldn't pay." So he refused that. And then, of course, that was what led to coming south of the border. Because they were in Dallas for many years.

Ty: What would you tell Harry if you could talk to him?

Pam: I'd tell him, thank you, thank you, thank you. You saved my life. I wouldn't still be alive.

Ty: Well thank you, Pam, for sharing your story. Very inspiring.

Pam: Thank you, Ty.

Ty: Forty years out.

Pam: I just want to encourage anyone to come and send their records. Dr. Gutierrez is even available by telephone.

Ty: Good people here.

Pam: Very good.

Ty: Thank you so much.

Pam: You're welcome. ***[end of transcript]***

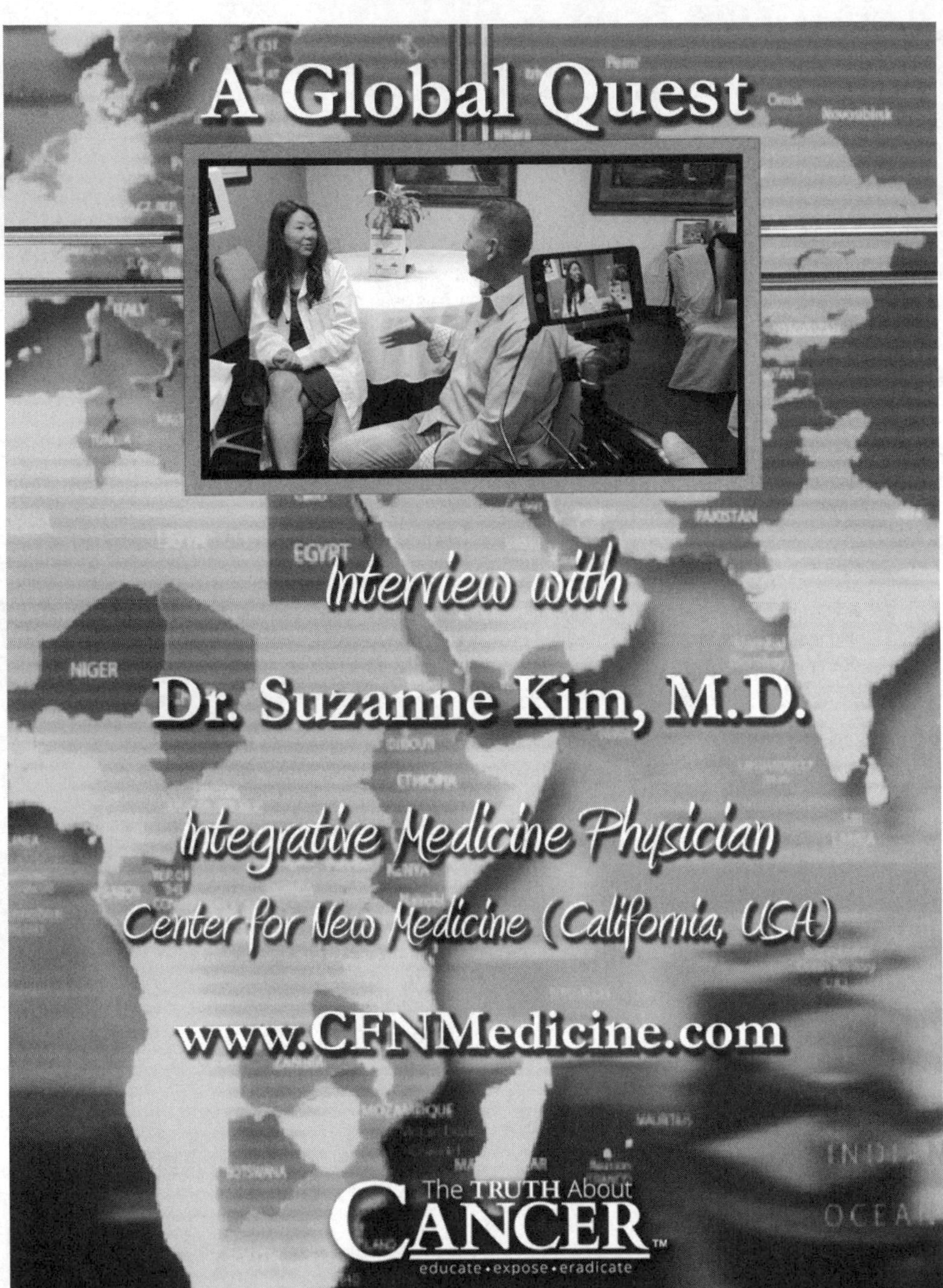
A Global Quest
Interview with
Dr. Suzanne Kim, M.D.
Integrative Medicine Physician
Center for New Medicine (California, USA)
www.CFNMedicine.com
The TRUTH About CANCER™
educate • expose • eradicate

Ty: I'm here at the cancer clinic here in Irvine, California. It's the Center for—what's it called? The Center for Cancer Healing?

Dr Kim: Cancer Center for Healing.

Ty: Cancer Center for Healing. Irvine, California with Dr. Kim. Thank you for joining me today. Really looking forward to getting a live shot of this UVLrx machine. So, what does UVLrx stand for?

Dr Kim: UltraViolet Light treatment. Rx is treatment. This is actually ultra violet blood irradiation which I think is not actually a new technology, that's been around for a long time. But this device is actually a new device that's come out in terms of the ability to transmit the light directly into the vein. So this is what we'll be showing you.

So previously we've been doing ultraviolet blood irradiation for many years here. The previous device, you have to actually remove the blood and then we add it to a saline bag and then it is runs through the ultraviolet light externally and then back into the person. You can only treat about 60ccs of blood that way. This way, with the catheter directly into the vein and the light emitting, it's going to treat 50 to 70 percent of the blood in one hour treatment

Ty: So why is the ultraviolet light so important?

Dr. Kim: Well, ultraviolet light has been known for a long time now to be a disinfectant. It is able to kill viruses, bacteria, and fungus. So the ultraviolet light, in the same way, will be able to kill the viruses, bacteria, and fungus in the blood. This is very important for, as you can imagine, for infection.

So anyone with an infection can be treated with this treatment. But as well for our cancer patients. We know that many cancers have their root in one of these. So this is why most of our cancer patients do get this treatment.

Ty: Great. So we're really looking forward to seeing this in action, so go ahead and walk us through the process and if there's anything as you're going that you want to describe it, feel free.

Dr. Kim: Okay, sure. No problem.

[demonstration sounds: latex gloves and equipment]

Ty: Now doctor, you had said before with the UVBI you've only been able to do about 60cc of blood?

Dr. Kim: We did about 60cc of blood. Correct.

Ty: As opposed to over 50 percent?

Dr. Kim: Right. About 50 to 70 percent of blood in one hour is going to be treated with the UVA. Now this actually we'll talk to you about, as you can see and hear, there's not just ultraviolet light, there's visible one and two and I'll tell you about that. So it's actually three treatments in one. So, this is actually the fiber optic that's going to go into the vein.

Ty: Wow, that's fascinating. We're running cable into the veins here.

Dr. Kim: Okay. We're just going to be running some saline.

Ty: So the fiber optic then is used to transmit the light into the vein?

Dr. Kim: Exactly, so this fiber optic cord you could see, I'm going to be attaching it right now. This is just the saline. Now I'm going to attach this right over here. So then you push this, okay. And then, you can't see it, but the timer will run for 60 minutes. And you can see, because it's light here, you can't really see the light as well but the light is transmitting directly in.

Ty: I can kind of see it.

Dr. Kim: Can you see it?

Ty: Yeah. Sure.

Dr. Kim: When it's darker it's more visible. So the first half hour, the ultraviolet light is running which is about 365-nm UVA light and the visible light one is red light which is 630-nm. And what the red light does—red light's been known for a long time to help with increased production of ATP and also to help with immune function. So the red light is going to run for the whole hour. The green light will run the second half hour.

The green light is 535-nm light and that one helps to increase flexibility of the red blood cells and also allows them to deliver oxygen more efficiently. So the combination of this, and this treatment is actually three treatments in one. So it's a really great treatment. We've really been enjoying using it. We have been using it since about February. It has kind of replaced our old ultraviolet blood treatment that we used to do. It is very good because it's helping not just with the ultraviolet light but also at the same time helping to increase the immune system function, increasing production of ATP as well, and then also helping to improve the function of the red blood cells. So it's got three functions in one.

Ty: And the ultraviolet light you said kills the pathogens – the viruses and bacteria that can lead to further immune compromise.

Dr. Kim: Exactly. As we know in cancer patients, they have a compromised immune function. So whether or not that's a causative problem of their cancer or as a result of a cancer—they have issues with a virus, or bacteria, or fungus—either way this is going to help them.

Ty: So the amount of blood, you said over 50 percent of the total blood volume, is able to be treated with this. Is that because over the course of the next hour, 50 to 70 percent of the blood passes within the certain area of the vein that's been hit here?

Dr. Kim: Right, right. Because actually, it's only during the first half hour, that's why probably it's only about 50 percent. If it was running the whole hour, it'd treat 100 percent. But they have it so that this actually initially runs for the first half hour and then allows the ultraviolet light to—it's ultraviolet UVA light, it is different than the other one that has UVA and UVC, the other ultraviolet machines.

The reason why they didn't include the other ultraviolet lights in this therapy is because they felt that it actually may be too strong and could actually damage some of your normal cells. So they chose to only include UVA, so it's a little bit milder. It can stun the viruses, bacteria, and fungus, but it's not so strong that it may damage our own cells.

Ty: So the UVA is chosen because it only hits the pathogens.

Dr. Kim: Exactly. And then again, you're coming in and having these two other fabulous light treatments that have been known to help improve the immune system. So together I think it's a great system.

Ty: Yea. And you've been using this for just a few months now?

Dr. Kim: Yes, since about February.

Ty: Okay. Before that time, how many treatments would you have to give? Not everyone will have access to this machine. Say somebody is doing a UVBI where you can get 60cc of blood, how many treatments of that would you need before when you used that to get marked improvement?

Dr. Kim: Typically patients will do this treatment anywhere from two to three times a week. We still use it similarly, the same way. We've seen patients after one treatment have an effect and some people take a couple of treatments to have an effect. It varies. The wonderful thing about this treatment is that we can use it for not just cancer but we use it for other infections as well. So it's been very effective.

Ty: Yeah. Well while it's working let me get a little of your background, Dr. Kim. Where did you go to school? How did you get involved with the practice here?

Dr. Kim: So, I went to undergraduate at Cornell and then I went to Hahnemann Medical School.

Ty: Hahnemann? Samuel Hahnemann.

Dr. Kim: Samuel Hahnemann, I know.

Ty: The father of homeopathy.

Dr. Kim: Exactly. The ironic thing is I had no idea what homeopathy was when I went there. It is kind of ironic but I think it was meant to be though, in some ways. So, and then after, I came out to White Memorial [Medical Center] in Los Angeles and did family practice training. I was practicing for about nine years in a traditional family practice office and started to feel a little dissatisfied as far as what I was able to do for patients. I truly wanted to go into preventative care but I felt that the preventive side was not very good. Mostly what I was seeing was a lot of chronic patients and just giving them medications.

A lot of these patients were not getting better and were already seeking alternative treatments. So I was open. They would tell me what they were doing and I was very open to that, but I didn't really know. So I just told them, "Honestly I really don't know enough to tell you either way, but since you're having problems"—and I sent patients to every specialist. They were having problems and I sent patients everywhere to every specialist and they'd come back to me and they tell me that they're still having the same problem, "Can you help me?"

So that was one factor. Another factor was probably some health issues that I had of my own that also were not addressed through conventional medical treatment. And so I think that led me to starting initially with nutritional medicine; started learning about that because you know in medical school they don't teach you anything about nutrition. So when I started learning a little bit about nutritional medicine that was really very, very helpful. I mean that's the foundation, I believe, for all health.

So that then lead me into homeopathy. As I learned about homeopathy, it kind of expanded my thinking. It challenged me because it really was very far off from what you learn in medical school. So after that I just said I'd try it and it just worked amazing. I tried it on myself. I tried on my family first before I tried it on patients and just found it to work amazing. After that you start to meet people and so I then went into and learned about some kinesiology.

That challenged me even further and pushed me way out of my comfort zone. It was very fascinating and it was very exciting because I felt that there were some answers here that I hadn't found before. Also for me, it started to help me personally to feel better and get on a track of getting off of some medication.

So after that is when I was introduced to Dr. Connealy, and I met her and came here and I felt that this was just the right place. This was definitely. She was way ahead, she was doing what I wanted to do. So I was so excited to come here and just continue my journey of learning and being able to really help patients and it's been so exciting. It's really enjoyable.

Now medicine to me is so much more enjoyable. I am able to help patients, really help patients who before I didn't want to see those patients: your fibromyalgia patients, patients with all these chronic diseases, and I didn't really enjoy seeing those patients.

Ty: Because you didn't have any answers.

Dr. Kim: Because I didn't have answers for them, exactly! And now those are the patients that I really *love* seeing. Those are the patients that generally tend to seek us out I think. Which is great because I think we have answers for those patients.

Ty: I think it's ironic, Dr Kim, that you went to Hahnemann Medical School and you didn't learn anything about homeopathy from the father of homeopathy.

Dr. Kim: You know I was just thinking about that the other day. I really think that the journey and my path—when you seek out truth it comes to you. I feel like I was put there—and I was just thinking about that, how it is so ironic. They have since then changed the name, it's not Hahnemann anymore which is unfortunate I think. But, exactly, I had no idea, absolutely no idea. I had an idea in my mind what I thought it was, but it wasn't anything what I thought it was.

Ty: I think that what you just said is true, especially for the viewers that are watching this documentary. When you seek out truth, you'll find it, right?

Dr. Kim: I absolutely believe that.

Ty: We're trying to provide bits and pieces of the truth so that people can put together this picture that they can use to get on the path to health. A lot of the pieces of truth that we need, we're not taught. You went to Hahnemann Medical School and did not learn about homeopathy, a big piece of truth in medicine that you didn't know about. We're not taught the truth in a lot of these areas.

Dr. Kim: Right. It was so interesting when I went to an Ozone conference and the speaker there referred to Hahnemann hospital and he showed an Ozone therapy that was done at Hahnemann hospital. He had records of it. I was blown away because I said that I can't believe that was actually done at the hospital a long time ago. At the hospital that I trained at. It was just ironic.

Ty: And now a lot of times, you'll read about that and think that's just a bunch of quackery, but it was mainstream until recently.

Dr. Kim: It was. It was actually at one point done in the hospital, but nobody knows that. I didn't know that.

Ty: As a matter of fact, ozone is frowned on a lot of times today by mainstream medicine. As are, what I was going to say, coffee enemas, right? Dr. Nicholas Gonzales talked about that last year. Until the 1970s coffee enemas were in the MERCK manual as the best way to detox the liver.

Dr. Kim: I heard about that.

Ty: But now you hear about people using coffee enemas as if it's nutty. So we've turned truth on its head.

Dr. Kim: Exactly.

Ty: We're trying to get back to the truth where with this.

Dr. Kim: Exactly.

Ty: And so thank you Dr. Kim for sharing this with us today. This UVLrx machine. Thank you Ronnie, the man with the good veins, we appreciate it.

[end of transcript]

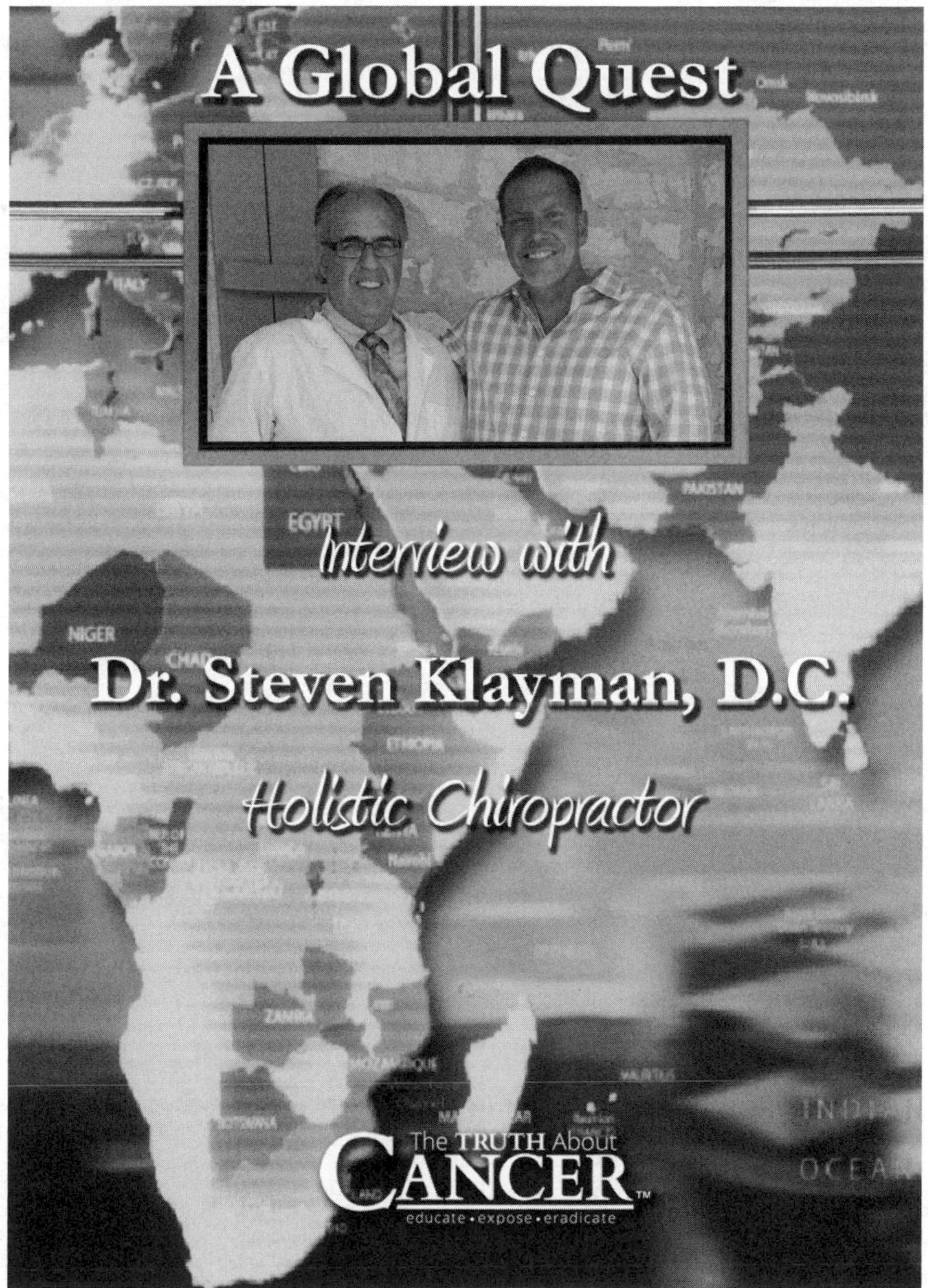
A Global Quest
Interview with
Dr. Steven Klayman, D.C.
Holistic Chiropractor
The TRUTH About
CANCER
educate • expose • eradicate

Ty: Really happy to be here with Austin, Texas, today with Dr. Steve Klayman. Dr. Klayman thanks for having me and the camera guys in the office here.

Dr. Klayman: My pleasure.

Ty: Really happy to be able to talk to you today about several things, number one the importance of the spine in overall health, but then we're going to get into some other nitty-gritty issues, like genetically modified organisms, vaccines, and might even talk about a few natural treatments for cancer.

Dr. Klayman: Okay.

Ty: Initially, if you could share with our viewing audience a little bit about your background and how you got involved with health.

Dr. Klayman: I've been in chiropractic for over 30 years, and the more I got involved in it, and the more in depth I got involved, I realized how much we could do for people's health with chiropractic and with nutrition, and proper rest, and proper exercise, and meditation. All of those are part of my practice—what I call a holistic practice.

Ty: Did you initially—when you got interested in health up front—have you always been holistic or did you go down the mainstream route initially and have some kind of a wakeup?

Dr. Klayman: No, I was pretty mainstream for most of my youth and then when I got into chiropractic school, I started hearing about why we shouldn't vaccinate. I was quite surprised. And I realized that I was getting involved in a profession that was really very much interested in people's health and had a different model—had a health model as opposed to a disease model. It was about preventing disease, not waiting for it to come on the scene and then trying to deal with it.

Ty: You mentioned you began to learn in chiropractic school about why we shouldn't vaccinate.

Dr. Klayman: Yeah.

Ty: Why should we not vaccinate? Because haven't they been proven safe and effective?

Dr. Klayman: You know the answer to that, Ty. No they haven't been proven safe and effective. Matter of fact, there's never been a study with multiple vaccines given to a child at the same time. It's all experiment, and we can see now the results of the experiment has been disastrous because now you have over four and a half million kids in the United States who are autistic. Many of them—some of them—due to immediate reactions of vaccines, not to mention the ones that died.

In the US you have Mississippi, which has a mandatory vaccination rule for all kids. Mississippi leads the country in vaccination rate. It also leads the country in infant mortality rate. Funny coincidence, huh?

Ty: I wonder if that's not actually a coincidence.

Dr. Klayman: It is not a coincidence. And, unfortunately, the United States is way down towards the bottom of the industrialized nations in infant mortality. You've got a much better chance as a child of making it through the first year if you're born in Europe than if you do in the United States.

Ty: It's funny you mention that—it's not funny—it's sad that you mention that, but—ironic that you mention that I think is a better word. There's a study in 2009 maybe—by a couple of researchers, Goldman and Miller, I believe I read, and they analyzed the infant mortality rates in the top industrialized countries and found that the United States had the highest number of vaccines, and the highest rate of infant mortality. The other countries that had the lowest vaccines had the lowest mortality.

Dr. Klayman: Correct. Now South Korea is catching up to us, because they're really starting to vaccinate and now their infant mortality rate is skyrocketing. China, which has a 99 percent vaccination rate, is showing really nasty signs of infant mortality also. If you analyze the statistics and stop believing the pharmaceutical industry representatives and the shills in Congress, you'll see that it's not a one-size-fits all. For me, personally, if I go to a foreign country and I'm going into a country where there's a disease—cholera, let's say—I'm going to get the cholera vaccine. But to give a Hep-B vaccine to a little baby who's probably not going to have sex for a while and not going to use intravenous needles, to give them on the day of birth is a tragedy.

Ty: Yeah. A tragedy at best.

Dr. Klayman: At best, yeah.

Ty: Could border on criminal.

Dr. Klayman: Yeah. Yeah. And the interesting thing is the pendulum swings and now with this Disneyland outbreak, the pendulum is swinging back the other way. The pharmaceutical industry attacked and the parents in California got irate and they came out of the woodwork and they're fighting this SB-277, the mandatory vaccination rule that now passed—is supposed to go into effect on July 1st of 2016 in California. Of course, they'll fight on a lot of grounds, including its Constitutionality and it's a violation of the Nuremberg Codes, forced medical procedures without informed consent.

Ty: Right. And also that goes along with the Helsinki documents. I can't think of the official name, but right in line with the Nuremberg—forced treatments against…

Dr. Klayman: Yeah, that's what happened in Nazi Germany. You can see a similarity going on here in the United States. It's scary.

Ty: Yeah, it really is.

Dr. Klayman: A lot of people are contemplating moving from California or home schooling.

Ty: Right. Now, they're talking about catching up the adults that are behind, right?

Dr. Klayman: That's exactly right. Who thought it would stop with the kids?

Ty: What's going on there?

Dr. Klayman: They're trying to slam through this rule of SB 792, mandatory vaccination for all adults, or without that you'll have a criminal record. It will be considered a crime.

Ty: A crime not to get caught up on your vaccines?

Dr. Klayman: Correct. And so you'll either be fined or imprisoned.

Ty: Wow.

Dr. Klayman: Yeah. Pretty scary.

Ty: I think at that point you're going to get a lot of people moving from California if that ever goes into effect.

Dr. Klayman: Yeah. It will be challenged. Certainly, it will be challenged, but we'll see what happens.

Ty: Just a mere fact that we're even discussing it in the United States is bizarre, isn't it?

Dr. Klayman: Yes. Totally. And, of course, nobody died from the outbreak of measles in Disneyland. Nobody died. Was a good excuse to propel their cause and so they did. Of course, Dr. Pan who led the charge was given $95,000 by a pharmaceutical industry to his coffers.

Ty: And you know the interesting thing I just saw—one of the top people in Dr. Pan organization that was pushing—it's really a propaganda campaign, right?—was pushing these vaccines was vaccinated and he has Guillain-Barré now. Did you see that?

Dr. Klayman: Yes, I did.

Ty: One of the top people in his organization now is speaking out against it saying, maybe we should have thought this a little bit longer because…

Dr. Klayman: No, this hasn't been thought through very well and there are really no scientific studies. Matter of fact, the CDC classifies vaccinations as necessarily [sic], but unsafe.

Ty: Necessary, but unsafe.

Dr. Klayman: Yeah.

Ty: One of the things that we heard last year from Sherry Tenpenny, she mentioned the fact that no studies on carcinogenicity are ever performed on any vaccine. So if you look at the package insert, I checked it. I went and found package inserts for these different vaccines: "This vaccine has not been tested for carcinogenicity or mutagenicity." So it had not been tested to see if it causes cancer in cells or causes cellular changes. It's on almost every vaccine. They're not tested to see if they cause cancer. So, if they haven't been tested to see if they cause cancer, how can we show that they're safe?

Dr. Klayman: You can't.

Ty: You can't.

Dr. Klayman: That's absolutely true.

Ty: And how can you show that they're effective if there's never been double-blind, placebo-controlled study on it?

Dr. Klayman: Absolutely.

Ty: That's the gold standard. They tell us, your apricot seeds don't work because there's never been double-blind, placebo-controlled study. Well, neither have there been on their vaccines. So what's good for the geese should be good for the gander.

Dr. Klayman: Not when there's money involved.

Ty: That's true. So you think that's a lot of what's driving these decisions today?

Dr. Klayman: Of course. Why would somebody spend hundreds of millions of dollars giving gifts to politicians if they didn't expect something in return? That's the way the system is working and, hopefully, we'll get some president in there who will stamp money out of politics.

Ty: That'd be nice. Speaking of money, you see the big money trail going up to Monsanto's headquarters don't you?

Dr. Klayman: We certainly do. Yeah, you know what that's about and, of course, now recently World Health Organization has classified Monsanto's glyphosate as a probable carcinogen, which Monsanto got very upset about. But, of course, that's sprayed on lots of crops and we end up ingesting it and so it's strange that there's such a big cancer rate in this country. Not very strange at all.

Ty: Not very strange at all.

Dr. Klayman: People want to eat pesticides, you're going to have to expect you're going to have various diseases and malfunctions. Of course, to my patients, I recognize that some of them are eating those types of foods and recommend, go organic. It costs you a little bit more, but you can also support local growers and you could have a better chance of being healthy if you're eating your vegetables and fruits organically.

Ty: Interesting—we were up in Virginia to interview Joel Salatin. Are you familiar with Joel?

Dr. Klayman: I am not.

Ty: He's a farmer. We interviewed him about the thing you just mentioned that it costs a little bit more to eat organic, but when you really boil it down, he said, if somebody told me I don't have the money to eat organic, I'm sure if I went into their house I wouldn't see any chips and Cokes and lottery tickets and all of these things that are just a waste of money. He said, "I'm sure I wouldn't see that, right?"

Dr. Klayman: Of course you will.

Ty: We waste money.

Dr. Klayman: Yeah.

Ty: He said, you could literally could go out and buy the most expensive organic potato in the world, slice it up, and make your homemade French fries with coconut oil and make them healthy and it would be cheaper than the ones you buy that are packaged, per ounce. It would be cheaper. But it's not as convenient. And so I think a lot of what—a lot of the reason we are sick is because we're so busy that we don't take the time out to make our own healthy food because we could, right?

Dr. Klayman: Certainly. Yeah, and a lot of us are lazy and a lot of us just want to save $.35 or $.40 cents on a pound of cherries, by buying the sprayed ones instead of organic ones.

Ty: Sure. It's convenient and I got to admit, a lot of the food is tasty, right?

Dr. Klayman: They make it that way so you'll eat it again.

Ty: They do.

Dr. Klayman: Cheetos—they don't have those great-tasting Cheetos for nothing. They make them so you want to buy them again.

Ty: They have the chemicals in them. Sure.

Dr. Klayman: Yeah, it's true.

Ty: So what do you think about, not just the glyphosate, but just the whole genetically engineered topic at hand—we're looking at all of these GMO crops…

Dr. Klayman: It's interesting because back in 1996, I ran for office—I ran for Congress here in Texas against Lloyd Doggett, who's been in office for a long time. One of the parts of the platform is labeling GMOs. Even Obama campaigned on in 2007—he said people have the right to know what's in their food. Of course, he turned around and signed the Monsanto Protection Act, like Monsanto needs protection from me or you, right?

Ty: Right.

Dr. Klayman: So I've been on this issue for a long time and I realized back in the 1990s as this issue was getting heated up—that the scientists were really playing God and they didn't know what they were doing. And now, of course, you have a whole industry that's sprung out called "gluten-free." They have so distorted the chemical makeup of the wheat that people can't digest it or it causes illnesses, so they have to buy gluten-free wheat.

Ty: Sure, and that's because the wheat used to be what we call natural grains and now it's not. It's been changed as well.

Dr. Klayman: Correct. So you don't mess with nature. Man, in his attempt to improve on nature, is creating a disaster and this disaster now is banned in many countries around the world because they recognize what it is. Unfortunately, in America, politicians have been paid off and they won't ban it. Even though 90 percent of the people want GMO-free foods. They want them labeled GMO-free—labeling hasn't taken effect yet.

Ty: Right. At least tell us what's in there.

Dr. Klayman: Too much money. Too much money's going into these politicians' pockets and so—we're seeing some backlash.

Ty: Interesting. Remember back in the '50s they had the little signs, "DDT is good for me."

Dr. Klayman: I don't remember that.

Ty: Well, I wasn't alive then either. In the magazines, I've seen the old ads.

Dr. Klayman: Okay.

Ty: "DDT is good for me." I've seen some ads recently, "GMO is good for you" or something like that. Saying that GMO foods are healthy, but my question is this. If they're healthy, why don't they want them labeled?

Dr. Klayman: Because they know they're not. Of course, the answer is obvious.

Ty: Yeah.

Dr. Klayman: And people know it. People aren't even buying that propaganda.

Ty: Yeah.

Dr. Klayman: I mean 90 percent of the population polled wants GMOs labeled.

Ty: Talk about—share with us the story that you shared with me earlier about Essiac tea, which is an amazing tea that has blood purification properties and might even cause cancer to go away.

Dr. Klayman: Well, throughout the years, I pay attention to various things that are cropping up in the medical journals, in my chiropractic journals, and one thing I got turned on to years ago was Essiac tea. I read about this nurse, Rene Caisse up in Canada, back in the 1920s, many of the cancer patients who were referred to her who were terminal by the doctors and she gave them this tea called Essiac tea—E-S-S-I-A-C. Essiac tea. It was a blend of herbs given to her by an Indian medicine man. Lots of people were getting cured.

Ty: What were the herbs, do you know? I had known it had sheep's sorrel and I think it has turkey rhubarb, but, I'm trying to think—burdock root maybe?

Dr. Klayman: Yeah, I think that's another one of them.

Ty: And maybe another, okay. I wondered if you knew.

Dr. Klayman: There's four main herbs.

Ty: Four main herbs, yeah.

Dr. Klayman: About 15 years ago, 18 years ago maybe, my secretary said to me one day, she said, "Dr. Klayman, my aunt has cancer of the spleen. What would you do if you had cancer of the spleen?" I told her I'd start drinking Essiac tea. She said, "Where can I get it?" and I said, "Go down to Whole Foods." So, about a month later, she tells me her aunt has been drinking the tea, goes into her medical doctor, medical doctor says, "I can't find any cancer in your body. I think you've had a healing." She said, "I've been drinking that Essiac tea." And he said, "That has nothing to do with it. You're in spontaneous remission." You've heard that term right?

Ty: Many times.

Dr. Klayman: That's a word that means, I don't know why you're better. We call it spontaneous remission.

Ty: All right.

Dr. Klayman: So she goes on, comes back to the doctor a couple of months later and he said I'm sorry to tell you the cancer has returned and I think you have about six to nine months to live. So when she goes home Angie asks her, "Are you still drinking the tea?" She said, "No, the doctor said it had nothing to do with my cancer disappearing." She said, "You start drinking that tea." And she did. I spoke to Angie a couple of years ago, which is about 15 years after this incident, and she said my [sic] aunt told her, "The next time you talk to Dr. Klayman, tell him, 'Thanks, I'm still drinking the Essiac tea, and I still have no cancer.'"

Ty: My grandmom was I think she had colon cancer. She drank Essiac tea as well. I think she was initially diagnosed back in the late '80s and she drank that tea for a good 10 years.

Dr. Klayman: Oh, really?

Ty: She died 10 years later, but she had stopped drinking the tea.

Dr. Klayman: Hmm...

Ty: She was supposedly terminal and lived 10 years after she was terminal.

Dr. Klayman: There's a lot of natural cures out there, unfortunately, most of them you have to go to Mexico for because in the US the AMA controls everything in the health field. You can do surgery, you can do chemo, and you can do radiation, if you're an oncologist. Otherwise, you're practicing outside your scope if you are doing other things like apricot seeds or Vitamin C therapy or Essiac tea or hypobaric therapy, etc. You know, of course, of all of these.

Ty: Sure. I saw some apricot seeds up at the front of your office here.

Dr. Klayman: Right. That's exactly right.

Ty: That's for people to munch on when they come in.

Dr. Klayman: It's for them to munch on; it's for me to munch on, also.

Ty: A little healthier than having a candy dish, isn't it?

Dr. Klayman: Absolutely. Absolutely.

Ty: So, you have any patients here that are eating apricot seeds regularly?

Dr. Klayman: I do. I do. Yep.

Ty: Okay.

Dr. Klayman: And I don't know if it's preventing any cancer in them, but I know the studies about the Hunzas in the Himalayas and they eat about 30 or 50 apricot seeds a day, and cancer is unknown amongst those people.

Ty: Yeah. We actually were privileged to interview Jason Vale last year who was thrown in jail for five years in New York for selling apricot seeds on the website. He cured his own cancer. Pretty interesting story. It's amazing how you can be an organization like the FDA that admittedly approves drugs that kill 100,000 people a year and nothing gets done. But you have somebody like Jason that's trying to help people and never harmed anyone with these seeds, but he gets thrown in jail for five years because they weren't approved. It's bizarre isn't it?

Dr. Klayman: It's really bizarre. It's called medical tyranny. I think that's where we are at in this country right now.

Ty: I think it is, yeah. We interviewed, earlier today, a young lady, 17 years old, that was literally strapped to a gurney and forced chemotherapy against her wishes. That's tyranny. That's criminal. It's assault.

Dr. Klayman: Yeah.

Ty: It's assault. And I could be literally assault with a deadly weapon. Right?

Dr. Klayman: Yes.

Ty: Chemotherapy—it used to kill the soldiers in World War I and World War II with the mustard gas. So it's the same derivatives.

Dr. Klayman: It's too bad and it's too bad this country has gotten to a place where it's at. Maybe now the pendulum is going to start to swing a little bit the other way because the industrialists have gotten pretty strong.

Ty: I think the pendulum is swinging the other way. I think we're making a lot of ground—making a lot of headway, gaining ground. And I'm actually really encouraged about where we're heading. Because people seem to be waking up to the fact that they do have control over their health if they make good choices.

Dr. Klayman: Yeah.

Ty: So somebody that's been recently diagnosed with cancer—I know you don't treat cancer; you can't treat cancer.

Dr. Klayman: Legally.

Ty: Right? But, if somebody is diagnosed with cancer, what word of advice would you give them? What questions should they ask their oncologist or what should they be doing once they're diagnosed with cancer—theoretically?

Dr. Klayman: Well, if it was me, I would certainly start taking some of the alternative treatments. Some of the cancers they've done very well with, like skin cancer. Medical science has done really great with that one. Cancers outside of the body, like in testicular cancer, they've done quite well with that. It's the internal cancers, the organ cancers that really have become a problem. And how are you going to clean up the body so that the cancer dies off? And, personally, because most of the oncologists won't do their own treatment, I would go to another type of cancer clinic, where they do alternative treatment maybe in conjunction with some of those surgical procedures, but certainly with, like in Tijuana, there is a number of clinics in Tijuana that will do alternative procedures where you have the Gerson Clinic and you have—what's, Dr. Garcia, is it Dr. Garcia down there in Tijuana has a clinic?

Ty: Let's see, Gutierrez has the Hoxsey clinic. Garcia—you thinking of Voices of Hope maybe?

Dr. Klayman: Maybe it is. He took over for his father.

Ty: Contreras.

Dr. Klayman: Contreras.

Ty: Voices of Hope, yeah.

Dr. Klayman: I would certainly check out some of those and even the United States there are cleansing clinics that you can go to so there's a variety of things that you have to investigate—but you have to recognize you are on your own because your local oncologist is probably not going to support that.

Ty: Because they can't.

Dr. Klayman: Because they can't.

Ty: They're not allowed to.

Dr. Klayman: Exactly.

Ty: What do you think about childhood cancer? Why do you think we're seeing such a rise in childhood cancer over the last 20 years?

Dr. Klayman: You know it's really a shame, but there's so many chemicals and so many toxins. And, you know, if you examine mother's placenta, you'll find sometimes in the number of hundreds of chemicals in the placenta at birth. So the parents are exposed either through the air, to the water, to the food, to all sorts of toxicity already so the child is inheriting that. We've got to do a much, much better job starting to clean up and not allow all of these sprays to be sprayed on the food—parents have to watch what they eat. They've got to get their body in shape before they have any kids. It's a big responsibility.

Ty: It is.

Dr. Klayman: Yeah.

Ty: I think somebody else said that a few weeks ago that we interviewed. Nowadays, it's important that the parents detoxify before they have a child.

Dr. Klayman: Totally.

Ty: Because of the toxicity flows through the umbilical cord to the child.

Dr. Klayman: One thing I see a lot in my clinic is childhood allergies and you have a lot of nut allergies. One of the ingredients—one of the adjuvants in vaccines is peanut oil. So when you inject—see people think that eating mercury is the same thing as injecting it. It's not the same. Of course, you're not to eat too many fish because of the mercury that's found in the fish. That's nothing compared to injecting it directly in the bloodstream. At least when you eat something, it goes through the digestive system, gets purified—

a lot of the stuff gets pulled out by the liver and it's dumped. Here, you're injecting it directly in the blood, so now the little child is getting a full dose of mercury or aluminum or MSG or peanut oil right in the blood. You have a foreign protein right in the blood. Not supposed to be there. So now the body notices it and reacts to it and it's alerted. So, the next time that child has some peanuts or some nuts, the body reacts and does what it's supposed to do, which is defend it and try and kill that. When so doing it, it puts the child into anaphylactic shock, and sometimes the child dies from a peanut because there's peanut oil in his vaccine. That shouldn't be in there. You shouldn't inject things like that directly in the bloodstream because we know aluminum, mercury, MSG, polysorbate 80, those are all neurotoxins. Neurotoxins means it's damaging to the brain. It crosses the blood–brain barrier and you have health problems, including autism.

Ty: Also in many vaccines is formaldehyde which is a...

Dr. Klayman: Formaldehyde. Yeah.

Ty: Don't want any formaldehyde in me until I'm dead. That's embalming fluid.

Dr. Klayman: That's right. That's right. So why it's in there, why they could not put something innocuous in there. That I don't have the answer to.

Ty: So, if somebody's been diagnosed with cancer and their oncologist has told them that they're terminal, should we listen to the oncologist?

Dr. Klayman: He's probably not going to do his treatment; why would you? Fifty-eight out of 64 oncologists said they wouldn't do their own treatment.

Ty: That's good advice. If he's not going to do his own, why would you? Well, Dr. Klayman, this has been a great interview. I really appreciate you covering what you've done today and I've not heard the peanut allergy analogy from anyone, but, you're right, peanut oil is in many vaccines.

Dr. Klayman: Yep.

Ty: Never put those pieces of the puzzle together.

Dr. Klayman: Yeah. One of the things that people don't put together—they say well, what's the big deal of a little mercury? But they don't recognize eating mercury or injecting it is two completely different things. Completely bypasses the liver, it goes right into the blood.

Ty: And if you do a web search, I think something like 670-something studies I've seen relating mercury to cancer.

Dr. Klayman: Is that right?

Ty: It's huge. Huge. And it's all of these vaccines as a preservative and they don't have to use thimerosal in vaccines; they could use something else. And even ones now, I'm learning they say that they are mercury-free—that's because the mercury—that thimerosal wasn't added, but it was used in the manufacturing process so it still has mercury. They're telling us that they're mercury-free and they're not. Anyway, does it surprise you that they're lying?

Dr. Klayman: Not a bit. Not a bit. One CEO of a pharmaceutical company speaking to his sales people and he said to them, "The worst thing we can do is kill somebody. The second-worse thing we can do is cure them." That tells you where the whole situation is at.

Ty: It does.

Dr. Klayman: It's a business. It's a business and there are casualties and, unfortunately, we've had a lot of casualties in the United States now.

Ty: So, Dr. Klayman, you ran for Congress?

Dr. Klayman: Yes.

Ty: Back in the '90s?

Dr. Klayman: Yes.

Ty: You understand about kind of getting the teams together?

Dr. Klayman: Yep.

Ty: And getting the people to support what you're doing?

Dr. Klayman: Yep.

Ty: What can we do now to help keep this momentum going in the right direction and regain our health?

Dr. Klayman: You know, I wouldn't be completely disheartened. Even though things look pretty bleak, because there's an old saying, "As negativity rises, positivity also rises," and we're seeing also some fantastic changes in health care.

In all areas of life—you use the word "awakening." People *are* awakening. They're realizing that most of the politicians are probably in the pockets of either Big Pharma or Big Oil or Monsanto, Dow, etc. People are waking up to this now and they're not accepting things as it was or as it's been lately. So people recognize that have to take more responsibility for their own health because, ultimately, the one who cares the most about their health is not the doctor, it's them. Even in my office, if a person cares about thoir hoalth, I'll caro. If thoy don't care very much, I won't care very much.

So nutrition is extremely important. We're the fattest country in the world. Exercise is really important. Stress control is really important. When I was a kid, there was no such thing as a yoga studio or a meditation retreat. Now, even the—*all* of the cardiologists are recommending that you do exercise, you do yoga, some stretching and do some meditation because the mind is really important and if you can calm down the mind, you calm down the physiology. And it's really an anti-stressed state what meditation is—by going inside and being quiet and if you look it's part of every religion, it's part of every culture—it's just not taught very much openly until recently in the United States.

Keeping your spine healthy and not having nerve impingement is really important because it's recently been found that having pinched nerves in your spine is actually mimicking a chronic fight-or-flight state. Fight or flight is really good if you have to run away from the dragon, or fight the bear, or whatever. That is what the fight or flight was designed for. It was not designed to be cursing at the guy in the car next to you because you're in traffic, continually. That increases output of adrenal glands, it damages your immune system, it produces chemicals in the brain that are not helpful. So you have to have some of this relaxation and you have to have it every day.

Ty: That's interesting. Nerve impingement causes you to be in constant fight or flight.

Dr. Klayman: Correct.

Ty: Wow.

Dr. Klayman: Correct. It sets up this adrenal gland secretion in your body and your adrenal glands are your stress glands. You need the adrenal glands for energy. Without adrenalin you don't survive. So when you wear those out, then you go into exhaustion. So it's important that there be some reversal of the stress process every day and meditation is a great way to do it, exercise is a great way to do it, yoga is a great way to do it, going into a bar is not a great way to do it.

Ty: Unless it's a juice bar, right?

Dr. Klayman: Unless it's a juice bar, there you go. Yeah. Taking a fuller look at your life, it's important to see where you're going because if you keep doing the same thing—if you're just a pizza and football type of guy every night, and you watch football and eat your pizza, drink your beer if that's what your diet is, you're not going to live very long. You're going to have to recognize that. You're going to have to make some changes.

Ty: Well, Dr. Klayman, thanks. I really appreciate it.

Dr. Klayman: My pleasure.

Ty: All right.

Dr. Klayman: Thank you, Ty.

Ty: You bet. Keep up the good work.

Dr. Klayman: Yeah.

[end of transcript]

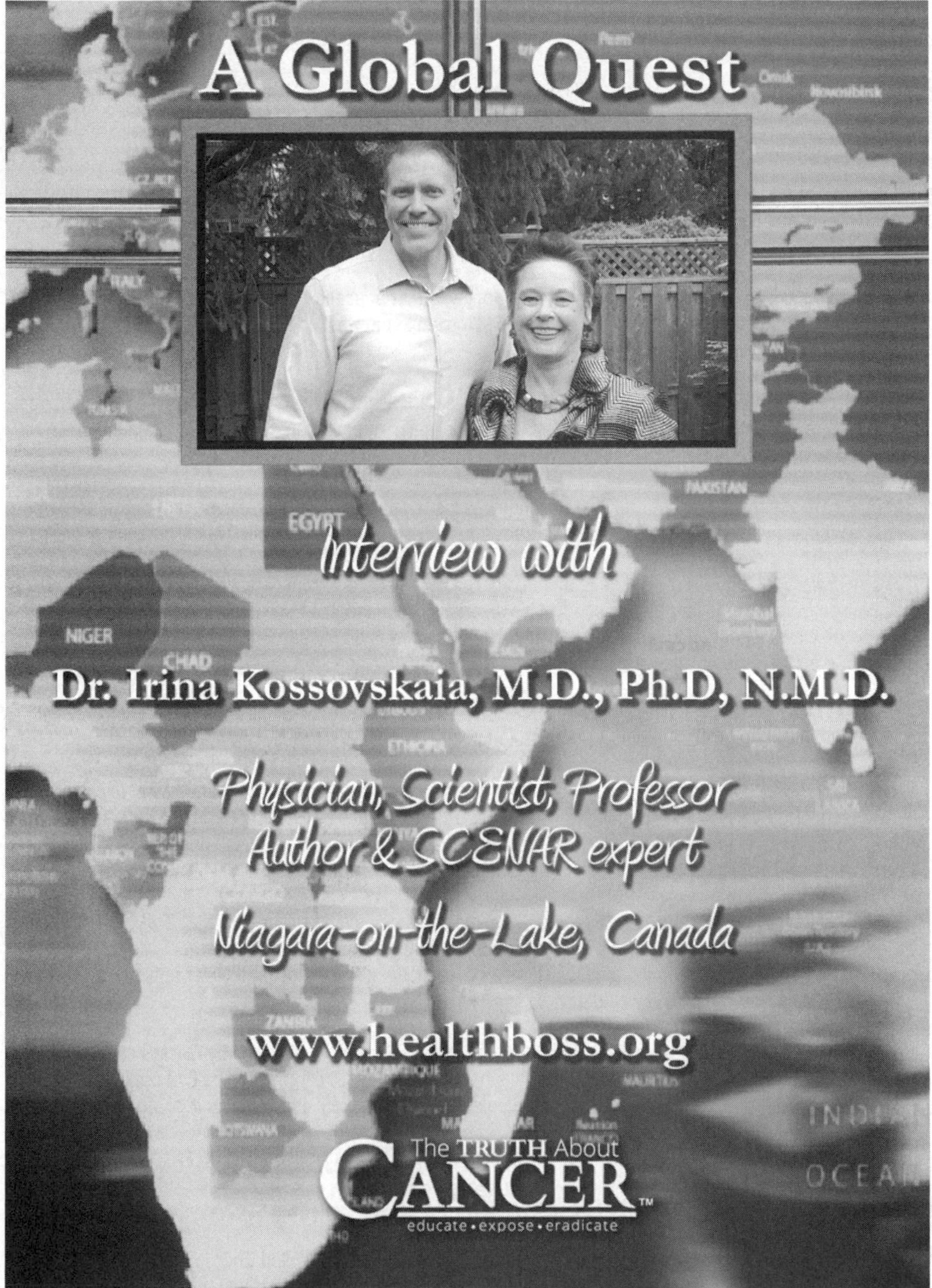
A Global Quest
Interview with
Dr. Irina Kossovskaia, M.D., Ph.D, N.M.D.
Physician, Scientist, Professor
Author & SCENAR expert
Niagara-on-the-Lake, Canada
www.healthboss.org
The TRUTH About CANCER
educate • expose • eradicate

Ty: Well, I'm really excited to be here in Niagara-on-the-Lake, Canada, 15 minutes away from Niagara Falls. Here with Dr. Irina Kossovskaia?

Dr. Kossovskaia: That's correct.

Ty: Thanks for joining today and inviting us to your home here.

Dr. Kossovskaia: My pleasure.

Ty: So, I'm really excited to get your input on a lot of these topics that we've been discussing regarding cancer and natural medicine. But first of all, could you tell the viewers a little bit about your education and your history.

Dr. Kossovskaia: I'm actually a former eye surgeon. So, my former education and practice is in Russia for almost 20 years. Actually, exactly 20 years. In 1997, I moved to the west, in North America. I'm a doctor of natural medicine.

So, I'm a holistic physician or an enlightened physician, as they say now. You know, the transition from you're a doctor, then to a quack, then you're an enlightened physician. So I went through the entire evolution.

Ty: You're a medical doctor from Russia. What was the "aha" moment or your moment of enlightenment that made you decide that you need to transition from the old school to into this enlightenment?

Dr. Kossovskaia: Well, I guess the enlightenment comes from, most likely, from personal tragedy. When you meet personal challenges, especially if it's a serious challenge, then you have to look outside the box. And that's happened to me when my only son, Dennis, was diagnosed with Tourette Syndrome at the age of four. Actually, he was diagnosed at the age of nine when it became pretty bad.

So, obviously, I was facing his pretty bleak future. And conventional medicine—and I had access to the best medical care I could possibly imagine at that time, and I couldn't find any answers.

So, I had to look outside the box and I came across a very interesting technology, a very exciting technology, holistic in nature. It is called SCENAR. And the device SCENAR was invented for Russian cosmonauts to support them well while they are in space without the facilities, diagnostic facilities or treatment facilities.

Basically, this was a little device that, at that time, t looked as a prototype of a *Star Trek* healing device from the *Star Trek* series, that Dr. Bones used. So, that was very fascinating to me. I started using it in my own practice as an ophthalmologist, as a conventional medical doctor. It was pretty amazing, almost healing-miracles, I would say.

After that, of course, my colleagues in SCENAR helped me with my son and by the age of 15 or 16, he almost had no trace of Tourettes. And that's how we, I guess, all come to the field of natural medicine if we were shaped, if we were formed and moulded into the conventional medical thinking.

So, you have to look outside the box and unless you get a good kick, you will do that.

Ty: Now, you said it's SCENAR? Spell it.

Dr. Kossovskaia: SCENAR is actually an acronym and it stands for Self-Controlled Energo-Neuro and Adaptive Regulator. So, it's S-C-E-N-A-R. SCENAR is a technology that started in Russia in about in the end of the 80s, let say. And it went through several stages of evolution and right now, it evolved into a very fascinating technology which we called Cosmodic. And it's not from the word cosmetology, it's from the word cosmos, actually.

Cosmodic is still SCENAR but it is much more evolved SCENAR. It targets regeneration. So it jump-starts regenerative processes in the human body. And it is capable of supporting and maintaining those processes to the extent that the body can actually regenerate tissues. Not completely organs yet, but it can regenerate tissues in many situations when conventional medicines are hopeless.

Ty: Really? So, like, maybe a finger has been amputated.

Dr. Kossovskaia: Fingers, yes, definitely. Like if you're looking at, say, body developing scaring—let's say you had a heart attack. Heart attack always results in scar tissue. Because the body losses blood supply and scar tissue is a compromise of the body. So scar is not that tissue as it should be, but it is something that the body puts on the place of a normal tissue just to keep functioning.

Because the body is not concerned with the structure, the body is concerned with function. So it is basically paying attention to keep working, whatever structure supports the function. In order to regenerate the original tissue, the body needs a lot of energy and needs right programs which we, as we age, we lose. They say an embryo can actually grow a finger but when we, adults and even children, we lose that ability. A salamander can grow a leg, we can't. Why not?

The programs are there but they locked. So, Cosmodic to a certain extent, can unlock those programs and give the body enough information and energy in order to run those programs and regenerate a normal tissue on the place where normally a body would form a scar.

So let say, after a heart attack you would have a normal heart muscle instead of a scar. With the internal organs, like a liver or a heart or a stomach—let's say a stomach ulcer, you can actually see it with fiber-optics where on the place of stomach ulcer, there is no scar. So, it is just nice stomach lining. It is more difficult to view the skin, believe it or not, but it is still possible.

So this technology is like the next step towards the *Star Trek* healing device.

Ty: *The Star Trek Healing Device.*

Dr. Kossovskaia: That's how I think of it.

Ty: It sounds like it would have some practical applications for cancer treatment.

Dr. Kossovskaia: We do. However, as you are probably well aware, cancer is an industry. And being in an industry it's well regulated. We can only work with people who come to us and consciously chose a certain way of dealing with their problem. So a lot of people just choose a natural way, alternative way into their way of searching plans in looking for answers.

Of course, even technologies that we use—the SCENAR and Cosmodic, are not only the technology that we utilize in our practices. They cannot give you all the answers. Technology is technology. High-tech energy healing is something that I am expert in and I run for many years. And yet, even our high-tech gadgets cannot provide you with answers when cancer is concerned. Because cancer, by nature, is the major breakdown in systemic communication.

So what happens with the cancer, as you probably know, the body just does not see the growing tissue. We all grow a little cancers in our bodies many times a year. Me, sometimes, once a day.

However, this growth is always controlled by the general regulation and management system of the body. The body is computerized. So when the communication is running correctly, our lines of communication are open, then the body detects that growth in early stage and suppresses it. However, when the lines are broken, that's when it happens that the body does not see the developing tissue until it is too late.

And cancer is a young—they are healthy, normal young cells. They are just very aggressive and they live for self-support. It's almost like a gang in a city. It attracts energy, grabs energy, any energy it can reach. And because of that energy, it just keeps growing. The body doesn't see it until it starts producing symptoms and when symptoms it's pretty late at that stage to suppress, so it is very difficult to do.

We try to support the body to start seeing the growing tissue. And when the body is aware, and it's all about awareness—so when the body becomes aware, then we can do something about it. We utilize technology that do two basic things, that give the body awareness so they serve as a mirror for the body. You know, when you look in the mirror and you don't like something, you will correct it, so the body does exactly the same thing. It looks at itself, at its energetic signature, energetic portrait. And when it doesn't like something, like a growing tissue, then it decides to do something about it.

Sometimes it doesn't have energy to do that. Then we have a different technology to supply the body with that energy, with coherent energy, structured energy, harmonized energy. And when the body has that energy, then it can deal with the problem. However, you need to support the workings of high-tech energy healing gadgets with the lifestyle choices, with correct nutrition, with anti-oxidants. Well, you know that. You know that cancer treatment always is systemic. So, it affects all sides of personal life and physical, as well as mental, spiritual, and emotional.

Ty: That's a good point. That a successful cancer treatment needs to be systemic. Isn't that where the conventional treatment protocol really falls flat? Because they don't treat it systemically. They treat the tumor and as long as they shrink the tumor or they cut-out the tumor, they say it is a success without looking at all the variables that have to do with cancer.

Dr. Kossovskaia: Definitely that. But I would also say, would dare to say, that conventional medical approach is flawed by its very principal, its very core. The conventional medical approach, not just to the cancer, but to almost all diseases and disorders in human body. It's a war on disease.

So, when you are fighting the disease which has been identified, you select the enemy, you give the enemy a name, you identify it, you name the disease, you have a diagnosis, and then you have the prescribed sequence of actions to deal with that enemy.

See, the disease is not an enemy. The very nature of the disease, if we'll look into the functioning of the body as a system, the disease is an adaptive reaction of the body to some change in outside world. So the body is trying to adapt to something.

Let say flu virus. Flu has all of these unpleasant symptoms, but it is bad? Well, the body is trying to adapt to flu virus through developing a fever and suppress the growth of the virus by developing a fever. By the very nature of it, if we wouldn't have a fever, the virus would spread all over and kill us.

Ty: So the fever is a good thing?

Dr. Kossovskaia: Fever is a good thing. Fever, and runny nose, and the cough, it's all attempts of the body to clear itself. To have a detox, to fight the virus and develop the immune response to the virus. So it is an adaptive reaction response of the body and so are all the other diseases. All except for the cancer. Cancer has no adaptive reaction. It is more, as we already said, disease of miscommunication.

But most of the other diseases, they are diseases of adaptation. So adaptation fails. Adaptation tries to come up back and then we have chronic diseases and relapses of chronic diseases. Because the body attempts to run the cycle of adaptation again, and again, and again, and finish it because any adaptive reaction is a program. So it starts from zero, have to go through the crisis. Remember what the old doctors used to say, "The crisis has passed?"

And it is. The crisis is the top of the cycle. So it has to pass through the crisis. And you're on the new regeneration cycle, then you're on the recovery, you come back to zero and the system actually gets into a different state of evolution. It evolved, it adapted, it restructured itself. So, it's zero again but it is already a different zero. So it's like a spiral. The body always adapts to something.

By the nature of it, the cycle of adaptation needs to be finalized. If it's not finalized, the program will linger in the system forever unless it has a chance to finish itself, it's a program. The program needs to run disease, needs to live its life through, that's how we call it. So fighting the disease, stopping the program, is not going to solve the problem. Yes, antibiotics can suppress the symptoms but the program is not finished. So it will be sitting in the body unless some circumstances develop. And it will flare up again because disease has to live its life through.

By the nature of the conventional approach. fighting the disease, trying to stop it, is not going to help the body. What's going to help is if we help the body go around the cycle to make it as fast as possible and as easy for the body as possible. And let the body finish the disease. And that's the basis of the SCENAR therapy and Cosmodic therapy and all the holistic medical technologies that we actually work with.

With the cancer, it's the same thing. The body needs to deal with the problem on its own. It needs to be aware. If the body is not aware of the growing tissue, if the communication is broken, burning the cancer out of the body is not going to help. Because if it is burned in one place, it will come up somewhere else.

Ty: Because the communication hasn't been fixed.

Dr. Kossovskaia: Of course. And you probably met many cancer survivors or sufferers, who had cancer several times. Treated conventionally, it will come up somewhere else because it is a systemic thing. Unless you restore the systemic communication, unless you make the body coherent. And cancer is one of the most incoherent diseases in the human body—or conditions I would say, conditions, it is not going to help.

So the approach that conventional medicine has towards cancer and other diseases, to my opinion, is flawed in its very principle.

Ty: Dr. Irina, what can we do to restore the communications in these cells? You mentioned that cancer is a result of a miscommunication in the cell.

Dr. Kossovskaia: Or broken lines of communication.

Ty: How can we restore that?

Dr. Kossovskaia: Well, that is a systemic approach. Consider a human being as a multi-layered system. A system that is not just physical, it is energetic and it's in unity of emotions, in unity of thoughts as well as our spirit. So we have the physical layer, we have the energetic layer, and then we have the informational matrix. So the core of our being is in the informational matrix.

Information dictates how energy is directed. So energy doesn't just run chaotic in the human body. It is a structured system. What directs energy? Informational matrix. So when informational matrix is distorted, then the computer doesn't work. When the programs are corrupted, the computer doesn't work. So the first thing to do is to actually restore the informational matrix then help the energy run the correct way. And the energetic system, the energetic structure, will affect the physical.

So the physical body is the last and the least of our concerns, actually. The major is the informational matrix, it's the core. And here, we actually have religion meet science because our informational core is our spirit. It is our system of beliefs, it is our understanding of who we are in this world, acceptance of our place in this world and understanding of what we are supposed to do.

Those who actually know exactly who they are and what they are here for, and what they do, they are happy people because they have a program. They know what to do. If we do not have that core set then we are always unsettled. Then we're always in search and it ends up in the chronic stress. And chronic stress is our killer because the chronic stress is what corrupts your programs.

When you are under the condition of chronic stress, everything goes to whack. And you know, chronic stress has so many faces. If you scratch almost any chronic disorder that human kind has, in the core of it, in the bottom of it, it will be chronic stress. And chronic stress mostly comes from the deep core. It comes from person not having good self-esteem, person being hopeless, helpless, worthless victim of the circumstances. And when you have that victim mentality—and you will not believe how many people have that victim-mentality, we mask it but almost all of us have it to one degree or another.

So you have to deal with that. Unless you deal with that, you cannot get out of chronic stress in our very hectic and very demanding environment.

Ty: On the way over here today—it just makes me think of a story. We were driving over here from Toronto and behind us was this guy and he was just so mad because he couldn't get around us and the other cars. And he was literally throwing his arms up in the air and making obscene gestures and screaming. I mean, I could see him in my mirror. Literally, he was the only one in his car but he was yelling in his car.

Dr. Kossovskaia: So obviously he has problems. He does not have the balance that we all need to find and it is difficult to find. But when you have cancer, that's the first thing you need to do. You need to find your place in this world and you'll have to get rid of the victim mentality. And you have to grow your self-esteem.

Cancer is not an enemy. Cancer is actually a process. A lot of our clients who successfully overcame cancer and, as we say now, "get into remission process" for many years—but we can't say cured, only remission. They have the attitude towards cancer like it is a challenge. It's not a death sentence that is written over their forehead, it is a challenge that they face and they need to learn something, they need to overcome it. And those who did overcome it, usually tell us—and that's actually very common—that, "cancer was my best teacher because in dealing with cancer, I learned so much about myself. I learned so much about the world. I learned so much about people. I changed the attitude and now I'm a much happer person than I was before I got cancer."

And some of them even say, "I'm 'cancering'." Those who are dealing with cancer, don't look at it as, "I have cancer." They say, "I am 'cancering.'" So it's a process. It's a learning curve for them. And those who have that attitude, are those ones who actually beat cancer. If you still have a victim mentality, even if you burn cancer out of your body, it will come up somewhere else.

So you need to fix your informational matrix first. Only you can do it. No one can do it for you. It is not something that is applied from the outside. Only you can grow your self-esteem, only you can find your place in the world. Your informational matrix it completely and totally depends on you and you only.

On top of that, of course, you apply energetic technologies that give you energy to do things. Give your body energy to run the programs. Give you enough bio-energy structured, coherent bio-energy, which we usually supply with low-level lasers of different types. But that is a technology that by definition is coherent.

So, it's a coherent light that is given to the body so the body can—the cells can—drink that light, can actually collect and accumulate ATP which is the energy molecule of the cell in order to fight cancer, in order to do many other things in your body.

So we supply the body with energy. We direct that energy correctly. We clean the blockages of energy, that way we structure the energy system of the body. And when that is done, we don't have to deal with the physical cancer because the body does it on its own. It actually starts seeing it and starts doing something with it, doing something about it.

So if you ask me, even though I do work with energy-healing technologies and high-tech equipment—but when you are dealing with cancer, the first thing to do is to deal with your informational matrix. Your very, very core.

Ty: So once you get the informational matrix corrected, once you get the energy that the body needs, then the body knows what to do with the cancer at that point.

Dr. Kossovskaia: Exactly.

Ty: You're not treating cancer.

Dr. Kossovskaia: And because it is aware, it sees it.

Ty: Right. So in other words, you're not treating cancer. You are providing the body with what it needs to be healthy.

Dr. Kossovskaia: Absolutely. As with many other diseases and disorders, we help the body to help itself and that's what we do. We do not fight disease. We don't even have to identify the disease. See, the diagnosis is only needed in conventional medicine, where you need to know the enemy. We don't because we don't view disease as enemy. All we need to do is to make the body stronger, make the body more aware. Make the body happier, make the body have more energy.

Ty: And that is what these machines will help do.

Dr. Kossovskaia: And that's what these machines are all about. They are mirrors for the body and they are energy donors.

Ty: So, contrast fear in stress against happiness and joy and laughter as far as the body's response.

Dr. Kossovskaia: Exactly right.

See, we create heaven and hell for ourselves in this. And love is our heaven. And vibrations of unconditional love are the most healing vibration that you can have. So the more unconditional love you experience and you have in you, the more coherent your system is going to be. And the opposite to love is not hate, as most people think, it's fear.

So, fear is your hell in earth. Fear destroys communication in the body. Fear destroys your personality and when it starts ruling your life, that's where you expose yourself to the potential dangers of developing cancer, as well as many other disorders. Some people will develop cancer and some people will develop a mass, other people develop chronic arthritis. Different manifestation. But in the core, in the root of it, it is usually always the same thing.

Ty: So then, that makes me question when someone is diagnosed with cancer and their doctor says, "You got terminal cancer, you're going to die." They just scared them, they just implanted fear into their whole being.

Dr. Kossovskaia: Absolutely. And that's what we try to explain to our community of home healers. That no matter what kind of diagnosis they are going to give you, what kind of label you're going to have, it is never a death sentence. It's a challenge. Yes, sure, cancer is a challenge, arthritis is a challenge.

Ty: But it is not a death sentence.

Dr. Kossovskaia: It is not a death sentence. It's something to be aware of, something to deal with but definitely not to put yourself into a situation where you live in constant fear.

Ty: So what would your advice be to a person who has been recently diagnosed with cancer and they've gone to their oncologist and the oncologist said, "Do chemo and radiation and you're going to die anyway but this will give you few more months." What's your advice to somebody that has a doctor like that?

Dr. Kossovskaia: You know I can't say, "Don't go to that route." Because cancer is an industry. But if it would be my friend, I would say, "Well, that's a wake-up call for you. It's not a death sentence, it's a wake-up call. Look at what is not going correctly in your life. Look at yourself. Look at your belief system. Look at your core. And see how much fear you have in your life, how much love you have in your life. Start with that. But now that you know that you have that challenge, let's deal with the challenge."

First of all, your body needs energy. So, the body needs correct nutrition and live food, of course. So change what you eat. We are what we eat. So change your life style. Get some exercise, get outside. Get the normal bio-energy. We are all so depleted of bio-energy because we do not walk barefoot on the grass. We do not sit under the tree. We do not hug the trees. We do not swim in the ocean enough. We do not sit on the sunshine enough. We are not getting the electrons that we are supposed to get from the environment.

As our ancestors were supplementing the energy that they are using for their different life processes, they were supplementing it from the environment. We don't do that. And because of that, our battery—biological batteries—are running really low. So get your biological battery charged. So start doing the right things. Start thinking about what you are putting in your body. Every time you put something in your body or you expose yourself into something, ask yourself one question, "Is it going to be giving me energy or taking it up? Is it going to give me energy? Or is it going to take it out?" In order to digest the food that we have in supermarket, which is genetically-modified, we waste so much energy and we are not supplementing it.

Yes, organic food is more expensive but at the end of the day, you're exposing yourself to huge dangers. First of all, you're not getting anything out of it, it's wax. And second of all, you're exposing yourself to GMOs, which is actually a really dangerous thing, and many other chemicals. So that's one thing.

And then, nature provided us with the sources of coherent energy. And it did provide us with the help when our system experiences the difficulties and it needs help. And help comes from other systems which are similar to us in complexity of organization. And that could be our support system as our friends and family and our loved ones, or it can be animals, it can be a pet. Think about yourself when you come home, all stressed out and tired at the end of the day and your dog runs to you and put its head on your lap at looks at you.

You're getting this energy of love, an unconditional love from them. This most coherent energy charges you up and your headache disappears at that time.

There were studies done that actually show blood pressure going down 10,20 millimeters just from petting your cat. It's that help that they give us and we communicate with our systems that help us become more coherent, help us become more structured. And when we are coherent and structured, then communication goes freely. Then we are open, we become self transparent. And when we become self-transparent, then cancer has no place to live.

So I would say to people who are diagnosed with cancer just now, open yourself up to the world. Get organic stuff, get stuff that gives you energy. And start opening yourself to communication with other systems on different levels, not just on the physical level, but on emotional level. Open your heart. Your heart is your compass. Your heart is something that connects you to others, not your mind. Your mind is actually an enemy sometimes. So calm down your mind and open your heart and start loving more. That would be the first thing.

And then, of course, get the technologies. Because without the technologies, it all can be done, but it will be a long process. So get the laser, get the SCENAR, get the Cosmodic and start healing yourself and cleaning your programs. That is what I will tell to my friends.

Ty: And when you mentioned energy, you say it's coherent. What exactly do you mean by coherent energy?

Dr. Kossovskaia: Coherence is an interesting notion. Coherence is a very fragile balance between total chaos and perfect order. Let say perfect order are marching soldiers on a bridge. You know how marching soldiers on the bridge can break a bridge if they got (inaudible - 31:24).

Ty: Or a cat walking.

Dr. Kossovskaia: Yes. It's a perfect order. Chaos on the other hand—chaos, there is no structure in chaos. So coherence is a balance in between. Neither is good enough. And when people ask me, "Well, explain what coherence is." I usually give them an example of an orchestra.

Let say every instrument in the orchestra is an individual. It has its individual frequencies and it plays its own part which is different for every instrument. So, they are all individuals. They are all different and yet when they all listened to each other and work in harmony and synergy, then you have a symphony. If one of the instruments fall out of the general harmony, it becomes a cacophony instead of a symphony.

So when everyone listens to each other and works in harmony, that's the state of coherence. You have individual units with individual vibrations and frequencies, all communicating and listening to each other and supplementing, complimenting each other for the common goal.

So you have a system working for the common goal where the system comprises of different elements which are individual. So, that's coherence. And our body is the same way. It has the organs and tissues. Each cell in the body has different vibrations, has different tune and different role. So our orchestra of our body needs to play the symphony of life. And when it does play the symphony, that's the state of coherence.

Ty: Great explanation. Thank you. So then, it makes less sense—the conventional model for treating cancer when we have a diseased organ and when we cut it out.

Dr. Kossovskaia: You said it.

Ty: Right? Because then, there's no coherence.

Dr. Kossovskaia: You're taking an instrument out of the orchestra. It still can play symphony but it will be much less beautiful. And, of course, when you supplement it with something else, then it's a different vibrations, different frequencies. We don't know what's going to happen. And sometimes, the body just doesn't take it.

Ty: I think we go back to the same old adage with this conventional treatments that we are really treating the wrong thing. We're treating the symptoms. Let say somebody has a big tumor, it's a symptom of something else in the body.

Dr. Kossovskaia: Absolutely. It's a wake-up call.

Ty: It's a wake-up call, right? And it's a symptom that something needs to be fixed, right? But it doesn't make sense that we could ever cure that with toxic poisons or with pills.

Dr. Kossovskaia: We can't.

Ty: Because we don't have cancer, because we are deficient in poison or pills, right?

Dr. Kossovskaia: Absolutely. We have cancer because our systemic communication is broken and we cannot restore systemic communication by burning something out or removing something. We can only do it by adding something and making the body aware.

Ty: Why do you think we have had such a large increase over the last couple of decades in childhood cancers?

Dr. Kossovskaia: Well, I contribute that to—obviously, cancer, as I already said, is the most incoherent disease or disorder in the body. So incoherency of the system. We all born coherent, harmonious, structured and happy. And then something happens. Your body is introduced to vaccinations, the heavy metals, genetically modified food, through the formula, milk, from the beginning to dysbiosis in the child's intestines and immune system suppressants in various forms.

Then the immune system is not fighting and not identifying the cancer cells. Then it's not going to work. Then somewhere in the body, the cancer is going to grow. Immune system function is not to only identify the viruses and bacteria, it is also to identify cancer cells. So, immune system is a major part of our system of adaptation. So when immune system is compromised from the childhood, and it is when you start pumping vaccines to the newborns, your immune system is going to be compromised.

Ty: It's kind of the opposite of what they tells us vaccines are going to do.

Dr. Kossovskaia: Yes. It is. But think logically, it just makes sense. I know, of course, there are dangers out there and different infections, could be life-threatening infections. But does that danger outweigh the dangers of the vaccines, I don't know.

It's an individual choice parents have to make. Yes, I did vaccinate my child, because I didn't know any better. And now, I think, if I knew then what I know now, I would never ever do that because that contribute to his Tourettes to actually one of vaccinations. I could even trace it chronologically. So, I would never do that again. And my grandchildren are not going to be vaccinated, no way.

Ty: We're a lot alike. We vaccinated our first two children because we didn't know any better. Our last two, our youngest have never been vaccinated. So you act on the knowledge that you've been given, right? And so, if somebody out there has never heard about the dangers of vaccines, it is not their fault at this point.

Dr. Kossovskaia: Of course not.

Ty: We're just trying to educated them.

Dr. Kossovskaia: Of course. But when the government starts pushing it on you, then I object.

Ty: Right. Like what's going on in California. I object heavily to that as well. Especially in light of the fact that, vaccines—there has never been a single vaccine that has been ever tested for carcinogenicity.

Dr. Kossovskaia: Exactly.

Ty: So how can they tell us they are safe and effective if they've never been tested if it cause cancer?

Dr. Kossovskaia: But again, logically, vaccines would attack your immune system. Immune system goes in overdrive and then it starts overreacting to the things in the environment that normally would be just normal and we have the explosion of allergies. How many children we know that do not have allergies?

Ty: Right. Everybody has allergies now.

Dr. Kossovskaia: Everybody has allergies to everything. Starting from peanuts to pollens to air or to sunlight. How strange is that? Allergy to sunlight.

So when you have that, you cannot expect your system to function directly and immune system to actually identify the dangers and the cancer cells in the body. So, yes, children are actually stronger. The programs are still running pretty good. But as we accumulate what we call the "energy cyst"with age—the "energy cyst" is our unfinished programs, all those suppressed by antibiotics or something else which the body never had a chance to finish so it attracts the body energy resources. And with age, we accumulate the cysts everywhere.

It breaks the communication down. It creates blockages on the energy flow. And when you have blockages in information on the energy flow that is setting the stage for cancer in the future. That's my opinion.

Ty: Well, I really appreciate you sharing your opinions today. This has been great information. I know that the people watching have been enlightened by what you shared. So thank you so much for your time today.

Dr. Kossovskaia: You are very welcome.

Ty: Awesome.

[end of transcript]

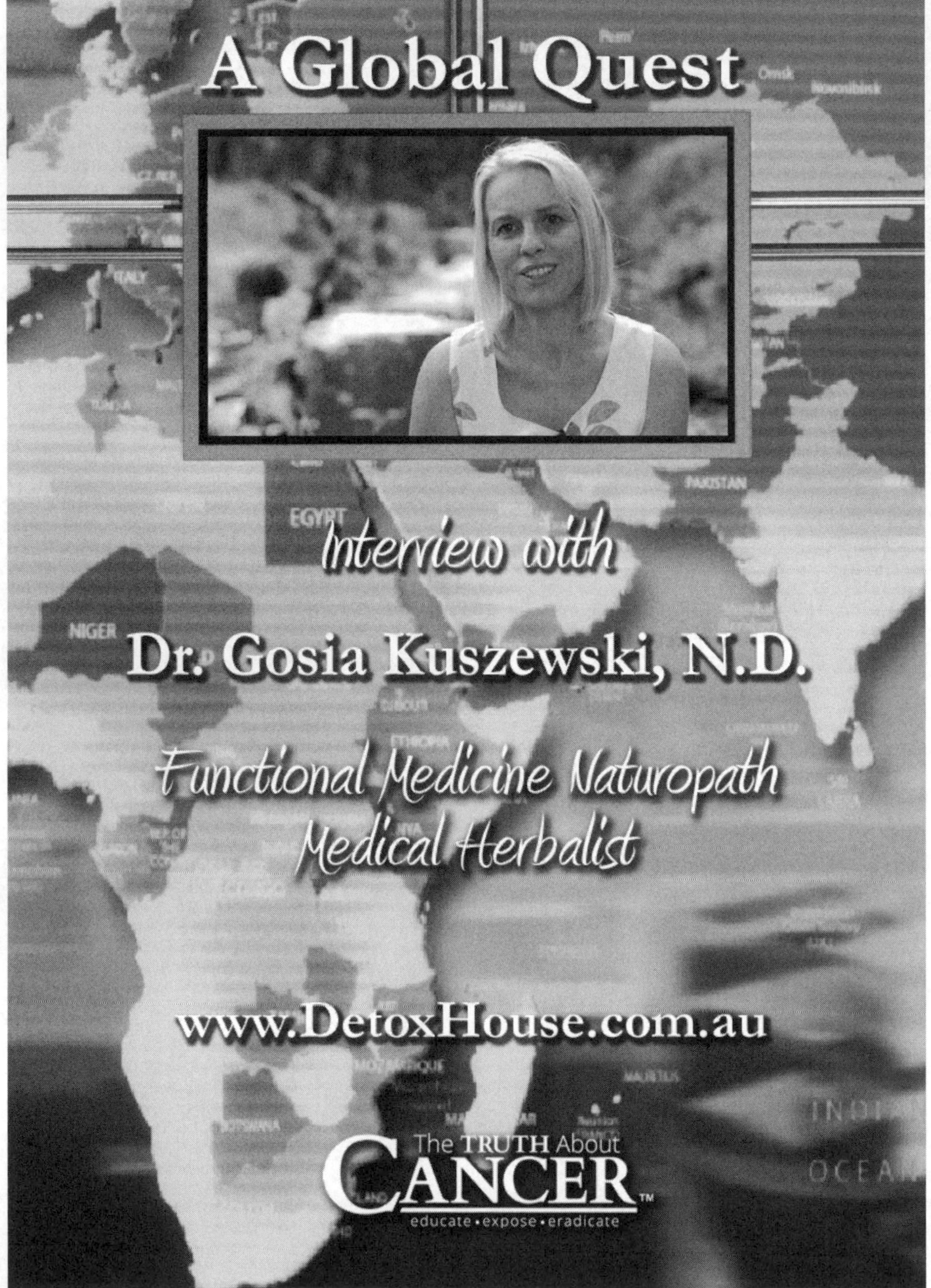
A Global Quest
EGYPT
NIGER
PAKISTAN
Interview with
Dr. Gosia Kuszewski, N.D.
Functional Medicine Naturopath
Medical Herbalist
www.DetoxHouse.com.au
The TRUTH About
CANCER
educate • expose • eradicate

THE TRUTH ABOUT CANCER

Gosia Kuszewski: The day my mom was diagnosed with cancer, on the same day my daughter was born, so I had two big news in the same day. So one beautiful news and the other one pretty sad. It was very sad, but at the same time, I was determined and I believed that I can do something about it, that we can beat the cancer. I believed that I could save my mom.

Although, everybody around me was panicking and really scared that mom was diagnosed. By the way, they told her there was nothing she can do and it's only that she has six months to live. I was determined that something positive will come out of this, that we will save her with natural treatments. However, when I was talking to my mom, I understood that she didn't want to try natural methods that she was ready to go the conventional path and go through chemotherapy and I knew what that meant. I knew that once she had the conventional treatment that was bad news. I knew the consequences of that. So that was devastating.

I had a baby and at the same time, I was watching my mom just getting worse and worse every day. Injecting chemicals into someone's bloodstream, even if you're the healthiest person, fit, healthy person – if someone would inject chemicals into your body that would make them sick. Cancer patients are already unwell and on top of it, they inject—they are given the chemicals. So I can't find any sense in it unfortunately.

I feel that both experiences were taken away: experience of my mom bonding with her granddaughter and for my daughter to just remember, just a little bit of her grandma. That was taken away. Because I couldn't save my mom's life, I felt with every patient after I did everything I possibly could in order to save their life.

Because of that you had countless cases of people recovering from cancer and that means everything to me. The experiences that I didn't have with my mom – I thought that I lost them – that I will never get them back. However, helping other people regain their life and watching grandmothers with their grandchildren, and husbands and wives, and the families being together is just beautiful and I'm really grateful that I can experience that moment looking at the families being together and lives saved. So I'm very grateful for the experience.

So the very thing which I thought I lost forever, now I found in experiences of other people. Watching them going through life, happy lives, with the families loving each other and experiencing life together.

[end of transcript]

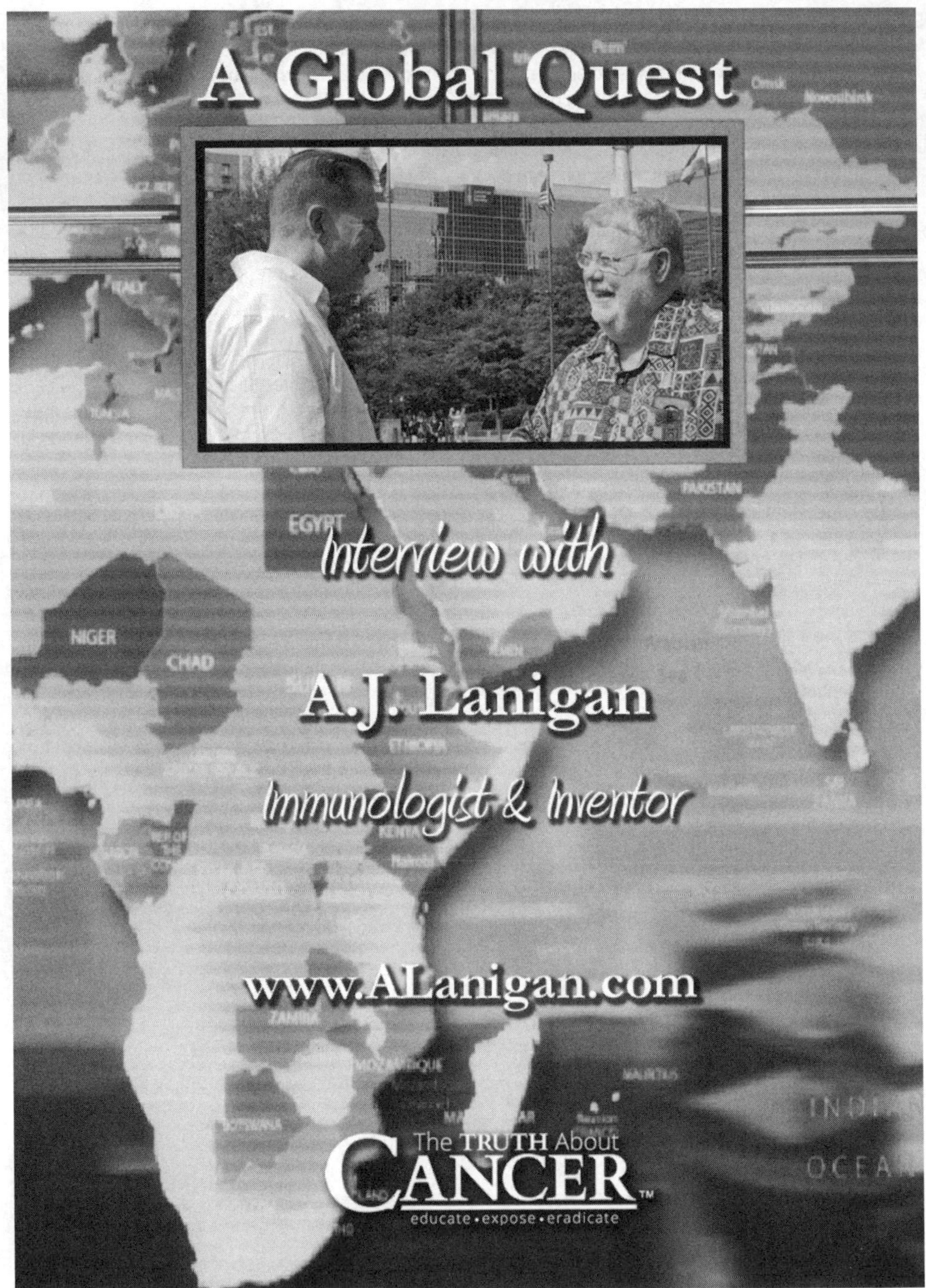
A Global Quest
Interview with
A.J. Lanigan
Immunologist & Inventor
www.ALanigan.com
The TRUTH About
CANCER
educate • expose • eradicate
EGYPT
NIGER
CHAD
PAKISTAN
INDIAN
OCEAN

Ty: So, A.J., thank you for joining me here today in beautiful, sunny, Atlanta, Georgia.

A.J.: Beautiful spring day, brother. Always great to see you. I don't need an excuse.

Ty: We got lots of excuses today, but you don't need anything, do you?

A.J.: That's right.

Ty: So what's this building I see over here behind us?

A.J.: Well, I tell you what. It's a testimony to a tremendous amount of money being spent and a long list of failures. I can remember just it was like yesterday, my grandfather dying back in the 50s and the tremendous amount of effort and time that my mother and other family spent taking up money, I guess, to help build that building.

And I hate to say it, but I don't see us any closer to any kind of a cure for cancer than we had way back when Tricky Dick said, well it'll just be ten years. So, that being said, it's kind of interesting that you and I would be standing here in front of this place—

Ty: It is. It is.

A.J.: —instead of some other setting that would be more, shall we say, inspiring to people that might watch this piece.

Ty: Right. So, the American Cancer Society here in Atlanta, Georgia, the headquarters, this is just the American version. There are global entities in every country that basically do the same thing as the American Cancer Society. So here, what the American Cancer Society tries to do is they push chemicals on people to treat a disease that's caused by a compromised immune system. You should know better than anybody as an immunologist, that these chemicals then devastate the immune system.

Tell me is that logical to you as an immunologist?

A.J.: Well, it never was and frankly, you know, over the last 40 or 50 years, this revelation has really come into more of a material state. We didn't know 50 or 60 years ago the role that the immune system played like we do today because we didn't have the technology to measure it and identify it.

But today, a person who is paying attention will see more and more medical articles. They'll see more and more stuff come out on the investigative news shows talking about breakthroughs in immunotherapy and how they are in fact tapping and harnessing the immune system to ferret out cancer and kill it in a very specific manner instead of this global napalming of the body with chemo and radiation. Which, I don't know if it's ever been successful at any level except to provide more money for the administration and I guess the folks that are coming out with that.

I mean if the money had been forwarding the immunotherapy over the last 50 years as it has been these other attempts that ended up failing, I have to believe that the results would be a whole lot better but certainly, there would have been a lot less suffering. I think anybody who has met or been close to someone undergoing chemo and radiation will admit that it is a suffering instead of a treatment for individuals. I'm hoping that in the next number of years that will change.

Ty: One of the things that you've done as a scientist and as an inventor is that you invented a product that helps people's immune system to work the way that it is supposed to. Tell us about that.

A.J.: Well, the invention or the conception of Beta-1, 3D Glucan actually came 50, 60 plus years ago but it was $200 a pill. Most of my friends, and I'm sure a lot of your friends as well, would just have to do without it if they have to pay 12 grand a bottle. My contribution has been able to manufacture that material effectively and actually at a more highly purified level so that the dose cost is more like a dollar in change a day as opposed to 200. What I've done, also, because I could have gone the private laboratory route but I wanted to go in to disinterested third parties, as I say, universities, teaching hospitals, to evaluate this product and not have any interest in the outcome of the work.

Just a couple of weeks ago, yet another study has been published, ironically, in the *Journal of Tumor*.

Ty: *Journal of Tumor*?

A.J.: *Journal of Tumor*. Demonstrating that even if people are going standard of care – chemo, radiation and so forth – which would typically drive white blood cell counts down, then this material will actually mitigate and keep those white blood cell counts up.

Ty: So Beta-1, 3D Glucan is a substance that you can use if you're currently undergoing chemo radiation to help your immune system stay strong and so that it won't be crippled by the treatment.

A.J.: That is correct because one of the things that we do know, without that compound, the chemo and the radiation basically wipes out everything. And if it's not successful, we know that only the bad guys are left behind and the cancer is going to come back with a tear and you have no defense at all. So keeping that immune system properly supported is really critical even if standard of care happens to be a choice.

You know, I think the more that this work gives people the understanding that options are out there. They just don't have the couple of two or three choices of the chemo, the radiation, and the knife. That there are other things out there that have been and are being used.

Immune therapy being, again, more and more important. Detoxing the heavy metals, the non-GMO and all these other steps are key but right up there in the forefront, keeping that immune system. I kind of talk about the people out there herding sheep and they feed those sheep and they give those sheep vitamins and water and they go to town for a long weekend and come back and nothing is left except sheep parts. Well they forgot to leave the sheepdog and that's your immune system, brother.

So let's keep a good, strong sheepdog in charge.

Ty: I like it and I appreciate you, A.J. because you have done what you can to provide that sheepdog for people so they can be healthy. Thank you for your contribution. By the way, I take your Beta-1, 3D Glucan every day.

A.J.: Well, I saw a movie, I don't remember the movie but the father was talking to his son and he said, "There's three kinds of people out there – you got sheep, you got wolves, and you got guardians. Be a guardian." There we go, brother.

Ty: Thank you, brother.

A.J.: I love you.

Ty: I love you, too, A.J.

[end of transcript]

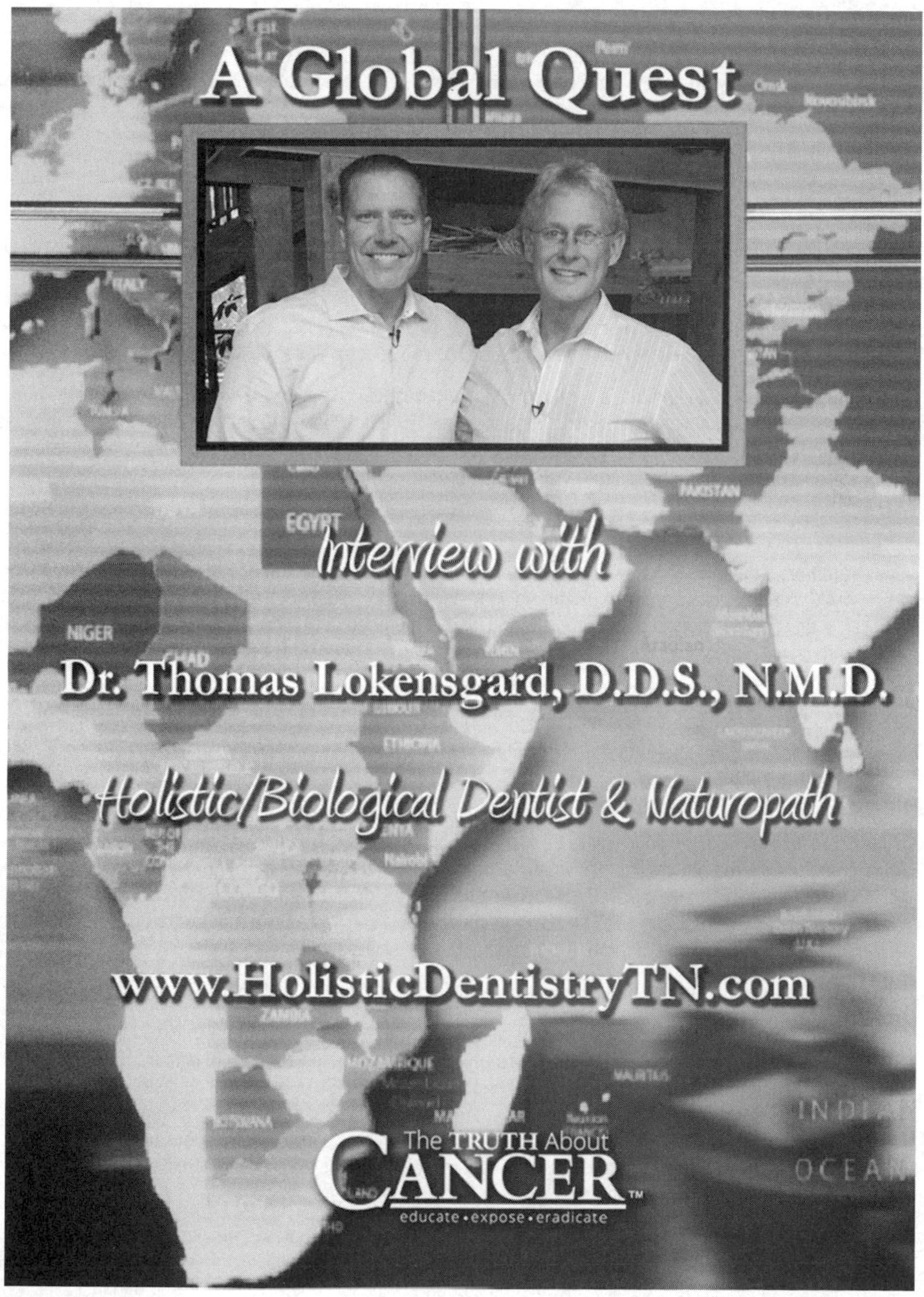
A Global Quest
Interview with
Dr. Thomas Lokensgard, D.D.S., N.M.D.
Holistic/Biological Dentist & Naturopath
www.HolisticDentistryTN.com
The TRUTH About
CANCER
educate • expose • eradicate

Ty: I'm glad that you agreed to an interview today, Dr. Tom, because the mouth is so important in overall health.

Dr. Lokensgard: True.

Ty: And it is actually one of the areas that many people are undereducated, right? You hear people talking about what you need to do to be healthy. You have to eat healthy, you have to exercise, you have to diet. You rarely, if ever, hear somebody say, "You need to clean up your mouth."

So, Dr. Tom, give us a little bit of your story. I know that you started out just as a general dentist, and how you became a biological dentist.

Dr. Lokensgard: When I first started out, I had just graduated from dental school and really didn't know very much. I didn't know what I didn't know, which is true with a lot of practitioners today. So it always bothered me that my patients would have all of these other issues, and the only thing I could do is to do a filling. And at that point in time it was mercury. So then—and I just had this overwhelming feeling that nutrition had something to do with health, but I couldn't put my finger on it.

So I started going—and that's what brought me to Nashville, Tennessee—is I went to an ANA, American Nutraceutical Association, meeting. I met Dr. Mark Houston, and just realized that there was a group of guys that did nutrition along with medicine—there were chiropractors, dentists, and MDs. And I thought, "Well, this is kind of a novelty here."

And so then I got my NMD degree because I wanted to pursue it, so I did a three-year stint in Birmingham, Alabama, and I got my NMD degree, and then I met a lady in Minnesota, which is where I am from. She said, "Tom, with all this stuff you are doing with nutrition and dentistry you should join the A4M, the American Academy of Anti-Aging Medicine." So I did; I got boarded by the A4M and got into the anti-aging protocols and therapies. So I kind of morphed from a dentist into a nutritionist and then into an anti-aging guy. So I kind of morphed out of the box. And it took me down here to Tennessee, and so here I am.

Ty: You saw the importance of nutrition, right? Something clicked, you said, "Hey, that's got to be important." Even though we're not told that very often, nutrition has to have something to do with the equation, right?

Dr. Lokensgard: Nutrition is at the source of everything. Nutrition is the key. And I knew that intrinsically, but I couldn't really put my finger on it. So once I got into all the nutritional therapies, with dentistry and medicine it's the bottom line. It's what He created. And He created it for our good and we've taken the food supply and we've messed it all up. And so what we do here is we talk about nutrition, we talk about biological dentistry, we talk about mercury detoxification, heavy metal toxicity, and how that can mess with the systems of the body, including and especially the immune system.

Ty: So, Dr. Tom, you just mentioned biological dentistry. Can you explain? What's biological dentistry?

Dr. Lokensgard: That's a great question. And we say here that your mouth is the window to the rest of your body, or the doorway, if you will. Because what happens here in your mouth, intrinsically, will affect what happens in the rest of your body. It becomes systemic. So in biological dentistry, we also call it functional integrative dentistry. So what we are looking at is cause. We are looking at cause and effect. So instead of just filling cavities, we are looking at heavy metal toxicity, we're looking at functional orthodontics, we are looking at the growth and development of jaws, we are looking at how the TM joints work, and how they operate.

And we're looking at how nutrition affects the dentinal fluid transport system, we're looking at how nutrition affects osteoporosis in bone, and periodontitis, and gingivitis. Gingivitis is just an inflammatory disease but it can very quickly become a periodontal situation where you are losing bone.

And so there are all these parameters that we have to look at because everything that happens here becomes a chronic inflammatory situation that affects the systemic circulation, the heart, the pancreas, into cancers.

Ty: So inflammation—you mention inflammation...

Dr. Lokensgard: Correct.

Ty: Talk about inflammation as it relates to the diseases that you have seen, including cancer.

Dr. Lokensgard: You remember back in the days of essential hypertension? You talked about—you have high blood pressure, it doesn't hurt, you don't feel it, you don't even know you have it, but there is something insidious about it. Well, today—we used to have the germ theory, which was one germ, one bug, one disease, one drug. And now what we have is we have chronic inflammation affects most all chronic degenerative disease. And we call it oral inflammation; we say it starts here.

Essentially what it is, is there is a switch called nuclear factor kappa beta, NFKB. I go around and I talk to dentists, I talk to physicians, and I say, "How many of you guys out there understand and know what nuclear factor kappa beta is? And I usually get these blank stares. What it is, it is a genetic transcription cytoplasmic switch that turns on inflammation. It's a genetic switch. The body is so intricately and amazingly designed, I don't know how anybody can look at the human body and not see a miracle, especially a little baby.

But what happens is inflammation, is, in its nascent state, is good for us because inflammation is what causes the voltage drop and it causes healing to occur. But when we are constantly chronically inflamed and we have this saber-toothed tiger behind our back, it ramps up the sympathetic nervous system, decreases the parasympathetic nervous system, it turns on the nuclear factor kappa beta, and it turns on all of these pathways—all these inflammatory pathways that affect hypertension. It affects stress levels. And stress is a killer. We all know this. But it affects every organ system in your body, so you have to control inflammation. And, as I said, inflammation starts here. It starts in the mouth.

Ty: Wow. That's a great connection. Another connection that we have seen over the past couple of interviews that we have done over the past couple of years is the link between root canals and cancer.

Dr. Lokensgard: Exactly.

Ty: So could you touch on that? As a biological dentist, talk about root canals.

Dr. Lokensgard: Root canals have been—there has been a lot of information and concerns about root canals. Root canals are—they fail quite often—they fail most of the time. And we have a problem with leaving—and it's been said that dentists are the only doctors that leave dead tissue in the body. So when you do a root canal there is the pulp tissue that you have to seal off, and when you do that you leave the dead tooth in the mouth, because if you want to keep your tooth in your head, you have to pretty much do a root canal, otherwise you have to extract it.

But the problem is there are these dental tubules called canaliculi that you can't—once you fill the root canal, they become dead space. And so then they fill up with anaerobic bacteria. So here is, basically, essentially, what happens. You have a tooth that goes bad, and so then the voltage drops in that tooth. And when the voltage drops, then the pH drops. When the pH drops, then the oxidation goes out of the tooth and out of the area. When the oxidation drops, then the bugs come in. And the bugs come in and they set up housekeeping. Well, bugs don't have teeth, but they need to eat, they wake up and they're hungry and they want to eat, so what they do is they begin to produce all kinds of enzymes. And they begin to liquefy you and me and they start having us for lunch.

So that begets an infection and an infective process that you cannot leave in your body because then it crosses the gingival sulcus barrier, goes right into the cardiovascular system, goes right to the liver, produces high specific C-reactive protein and some other—that's a general inflammatory marker—and it says to your body, "Hey, we're chronically inflamed. We have all this inflammation." So then all of these pathways get turned on.

So then what you have to do, is what we've started to do, is bio-oxidative therapies for root canals that are failed, because sometimes root canals in the anterior segment would be okay because they are single-rooted, but you leave all these dentinal tubules and all these canaliculi that are open to bacterial infection, and you can't have bacterial infection, which becomes systemic. It's a real problem.

Ty: Yes, a real problem. Now the solution—or one of the solutions—you mentioned bio-oxidative therapies. Can you explain what that means?

Dr. Lokensgard: Yes. Bio-oxidative therapies is [sic] oxygen. If you ask me what causes cancer, I would say—well, I would say a couple of things—but I would say lack of iodine, and I would say lack of oxygen. And so bio-oxidative therapies—when you increase—when we are—we talk about oxidation, oxidation is rust. When we talk about oxidation, the body, we need oxygen every day. We can live without water for a while, we can live without food for a while, but we cannot live without oxygen for more than three to five minutes, or we're dead.

So when we become oxygenated and we breathe in, then that keeps the bacteria at bay, because most bacteria that are bad, that are pathogens—we call them pathogenic bacteria—are what we call anaerobes—anaerobes meaning "without oxygen." And they can live in areas that have no oxygen. Once you introduce an oxidative burst of oxygen into an infected area, anywhere in your body, it doesn't have to be your teeth, but anywhere in your body, what happens is you kill—you drive back the oxygen levels and you drive off, you kill, oxidatively, you kill all of the anaerobes, all of the bad bacteria.

Ty: When you say oxidatively, it just means you are doing it with oxygen.

Dr. Lokensgard: With oxygen, right. We talk a lot about free radical oxidative stress, right? And free radical oxidative stress is bad. So you say, "Well, wait a minute. So you are saying now oxidation is good?" Well, when you give an oxidative burst into an area, the bacteria can't handle it and they die. And so what we do, and we have had people that, on a daily basis, and we're going to get this machine very quickly, I'm taking a course this weekend on bio-oxidative therapies, but this is very commonly done in Europe, and in England, Switzerland. They've been doing this for years. They are curing all kinds of diseases with bio-oxidative therapies.

Now, our "Food and Death" administration, bless their hearts, in Tennessee, they don't really get into therapies that really cure a lot of things because that interrupts the monetary flow. And I'll stop right there [laughs], but you know what I'm talking about.

Ty: Exactly.

Dr. Lokensgard: And I try to leave the politics out of this, but we know that there is a political component when it comes to cancer, or root canals, or mercury toxicity. Because that is a huge problem, because that affects a lot of systems in your body.

Ty: Talk about mercury toxicity because, thus far, we have interviewed with doctors that have talked about the toxicity that are in vaccines, the thimerosal...

Dr. Lokensgard: Thimerosal.

Ty: You talk about—you are a dentist, so you deal with the silver fillings that aren't all silver, right?

Dr. Lokensgard: Exactly.

Ty: So could you talk about that?

Dr. Lokensgard: Yes, you bet. The silver fillings, you are right, they are about 40 percent silver. The rest is copper, tin, and mercury—43 percent to 55 percent is the mercury in a silver filling. So it's a huge problem, and the question is, do they outgas? The ADA's position, the American Dental Association's position, is that they do not outgas, is that they are inert. Well, I have news for the ADA; this is not true. They do outgas, and they outgas from the time they are put in to the time they are taken out.

So what we do here is we take them out in a correct way because when you drill an amalgam filling, most of them have been in there 30, 40, 50 years. The problem is there is still 50 percent of the dentists, or I would say 40 percent now, that still put mercury fillings in your mouth. So when they outgas, what happens? Mercury is a known toxin, not a dental toxin, it is just a known toxin. It is very toxic to the neurological system, it is very toxic to the gastrointestinal system, it ties with *Candida*—*Candida* some people will call it. And so if you have a candidiasis or *Candida* infection, or you have gut dysfunction, it is going to mess with that. It is going to be very difficult to fix your gut.

It also has an affinity for fat tissue and since we are all fatheads, it goes to your brain. It has a great affinity to cross the blood–brain barrier, to cross the placental barrier. That's really bad news because that's supposed to be a sterile environment. And it causes memory loss, it causes fatigue, it causes brain fog. And it's an—we say it is an uncoupler. Mercury, as an element, is an uncoupler. It gets involved with co-enyzme reactions and it screws everything up.

One of the biggest offenders—when you talk about mercury you can talk about fluoride, you can talk about chlorine, you can talk about bromine, and I know Dr. Bronson talks a lot about this, where you've got all these lesser halide molecules that will get into the tyrosine ring, which is the iodine, which is the thyroid molecule. The biggest precursor for the thyroid molecule is tyrosine. Then you have an iodine molecule and you have a conversion factor where an iodine gets knocked off, and then you get T3 and that's your active thyroid hormone.

Well, mercury messes with that, it messes with ATP production, and when you have low oxygenation and when you have mercury binding with ATP, now instead of getting 38 molecules per ATP when you have proper oxygenation, and you introduce mercury, now you get two. So you become very fatigued. And people they come here all the time and they say, "I have all these symptoms, and my doctor says I'm normal, and my tests say I'm normal." Well, basically, because these ranges are so big today, and they throw all of these sick people in these ranges, what they are really saying is, "You're normally screwed up like everybody else your age."

Ty: Yes, that's what I was going to say. Sick has become the new normal.

Dr. Lokensgard: Exactly. Exactly. That's exactly...

Ty: And that's because of what? You have mentioned poor diet, you have mentioned mercury toxicity.

Dr. Lokensgard: Poor nutrition, all of these chemicals that we dump into the atmosphere, the mercury. But one of the biggest drivers is stress.

Ty: Stress.

Dr. Lokensgard: Stress levels. Stress screws up everything.

Ty: So, Dr. Tom, you just mentioned stress. In *The Quest for the Cures Continues* last year, I remember, it was I think Dr. Patrick Quillin, said that stress is a killer and laughter is a healer.

Dr. Lokensgard: That's right.

Ty: Let's talk about the stress part of that.

Dr. Lokensgard: Well, that's true, laughter increases natural killer cells. Your basic—your immune system is what I call your Navy Seals SWAT team. It is out there, it's detecting self or non-self. And it does it in a very efficient way. But when we introduce stress into our lives, when we get back to the chronic inflammation and the oral inflammation, stress—we are designed to handle very short bursts of stress, kind of like a sports car engine. You know, you give it high-octane gas, it runs, it does its thing, and then it shuts down.

With us, stress is the same way. We're designed to—our basic nervous system is designed to handle short bursts of stress and when it's chronic—when it becomes chronic, much like chronic inflammation, it causes chronic inflammation. And when you are chronically—you're worried about work, you are worried about what you are going to wear today, you are worried about your mother who has maybe developed cancer, you are worried about the finances, maybe your wife and you didn't have such a good night last night, you are worried about the kids, you are worried about all this stuff—you are chronically worried about things.

Ty: Right.

Dr. Lokensgard: And so what that does is it taxes our immune system and it drives our sympathetic nervous system into high gear. So what we are talking about here is the sympathetic and the parasympathetic nervous system. The sympathetic nervous system is your fight or flight. That is when somebody runs over their kid with a car and they pick up the car. That is your sympathetic nervous system. And then your parasympathetic nervous system is sleep, digestion, and just all the basic functions of life.

But when we are in sympathetic overdrive it screws up our neurotransmitters, and our neurotransmitters are brain chemicals that are produced in the gut, so if you are having depression, you have to take a look at the gut. And one of the first questions I always ask my patients is, "How's your gut?" And they go, "Well, you're a dentist, right? Why would you care about the gut?"

Ty: It all goes back to the gut.

Dr. Lokensgard: It *all* goes back to the gut. Digestion and disease starts in the gut. There are numerous, millions of articles written about this. But that's where your neurotransmitters are made—in particular, serotonin is made, 90 percent, in the gut. So if you are having issues with stress and you have gut dysfunction, and you have neurological dysfunction, it is all connected.

And what I didn't understand as a young practitioner is that everything is connected. So I didn't understand the big, main plan, like I do now. He has put everything on this earth for nutrition, and we've taken it, like we said before, and we've kind of messed it all up. So now we have to get away from the GMO foods. People say to me, "Well, it's organic." I say, "Well, that's great that it's organic, but is it genetically modified?"

Because when you talk about the immune system, your immune system is trying to identify, is this self or is this non-self? Well, when you put all this propylene glycol, which is antifreeze, by the way, into your system, and the immune system is saying, "What do we do with this? We don't recognize this as anything." But your liver has to deal with it. Your liver and your kidneys have to deal with an incomplete burn, an incomplete protein burn, and all these chemicals. So then we talk about the liver, we talk about cytochrome P450 system, boosting enzymes so we can detox and all that kind of thing.

Ty: One of the things that you just mentioned, Dr. Tom, was that everything is connected, right?

Dr. Lokensgard: Sure.

Ty: One of the things that we have seen over the last couple of years with the documentaries that we've done, is the common thread is one of the main differences between the conventional way to treat disease, specifically cancer, and the natural way to treat cancer, is that those that are doing it naturally look at the body as a whole, and the conventional, they say, "Okay, you have cancer of the ear, we'll cut your ear off." They look at it compartmentally, but they don't look at the body as a whole. Could you talk about that?

Dr. Lokensgard: Sure. Traditionally, because of the way the whole medical system is set up, drug companies cannot—and they do a lot of good, I'm not going to sit here and just completely trash drug companies because they do a lot of good things, and in acute care we do wonderful things. But what we are looking for is the silver magic bullet for cancer, and I'm here to tell you, it ain't there. It's not there.

So what we have to do is we have to look at things like glutathione, superoxide dismutase. We have to look at antioxidants. What amazes me so much is that each cell that the Lord has created has a cellular membrane, it has a certain voltage and potential, and each cell is genetically prepared and designed to fix itself, *if* we give it the right materials. That's why I was drawn to naturopathy, because naturopathy says if we give the body the right stuff, it's already pre-programmed to fix itself.

And so we're out here over in medicine trying to figure out all these—trying to find out the cures for cancer when we know that 80 percent of them are lifestyle. So if I went into Congress and I said, "Hey you guys, I have a fix"—let's talk about Obamacare, or whatever—"I have a fix that could fix 80 percent of chronic degenerative disease. Are you interested?" And they would say, "Sure." And I would say, "Guess what? You're not going to make any money off of it, but it's nutrition, it's antioxidants, it's bio-oxidative therapies."

Ty: Interest just went down the tube at that point, right?

Dr. Lokensgard: It's like, "Sorry, not interested. Not interested." Which is a shame, because, really, we need to exercise. Oxidation, all that kind of thing that we are talking about, is really the answer for cancer.

Ty: And I'm glad you say that because there is an answer, there are many answers, but we're not going to find them conventionally. And the reason is that conventional medicine and the doctors in training—they aren't trained about these things. One of the common threads…

Dr. Lokensgard: We're not trained in using—here is an interesting story. When I was in biochemistry, my first year in dental school, there was a world-class biochemist, his name was Dr. Leon Singer—don't even know if he is still around. He said to our class, and I will never forget this, "In America there will never be any micronutrient or macronutrient deficiencies because we have vitamin-enriched bread like Wonder Bread." And I wrote it down. I'm like, "Well, cool. Cool, so there can be no micro- or macronutrient deficiencies."

Ty: Because it is enriched.

Dr. Lokensgard: Yes, it is vitamin-enriched.

Ty: So the solution is Wonder Bread.

Dr. Lokensgard: Well, never mind it's all white bread, and it is high-glycemic, and it's right spin and all that kind of stuff. But we haven't really been taught.

Ty: That's it. The doctors have not been taught. And it's not just America, this is worldwide.

Dr. Lokensgard: Well, they are a little more—I hate to use the word "progressive," but they are a little more open to bio-oxidative therapies and functional orthodontics like we do here and some of the TMJ therapies that we use here, and endodontic therapies, too. And, in fact, overseas they have banned mercury. There are not many countries that use mercury. We still use mercury, and I think what is going to happen there is, what they are going to say—the ADA, or the AMA, is never going to admit that mercury is bad for your health. What they are going to do is they're going to say, "We have an environmental concern. Mercury is bad for the environment. So we're not going to use mercury anymore, we're going to switch over to these other…"

Ty: So that will be their cover story.

Dr. Lokensgard: Exactly, because they know if they do they are going to open up a Pandora's box, because with people with MS, and autism, and autistic spectral disorders that are having trouble understand and they come here because—not that it is cause and effect, I can't say that for the FDA—but I can tell you story after story after story of patients that have had their mercury fillings removed the right, the proper way—we put all the garb on them, we make sure that there is no vapor escaping and crossing the blood–brain barrier or the placental barrier, and they come back months later and we say, "How are you feeling?" They go, "I feel a whole lot better." What did we do? We just took out a toxin and then they went and they detoxified. And I'm telling you, it works.

Ty: Are there ways that someone that is watching this could detoxify mercury at home? Are there natural herbs or substances that they might be able to use?

Dr. Lokensgard: Yes, there are a lot of foods that will increase the cytochrome P450 system, the conjugation and the bio-oxidative bioconjugation of the liver. Because the liver is the organ system that has to up-regulate and has to prepare the toxin to be removed from the body. Foods like garlic are great. Foods like cloves are really good. And I'm not a cook [laughs], but any of the broccolis, any of the sulfuraphane, watercress—those types of…

Ty: And they help to detox the body of mercury.

Dr. Lokensgard: Yes, they will help because they help up-regulate the genetic switches. You get into what we call epigenetics and epigenomics. There is a term I call dietary endocrinology. You eat specific foods, and there is a ton of them out there, there are also a lot of nutrients like trans-resveratrol, and if you are talking about cardiovascular supplementation then you are talking about d-ribose and acetyl L-carnitine. And so, our patients are very aware of these types of nutrients.

Ty: Could that be of the reasons that a lot of mouthwashes that you see have cloves in it?

Dr. Lokensgard: Yes. Oh, yes. I've just met with a compounding pharmacist and we are developing our own line, but too many of these commercial brands have all this junky stuff like sodium lauryl sulfate and propylene glycol and all these different FDC-type coloring agents and this kind of thing. But when it comes to mouth rinses and mouthwashes and remineralization pastes, you are talking about calcium. The real thing is, what you have to do is get the mineral balance right. You have to get the phosphorus-to-calcium ratio, the sodium-to-potassium ratio. The sodium-to-potassium ratio should be one-to-one—it is five-to-one in this country. Omega-3 fatty acids, it should be one-to-one. It is like 20-to-one in this country. That's why we have so much inflammation. We eat a highly inflammatory diet. Almost everything we eat in the standard American diet, SAD, is very, very inflammatory.

Ty: Wow.

Dr. Lokensgard: And it's killing us. I'm sorry, but it's killing us. And so this brings me back to another thing. I attended a seminar when I first started getting into this. There was a nutritionist there and he said, "You guys, I have news for you. There is a battle out there, but it's not between you and your doctor, it's not between you and your insurance company, it's not between you and the hospital. It's at the grocery store. The battle is raging at the grocery store." And I thought about this for quite a while, Ty, and I said, "This guy is right. He is absolutely right."

And my mother taught me to go around the outside aisles. Well, it turns out she was right, too. So there is all this ancient wisdom, like oil-pulling, and all this stuff, that people come to me and say, "Do you know about oil-pulling? Do you believe in that?" And I say, "Yes, absolutely."

There is another therapy, called, it's a bio-oxidative therapy. It's called honey. And they have found this in the Egyptian tombs. Honey is a bio-oxidative therapy because it produces hydrogen peroxide. You can put it on your skin and put a bandage over it or anywhere on your body, anywhere you have a lesion, and it will heal it with no scarring at all.

Ty: Honey.

Dr. Lokensgard: Honey.

Ty: Wow.

Dr. Lokensgard: So, like I said, He has put everything here fit for our use and we have either ignored it, or we just don't know anything about it, or we've tried to develop drugs. And all drugs have side effects; they just do. All medications are acidic and they all have side effects. And they all up-regulate the wrong stuff, and down-regulate the wrong stuff. And naturopathic and nutraceutical supplementation up-regulates the right enzyme systems. So does food. That's why you call it dietary endocrinology. And people say to me, "Well, you mean, I can eat something and it will affect my genes?" "Yes." "Well, how long is that? How long will that take?" "Two minutes, three minutes." "You mean, I can eat foods, I can eat supplements, and they will up-regulate my hormones?" "Yes, absolutely."

One of the best ways to control cancer is to balance your hormones, we all know this, but we try to balance it on the medical side with synthetic hormones. Well, we found out through the Natural Women's Study that didn't work very well. They had to stop the study.

Ty: Bio-identical...

Dr. Lokensgard: Bio-identical is exactly that. You hang an OH molecule in the wrong place, your receptors shut down. It's called receptor-site sensitivity. It's like a lock and key. These hormones have to hit the right receptor, and they have to hit it exactly, otherwise they up-regulate or they down-regulate the wrong thing. So, in A4M, in anti-aging medicine, we are very big on bio-identical hormones. The rest of the medical world says, "No, that doesn't matter—synthetic or 'schminthetic,' it doesn't matter."

I used to argue with my wife about this. When I first got into dentistry she came in and said, "Tom, I don't want the kids to have fluoride." I said, "What? What do you mean you don't want the kids to have fluoride?" To a dentist this is heresy. [laughs] It is. I said, "You're telling me I'm not supposed to give my kids fluoride?" Well, it turns out she was right. She's always right.

Ty: Talk about fluoride. And yes, that's a good point; they're always right.

Dr. Lokensgard: Right.

Ty: My wife, Charlene, is here.

Dr. Lokensgard: Right, Charlene?

Ty: And one of the things my dad said before he died, when we were getting married, he said, "Remember, your wife is always right."

Dr. Lokensgard: Yes, sir.

Ty: And that was good advice.

Dr. Lokensgard: Yes, ma'am.

Ty: But talk about fluoride, because this is the sacred cow of modern dentistry, right? Fluoride.

Dr. Lokensgard: Truly it is. Truly it is.

Ty: So talk about that. You mentioned the fact that the choices that we make at the grocery store are killing us. Are we drinking ourselves to death with fluoride?

Dr. Lokensgard: Well, yes. Yes we are. Fluoride will down-regulate iodine. Fluoride is a—well, I'll just say this. The journal of—*The Lancet*, the very prestigious medical journal, *The Lancet*, has just labelled fluoride as an excito-neurotoxin. Excito because it excites brain chemistry, and neurotoxin because it screws up the—we know it is a neurotoxin. It causes cancer. It causes osteosarcoma. Kids have died from the stuff.

Ty: It is a toxic waste

Dr. Lokensgard: It is very much a toxic waste.

Ty: And they bring it in HazMat material.

Dr. Lokensgard: Exactly. It is okay for me to put mercury in somebody's mouth, but if I drop it on the floor, or you break a thermometer or a fluorescent bulb, God forbid, you have to call HazMat and you have to do an environmental impact statement and study, and it's crazy. It's ridiculousness.

Ty: Right. I was doing a question/answer session recently and one of the questions was about the fluorescent bulbs. On EPA.gov there is actually a step-by-step process that you are supposed to follow if it breaks.

Dr. Lokensgard: Exactly right.

Ty: Because it's so hazardous.

Dr. Lokensgard: Right. But yet, dentists can put it in the mouth, next to the blood–brain barrier, when you have all this autism and autistic spectral disorders in these kids? It's crazy.

Ty: Makes no sense whatsoever.

Dr. Lokensgard: It makes no sense at all. Just from a thought process whereby you just go, "Is that even rational?" It just doesn't make sense.

Ty: It makes no sense at all. Last question for you, Dr. Tom. It's been a fascinating interview thus far, by the way.

Dr. Lokensgard: Thanks. And, by the way, thank you for what you do. What you're doing is amazing. I got a copy of your book, thank you very much, and I watched part of your first series, and I just think what you are doing the world needs to hear. And I am honored and privileged to be a part of this.

Ty: Well the honor goes right back at you.

Dr. Lokensgard: I really am, my man. Thank you.

Ty: Thank you. Last question.

Dr. Lokensgard: Sure.

Ty: Children with cancer. We are seeing an epidemic of children with cancer.

Dr. Lokensgard: Yes, we are.

Ty: What is your opinion as to why the explosion of these last couple of decades with children?

Dr. Lokensgard: My opinion is toxins and excito-toxins and the—well, let me just put it this way. They have done studies on cord blood, placental cord blood, which is normally a sterile-type environment. They have found over 256 toxins in cord blood, coming from where? The mother. So before the baby even gets out of the womb, they are already fraught with 256 different toxins, half of which are carcinogenic.

And so now you have a developing immune system, and then we put them on Similac, and we put them on Enfamil, instead of breast milk, which has lactoperoxidase, which is another bio-oxidative therapy. Lactoperoxidase, which is in mother's milk, will break down into hydrogen peroxide. Well, we have already said that kills anaerobes, right? So that's a good thing. But what we do is we put them on high-fructose corn syrup, or we put them on some type of modified corn syrup, and whenever you see "modified," forget about it. We are modifying everything in our food supply and I think it's killing our kids, and it's causing—plus the fact that we are depleted of magnesium, we're depleted of iodine.

Iodine is the big protector. It is the biggest protector of cancer, and we all have low iodine levels. If you compare Japanese studies—Japanese populations to American populations in breast cancer, you will see far more breast cancer in America than you will in Japan.

And I think that that transfers into our children's population. They are young, they are developing, we are giving them, like you said, shots with thimerosal for immunity, instead of letting their own immune systems develop. I mean, we've done wonderful things in medicine, we really have. I don't mean to sit here and trash all that. We really have, especially when it comes to acute care. If you or I were in a car accident, there is no place that you would rather be than in an American trauma center.

Ty: Yes.

Dr. Lokensgard: Having all those surgeons around, keeping you alive. I've seen it at Vanderbilt, where they have kept people alive. They do amazing stuff.

Ty: It *is* amazing.

Dr. Lokensgard: But when it comes to chronic degenerative disease, which is lifestyle, we have failed as a country, and we need to turn this around. And you, my friend, are doing a great work in doing that, so thank you.

Ty: Well, you are, too, Dr. Tom. I appreciate all you are doing, and thank you for your time today. God bless you.

Dr. Lokensgard: Thank you. God bless you, too.

[end of transcript]

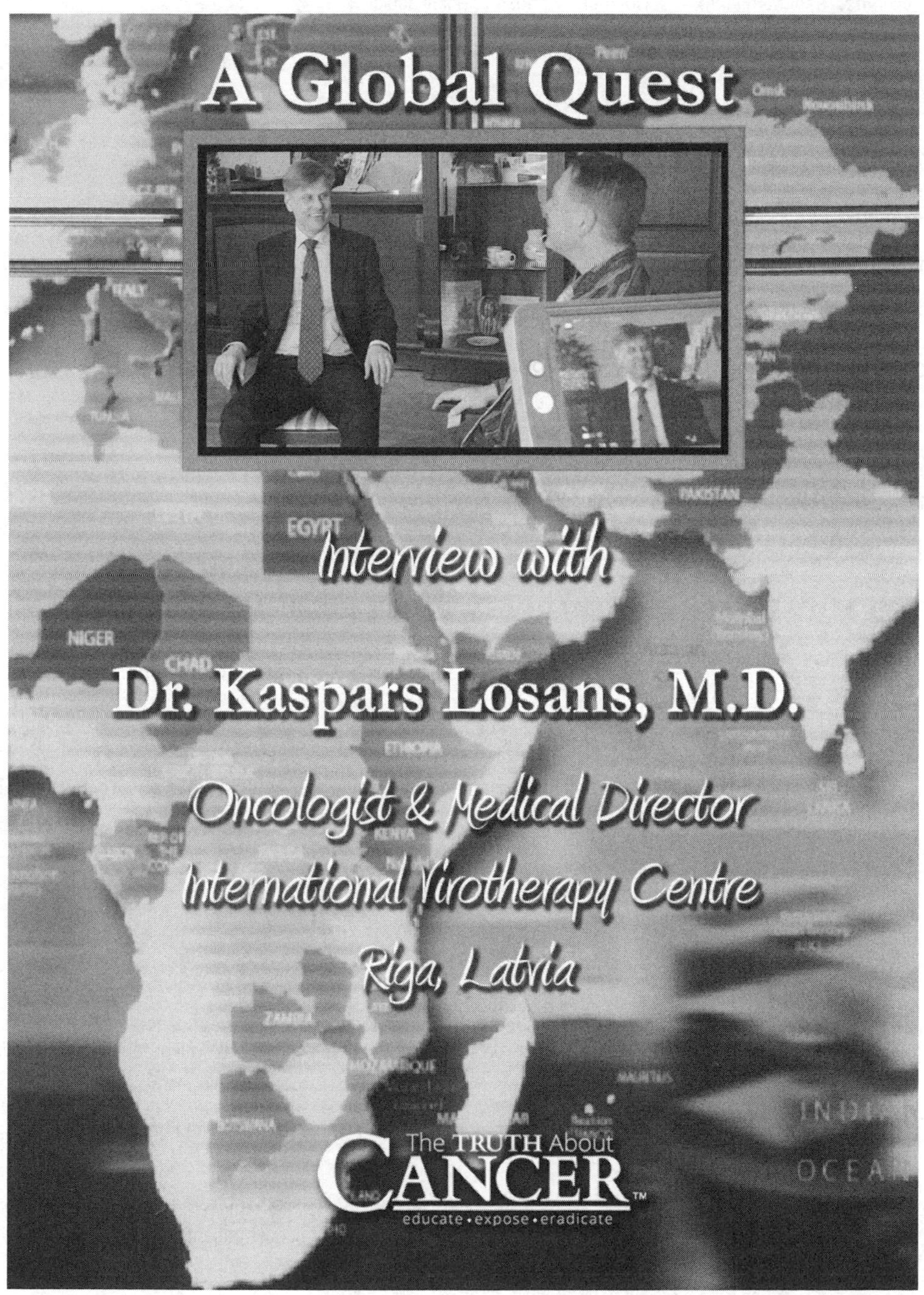
A Global Quest
Interview with
Dr. Kaspars Losans, M.D.
Oncologist & Medical Director
International Virotherapy Centre
Riga, Latvia
The TRUTH About
CANCER
educate • expose • eradicate

Ty: I'm here at the Latvian Virotherapy center with Kaspars Losans, not Casper the friendly ghost. Kaspars Losans. Very nice to be with you today, Kaspars.

Dr. Losans: Thank you, thank you. Not friendly ghost. Friendly doctor.

Ty: Not friendly ghost. You're a friendly doctor?

Dr. Losans: Yeah.

Ty: And you're alive, so you're definitely not a ghost.

Dr. Losans: No. I'm real.

Ty: You're real, and you're going to be spending the next few minutes telling us a little bit about this incredible virotherapy center that we've been filming in thus far today. How long since you've been involved with this particular location of the Latvian Virotherapy Center?

Dr. Losans: Actually, I moved quite recently. But the center is working already for eight years, and doing it real successful.

Ty: What is your position here?

Dr. Losans: I Medical Director for International Virotherapy Center.

Ty: Okay. So what is your education?

Dr. Losans: I medical doctor. In past I've been oncologist, surgeon, now I'm here working for virotherapy.

Ty: Okay, so medical doctor, oncologist, and surgeon. I'd say you're qualified to be the Medical Director then.

Dr. Losans: Sure. Sure. For being qualified a lot.

Ty: How do the therapies that you use here compare to the therapies that you learned about going through medical school?

Dr. Losans: Actually they complete each other. And here, in International Virotherapy Center, we are using virotherapy, which is proven and unique method, and we are using Rigvir, which is first virotherapy medicine proven in clinical practice.

Ty: What do you mean that it's proven in clinical practice, this Rigvir?

Dr. Losans: So that means this is medication, this registered medication, and we apply for cancer patients to treat cancers with Rigvir. And one is proof for registration, proof of registration, as well great experience is in our center to work with Rigvir.

Ty: How does Rigvir, you said, complete the therapies that you learned about going through medical school? How does it work to complete these therapies?

Dr. Losans: Actually for majority of cancer patients, it's good to have operation to remove as much as possible tumor, and then to give either adjuvant or treating virotherapy for cancer patients.

Ty: Okay, so you said it's good to have, give either an adjuvant?

Dr. Losans: Yes. That means for patients who are at early stages, it's great to avoid re-occurrence and metastasis. And for patients in later stages, it's really good to get rid of cell tumors.

Ty: So when you say you add the adjuvant, you're talking about Rigvir?

Dr. Losans: Yes.

Ty: Rigvir is the adjuvant. What is an adjuvant?

Dr. Losans: So that means, for patient which is from examination point is clean of tumor of cells, they are not visible in any examination, it's good to add virotherapy with Rigvir to make sure that this patient will not get metastasis or disease re-occurrence in coming years.

Ty: Is Rigvir a vaccine?

Dr. Losans: No, no. Rigvir is not vaccine. Rigvir is live virus, live, and frozen virus to keep Rigvir alive. And it works as a live virus, which finds in human body cancer cells and destroys them.

Ty: So you could think of it as a good, or healthy, virus?

Dr. Losans: It's exceptionally, a really good virus. We get use to that name virus means something bad. Here we talk about opposite situation. We know of at least one really good virus which helps patients to get rid of cancer cells.

Ty: I think that's an important point to stress about this particular treatment, because as soon as someone hears virus, they're going to think, "Oh, it's bad. Bad virus." I know I did, that was my first reaction when I learned about this a year ago, was, "How can this be good for you? It's a virus."

And it's the same perception that most people have about bacteria. They don't realize that there are good and bad bacteria. There are also good viruses. This is, as you say, the best virus for treating cancer. So how does Rigvir work as a good virus to attack cancer cells, and to help control cancer?

Dr. Losans: Actually as you told, my story about good bacterias and bad bacterias. The same bad viruses and this exceptional one, good virus. And this virus has two abilities. Oncotropism, which means that virus able to find [sic] cancer cells in patient body. And oncolysis, which means that this virus can destroy the cancer cells.

Ty: So Rigvir treatment contains both of those properties, oncotropism, it finds the cancer cell, and oncolysis, it kills, destroys, the cancer cell. That's pretty impressive in light of the fact that cancer cells, do they not have some kind of a mechanism that renders them invisible to the immune system?

Dr. Losans: That's true. And then comes second mechanism of Rigvir. Whenever those Rigvirs are attracted to cancer cells, those cancer cells become visible for human immune system. Until that time they are invisible, they have natural ability to be hided [sic] from immune system, and due to Rigvir guidance, because Rigvir is attached, virus is attached to cancer, and this Rigvir is inside the cancer cell. So immune system, due to Rigvir, recognize cancer and start react against this cancer.

Ty: So the Rigvir has an effect on the immune system, it allows it to begin to attack the cancer, if I'm hearing you properly.

Dr. Losans: Yes.

Ty: And let me ask you this, though. Concerning the cancer cells, does Rigvir have any effect on the stem cells?

Dr. Losans: Actually, we don't know how Rigvir works on stem cells. We know the great ability of Rigvir to destroy cancer cells. So we based on this effect, ascribed our patients virotherapy, and they are getting great life expectancy due to Rigvir.

Ty: Many of them I've interviewed today, with exceptional stories. The, one of the ladies that I interviewed today, actually had to be carried here. She couldn't walk. Another man, given weeks to months to live. These exceptional stories of late-stage cancer patients that are using Rigvir successfully. So we know that it's working. Do we have any scientific studies to back up the fact that it helps the immune system, and it attacks cancer cells?

Dr. Losans: Yeah there are multiple studies performed before registration. Both proved efficacy and safety. Actually, you just talk about efficacy. But the safety profile is exceptional among all oncology treatments, because in the field of oncology, where all treatments usually faced like aggressive and full of damages [sic]. Rigvir treatment goes mostly with no side effects. Since Rigvir registration, there are no serious adverse events registered for Rigvir.

So the story about efficacy, of course we know from clinical studies. Efficacy is proven. But we are much more grateful for our patients who we saw with really bad stages, bad diagnoses, and we see them alive for five years, for 10 years, for 15 years. So they are cured. They are living healthy life for themselves and for their relatives as well.

Ty: And it's no doubt that it's changed their lives. I've interviewed them here today, many of them brought to tears telling their stories about being sentenced to death and then still being alive because of this amazing treatment. You mentioned two things, Kaspars that I want to touch on. Number one you mentioned registration, and number two you mentioned no side effects. So there's no adverse side effects from Rigvir, which is very odd, in light of the fact that other conventional treatments have a lot of side effects.

Dr. Losans: From first year it's surprising me how medication can be without side effects. But listen, this is live virus, and as a live virus, the only side reaction could be a bit sufferable temperature, which is quite normal. When we are getting flu, we are getting a bit temperature [sic]. The same happens with Rigvir treatment, when live virus injected, patient is getting in body live virus, a bit temperature reaction starts, because human immune system reacts versus this virus, which shows where cancer cells are hidden.

Ty: So really, the one side effect, the potential low-grade fever, is actually a good effect, because it shows you that your immune system is responding to the virus.

Dr. Losans: That's true.

Ty: Now you mentioned registration. Is Rigvir approved in Latvia as an official medicine for cancer?

Dr. Losans: Yes. Rigvir is registered in Latvia, in drug agency, as an official medicine approved for treatment. Actually, in Latvia, patients happy, for skin melanoma, Rigvir is compensated by country, so patients should not buy it. It's free of charge for them. So treatment is cure it in best possible way.

Ty: Wow. So it's approved here in Latvia, any other countries that it's approved as a treatment for cancer, or for melanoma?

Dr. Losans: Actually yeah. We are looking for new registrations right now in the world. Actually a producer is in charge of that.

Ty: Okay. You mentioned melanoma. Are there any other types of cancer that Rigvir works well with?

Dr. Losans: Actually, here in our center, we have good experience with many types of cancer. The best prognosis we see for melanoma, then for gastrointestinal cancers, as well for some cancers with bad prognosis, we see good effect of Rigvir as well. Like lung cancer, uterus cancer, many others, as well, is treated in our center.

Ty: So it works on a multiple different types of cancer. And just today, I've seen patients from Ukraine, Lithuania, Russia, Latvia of course, who else? Chechnya, part of Russia. I've seen patients from all over. Is this becoming a place where people come from all over to get this treatment?

Dr. Losans: Actually, here in International Virotherapy Center, we have largest experience yet accumulated for virotherapy with Rigvir, so patients today more than from 40 countries are coming to Riga to get this treatment and to be cured from their cancers.

Ty: So Kaspars, this treatment, Rigvir, is this something that it works best with somebody that's been diagnosed with an early-stage cancer, or kind of rhetorical here, I've seen the late stage today. Is this something that could work for late-stage cancers as well?

Because you know, I've interviewed several people today, and they've come in from being bedridden to being given several weeks to live, and really being diagnosed as terminal, given no hope by their oncologist, is this a place that might offer some hope for them?

Dr. Losans: Yes it gives hope to everyone, to every stage. Of course, we are doing a lot of educational job, to educate people about early detection of cancers. Of course, for early stages, results are much, much better. But for late stages, in many cases, there are no other option. And we are so happy for patients in late stages when they are cured from cancer even in this situation without no solution. And they are cured and they stay alive for many, many years.

Ty: So the treatment's very effective for even late-stage cancer. The location is beautiful, I'm really impressed with Riga, Latvia. I honestly had no idea what to expect before coming, but I have to say, it's one of the prettiest cities that I've seen.

Dr. Losans: Thank you.

Ty: So you're in a great location, a lot of really caring doctors here in the center, a great staff. So I think you've got a great thing going here, and I appreciate what you're doing, because what you're doing is you're offering hope to cancer patients who have really not been given any hope by anybody else. So you're doing invaluable work. Thank you so much.

Dr. Losans: Thank you friend. Thank you.

[end of transcript]

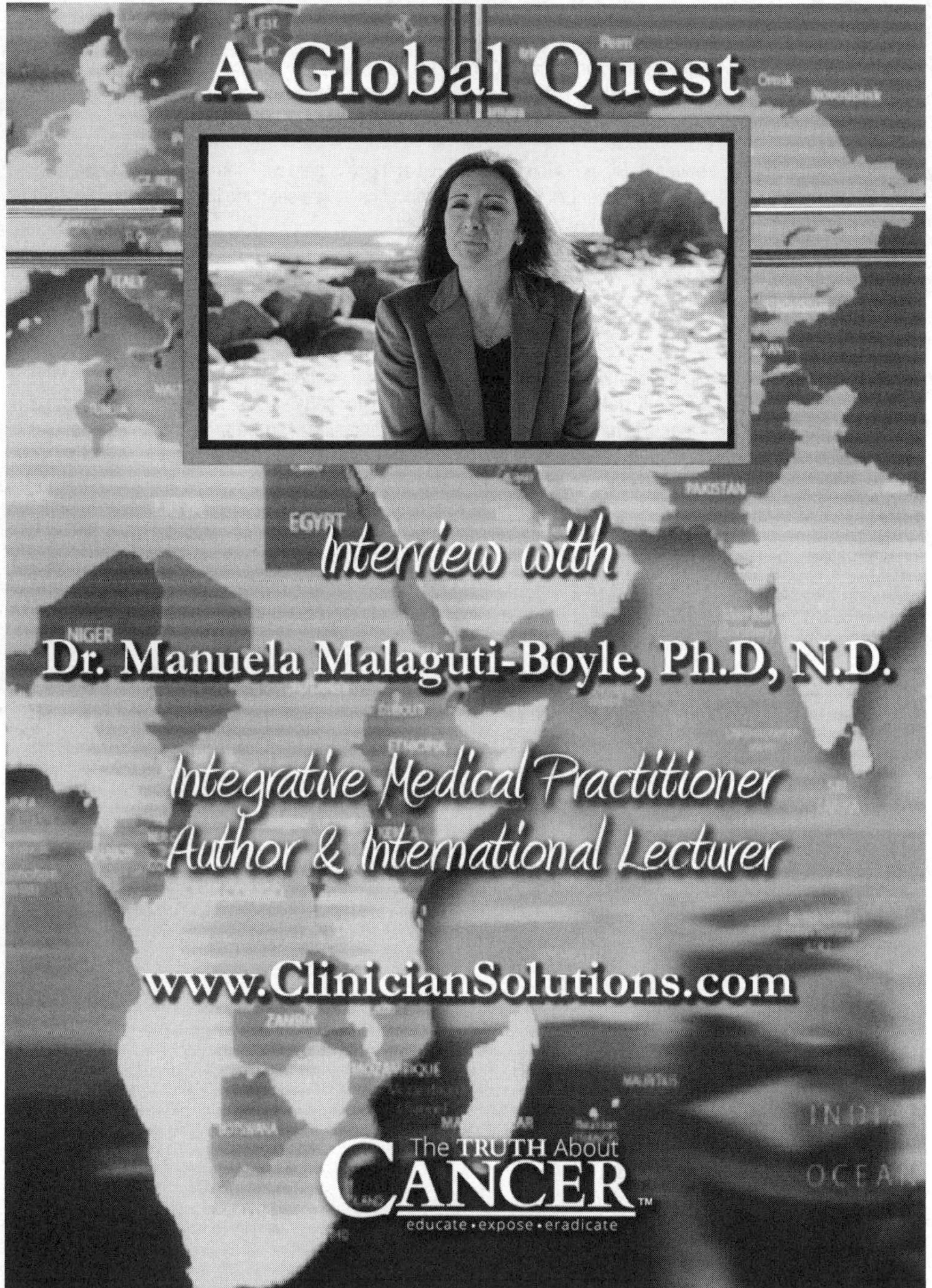
A Global Quest
Interview with
Dr. Manuela Malaguti-Boyle, Ph.D, N.D.
Integrative Medical Practitioner
Author & International Lecturer
www.ClinicianSolutions.com
The TRUTH About
CANCER
educate • expose • eradicate

***Interviewer*:** What was your "aha" moment when you realized that conventional medicine wasn't working?

Dr. Malaguti: Right. Well I realized that when I kept on seeing patients who had gone through a conventional treatment, however throughout remission they had, in fact, had a reoccurrence of cancer or perhaps a secondary cancer, meaning that the first approach hadn't worked.

And beside that fact, they had experience throughout the first treatment was so horrific that they were really not wanting to go through the same process again. So recurrence of another cancer throughout the time between two to five years post treatment as well as of course the side effects were accompanying all these patients and unfortunately were going to pretty much affect them for the rest of their lives.

I realized that, yeah, there wasn't quite enough. And of course these patients clearly were reaching out for something different to help themselves overcoming cancer once again.

I also had a chance to spend some times in cancer ward hospitals. Some of my patients asked me to support them there as well and I really got in touch with—realized the horrible treatments these patients get, receive. Just the smell in a chemotherapeutic ward of hospitals is something you'll never forget.

The acetyl toxic drugs used in those cancer wards are so extreme that nurses, for example, wear masks or gloves and it's just, yeah, something that people don't realize. It's really, really quite confronting and difficult to see patients being injected with so much drugs and toxins and poisons and you see them just fading away.

On the observation point of view, yes, absolutely. You see these people are going through the nuclear war in many ways. And on the science point of view, since I am also very much a scientist—I'm doing a PhD study on use of a particular type of amino acid to prevent a secondary effect from the chemotherapeutic drugs—so from the science point of view also it shows that there are many other agents that can be used to help these patients and these agents are highly likely to be as effective if not more effective, without the side effects.

Interview: Why does cancer develop? What are the main causes?

Dr. Malaguti: That is a very good question and a question that perhaps could deserve hours and hours and hours and hours of explanation. There is no one only theory why cancer develops. It can be seen in a variety of different ways. From the nutritionists point of view of course it is absolutely an issue with metabolic disturbances, with the particular type diet, with high sugar, with all sorts of very poor nutritional status.

From the immunology point of view, there is a very broken down immune system that is not able to cope well, or well enough anyway, to get rid of or keep on track what the immune system is supposed to do.

There obviously are from the virologist's point of view, there are viruses that become viral of the genes and they can create in fact disruption, to a degree, of creating cancer. And from the cognitive, from the psychological side of oncology point of view is really a breakdown of core beliefs and purpose in life.

There are many theories really. All of those are in my opinion very valid, they are all part of a big puzzle, and if we have had just one clear explanation why cancer happens to some people and not to others and a solution to it, we wouldn't be talking about cancer. Cancer is a very complex issue that requires a multi-specialist approach and one is not exclusive to the others.

All of these elements participate and work together and that's why I work within an integrative model. I work with all different specialists when a patient comes to me. There is the nutritionist, there is the naturopath, there is the doctor, the nurses, there are psycho-oncologists. There are specialists, massage therapists. There are all kinds of people and all kinds of people do their very best to help patients.

But why cancer comes? Why some people and not others? Well there also is the genetic understanding that some people are more susceptible than others to develop cancer. Yeah, from the genetic point of view of course it is also important to understand that some people are susceptible, more susceptible than others to develop cancer and some patients of course carry genes. Certain genes makes them more sensible to develop cancer, but our genes are not our destiny.

There's a lot of things that can be done, a lot of things that can be done. The knowledge that we have today is so much more advanced compared to what it was five years ago, ten years ago. In the world of integrative medicine, there has been heaps of new research coming out which has been translated into clinical practice and I'm happy to be part of it.

Interviewer: Talk about the link between stress and cancer. What emotions are important in the cancer equation?

Dr. Malaguti: Of course. Yes, this is also an excellent question. We can see this in two different ways. From the biochemical point of view there is a shift in the pH of the body. The body becomes instantly acidic. And when there is acidity, there is inflammation, there is absolutely the great terrain for cancer to develop and to metastasize, we know that. There is a shift in acidity and calcidity of the system.

From the emotional, psychological point of view, well, people don't have any purpose in life. When there is a major stress, a major breakdown, there is lacking of purpose, of joy of living. When I see my patients, I always ask them. "Okay, say you were diagnosed six months ago, three months ago, a year ago with cancer. What happened then? What happened at that point in time in your life?"

There is always some major stress or some major trauma, and unfortunately when there are unresolved... It becomes—the joy of living, the emotional distress continues on and there is just no reason to live. So regaining that, making sure that people can—I suppose they have been overcoming the stresses—it's very important and moving on.

The key—one of the key person in my team is an excellent psycho-oncologist who absolutely helps greatly, helping these people really facing the distress they are going through right there and then, but also going back a bit to the time when this stress culminated and it was concomitant to a diagnosis of cancer. It works great. So stress has a significant impact on people's lives. Yes.

Interviewer: How does it feel for you to help people get through those stressful—like that stress, that thing that is causing them so much difficulty? A lot of the people wouldn't even have identified that it was a causative factor and then you help them identify something. You've given the steps by which they can change that scene and increase their level of happiness. How has that felt for you doing that?

Dr. Malaguti: Oh, it feels absolutely fantastic. The point is, every time I have a patient, it is always clear that this is our team effort. He or she is very much the center of the attention and care. But it is a team effort. This team, even if though I'm the coach of this team, the team has to perform and work well together to be successful.

Their success is my success. I rejoice in seeing patients who thrive and I have, I don't know, hundreds of testimonials of people who are happy to write their gratitude to witness that. But most of all what is important is that once the healing has taken place, then they are happy to tell others and there are hopes. There is hope and there are options available.

My youngest patient is three and a half years old. She's a little girl with brain cancer. My oldest patient is about 83 years old. She's an old lady with breast cancer, and I've seen everybody in between. I've seen young guys and girls and older people and they all obviously have their own story and their successes and their failures and their tough times and good times.

I always make sure that they know that they are not alone and we can go through this together. So it makes me feel very happy when there is success and when they thrive and they put their lives back together really.

Interviewer: That must be amazing. That must be an amazing feeling.

Dr. Malaguti: It is, yes. Very much so. Cancer is an extremely stressful, in fact beyond stressful, a distressful time and very traumatic for a lot of people.

I've been in practice for almost 20 years. I'm originally from Milan, from Italy. I worked for a number of years in London, a very big clinic in London. I used to see over there also cancer patients. I worked in Singapore as well, so over there same thing, and in Australia. Overall there would be oh, a lot of people.

I see new patients. There is a certain waiting list to see me but overall I'd say I've seen a few hundred patients. The majority of them are people who came to me—or come to me while they are undergoing chemotherapy and radiation therapy. Those are people who have chosen to go through conventional treatment but also to seek out somebody who can help them through overcoming the journey.

But there is also quite a large population there of people who have decided to take an alternative approach. I want to make sure that they go to see somebody who knows about biochemistry, about how to use and what to use throughout their treatment.

I see a lot of people in my two clinics. I have a clinic on the Gold Coast and a clinic in Brisbane and I also see people overseas as well. I have a guest practitioner in a couple of centers overseas as well. Very much of my experience overseas and my experience in Australia has brought me to the understanding that cancer is very much an international issue.

There are some differences in perhaps, obviously, cultural background, beliefs and diets, but at the end of the day, the patient who is undergoing chemotherapy at the local hospital here on the Gold Coast will be receiving exactly the same type of drug that a patient in Sri Lanka right now with breast cancer will be receiving, and the person in America will be receiving and in South Africa will be receiving, which means basically the conventional treatment is still one size fits all.

In terms of integrative approach, we know that this is obviously a very significant shortcoming. One size doesn't fit all, at all. We have the opportunity to use botanical agents and nutritional supplementation that is designed for each and every individual.

We have about 220 different cancers that have been identified. Those 220 different cancers are again different for each and every person. Individualized treatment is absolutely essential for the successful treatment of an individual patient. This is something that hopefully, one day, perhaps still in my lifetime, we'll be able to see in integrative hospitals.

If you have two patients with the same cancer, same age, same name, dietary background, they'll have two completely different responses to treatment. Therefore making sure that there is an individualized approach, that there is a really deep understanding of the biochemistry of each individual is very important. This is what we do.

My team and I have the ability to use cutting edge technical, amazing machines. We have a hyperthermia machine, hyperthermia chamber. We have IV, Vitamin C, glutathione, alpha Lipoic acids. We have dendritic vaccine injections.

All this is absolutely evidence-based, it is supported by human clinical trials and it is very successful. Each and every time it's modified and tweaked according to the presentation of each patient. I'm very happy to be able to use all this knowledge and to help people.

My first experience of cancer was when I was about 14. My grandmother had... At the time I was living in Milan and my grandmother had been diagnosed with breast cancer.

At the time, the treatment required to have very invasive surgery. She had a mastectomy and most of her lymph nodes were removed. The result of that was a significant scar and also her right arm became very swollen, very big and she was very much ashamed of all of it.

She was a simple woman, she was a country woman and she felt that the whole experience had taken such—her feminine attributes away from her. She spent her life really hiding and covering and being very shy about the way in which she looked.

I remember the time also that she hadn't had any support post-surgery, once she was obviously dismissed from the hospital, released from the hospital. She was very much severely sore and sad for a very long time. She survived that cancer. She died many years later and when she died her... After the surgery she had chemotherapy and radiation therapy and she died some years later.

When she died, her bones were still radioactive, so a significant amount of chemotherapy and radiation therapy that had been given to her, let alone the surgery which disfigured her in many ways and the lack of help and support from the medical team made me realize that it was the most horrible experience anyone could go through. From that fear to then realizing there were other people I got to know in life who had been affected by cancer made me realize that surely there would have to be a better way to go through this and so my interest in studying more.

I had two wonderful mentors in my life. One is Dr. Jeffrey Bland from the Institute of Functional Medicine whom I'm very happy to know and correspond with. The other one is Henry Osiecki who is very much one of the greatest biochemistry and nutritionists in Australia and overseas as well. They taught me a lot.

I studied in Australia, in England and also in the United States and I am a Fellow of Integrative Oncology. My learning and studying is ongoing and hopefully I will conclude my doctorate at the end of this year and we'll be in a better place then.

Interviewer: Wow. That's incredible. Manuela, with your grandmother, when you were watching her go through that, was that hard for you? Was that painful seeing her like that? You obviously would have seen her when she was happy and well.

Dr. Malaguti: Sure. She transformed completely. Women of that generation, again so many years ago, had absolutely no emotional or psychological support. You can imagine that they hardly knew what cancer was about and from one day to another they were put through such a significant and horrible treatment and the operations at the time weren't done in a way to preserve the breast as much as possible.

Those were extreme surgeries from taking as many tissue as possible out, it was what we call an aggressive treatment from the surgery point of view. That means that women were scarred immensely. So her change of life from again a happy go lucky, lovely lady to being very withdrawn, reclusive, suffering, ashamed of herself, covering the part that she had been obviously missed... Yeah, there was a significant change. So she, yeah, very much suffered for the rest of her life because of that. I think that, look. If surgery is necessary—if it is necessary—I understand that, but the methods and the way in which it was done was really pretty much not okay, nonhuman.

Interviewer: You think that was robbed from her?

Dr. Malaguti: Yeah, very much so. Oh yeah.

Interviewer: That femininity?

Dr. Malaguti: Very much so, yes. Yes. Yes, absolutely. At the time there was no reconstruction, breast reconstruction. They weren't small surgeries that I'm talking about, extensive surgeries.

Interviewer: So now you're able to help women, have you ever seen women that recover without having to do surgery and they come—patients that you work with personally?

Dr. Malaguti-: Oh yes.

Interviewer: How does that feel now that you give to them what you would have loved to have given to your grandmother, that you had to live it out in the lives of your patients?

Dr. Malaguti: It's a wonderful possibility to be able to see people thriving. Everyone who is within or works within a medical system whether it is conventional or integrative, is obviously—aims at improving people's lives and supporting their quality of life. I certainly do that. I know a lot of colleagues and a lot of other doctors and naturopaths and nutritionists who do that too.

It's the joy that you see in the faces of these patients who are able to overcome the biggest fear in their lives. It is priceless. The gratitude and the happiness that... Also the family members is just amazing. And this is at the end of the journey.

Throughout the journey there are moments that are really difficult, difficult for everyone. As a healthcare practitioner I have to make sure to keep the information clear, focused and just to move on in such a way that patients are supported and the families are supported and they know a clear way where to go and what to expect.

Interviewer: What treatments do you use for cancer?

Dr. Malaguti: I have a six steps protocol which, again, I individualize absolutely for each and every one. I use a number of steps. I use pancreatic enzyme therapy, I use obviously, hormonal blockade. We use detoxification of heavy metals, reconstruction of GIT tract integrity and lots of machines and herbal medicine as well as nutritional medicine.

Interviewer: And what results does that get for people?

Dr. Malaguti: Great. Great results. Look, I'm so lucky I have witnessed spontaneous remissions. I have witnessed people who had a second or third cancer to thrive and come out of it. I've had people who were able to go back to their oncologist and say, “Look, I'll show you here. These are the tests. I don't have this cancer anymore” and be triumphant about it.

So the oncologists always scratch their head and think, “What's going on? How is this possible?” and then they come to the conclusion, “Yes, there are lots of things that can be done. Good.” So I'll cooperate with a lot of oncologists. And it works okay – most of the time.

Interviewer: It must be a great feeling when they come in with having had success and going back to have that conversation and then...

Dr. Malaguti: Yes. Yes.

Interviewer: Does it make sense to treat cancer by suppressing symptoms and the body's immune system?

Dr. Malaguti: No. That's the biggest fallacy of all times. The immune system is the cancer patient's best friend. In fact, conventional oncology is moving towards embracing immunotherapy as part of their treatment. We've been saying that for a long time.

Interviewer: For those who have undergone chemo, how can they rebuild their immune system?

Dr. Malaguti: They need a lot of help from integrative support. There are specific botanicals, specific nutrients and those dependent methods that can certainly help them through a lot.

Interviewer: That's great. Do you ever wish that people would come to you after they go through chemo a lot, do you ever wish they had come to you first?

Dr. Malaguti: Yes, I do, for the simple reason that even if they do choose at the end to go through chemotherapy, for whatever reason, and sometimes it's family pressure believe it or not, but even if they decide to go through that, it is essential to prepare the patient for that event.

When somebody is diagnosed with cancer, there is this quickness in wanting to schedule surgery or chemotherapy or radiation therapy almost immediately, almost instantly. This is from the oncologist's point of view.

There is absolutely no rush with this. Scheduling the patient six or eight weeks after the diagnosis, in most cases, makes absolutely zero difference, but what it gives integrative oncologists the opportunity to do is to build up the resistance, the nutrition, the immune system and everything else to prepare the patient for treatment.

If we do that, if we are able to do that and the patient still wants to go through chemotherapy, first of all he will receive less chemotherapy, less drugs simply because his resistance are high and also will bounce back in a much better way. So yes, I wish they came to see me before they choose to go and do whatever they want to do at the end. It's still the patient's decision and I support whichever decision they make.

Well I love Ty. Ty is a friend of mine. I admire his work. He is awesome and he starts with education and education is empowerment. People can make better choice, better options and feel secure about their options and their choices.

I owe Ty a lot. I think all of us do. He's a very courageous man and good on him for doing so. He's really great.

The Global Quest is saving lives, no doubt about that. Ty is not only a celebrity in the United States but also here in Australia. I know a lot of people who know of Ty, who obviously have been following him and listening to him and reading his blog and so on and so forth.

Absolutely what Ty has done is something that not many others have attempted so far, making sure that the truth is out there, the truth is available. There is a lot still to be learned, to be explored, but by and large by giving some tools and educational tools, some motivational tools to people, the fear factor all of a sudden goes, and if the fear is out of the way, well, there is a lot of room for a true quest and a true recovery and true healing.

Look. I think that if one in three people in the US as well as in Australia will be diagnosed or has been diagnosed at some stage with cancer, one in three, it pretty much touches everyone. Everyone knows somebody who has had cancer or who has cancer right now. I invite people to log on or connect with Ty. The website is amazing. The newsletters are amazing. The knowledge is there, is available, is up to date, is cutting edge, is there. Just a list of gifts of informations.

I have patients who come to see me and they've been diagnosed with a cancer and I ask them, "Well do you know what that means?" and they say, "No, because the oncologist didn't have time to explain." "What do you mean? That's all about you and your life and he hasn't had the chance to explain that to you?"

Well, it's difficult. Teaching, giving the options, giving the tools is number one and Ty is doing that for us all and that's fantastic. So my advice is don't hesitate to own the series. It can absolutely save your lives, save the lives of your loved ones, save the lives of somebody you know. Like I said before, one in three people will be diagnosed with cancer or has already been diagnosed with cancer. It makes a lot of sense to own the series. Have a look, take a look. You'd be very amazed, impressed.

[end of transcript]

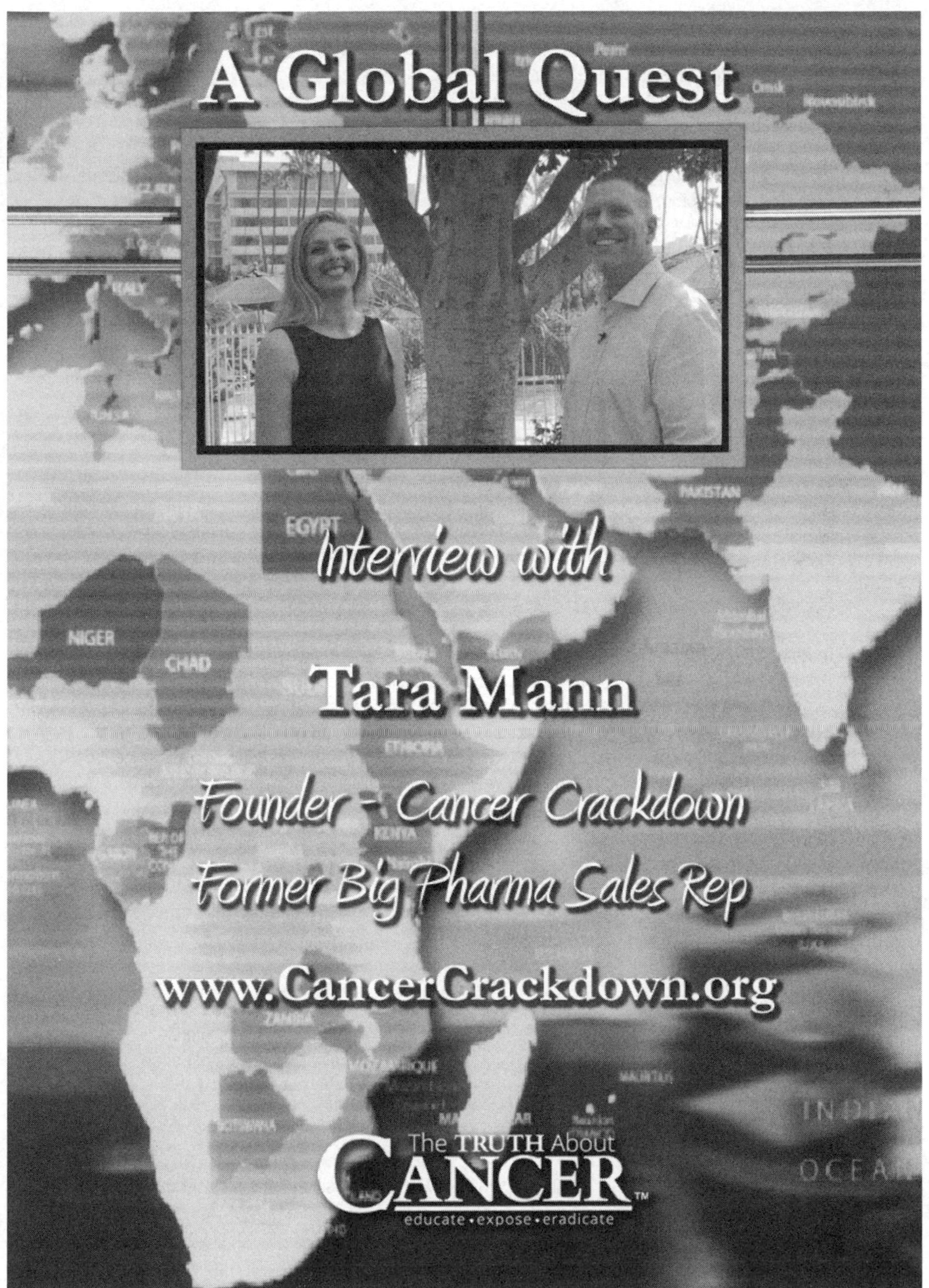
A Global Quest
Interview with
Tara Mann
Founder - Cancer Crackdown
Former Big Pharma Sales Rep
www.CancerCrackdown.org
The TRUTH About
CANCER
educate • expose • eradicate

Ty: So, Tara, tell me about your time as a pharmaceutical rep and how you got started in that?

Tara: Well, my background is science and my degree was in Medical Technology. In my senior year in college, I was in the lab constantly. By 10 o'clock in the morning, I was bored to tears and said there is no way I can do this for a living.

When I got out of college, I went directly into outside sales and a lot of different sales positions, first aid, and even sold custom made clothing.

A friend of mine approached me that worked for the pharmaceutical company and said you really need to consider this. It's a good job. I said I'm good now and she came back later and said, "I'm about to launch a blockbuster drug. You need to put your resume in."

I put my resume in, interviewed and got hired and I started back in 2000. I can't remember exactly. Started there and you go off for three weeks of training and you learn tons and tons about products you're going to sell and I ended up doing that for 11 years.

Ty: You apparently were part of the team that launched several big drugs.

Tara: I launched five or six blockbuster drugs. I worked in central nervous system, so anti-depressants, anxiety medication. I worked in cardiovascular. I had blood pressure medication, I had Alzheimer's drugs. I worked in a lot of different areas of pharmaceuticals with that position.

Ty: So, you said you did it for 11 years. Why are you not still doing it today?

Tara: In 2011, by chance, I found a documentary and the title caught my eye. It was called, *Dying To Have Known*. It was one of the documentaries about the Gerson Therapy. I remember watching it, it was almost stages when I was watching the video. First it was, what in the world are they talking about? They were talking about people that had late stage cancer and they had somewhere to go and they were surviving. I'm like, I have never heard of this. So, I kept watching and as a pharmaceutical representative, the doctors teach us very well that we practice evidence-based medicine.

Ty: Right.

Tara: I'm watching and I'm thinking, this all sounds really good, but I wonder what kind of evidence they have?

Ty: Right.

Tara: They switched to the physician and I believe it's China that is doing the Gerson Therapy and I just remember him sitting in front of this huge filing cabinet. The person that was interviewing, he told him, "Just pick files," and he just started opening these drawers of all of these files of patients, all of this evidence.

Ty: Okay.

Tara: All of this evidence, right? So I'm going, "Wow, how is this possible, there's evidence?" Then the documentary goes on to talk about Max Gerson, the way that the therapies were suppressed and I remember sitting up on the edge of the couch—it was like the Band-Aid being ripped off, that moment of just disbelief.

Ty: Right.

Tara: My whole life—my mother is a nurse. I mean we grew up at the doctor's office and at the nursing home and I had no idea. I worked in the hospital. I was a phlebotomist. I worked in the lab. My whole life was medicine.

Ty: Right.

Tara: And so it was shocking in a really impactful way, immediately. Immediately, it changed my life. I wanted to research, but I really thought that my research would disprove it. I thought this is really awesome, but it's hard to believe. I started researching and I felt really strange. I felt like I was alone and I'd go to work every day in this industry and I'm thinking, "Do they know this? Do they know what I know?"

So I mentioned it to a couple of people—one of the reps that I worked with, her 16 month old daughter had cancer. I told her, I said, "I'm still kind of wrapping my head around this, but I saw this documentary about this therapy for cancer where they drink juice and they do this detox and these people live that are dying." I just told her that and I left it. I didn't even know how to approach people with it.

A couple of months went by and she called me and she said, "I want to know everything about what you know." I told her and she was angry that she had been giving her daughter Popsicles and sugar and candy. Put her on a probiotic—really fought with the doctors. She was very good with her scientific data. It was amazing what she did. Her daughter is alive and thriving today.

She and another caregiver that was really begging for someone to give him ideas for his girlfriend that was dying. I wanted to connect them. I thought, well, I'll just start a little support group that was easy on Facebook and I pulled it up and "Cancer Crackdown" just came—I don't know where it came from. I started that as a support group just to connect people. That grew and the group grew. I just saw the need.

For me, in doing all that research, I have a science background. I've done tons of research. It came really easy to me and I was healthy, but I was confused. Healthy, no diagnosis, right? I'm confused, there's all of this information. They don't all agree and I'm thinking, what if I had cancer and I was learning this. I don't have a research background. I don't have time.

Ty: Right.

Tara: And I don't have the resources. What would I do?

Ty: You basically took that as your impetus to begin researching on behalf of other people, because you do have a research background. You do have the medicine background.

Tara: Yes.

Ty: You saw that this was an area that we're not necessarily being fed evidence based medicine when they teach us to go treat cancer with chemo, radiation. That doesn't really have the support that these other treatments.

Tara: Right.

Ty: You wanted to put that out there for people.

Tara: Absolutely.

Ty: That's admirable that you've done that, but let me ask you this. How did it make you feel when you realized that we've been snookered for lack of a better term?

Tara: It was so personal. I mean it was really personal to me. I had never really had a close loss to cancer, but I did lose a friend that was a nurse practitioner and I knew she would have done anything. She had young kids, same age as my kids, and it's changed personally. I've been vegan now for a couple of years. I went off of every pharmaceutical because I was drinking the Kool-Aid. I was taking three things, synthetic hormones, with birth control for many years. I got off all of that. Went vegan, started detoxing. From a health perspective, it's been very empowering.

I always struggle a little in my little corner of the world with feeling alone and feeling that there's not a lot of places to go out and eat anymore. It's affected me and my family tremendously. It's changed our lives in a lot of ways. My husband and I both stepped away from the corporate world to really do something that matters and to help these people that have been given death sentences and been told that they have cancer and scared to death and help them find their way, to give them comfort and let them know they are not alone. Our slogan is, "We fight with you and we fight for you."

Ty: What you're doing with "Cancer Crackdown" is really admirable.

Tara: Thank you.

Ty: With "The Truth About Cancer" we really are thankful for what you're doing. We've donated to your charity last year.

Tara: Absolutely. We really appreciate you so much.

Ty: What you're doing is great work. For those who don't know what they do, they actually connect cancer patients with doctors that are able to help them go down a natural treatment path. Tara and her husband, Steve, the founders of the "Cancer Crackdown," are really great people and we really support people like you and your organization because it does give people not only the knowledge that we're giving, but you really are able to connect them with the proper protocols and the proper doctors to where they can get down that path and succeed and be healthy.

Tara: Yeah.

Ty: What you're doing is great work and we're really honored to be associated with you.

Tara: Thank you.

Ty: You're not alone. We're all part of a greater thing. This is a worldwide movement and it's just starting.

Tara: Thanks to you. And a lot of great people.

Ty: I'm just honored you're with us from the start. It's going to be bigger and bigger in the future and greater things to come for all of us—

Tara: Yeah, absolutely.

Ty: As we help to enlighten the whole world about these treatments. Tara, you are really inspiring to my wife, Charlene and myself, because we know you were raking [in] a lot of money. You were living the high life. You've told me about the houses and the cars and all of these things the sales of drugs were giving you.

Tara: Absolutely. Yes.

Ty: To me that's just an admirable thing that you've done.

Tara: Thank you.

Ty: Many people are making the money and they realize what they're doing is not helping people, it's hurting people, but they don't make the noble choice that you did and step down. They continue it because they put their lifestyle over top of the health of the people that they're dealing with. You didn't do that and so to me, you've got true wealth because of what you're doing. The things that you're doing now, you're going to reap eternal benefits for because you're helping people. That's a huge inspiration to us.

Tara: Well, thank you. You are a huge inspiration to us.

Ty: Thank you Tara. You and Steve are great and we support "Cancer Crackdown."

Tara: You do. You're a big supporter. We don't think we'd be here with y'all. And your book, like I've told you in the beginning helped me in my confusion to find someone like you that was giving people answers that are so important.

Ty: Thank you Tara and you and Steve keep up the great work.

Tara: Thank you.

Ty: Thanks for talking to us today.

Tara: Thank you.

Ty: All right.

[end of transcript]

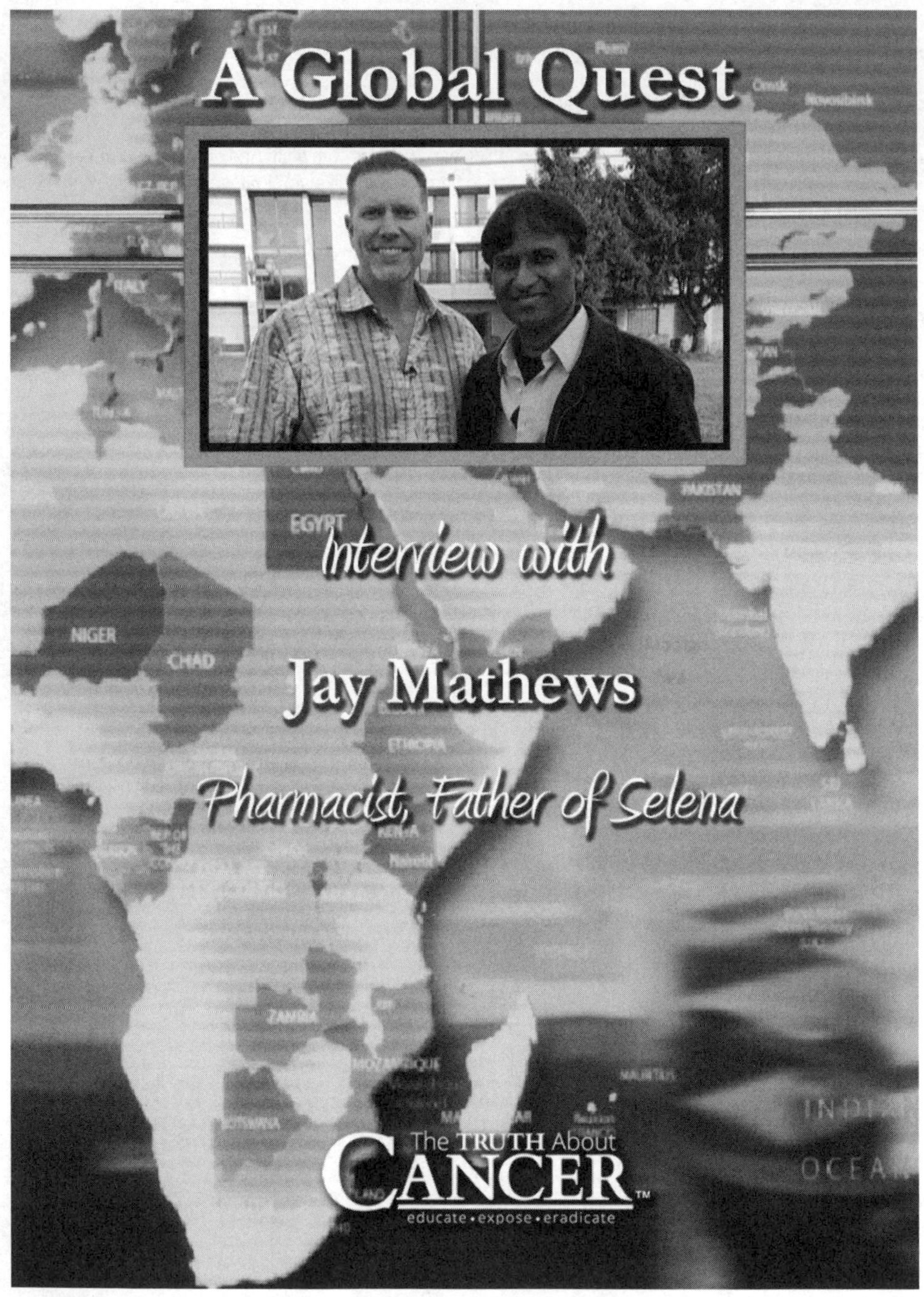
A Global Quest
Interview with
Jay Mathews
Pharmacist, Father of Selena
The TRUTH About CANCER
educate • expose • eradicate

Ty: So, I'm here in Troy, Michigan, with Jay Mathews. Jay, thanks for joining me tonight. I want to talk to you about something. It's a personal story for you. It's become personal for me over the last few years. Let's go back to maybe four years ago, maybe 2011—I think it was that you initially contacted me and your daughter, Selena, had been diagnosed with osteosarcoma.

Jay: That's right, yeah..

Ty: And at that point, weren't you—you were down in Arizona?

Jay: That's correct. Right.

Ty: So give us the story of what had happened with Selena and tell the viewing audience a little bit about yourself, what you do for a living, and then we'll work up to current day.

Jay: Okay. Well, I'm a pharmacist by my profession. So I have been practicing that for about 20 years. So when my daughter was diagnosed—it's about three years ago, we decided—the whole treatment was huge—it's barbaric and the options were just very limited and I think I ran that by you at the time. The prognosis was less than 20 percent. Amputation was almost definite.

Ty: So, you're a pharmacist, so you read about the efficacy of the drugs they proposed and determined that they were ineffective.

Jay: Correct. Right. They may mix it around and cut everything out and then at the end of the day, they'll say it's effective, but when you call the Children's Oncology Group, they're the group that collects all of this data for children's cancer, they'll tell you that they're making advancements in pediatric cancer. But I think they're mistaking surgical advancements for oncological advancements.

Certainly now, surgically, like in emergency medicine, there are advancements, but getting to areas are now much more possible and I think that's where the advancements are. So at that point when we saw that the options were very limited in the sense that we hadn't seen any successes with the other patients. Some patients started chemo within three months, maybe amputation was done, another three months they weren't here. So, we had gone to Arizona at that time. We were doing treatment, but of course, we have four kids.

Ty: How old was Selena at the time?

Jay: She was eight.

Ty: Eight?

Jay: Eight years old. And so I had the other three kids with our grandparents, my parents were watching two of the kids and my wife's were watching one in different parts of the country. We had come back home and at that point—right after that last bit of treatment, and it's not like we're completely against conventional treatment. We did Cyberknife radiation on her because the tumor was getting larger.

There are certain things you need to do at that point where aggressive therapy is needed, and at that point it was needed. I think that did a lot. It did stop the cancer at the foot, but when we got home, we noticed—this is where the mistake happened—is when we got home I'm trying to aggressively get the kids ready for school because school starts the following day. They're all over the country, and I get home, there was a little bit of a swelling. My wife was concerned. I was concerned.

We didn't know what to do at that point. Certainly we could have flown back to New York. We were being treated at the time in New York. We could have certainly done that. In hindsight, that might have been the best option.

Ty: You went from Arizona to New York.

Jay: Correct. Yeah.

Ty: Doing natural treatments or a combination?

Jay: Combination.

Ty: Okay.

Jay: Combination—natural …

Ty: And Cyberknife.

Jay: Cyberknife. Cyberknife was sort of—get some of the holistic treatments under control—sometimes it takes a little bit more time. Anyway, when the swelling happened, that's where we made mistake number one. We went to the emergency room. At that point, I thought they didn't have too significant successes with that, and I thought at an ethical standpoint, if you don't have very much, you shouldn't be doing that much. That's what I thought. I didn't think they would pursue such aggressive means to get it and at that point, the doctor, was again, depending on who you get, we had a physician who was very stubborn—thinks that he has all of the answers. Didn't know anything about our approach.

Ty: What did the physician tell you? So you take her to the emergency room. She has some swelling. What was going on there?

Jay: The swelling—we don't know. It's naturally subsided. Maybe we overreacted. I don't know. We sort of felt like it might have been just the reaction from the radiation. Ultimately, they kept her for days. and then they knew that we were in the middle of treatment and we had appointments already set for her. They realized that this wasn't standard care and so they pushed us into —.

I already said, show me a patient that you have treated, since it's such a big facility in Chicago. Show me a patient who has great success that you've succeeded on. They proceeded to give me a couple of numbers, and I certainly have their numbers until today. One is on dialysis, one is in kidney transplant—one of the side effects—the other had a recurrence. The other child was there for the second time. Where are the successes there? They seemed to be attached to the hospital for the rest of their lives.

Ty: That was the two successes that they gave.

Jay: They gave me—yeah.

Ty: Okay, so they didn't like the fact that you were treating naturally—and so they kept Selena …

Jay: Selena was guarded. They had armed guards at that point because they knew where my mind was at.

Ty: They had armed guards in her room?

Jay: In her room. They knew where my mind was at. My mind was to take her back to the facility of my choice.

Ty: Right.

Jay: And the facility would give her a chance to have some sort of a normal life.

Ty: She was eight years old at the time, and you looked at the five-year statistics and it showed she had what less than a 20 percent of chance?

Jay: Exactly.

Ty: That's not good for an eight year old.

Jay: Absolutely not. Even if you happen to be one of 80 percent that did survive, you have such a quality of life significantly diminished. Amputation is almost certain. I mean, they'll do prosthetics and they'll call it a limb salvage, but it didn't seem like it would be the way I would have done it for myself. I felt like we owed that to her to do what I do for myself and my wife would do for herself.

Ty: They had armed guards at her hospital room door …

Jay: At her door.

Ty: To keep you from taking your own daughter.

Jay: Right.

Ty: Did they threatened you at all as far as if you took her, if you didn't follow what they were going to do or what they wanted to do?

Jay: It was kind of somehow in the air—if you figured out that DCSF was going to be involved.

Ty: DSF, what's that?

Jay: DCSF. The CPS, the Child Protective Services.

Ty: Child Protective Services.

Jay: Yeah. So they came—the first time they wanted me to sign consent to do another set of CT scans. I was refusing because she just had one just a month prior. And just that much radiation for a child, in particular where cancer is involved, is something we didn't want to do. In a holistic sense we wouldn't do that many CT scans.

Ty: Because the radiation can do much more harm.

Jay: Harm—correct. So they said they'll file for taking custody at that point. I signed consent. They did the whole set of CT scans. They came again. I knew it was coming—the hospital lawyers and the DCSF, the CPS. They came with their lawyers and they said, "If you don't sign consent, we're going to take custody of the child. You're going to lose custody of the child."

At that point we were going to go in front of a judge, we knew that. So I thought that if I showed the judge—this was mistake number two, mistake number one was going to the emergency room—if I showed the judge we have a protocol in place, this is where we're going. This is where we want to go. At that point, I thought that would stand.

But what happened when we went to the judge, you have a public defender, you converse for maybe 20 minutes, you have 20 minutes converse with the public defender. I still thought I'd have more of an opportunity to speak. Ultimately the judge said, "You're not an expert, he is, the oncologist. He's the expert." There's nothing he can do, and the custody was given to the state and then —

Ty: They took custody of Selena.

Jay: Yeah. And then they started aggressive chemotherapy at that point.

Ty: So this was what time period?

Jay: It started in September of '12.

Ty: 2012, okay.

Jay: Until about June—the beginning of June, end of May the following year.

Ty: So aggressive chemo.

Jay: Yeah.

Ty: How did she progress on these treatments?

Jay: There was so many treatments that it reacted, some of the chemo treatments, it's written in their compendium, this thing called radiation recall, when you give this drug, the radiation just goes out of control. It's like a synergistic kind of massive response. Whatever radiation you get before—who knows how many times ...

Ty: This is documented.

Jay: It's documented. Documented. So they knew that, but they continued with the chemo. I think that any adult would have been just saying, "Look at my arms deteriorating every dose you give. My arm is opening up—just opening up and the wound is getting bigger." I pleaded with the physician. I have no way to even get second opinions at that point because the state's got custody. I can't go to a physician and say, "This is wrong, You have to take a look at it," because they wouldn't approach us because we don't have custody.

Ty: Right.

Jay: We're not the legal custodians —

Ty: You don't have custody of your own child.

Jay: Correct.

Ty: The State of Illinois did.

Jay: State of Illinois. So I pleaded with them. I said the arm is not going withstand—it's not going to make it. All I could do. And every time about eight white coats come into the room, look at her wound getting bigger and bigger with every dose. At one point, we pleaded with the mediator to say at least let us have her between treatments. You can't put her in a home. We won that.

Thank God they sided with us on that. It was sort of a plea for humanity. You can't take a child that's been taken in this fashion and then put in another home. How is she going to deal with it conceptually?

Ty: Right.

Jay: I had to convince her that this is the best thing for her although, I wasn't saying that in the first round when we were holistically being treated. I had to convince her that this is the best thing. So, that's where we were at. When she came home, we did all kinds to try to get that wound to heal, but we had her for two days and back in the hospital because it's neutropenic, she's got no white blood cell count, they have to start the next dose.

I pleaded with the doctors, to give us a few more days—maybe the wound—just got bigger with every dose and in the end—as much as I pleaded with them, as much as they saw the wound got so big—got infected with MRSA. They did all these cultures at that point. The wound if you see it's horrific—it's so graphic—you will not believe that's a human arm the way that it deteriorated over time. It was incredible. It was graphic for her. That's post-traumatic stress for her, for us certainly it is.

Ty: Sure.

Jay: In the end, an amputation was required. I knew it. There was no way she can move the arm, it was pretty much going to fall off.

Ty: You'd been telling them that all along.

Jay: All along.

Ty: The arm's not going to make it.

Jay: Not gonna make it.

Ty: When did they cut her arm off?

Jay: They couldn't do it, so we're running around the rest of the State of Illinois trying to find another physician…

Ty: This is unbelievable. They take custody, they give chemo and radiation, and they know that the synergistic effect is going to cause the radiation to destroy the arm. Then they give her to you and say, go find somebody else to cut her arm off.

Jay: Right.

Ty: Because we destroyed it.

Jay: Correct. So we go to the other two hospitals, and the only option they were giving us at that point—this is the most graphic one of all —is a four-quarter amputation. If you look at it, it's the most disfiguring kind of amputation possible. They don't just take your arm off, they take it right up to the shoulder. These were all the things we were trying to avoid. This is why we didn't want to go this route. This is almost standard in a lot of cases and being stuck to the hospital.

Ultimately, the only option, the only physician—the only way to save her life now —was an amputation. I'm hoping and I'm begging these doctors to look at—you can go low, can you go to the elbow—give her at least a stump so that she has an option. They are all wanting to go not just to the shoulder, they're taking the shoulder off. So it goes right to the neck. It's the most horrific thing you could see. If you look at it, it's the most horrific thing you can think of.

I think the Good Lord was with us because we pleaded and some unforeseen circumstances —. What happened was the arm was just about to fall off. Literally it was almost in two pieces. I took her to an emergency room at another hospital. So we've got all of the hospitals covered here. They just did an emergency amputation just to resect it because the arm wasn't going to make to the appointment date for that four-quarter amputation. So, I wish we could have more, but they did a disarticulation right up to here —

Ty: Okay.

Jay: She still has her shoulder. The initial doctor who was going to take the shoulder off as well, I have a gripe with him. I told him, "Look, I know you're trying,"—because doctors will try to get everything to say that they tried to get everything. I think I might have upset him when I asked him, "Do you get a notch on your belt if you get full successes? Is that why you're trying to take so much?" That really offended him. He looked at me and said, "This is the most humane thing you can do for her, is to take the shoulder". She has her shoulder.

The point is that doctors don't really know everything. She does have her shoulder, still. So we went there at another hospital in Chicago, they took the arm off. She has her shoulder still and things are going good and since we've had—after that point, we still didn't have custody after the amputation for another six months. We have custody of her now.

Ty: You have custody now.

Jay: We have custody now. We've certainly incorporated a lot of the nutrition. One of the things that worked for us was the fact that she did have the opportunity to come home, and we employed nutrition as much as we can. We had to get some of the side effects. We did all the stuff that we could to get her to as close to—as best as we could do under the circumstances.

Ty: Is she able to potentially have a prosthetic in the future?

Jay: Yeah, we're working on that.

Ty: Okay.

Jay: Yeah. We had the best insurance and I think really it's the worst thing you can have. We had the best insurance. To have the best insurance means every drug that is covered will be used and was used. Every drug that wasn't covered, he would have used Avastin. Avastin is another $400,000.00 drug. He would have used it if it was covered. Ultimately, I was in a position where I could have dropped her from my insurance—the state didn't pay for it. All of this, $2.2 million, was paid out to the hospitals.

Ty: $2.2 million?

Jay: Yeah. And it was all paid from my insurance. It wasn't paid from the state insurance.

Ty: Okay. Even though they took custody of her?

Jay: Yeah, the state didn't pay the $2.2 million. The reason—and my standpoint is, I don't to use that use those drugs particular—those were my arguments because we had all kinds of other tests done, but what would you do? If they have custody, would I take her off of my insurance? I could have done that. I could have done that, but then I knew that at the end of the day, there's no one to come out, the need of ancillary services. I knew we would need those.

Ty: Right.

Jay: Right now, the prosthetics are over $110,000, the part the insurance is picking it up. If I had dropped her, and we might have not been able to afford the prosthetics. That's it. I think that—if your video or this video gets out to the general doctors and stuff, they might think I have a gripe with this and I should be happy, but I really want to say one thing is that—I don't know if you know this, he's a hero of mine—his name is Terry Fox. Have you heard of him? Terry Fox, he's a Canadian and he ran across the country with—he had the same cancer as my daughter.

Ty: Yeah, I do.

Jay: With the one leg and he was running across the country. He had a four-quarter amputation too. Same cancer as Selena. I grew up in Canada, and he was our hero. I really believe that Terry—he raised billions of dollars now. Thirty-five years later, my daughter had the same chemo treatment as he did 35 years ago. My daughter had the same amputation like him.

Ty: No progress.

Jay: No progress. I really want to say this is that—Terry Fox would agree with me, I am convinced of that — is that this sort of treatment is not progress where we're taking funding. He wanted to do the right thing, he funded a charity that raised billions of dollars, raising it and doing the exact same thing we did 35 years ago.

That's it. That's my story and we have her back. She's doing great, thanks to some of the options that you presented. There are plenty of options that I think we do believe in nutrition and we do believe that there are other options out there.

Ty: It really seems surreal to me. I'm sure it seems surreal to you that you've gone through this this last few years with her basically being kidnapped from you by the state, forced treatments that were against your better—and you're no dummy, you're a pharmacist. You understand drug interactions, you understand the way that chemotherapy works. You understand all of these things.

I would argue that many pharmacists, including yourself, understand better than many of the doctors because that's all you do. You presented that to the court and they didn't care. They said, "We'll take her anyway."

Jay: That was my other mistake—I needed an expert with me in court.

Ty: What exactly is an expert is my question.

Jay: Someone who can compete with the status quo. If an expert were to come with me, what would happen? What would happen is that option would be eliminated because they would call the medical board and get his license kicked out. If someone else had to put their livelihood on the line. So this monopoly way of thinking on this, progress is not going to be possible.

Terry Fox would agree with me, I know it, I believe wholeheartedly. I believe that and so that's the option. There is one way of thinking. I'm sure other parents are going to go through this and may come to that awareness that we have. They would probably end up having to flee the country. I don't think any kind of holistic practitioner would take a child anymore after our situation. They're yanking people's licenses that way if you do anything other what's standard—and the doctors will tell you, well this is the best we have—and that's not true.

Ty: That's not good enough.

Jay: That's not true. It's the best profitable thing that they have or it's the best thing, putting up economic barriers that you can't try other options. Well, they continue to take people's body parts and limbs off, they're going to continue to do that. That's the option that are left for kids that are faced with this kind of a cancer. It's sort of the situation I think the country is running into, but nobody sees it this way.

Ty: It's really unbelievable to me that—I think you're right. It may be the best option is to leave the country and go somewhere else if you have a child.

Jay: That's the only option left now if you had to. There isn't anyone who wouldn't consider—a caretaker that would take you because their livelihood is on the line.

Ty: Jay, I've interviewed parents over the last few months that have told me the exact same thing that once the clinic found out that their child was under the age of majority, they said we can't help him.

Jay: Yeah. Right.

Ty: Unreal. I'm so glad to have finally been able to talk to you about this and I'm glad that Selena is doing well. I'm hopeful that she can have a prosthetic limb soon and I'd be able to meet her soon. I'd love to be able to do that. I really appreciate you taking the time with me today.

Jay: Thanks, Ty. You've been a great support for us.

Ty: Thank you. God bless you and your family.

Jay: Thank you. ***[end of transcript]***

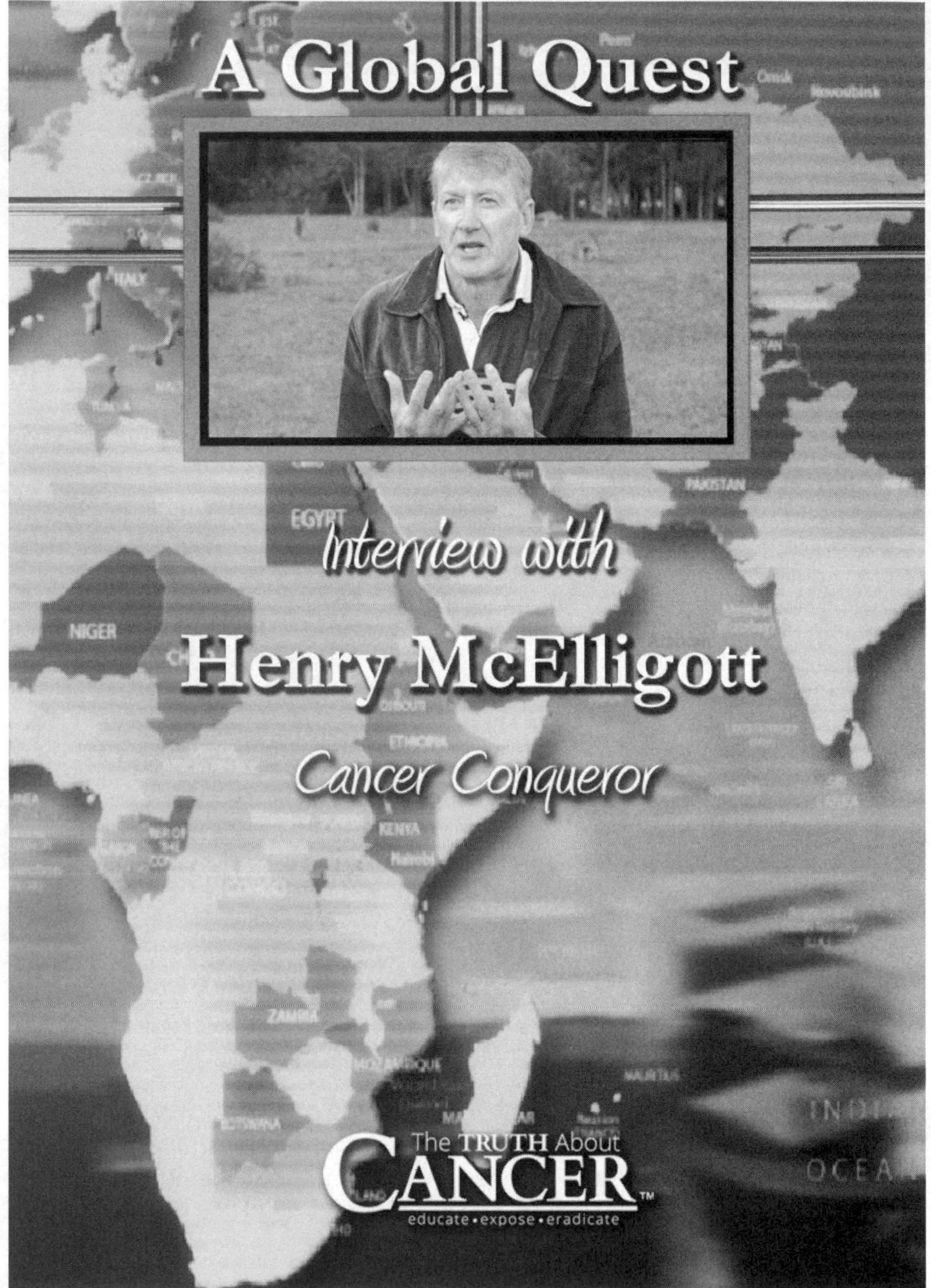
A Global Quest
Interview with
Henry McElligott
Cancer Conqueror
The TRUTH About
CANCER™
educate • expose • eradicate

Henry: During last year, Jonathan, a lump started appearing here, at the left side of my jaw. And it got bigger and then it spread back to here. And then, a lump started here and I began to notice difficulty swallowing, as if there was a chicken bone in my throat, and my tongue began to swell.

So I went for a CT scan on the 1st of December 2014, and I got the results back on the 2nd of December. I was sent to see an oncologist, an ear and throat specialist, at one of the major Sydney hospitals. And I was told that I had base of tongue cancer tumors that had spread to my lymph nodes on my neck. They were worried that it had already spread to the rest of my body and my organs.

So they put me in a room with about 34 oncologists at this major hospital, and put a camera down through my nose to have a look at the tumors that were at the base of my tongue. A copy of the tumors all appeared up in a screen behind my head, and my wife saw them. She said, "They look scary." The head oncologist at the hospital said to go in the next room and wait while they discussed the best treatment for me. So my wife and I went to the next room and waited.

The head oncologist came to us, and he said, "You need to start radiation and chemo immediately," because they were worried of it spreading, or else I would not survive. We were in total shock at the time. We lost words and we just looked at each other. Then my wife said to the oncologist, "We're booked in to go over to Asia in January for the holiday." The oncologist said, "You got to cancel. This is too serious. If Henry doesn't receive radiation and chemo straight away, he will not survive." I said to the oncologist, "Could I get a second opinion or would you transfer me to another hospital which is about ten minutes from my home?"

He reluctantly agreed, so a few days later I went to see another group of 11 oncologists at another hospital near my home, and they said the same thing. They said, "Immediate radiation and chemo, or you will not survive very long, because this is a very dangerous type of cancer. It's already spread to your lymph nodes. We don't know where it is at this stage without further PET scans, MRIs," things like that. I went home with Joy just in total confusion, hopelessness. Despair set in for a few days, I didn't know what to do.

I decided to start looking on the Internet what are the side effects of radiation and chemo, and what exactly is chemo and radiation. I discovered that chemo basically destroys the immune system, and radiation just burns the tissue—burns the good cells and the bad cells in the body. For treatment with chemo and radiation for the type of tumors I had, I would need a tube to breathe. They wanted to insert a tube in my stomach for food.

I got a bit scared at that stage and I said, "I've made up my mind," then and there to my wife, "I will seek natural treatment for this cancer diagnosis." So I rang the hospital and sent them an email—both hospitals—and I said, "I refuse the chemo treatment and radiation. I'm going to do some research myself and seek a natural alternative to the chemo and the radiation." That was it for a couple of days. Then they started ringing me, creating fear over the phone, and saying things, "You won't live very long."

I remember being in church eight years ago and I heard a friend of ours in church by the name of Leanne, share her testimony how she used these isotonic vitamins and minerals from Market Australia and Market America to build up her immune system. It totally healed her thyroid cancer. These vitamins she was sharing were very high in antioxidants and selenium. She was very excited about what they did to her immune system. Then the immune system healed the cancer tumors that were on her thyroid.

So I said to my wife, "We'll get in contact with Leanne over in Singapore." And then she sent us a heap of vitamins and minerals—isotonic from Singapore like OPC-3, beryllium, resveratrol, combination B, vitamin C, isochrome, (inaudible - 00:06:38), antioxidant, curcumine, and Oxygen Extreme. She had another friend here in Sydney she put us in contact with to mentor me on how much to take. And this friend here in Sydney, her name is Juno. She used these products to build up her immune system and heal her colon cancer about seven years ago, and she's still healed today.

I was very encouraged to hear these two testimonies, so I started taking these isotonic products and mega-dosing on the OPC-3. Every six hours I was taking six spoons with vitamin C and the other products periodically during the day. I went on total vegetarian food. I had a lot of fruit and nuts to eat, and I went on a three-week fast, just water and taking these vitamins. After the three-week fast, I had lost about 10 or 15 kilos.

However, I was feeling good and what I noticed after taking these products for about six weeks, the swelling at the left side of my neck began to decrease in size. And the swelling of my right decreased, and I was able to swallow much more easily, and my tongue was not swollen so much. So I got really encouraged by this because I was under no doctor's care whatsoever.

I continued this treatment until March and I discovered on the Internet, Ty Bollinger's *Quest for Cancer Cures*. I listened to all his interviews with various cancer specialists all over America. And I was especially intrigued by some of them, and I learned so much. So at that point, I decided, "Are these tumors decreasing or has the cancer spread already?" That was my major concern.

I was listening to a doctor in America that does vitamin C intravenous treatment. I think it was at O'Reardon Clinic. I think his name was Dr. O'Reardon. I also listened to some video about Dr. Linus Pauling who discovered vitamin C intravenous as a treatment for cancer. I checked around Sydney for clinics that do IV vitamin C, and I found one, and I made an appointment to go and look at—and I have a chat at the doctor.

When I got there, I showed him all my reports that I had—the CAT scan, the ultrasound, the biopsy. And he looked at me and he said, "Henry, if these tumors have spread through the lymph nodes to the rest of your body, you are finished and I can't help you." I said, "Look, Doc. I don't want to hear that. I want to know if you can put me on vitamin C intravenous." He said, "Yes, I can, but I need to get you a blood test first to check if your kidneys are well enough to have the high doses of vitamin C, like 75 grams a day." So I said, "Okay, Doc." So I went for the blood test and the result came back a few days later. My kidneys were very good. Then, every week for the next 6 or 7 weeks—he put me on the first week 15 grams IV. The second week he put me on 30 grams IV, and he kept going up 45 grams the next week, 60 grams, and 75 grams.

Then he said, "You got two choices now, you can go for a PET scan or send a blood test to the Genostics Clinics in Germany to determine where the tumors are and how big they are. And I want a cancer bar to see where you're at with this treatment." So I said, "Okay Doc, I don't want the PET scan. I don't want any radiation and sugary substance put in my blood. I don't want anything to do with CAT scans, MRIs, no radiation whatsoever." So he said, "Okay, we'll send your blood to Germany to Genostics Clinic. It's a very accurate clinic. It can determine the size of a cancer tumor to half a millimeter, where it is in the body." I said, "I'm happy with that, doctor."

I continued on my vitamin C. All I had was about six treatments—not much. And I continued on the mega doses of the OPC-3 isotonic vitamins in the same time, and drinking heaps of water, exercising, getting plenty of fresh air out in the sun every day, eating vegetables. My wife used to make very good organic juices for me with kale, broccoli, carrots, apples, with cayenne pepper, with oregano, with curcumin, with lots of stuff, these power drinks.

Jonathan: Is it good? Did it taste good?

Henry: It tastes great. And vegetarian food. So I was feeling good, even though I had lost—I was 108 kilos when I was diagnosed with the tumors that were spreading. And now I'm 88, so I've lost 20 kilos in that six months. But I'm feeling great, full of energy.

My blood test went to Germany at the end of April. And I got a call from the doctor's secretary on the 8th of May. She said, "Your results are here from Germany. Would you like to come in and see them?" I said, "Of course I do." I got really excited. But yet, I was never so scared. I was reading my Bible that morning—I was a Christian—the Lord led me to a scripture about, "My peace I give you. Do not let your heart be troubled. Do not be afraid." So I just kept meditating on that scripture as I went to the clinic, and when I got there, I had to wait in the room for about 20 minutes for the doctor to see me. It felt like the longest 20 minutes in my life. I just kept twiddling my thumbs.

Eventually, he called me upstairs to his office and he opened this envelope. He looked at me stunned. I said, "Doctor, what's the result? I'm sweating. What is the result?" And he said, "Henry, this is a miracle." He said, "I've been a doctor since 1979. You are the first person that has come to this clinic that hasn't messed around with chemotherapy, radiation, or surgery as a cancer cure." And I said, "Am I?" He said, "These are marvelous results. This report is a miracle." He said, "It says, 'Numerous fragmented dead cancer tumors floating all over the blood.'" And then he said, "It is the same result as if you've been having chemo and radiation treatment for the last six months."

I was in total shock. I just relaxed in the chair and I said, "What does that mean, doctor?" He says, "Your cancer marker is barely registering on the scale, on the radar scale." He said, "I'm very shocked." I said, "Well, what will I do now doctor?" He said, "Whatever you're doing, just keep doing it for the rest of your life and you'll live another 100 years." And I said, "What?" I said, "Will I continue the IV vitamin C treatment?" He said, "If you like." He said, "The IV vitamin C treatment, you haven't had much. You've only had a few grams over the last six weeks. It was the (inaudible - 00:15:43) you using the IV for a few weeks and see how I go." He said, "Go for another test in three months and then we'll see if that's okay with the same results as these; have another test six months after that."

Jonathan: Isn't that something? That's incredible. How did that feel for you? You heard that and you thought there was chance you were going to die. Obviously, you grappled with the reality that you could die. You're a sober personality. Then you went from, in a sense, having a death sentence. You would have to second guess yourself. I mean, "Are these people right?" And because most people cave, you must have considered the thought that you could've been wrong and you were putting yourself in a really precarious position. And then to get the feedback that you got, how did that feel for you in that moment?

Henry: The doctor said, "You are a really brave person to refuse chemo and radiation at that point." And I said, "I don't think so, doctor. I think the people that have chemo and radiation are a lot more brave than me." He said, "What do you mean?" I said, "When the oncologist told me at the hospital I would need to breathe through a tube and I would need to eat through a tube in my stomach, that was scary, doctor. Taking these natural products every six hours was easy. I don't need much courage for that." And he was in shock. He said, "I never thought about it like that, because I've never dealt with a situation like this before."

Jonathan: And the lighting is fine, by the way. It's beautiful. It's like ambient—

Henry: The Lord is here with us, Jonathan. You don't have to worry about anything. He's here.

Jonathan: Wow. Do you think God wants people to know this truth?

Henry: Yes. When I was saved in '96, the Lord spoke to me and He said, "I will lead you into all truths and show you things to come." And He's done that for the last 19 years, and He led me to these cures for cancer. Now I'm helping hundreds of people.

Jonathan: Something else, man. Something else.

Henry: I'm writing a book at the moment. It will be published by Christmas, *23-week Cancer Cure Through Nature*. It's all happening.

Jonathan: Henry, God has been in your life before, and obviously you cooperated with God's power. In the case before, particularly in this case, you've taken something that was like a curse on you and you turned it into a blessing. How does that feel being able to take something that could've taken away everything that you longed for and it's actually given you the things that you've been looking for?

You love to inspire people. You love to help people and bring people hope and healing. How does it feel to have taken that thing that could've taken away everything you wanted and it gave you so much more?

Henry: I just look at this experience of the last six months as a wake-up call. It's just a wake-up call. It's just another chapter in my life, and I take it as a challenge. Through the last six months, I had to be mentally very strong. And that has helped me—being mentally strong—because the first, say, two thirds of my life were very difficult, if you know my background. So that has prepared me for what I've been through in the last six months.

It's like in the Bible with David, God—it was the same God that helped him to kill the bear and the lion. So that same faith in God that helped him to kill the lion and the bear, it was the same God that was with him killing Goliath. With me, it's the same God that helped me through my past experiences and the experience of cancer over the last six months. It's just another challenge. It's another opportunity for me to help people worldwide through this testimony and through what I've been through for the last six months.

Jonathan: It's awesome, man. Tell me about when your wife first—when you both heard the news. What I'm going to do, Henry, is I'm going to give you—by the way, it's been incredible. This is awesome. I've been up until 12:00, 1:00 the last couple of nights, looking for information to create something like a promotional material. I just got some of the things I've been looking for a very long time, so thank you. Thank you for blessing us.

Henry: That's okay.

Jonathan: One thing that I'm interested about is when you first found out the news, did you ever wonder what you did wrong to have that happen, what you might have neglected within your body? What did I do? What didn't I do to make it better?

And then, obviously, you have a wife that's depending on you and a daughter that is just starting her life. She's doing the HSC and she needs support rather than to be supporting someone. It's not the age for it nor is it the time in life—and then you, in a sense, brought a burden to the family. Was that ever hard for you to grapple with? And it may or may not have been, but was there ever any guilt or something like that you've done something wrong? Or that the family were going to be hurt as a consequence of something that was going wrong with you?

Henry: I read somewhere once that you get cancer from what's eating you, not what you're eating. So over the years, I've had a lot of difficult times. There was a lot of unforgiveness and bitterness deep inside my heart, and pain that I never had dealt with.

Looking back then and looking back now, I didn't really have peace, even though I was a Christian for 18 years at the time. I didn't have any real peace inside. There was a lot of confusion, and unforgiveness, and bitterness, and pain in my heart. I decided then and there that I wanted peace in my heart. I asked the Lord for forgiveness and to bring healing deep inside me.

Slowly over the weeks, I felt a big release of the pain, the unforgiveness, the bitterness, the anger, the resentment. As that was lifting from deep inside me, I could feel the flow of healing to my body as I took more and more of these natural vitamins and minerals to nourish my immune system and build me up.

Jonathan: That's something else, man. That's unique. Some of the stuff in the past that you felt like you hadn't truly forgiven it, eh?

Henry: I hadn't truly dealt with it in a deep and meaningful way, and I feel that contributed to my physical state. Because I was reading in some website by Dr. Lorraine Day that healing begins in the body when we let go of our bitterness, and anger, and unforgiveness. I was reading that 90 percent of cancers and other major illnesses are caused in the body by unforgiveness, and bitterness, and anger, and resentment, and all the evil that is within you, through these things. So I just dealt with everything, and just humbled myself, and just prayed, and just as all these things lifted, I could feel healing and restoration deep inside my body.

Jonathan: Did you change as a person?

Henry: Changed completely. One hundred percent. I gave up alcohol. I used to have drinks, maybe two or three glasses of wine with dinner, a couple of beers after that. Weekends, I might have half a bottle of wine or a few beers at a barbecue. I gave up all the beer. I gave up the wine. I haven't drank for six months, more. I gave up coffee. I gave up all sugary products. I gave up all processed foods, processed meats.

And now I've just got a very basic diet of vegetables, fruit, my vitamins and minerals. And I might have meat now once a week, organic meats, since I got my results on the 8th of May. And I have fish maybe once or twice a week since I got the results. But I have no grains.

Jonathan: That's incredible. Henry, what do you think about the *Quest for the Cures*? What impact did that have in helping to help save your life? How did that information help you to actually have your life from going down that path to whatever that could've been—and you know what that was—to having the life you have now? Do you feel that *Quest for the Cures* did that and how do you feel towards that?

Henry: I learned so much. I learned so much. It was just a miracle that my wife and I came across Ty Bollinger. We just loved all the interviews he did with the different medical specialists right through America. We learned so much from each one. At the time, I think it was one of these videos that I learned about the IV vitamin C. It was through one of these videos I learned about the IV Vitamin C also. I learned from Dr.— in New York, Dr.—about the coffee enemas. Dr.—

Jonathan: Nick Gonzalez.

Henry: Nick Gonzalez. I've learned so much from him. I just combined all of them and now my wife and I have got a whole book of notes that we've learned from Ty Bollinger's interviews on *Quest for Cancer Cures*. Now I'm sharing this information to people that were diagnosed with cancer all over the world. It's just so brilliant and I'd like to congratulate Ty on the brilliant work he's doing to bring the truth to the world about cancer cures. He's doing a brilliant job, and I admire him, and I want to thank him on behalf of everybody around the world, and my wife, and daughter, and myself.

Jonathan: It was actually what you learned inside the Quest for the Cures that you used that then saved your life?

Henry: Not everything, no.

Jonathan: Not everything, but as in one of the things that was in the *Quest for the Cures*.

Henry: I learned about the IV vitamin C in *Quest for Cures*. I learned about the apricot kernels and the B17 in *Quest for Cures*. I learned about the coffee enemas for detox in *Quest for Cures*. And numerous other things I cannot—about the vegetarian food, about organic food, so many things. I've got a whole book of them at home. So many, I don't know how to touch on them all.

Jonathan: That's awesome.

Henry: But I can say the IV vitamin C, the apricot kernels, the B17, the coffee enemas for detox. From Quest for Cancer Cures I could see hope for myself. I could see hope for the future, and it was like I could see a light at the end of the tunnel. Knowledge is power and I used some of the knowledge for total healing. I'm totally healed today [chuckles] of base of tongue cancer that had spread to my lymph nodes. The doctor said I would only live for a few months ; it's six months ago. I can swallow properly again. The lymph nodes are still a little swollen, but nothing like before. I've got doctors confused here in Sydney by my results.

I used the Truth About Cancer Global Quest as a vehicle to bring total healing to my body. I learned a handful of different techniques and methods like the coffee enemas, the IV vitamin C, the B17, the apricot kernels and lots of other stuff. I'm so excited about it because today I'm totally free of cancer. My tongue is back to normal size. The lymph nodes in my neck have gone back to the normal size almost. I am so excited about the future and I am so happy to have come across the Cure for Cancer Global Quest. It helped to change my life completely.

Jonathan: That's awesome. How do you feel towards Ty and that work that they've done and the Truth About Cancer? That's really Ty and Charlene. How do you feel towards them for giving you information that saved your life?

Henry: I cannot put it in words, Ty. I really cannot put it in words because what they're doing is just amazing. Because the pharmaceutical industry is a multi-billion dollar industry. The work that Ty is doing and his wife Charlene is like a little voice of truth in the wilderness that's giving people around the world hope for a future without the chemical poisoning of chemotherapy drugs, or burning through radiation and destroying people's bodies, and giving them an early grave instead of a long, fulfilling life with perfect health like me.

I was diagnosed to die in a few months. I'm fully healthy. I'm leading an active life. I'm helping hundreds of people. Through information I learned, I'm teaching hundreds of people and helping them with their cancer cures through the information I got from Ty's show.

Jonathan: That's awesome. What would you say to someone that was thinking about getting their hands on this information right now? What would you say to that person?

Henry: Getting their hands on this information is like winning lotto. That's how I look at it.

Jonathan: When should I do it? So I might want to put that off and think maybe I could do that later. Imagine you're speaking to me about my urgency. What should I do right now, Henry?

Henry: I think everybody should be equipped with this information, whether they've got cancer, whether they're a normal human being. Everybody has got aunts, uncles, cousins, friends, relatives that have cancer. Fifty percent of males in America right now have cancer and 33 percent of females have cancer. In Australia, the numbers are slightly less.

So I believe it's a very important tool to empower a person to deal with healing cancer and treating themselves, and then helping their immune system to grow stronger. If you are considering owning the DVD series, now is the best time to equip and empower yourself with the information on them.

[end of transcript]

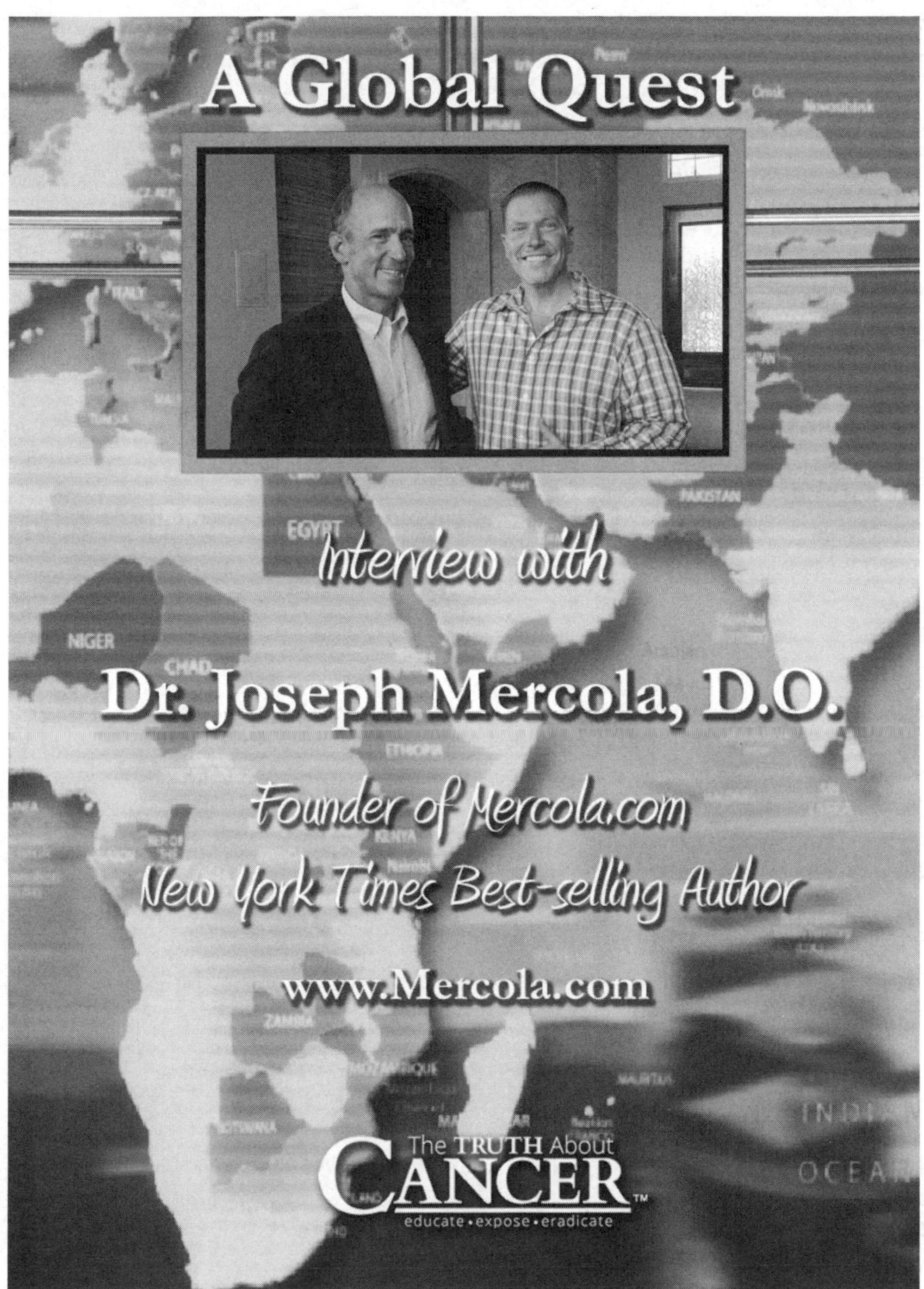
A Global Quest
Interview with
Dr. Joseph Mercola, D.O.
Founder of Mercola.com
New York Times Best-selling Author
www.Mercola.com
The TRUTH About
CANCER
educate • expose • eradicate

***Ty*:** Dr. Mercola, thank you for inviting us today.

Dr. Mercola: Thank you for having me.

Ty: Yes, really glad to be able to talk to you today about several subjects, health-related. But before we get there, I would just like you to share with your viewers a little bit about yourself and how you got to be Dr. Mercola. Did you grow up in a home that focused on medicine?

Dr. Mercola: No, that wasn't the case. It was a typical American home. My father was a parcel delivery person, my mother was a waitress for many years. And we ate typical foods, the processed foods, and as a result of that I suffered a lot of health problems—not significant ones but dental decay. Half of my mouth was filled with mercury fillings by the time I was in high school. That's what happens when you don't eat healthy food. That's the logical consequence.

My parents weren't educated and informed, they were typical American consumers. Toward the end of grade school, I've always been an avid reader, and I read Dr. Cooper's book on aerobic exercise, and back in the late 60s exercise wasn't a fad back then. In fact, if you had a heart attack, you were typically given a prescription of bed-rest for six weeks, which now, of course, would not be done. So, it wasn't widely adopted. In fact, when I first started running people would throw rocks and beer cans thinking I was running away from a crime.

So that was my initial interest. I was also interested in science. I wanted to be an astronaut but then I decided with a little experience with the military, that was definitely not a wise choice and I'm so glad I did because now we know the dangers of being in space. It is not really conducive to being healthy. So I went to medical school, primarily as an effort to understand more about health and how to be healthy. Which is interesting because most of my fellow students who were in school were there to treat disease, not to understand how to be healthy, so it is a little different motivation.

Ty: And that is kind of still the same paradigm, isn't it?

Dr. Mercola: Yes.

Ty: In medical school. Doctors are taught how to treat a disease but not really give them the foundational building blocks that they need to learn how to be healthy, or to teach someone else.

Dr. Mercola: No, and that's by design, specifically. Over a century ago, there were foundations, the Carnegie and the Rockefeller Foundations, who sort of engineered the curriculum through their grants and donations.

Ty: Yes, the Flexner report, and so forth. Sure. And how can a doctor teach you to be healthy if he doesn't know anything about nutrition, right?

Dr. Mercola: (laughs) The common basics.

Ty: Yes. You mentioned Dr. Cooper. I used to live in Dallas, there's a Cooper Aerobic Center in Dallas, that's the same Dr. Cooper?

Dr. Mercola: That's right. Dr. Ken Cooper. He was a colonel in the military. He developed the exercise program for the astronauts. He was a rebel at the time and probably still is somewhere. But he coined the term aerobics and I think most people would attribute the increase in interest in fitness and exercise in this country as being attributed to him.

Ty: Yes. I know, at least in north Texas there, everybody looks at Dr. Cooper as really the one that brought exercise fad to the Dallas/Ft. Worth metroplex.

Dr. Mercola: And he inspired my initial interest in fitness, no question.

Ty: Let's go back before Dr. Cooper then, maybe 20 or 30 years, and let's discuss some happenings at Memorial Sloan Kettering Hospital.

Dr. Mercola: Sure.

Ty: It's up in New York State, right?

Dr. Mercola: Yes.

Ty: And there was an issue with a substance called laetrile.

Dr. Mercola: Right.

Ty: And you've written about this on your website. But this is an example. One of the things that we've discussed with several doctors on this documentary series is just the different ways that certain natural treatments have been suppressed, and I think that this laetrile story at Memorial Sloan Kettering is a good example of that. Could you kind of describe what happened there?

Dr. Mercola: Well, first of all, what is laetrile? Laetrile is also called amygdalin, and vitamin B17, and there actually have been investigations showing that it has some benefit to the use of treatment of cancer, and it may be because cyanide is a component of laetrile and it may also be a nutritional deficiency, that it provides some benefits, some nutrients that the body needs to fight these malignancies.

But anyway, there was a Japanese researcher at Sloan Kettering who was studying this, and Dr. Ralph Moss was an investigative journalist there at the time and started covering it and he appeared to have beneficial results. But then for some unbeknownst reason the information was suppressed. And that information was not allowed to be disseminated, and Dr. Moss wrote extensively about that. That was the mid-1970s.

Ty: 70s, yeah.

Dr. Mercola: And about the same time, too, there were two other investigators. One was G. Edward Griffin, who wrote the book, *A World Without Cancer*, and goes into great detail about that. Actually, Mr. Griffin is better known for his other book which is *The Creature from Jekyll Island*, which is an expose of the Federal Reserve in the United States, a very interesting story, it goes back to 1910.

Then there was another investigator, interestingly, Dr. Harold Manner, who was a professor of Biology at Loyola University in Chicago who also wrote extensively, did a lot of lab research on rats and mice and showed pretty impressive results with the treatment of laetrile and cancer. And interestingly, two of his graduate students wound up being my classmates in medical school, and one of them was my roommate, Steven Desanti, and then Tom Michaelson helped write his book on laetrile.

We never really discussed it extensively, and I'm not sure how beneficial laetrile is, I have no experience with it, but it is an interesting example of how these types of alternative approaches are routinely suppressed when they are opposed to the traditional conventional approaches, because there is such a significant amount of funding that is involved.

Ty: Right. So in your opinion, then, it is really the money that was driving those decisions to try to suppress this potentially good treatment for cancer, because it is not standard of care?

Dr. Mercola: That's what it is viewed as, and then the big agencies, the FDA, of course, the AMA, the American Cancer Society, which are all in some way influenced by the drug cartels, and they are funded to oppose these and essentially classify them as quackery. It is a common strategy that is used for many alternative treatments, and laetrile being one of the earlier ones they targeted, but there are dozens and dozens since then.

Ty: Yes, and that is a popular technique, isn't it, to name call?

Dr. Mercola: Yes. They discredit you. It's their modus operandi, to really target them, discredit and vilify in every way that they can.

Ty: Yes. Isn't it interesting, though, that the things that you and I would consider quackery today, and even many mainstream people would consider quackery, they used to be the standard of care?

Dr. Mercola: Right.

Ty: One of the things that we mentioned earlier, not in this interview, but another interview, was George Washington, our first president. He died as a result of bloodletting. Now that was standard practice then. Now we look at that and we say, "That's quackery. Are you serious? You are going to leech somebody? Put leeches on them?"

Dr. Mercola: Well, actually, it may be beneficial.

Ty: It can be, you're right.

Dr. Mercola: Because there are so many of us who have elevated iron levels, and that can radically increase your risk for cancer.

Ty: And it can also, actually, help you with heart disease, with heart attacks, as well, yes. But I'm just saying, we look back at things—let's use Dr. Semmelweis, who recommended that physicians wash their hands. He was considered a quack for recommending something that today makes sense to us.

Dr. Mercola: Yes, I believe he wound up dying in an insane asylum.

Ty: He did die in an insane asylum. So it is just interesting the things that now are looked upon as quackery. For instance, an oncologist that does not use chemotherapy today is looked at as a quack. And so it is just interesting the way that the definition of that term changes.

Dr. Mercola: And that is a challenge because there are many physicians who are truly, authentically motivated to want to help people, but there is this pervasive fear that they are going to be discredited and ostracized in their own community when they start to embrace some of these alternative philosophies, so that is a strategy that is used to suppress this type of information.

Ty: Yes, and it works really well.

Dr. Mercola: Very effective.

Ty: Because it makes a lot of people back off.

Dr. Mercola: Yes.

Ty: Edwin Bernays wrote *Propaganda*, and that was the techniques that were used back when they—

Dr. Mercola: The cousin of Sigmund Freud.

Ty: Sigmund Freud.

Dr. Mercola: Yes.

Ty: So those techniques were made popular 80 years ago.

Dr. Mercola: Yes, they have even better ones now. When you have tens of billions of dollar of revenue, there is no limit to the clever and sophisticated techniques that you can acquire to manipulate the masses.

Ty: Sure. Yes, and they are very good at it. Dr. Mercola, the ketogenic diet is a very popular diet as far as losing weight. It also can be good as far as cancer is concerned, in many people's opinion. But what is your take on the ketogenic diet and cancer?

Dr. Mercola: Well, I believe it has great value and in my view should be seriously considered as an adjunctive therapy in the treatment of most malignancies. And you might say, "Well, why?" Because of the basic understanding that we have of the physiology of cancer cells. Otto Warburg was awarded a Nobel prize, I believe in the 30s, for the understanding that the primary fuel for cancer cells is glucose, or sugar. Our non-cancerous cells have the ability to use glucose or fat. Those are the two primary fuels. And cancer cells seem to have lost this ability.

The unfortunate challenge in contemporary Western countries is that most of us are not very well adapted to burning fat effectively, and this is an artifact of the way we eat and the timing of the food that we eat. Primarily, it is both. Many people don't understand the timing. We'll talk about the timing in a moment. The problem is that we eat regularly, pretty much three meals a day, and then snacks in between, and about the only time we aren't eating is when we are sleeping. So our body can store sugar as glycogen in our muscles and in our liver, and we have about a 12-hour supply, some people less, some people a little bit more, but in that range. Not a very long supply. Whereas our fat stores can last us for months.

So if we are given sugar all the time and we have that fuel available, then there is really limited reason for our body to have the ability to burn fat. So it suppresses those enzymes and we just eventually forget how to burn fat efficiently or effectively. So when we shift our diet, primarily through restricting processed foods and especially processed sugars, and change the timing of the foods so we have these regular periods where we are not eating for a while, something called intermittent fasting, then we up-regulate those enzymes that burn fat, and we can really shift away from having high levels of sugar in our blood which also has the additional benefit of improving insulin resistance and insulin resistance, many experts believe, may be at the core of many of these degenerative disease and many malignancies.

So it's really a challenge to treat a cancer if you have high insulin resistance. How do you know if you have insulin resistance? Typically, clinically, if you are overweight, if you have high blood pressure, diabetes, or if you are taking a statin drug, that is a good suggestion. Or higher blood pressure.

Ty: And how many—that's like 70 percent of people.

Dr. Mercola: Well, it's about 70 to 80 percent. And the other way to know for sure, objectively, is to draw a fasting blood insulin—not blood sugar, but blood insulin level. If that is below three then you are fine. If it is above four or five then you probably have it, and the higher it is the worse it is. A simple test to do, very inexpensive, available at any commercial lab across the world, and to me, it should be the standard of care in the treatment of anyone with a malignancy to understand what your fasting insulin level is and to control that.

Because if your fasting insulin level is low that's going to be highly correlated with your body's ability to effectively metabolize fat as a primary fuel, and that is what you want, to be able to have that metabolic flexibility, to be able to burn fat or sugar, not just be able to rely on sugar. Because that is going to potentially, more than likely, feed into the growth and acceleration of the malignant cells.

Ty: That's a great explanation. So how would somebody get their body into the state of ketosis where you are burning fat instead of sugar?

Dr. Mercola: Well, I don't know that it necessarily has to be ketosis. And it is my understanding that it has actually been shown there are a number of good studies that show it is quite effective for treatment of certain types of malignancies, specifically brain cancers. It probably is generally used for most malignancies, but the typical strategy one would do, I think, is to really focus on the quality of the food and the timing of the food. So, I like to call it the 3-8-3. That is, basically, don't eat for at least—at least—three hours before you go to bed. Sleep for eight hours, because sleep is another crucial component for healing, and if you are only sleeping four or five hours a night, your body's immune system is not going to be optimized to fight these malignancies. And then, wait for at least three hours before you eat.

Now, you can modify that, too, basically by moving your breakfast forward. But the other approach is you can eat your breakfast, especially if you are going to have an active work day, like a farmer, or some vigorous occupation that you are involved in, and then have a pretty big breakfast, and even a bigger lunch, but then skip your dinner. So then, actually, even extend it, instead of three hours, maybe four, five or six hours before you go to bed. And I think that may be more beneficial for a really good reason, in that it tends to improve your mitochondrial function.

You might wonder what mitochondria are. They are derivatives of bacteria, ancient bacteria, that are embedded in just about every one of our cells, and each one of our cells has about 100 to 100,000 of these things. You might say, "What are they?" Well, these are the powerhouses where our body is actually able to burn fuel. When you eat food, whatever type of food it is, it doesn't magically turn to energy, it has to be converted in some process, and the primary process is using the mitochondria. And the mitochondria have these electron transport chains in there where they actually incorporate the oxygen from the air you breathe, and the broken down fuel substrate, such as fat and glucose, and they combine those together in these electron transfer chains, and they basically produce electrons, get transferred to substrates like ATP, adenosine triphosphate, that circulate around and transfer this energy into your body.

Here is the problem, though, because if you are not able to burn fat effectively, and you have this excess of sugar, or if you eat before you go to bed, one of the worst things you can do, what happens is you have this inefficiency in your mitochondria. So when you produce energy in your body it doesn't occur there magically, there is this process that occurs, and you take these substrates, the fuels that are broken down to either the carbohydrates or the fats, and it combines it with the oxygen.

And there is usually some residual. When you are burning any fuel for energy there is a byproduct. There are waste products. Some fuel is minimal, like water would be the waste product when you are converting hydrogen for fuel. That's a pretty innocuous byproduct. But in our own mitochondria they have the potential to produce excessive electrons, and when you do that, your body has to compensate for that with antioxidants. And if you are using the energy, then it is no problem because you generate it, you use it, and it flows, and there is very little excess waste product.

But when you don't use the energy, if you are not being able to be able to burn fat, and you have a lot of sugar that you are building up, then you have this excess energy, and then these electrons build up, it causes massive amounts of free radicals which can damage your tissues, your cell membranes, your DNA, can actually prematurely kill your mitochondria, and certainly, prematurely age you. There are many experts who believe in the mitochondrial theory of aging.

So we want to preserve the function and the health of the mitochondria and one of the best ways you can do this is by simple strategies like delaying the time, or not eating before you go to bed. Simple concept, right? But we didn't know that if you eat right before you go to bed it's one of the worst things you can do because you have all this excess energy that is generating. You don't need energy when you are sleeping, that is when you recover and repair. Your body has more than enough fuel to compensate for that.

When you have extra and surplus energy running around, you actually cause free radical damage, excessive, and you don't want to compensate for that with antioxidants, because you can take too much anti-oxidants, and how do you know it's enough? You just want to rely on your body's own way to do it.

That's the simplest strategy, and I like to keep things simple and, really, follow patterns that our ancestors did. And our ancestors really never had access to food 24/7. They never did. So they regularly went through these periods where they weren't eating food for a while. So our physiology, our genetics, our biochemistry has adapted to that way of eating.

Ty: Wow, that's a great suggestion for people. Just eat dinner earlier, or skip it.

Dr. Mercola: Yes.

Ty: Because then you reach that period of intermittent fasting that you are talking about.

Dr. Mercola: Yes, it doesn't mean you can't ever eat three meals a day, or even four. I personally don't eat more than two meals a day, with rare exception, and I think it is a healthy process, and I think you can do just fine with that, and it just helps normalize the way you do, and really optimizes your genes and biochemistry because we are based on—I mean, these genes have developed over time, over many generations, and you don't change them in one or two generations, you change them in hundreds of thousands because of the genetics. So we have to honor what our genetic ancestry was exposed to, and that is, in other words, like a Paleo concept, and try to replicate some of those patterns.

And we were never designed to sit down all day long. This is *another problem*. When you are sitting down it causes massive challenges in your system, which it was never designed to do. You were never designed to sit for eight or ten hours a day, so that is why I think it is really good to get up and walk a few miles a day, 7000 to 10,000 steps a day or more, in addition to an exercise program. It is not just exercise, it is movement that is so critical. And it doesn't have to be walking, just as long as you are moving is the key. But typically, it is easier to monitor and track it if you track your steps.

Ty: Yes. So we've got a double whammy today, right? We're sitting—most people sit all day.

Dr. Mercola: I hardly ever sit anymore, I literally sit less than a half-hour a day.

Ty: You're always moving. But the typical American, working at an office job, sitting, and has access to food all day long and all night long.

Dr. Mercola: Yes. And I was confused, I think, as many people are, and it was really a shock to me, because as I mentioned earlier, Cooper was my hero and it really motivated and inspired me to an exercise program. I have been exercising for nearly 50 years now thanks to Dr. Cooper. And I thought that provided me protection from sitting down. Boy, was I surprised when the studies started coming up, it doesn't matter if you are a professional athlete, world class, Olympic caliber, and you're sitting eight to ten hours a day, you are going to die prematurely. You are going to suffer morbidity and complications from that lack of activity. So, we need regular movement throughout the day, not just one hour a day at the gym. That's not going to cut it. It *will* not cut it.

Ty: That will be good news for my son, he counts his steps and he tries to move for hours a day.

Dr. Mercola: You're raising him well. That's good.

Ty: Trying to. Now, one of the things that goes against what I used to believe, I was a competitive bodybuilder for many years, and as competitive bodybuilders we always ate a huge protein meal right before we went to be bed.

Dr. Mercola: Well, that's a different strategy, and if you want to be a competitive bodybuilder and that is your goal, and everyone gets their choices, then you are going to have to eat differently. But a meal and an exercise program for a competitive bodybuilder is not going to be optimized for longevity or treating cancer.

Ty: Right.

Dr. Mercola: Especially with protein, because protein is metabolized very similar to glucose—not identical, but similar, so in other words, if you are going to go on a low sugar diet, and high protein, your body will convert that protein to sugar and you will raise it. So you have to be careful of your protein intake. And in fact, there is some literature to suggest that high protein content will stimulate the MTOR pathway which will increase malignancies. So excessive protein can be a problem. But you are right, you are *not* going to build muscle mass without protein, it just will not work.

Ty: Right.

Dr. Mercola: And I'm a firm believer in strength training. I strongly recommend it to everyone. It is something that I do, I've adopted myself personally, too. In fact, I love the dead lifts.

Ty: And the rows?

Dr. Mercola: The rows—dead lifts more, I think, just because I think it's a great strength-building exercise.

Ty: Yes. So with the ketogenic diet then, the healthy fats are a key, aren't they?

Dr. Mercola: Yes. You have to pay attention to the quality of the food.

Ty: So give me an example of what somebody would look to eat on a ketogenic diet. What would they eat? What would be the—

Dr. Mercola: Well, I think you don't want to make the mistake that I think Atkins made, and I have enormous respect for Dr. Atkins because he helped us understand the dangers of too many carbohydrates. But really, he didn't pay much attention to the quality of the fat, so you have to be really careful of that. So high-quality fats, and examples would be avocadoes, coconut oil, grass-fed, pastured, organic butter, ideally raw, olives. Nuts would be another good source, and you want to be careful to have relatively low protein nuts, so macadamia and pecans would be the two best because they are high in the fat and very low in the protein. Those are some of the top ones.

Ty: Good oils like maybe olive oil? Is that good?

Dr. Mercola: Olive oil, yes, olive oil would work, too. You want to be careful to avoid other oils, the omega 6 oils, the processed oils, the industrialized oils.

Ty: All the vegetable oils that people think are healthy because it says "vegetable."

Dr. Mercola: Oh yes, that is absolutely the worst, because the other factor that is a variable that is really important in the treatment of cancer is something called the omega 6 to the omega 3 ratio, omega 3 being the good fats, of course, like fish oil and ALA from flaxseed and chia seeds. These are beneficial ones, and normally that ratio should be anywhere from one-to-one to five-to-one. The problem is when you have a processed food diet, which is loaded with these Omega 6 industrialized oil, that ratio can go to 20-to-1 to 50-to-1, literally 75 to 100 times what it was last century, around 1900, all because of this industrialization process that allowed us the opportunity to have access to this food. You could not create that food prior to that time. This is really an artifact of modern industry.

Ty: Yes, the technology wasn't even in place.

Dr. Mercola: It did not exist, so it was not a choice. You could not—so it's not a big leap of faith to understand that our bodies weren't designed to be exposed to that type of food. So you have to be careful because it's easy—anyone can easily do that today. And how do you avoid it? You just stay away from processed foods. There are three words that I strongly recommend, three easy words to remember, and that is: Eat real food.

Ty: I love that. Eat real food.

Dr. Mercola: Eat real food. Because when you do that, you know what you accomplish? You avoid the artificial ingredients that are inserted into your food, and most people are not aware that there are over 10,000 chemicals that are labeled GRAS, Generally Recognized As Safe, by the food industry themselves. And by labeling them as GRAS, they are able to penetrate a loophole that allows them never to be tested for human safety, not just singly, but let alone when combined with all the others, so there is synergistic toxicity.

So when you eat real food you avoid the chemicals. You avoid the exposure to these untested chemicals that essentially are making the population a guinea pig, because we have no idea what the chronic exposure to many of these combinations of chemicals will do.

Ty: Because of the fact that these chemicals are generally regarded as safe, but they are not tested.

Dr. Mercola: Never tested. They have been labeled by the food industry.

Ty: So you're right, we are the guinea pigs on that.

Dr. Mercola: Yes. And you could say, "That's okay, I'll just read the label." Well, if you had the eyesight and the glasses to be able to read the 2-point font, and the chemical understanding to read the label, because those are complex chemical terms, *they're not even there!* The loopholes says because they're GRAS, you don't even have to put them on the food label.

Ty: Really?

Dr. Mercola: Yes!

Ty: Wow.

Dr. Mercola: Yes. So there is no way a conscientious consumer could possibly choose the right food in packaged food. So just play it safe, eat real food, which means you, or someone you know or love, or pay, prepares the food. Now, does that mean you have to do it 100 percent? It's almost physically impossible to do that, because you're going to go out to eat at restaurants, and obviously, you are going to delegate that responsibility, but your general pattern, 80 to 90 percent of the time, is to eat real food that is prepared by your or someone you know.

Ty: Think about the way your grandmom and grandpop ate, and eat that.

Dr. Mercola: Absolutely. Or, you've been around the world interviewing experts and you go to places like Eastern Europe where they are still doing that. When I was seeing patients, I was just absolutely delighted when I had patients from Eastern Europe because this is the way they operate. They have hardly any exposure to these processed foods. They get it, at a foundational level. You don't have to try to teach or preach to them or convince them that this is the way we were designed to eat.

Ty: Yes, it was refreshing for us.

Dr. Mercola: Yes, and you are so much healthier, you just avoid so many challenges when you take this approach to a lifestyle and feeding yourself, and then you can avoid all the challenges, because your body is designed to stay healthy. It wants to be healthy. It never was designed to go toward disease so that you have to see a physician who is going to prescribe a medication to treat that. That is not the design. The design is to be healthy. You can easily do that when you are eating real food, exercising the right way, sleeping, getting movement, and your body self-regulates, it heals. And sleeping. And exposure to sunlight, which is why I moved down here so I could have more sunlight in the winter and get vitamin D.

Ty: Talk about that, sunlight and vitamin D.

Dr. Mercola: Vitamin D is literally nothing short of a miracle. It is a God-given miracle, it is a part of the natural plan. We were designed to be exposed to the sun. Unlike most any dermatologist you will see who will warn you and plead with you to stay out of the sun because of their fear of getting a skin cancer, which is most unlikely—yes, people die from skin cancer, but not many. It is a small fraction, probably less than one percent of the people who die from lack of sun exposure and getting other cancers, like prostate and lung cancer, and all these other malignancies—breast cancers.

So vitamin D, we did not understand or appreciate its full value until this century. Last century we didn't know, we just knew that it was available and was primarily thought to treat bone diseases, like Rickets and osteomalacia. But in the late 1990s the commercial labs became available to actually measure this. So they were able to do studies and they found out, "Oh my gosh, 90 to 95 percent of people don't have ideal levels of vitamin D."

And not only is it good for bone disease, but it is good to reduce the risk of the two biggest killers of the human race, which is heart disease and cancer, and the epidemiological studies show that you reduce all cancers by 50 percent when you have adequate vitamin D levels. If that is not almost magical, I don't know what is.

Ty: Can you imagine if big pharma had a drug that reduced all cancers? I mean it would be on every commercial, wouldn't it?

Dr. Mercola: Now, the devil is in the details, right Ty? The danger that we could have is to say, "Okay, let's just swallow this vitamin D and get our vitamin D levels up." And that is one way you can do it, and in many cases it's the only way you have, the only practical option. But that's not the ideal way. The ideal way is to follow the natural pattern, which is to go outside with very little clothing, and so, obviously, you have to be in a very moderate climate, that's usually subtropical or tropical, at least in the winter, and have the sun shine on your skin, because the sun converts a cholesterol precursor to vitamin D, and then vitamin D gets transferred and converted in your body to active metabolites where it does its magic.

And it affects, literally, 10 percent of our genome. It's called an epigenetic influencer, so it optimizes 10 percent of our genes. It's not so much that we are born with this gene that is going to give us breast cancer, it's that our epigenetic, our environmental influences, the food we eat, the exercises we do or don't do, the toxic exposure rates, turn those genes on or off.

And vitamin D is one of the most profound epigenetic influencers of the genetic code. So you don't have to worry about these inherited genes that may cause you to do a prophylactic double mastectomy, that's just insanity from my perspective, and it is an irrational fear, if you appreciate and fully understand the amazing regenerative capacity our body has if it is given the proper tools.

Ty: That's great stuff on vitamin D. And the thing that is really absurd to me is that if you do go out in the sun, be sure you put the sunscreen on that has known carcinogens in it.

Dr. Mercola: And it's even worse than the carcinogens, because the intention was to decrease the risk of skin cancers. Here is the paradox. Sunscreens screen out—there are three types of ultraviolet radiation: UV A, B, and C. C hardly comes down because is it usually filtered out in the atmosphere. But UV A and B. UV A is really the dangerous one, the one that causes most of the cancers, and UV B is what causes our body to make vitamin D. Well, these sunscreens—they filtered UV B so your body couldn't make vitamin D, they essentially stop vitamin D production, and they let UV A light through. So it actually increased the rate of skin cancer, and that's what the studies show. If you use sunscreen you increase your risk of skin cancer. (laughs) So it was just a wacky approach. When we try to use our limited understanding rather than just try to replicate what our ancestors were doing all along. And that's the way I approach natural therapies, is to look in that context, because otherwise, no one is smart enough to figure it out, there are just too many variables involved. And so if you use this natural context, it really helps focus your vision and understanding and helps you have a deeper appreciation of what is going to be beneficial.

Ty: You mentioned earlier the fact that we are sitting all the time and it increases your risk of obesity. So let's talk about obesity, and is there a link between obesity and cancer?

Dr. Mercola: Well, I think it goes back to insulin resistance. There are some studies that show a correlation, and correlation, of course, is not causation. So the central roles, or whatever contributes to obesity, most likely contributes to other diseases. And it could be all the other chronic degenerative diseases like heart disease, and Alzheimer's and diabetes. So cancer is just one of those. That is exactly what you would expect when you are not giving your body what it needs. But insulin resistance is the core, absolutely the core.

And I've known this for 20 years, I'm grateful to Dr. Ron Rosehills, a physician who taught me and helped me appreciate and understand that. And that really has been one of the primary focuses of the way I have treated patients is to understand strategies to address insulin resistance, and there is just no question in my mind the single most effective intervention I have ever seen to address insulin resistance is intermittent fasting, with the right foods, ideally, but intermittent fasting.

Well, you might say, "Well, I can't, I've got to eat every two hours otherwise I will pass out, I'll have no, or low energy." And yes, that's what happens because your body is used to that sugar high and you can't burn fat. But once you make that transition it literally is nothing short of magical. Your body is not hungry anymore, it just isn't hungry. And I've just seen it time and time again, it has changed so many people's lives. I have recommended and encouraged and mentored to apply and adopt that type of eating.

And I really think there is indisputable evidence, if you are interested in longevity, and as you get older most people are (laughs), you know, in living a long, healthy life, so you are not disabled and crippled. You will find that the science is really clear that calorie restriction seems to work. The problem is, who is going to do calorie restriction But you can get most all the same benefits of calorie restriction from intermittent fasting, and none of the pain.

Ty: Yes.

Dr. Mercola: And I don't think we were designed to eat a small amount of calories. In fact, there have been unintentional experiments done, like starvation famine experiments, like during World War II where certain countries didn't have access to food because of the war. And when they go back and review that evidence, those people wound up living a lot longer because they went through periods of time when they didn't have access to a lot of food.

Ty: Yes.

Dr. Mercola: A lot of people are confused about the importance of eating regularly. Your body is designed to survive that and do just fine. Of course, you don't want to be underweight and malnourished, but having a pattern where you are not eating food on a regular basis for at least, I think, 12 to 16 hours a day, is a really powerful strategy, and virtually doesn't cost you anything. In many cases it saves you money because you are eating less food.

Ty: Yes. I'm nodding so vigorously here because the last documentary last year that we released, my college roommate named Dr. Irvin Sahni—he is a medical doctor, we graduated from Baylor 24 years ago—he went to medical school. And he learned some stuff from "The Quest for the Cures" last year about intermittent fasting and a ketogenic diet. He went to a ketogenic diet with 18 hours of intermittent fasting every day and within a period of about four months he dropped 50 pounds and he looks as good as he did in college.

And he just texted me this morning while I'm thinking about this and he's in the gym hitting the punching bag. He's 48 years old now. And he said a little 20-year-old guy said, "Man, you look like you're going to tear the bag up." He was in as good a shape as anybody in the gym and he is almost 50 now.

Dr. Mercola: Exactly what you would expect.

Ty: Yes.

Dr. Mercola: Yes, if you're seeking the truth, eventually, honestly, objectively and sincerely seeking it, this information will hit you. And it is just sad from my perspective that so many physicians fail to seriously investigate this or acknowledge it, or implement it in their practice, because it is a pretty well accepted fact that really, there is very limited, virtually no influence on their medical boards for applying intermittent fasting in their practice. It may be hard from a compliance perspective, or it would require more time to convince people to do it but the effects and the impact on their health would be pretty dramatic. And your friend's example is a really good illustration of that.

Ty: And I think you are dead right, too, that you do it without the pain.

Dr. Mercola: Right.

Ty: Because here, you have a six-hour window each day when you can eat, and you can eat good-sized meals.

Dr. Mercola: Pretty much there is no limit on the amount of calories—none.

Ty: If you are trying to do a two-week fast, you're like, I can't do this.

Dr. Mercola: Oh, no, no, no. I don't even think that's healthy, truthfully. Not even these long, prolonged fasts like water—I think that you may cause more damage than good.

Ty: Sure.

Dr. Mercola: I mean, if you don't have a choice, fine, and maybe it is best in the long run, but…

Ty: Maybe occasionally.

Dr. Mercola: Yes.

Ty: But yes, this is a diet without the pain because you know you have a six-hour or eight-hour period each day that you are going to be able to just pig out on good, healthy food.

Dr. Mercola: Yes.

Ty: But then you have to wait till the next day, but you get to eat again.

Dr. Mercola: Yes, and the kind of question that people have on that time when you are not allowed to eat, essentially the fasting portion is, "Can I have coffee or tea?" And you can, as long as you don't put sugar or cream in them, because essentially, it is water. You could take supplements during that time, too.

Ty: When I do intermittent fasting I'll do a hot tea with stevia.

Dr. Mercola: Yes, that's perfect.

Ty: It's good. It satisfies you.

Dr. Mercola: I didn't show you my stevia out there.

Ty: Oh you have stevia out there—awesome.

Dr. Mercola: I have stevia bushes, yes.

Ty: Well, that leads me to my question. One of the things I wanted to ask you about is for people that don't have an acre where they are growing their own food. I live in Tennessee, we have 15 acres, we grow a lot of our own food, but people may not be able to.

Dr. Mercola: No. Or if you are renting, or you are in an apartment.

Ty: Let's say you are in an apartment, so name something that people can do to provide nutrition that is easy to do in an apartment, let's say.

Dr. Mercola: Well, one of the best strategies, and I learned this at the Hippocrates Health Institute here in Florida, is growing sprouts, and there are a number of different sprouts, there are dozens and dozens of different ones that you can use, but the most efficient and effective one that I've found that seems to provide the best value is sunflower seed sprouts. You can purchase them at many health food stores, or even Whole Foods, but you will pay $30 a pound. But you can grow them yourself for about 10 to 20 cents a pound, which is really a simple strategy. You grow them from seed to harvest in about a week, maybe ten days.

Ty: Really?

Dr. Mercola: Yes, that's all it takes. And you may say, "Well, why would I do that?" Well, it's easy, it's simple, it's fun. Your kids love to see that, it kinds of catalyzes and piques that interest in gardening. But also they are 30 times more nutrient dense than the organic vegetables you grow in your backyard. So it's really a powerhouse of nutrition. It is all condensed and concentrated in those sprouts.

Ty: And you can grow it in your own house.

Dr. Mercola: Yes. Easy to do, simple to do. Ideally, you would use organic seeds, and there are little tricks to it, I've got some details how to do it on the website to give people the specifics, but it's a pretty simple process. You could look on line, too, to figure it out. But I would encourage everyone to do that, and then once you get comfortable with that and you start enjoying that, that is actually the biggest component of my salad is the sunflower seed sprouts. That is the base, and then I add other things to it.

Ty: Yes, we love to put sprouts on our salads, as well, but we haven't done the sunflower seeds.

Dr. Mercola: Oh, sunflower seeds are great.

Ty: Okay.

Dr. Mercola: Yes. They are high in omega 6, but when you sprout them it turns into a plant so it is actually relatively low in fat. If you just eat a half a pound of sunflower seeds you are going to get a lot of omega 6 fats.

Ty: Okay, so by sprouting them you have also activated the enzymes, as well.

Dr. Mercola: Oh, absolutely, and not only the enzymes, but you increase the nutrient density like 30-fold.

Ty: So that is a great, very inexpensive easy way that people can start really packing their meals with nutrition without—

Dr. Mercola: Simple.

Ty: Especially somebody who is on a ketogenic diet, because you don't have a lot of cost there.

Dr. Mercola: I really focus on simple, inexpensive strategies to get people healthy, and what better—why couldn't it be this? I mean, it takes a little time, but not much. We're talking maybe a five to ten minute a week investment. That's not a lot of time.

Ty: They just grow on their own.

Dr. Mercola: Yes, they do. And it's fun to see them grow.

Ty: Yes.

Dr. Mercola: Yes.

Ty: Okay excellent. That's a great suggestion that we're going to add to our salads, because we eat a lot of sprouts, but not sunflower.

Dr. Mercola: And it is *real* food.

Ty: It's real food. Not any of the thousands of chemicals, right?

Dr. Mercola: Right. Totally chemical free.

Ty: Okay, excellent.

Dr. Mercola: These studies show us the dangers of sitting all day long, and I was every bit as guilty, for literally 40 years, I was sitting eight to twelve hours a day. And actually, the last five or six years, mostly, it went up to over twelve hours a day. For the average officer worker it is eight hours a day. Some people don't have a choice because they have an occupation like driving, a taxi driver or a truck driver, where there is just no other real practical option.

But for most of us the simple strategies are, if you are an officer worker is that you can have a stand-up desk. And you might say, "Well, my boss would never do that, my company would never do it." Well, you might be surprised. There are many Fortune 500 companies who are making the shift. And why are they making the shift? Because their employee productivity goes through the roof, for a relatively small investment, not only their productivity, but the health of their employees—their sick time goes down, their efficiency, their energy levels, their ability to produce whatever the product is, or information that they are putting out, increases dramatically. So that's a really strong incentive.

And these stand-up desks—you can get a motorized stand-up desk that comes up and down or you can get a desk that you can put your keyboard and monitor on, and use with your existing desk. So those are both types of strategies, and we actually purchased stand-up desks for our entire office because we so strongly believe in that. So that is one. That will stop you from sitting down. But standing is clearly better than sitting because it radically increases your metabolism and structural forces. But you still want to move and get in different positions and walk.

That's why getting a fitness tracker—you could use your phone, any smartphone has an ability to record your steps. If it doesn't directly, you could download an app that would do that for free. Then you'd have to wear your phone all the time and I'm not a big fan of keeping my phone on my body, so you could use a fitness tracker which is less radiation exposure. And they're easy to do. The typical recommendation is about 7000 steps a day. I'm obsessive-compulsive, so I do about 17,000 steps (laughs).

But I really decided to optimize my lifestyle for health, so I moved down to Florida and I was able to walk about two hours on the beach every day and not only satisfy my movement requirement, but also my sun exposure, and grounding, because that is another component that we didn't really mention but may have some benefit to health, and maybe even the treatment of malignancies. It certainly would only be beneficial.

Ty: When you mention grounding, what do you mean?

Dr. Mercola: I mean connecting to the earth, and again, replicating ancestral patterns, to follow what our ancestors did because typically they were connected, either sleeping or walking on the earth, not in rubber soled shoes. They were directly connected. So you say, "Well, what happens when you do that?" Well, what happens when you are at the beach, or in the ocean? The earth surface has an abundance of electrons, and we need electrons to stay healthy. And when you are connected to the earth those electrons go into your body and they squelch free radicals, and they optimize your health. I mean, they really are required for metabolic processes.

So this grounding is really important, and with our stand-up desks, we have stand-up desk grounding pads that people stand on without shoes, because if you stand on them with shoes it won't work. So that's another thing that you can do. But it's just magnificent. So movement and grounding, just following ancestral practices. If you are replicating what our ancestors did, odds are you are going to be fine-tuning and optimizing the genetics in your biochemistry. It's not rocket science, if you think about it.

And I've studied health for nearly 40 years now, and the more I study, Ty, the simpler it becomes. God was great, he made up a simple plan, just follow the plan. It's not complicated. We make it complicated. Now, it's not that way in every case, and you certainly are going to need qualified, competent healthcare coaches and clinicians and physicians to guide you through and fine-tune and tweak it, but 80 to 90 percent of it is pretty simple. It really is.

Ty: So I guess that pretty much rules out RC Cola and moon pies, then.

Dr. Mercola: Well, you can have almost anything occasionally.

Ty: Every now and then—

Dr. Mercola: Yes, as long as the bulk of your practices are healthy you're going to be fine.

Ty: Now like Casey Craychee mentioned in an interview last year with him. He said, "You know, everybody loves sugar, but it should be one of the fun foods that we eat occasionally, and not a staple." So I think that's a good principle, isn't it?

Dr. Mercola: Yes, you have to enjoy life, and I certainly eat sugar occasionally. It's certainly not my rule. And if you have a healthy lifestyle—I'll give you a little tip. If you want to enjoy sugar, and this is actually another tip for fine-tuning the movement, and you're eating, and integrating them together in a seamless method, is to have your biggest meal before you do your most movement. And if you want to engage in sugar and have that treat, then eat the sugar before you move, because you will burn that sugar as fuel rapidly rather than going through this complex metabolic processes of storing it as fat and causing damage from that.

Ty: So then a good rule of thumb, as you mentioned earlier, don't eat a big meal right before you go to bed.

Dr. Mercola: That's one of the worst things you could do.

Ty: And that's one of the reasons why.

Dr. Mercola: That is one reason why for sure. I mean, to have an ice cream before you go to bed it's like, oh my gosh. Yes, it's not that ice cream by itself is bad, especially if you have it before you do an activity, and if it is a high quality one, not one loaded with a lot of toxins and junk, or if you make it yourself, it would be even better.

Ty: Yes. Well, we do. I've got four kids.

Dr. Mercola: Yes, there you go.

Ty: We get the raw cream, and the organic non GMO sugar, and whatever else she uses in it. It's all natural. Fresh fruit.

Dr. Mercola: There you go. Stevia.

Ty: Stevia. Yes, sure. Well, she'll use honey it a lot of times, raw honey.

Dr. Mercola: Yes, sure.

Ty: So, yes, it's a good food, if you make it. I guess, a lot of things, what you said, though, with these Generally Regarded As Safe chemicals, we don't even really know what is in some of the food that we are eating.

Dr. Mercola: It's literally physically impossible to know. By design. I didn't realize how nefarious the food industry was until I read Marion Nestle's book which will be out in October 2015 called *Soda Politics*. And they are every bit as evil as the drug companies with respect to their political lobbying, they are a revolving door between industry and the federal regulatory processors. The whole system is stacked against you.

But the good news is that you can easily avoid it by eating real food. You don't have to worry about it. They are counting on the fact that you're not, that you're going to be what the typical American, who has 95 percent of his calories—95 percent of his calories is processed food—95 percent.

Ty: Wow, that's amazing. I didn't know it was that high—95 percent processed.

Dr. Mercola: The typical American. That's not you and me, but the average American, it is 95 percent. So they've got a long way to—now does it have to be 100 percent real food? No. You can have 5 to 10 percent, it's probably okay. The lower the better, of course, and the less pernicious the better. But that's the strategy, is to eat as healthy as you can.

Ty: I think that's a great take-away from this interview. Eat real food.

Dr. Mercola: Eat real food. Keep it simple.

Ty: I love it. Yes, keep is simple. Dr. Mercola, thank you so much.

Dr. Mercola: Thank you.

[end of transcript]

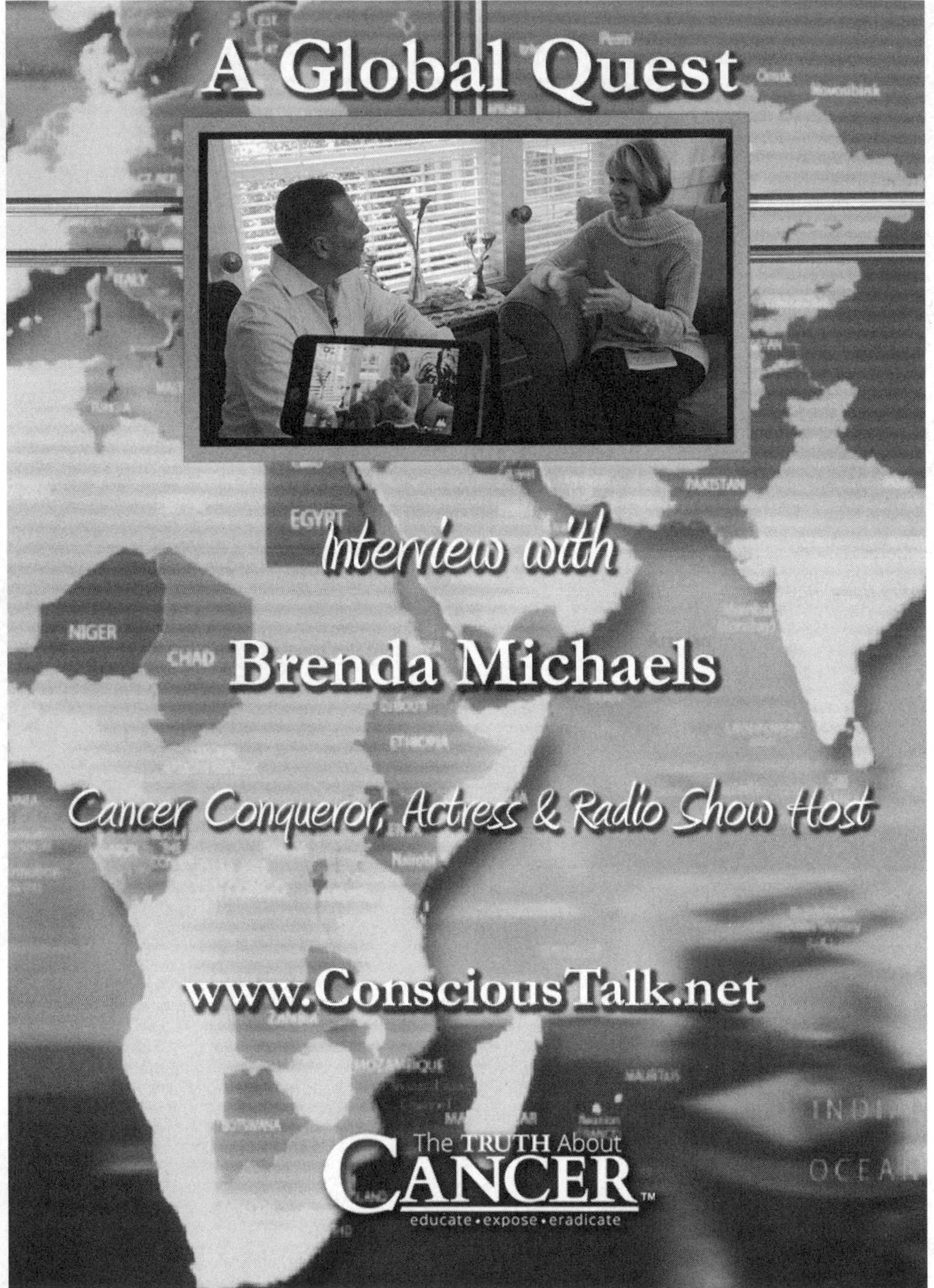
A Global Quest
Interview with
Brenda Michaels
Cancer Conqueror, Actress & Radio Show Host
www.ConsciousTalk.net
The TRUTH About
CANCER
educate • expose • eradicate

Ty: I'm really excited to be here today in Issaquah, Washington with Brenda Michaels at her lovely home. Thank you for joining us today.

Brenda: Thank you for having me.

Ty: Thank you for the invitation out here. It's really lovely here.

Brenda: Isn't it great? It's a beautiful area.

Ty: It is. It's a little bit different than I was expecting because you hear Pacific Northwest, I was expecting rain and clouds, and gloom. And it's really beautiful up here.

Brenda: We tell everybody that so they stay away.

Ty: That's a good technique, right? I think you're going to have some people coming from California here shortly. I've got a feeling.

Brenda: Oh I think so. Definitely.

Ty: Really beautiful.

Brenda: Yeah, it's lush. That's why we're here.

Ty: Well, I hear great things about you from Dr. Nick Gonzalez. You come highly recommended as an interviewee, so that's why we're here. Nick recommended that we talk to you about your cancer journey. So I want to get all of that information from you today. But let's walk back to when you were a child. You mentioned that you had some issues growing up that you think might have contributed.

Brenda: You know, we all grow up in dysfunctional families. And if I knew then what I know now, I could have handled myself differently. But as children, we only know what we see and what we're taught by our parents, and what we hear. And I came from a family that was very chaotic. There was a lot of yelling and screaming in my house, there was a lot of bickering. There was a lot of anger. My dad was very rageful. He did a good job of sitting on it but when he got triggered enough, he would explode. And you know, he was raised as a young boy to be disciplined with whatever was handy, a stick, a belt, whatever.

So he disciplined us that way as well. And so there was a lot of that physical type of abuse in our house. And sometimes it went over the top. My mother was emotionally unavailable for the most part. So it didn't feel like we could go to her to be really protected. She did her best, but my dad was a very strong, a very dominating male. His home was his castle, and he ran it like a castle, and he was the king. That's kind of how I grew up. I was the sensitive one in the family. I was sensitive to the environmental issues.

I grew up in a farming community, lots of fertilizers, lots of pesticides, that kind of thing. So I was really exposed to all of that. But I was also the sensitive one when it came to emotions and that type of thing, so I took all that in really deeply. And I was affected by it. I was the kid that was sick all the time. I was also one that broke out with acne and didn't realize how toxic I was. Living in that environment was really harmful to my health. I had to learn all of that. And I learned it as I looked back but when you're a child that's all you know. So I really feel all of that emotional degradation I went through, the physical abuse, the chaos all the time. I'm one that loves peace. I was the middle child, so I was a peacemaker. It was really difficult for me to navigate, and it affected my body, my immune system, all of it.

Ty: But I guess one of the positive things that came out of the fact that you were the emotional one, or one of the emotional ones, was your acting career, correct?

Brenda: Oh yes.

Ty: I mean, so that's one of the things that most actors and actresses have in common, is that trait.

Brenda: Yes. Well, I also learned to protect myself. You become who you're not. You take on certain patterns, certain behaviors, that are not who you are. And I was very good at that. I was a chameleon. I was also a people pleaser, I wanted people to like me. I did everything I could to get my dad to like and accept me, and my mom too, to pay attention to me, to give me what I needed and I wasn't getting. So I think all of that probably contributed to the actress part of me as well.

Ty: So when you moved to LA, you worked on some soap operas. What did you do out there?

Brenda: Oh, yes. And commercials. I was on, what is it called now? I never watch these anymore. I think they're still on, the hospital one. There's one on.

Ty: General Hospital?

Brenda: Yes. General Hospital. I'd have to pull my resume out. I was a day player on several of those. I did commercials. I did a couple of plays. But probably the most exciting thing for me was when I did my own television show with another lady. We started interviewing Deepak Chopra when he first came out with his very first book. That was really fun for me, to interview people that had that spiritual wisdom and that deepness. I just loved doing that. And then I went from that at one point, to doing some radio, which is what I do today with my husband. We do our radio show, *Conscious Talk Radio*. We've been doing it 14 years now. My dream is to actually get back into television again one day. But to do really meaningful things.

Ty: What was it you said before we sat down? I should have made a note of it. You said now you're doing things that are more meaningful.

Brenda: Yes. I used to do it for fame and money. Now I'm doing it for meaning. I'm making meaning in my life and the lives of others. I feel like it's sort of a service, to help people. And that has brought tremendous amount of joy into my life.

Ty: Well that's great that you're able to do that now. It's a great transition. But one of the things that started the transition was when you were diagnosed with cancer, right? So let's go back there.

Brenda: Well, that's really what brought it all forward for me. I say to a lot of people when they have that disease that they don't realize yet what a gift that can be in their lives. Because it is a wake-up call if you take it that way. It's all how we perceive things, Ty. My perception was not quite there when I was diagnosed the first and second time.

But the third time, when I was told that I had about a year to live if I was unwilling to do the chemo, which I'd been all along, and that the cancer would metastasize, and maybe within a year there would be no hope for me. That stirred something very deep inside of me, and I began to awaken. And it was not an easy journey.

I still had my fears. I still had days where I felt like maybe it was easier to die than it was to live. I went through all of that. But all along, underneath all that, was this guidance that I had never opened up to before, that I was beginning to follow. And that guidance, just step by step, day by day, it led me, and it saved my life.

Ty: Well, talk about the type of cancer that you had, it was late-stage, was it stage four?

Brenda: It was, oh boy, I wish Dr. Gonzalez would say it was stage four, whatever it was. He told me what it was. It's a very long name. It's a very aggressive breast cancer. I don't know if it was stage three or four. I don't know that. I do know that he said it was very aggressive and the name for it I can't even pronounce.

Ty: Okay. But they said it was late-stage.

Brenda: Yes.

Ty: And supposedly terminal, you had less than a year to live.

Brenda: Yes, they were saying that I had, without chemo, they thought that they could maybe give me five years. That was a maybe. But without it, they thought that within a year, they were pretty sure it would metastasize and there would be nothing they could do. Remember, it started with cervical cancer at the age of 26.

Ty: Oh, that's how it began. Okay.

Brenda: Yes, that's how it began. I lost my ability to have children then. And then they told me if I went five years, more than five years, that I was cancer free. Well, I went 13 years between the first diagnosis and the second, which was in my left breast. I discovered the lump and I had it checked by three different physicians. And I was told that it was an infected milk gland. There was a red ring around the lump and the lump was sitting right on my nipple. It was protruding, so you could see it, but it burned like fire in there.

They'd give me a course of antibiotics, and the burning would go away, but the lump never did. I moved to LA at that time. I was living, for a short time here, and had doctors checking it here telling me that. I moved to LA, and one of the things that I pursued in LA besides acting was modeling. I was doing the modeling job for a lady in Beverly Hills. I was up doing a trunk show one day, which is you walk out and you model the clothes, and they have people sitting there, the buyers are there. She pulled me back to the back room and pulled me to the side and asked me why my sparkle was missing.

She said, "You're not sparkling out there. Are you okay?" And my breast was really hurting. It was burning and hurting, and throbbing. So I told her and she panicked. So after that trunk show was complete, she called her surgeon in Beverly Hills and he said, "She has to come in right away." And they got me in the next day. It was a really wonderful surgeon there. The first thing he said to me, he just felt the lump and looked at it, and he said, "Why haven't you had something done about this?" And I just broke into tears, because I had been trying for nearly two years. So I'm sitting with this cancer in my breast for two years.

He took a biopsy of it. No one had ever done that, out of there, and had it diagnosed right away. He made me wait in his office, actually. He wanted to get the results that day and he did. And it was cancer.

Ty: And so, at that point, was that the recommendation from him, chemotherapy immediately?

Brenda: That tumor was contained which he felt good about. He thought he got clean margins. He offered it up, it wasn't a must-do, but he wanted me to consider it. And I said no. I really didn't want to. So he put me in touch with a doctor that put me on Tamoxifen.

I was on that for a time. I actually stopped taking it on my own because one of the side effects of Tamoxifen is that it vaginally really dries you out. I kept getting yeast infections and they couldn't seem to control that.

Ty: What year was this? I guess this the first diagnosis of the breast cancer right?

Brenda: Yes, this is 1988.

Ty: So just a side note then, I don't know if you're aware of this but in 1996 the World Health Organization declared Tamoxifen to be a known carcinogen.

Brenda: I know. I was, but see I was kind of tuning in a little bit then and listening. I was actually listening to my body then. I just couldn't deal with the yeast infections, so I just stopped taking it. I didn't tell my doctor. I just stopped on my own because he would have been very upset with me. But one year later, I was sent in to have a mammography on my right breast.

And here's something interesting. When they were doing the surgery on my left breast, I had asked my doctor to maybe take a look at my right breast. Number one, I'd been reading up on things, and I knew there was a possibility that breast cancer could be bilateral. Okay, that was one possibility.

But I had had a lump in that breast 15 years earlier that was deep in the tissue and they couldn't aspirate it with a needle so they had to do some surgery. When they got in there it was filled with fluid. But I had scar tissue there from the surgery. And I have learned that you can often have cancer in a scarred area and not even know it.

I felt intuitively something wasn't right. So I told my surgeon this and he did another mammography. He felt around, and he said, "No, I don't think it's necessary that we invade this breast when we're taking off the other one." So he didn't do it. And a year later they did find cancer, not only in that scarred area, but now it had spread below, the cancer, and into lymph nodes at this point.

That was a year after they removed my left breast.

Ty: So this was 1989?

Brenda: Yes.

Ty: Okay, so this is how many years after the initial cervical cancer diagnosis?

Brenda: Well, I was 26 years old, and this was, that was 13, 14, years later that I had that second, that third diagnosis.

Ty: Okay, so now we're sitting here over 30 years later.

Brenda: We're sitting here from the time that I felt I was really on my feet and really healed, it's been 14, it's been 25 years since then.

Ty: Twenty-five years.

Brenda: Yes. But that whole thing happened almost 30 years ago.

Ty: So then, let's go to the third diagnosis then.

Brenda: This breast.

Ty: The right breast. And then talk about how you chose to treat the cancer and the prognosis at that point.

Brenda: Right. That's when something in me began to awaken. And I realized that I had a systemic problem and I wanted to know why. I asked my surgeon and the oncologist that had diagnosed the Tamoxifen for me and they didn't know. They didn't have concrete answers.

So what I did is I began a lot of prayer, a lot of meditation, I started journaling, I started asking questions, and I started getting answers from inside instead of outside of me. And that changed my whole world.

I was really getting connected, I feel, to my higher self, my spirit, whatever you want to call it. I was calling all that information forth. I was willing to trust that information, and trust my body. And my body was giving me signals.

Because when I asked about chemotherapy, Ty, I would get this sort of real deep clenching in my gut. Sometimes almost painful, and then when I would say something because I didn't know what to do, I had no idea there was an alternative out there of any kind. I would say something like, "If there was something out there better for me, would that be helpful?"

And that clenching would just completely release. So I knew, even though I didn't know where to go and what to do. I knew I couldn't walk the path they were asking me.

Ty: You knew there must be a better way.

Brenda: I did. I intuitively knew that.

Ty: Right. I think you hit on one of the key points. You talked about the fact that it's systemic, right? So, talk about that. The fact that with modern oncology, we don't really look at it as a systemic disease, as cancer is more isolated, so they see a tumor, they cut the tumor out, but they don't look for the underlying causes.

Brenda: Right, absolutely. They don't look at the body as a holistic body. We have a spiritual body, an emotional body, a mental body, and a physical body. And in the Bible it says, "As above, so below."

In fact, I wrote a book I titled it *The Gift of Cancer*. I didn't write it alone. I wrote it with my co-writer, Marsha Mercant, who's an incredible lady, and she has a whole great story of how we came together. But I had thought about when the subject of writing a book came up, I thought about titling it *The Final Messenger*, because the body is the final message for us.

Everything starts in our spiritual energy. Patterns, our energetic patterns, lay in that energetic field. And then those patterns move down into mental fields, emotional fields, and finally, your physical body. So, I knew just from—if you're asking me how I knew all this, I was getting almost like downloads of information.

Because I was reading, and I was passionate about learning, and I was sitting in meditation, and I was doing a lot of automatic writing and journaling. So these answers were coming to me and if I couldn't get the answer inside, all of a sudden, a book would show up. Some of the things I'd been asking about were written in the book.

I realized that there is a spiritual and an emotional component to all illness and that if we don't address those, and clear those patterns, we re-manifest. I had re-manifested this disease three times. I know that they look at original incidence of cancer, but I also know that they're looking at the number of recurrences that happen with people.

Why is that happening? If the chemo puts you into remission, and if it's five years or more, and you're supposed to be cured, why are some people, a lot of our clients that we work with, have had it come back after 10 years, 6 years, 8years, 20 years. Why is that happening? Well, I feel and believe, the pattern is still in the field. Those dysfunctional patterns that open us up for illness and disease to be present, are still there.

If we go back and trigger those through old ways of thinking, through old beliefs that don't serve us, through things that we hold on to, that we're not willing to let go of, maybe old angers and resentments, and un-forgiveness, all of that is part of that pattern. And all of that manifests in the body in forms of illness and disease and for me it was simply cancer. I don't look at it as a disease. I look at it as a symptom.

Ty: Symptom, right. Symptom of something that's wrong.

Brenda: Yes, something deeper. Something that's calling out to be healed, calling out for your attention. To want to fight it the way we're taught, to want to get rid of it the way we're taught,we're in a contracted state of energy doing that. We're in fear and contraction, and we're going to fight this thing, and we're going to beat it with all we're worth. Is that really a healing environment? That didn't make sense to me.

I'm looking for healing. I'm not looking for a cure per se because they told me once I was cured and I wasn't. So I was out after healing. And you have to create a healing environment. And that means emotionally, spiritually, mentally and physically.

Ty: You're making way too much sense. Right? Because it does make sense, right?

Brenda: It does make sense.

Ty: You've got to cure, you've got to treat the whole person. And so does it make sense to treat a sick body with a chemical that can kill you?

Brenda: No. And just on that practical level, I have to tell you, my little mind said, "Does it really make sense to make me sicker to get me well?" Everything in me screamed no. And that was just on a practical level. That was at the beginning of all this, some of those things were already showing up for me.

But it's because I was willing to walk into it, to face it, to embrace it, to discover, and I went into it with a lot of curiosity. I wanted to explore this, and learn. And we're not given much time to do that, because the doctors tell us we have a certain amount of time to live, and we're known as a culture, when cancer comes up, even the word, the c word, people go into this paralysis and this deep fear.

I really understand that. But we cannot heal something, we can't be with, and own, and learn about, and move through. We can't heal something we're pushing away from us. We can only heal what we embrace and own.

Ty: Right. I think one of the problems, let me know if you agree with this, is the fact that there's such a spirit of fear that's created today when somebody has that diagnosis. They're paralyzed.

Brenda: Oh they are. And then the mind grabs a hold of it, of that fear, and the mind begins to create a story, or a multitude of stories around that. Then we input those stories with our emotions.

So we put in the fear part, and then we put in the really sad part, because we're sick, and then we might put in the angry part, "How could this happen to me?" We infuse that story with all those negative emotions. And that isn't a healing environment. It's also a way that we suffer. We suffer because of the stories keep playing and replaying, and playing and replaying.

Ty: I think the stories start when you go into the oncologist office, and they say, "If you don't do what I say, you're dead." And that would create fear in almost anybody.

Brenda: Of course.

Ty: Because we're taught to trust their—

Brenda: And to give someone a death sentence, it's—

Ty: We're taught to trust their judgement, right?

Brenda: Absolutely.

Ty: And talk about that, you mentioned that they're giving a death sentence.

Brenda: Yes. They give you a death sentence and people in that vulnerable place, they take that in. They take it in with every fiber of their being. And what does it become for some people, and a lot of people? A self-fulfilling prophecy.

Ty: Yes. It becomes reality, doesn't it?

Brenda: It becomes a reality. Our thoughts and our perceptions, and the beliefs that sponsor all that are how our experiences are going to be. We're going to live through those experiences with those thoughts, those beliefs, and that perspective. Because we are co-creators here. We do create our own reality.

We create it with those instruments that we infuse with all this emotion. A wonderful mentor of ours, Jim Self, he said, "Thoughts are electrical and emotions are magnetic." So you get a thought, and it goes through the electrical system of the body, and it recruits an emotion or a group of emotions, and those emotions magnetically draw to you your experiences.

So if you're not aware of what you're thinking, if you're not aware of what emotions that you're infusing those thoughts with, then you're unconsciously creating. So it's really about being aware. That awareness is the beginning, to me, of healing and waking up.

Ty: So talk about the first time that you walked through the doors of Dr. Gonzalez's office.

Brenda: Oh, I loved him, and it was scary as hell, I have to tell you. I was married to my second husband, who really supported me through this whole time. I walked into his office, it was very cold that day, and I saw about five or six people in there. And honest to God, Ty, they looked like death warmed over. These people were not living.

I could tell these people were dying. I was terrified, and I thought, "Oh my God, if these are his patients, I'm in trouble here." So I sat down, and I was clammy, and I was shaking. I was so scared, and so nervous. I couldn't settle my system down. Because I wasn't sure on that physical level what he was going to report back to me.

I'd never met him before. So it was the newness of that and it was just being in that energy. But that's very difficult energy. It's very dense, heavy energy to navigate and I'm sensitive to all of that.

What I loved about him is he came out and he introduced himself to his patients and took them in. He didn't have a nurse leading them in there. I really thought was a very nice thing for him to do. It made me feel more comfortable with him. I sat down across the desk from him and he talks very fast, as you know. You know who he is. He was just a fount of information about the physical body and about cancer in relationship to that. Things that no other doctor had ever shared with me before.

I immediately liked him. I immediately appreciated what he was doing. I was so inspired by his courage to do what he was doing, because you know, like Burzynski and a lot of other doctors have been attacked in this field, and put out of business, a lot of them. So I was very stirred inside by him.

My heart opened to him and I just knew that for me physically, that he could really help me physically. I was going to work on the emotional, mental, and spiritual sides. I had already made the commitment to do that.

But I knew that particular program that he was offering, I just intuitively knew that was going to, again, change my life. Change the way I eat, change the way I think of food, change the way I think of our environment, all of that. I was elated. I was so excited about this.

I wanted to learn all I could about it. And that, again, that sense of curiosity. I wasn't focusing on beating cancer, I was focusing on wellness and well-being and what I could learn from that. It was a passion. I was very passionate about it, I am to this day.

Ty: So you mentioned that Dr. Gonzalez did a really great job of the physical healing, getting that going for you. But the emotional and the mental was something that you had to undertake? Can you describe the process that you took control of those healing aspects of your journey?

Brenda: The very first step I took was prayer, and then learning to meditate, and then I'm starting to want information. And literally, I have to tell you, this was sort of a magical journey for me because I was so committed. I'd made that internal commitment to find out what was at the bottom of this for me.

That's an important point I want everyone to understand. You have to commit to something in order to draw to you what you need to learn about it. So I really made that deep commitment, and I started receiving books, and I started receiving information. I was learning to journal and do automatic writing. I did that as well.

I did my prayers and meditation. I asked questions and waited for answers. I was waking up and becoming aware that I may not hear that answer in meditation but I might hear it from someone like you, that spoke something. And, oh my gosh, that's answering one of the questions I asked.

Or maybe the answer showed up in a book. Or maybe it showed up on a billboard. Maybe it's in the music, in the verse in the music. I stayed open and aware, but I didn't stop until I got my answers. I asked with all my heart. You have to get your heart and soul involved in this process, and when you do, everything you need is given to you.

Ask and you shall receive. We have a hard time receiving a lot of times, because we don't believe we deserve to, or we don't believe it's really going to happen to us. Who are we to get that kind of knowledge or wisdom?

There are a lot of things that you have to be willing to surrender and move and heal in your life, so you can be open to that wisdom. And I wasn't going to stop until I was.

Ty: What did you learn, Brenda, about the treatment protocol that Dr. Gonzalez uses to treat cancer?

Brenda: Well, I learned that I was eating a lot of the wrong foods. I learned that I wasn't eating organically. What I was eating was smothered in pesticides, and herbicides, that type of thing. I learned that I wasn't eating particularly right for my body at the time, and for the condition that I was in.

I learned that I was extremely toxic, and that I needed to be detoxified. He had these amazing, very difficult, detoxifying procedures. But I learned about that. I learned about coffee enemas, something that most people go, "Oh my God, don't tell me, don't share that with me."

But when I learned about what the coffee bean holds and how it helps to open up those pores in the liver, to draw the toxins out of the liver, it made sense to me. So instead of pushing all that away, because for a lot of people the diet is so strict having to take the pills every so often and waking up in the middle of the night and having to do coffee enemas.

Because I had met some of his patients after that who were in such resistance to it, I made the decision that day to go for the gold with it. And that was it. It was going to become my life now for however long it needed to be and I was going to be with it. I was going to make the very best of it. And I did.

I was an actress then and I was going out on a lot of auditions. When I got jobs I brought a cooler of my own food with me. I brought all my vitamins and stuff. I brought it all and when people would ask me I'd share with them what I was doing.

Ty: And when you'd say the pills, the enzymes, a lot of enzymes?

Brenda: Enzymes, vitamins, minerals. I was taking 143 different vitamins, minerals, and enzymes a day. Five days on, two days off. And then, in between, I was doing these very heavy detoxifying procedures that he has his patients do.

Ty: Can you describe those detox regimens that Dr. Gonzalez had you on?

Brenda: Well, there's one where you have to drink oranges and grapefruit juice, and lemons, all together, in a big jar, a gallon of it. You have to drink it. And that's all you can drink. You're on a fast with that for a couple of days. And what you do in between, which is Godawful, is you have to take, oh what's it called? Epsom salts in warm water and dissolve it and drink it down. Oh my God, that was torture.

Ty: I can see it in your face.

Brenda: Oh, that was just torturous. And I would do everything I could to psych myself up for it because I had to do it. Once a month, we had to do these different detoxifying procedures and intestinal cleanses where you have to drink the strawberries and the raw milk and drink that down. Then you have to drink olive oil and you have to do the Epsom salts. So those were some of those things that I had to do beyond the coffee enemas.

Ty: So Brenda, was it all worth it?

Brenda: Oh my God, yes. I learned so much. I mean, I'm in my 60s, I'm the healthiest I feel I've ever been. My life works, and it works because I started to heal those emotional and spiritual wounds that I carried and started to adjust my thinking and become aware and wake up. I went for the gold in that arena as well.

And combining it all, it was a gift. That's why I said, *The Gift of Cancer*. I couldn't be here today, where I'm at, had I not traversed that particular disease. It was perfect for me. I know that sounds weird, in a weird kind of a way, but it was exactly what I needed.

Ty: What is your message, Brenda, to somebody that might have been recently diagnosed with cancer, maybe even terminal cancer, according to the oncologist? Is there always hope for them?

Brenda: Oh, always. First of all, there's always hope. But I do know one thing. We don't know what our walk is, Ty. When I have cancer patients that come to me for coaching and they want to know, "Am I going to live?" I don't know. And neither do they really. You don't know.

But what I offer is the hope in healing whatever is at the core of that for them if they're meant to be here they will be and they will have a blessed life. And if not, they can still heal the dis-ease, the wounding, and have a very incredible quality of life until that day is there.

We're all going the same direction, we're all leaving at some point. I don't mean to make light of that. But I work, and my husband is with me on this, we work with our clients to help them move through some of that fear of death so that they can be engaged in their healing and not focused over here on the disease and the death part.

Because what you give thought to, you flow energy to. So if that's all you're focused on, you're giving that a lot of power in your life. That's not where you want to be. You want to be over here giving power to what you want. So we help them to stay here.

Ty: That's a great message for people to remember.

Brenda: Absolutely. What we focus on is what we get. And when we focus in a direction of getting rid of something, it's like trying to get rid of weight. What are you focused on? You're focused on the weight. What message does that send the universe? "Oh wait, we're getting more weight."

They stick with the thing that they're resisting the most. It's like this, and they judge it, and that even sticks it even harder to them. Where you want to be is you want to acknowledge the problem and be able to be with it, and squarely look at it, and examine it, and explore it. And then you want to move over here.

"What am I going to do about it? I'm going to focus here. I know about this. Now I want to learn about this. And this energy, this is what I'm going to give my energy to. This is what's going to create the new story in my life." We live and die by our stories. So that's what we do with our clients.

I want them to focus and to write a vision for themselves. I wrote a vision for me, and when I was finally able to work out, which Dr. Gonzalez did not let me do very much of in the beginning. But a couple of years down the road I got to start working out again. I would just, in my vision, see myself, that healthy person, walking right toward me.

What did she look like? How did she feel? What was the texture, and the colors? I was very vivid with my imagination. I could see her. Because I was her, I was becoming her. That's where my focus was.

Ty: So how many years ago was it that you began to write this new story in your life, this new vision?

Brenda: About 27-28 years ago.

Ty: And that was about when you were told that you would be dead within a year?

Brenda: Yes. It was. I did see my one oncologist, who I really admire and respect. I know he's retired now, but I still really admire and respect him. I saw him at a black tie function in LA and he spotted me, I didn't spot him. He came across the room and I kind of felt his presence and I turned around and there he was.

He was just smiling at me. He hugged me and he said he was shocked to see me. And he said, "Oh my gosh, Brenda, you look wonderful. Whatever you're doing, keep doing it." And I said, "Would you like to know what I'm doing? Because I have a tape from my doctor that could help you." And he said, "Nope. Nope."

And the energy sort of went up. The shield went up and there was a little bit of small talk and then he walked off. So I got it. I get why he's invested there, that's what he knows. That's his livelihood.

Granted, he helped a lot of people in a lot of different ways. But I knew I could help him learn about how to help his patients detoxify while they're going through their treatments, to eat better, to eat organically. I was hoping he'd be open, but he wasn't.

Ty: He wasn't.

Brenda: No.

Ty: Too much of a vested interest in the status quo.

Brenda: Well, he had been practicing it for 30-some years. At the time, I got it, I understood.

Ty: That reminds me of a quote from Mark Twain that it's easier to fool people than to convince them they've been fooled. And I think that applies for the oncologists. You know?

Brenda: Yes. Well, I knew Dr. Gonzalez. I was in touch with the producer of Michael Landon's shows and when Michael had his pancreatic cancer I was able to set up a meeting for Michael Landon and Dr. Gonzalez.

And I think Michael was a little surprised when Dr. Gonzalez shared with him that a lot of his patients were actually oncologists. A lot of Dr. Gonzalez's patients were oncologists. Medical doctors that had exhausted that model and were still having the problem. He was kind of their last ditch effort.

Ty: What ended up happening with Michael Landon? I'm not aware.

Brenda: Michael brought his, not his producer who I was in touch with, but another very close friend that worked with him on the set. This person was very skeptical of Dr. Gonzalez and his program. Michael never did get on the program. I think he listened to his friend, and his fear was talking.

It takes a lot of trust and it takes a lot of courage. I don't want to make light of that. To step out of a model we've all been conditioned to believe is the only answer, to step away from that into unknown land, is very scary. I have great compassion for people who simply are not able to do it. Because not everybody can.

Ty: It does take a lot of courage, doesn't it?

Brenda: It does. You bet. I mean, I was kind of flying by the seat of my pants back then. Because I didn't know about Dr. Gonzalez. I didn't know about alternative therapies. I had no inkling that I had something to do with why I was sick. No inkling.

I just thought I got cancer. You know? You catch a cold. Well nothing happens randomly, nothing. Everything expresses for a great purpose and it's a purpose much greater than our small minds, I feel, can even comprehend. But we have to dig for that gold.

Ty: I think you actually dug for it, you found it.

Brenda: I did.

Ty: Well, I really appreciate you taking the time to give us your story today, because, I wouldn't listen to an obese person talk about how to lose weight, because they don't know, obviously. But you know what you're talking about. You've walked the walk here for 25 plus years and you're alive when you were supposed to be dead.

So I think that this interview's going to be some really great information for people to listen to, to learn from, and they can believe in. Because you're walking the walk.

Brenda: I am, and I'm loving my life. I have a great life. I have an incredible husband. I have a job that, I mean, like you, doing interviews and talking to people that have that wisdom and that courage, and life can't get a whole lot sweeter. Maybe it can. If it does, I'm open to it. But I am, I'm feeling really, really good in my life.

Ty: Well, I appreciate it. You made my job as an interviewer easy today.

Brenda: Thank you.

Ty: Because you're such a good interviewee. So thank you for the time today and for your story.

Brenda: Oh gosh, thank you, Ty. I really appreciate what you are doing so much.

Ty: Thank you.

Brenda: And we're going to have you on our radio show tomorrow.

Ty: I'm looking forward to it.

[end of transcript]

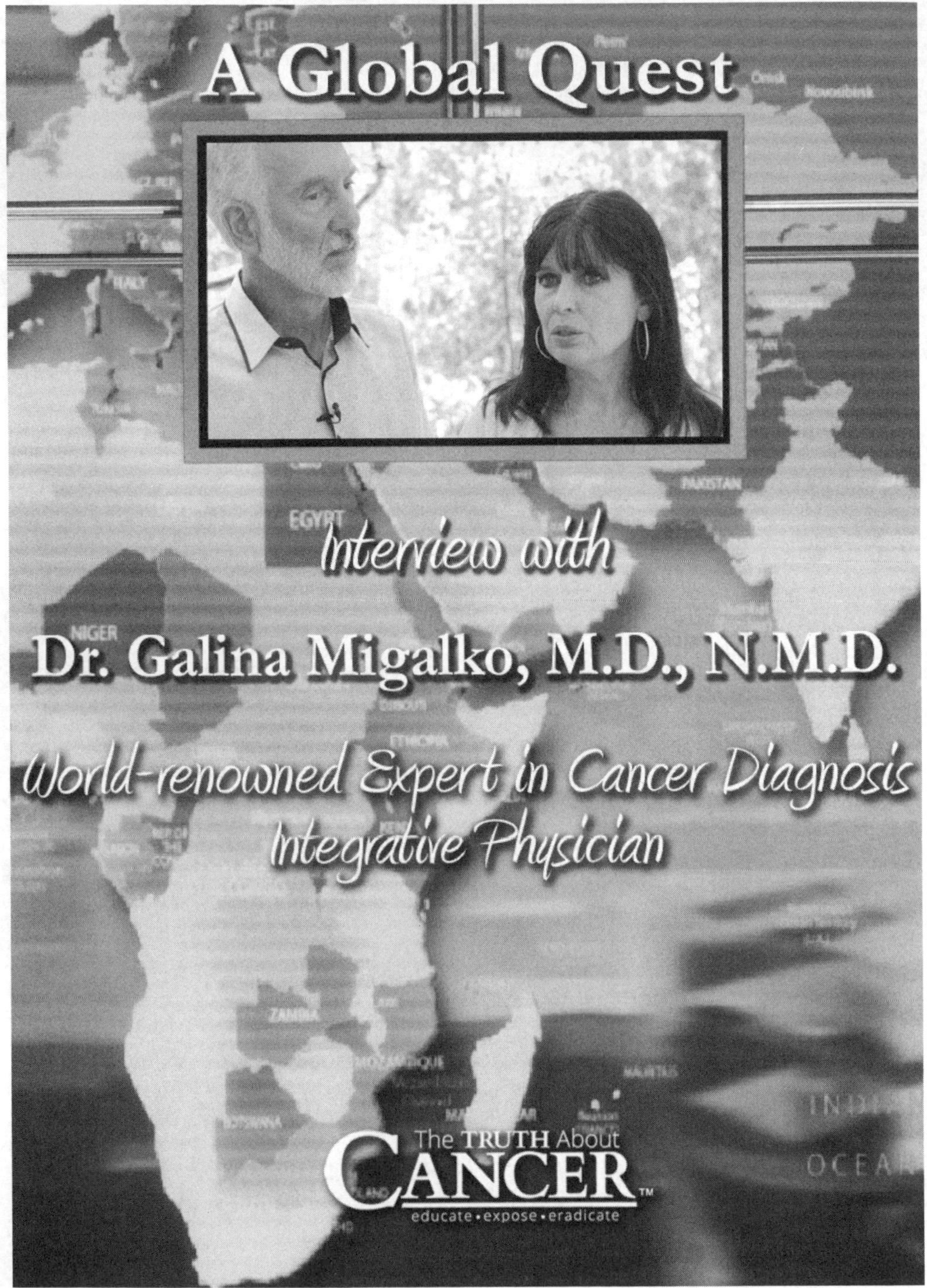
A Global Quest
Interview with
Dr. Galina Migalko, M.D., N.M.D.
World-renowned Expert in Cancer Diagnosis
Integrative Physician
The TRUTH About
CANCER
educate • expose • eradicate

Dr. Ben: This Dr. Galina Migalko, she is the most amazing imaging specialist on the planet. She has invented the triple scan, which combines full body thermography, full body BioScan and full body ultrasound and synthesizing those together.

So I require all of my cancer patients to go to Dr. Galina because she gives me more information about them than all of the blood work and all of the CTs and MRIs could ever, because she is looking at the physiology, the function, and the anatomy, not just anatomy. Those others are all tests of anatomy.

Tell us a little bit about what you do, Dr. Galina.

Dr. Migalko: Thank you Dr. Ben. I really enjoy working with you and with your patients and I really appreciate you for your referrals to help your patients understand the cause of the disease and the issues.

After maybe 25 years of experience with diagnostic medical imaging, I realize that it's really good to have noninvasive, nonradioactive ultrasound imaging, but it's not the answer to all questions we have.

We want to know not only about anatomy, but also physiology and functional information. That's why I created the full body scan, which includes full body ultrasound, full body thermography and full body functional scan we call BioScan to give this information not only to a patient, but to referring physicians.

We believe it is very, very important because the information we are getting is unbelievable and equal to maybe 15 doctor's appointments. Because we see if there is a tumor present in the body, if there is a calcification or dilated duct or physiological changes like inflammation.

We only can see inflammation with thermography. We can see information from functional tests, very unique information, for example like electrical potential of your cells, conductivity of your cells, the pH of your interstitial fluid. Doctors usually don't even look at that information.

Dr. Ben: Phase angle.

Dr. Migalko: Absolutely. We have patients 16 to 20 percent of interstitial fluid in our body and a patient can come with normal blood tests showing normal pH and normal calcium and magnesium, but interstitial fluids showing a spike of calcium.

Why is that? Because the patient maybe is in metabolic acidosis and the body is using calcium from the patient's bones and magnesium from muscles to compensate the delicate pH of the blood.

Dr. Ben: I require all of my patients to go to see Dr. Galina at Universal Medical Imaging because she always finds something else significant that I need to fix to help get them well. There may be another tumor, it may have spread, and they didn't even know it.

The thymo erythroid may be not functioning. Their adrenals may not be functioning. There is so much more information and I need that to get patients well. She gives me a huge amount of information that I can't get anyplace else.

Dr. Migalko: Yes, please visit UniversalMedicalImaging.com and if you would like to learn more about this revolutionary, noninvasive, nonradioactive, painless, comprehensive, full body scan when you can spend two, three hours with us and learn about your body, get motivation for how to change your life, how to change your diet, maybe hydration and much, much more based on your result.

It is not theoretical information, it's about you and we want you to be aware of that: health education instead of medication. Don't wait until it's too late because cancer is curable if it's detected early. And thermography, ultrasound, a functional test—this is early detection and can save life and this life can be yours.

Interviewer: Have you been able to stop it in its tracks before it became something that even became life threatening? Have you seen any experience that you can look at here?

Dr. Migalko: This is a very good question. That is why we do diagnostic imaging like thermography. Because thermography can see pathology eight to ten years before we see it with anatomical tests like MRIs, CT scan, or ultrasound. Just think about it: eight to ten years before!

This is early detection and truly, when we see it, we can give suggestions and the patient can prevent a serious, serious condition. Then the patient can come for a follow up scan, and based on what the patient did, they can see if that program works for them or it doesn't work for them and they need to adjust it or add something else. Absolutely we have many, many cases, and we have documentation. It's not like we talk about it, we can show pictures. We can show slides.

A lot of patients will come and say, "I believe that my diabetes or heart problem or cancer is genetic because my mom and my grandma had the same issue and that's probably why I have it."

But when they see their body, when they see where the inflammation is, when they learn how to reduce this inflammation which is a precursor to cancer—when they learn about lifestyle and diet change and they see that they can reverse and eliminate that issue, they understand it's not because their parents had it. It's because they are just repeating the same lifestyle and diet their parents had and that is why they have the same problem.

So yes, we do have a lot of cases to share with anybody who would like to learn and that is why we say health education instead of medication and radiation.

Interviewer: Yeah. Great.

Dr. Ben: Share with us a specific patient that we had that you saw a condition and, by your counsel and recommendations and then the follow up and how that changed their life.

Dr. Migalko: Yes. I had an amazing patient's case. This lady came from Russia, from Moscow. She had a diagnosis of ductal cell carcinoma and the only choice she had in Russia is a complete mastectomy with the possibility of a double mastectomy and radiation and chemotherapy—horrible surgery, which affects everybody on an emotional level, a physical level, a spiritual level—and she came to America to see if there is anything possible she can do.

She was under an alkaline diet, under a pH Miracle Diet guided by Dr. Robert Young and also other medical doctors. It was complementary medical treatment. I was driving to that Center every Monday to do a follow up scan just to see how physiology changed, and thermography, and how ultrasound is showing changes.

And it was an amazing experience because she had a tumor of 14 centimeters and every week the size of the tumor was decreasing, decreasing, and in the end of the eight weeks the tumor from 14 centimeters went down to 2. I think this is the very amazing case and when that tissue was sent to pathology, the result came negative.

We have a series of images showing how inflammation was reduced, how the size of the tumor was reduced based on the certain protocol, which complements the patient's not only physical body, but also spiritual body.

It is very, very important because sometimes we have patients with the same diagnosis going under the same treatment and they have different results or they have the same result, but some patients can achieve that result in a month. Other patients will achieve it in maybe a half a year or a year.

Why is that? Because, from our observation, if the patient has a strong motivation, if the patient has family and friends' support, if the patient will believe, truly believe that that is the way to go... Belief comes from education because if you have the opportunity to educate yourself from social media, from doctors who have results and—

Dr. Ben: Ty Bollinger Series.

Dr. Migalko: Yes! Share those results with you, then you are empowered because knowledge is power. That is why, when there is a reduction of stress, there is a right diet, when there is physical activity, maybe infrared sound, maybe a lymphatic massage and much, much more, then we see results and we are always happy to see it.

We believe that every patient can be our teacher or student because if the patient wants to learn something from us, the patient can be a student. But every time we see a new patient, we will learn something from this patient. That is why we think like doctors and we think like researchers. We believe that we need to learn every day.

Many years ago we finished medical school and we didn't have technology that we have right now. That's why we need to use this technology and we need to help patients to learn about it.

Dr. Ben: Absolutely.

Dr. Migalko: I think it is great. I think that every piece of educational material specifically based on the natural approach is very important because I'm a medical doctor and also a naturopathic doctor. I'm working on my dissertation right now to show people that this combination of two worlds, combining Western medicine with integrative alternative medicine is the best.

Because we can use emergency medicine, which is very powerful when it is needed. We can use a dietary approach and this is very important. This is something we never learned in medical school!

We have thousands of hours of information in medical school how to fight off disease and death, and we didn't have any hours of how to live a healthy life. I think it is great what you guys do and I think that it is very important for everyone who has an opportunity to see these videos.

Interviewer: We believe that those people that have gone against the grain, like yourself, deserve to have that publicity pointed towards you because we believe that you've earned that respect and you deserve people to come to you.

Is it nice for once to have people support you in your mission and say, "Look, we believe in you, we support you and we want people to know about what you're doing"? How does that feel for you, Dr. Galina?

Dr. Migalko: It feels incredible because this is our mission. In medical school, we truly believe that after getting all the knowledge from this institution, we will help so many people.

But we also believe that we need to learn on a daily basis about all the new science, all the new information and spread it with everyone we see to help as many people as possible. That is why, when we have an opportunity to share this information with thousands, with millions all over the world, it feels good, specifically when patients come to us and say, "Thank you, Dr. Ben. Thank you Dr. Galina. Thank you doctors, all doctors who work with us. You really helped me to change my life."

I believe that every person who will not only to learn how to take a pill and reduce pain temporarily, but if they will learn how to change their life, how to eat healthy, how to get more energy, how to live longer—not only longer, but happier, with joy and love in their heart—what are they going to do?

They are going to share this information with their friends, with their family and most importantly, with their kids so kids can grow up healthy, happy, with joy in their heart and teach their kids. That's what we need to do. We need to spread this information to medical schools, the hospitals. Hospitals! Look at what food they serve to their patients.

Dr. Ben: Oh don't get started there! It's nutritionless, it's like cardboard.

Dr. Migalko: Yes.

Dr. Ben: No value.

Dr. Migalko: But you know what? If you, as a patient in that hospital and you know it's not good for you for your condition, you are not going to eat it. Right?

Dr. Ben: You're going to have somebody bringing food into you.

Dr. Migalko: It's inevitable. But knowledge is power, okay, so it doesn't matter. It can go to the restaurant where they serve meat and everything maybe you don't want to eat. But you can choose something healthy from the menu. You can choose a side dish of spinach or broccoli or something you believe is good for your body because this is your temple. We need to take care of our temple.

Interviewer: Dr. Galina, when I just asked you that question before and I saw you respond, I could see a fire inside that heart of yours. I could see a strong motivation that you have worked for a long time to fulfill your original mission to help heal people's lives and to help alleviate suffering.

I could imagine you've seen so much of that and that you have wanted to dedicate your life to that, to be in this place right now and to just be doing what you're doing, and seeing lives change, that's enough for you, that's your reward.

But what is it like for you to have that sense of peace that you know you're doing the right thing? There's a lot of things you could be doing. You took a road less traveled, you could have taken an easier path, but you took this one because you believe that that's the way that you can help heal people.

Yeah. For you, what is it like seeing the results, seeing the lives change, seeing that you are a part of that and those people are thanking you for helping to shine that truth to them. What is that like for you?

Dr. Migalko: Thank you so much for your question. I would like to answer this. When I went to medical school, I had a problem I wanted to fix for myself. I had occasional headaches and doctors couldn't help me, so I wanted to learn what to do with that.

But after finishing school, I realized that taking a pill is not the way to do it. There is something more. That was many, many years ago, okay? That was my motivation. But later, actually during medical school, I lost my father due to cancer. Then later I lost my brother because of pancreatic cancer and I lost my best friend because of colon cancer. They literally left this earth in my hands.

By analyzing later what was wrong in their diet, maybe in their stress level, and much, much more, a combination of everything, I understood that if they would have this knowledge, if I had this knowledge before, I probably would help them to stay alive. They would probably be here with us.

Right now, every patient I see I think about them like it's my father, it's my sister, it's my brother. It's someone I really care about. That's why we're doing what we're doing, not just because of money or fame or something else, because if we save one life, this is the biggest reward for us.

Interviewer: Wow. You see, it's like all you want to be able to do is turn back the clock so you could go back and give your father, your brother the thing that they needed, and that moment was taken from you.

But then these people come in and you look into their faces and you see your father and you see your brother. What does that mean to you to be able to give that gift that you longed to give to them, but you give it in the person of these other people that need your help, that are fathers to somebody, that are brothers to somebody, what does that mean to you?

Dr. Migalko: Because we are all here on this planet to learn and grow. It is good if we understand why we're here, what is our mission. I think I found mine and I want to continue to learn and grow to help others to save lives. I think if I can help someone who has relatives, kids, and those people help their father, their brother for a long period of time, to enjoy their family... Like I said, this is the biggest reward. Money cannot buy it! It is hard to explain what we feel at that moment, but this is the moment of joy! It's priceless!

I think the key here is to have a personal experience. When you have this personal experience—not theoretical, not just from someone telling you that this is the right way to do or that's the way it's supposed to be—but you live through it, you have this passion! And when you have this passion, you understand, you feel what is the meaning of what you're doing and it's natural. For me English is a second language and sometimes it's in my head not only what to say, but how to say it. But everything goes on the second plan when I'm engaged in my work.

That's why, when we see a patient for a full body scan, the reason we use technology which is not only noninvasive, without radiation, but very visual, it's not just like to have a boring doctor's appointment. You know, you have these symptoms. I think that's what you have from my experience. Now it's all about this patient. Two or three hours, it's all about this patient, showing them their body and saying, "This is where the inflammation is. Can you see it?" "Wow, I see it! This is where lymphatic congestion is. This is where probably nerve damage or poor circulation. Did you know that?"

"No." "Look at your legs, look at your fingers. You need to improve your circulation." When they engage in the conversation with you, when they feel that you really care, when they know that they are here because you want to help them, they can learn, that's why we do what we do.

Dr. Ben: And your metabolic calculosis, your thyroid is not functioning, your adrenals aren't part—functioning.

Dr. Migalko: It's all about the patient. It's about the patients.

Dr. Ben: Empowering them with knowledge.

Dr. Migalko: It's not like "Oh, my experience" or "Statistics will say...." No! Because we don't know where this patient, in that statistical number, is! It's on the left or on the right. This is the individual. Many times a patient will go to the doctor's office and, by having conversation with their doctor, they hear—the doctor will say, "Statistically, we know that this drug works better for your condition, or this approach works better."

But how do we know where this patient in this statistical group, in this 90 percent or 10 percent? We talk about it with Dr. Ben very often because he has a very individual approach how to treat his patients by taking blood and examining which natural substance works exactly for this patient, not somebody else, statistically, but for this patient, just to really help this particular individual I think is very important.

I really respect what Ty Bollinger does because after experiencing this pain, after going through all this suffering by losing loved ones, he has this courage and strength to stand up and talk to so many people around the world and learning by himself because every time he interviews someone it's additional knowledge for him how to help his family and loved ones and everybody who can listen to this beautiful series. That is why we have to do this. We don't have to sit in our small offices just helping one by one patients. This is great, but if we have the opportunity to educate millions, when we have the opportunity to stand up without any fear that someone will be jealous or someone will say that "No, that's not what medical school teaches, that's not what a pharmaceutical company wants you to know."

If we have this strength, if we have this will power to empower everyone and encourage them to spread this message, I think this is very, very important. I think that everyone who has something to say to help others is supposed to stand up and say it.

Some opinions can be not acceptable by people, but it's good to know. It's good to know. That's why we send patients, after our scan, for other opinions. Don't trust only us. Educate yourself. We want you to go to another doctor and listen to what that doctor will say to you, and a third doctor and fourth doctor. Then combine that knowledge together, then go to social media, watch this series and make your choice because this is your body, this is your health and this is your life.

Interviewer: Awesome. You guys are great. You guys are excellent. What a blessing.

Dr. Migalko: This is the case I was talking about, the lady who came from Moscow with ductal cell carcinoma and the only choice she had—to have a complete mastectomy of the left breast. The treatment progress, by using thermography and ultrasound... This is the picture of thermography. You see that every week the picture was taken and we can see reduction of inflammation, lymphatic congestion, and anatomically ultrasound was showing reduction of the tumor from 14 to 2 centimeters.

This is a beautiful demonstration, a very visual demonstration of the treatment progress. It is not only for us as doctors and scientists, this is for the patient to see. This is for the patient to understand that she is on the right track, that she needs to continue, that she needs to have motivation. "Don't stop, because you are doing good. Even sometimes you cry, even sometimes you feel pain, but don't stop because you see and we can show it to you that the result is really positive."

Interviewer: That's great, and did the tumor end up going away?

Dr. Ben: She couldn't let it go. There's two centimeters of lump there and so she got back to Moscow, she wanted it removed, but there is no cancer in the mass. All the cancer was gone.

Interviewer: So they didn't need to—

Dr. Ben: No, but you know people get stuck and they go "Oh, there's still a lump there. I want it gone." So she got it gone. The good news was there was no cancer left in the lump.

Dr. Migalko: So anatomically, using ultrasound, we detected that mass from 14 centimeters was decreased to 2 centimeters, but that was the time for the patient to go back home to Russia and she didn't want to keep that 2 centimeter mass in her body, even when the condition was improved dramatically, so she asked the surgeon to remove it.

Actually it was another positive news because after removing that mass which was sent to pathology, she learned that there is no cancer activity in that tissue. Yeah.

Dr. Ben: Scar tissue which she could still feel which she perceived as a lump, so she wanted it out. But there's no cancer in it.

Dr. Migalko: Yes, that means that you can still have a tumor in your body. It doesn't mean that tumor is cancerous. Sometimes we do benign tumors and they can stay in your body for the rest of your life if you can maintain the right pH of the body, if you can eat right, drink right.

When I say drink, I don't mean alcohol. I mean good quality water in the right amount for your body so you stay hydrated. It is very important for your cells. And the most important, when we say positive thinking, it's kind of like I don't know what you mean.

We can talk a lot about this, but just create a strong motivation whatever it is. For this particular patient, when I was seeing her every week, I was asking her, "Wow, I never saw such a quick result in my practice. What is your motivation?"

She was sharing her story with me. She said, "I was raising my son as a single mother and I was asking him, "Please get good grades. I want you to achieve this beautiful result. I want you to go to that prestigious university. I want you to take care of yourself when you grow up. I want you to do this." And he did everything what Mom was teaching him.

Now when she was diagnosed with cancer, her son came back to her and said, "Mom, I did everything you asked. Can you do something for me? I want you to get healthy. I want to enjoy you for a long, long time. Can you just do everything what this doctor's natural approach teaching you what to do? Just do it religiously every day."

And she did it! She did it very quick because she had strong, strong motivation. She believed in what she did. Using diagnostic medical ultrasound, we learned that mass from 14 centimeters went down to 2 centimeters. The size was reduced.

And the patient requested surgery to remove the mass from her body because she was not comfortable to go home knowing that something left. That was actually a good decision because we learned, after sending that tissue to pathology, that the cancer was completely gone.

The pathology result was negative. So she made not only her son and her family happy, but she gave us knowledge that it's possible not only for her, but for anybody else.

It was ugly. It was sticking out from the chest. It was a huge tumor. It hurt.

Dr. Ben: 14 by 8 by 6, it was huge, sticking out of her chest. Biopsy proven that this wasn't...

Dr. Migalko: Everything was documented.

Interviewer: How long did it take for that to go from 14—

Dr. Migalko: Eight weeks.

Interviewer: Wow. In eight weeks she got something that had been growing probably for eight years.

Dr. Migalko: Oh absolutely, maybe more because when we see anatomical pathology in the breast, a one centimeter tumor already has billions of cells in it. Her tumor was 14 centimeters so it is years and years of development. It was years of developing that tumor and she was able to reverse it in eight weeks, with our help to educate her with scientists who were showing her life in lab results, thermography and ultrasound, functionality, with doctors who form IPT together with lifestyle and diet at the pH Miracle Center with nutritional colonics, with lymphatic massages, with infrared sauna and much, much more.

Even when I talk about colonics, we think about it different. People think colonic is something, some procedure to remove stuff from your body. We actually give you nutrition through the colon. Why? Because hemorrhoidal veins will pick up all the nutrients and transport throughout your body very, very quick.

We know what to do and how do we know what to do? Because we are using diagnostic tests to prove on a monthly basis, on a weekly basis which therapy, which approach works.

It doesn't matter if the patient will go to Vester Medical Center and wants to know if whatever they do there works, we will tell the patient "It works." If everything is the same or it doesn't work or if they will take a natural approach, which is usually the case.

Interviewer: Excellent. Good job.

[end of transcript]

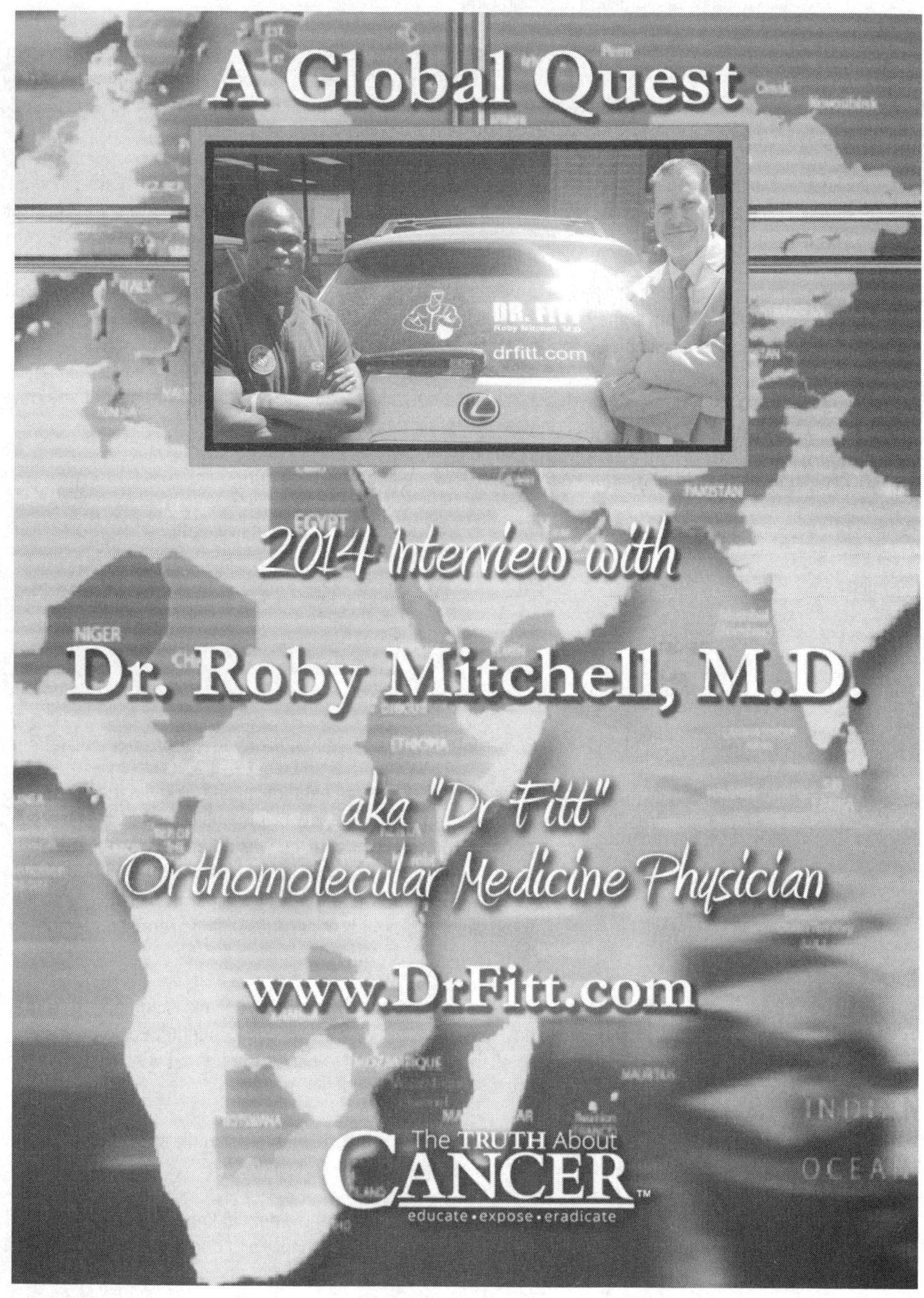
A Global Quest
DR. FITT
drfitt.com
2014 Interview with
Dr. Roby Mitchell, M.D.
aka "Dr Fitt"
Orthomolecular Medicine Physician
www.DrFitt.com
The TRUTH About
CANCER
educate • expose • eradicate

Ty: Today we have with us Dr. Roby Mitchell. Dr. Mitchell, thank you so much for being with us.

Dr Mitchell: Glad to be here.

Ty: I appreciate you taking the time to spend with us today, really looking forward to picking your brain about cancer. But first of all, I want you to tell us a little bit about yourself, about your background, your experience, and then I want to get into your "Doctor Fit" moniker. But first, tell us a little bit about yourself.

Dr. Mitchell: Well, so I'm an AMD so I went to Texas Tech Medical School. I did their first MD/PhD program. And my proctor, Dr. Peter Pang, was from Hong Kong. And he had for some time been wanting to send a student over to China to study oriental medicine or he wanted to establish a student exchange program. So it just so happened while I was working on my PhD under him the opportunity came for me to go over to China and study acupuncture and oriental medicine. This was back in '85 when this stuff was really considered voodoo. But I had been in the Marine Corps, been a karate instructor in the Marine Corps, and had been very interested in trying to meet Bruce Lee. So this was my—I saw this as my opportunity to get over to China maybe to meet Bruce Lee. And so I said sign me up, didn't really know anything about alternative medicine or acupuncture or any of this other stuff except that it was classified as voodoo. But got over there and in that first week saw some things that opened my eyes a little bit. And as I stayed there and saw what they had was a marriage between conventional medicine and oriental medicine. So one wing was conventional medicine, one wing was oriental medicine. And there was just a unrestricted flow back and forth. If they couldn't help you they sent you over here and vice versa.

What they did have over on the western wing were the parametrics that I was used to that measured before and after whether things were working or not. So we could have a kid that came in with asthma and we could put them—put this little device that we use to measure the restriction of the airways so they blow in this thing and there's a little ball that goes up, right. And so the worse their asthma is then the less that ball goes up. So they would get tested over here and we documented their airway restriction and then they'd go over here. They'd get the needle stuck in them and then they'd come back over here and then they're blowing the top off the thing. So for me that was important in my belief system, right, to establish that really there was something happening and this was not mind over matter. And the last thing that really confirmed that was a cholecystectomy, which is a gallbladder extraction, and the only anesthesia was the acupuncture, right. So I came there, you know, with a pretty firm belief that there is some healing ability in the body but went on back and finished up my training and became an emergency room doctor. And as it happens with a lot of us, particularly doctors, you know, the drug companies bring in all the food and you're working all kinds of hours, and my weight went up. And with that my blood pressure went up, cholesterol went up, blood sugar went up, and I was 35 and I had a 37-year-old come in with a heart attack. And that got my attention and made me think I need to start doing something to address these, what we call, metabolic syndrome with the high blood sugar, high cholesterol and high blood pressure.

So I took a blood pressure medication, right. I just asked one of the cardiologists, you know, what's the flavor of the day pharmaceutical for blood pressure. And I took that and I had all these side effects, right. So that got my attention and made me think back to that experience in China where these people were using the innate ability of the body to heal itself. And so I said, well, let me give that a try. So now I started the fruit and vegetable stuff and changing my diet and lo and behold, you know, blood pressure, blood sugar, cholesterol all came back into order. And they also discovered that I had thyroid deficiency so addressing those things, the weight came down, everything came back in order so I started doing that more and more with patients. And I found out that there were a lot of people out there who were really interested in not having the pill for every ill, that they really wanted to address the root cause of the problem and get healthy again. So as I saw that more and more then I just kind of eased my way out of the emergency room and made this the type of medicine that I practice. In that evolution I looked for mentors and found some good ones. So Dr. Jonathan Wright out in Washington, I studied under him, and then Hugh Reardon in Wichita, Kansas, studied under him, Christiane Northrup taught me about bioidentical hormone replacement for women. And then there were several other mentors, Carolyn Dean, I got with Doug Kauffman and he mentioned to me about this yeast thing. And I did my due diligence on that.

So, long story short, I got very good at looking at what symptom a person had and being able to delve into that with my background in biochemistry and physiology and so forth and kind of like an investigator at an airplane crash—FFA. You know, I put all the pieces together to find out what went wrong and we put back the things, you know, the body needs to heal itself. And that's what happens, right. And so that's what I have been doing since maybe around '92.

Ty: Great! Great synopsis there. I liked your pill for every ill. That's indicative I think of a lot of the things that we see, a lot of the protocols that we see. So what you got a chance to visit firsthand in China was, what we call, integrative medicine.

Dr. Mitchell: Right. And it was really—I mean I think it was very important for me to not hear that third hand but to be there firsthand and to be able to witness it eye-to-eye because if I was over here and I heard that from somebody what was going on in China I would not have accepted it.

Ty: Firsthand knowledge, that will persuade you, won't it?

Dr. Mitchell: Right.

Ty: So you were in the Marines.

Dr. Mitchell: Right.

Ty: And you came out and you learned how to—apparently you learned how to get healthy through nutrition…

Dr. Mitchell: Correct!

Ty: …primarily changing your diet. When did Dr. Fit, your nickname Dr. Fit, come about?

Dr. Mitchell: So just as—I mean even through before—well, of course, you know, I came out of the marines and was just kind of an exercise, some people would call it a fanatic but I kept my body in shape. And as I got into medical school, got the health nut moniker and as I became—started doing this with patients someone just said, oh, you're Dr. Fit. I thought that was a pretty good nickname so I kept it.

Ty: It kind of stuck.

Dr. Mitchell: Right.

Ty: Okay. I like it. I like it. So let me ask you this Dr. Roby, what is cancer?

Dr. Mitchell: So cancer, when we look at it deductively and, of course, the oh, the conventional paradigm in the past was that cancer or these cells that have damaged DNA and its damaged in such a way that it incents them to multiply continuously. So normally a cell will be one cell and it'll multiply into two and then it'll multiply into four. So there's this exponential growth but at some point it will shut off growth, right, and it will just stay so your liver grows to a certain size and it stays that size—your brain, your heart, all these other cells, they grow to a certain size and they stay that size. So they have a built-in regulator that keeps those cells from growing more than a particular number. In cancer cells that regulator is turned off and so they just keep multiplying, multiplying, multiplying, multiplying, and because of their physiologic makeup that they absorb sugar and they absorb sugar better than your human cells then they suck up everything around them and people with cancer die of starvation. What we find now is that—and we've got very good documentation to make this a valid hypothesis—is that cancer cells are normal cells that have pleomorphed, and when I say pleomorphed I mean changed over a period of time, from a normal cell into a cancer cell and that pleomorphism is reversible. So there's an intelligence there that says that these cells are trying to survive a toxic situation, right.

And so when we look at—for instance, if you look at my prostate biopsies, right, when I had prostate cancer, you'll see prostate cancer cells, right, we'll say adenocarcinoma right on several of the biopsies. But then you'll also see normal cells and then you'll see what's called PIN or prosthetic inflammatory neoplasia, which is the link between normal cells, that's the transitional cell between cancer and normal cells, right. So what happens with cancer is that it's in that toxic environment, right. So let's say the colon for instance, so you create a toxic environment in your colon by eating the standard American diet. The first thing that happens is a process that we call hyperplasia. So we get more cells than normal, right. Look at the DNA of these cells, the DNA is normal DNA but there's just a lot of them. I mean like you would have a callous on your hand, right, if you were working hard you'd build up a callous. So those cells are not cancer cells, they're normal cells but there's a lot more of them than normal because it's trying to protect itself. Well, in the colon that happens to be a polyp, right. So in the colon there is this polyp. It happens, again, in the hyperplasia, right, more cells than normal. And that is the first stage. That polyp then will go onto another transitional stage, right, what we call neoplastic stage and then that will—if that situation stays there then it will go on to cancer, right. So this is why it's really helpful for us to understand this concept because if that red light comes on, if you were down in the coal mine and one of those canaries dies, right, then it's a signal—you have a chance, right, to get out of that situation. So if there's a polyp, if there's benign prosthetic hyperplasia, if there is fiber adenoma in the breast, if there's just what we call Barrett's esophagus in the esophagus, right, those are all red flags, right, telling us that there's a toxic situation that's making these cells try to move into a cell form that will be able to survive a toxic environment.

So we know now that if we change that environment—so one of the—most any cancer doctor now that uses this, what we call, alternative therapies, to any degree of success, the first thing that they will have patients do is change what you eat. You've got to change that internal environment, right, so you can give these cells the heads up that you're not going to have to try to survive in a toxic environment anymore. When that happens then they start to pleomorph back into normal cells because it's much easier physiologically to live as a normal cell, right. Normal cells go through what we call oxidative phosphorylation which means you take oxygen, you take sugar, and you make 32 molecules of this ATP, which is our energy currency, right.

Ty: You said oxidative phosphorylation.

Dr. Mitchell: Oxidative phosphorylation, right, so we put—take oxygen and through this process we add a phosphorous to this ATP and that's our energy currency, right. That's how we move about. And the more ATP the better, right? So if you're a cell that is able undergo oxidative phosphorylation, and again you're able to do that because of cellular genes is turned on you have to go through what's called the Krebs cycle. Then that's a happy state, right. If you have to move to this anaerobic, what we call anaerobic, metabolism for every molecule of glucose, you can't get 32 ATP anymore. You can only get two molecules of ATP, right.

Ty: Right. And anaerobic means…

Dr. Mitchell: Anaerobic means you don't have to have oxygen, right.

Ty: Okay.

Dr. Mitchell: That means that I can survive without oxygen, right, which makes me able to survive in a more toxic environment but it makes my energy level a lot more restricted. So then that's why cancer cells are so ravenous about having to absorb sugar, right, because they can only make two ATP per molecule.

Ty: Okay. Yeah. Because you hear the phrase "cancer loves sugar" so that explains why.

Dr. Mitchell: Correct! You know, one of the tests that we use to diagnose cancer is a PET scan. So with a PET scan we take radiated sugar, right, and we inject it in you because cancer cells take up sugar so much more efficiently than normal cells, they will take up that radiated sugar, and then we're able to see on the CAT scan where the sugar is, which that tells us is where the cancer is, right? So yeah, so we're very aware of the dependence on cancer cells for prodigious amounts of sugar. And that's why, again, cancer—I mean cancer patients die of starvation is because the cancer cells will suck up all the sugar from human cells—I mean from normal cells.

Ty: That leads me to the question then when you see a cancer patient, and what is it called when a cancer patient dies of starvation. It's…

Dr. Mitchell: Cachexia.

Ty: When you see a patient that has cachexia and let's say their oncologist says you're wasting away, go out and eat anything you want. Is that wise advice?

Dr. Mitchell: That's like you being stranded in the middle of the ocean and thirsty and you drink salt water.

Ty: Great analogy.

Dr. Mitchell: Yeah

Ty: So I mean I don't know how many patients that I've dealt with over the years that have come and said, you know, I'm losing weight. I'm in the cachexia cycle. And my oncologist has told me to go eat ice cream, cake, whatever will put the weight on me.

Dr. Mitchell: Right

Ty: So in other words…

Dr. Mitchell: That's gasoline on the fire.

Ty: Well put, gasoline on the fire. So Dr. Roby, would you talk about the relationship between fat cells and cancers?

Dr. Mitchell: So fat cells. we have to delineate normal fat cells that are fat cells because of the inflammatory process, right? So you know, normal fat cells, per se, are not necessarily carcinogenic. Inflammation is carcinogenic. And what inflammation is, basically a war between your immune cells and some critter, right. It can be a virus. It can be a bacteria. It can be a fungus. It can be cancer, right. So if you remember back to the beginning of the Iraq war and that shock and awe. So that's very analogous to what happens in the—with the immune system when its trying to fight off a bacteria, virus, or a fungus to some degree. So as your immune system, and it's a very apropos analogy to compare the immune system to the military because you do have all these different soldiers, T-cells and killer T-cells and macrophages and macrocytes and so forth for cells in the liver and specialized cells in each tissue in the body that are sentinels that are surveying the area and then if something goes awry they let loose. They have all these weapons of mass destruction to make things happen. So when your temperature goes up, when you get red, when you have diarrhea, when you have the sniffles, and the watery eyes, and all that, so all of that is not because of the critter. That's because of these chemicals that your immune system is able to release.

And these—you know, I was an emergency room doctor before and I can tell you that these chemicals are so powerful that they can kill you very quickly in a process that we call anaphylactic shock. So if you go into anaphylactic shock and, again, that's a consequence of the production of these weapons of mass destruction of the immune system—you die very quickly if you're not in my emergency room, right? So we have to respect that the immune system has some really powerful weapons. And so in a condition less benign than anaphylactic shock where you've gotten fever and red and that type of thing, then the immune system is just spitting out some chemicals that make the environment not so hospitable, not so hospitable for the bacteria, but also not so hospitable for human cells either, right? And so this is what creates that toxic situation that over a long period of time the human cell will try to protect itself from. The chemicals that are produced during this inflammatory process are called growth factors. So growth factors have an estrogenic effect and estrogens, in general, make cells go into hyperplasia that we talked about before so making one cell faster than normal changed to two, changed to four, changed to eight, again, exponential growth, right? So those fat cells that are born of an inflammatory situation, right, those then are linked the formation of cancer.

Ty: Now you mentioned estrogens, is estrogen the hormone that females have and males have testosterone or do we both have both? What is the difference between the hormones in females and males? And then I want to get to a question concerning the effect of estrogens on cancers.

Dr. Mitchell: There's no difference in the molecular aspect of the hormones that are in men and women. Women have testosterone, men have estrogen, both have progesterone and corticosteroids and all these. What's different is the amount, right? So women have a higher amount of estrogen, men have a higher amount of testosterone. Women have a higher amount of estrogen receptors. And men have a higher amount of testosterone receptors,. And so that's key, that marriage between the receptor, the hormone, such that a woman—I can give a woman testosterone injections. She will never get as big as a man because she doesn't have the receptors that a man has. We can put estrogen into a man and you're not going to turn him into a woman, right, because he doesn't have the receptors for those estrogens, right, so. But we all have the same—we all produce the same, exact molecules as for, as estrogens and testosterone and DHEA and progesterone and these other hormones. It's important that we understand for these estrogens, the human ones anyway, that again the—one of the pharmacologic characteristics of estrogen is that they make cells multiply, right? And this is very important in pregnancy, right, because that fetus has to grow so much. And so during pregnancy estrogen levels go way up and we get, again, we get exponential growth of a fetus.

Other cells, if they get exposed to higher levels of estrogen, right, then they can grow faster also. So in breast cancer, in prostate cancer, and in other cancers if estrogen levels are elevated, right, or if we're exposed to a more potent estrogen, right, and this is where we're getting into environmental estrogens, then that cancer can grow faster. And it's not necessarily that indigenous estrogens cause cancer, right, but they can certainly like insulin, right? That's the other cancer promoting hormone. They can make the fire burn hotter.

Ty: Okay, great analogy. So it's like more gasoline on the fire when you have a higher level of estrogen than you should have …

Dr. Mitchell: Correct!

Ty: …which lots of articles today that we're reading about the effect of what they call xenoestrogens, which are fake estrogens in the environment. So can you talk about that in relationship to cancer?

Dr. Mitchell: Right, and then, so that's one of the reasons why we see such a proliferation of cancer in the West. We're seeing it more in third-world countries now. But because of our exposure to environmental and pharmaceutical estrogens that has the effect of throwing more gasoline on the fire. So some of the insecticides, pesticides, fungicides that we use, they have an estrogen effect, right? These are what we call xenoestrogens, xeno meaning foreign. So those, again, long-term exposures, so we have to think about estrogen exposure and lifetime exposure as we do like with radiation exposure. So if you're a radiation technologist, right, you wear a little badge on you that gives us a Geiger counter amount of radiation that you are getting exposed to over a lifetime and you get to here, in other words, to where you can't be exposed to anymore radiation. The same thing with these estrogens, right, so there is a lifetime exposure of estrogen that dictates your risk for different cancers, right. So you are producing estrogens as a human. As a man, you're producing estrogen, as a woman, they're producing estrogens. Women produce more. So if we go adding on top of that environmental estrogens, then that increases your lifetime exposure of estrogen. If you take birth control pills, that increases your lifetime exposure of estrogen. If you take synthetic hormone replacement after menopause, that increases your lifetime exposure of estrogen. If you stay overweight with these fat cells that are born of inflammation, these growth factors, right, that is increasing your lifetime exposure of estrogen.

Ty: So it's really a cumulative effective when we're talking about the exposure to estrogens…

Dr. Mitchell: Exactly! Exactly!

Ty: ….as opposed to just one off.

Dr. Mitchell: Right.

Ty: Okay. So if you could tell us a little bit about your personal experience. You mentioned prostate cancer. What did you do to treat your own cancer?

Dr. Mitchell: So I had been vigilant about prostate cancer because my dad had prostate cancer. And I saw what he went through. So he had the prostatectomy, and I saw the results of that. So I started evaluating or started being vigilant about my PSA as most men should around about—well, probably in my 40s, mid 40s. And so I would go every year and have a—I did a rectal exam, again, as all men should, and a PSA. At around age 49 I think I saw my PSA go from 1.-something up to 3.-something, right, which was a fairly dramatic increase. And that got my attention. So I didn't do anything initially, but then when I went the next year it had gone up to 4.0. And four is kind of the cutoff point in conventional medicine for when you need to do something, so kind of the, what I now call, the boiling point. So in medicine we treat boiling points, right? So I'll give you this little analogy, that if you were to take a pot of cold water and put it on the stove, and then stick your hand in it, and then turn the heat on high, at some point you would take your hand out of that water because it's getting so hot, right. And that may be a 130 degrees, it may be a 140 degrees depending on your pain tolerance. One, you take your hand out of that water and it stays under there once it gets to 212 degrees, right, if we're talking about solute-free water at sea level then at 212 degrees it's going to boil. Now if you stick your hand in that water at 212 degrees, you're going to get burned. If you stick your hand in there at 211 degrees it's going to burn, 210 or 200. So it's not a good idea to wait till the boiling point to make that an actionable time for you to intervene. But that's what we do in conventional medicine, right?

That water's getting hotter and hotter and hotter here and your A1C gets up to 5.7 or 6.0, or whatever the number is, and that's the boiling point. Now all of a sudden you have diabetes, right? Let's say your hemoglobin A1C is at 6.0. Well, what were you at 5.9, right? You weren't boiling but you were still hot enough that you're getting burnt, right. The same thing with high blood pressure. So with the PSA the boiling point is four, right. So that's when they say you need to get a biopsy or whatever. Well, what was it at 3.9, right? We should be looking or investigating why PSAs are elevating when they get anything above 2.0, right, so above 2.0 you've either got some type of infection or you have—or you got cancer, right, if you haven't had trauma or some of these other things. So when it got to a 4.0, I approached, actually, one of my instructors here—you know, I've lived here, I went to medical school here, finished up medical school here in Amarillo so I know many of the doctors and many of them had been my teachers in medical school. And Mike Wilkerson is a local urologist that I had studied under, really good guy. So I went to him. And I was only 50 years old and very good-looking. And so it's hard to believe looking at me that I've got cancer. So he didn't believe that I had cancer and told me most likely this was an infection, you know. Let's take some antibiotics and then we'll check it again. And so I went with his recommendation and we did that and the number had went up. And so I said, "Mike, I think it's time for us to do a biopsy." He agreed. And there was cancer and there was, not just cancer, I mean it was widespread cancer as you'll see on the documentation.

So I had taken care of my mother. She had been diagnosed with colon cancer back in 2000 and we did the natural immune boosting therapies on her. They had given her six months to live and she lived for six years. And so I started doing the same thing with myself. At this time I was headed on my way actually up to be with Dr. Jonathan Wright to work with him in the clinic up there in Renton, Washington. And so he and I put our heads together—we're able to put our heads together and to start to do some things in order to one, boost up the immune system, two, maybe to kill off some of the cells because there will be some cells that refuse to change. And so we started doing those things. And you know, made the numbers come down. One of the things that we did out there—I was able to do it out there because of the laws out there, medical marijuana is legal. So we did the medical marijuana, we did high-dose vitamin D. We did this immunotherapy called the universal oral vaccine, of course, the diet was very important, so did the juicing and stayed away from any kind of grains, sugars, and that type of thing. And you know, and I saw that I had symptoms that let me know that my cancer had progressed. So I saw those symptoms reverse.

But it really had gotten up to a point, you know, where I had said my good-byes to everybody and let people know that this is, we're in kind of in a no-win situation here. But then things turned around and, long story short, you know, went and had a repeat PET scan here back in, I guess, November, that we'll be able to get a shot of also, that, again, showed no cancer. And I've done this with person after person after person if they are willing to do what it takes to get off this toxic diet, right. That's usually kind of the stumbling block for a lot of people. They're just so addicted to the sugar and the wheat and so forth. You know, they just can't get off of it. But when people do we certainly do see, again, a reversal of his pleomorphism and cancers not there anymore. I mean the cells are still there but they have just chosen that they don't need to be cancer cells anymore.

Ty: Right. So in other words they reverted back into normal cells that live on oxygen.

Dr. Mitchell: Right.

Ty: Okay. Wow! That's impressive. I'm impressed with the protocol. I'm also impressed—I can't believe you're how old? You're over 50—older than 50…

Dr. Mitchell: 58

Ty: 58…?

Dr. Mitchell: Yep.

Ty: Okay. Well, whatever you're doing keep it up because I had no idea that you were 58. You look fantastic. Talk a little bit, if you could, you mentioned conventional medicine tends to treat when you get to a boiling point.

Dr. Mitchell: Right.

Ty: So when it comes to cancer typically conventional medicine will treat with either chemotherapy or radiation or surgery or a combination thereof. What is your opinion on the efficacy of the conventional treatments? Would you recommend that people go down that path or would you recommend that they go down what you went or would you recommend maybe an integrative approach?

Dr. Mitchell: So each situation is different. And so we have to approach each situation as different. Unfortunately, in a lot of conventional medicine, like I said, I was just down at MD Anderson. People are treated more like a feedlot situation where if you have this, you know, colon cancer, right, this is the protocol that we use. If you've got breast cancer this is the protocol that we use. And obviously, you know, that has failed.

So for instance with my prostate cancer had that been isolated to just the prostate, right, then I could have selected the treatment that my father did which was have a total prostatectomy and the prostate taken out and that would have been curative. There are other modalities with using radiation or proton beams or ultrasound that can pretty much accomplish the same thing. So with prostate cancer I mean you have lots of alternatives. So if it's confined just to the prostate, that will be curative. So it's just a matter of what side effects you're willing to live with, right, incontinence or impotency or some of these other things. So in that particular case the conventional therapy can work. I mean, it can cure cancer. If you're a breast cancer patient and you have a lump in your breast that is circumscribed and hasn't invaded the lymph nodes or any other tissue then with a lumpectomy you can get rid of that, right, and you can survive. Our problem with conventional therapy is when cancer has moved from one place to another when there is a metastasis from the prostate into the bone or from the breast into the brain or from the colon into the lymph nodes, then conventional therapy doesn't work so well, right? So it does depend on what type of cancer there is. There are lots of rarer types of cancers like the cancer that Lance Armstrong had that was amenable to the conventional approach, and he goes on to be able to cheat and win some races.

Ty: And that was testicular cancer...

Dr. Mitchell: Right, testicular cancer.

Ty: So cheating, yeah, cheating to win some races.

Dr. Mitchell: Yeah. So it does—and there are some blood cancers, some blood-borne cancers also that respond to the conventional therapy, so. But for the most part the bread- and-butter cancers, so when we're looking at ovarian cancer, pancreatic cancer, prostate cancer, breast cancer, colon cancer, uterine cancer, once the barn door gets opened with any of those then the conventional therapeutic model doesn't work.

Ty: One last question for you Dr. Roby. You've talked about the importance of the environment for cancer cells to be able to revert back into normal cells. So what is an optimal diet that you could recommend people eat just generalities, of course, to make that environment in the body so that it would not be a good host for cancer cells, so that it would be a good host for normal cells and it would keep cancer at bay? What would be a diet that you—a general diet that you could recommend that would keep the immune system strong and prevent cancer?

Dr. Mitchell: So when I started working with Dr. Wright, one of the things that I have been involved with was treating people for the fungal overgrowth that happens in our body. And the thing that I started to realize—one of the things that I realized years before that was that the common denominator of any of these natural herbal plant, exotic fruit, superfood remedies that work, the common denominator with them was that they had some powerful antifungal in them, right, and that's what garlic, that's with aspirin, that's with these polyphenolic compounds in the skin of red grapes, the resveratrol. So I went into the lab and I started investigating, well, which foods are the highest in these—or not necessarily which foods are the highest but which foods had the most impact on controlling candida overgrowth. And so I set up petri dishes right there in the lab. And we inoculated them with candida. And then we just went about inoculating them then with extracts from different fruits and vegetables and so forth to see which ones made the biggest, what we call, zone of exclusion in the petri dish, right? And so we had the petri control down here with a medication called Diflucan that we know kills yeast, right? And so we knew that it was going to leave a big clear space in there, right, where it didn't allow yeast to grow. And then down here we have just water, right. And so that plate just grew white with yeast overgrowth because there was nothing to inhibit it. And then all these other plates I was able to see, you know, which ones worked better or worse at keeping yeast under control. So with that, that was the springboard for what is now called the BALI eating plan—B-A-L-I. And BALI's standing for—that's an acronym for basic antioxidant/antifungal, and then low insulin.

So we want to—and regardless of the name that you call it, right, whether it's the Gerson therapy or the paleo diet or Mediterranean diet or whatever, what is going to work as far as keeping cells out of an environment that incents them to pleomorph into cancer cells is one that keeps the yeast under control. It keeps you from developing fungal overgrowth because when that fungus gets up to a certain level then your immune system is going to respond with the weapons of mass destruction and it's going to create a toxic environment and your cells are going to cough and choke and they're going to start changing into a cellular form that will allow them to survive that toxic environment. So again, regardless of what you'd call it, the food that you eat has to be food that keeps fungal growth under control and doesn't throw gasoline on the fire. So when we eat foods that have, what we call, a high glycemic index, right, so the grains and sugars, right, in corn, wheat, rice, those things, then we're creating an environment, right, that promotes fungal overgrowth, right, and that's going to cause inflammation and that's going to, again, incent cells to turn to cancer cells, right. So we have just seen that more and more as our diets have gotten more and more refined. That was over here—it started over here in the western world. Now we see it as we have outsourced all of our computer jobs and manufacturing jobs over to these third worlds, right, and they get money in their pocket and then we send Coke and McDonald's over there. Now we're seeing breast cancer, for instance, in women that we didn't see breast cancer in before. We're seeing prostate cancer in men that we didn't prostate cancer in before in these third world countries, right. And its again, because they're eating the same food that gave us the problem over here.

Ty: Very, very good explanation of the relationship between fungus and cancer. I've read—some people take the position that cancer is a fungus. But if I understood you correctly, what you're saying is that fungal overgrowth creates the internal environment then that cancer feeds—that will then cause the immune system to respond in such a way that then could create cancer.

Dr. Mitchell: Correct! We know that cancer is not a fungus because a fungus could never turn into a human cell, right. So if these cancer cells are pleomorphing back into human cells they can't be a fungus, right? That would be an impossibility, so. But what fungus does it can be a facilitator in that fungi, they are not passive, right, so they product what are called gliotoxins, gliotoxins or—they're kind of weapons of mass destruction that incapacitate the immune system. And so with the weakened immune system then that allows cancer cells to grow better. So they do work together, right, and so and that's another reason why a lot—one of the protocols for many physicians that treat cancer is to bring down the fungal load because if you bring down the fungal load then the immune system gets stronger. And one of the—and the one thing that does kill cancer or cure cancer is your immune system. Chemotherapy, radiation, these things, right, they—if you go to the cancer 101 book it will tell you that they can't cure cancer. The cell kinetics are just against it. That will never happen. It's basically the same effect as when we give antibiotics. Antibiotics can't cure anything. They can bring down the number, the cell count, such that then your immune system can take over but it's your immune system that does the curing right? So if you've got HIV and your immune system's compromised and you get an infection it doesn't matter what antibiotic I give you you're not going to survive because you don't have an immune system response.

So it's important to understand the—you know, whether we come to a conclusion that we can use maybe a little bit of chemotherapy or a little radiation to bring down the cell number. And I have a belief that that can be done. We have to understand that the thing that cures cancer is your immune system.

Ty: Excellent explanation because that is what then would give your body—your body really is what you're saying then would take care of the cancer if it's given the proper fuel. So if you fuel your body properly, if I'm understanding you right, then it can take care of the cancer via the immune system working the way that it's supposed to.

Dr. Mitchell: Correct! And again, you know, if we stay with the bacterial overgrowth analogy—I might need to give a bit of an antibiotic, right, to get the number down so that your immune system is just not overwhelmed, but then bring that number down and then your immune system can take over. There may be a role for chemotherapy, radiation therapy, in that sense. The overwhelming majority of physicians who treat cancer, though, with those therapies, depends solely on the radiation or the chemo. And the consequence of that is a weakened immune system. So the very system that you're depending on to cure cancer, right, we kill that off, right, and that's why so many people with cancer, they die of the treatment, right, rather than the cancer.

Ty: It almost sounds like at times the conventional treatments are the weapons of mass destruction.

Dr. Mitchell: Well no, there's no question they are. I mean that is their objective, right, is to massively kill off cells that multiply fast, and that's what cancer cells do. They multiply fast but that's the same thing with your immune cells and the cells that line your gut. They multiply fast, right? And so any cells that undergo rapid multiplication they are going to be in the cross hairs of chemotherapy and radiation therapy.

Ty: So would that explain why people get nauseated when they take chemotherapy because the cells in their gut...

Dr. Mitchell: Nausea—yes, right, esophagitis, right, all those problems with the gut from the esophagus on down to the rectum, yes.

Ty: Okay. So if I understand what you've been saying to us over this last hour, if we give the body the nutrition that it needs, the fuel that it needs, then it can respond, the immune system can respond, and can actually take care of the cancer the way that it's supposed to. So it's really our body that's doing the healing when we provide it with the necessary fuel.

Dr. Mitchell: Correct! So the necessary fuel, there are some hormonal balance issues you know that we address, some nutritional issues like with vitamin D. We see vitamin D deficiency a lot, thyroid deficiency a lot, but yes, if we just put the things back that a normal body functions optimally off of then it goes to work healing.

Ty: Okay. Well, Dr. Roby, thank you for the time that you've spent with us today. I love your analogies of weapons of mass destruction especially coming from a former Marine. Or actually, once a Marine always a Marine, right? So you're still a Marine. And I really appreciate your personal story that you shared with us about healing your own cancer and the protocols that you used and I really appreciate the influence that you're making on all of your patient's lives and in the lives of people around the world. I first met you just a couple years ago at the Cancer Control Society in Los Angeles, and you made a huge impact on me. I was telling you earlier after your lecture there, I went home and watched the DVD several times, specifically your lecture, because I learned so much of what you were talking about, things that I had not heard before. So I really appreciate what you've done and I thank you for your time today.

Dr. Mitchell: You're very welcome.

[end transcripts]

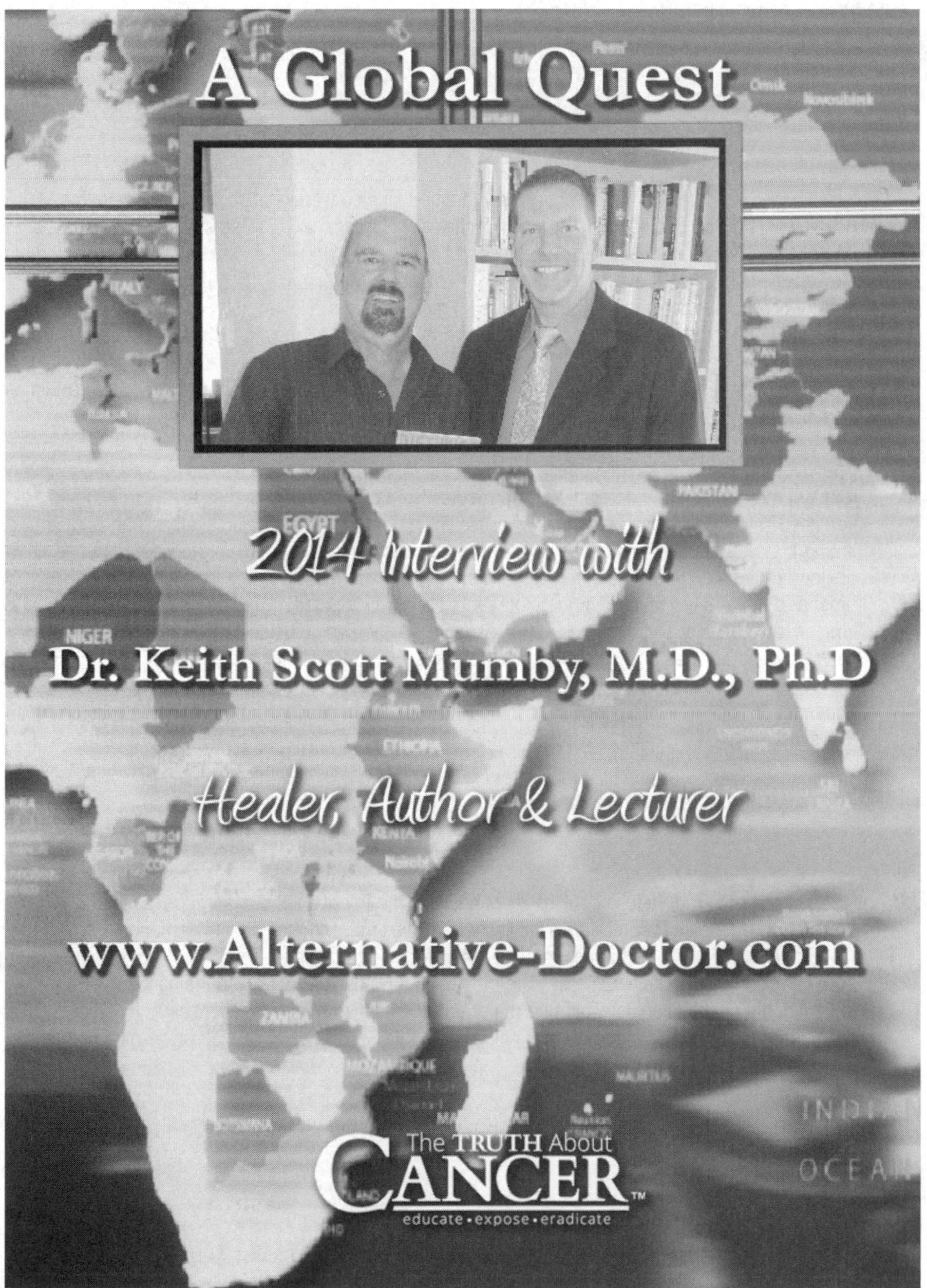
A Global Quest
2014 Interview with
Dr. Keith Scott Mumby, M.D., Ph.D
Healer, Author & Lecturer
www.Alternative-Doctor.com
The TRUTH About
CANCER
educate • expose • eradicate

Ty: I'm here today with Dr. Keith Scott Mumby and we're here in Las Vegas at his home and I just wanted to thank you Keith for taking the time to talk to us today.

Dr. Mumby: Pleasure, Ty.

Ty: So tell me Keith a little bit about your background, your experience, I know you're from the UK so how did you get to where you're at?

Dr. Mumby: Okay. Well first of all I should say I trained as a conventional doctor. Over there, the M.D., the equivalent is called Bachelor of Medicine, Bachelor of Surgery, so qualified surgeon. I won prizes. I was an orthodox model at one stage but pretty soon I jumped the fence and went into alternatives and sort of plowed my own furlough ever since. In the 80's I made my name quite strongly around the world with the subject of what we then called food allergies, I mean that's a relevant term but I made some amazing breakthroughs with a small group of colleagues around the world, maybe eight to ten of us, really pushed the envelope forward at that time. We found food allergies responsible for all kinds of things, like migraines, arthritis, eczema, all kinds of stuff would just improve like magic if you remove certain foods from the diet. It's important to say it's different foods for everybody.

The idea of a standard set diet doesn't really work. But you know there was some amazing recovery so it taught me nutrition in a different way. In medical school nutrition is kind of, what are you short of that you need? Whereas I came to realize, what are you eating that you shouldn't, rather than what you're not eating that you should? It produces more dramatic recoveries, certainly in the western world anyway, obviously third world countries, they're deficient, but we are mostly eating too much of the wrong thing, emphasis there is *too much*. Through the years I built my reputation, I published books, I spent a lot of time on radio and TV sort of carrying the message. The beginning of the 80's I was called a quack by my colleagues. There was an expression, "Mumby jumbo", in my town for all that kind of stuff. By the end of the 90's I was official. The British National Health Service was buying my allergy formulas to give to government health patients. So I went from quack to respectable to in less than 20 years. In medicine that's fast.

Ty: That is fast.

Dr. Mumby: I came over to the States about 10 years ago with the intention of primarily educating and writing and that's what I do mostly. I don't have a facility here at this time, although, that may change. I have a license here in Nevada and I'm reviewing the possibilities for using that because it's very sad, you know, people here can't get enough help basically. There's not enough people tuned into the right sort of approaches to health. It's all, as you know, big pharma oriented, and it's not about patient care. It's about profits so the more guys willing to stand up and help the better. So that compression alone may call me out of retirement, as you would.

Ty: Tell me about, before the interview today, you were telling me about a story that I think it was Brompton Hospital.

Dr. Mumby: Oh yeah. Well we are talking about cancer aren't we? I found, I mean I do a lot of research. We need a lot of stuff, I kind of have this sort of encyclopedia retention thing, which is very useful at times but I love following pathways, side pathways particularly. I was looking at early cases of cancer at the Brompton Hospital in Western London and I found a very interesting report. One of the consulting physicians there was taking his group of medical students to see this case and he said, now look, first of all it's a cancer case, which is very rare, you won't see many cancer cases, but this is a rare form of cancer. You'll probably never see this again. So what it was Ty, it was lung cancer, which is now the number one world's killer. So that was back in Victorian times. Cancer was virtually unknown then anyway. Today's number one killer was exceptionally rare. What's changed in our world? Well, of course, we all know it's lifestyle basically, which covers everything from how we live to what we eat and so on. Just such major, shocking changes that it's gone from that to being the number one killer. That was a very interesting story and I started to look for why would the Victorians be different and the answer is they ate a lot of food that on average there were no buses and cabs and nobody had their own vehicles in those days, so they walked, literally and the average Victorian walked more than 20 miles a day, which gave them a lot of calories to burn so they could eat a lot of food to make up, and that meant they got lots of antioxidants and nutrients, phytonutrients, so all the other good things that we like, so it fits our present model and I think it's sort of a moral story that if you treat it right... It's one of the things I teach, Ty, is that cancer is not native to humans. If you go back to primitive, or, we shouldn't say primitive, but you know, early aboriginal types of societies, cancer is virtually unknown. It's a disease among men, and as I like to say, it's you. You know cancer is not some alien thing that was dumped in your body from a spaceship or something. It's you. It's your body kind of gone a bit wrong and if you fix things your body will restore its health. It's not a runaway train that can't be stopped. I mean yes, it's a runaway but you can put the brakes on and then reverse it. I mean, that number, of natural cures now, are so vast that you'd have to be blind or dumb not see what's going on and not to realize that orthodox medicine isn't hitting the bar at all.

Ty: You mentioned the people in Victorian times in England they walked a lot and they ate diets that were high in phytonutrients and antioxidants. Just real briefly could you explain what is phytonutrients mean? What does antioxidant mean?

Dr. Mumby: Okay well let's go back to oxygen. Oxygen is a great paradox right? It's very poisonous and yet we can't live longer than three or four minutes without it. We happen to need this in our bodies but it will do damage unless it's controlled. So our body has a built in mechanism for suppressing the damage caused by oxygen. For example, you may not know, but the typical white blood cell, when it's going to attack a bacteria, will go bizz with some hydrogen peroxide, which is deadly, you know, it's like very strong oxygen and kills the bacteria, but then the cell has to very rapidly pour antioxidants on that otherwise it will kill itself. It's like having a gun that shoots all over the place and if you're not careful it will shoot you so you have to suppress it very quickly. That's what we need antioxidants for. It's just one of those things that oxygen is a great blessing and a great damage to our tissues that's why today you hear words like free oxygen radicals and things like that.

Phytonutrients, phyto is just a word that means green leaf or plants, so, nutrients that you get from plants. Well, of course, that's where we get all our food but what's become very clear is that there's a tremendous pharmacopeia in food, you know, with all kinds of effects. I mean, perhaps, one of the obvious examples is the poisonous stuff, you know, the alkaloids include things like mescaline and peyote, but caffeine is one of those, tobacco and nicotine, and tobacco is just a leaf, but nicotine is not good as we know. So not all compounds, in fact, let me tell you something else that I wrote in a couple of articles, somebody pointed out that if cabbage had to go through the tests that drugs have to go through so it's fit for humans, cabbage wouldn't pass. There are simply quite a number of toxic substances. Well, we don't mind, because we cook it and that disables the toxic chemicals. Carrot is another one that has a nerve toxin in it called carototoxin, which is quite like an organ or phosphate poison.

So it's a mixed bag but basically it's emerged. There's an awful lot of good stuff in food but it isn't all safe and that's a message that I will have recurring probably in this talk time, which is that foods can hurt and it depends on whether the person is able to metabolize them successfully or not. It might not be what we used to call an allergy in the old days but if somebody has tiny genetic variance and maybe they can't metabolize tomatoes like everybody else, that would become a toxic food and it is, in fact, in the toxic family, you know the nightshades, the deadly shade, tomatoes is one of those. So even though Steven Pratt put it down as a superfood, I put it down as an careful food. It's not really a superfood it's quite toxic, but anyway this is a very complex subject, but basically what I'm saying is that foods can be harmful, foods are very rich in good stuff too and you have to pick carefully. You must not assume because you read somewhere that this food is good for most people that it's good for everyone. I told you a story, didn't I, just now, about a lady with lettuce that had severe colitis, bloody colitis and slime in her stool, very old lady and she was doing all the right things and eating salads and being healthy and anyway, long story short, she came to me and I found it was lettuce that was making her sick. The only food. Stopped lettuce, she was totally cured and yet we perceive lettuce as a healthy food, don't we, as I say jokingly of course. I said, oh you'll be okay with the burgers and fries just stay off the salads, right, and she was.

Ty: That's amazing, though, because I think probably the people that are watching the show, I'd guess 99 maybe 100 percent of the people watching, would think that lettuce is always safe. As long as it's...

Dr. Mumby: Yep.

Ty: ...organic, lettuce is good for everyone.

Dr. Mumby: If I tell you it's in the mustard family, you might think, well okay maybe it's not that friendly, but look, carrots, you know, who doesn't juice carrots, right. I had a patient back in the early 80's who was a young kid who had epilepsy due to anything in the carrot family. Not just carrots but dill, parsley, celery, those are all in that family of foods, any of those would make him have epilepsy. If he avoided the foods, no problem, no drugs.

Ty: So what I'm hearing from you, and this is fascinating because this is not really mainstream, is that you really need to individualize a person's diet, because one person might not metabolize lettuce well. You just gave us an example of that, where somebody else might.

Dr. Mumby: Right.

Ty: So there's not really a one size fits all diet.

Dr. Mumby: Absolutely not.

Ty: You need to work with a doctor like yourself that understands that...

Dr. Mumby: Yes.

Ty: ...your intake of nutrients needs to be individualized to your own genetic type.

Dr. Mumby: Right. Well, I did write a book about this. A self-help book. So if you can't get to an expert or practicing physician, it's called *Diet Wise,* and it's hard to figure it out for yourself, and 99 percent of the people could figure it out for themselves using that book. I think it's very important and it's a journey, should—you know, whether you got cancer or not, listen, any—one of my sayings, Ty, is that any good health measure is an anticancer measure. Okay, I'm not sure you see them as that, instantly, so this is a journey that everyone should do at sometime in their lifetime, whether or not they've got cancer, but if you've got cancer, you better do it now. Which is to figure out which foods are safe for you, which ones you tolerate, and which ones you don't, because inflammatory foods will load up the immune system, they'll cause it to misfire, and we know that's the last thing you want to happen if you've got cancer. You want a purring, smooth, sweet running immune system. I mean we already know it isn't if you've got cancer but you know what I mean. You don't need to oppress it further. You need to lift the immune system, and getting rid of stressful inflammatory type foods. That's what they are, really. Food allergies is maybe not quite the right term. That's a specific type of reaction, but all these other foods, they cause inflammation in the body, and you can't make assumptions.

For example, this will shock you too. I know a lot of people who can't eat whole meal brown bread but are perfectly healthy if they eat white bread. You think, wow, that's crazy, that's not what we learned, but, in fact, this is the explanation, Ty, which is, white flour and white bread is just fluff, there's not wheatiness in it at all, so a wheat sensitive person wouldn't react to it, but me, for example, I'm sensitive to wheat. If

I eat whole meal bread I get a belly ache, I mean a belly ache isn't that intolerable, but if I had psychiatric problems or colitis or something, of course, I wouldn't do it, and I only do it very occasionally anyway. So there are a lot of quirks to this approach to things that I find out by trial and error over the years that are very different, except first of all, mainstream medicine is way off the page. They don't even think nutrition matters, but sadly, a lot of alternative holistic and health practitioners don't get this right either. If you mention food allergies, or Google it on the web, all that comes back is gluten and casein. That's all you ever see, but it can be anything. I've had people sensitive to spring water. They can drink Pierre and they can't drink Avian. It's not just water, of course, there are organics in it, and a person might react to one or the other or both, so it's a big story. A very important aspect of cancer therapy, you know, nutrition is one of the absolute crucial keys to beating cancer, as you know.

Ty: It's interesting that you mention white bread versus wheat bread. It goes completely against what we're told, that you should only eat whole grains, but some people are sensitive. I know people just like yourself, they can't eat whole wheat bread, but they can have white bread. They don't react to it. Not that it's a health food, but they don't react to it.

Dr. Mumby: ...yeah. If you want some toast, obviously you don't want toast that's going to give you a bellyache...

Ty: Exactly.

Dr. Mumby: ...but don't believe that having white bread is going to give you any nutrients. There are virtually zero nutrients...

Ty: Right.

Dr. Mumby: ...so you have to get your nutrients some other way.

Ty: You mentioned a couple of things that were fascinating. You mentioned inflammation, you mentioned the immune system and white blood cells a couple times, which are part of the immune system. Talk about white blood cells, the immune system and inflammation as it all relates to cancer.

Dr. Mumby: Okay. Well part of the question, Ty, is, what is the basic model for cancer. There's the stem cell model and the metabolic model and so on. Certainly at the core, if not the cause, many people, and I'm one of them, see cancer as basically a disease of the immune system. I don't think there's anyway you're going to stop cells firing off and going wrong and turning into rogue cells. There's just too many toxins. But a good immune system will pick them up very quickly, and eliminate them, so in a very strong sense, kind of sort of a disease of the immune system, so you want to do everything in your power to help the immune systems. That means the right kind of nutrients that will help it. It also means removing the stressors that will stop it working and they're all inflammatory in nature. I mentioned food, inflammatory foods, but that's chemicals, pesticides, pollutants, bisphenol all of these things, loads of those two, and don't forget heavy metal toxicity, mercury and lead and these things, not only have their poisonous powers but they're highly inflammatory too. So it's very important to unburden the immune system. I've got to say, emotions can be pretty inflammatory too. The immune system gets burdened even if a person is upset, sad, depressed or whatever, and I would like a minute to talk about that with cancer. I think it's a very crucial element in cancer, but really anything, that's what I'm saying, anything that's inflammatory is bad for cancer, and yet we can get a good handle on it, you know. There are ways, you can take your antioxidants, your phytonutrients, Omega 3's a brilliant anti-inflammatory, but removing the triggers likely inflammatory foods and heavy metals is better strategy anyway. That's something we should all do, and it's back to my saying any good health measure is an anticancer measure.

Ty: I like that saying. Talk about, you said you like to take a minute to talk about the emotional toxicity.

Dr. Mumby: Well okay. Now listen. This is the most undervalued and underperformed part of cancer therapies and everyone's running around talking about oxygen therapies and things like that and different kinds of herbal helpers and things like that. Physical stuff, in other words, right, but there is a cancer personality. No question. In fact, Galen, who was a Roman physician 2000 years ago, first spotted it. Basically, he said cancer doesn't strike happy people. In our times we believe that and we've examined lots of, you know, like a Type A driver heart attack person, there's a classic cancer personality, typically a woman but not necessarily but a person who is self-effacing, they don't fulfill their own needs, they put up and endure other people's rages and stormy emotions and they don't respond, they can't assert themselves and that's the kind of person who is likely to suffer with cancer. If you read Benny Segal's book about exceptional cancer survivors, he talks about the ideal survivor. He said they're ornery as anything and they'll spit and shout at their oncologist and that's the kind of person who's likely to survive, not the ones who says yes doctor, no doctor, I'm sorry doctor. So there are other ways to bring this in but do you know Hamer's work?

Ty: Yeah.

Dr. Mumby: ...Ryke Geerd Hamer, he had this thing called the Iron Rule of Cancer, to mean that all cancers are preceded, you know, three years, by some kind of shocking psychotic stress. Well he's very German, or German as I like to say, and everything's got to be a 100 percent otherwise, it's not satisfactory, and he's not quite right but it's very, very, very common and always there's a stressor element and an emotional element, but it may be back in childhood, you know, childhood abuse for example. Honestly I've done them all, on all the things I've done, I've done a lot of alternative psychology too. When you start working with people, especially when abuse is on the table, you begin to realize—and it's often women, isn't it—but somehow they sit on it, they suppress it and hold it down and hold it down for about 30 years and then in their 40's it's like, boom, and they just can't hold it back anymore, it bursts out, and so that's when a lot of women start remembering their abuse that they've been suppressing. All of that sort of bottled in hurt and resentment and pain and so is all very destructive indeed so it will often emerge—holistic expert in your own way, aren't you, and you know that if it don't come out one way it'll come out some other way. That's what nature does. If there's a disease process it has to come out. It's better if you shout and scream and fling properly across the room then don't, but if you don't do it sooner or later, you'll get something, whether it's warts or something serious like cancer. I must tell you actually I had a wonderful case that I encountered. This is in Utah not far from here. A girl's brain tumor, I went to interview, because she survived a brain tumor. Without going into all the details of how and why, it was uncovered that she had been a child abuse case. She was famously cold and unemotional and not responsive, though she was married, her husband was very much in love with her and she couldn't remember a thing before the age of six. She was totally blank. Well when all that changed she remembered abuse. Her grandfather leading her out to the woods and she was tied to a table and abused by adults, and if you ever tell anybody we'll kill you, that kind of thing. So the child, of course, shut it all down, result brain tumor. As soon as she discovered that, zoop, the brain tumor disappeared in about five, six weeks. All the markers went to zero.

Ty: Wow.

Dr. Mumby: She wouldn't even take vitamins and minerals and I say well that's going a bit far, I like your story but why don't you change some lifestyle things you know, maybe protect yourself against any future sickness. Anyway she remembered, that was it, cured.

Ty: So just the removal of that or releasing that memory?

Dr. Mumby: Yes exactly. It's just releasing it. I mean the painful memory was still there but she didn't have to suppress it anymore and it wasn't controlling her, so. So very crucial, and one of the things that we find with cancer patients is, if allowed, the cancer will literally heal a person's life. The person who gets cancer is in a mess. I mean I say it's not death now but it is a wakeup call. If you don't do something you're not going to survive. Most people have to face their issues and heal and that healing could just be bad diet, that's a kind of healing our toxic lifestyle, or relationships and family and things and lots of people who finally figured out that cancer is saying something good, you know, you need to deal with this situation with your parents, and so they do, and you know what follows is their love, laughter and tears and all this massive healing and so on. Actually, in a real sense, cancer will heal a person's life if they let it, but most of them are driven down a pathway of terror. The model of it is, you're going to die unless we get enough chemo in you to stop it, and this afternoon or you're going to die. It's not true. It really isn't true. It's very sad to panic people. Yes you got to take stock. Yes you got to figure out what you need to do but if you do it-it can be reversed.

Ty: So it's a wakeup call?

Dr. Mumby: True.

Ty: It's like I've heard people say it's like a check engine light in your car going off. Something's wrong and you need to take action to fix it.

Dr. Mumby: Right. That's right. Of course the orthodox signature's blanking out but the warning light doesn't work. You need to fix causes and of course cancer has causes. Here's another problem. It's a multifactorial disease. It's not like malaria where the cause is a mosquito bite and this plasmodium. It's not that simple. There are many, many—my three pillars, I call it the three pillars of healing of cancer, emotions, which I talked about. We barely mentioned chemical overload but our environment now is full of cancerogenic substances. We're awash literally with carcinogens. Some of them are choices best not used like cosmetics. I love to see the gals looking pretty, you've seen my wife, she's beautiful, so you like them to look good but most of what women put on their skin is dangerous. I think the average woman would probably do less if they realized that they absorb about two pounds, that's around a kilogram of cosmetics through their skin every year. That's two pounds of sludge and a slime, toxic sludge and slime that your liver's got to deal with. You weren't given a liver to deal with cosmetics, it's supposed to deal with foods and environmental factors not man made synthetics such as now. So there's the whole of that element and then I've talked about—well I mentioned food. I don't think I really go into it enough. Can I just say a bit more about that because...

Ty: Absolutely.

Dr. Mumby :...if you look at every simple, I'm using the word simple rather than primitive or aboriginal society, cancer is unknown. Now there was a famous Harvard Researcher called Vilhjalmur Stefansson I'm not sure how to pronounce his name, he's obviously Norwegian or Swedish name... I think, my best shot is Vilhjalmur Stefansson and he lived with Eskimos for about 30 years, I shouldn't say Eskimos, I knew it, but you know what I mean. He lived with them and he ate their food and lived their lifestyle and at first he couldn't tolerate the diet. It was about 50 percent fat, you know, it was just slopping with grease in the dish and so he said no, I can't take it. I'll eat more of the western way and within a few weeks he was pretty sick and he had to eat that way. Soon as he did his body recovered enormously and he was really fit and well. He was out on the ice. He could walk 50 miles in a day. He was a really fit man for his age and brought back a very interesting story and wrote a book. Basically in all his time in that territory he never saw a case of cancer. It's pretty well unknown amongst the—it's only when they came into the bases, started eating the burgers and the colas that they started to get diabetes and heart disease, cancer the same as the rest of them. That's a picture that repeats itself all over the world.

Albert Schatz is a famous humanitarian. He went to work in the Gabon in Africa and he said he never saw a case of cancer in anyone that was living the natural lifestyle. He directly attributed it to food. He was pretty sure that was the reason. They just eat differently and you've got your—it's tempting to think it's genetic, the argument's that just strong in the case of cancer. They do eat a lot of selenium from the seafood and we know that's a protectant. The real killer in the story, Ty, is they go and move into a different environment and eat somebody else's diet, they're sick as dogs just the same as the rest of them. So it's not really a genetic factor. You know that's pretty stark epidemiological evidence. You almost don't need any of the cause of the cancer if you know that people living the natural lifestyle in the Stone Age or the aboriginal way like a hunter gatherer and keeping their lifestyle pure never gets cancer. What does that tell you? It tells you it's probably the number one element anyway and why we get cancer because our diets are awful.

Ty: Now and I would agree with that. When you mention modern foods that we should stay away from as opposed to the Indians or the Eskimos that are eating natural foods what are you talking about? What foods should people look to stay away from?

Dr. Mumby: Well let's see. Let me flip it right the other way first, which is basically we are on earth as hunters and gatherers, that's what nature put us here as, which means walking through the forest, you gather nuts and berries, by the way a great joke on the old caveman hunter model is bring down a kill and feed the tribe. It's BS. About 70 percent of the calories were gathered by women in ancient societies. Those are the nuts and berries and roots.

Ty: Right.

Dr. Mumby: Occasionally some meat and occasionally some fish and you drank water. That's what we're supposed to do. Also included in that by the way is a lot of activity. Hunter-gatherers were all nomadic, they all walked. So we do the exact opposite. We have far too many, what I call, farmer foods. Those are really the last 10,000 years. In evolutionary terms what's 10,000 years, it's the blink of an eye when it takes millions of years to evolve a new animal or new lifestyle. So the farmer foods drastically across the grains, harvesting grains with dairy products too. Then you got all the weird and wonderful stuff like sugar, tea, coffee, alcohol, although I should be careful because alcohol technically is a Stone Age food. If you go on YouTube you can see animals eating fermented fruits and getting drunk. It's rather funny. So occasionally in the fall even man would probably eat fermented fruits and get drunk so there is kind of an argument of the fact of it being Stone Age but anyway you know what I mean.

Then we got non-synthetic things with colorings and flavorings. It makes you shudder really. It's vitiated food, vitiated means all the goodness gone, and then plasticized in cosmetic food with the all the fancy outward appearance put back on so that people are tempted to eat it. It's a sin but it's certainly a health disaster to do it that way. So unless we learn better ways—people who eat that kind of diet are going to join the average statistics for cancer, which you know, are now pretty scary. One in two men and almost that many women will get cancer at sometime in their lives. I don't mean it will necessarily kill them but as I like to say we're all battling cancer because if you are married to somebody it's a 50/50 chance one or the other of you might get this disease. So you could say the big C in movie is coming to a movie house near you sometime and you need to be ready. Of course, that's not true if you do the right lifestyle. So all the people watching this video, your series of videos they're in a great position because they've been told what they need to do and it's stupid not to because eating properly is very enjoyable, taking in exercise is good for you and a healthy lifestyle you feel great. I've got another saying you'll like. I got a lot of sayings but if you don't leap out of bed in the morning, burn some of that energy and bursting to get things done something is wrong. Who takes that point of view. Most people get out of bed like this and think it's normal. It's common but that doesn't make it normal.

Ty: Right.

Dr. Mumby: That means something is wrong. You're body's screaming at you in the morning, no you can't keep doing this, is what you're body is saying. You know, you fix your coffee, you fix your sugar and fix your donut or whatever way you go but that's again, the next morning. That's not health. That's a disaster.

Ty: It is a disaster and I would beckon to say that most people watching this might not be jumping out of bed in the morning ready to go.

Dr. Mumby: They will if they read my *Diet Wise* book and do it.

Ty: Talk about doctor interference and the fact that sometimes cancers will go away on their own.

Dr. Mumby: That's right. Well this is a very good point and I found a wonderful study a little while ago, I think was 2008, 2009, a Scandinavian study that showed very remarkably that if doctors don't get on the case that most cancers will actually, well let's say a large percentage okay, let's not get too exaggerating, but a large percentage of the cancers will resolve. Now this fits with Ryke Geerd Hamer's work, which I just mentioned it, he thinks cancer has a healing principle. I think that too by the way, but his idea is that it heals—cancer appears, something changes, the person heals, the cancer disappears and there's a very strong suspicion that the real problem is not the cancer, just leave it alone, take your hands off, in a lot of cases it will go away but doctors jump on it and then complicate the picture by saying you need chemotherapy, you have to do radiation, you know these are extremely stressful and give the cancer a real running edge so it can then break away and become out of control. I think that's very important and I think unless conventional doctors can learn a hands off, let's wait and see model than a lot of people are literally being sent to their death basically. I'll tell you another way, which I really don't like, I have a bee in bonnet about this type, which is doctors saying oh, you're going to die in six months, you only have six months, put your affairs in order.

Most doctors don't even know when they're going to die so it's totally arrogant to tell a patient when they think they're going to die. Let me tell you a lovely story I brought from a colleague in Reno a couple years back. The patient isn't mine it comes from a doctor colleague. She had a patient that came by who had been told by a doctor you're only going to live six months, 20 years later, she's still rocking and rolling. The doctor that said that, long dead. I think that's so funny. A doctor should not make these pronouncements. You know why, they become self-filling prophecies. Oh well the doctor, the expert knows all about this and says I'm going to last very long so the person just goes down, they fold up and give in. The one thing that you need is a bit of spunk and a bit of spirit to fight back, you know, I'm really going to beat this puppy and it trashes one of their main resources, which is their will to live and their desire to overcome the disease. So doctors, they're particularly bad news in this field because they're not getting competent results but they are standing firmly in the way of natural recoveries and good things and I what I would call proper healing and the things we've been talking about. Yeah a big issue for me.

Ty: That's a common thread that I've heard from other doctors on this series is that when a doctor says you're going to be dead in three months, six months, whatever, it does sometimes become a self-filling prophecy because I guess just the emotional trauma of having a medical doctor tell you that you're going to die…

Dr. Mumby: Right.

Ty: …is that what's considered geopathic stress?

Dr. Mumby: Oh, no, no, no, no I'll come to that in a minute. No that's a bit different but don't forget I talked about that cancer personality, the self effacing sort of, crushed, that can't assert themselves person, that would naturally be very obedient to an authority figure like a doctor, so if the doctor says, I'm going to die, the patient would naturally think, well it must be true then. So they're the worst person to say that to. No let's move on to another aspect. There's a couple of things I'd like to bring in here, but let me talk about this thing, then geopathic stress, okay? Geo means the earth or the globe, as you know that. I first encountered this back in the 80's. I had a clinic, I had several in London and Manchester but I went to Dublin and met some very interesting people there. It's a wonderful city, Dublin, I had a clinic there for a while. That's where I first announced, by the way to the world on the radio that I thought measles vaccine was causing Autism. I was practically the first person on earth to say it.

Ty: What year was that?

Dr. Mumby: 1983. I had a stream of cases coming in so, I mean I was certainly among the first. It was in Ireland, that was thing, I released the information. Anyway I met all kinds of interesting people and they're accounts. Listen I'm half Scottish so I'm Celtic, you know Scot means literally means Scottish from Scotland and Celtics are very deep into mysticism, should we call it lore. It's not Druids or Druidic but the tradition, the Druids were before the Celtics so they swept in and overran the Druids, but that kind of modeled into this kind of thing, and they told me about dowsing a house for black spots. I said, what do you mean, so they showed me some cases where they would draw a map of the house and a person with a pendulum would dowse it and say that's a dangerous spot, they mark a black spot on the house and time after time it would be where the kiddie's sleeping, his crib is over in that spot, and there was a sick kiddie, so you move it off the black spot, kiddie gets well. That's what we call geopathic stress, okay. Now since then I met lots of experts all over Europe and realized what a vast model it is for cancer. It's to do with the earth radiation. The earth, first of all let me just give you a little bit of the electric model, but the sun is a huge electrical plasma that's pouring all this energy towards us. The earth is kind of transmuting it. We have a plasma sphere around here. Lightning pouring every which way, millions of lightning strikes and it's a highly, highly electrical environment, and the earth's got an iron core so it's like, rotating like this, it's like a huge dynamo flinging off mega schoolings of gazillions of watts and—so we live in a strong environment like that. What seems to be the model is that the earth surface modifies this in certain places, it intensifies or depletes but certainly intensifying this earth radiation can prove extremely toxic to health. Now I—well I'm a professor. I've been a professor a couple of years and they do stories right. That's what I always thought a professor was for. Not for the knowledge you could just read that in a book but full of these stories, Wade Barney, right.

Ty: Yeah.

Dr. Mumby: So I've got one of these for this round, which is, back in Germany, in the 1930's, there was a German, Baron Friedrich Friar Von Pohl called, and he was a really hot dowser. Dowsing is very big in Germany by the way, about 40 percent of the doctors—don't know if you knew that but he was very good at it. He dowsed at a town called Vilsbiburg and he did it blind. He just took a mark, dowsed it, marked on what he thought was dangerous earth radiations. He had a scale of 1 to 16 and he thought anything 9 or above dangerous, marked them up. He then went off to City Hall to find out all the records of the deaths and interestingly every single cancer death in that town over 50 years had been cited over one of these dangerous radiation spots. He thought that was significant, and he was, that's what I'm just telling you, it's called geopathic stress, but of course all the other doctors, they scoff and said, well, do it again. So they took him to another town, can't remember the name of that town, but he did it again. Same result. Exactly the same result. Doing it blind he identified all the bad spots, which is where all the cancer patients died. He on to something you think?

Ty: Yeah.

Dr. Mumby: Then a guy called Dr. Hager in a German city called Schnity and he was no lightweight. He was president of the General Medical Association for something, no jerk. He did it the other way around. He took the houses and dowsed them and he dowsed 120 houses that had been cancer houses and found this bad radiation in all of them. What was wild—in five houses it killed 120 people. More than 120 people had died in just five houses over the years. Don't forget this is Europe, history goes back two, three or 400 years right. Again, wow, if that doesn't set your alarm bells going what would. Then one final character, a man called Manfred Curry, he was a brilliant dowser too, and he got this down to such an art he would dowse somebody's bed and say well, there's a strong radiation in the pelvic area or a strong intense radiation in the head area and he did this in front of a panel of doctors that are watching him do it and it was all blind. They would take him somewhere and say, all right, dowse that, and tell us what you find. Every time he was right, whether it was in the pelvic area, one of those was the beds he was dowsing. I didn't say that, but the dangerous places, the bed, because you spend a third of your life lying on the black spot right? So he dowsed the beds and if it was in the pelvic area, one bed he found had killed two women with uterine cancer. Where he said it was in the head had brain tumors, and so on, so it's a very fascinating phenomena.

It relates to the issues we've got with cell phones, microwave radiation and so on, but the name geopathic stress really reflects the fact that it's the earth itself that's doing it. Now, how to get an angle on this. If you've got cancer you should do this, but a good dowser is still the best tool we've got, and I've known one of the best dowsers in the world. I paid to have her book translated into English, published back in the 80's. Wonderful lady. She taught me how to dowse, but there are good ones and bad ones, and it's difficult to say how you'd find a good one, but they have to be good, but I followed around the very best and I would do things like take on a TV set, you know, they say this is a bad spot but I would walk across it with the TV and the TV is working fine and it would do shhh white noise and things while I crossed it and at the other side worked again. There was definitely strong electromagnetic radiation forces coming out of these spots. So that's the whole phenomenon and it's very important to a cancer sufferer to check if you're on a geopathic hot spot because if you are you need to move. The very least, move your bed, but we've had people moving out of the house. There are other sort of remedies, like putting in metal spikes around the house to try and deflect the rays and so on. It's not unscientific but no question would be the best thing to do is to just move. I tell a story in one of my books, Ty, about how this comes about, you know, farmers and vets know this. If you want to learn medicine go and look at farmers and vets because they know, they keep their animals healthy. They go bust if they don't, so vets know more about medicine and nutritional needs than any of the average doctors. So what happened is the farmer would notice these things called bad land and they're a tradition in, I doubt if you have them here, I know you have the word, but there's a tradition, if you turn cattle out onto this field they get sick and die at extraordinary rates, so you must not put cows on that area so, of course, what happens is the farmer says well, that land is no use to me, I can't raise livestock, so he sells it. Along come the real estate developers, cover it with houses and people live on this bad land spot, so it's the worst possible formula for health and a lot of modern subdivisions are put in the worst possible place.

Ty: You know that makes sense. I've not heard about geopathic stress before but the principle makes sense in light of the fact that we know the harmful effects of radiation on people especially with cancer. So that does make sense. You've mentioned chemotherapy a couple times. I know you're not a big fan of chemo but let's say—I'm sure that there are millions of people watching this that are already doing chemo. Is there anything they can do nutritionally to mitigate the side effects?

Dr. Mumby: That's a good point Ty. It's one of the best questions because I'm not, you know, I'm a holistic viewed practitioner, but I'm not part of the herd and, you know, I don't like the way—it's almost sneering and scoffing at people that do chemo, like you dummy, why would you do that. It has to be the person's own choice but it should be an informed choice and that they all take a look at the facts and figures, and I don't know why you'd choose to do it, but be honest, a lot of people get frightened. They want to hedge their bets. I'll do it and maybe I can take vitamins and I'll be okay. I don't think that's enough, but it is true that if you use proper holistic health approach, the kind I've been talking about, you know, change to really killer nutrition, take lots of antioxidants, I mean, antioxidants will protect you against chemo and radiation, that's what it does. It knocks off all kinds of free radicals. So it's possible to protect yourself. This is, perhaps, the best way of saying quickly. You can protect yourself against the damaging side effects of the orthodox therapy if you want to do that. As I told you before, Ty, over a ten year period not one of my patients lost their hair even though they were taking the chemo and things like that and yet they recovered so the oncologist's—silly story. That was stopped, they stopped chemotherapy working is nonsense. It did—it's just as poisonous as ever but the person was taking steps to protect themselves and didn't even lose their hair so that's a valuable tip if a person really wants to go that route.

Ty: Give us some maybe three or four different foods that people should look to eat if they are on chemo and they want to get the antioxidants...

Dr. Mumby: You're falling into the trap already. Remember what I said in the earlier part of this interview, a person must find their own good, safe foods—but you clearly need to remove the junk foods. They're not going to do you any good at all. There's not protective nutrients in something, synthetic manufactured food, white flour as we were saying, sugary foods, colas, anything cola flavored. Basically if it's in a tin or a package you need to just eat whole foods the way that nature made it but with the caution of what I said before, of being aware that they may not all be obviously safe. But that's very important. Then you got vitamin C. Vitamin C is a whole therapy in itself. You shoot an IV line loaded with vitamin C that is actually cytotoxic to cancers and I saw a very good study on that where at about three milligrams percent, it's called milligrams of a hundred of mills of blood, it was actually cytotoxic to cancer cells without doing anything harmful at all to healthy cells. So you know, the value of that, and it's an antioxidant, it's a detoxer. If somebody is in a toxic environment, vitamin C will help that too. So if you can't find somebody who will give you an IV vitamin C, is you can Lypo-Spheric vitamin C where 1 gram in a session one session will give you the equivalent of ten grams of oral vitamin C if you just took it as a powder. That's a pretty good dose, ten grams, 20 grams would be great.

Ty: Why does the Lypospheric vitamin C work that way. How does that deliver more than you would normally get?

Dr. Mumby: Well because basically vitamin C is a bit toxic to bile beyond a certain level. You get this phenomenon we call fill and flush. We used to use that as a measure back in the 70's and 80's. You take more vitamin C until it gives you diarrhea and then take less. So if ten grams causes diarrhea you take eight. That would be a limit that if you try and take any more of that you get diarrhea and you lose more vitamin C than you're swallowing so it becomes counter productive. The Lypospheric protective form does that because it's so complete, absorbed, it delivers almost all of the vitamin C—it's not just Lypospheric getting through the gut wall, but it's getting into the cells and you're now taking it where it counts in the body so it's a very, very valuable technique thing to use.

Ty: Talk a little bit about homeopathy. I know you're a homeopath.

Dr. Mumby: Indeed and I'm on a homeopathic advisory board back in Europe. The only thing is I can't talk a little bit about homeopathic. I can run out the camera batteries…

Ty: I'm sure you could

.

Dr. Mumby: No seriously I'll try hack it down okay, but first of all it's important to understand the model because a lot of people have probably heard the word and they're probably seeing all the scoffing and saying there's nothing in it. You know we proved there are no chemicals in it therefore it's a fraud and think, well it must be a fraud when, in fact, it's one of the most healing restorative modalities I know. The thing is, it's not based on the amount of stuff. It's based on an energetic signal and information signal if you like. So this is like homeopathy in two or three sentences. You pick a substance that copies the illness, not one that opposes it, but one that copies it, for example, if someone has scarlet fever you chose your belladonna, because if you take belladonna your face goes all bright red and your throat's sore, hectic temperature, you feel ghastly, taking belladonna is like having scarlet fever, so it's a good remedy for scarlet fever. It's called, like cures like. So you're looking for a mimic of the disease. A conventional adult would take an antagonist so you take your aspirin to lower temperature, different kinds of opposing ideas. This is, first of all, identifies something that copies your illness then you dilute it. Now this is the weird part that doctors and scientists can't get a hold of, it's called potentization and you can dilute it one in ten, one in ten, one in ten, one in ten, one in ten, and after 12 dilutions you've passed the Avogadro number so we know there is no belladonna left. Well interestingly, if you hitch it up to a spectrographic transmitter, you find that the more you dilute it the more it starts transmitting energies and now—I'll give you spectrograph, it's the most exquisitely sensitive scientific instrument we have. That's what tells you there's manganese on a star that's thousand billion light years away. You can't argue with a spectrogram and yet the homeopathic remedies actually start to broadcast the more you dilute them.

There's another series that goes a hundred, by a hundred, by a hundred, by a hundred. That's called a C sieve so you got the D or ten series or the C, 100 sieves, so get rid of any concern that you've removed the substance, that's true, but, of course, what's happened is that you've imprinted signal in each dilution and gets re-imprinted on the water and that's the third point of homeopathy. It's like cures like, then the dilutations, and then what we call succussion. In making the dilutions the homeopath will bang it on his hand like that a few times, then do the next dilution into plain water, bang it on his hand, that's called succussion and it enhances the transmission of the signal from each substance, and although you'll read all over the place that homeopathy has been proven not to work. First of all you can't prove anything doesn't work. You can only fail to prove it does work. There are thousands of studies showing it's highly effective. In fact there's a very good one that was published in 1994, they did it three times because they couldn't believe it was working. Three times it performed better than placebo. Well what I want to say—so that's what homeopathy is.

Now what I want to say is that you can take healing substances like pokeweed, or Viscum is one, that's the mistletoe, we'll talk about that it in a minute, mistletoe. You can dilute those. You can also dilute healthy organ signals so you if somebody has lung cancer you can administer them healthy lung signals using homeopathy. It can also look for historic shadows of diseases that call they call miasms and remove those. So there's many ways of tackling it. Your viewers I'm sure will be very interested in studies that were done in India originally but they were repeated here and they found that using three or four homeopathic remedies were actually effective. Listen to this. Glioma, you know the brain tumor's pretty deadly. They found two remedies, Phytolacca, and one cause, that's pokeweed and carcinogens made from cancer itself, actually resolved six out of seven gliomas and results showed all the tumors disappeared, the markers disappeared. There's not enough follow up on that to know, you know, this was famous five years or however it was but that's a pretty remarkable result for taking what the orthodox doctors say is just water. It's a fake. There's nothing in here.

Well, you know, the patients certainly did better. Then maybe I should just mention an alternative type of homeopathy sometimes called complex homeopathy or German homeopathy and it was invented by a guy called Hans-Heinrich Reckeweg and basically it's mixtures that classic homeopaths think that's all wrong, you know, you got to get the exact remedy. He said mixtures are good and so you'd have mixtures of things like drainage to drain toxins, mixtures of things that would help liver, mixtures of things that would help the brain and blood flow and all those things. I'm an international advisor in this particular branch called Homeotoxic Ecology, is the preferred. We got turned out of a hotel once for our meeting cause they heard the word homo and thought homosexuals and you're not going to, your people here. That's Europe for you. Homeotoxic ecology because it means auto toxins, our body's own toxins and the model here is not cells so much as extra cellular fluid. Cleansing it of toxins and you can do this with interesting mixtures. The most famous one is called Iscador. I'm sure you've heard of that on your travels. Somebody's got to be talking about it. Suzanne Sommers made it famous. In fact she took it. It's basically mistletoe, Viscum Album it's called. I think I have enough time on the camera to just tell a little story about mistletoe all right.

Ty: Sure.

Dr. Mumby: You'll like this. It's one of these little things back in Druidic times they used to have these sort of—at Christmas time they had, what's it called, the winter solstices they'd have all these big festival feasts and wild parties and what would happen is the women would drink a draft of mistletoe juice and it would render them infertile for a few days so they had all this wild sex and didn't get pregnant right. Fast forward 3,000 years so now we have a little sprig of mistletoe and you just kiss the girl under the mistletoe. You're not smiling. Have you got it Ty? It's the echo of the earlier orgies rite using mistletoe as a contraceptive but now it works as this little symbol of an affectionate kiss at Christmas time. Of course the winter solstice was the old Yule festival which how became Christmas.

Ty: What is the action though in the mistletoe to treat cancer?

Dr. Mumby: Well mistletoe is highly toxic. Now listen, this is, you got me going on another thing, but we don't want too much in alternative holistic treatments of the toxic stuff. You know that's what I call chemotherapy thinking. You know I take stuff and it'll kill the cancer and I don't even have to change my diet. That's not going to work. You got to do all the good things I've been talking about. Mistletoe, you can't say it's safe and natural and hololistic, it's extremely poisonous, but if you take it in the right dose and it's got a tradition of hundreds of years now—Iscador itself was developed by Rudolph Steiner back in Victorian times and it contained, there's a few things, it's a mixture. One of the important ones is mercury iodide and the iodine is great for the thyroid because that's something else I haven't got time to elaborate on but 20 years ago I noticed that many surfaced in all the literature, I keep seeing it, but I noticed it because I use those EAAV testing machines and it would tell you hidden signals. Time and again with cancer you get a signal on thyroid. The thyroid wasn't performing and the underperforming thyroid is one of the biggest reasons why the immune system goes down. You can't not afford to have an inefficient thyroid if you've got cancer so you need to beef it up and you need to have your thyroid checked, in fact, there's another hot tip. All that's built into Iscador remedy.

If you take it as it should be it's very safe and I got to tell you that something like 60 percent, it's the most prescribed oncological treatment in Germany now. You wouldn't believe that but 60 percent of the cancer patients will take it whether the doctor says to or not. They will, it's got a very strong tradition, and I said over here, if you don't think German means it could be could then Suzanne Sommers is your reference. She liked it. She claims it really, really helped her. I've used it a lot across—I used a slightly different variation. It's called Viscum compositum forte from a German company and I found it very, very valuable. So there's another tick. You see homeopathy is very safe because it's very diluted. The complex homeopathy depends on what's in it and how safe it is. We still dilute it. I mean Viscum you still dilute lots of times so you're not going to hurt yourself. That's the message. Yet it's got this powerful effect. It really does help shift body metabolism and body disease. It depends on the skill of the homeopath. Listen you go to whole foods and buy complex homeopathic remedies. Have you heard of Tromine? It's on sale there regularly. That's made by the same firm that's Viscum compositum, it's a German firm called Heel. It was founded by Hans-Heinrich. Anyway that's probably a good way place to shut up.

Ty: Well Keith your explanation of homeopathy there was amazing. I've read about homeopathy. I've had it explained to me but the way that you just explained the dilutions and the way that it affects the energy, something I've never heard before. So thank you for that. I know that the viewers gained a really important knowledge of homeopathy from that. Fascinating information about mistletoe. This has been great. Unfortunately we're out of time but is there anything that you want to leave the viewers with? Just a couple of quick tidbits that they take away from today's talk?

Dr. Mumby: Yeah well okay in one phrase it's like "life is like cancer cause only the fighters are going to survive right. Don't give in." Churchill, I'm British, let me quote Winston Churchill. "Never, never, never give up."

Ty: Well Keith thank you for your time today. Been enlightening and we really appreciate it.

Dr. Mumby: Pleasure.

[end of transcript]

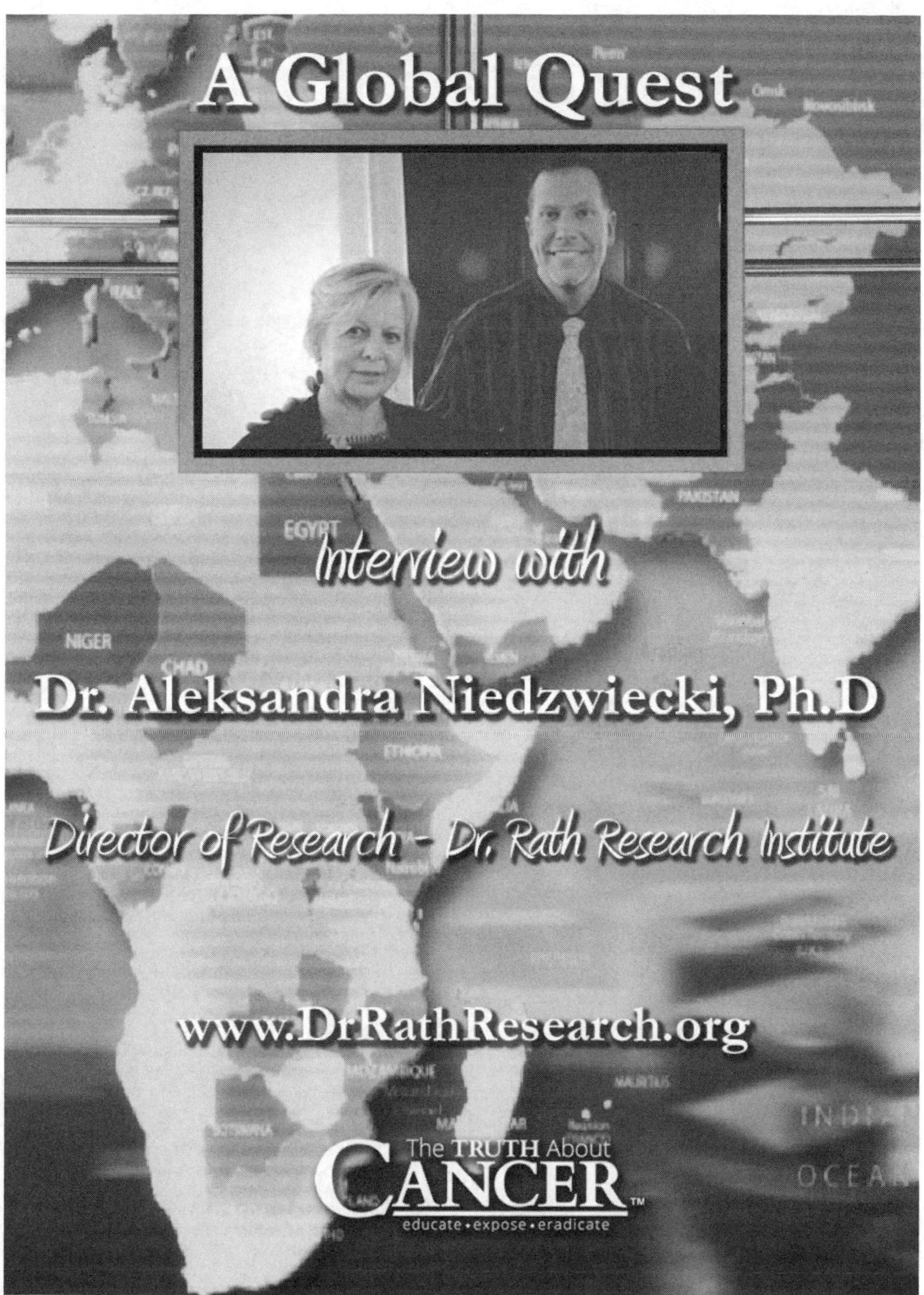
A Global Quest
Interview with
Dr. Aleksandra Niedzwiecki, Ph.D
Director of Research - Dr. Rath Research Institute
www.DrRathResearch.org
The TRUTH About CANCER™
educate • expose • eradicate

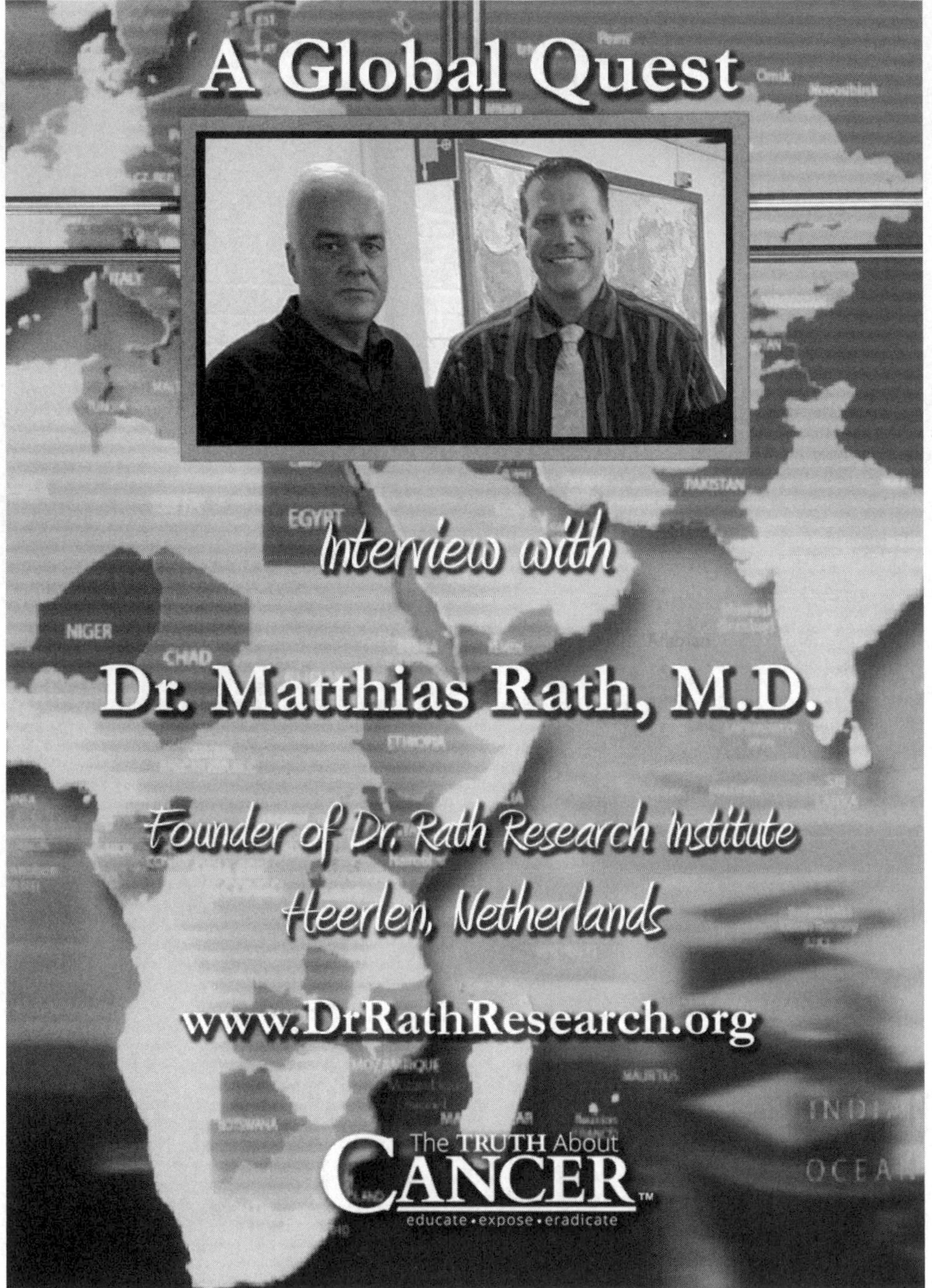
A Global Quest
Interview with
Dr. Matthias Rath, M.D.
Founder of Dr. Rath Research Institute
Heerlen, Netherlands
www.DrRathResearch.org
The TRUTH About
CANCER
educate • expose • eradicate

Ty: Matthias Rath, and Dr. Aleksandra Niedzwiecki.

Dr. Niedzwiecki: Yeah.

Ty: Thank you for joining us today. And I'm really excited to get your perspective. You've been sharing some things before the interview here with your treatment protocol. Before we get into that though, I'll start with you, Dr. Rath. Would you just share your education and how you got into medicine?

Dr. Rath: These are two different questions. I got into medicine because I come from a very humanistic family, and it was a vocation, an interest, to help others. As I moved along, I realized, of course, that medicine is something different.

But I tried to keep, to this day I try to keep, this very essence of serving others, as we will reflect on this interview. I graduated from the University of Hamburg in Germany for medical doctor. I held positions at the university there, the student clinic in Hamburg.

I later moved to the German Heart Center in Berlin, before accepting the position of Head of Cardiovascular Research at the Linus Pauling Institute, which of course led into various fields of research, including cancer. That's the sequence of that.

Ty: Dr. Aleksandra? Same question.

Dr. Niedzwiecki: Oh, okay. I have a PhD in Biochemistry from the University of Warsaw, in Poland. And later on, I did my post-doctoral work in the field of molecular biology of cell division at the Rockefeller University in New York.

And then later, I started my work in the area of mechanisms of aging at the University of Toronto in Canada. And the aging project actually brought me to work, to continue my work, at the Linus Pauling Institute in Palo Alto.

Ty: Okay.

Dr. Rath: That's where we met, and a few years later we decided to launch our own research organization, after the death of Professor Pauling. And that's what connects us, what has been connecting us over the past three decades.

Dr. Niedzwiecki: Then we started working on common projects, on the area of heart disease, all the micro-nutrients in heart disease. And expanded to cancer, and also infectious diseases and other chronic, mostly chronic health problems that people suffer.

Ty: You mentioned, Dr. Pauling, Linus Pauling. Most people realize that he was associated with vitamin C. Is this—when you mentioned micro-nutrients—is vitamin C a micro-nutrient? Or what exactly do you mean by micro-nutrients?

Dr. Rath: Yes, vitamin C is a micro-nutrient. Generally, micro-nutrients comprise vitamins, minerals, trace elements, certain amino acids, phytochemicals, or phytologicals as we call them, extracts from plants, small molecules that have a distinct metabolic role in the cells of the body.

Ty: We're fighting a war on cancer that began in 1972, I think, according to President Nixon. So does it make sense to you to be fighting a war, because in a war, there are people dying? Is that the right approach to have a war on cancer, Dr. Niedzwiecki?

Dr. Niedzwiecki: Yeah. There are so many casualties of this war, and the end of this war is not even in sight. And one of the reasons why this war continues is that money that are being made in this war. And this refers to the treatments, so-called treatments, that are being used in cancer, mainly chemotherapy and radiation.

Chemotherapy uses the most powerful toxins now known to humans. And these toxins, of course, are being sold to us as substances that can kill cancer cells. But these substances also kill, annihilate, healthy cells in the body, damage its organs, which make recovery from cancer almost a miracle, impossible.

And also this, they're very, substances that are being used to fight cancer are cancer-causing chemicals. So instead of eliminating cancer, or curbing cancer, we are inducing and generating new cancers.

Ty: Not a bad business model if you're in it for the money, big pharmaceutical companies producing the drugs to treat cancer that are then actually causing cancer. Dr. Rath, I've seen you've written extensively about big pharmaceutical companies. What do you think about that?

Dr. Rath: Unfortunately, Ty, you're right. We all think that the pharmaceutical industry has been around for ages to take care of the health problems of humanity, try to alleviate suffering, and prevent death.

As you know, that the birth hour of the pharmaceutical industry is actually a delivered dissension by a handful of people on this side and on the other side of the Atlantic Ocean, to define disease as a marketplace, and build what has now become the largest investment industry upon that simple thought. So cancer is just one element of this unspeakable business of defining diseases as a marketplace.

Everything else that you see today around the pharmaceutical industry, the tremendous profits, the inability to eliminate diseases, the propaganda war from that side that they are actually making progress in any disease, all of that comes from the fact that it's a business model. An investment industry that thrives on the continuation of existing diseases, and the launching of new diseases, as Dr. Niedzwiecki just mentioned.

One trick that they use, they produce patented synthetic drugs from which they know that, sooner or later, they cause new diseases by the mere side effects. So as you say, it's a fantastic business model. And maybe one aspect is important too for the audience. And that is the principle of patentability.

In other words, once you define a business as an investment business, you have to define the return on investment. In the pharmaceutical industry, these are patent fees, royalties. Then the next step is, how do you get a patent? You only get a patent if you do something new, and most of the patents in the pharmaceutical industry, therefore, relate to synthetically defined new drugs, artificially created.

In other words, the body doesn't know them, the small molecules, and treats them as toxins. And in many cases, our organs are not able to detoxify them, and there you have it. As a result of this business model, of being an investment industry, you have this avalanche of side effects factored into this business model.

Dr. Niedzwiecki: Yeah, and another aspect is that the majority of drugs that are being used to treat our diseases are the drugs that treat only symptoms, not underlying causes of diseases, just to make sure that your numbers looks better, and there is less cholesterol or sugar in your blood. But the disease continues.

So this is symptom-oriented medicine, contrary to what we've been working on, which is cause-oriented approach, where we look what is the underlying cause of diseases or health problems, and eliminate their causes. And the other aspect is also a monopoly on treatment.

Only pharmaceutical, conventional medicine is the medicine that is officially approved and acclaimed, and people who try to find other solutions have difficulties when it comes to insurance coverage and other problems. So maintaining monopoly on treatment is also another way to protect and grow this business.

Ty: Because it's an investment business.

Dr. Niedzwiecki: Yes. Of course.

Ty: Yeah.

Dr. Niedzwiecki: Yep.

Ty: It's sad that people's lives are being lost because of money, because of the underlying greed of the industry. You mentioned chemotherapy, and Dr. Rath, you were telling me before the interview, you were recently in Auschwitz. And is it true? I've heard that the origins of the first chemotherapy drugs were from the World Wars, the gasses that were used in the World Wars. Is this true?

Dr. Rath: It's very true. The first chemotherapy commercialized by Bayer was actually the same substance that they produced for the German army in World War I. It was mustard gas, with the replacement of one molecule in this gas molecule from being used as a tool of mass extermination. A chemical weapon is a weapon to kill thousands at one time, and a few years later, these substances turns up as a chemotherapy drug.

It underlines again, the principle of business. You can produce and make millions by selling weapons to the army, and then, when the war is over, you look for new applications of this drug. In this case, the unfortunate decision was taken to apply it for the alleged treatment of cancer.

In fact, as Dr. Niedzwiecki pointed out, this was a business model, it's not a treatment. The intention is to give the impression that something goes away. And it may go away for a few months, but the real mass mega death in the field of cancer patients is happening after six months, or nine months, when this initial effect of doing away with the tumor breaks down, and the cancer comes back massively, even more than before, because now the immune system is dead.

No one talks about that. So yes, we were in Auschwitz because we have a friendship with some of the survivors that are still alive from that time, and since you asked me this question, I may just spend a moment on something that is very little known about Auschwitz.

We've been told in the history books it was a camp that was built to annihilate the Jewish people, and the Slavic people, and people that the Nazis didn't like in the conquered countries. But what made Auschwitz the mega-death extermination camp was actually the decision by Bayer, Hoechst, and BASF to build the largest industrial plant of war time in Europe.

It is called IG Auschwitz, 100 percent subsidiary of Bayer, Hoechst, and BASF. And the plant was eight kilometers long, about five miles long, and two miles wide. So it's a giant industrial area. And the Birkenau concentration camp, the huge camp that was featured in *Schindler's List*, in that movie, was a deliberate decision to supply slave labor for the construction of this industrial plant.

So without the interests that we just touched upon, that put profits over lives, Auschwitz would never have had this meaning. The decision of one thing, which was the decision by the Nazis to exterminate the Jewish people, was taken roughly one year after the decision of IG Farben to build this plant.

So the Nazis used the death apparatus that was already existing because of the slave labor camp being in existence. The chimneys were burning, IG Farben was not taking care of the sick people. After three months on average, the people were immiserated, and so they were just put to the gas chamber and shut up in the chimney.

So I used a few more sentences than normal to exemplify. If we are talking today that there is an industry among humanity that sacrifices millions of lives, or puts them at risk for profit, we are sometimes, you included, being attacked as being out of this world, conspiracy people.

Now we turn around, we look at Auschwitz, we look at the industrial plant, we look at the concentration/extermination plant being built, initially built, to serve as slave labor camp for that purpose. And we look and say, "They've done it before."

Dr. Niedzwiecki: Yeah, to add to it. There were employees of Bayer, doctors, who were conducting medical experiments on prisoners, and testing variety of drugs that are being sold until this day. So they were tested on innocent people, in inhumane conditions, in the name of profit. At least we're not crazy and cruel as doctors who conducted those experiments.

These were employees, these were employees of the pharmaceutical company Bayer, and we have a website, Profit Over Life, that presents original documents from the Nuremberg trial of IG Farben, and where all this information is available, and we are encouraging everybody who watches this movie to go and learn about historic truth.

Dr. Rath: I'm a German. I didn't learn anything about that. I was 35 years old when I leaned about Bayer, BASF, the largest pharmaceutical companies at that time, were actually building, or responsible for, the extermination camp at Auschwitz. And then I wanted to know more, and there was nothing.

So we finally found, in the archives of the US National Library in Washington, the US National Library, the records of case number six of the Nuremberg War Crime Tribunals. We were told there was only one tribunal against the main war criminals, but in fact, there were 12.

Number six was against Bayer, BASF, and Hoechst at that time, they were forming a cartel by the name of IG Farben. And that whole case lasted an entire year, against 24 managers of these pharmaceutical and chemical companies.

And it showed that they were largely financing the rise of the Nazis to power, that they supplied 100 percent of the raw materials so that the Nazis could lead the war, including 100 percent of the synthetic gasoline and rubber, 100 percent of the explosives. The report came to the conclusion, the US process said, without IG Farben, World War II would not have been possible.

In other words, we have to redefine history, even if we talk about cancer today, we need to know those things. That these interests for expanding patented product markets worldwide, they were risking eventually, they were responsible for the death of 60 million people in World War II.

And that shows you the dimension of the topic that we are talking about today. There's nothing, absolutely nothing, that these interests will not do if the profit is high enough, then and now.

Dr. Niedzwiecki: Yeah, and those activities didn't end with the war, end with Nuremberg process, because the head of Bayer Pharmaceutical Company, who was sentenced to six or sevem years of prison, was released after two years, and for the next 10 years, he served as a Chairman of the Board for the same company, Bayer.

So there are many other examples. The head of the company Degesch, that was providing the gas, Zyklon B, used to gas innocent people, the same. Returned to his position.

Dr. Rath: But talking about making the connection our topic today, a doctor that we keep mentioning, Fritz ter Meer, head of Bayer, who was sentenced for six years in Nuremberg, and returned to the position of Supervisory Board of Bayer, essentially immediately after the war.

So a war criminal, a convicted war criminal, becomes head of the largest pharmaceutical company at that time. During the first half of the 21st century, no less than nine Nobel Prizes were rewarded, or awarded, for vitamin research, for the benefits of vitamins for human health.

In 1963, the German government, under pressure of Bayer, under pressure of then the Supervisory Board head Fritz ter Meer, launched what is called a Codex Elementarius Commission with the goal to make sure that vitamins, and the benefits of vitamins for human health, are being eliminated worldwide.

So you can see, it is not just you and us talking about cancer. There's a century long tradition of crime against human health, and when you follow that trek, a lot of things we will be talking about today will become easier to understand for the people that watch this interview.

Ty: Wow. So they've done it before, it shouldn't surprise us that they're still doing it now.

Dr. Rath: Very true.

Dr. Niedzwiecki: Yeah, chemotherapy business is also a wonderful example of multiplicator, because the side effects that chemotherapy produces is the reserve word for prescribing other drugs, bone marrow transplants. This is the results of chemotherapy, bleeding from the intestines, that requires drug. Anti-nausea drugs, and many others.

Changes in the brain. There's even a term for it, it's called chemo brain, because the chemotherapy affects so many organs in the body, and it's the reason for prescribing more drugs. So chemotherapy multiplies the business, and this is why it lasts until this day.

Ty: Wow.

Dr. Niedzwiecki: It's hard to imagine.

Ty: It is. It is. But thank you for sharing the history there, because it's really the history that's been re-written, right? The history that we are taught now, is not what actually happened.

Dr. Rath: Right. If we are not learning from history, and I'm quoting a philosopher, "We are sentenced to live it again." And I wasn't born as a historian. I was a scientist, a doctor, and after publishing these initial new concepts on cancer and heart disease with Linus Pauling, I felt the world will embrace us. They will say, "This is great." Fact is, we were being fought for every single advance in natural health.

There are more than 100 lawsuits that the state has scrolled, the pharmaceutical lobby has been bringing against myself, Dr. Niedzwiecki, our research, over the past 15 years. More than 100 times we were dragged into the courtrooms for one goal. These interests did not want us to talk today, they fought the matter to inform you of what we have found out about the most common diseases can be greatly reduced, maybe eventually largely eliminated with the knowledge we have today.

The fact that we're doing this interview now shows they didn't succeed. And the main reason why we succeeded, actually summarizing it in one word, was science. We could prove it. So if we will touch upon the scientific details later on of our research. They have been rejecting in more than 100 litigations for the validity, for the truth, and for the use, for the people on this planet.

Ty: So it's science based natural medicine, that's what it is.

Dr. Niedzwiecki: Yes.

Ty: Science-based.

Dr. Niedzwiecki: Mm-hmm.

Dr. Rath: Science-based, and to court validated, if you want it.

Ty: Oh 100 times.

Dr. Rath: Mm-hmm.

Dr. Niedzwiecki: Yeah, we call it cellular medicine.

Ty: Cellular.

Dr. Niedzwiecki: Because we look at the beginning, or development, of health and disease at the level of smallest units of our body, which are cells. And our study shows that the underlying cause of majority of chronic diseases, diseases that develop over years, or even decades, is the long term deficiency of micro-nutrients, vitamins, trace elements, some acids, or other active components which cause dysfunction, cellular dysfunction, that with time turns into a diseased organ, and disease.

And therefore, since we know the underlying cause of these health problems, we also can develop effective solutions to alleviate those.

Ty: So, with cancer specifically, you look over the last 100 years, the lack of micro-nutrients being one of the causes makes a lot of sense. Because look at depleted soils, the food's no longer food, it's being genetically modified, and so forth.

It makes sense that we would have a lack of micro-nutrients in our bodies now, and maybe that's one of the reasons that we've had this increase in cancer. Dr. Niedzwiecki, you were talking about the fact that even though the statistics might say otherwise, there's a huge explosion in cancer over the last several decades.

Dr. Niedzwiecki: Yes. Today I think everybody knows somebody who gets diagnosed with cancer, or died of cancer, maybe in our families or friends. So there is a tremendous explosion of cases of cancer that exactly relates to the pollution, chemical pollutions, of our environment, soil, food that we eat, all the processed foods.

When you read the label, you don't understand half of the ingredients that are in. But all of them have impact on the metabolism of cells. It is known that certain micro-nutrients, such as, for instance, vitamin C, protects our DNA against damage that can trigger development of cancer.

And many other micro-nutrients act at a genetic level, and there have been studies showing that micro-nutrients also help alleviate many diseases that are of genetic origin that stem from so-called pleiotropic effects, not the lack of gene, but small activity of certain enzymes, which are coded by the genes. Micro-nutrients, applied in larger quantities, are effective in alleviating those symptoms.

Ty: And even in cancer, correct?

Dr. Niedzwiecki: Exactly.

Ty: So, let's, you're talking about cells, what is a cancer cell? What exactly is cancer?

Dr. Niedzwiecki: What exactly is cancer? Cancer is a process that occurs in our body all the time. So as we are sitting and talking, there are cancer cells that are constantly created in our body. They do not always lead to the development of cancer, because our immune system finds them as abnormal cells and eliminates them.

And a cancer cell is a cell that escaped biological control. That is, to which all normal cells in our body are subjected. So cancer cells divides indefinitely. And also, cancer cells are immortal. They never die, because the genetic program that regulates life and death cycles in in those cells has been damaged.

And cancer cells also have another ability. They are not happy in sitting in one spot in our body. They invade our organs, and also they metastasize, which means that they escape to other organs. And metastasis is the most dangerous process of cancer, because nine out of 10 patients die of metastasis, not of primary cancer.

And metastasis is the stage of cancer, process of cancer, for which there are no treatment, and what is also interesting, there is not much scientific interest in studying metastasis, because about five, maybe now 10 percent of funds for cancer research from National Cancer Institute is directed to study metastasis.

Imagine that the process that kills 90 percent of cancer patients is not studied in the same proportion, a very small percentage is directed to study metastasis.

Ty: It's kind of the inverse, right?

Dr. Niedzwiecki: Exactly.

Ty: The largest percentages is used to fund the cancer that is not spread.

Dr. Niedzwiecki: Yeah. And find drugs that eliminate cancer.

Ty: Right. And I think it probably goes back, you were mentioning earlier, the difference between treating symptoms versus the cause, right? You treat the tumor, you can get a reduction in the tumor size, and everything seems to be happy. But then, as Dr. Rath said, it always comes back.

Dr. Niedzwiecki: Yeah.

Ty: Because you haven't really affected the cause. So when you're looking at micro-nutrients for cancer, Dr. Rath, do micro-nutrients have any kind of effect on a cancer that might be spreading, or metastasizing?

Dr. Rath: Well, yes, it does in several ways. Perhaps it is important to go one step back and explain how cancers spread.

Ty: Yeah, what you were telling me before. Absolutely. Yes.

Dr. Rath: It relates to what Dr. Niedzwiecki said. I believe that the largest contribution we make to the field was exactly that. That we said, "We are not looking at individual types of cancer, but we are looking at the key mechanism that unites them all." Cells, many cells, migrate within our body at any time.

White blood cells, the police cells, they need to leave the bloodstream and enter, for example, the lung to fight pneumonia, or any other organ. We have the egg cell in the monthly cycle of a woman that leaves the ovary, and migrates into the fallopian tube.

All these processes are extremely, tightly controlled, because they involve destruction of connective tissue, meaning destructing of tissue that surrounds the cell at that moment, mostly collagen or elastin. And this destruction happens with the help of an enzyme, or group of enzymes, which for simplicity we call collagenases, collagen digesting enzymes.

On a normal consensus, this mechanism is tightly controlled. Cancer cells use exactly that mechanism, exactly the same group of enzymes, to make their way through the body, to migrate through the body. First in their environment, called, we call this invasion, so the tumor grows and spreads, let's say, within the organ of the liver.

And then, ultimately, to migrate into other organs, and we call that metastasis. In each case, it's the same type of enzyme that paves the way of the cancer cell, or cancer cells, to migrate. It's probably like an expeditionary tour in the jungle with a machete, they pave their way through the jungle.

And what we found out is that we can block these collagen digesting enzymes, and we understand today the key micro-nutrients that are able to do that. Not chemotherapy, natural substances that are able to block cancer cells from doing harm to the body.

And therefore, the approach, we are going to talk about it a little bit more, is not related to an individual type of cancer, like breast cancer, or prostate cancer. It is a common mechanism that we understand today quite well. And that we have developed and tested a composition of micro-nutrients for, in over 50 human cell lines.

In other words, any commercial human cancer cell line that is available currently, we tested those micro-nutrients, and they are effective in each and every case. So we are not just talking about an experience of an individual or a test group of people.

We have been working on this for the last 15 years, and Dr. Niedzwiecki has been heading this research, and has developed it, the group has developed it, in many areas. And I'm sure that you can elaborate on this.

Dr. Niedzwiecki: Yeah. We've published over, let's see, 100 publications, scientific publications in the area of cancer. And like Dr. Roth pointed out, that our goal was to control the main common mechanism that cancer cells use to spread in the body, to metastasize, but also the same mechanism which is degradation of connective tissue, is being used in the process of angiogenesis, which is formation of new blood vessels that feed the tumor and support tumor growth.

So in our approach, we were looking at the substances, natural components, which, from one side, can inhibit the degradation of connective tissue, inhibit those enzymes that are involved in destroying collagen and other components. But also the substances which can increase the production of connective tissue, increase the strength and the structure of connective tissue in the body.

And the group of natural compounds includes, of course, vitamin C as the essential nutrients without which collagen cannot be produced in our body. And humans lost the ability to produce internal vitamin C, and also several amino acids in plant extracts and some trace elements.

So this is the group of natural compounds that work together in the synergy. And all our work also in other aspects of health, includes application of several micro-nutrients working in synergy. So our studies have shown that this composition of micro-nutrients is effective in inhibiting key mechanisms that cancer cells, or cancer uses in our body.

So these micro-nutrients can inhibit proliferation, or growth of cancer cells, inhibit formation of tumors. They can also inhibit the invasion of cancer cells in the tissue. They are effective in inhibiting metastasis. We tested in several cases the metastasis can be inhibited by 70, up to 80 percent.

And also they are effective in inhibiting formation of new blood vessels that feed the tumor. Interestingly, this natural, mixture of natural compounds, is also able to work at the genetic level in cancer cells, and convert them from cells which are immortal, into cells that start dying.

So these micro-nutrients can induce natural death of cancer cells, called apoptosis, and we also published a lot of studies supporting this type of finding. So if we can, what is the beauty of using nutrient synergy, is that several mechanisms that are involved in certain pathology can be effected at once, making in case of cancer, more difficult for cancer cells to escape this control.

Dr. Rath: We have mostly, here in Europe, more than 10,000 patients who are using this synergy program. And some of them have survived the predicted death now for 15 years. We have X-ray documentation for many of them, etc. And we've summarized this fantastic work that Dr. Niedzwiecki and her team were leading in a book called *Victory Over Cancer*.

So anyone who wants to get more details on what we're just explaining, it is available for free online. Everyone can read it anywhere in the world. There are, to our knowledge, to our understanding, there is no more precise mechanism that has been identified as being critical for the control of cancer than the one we just described.

There's no program that we are aware of in the field of natural health that is more effective in controlling cancer in vivo in humans. We are not giving a guarantee, obviously. That would be not what we ethically should do. But we are, we know that there are no science-based programs in natural health that are more effective as we speak.

Why are we not more outspoken about it? Well in many cases, patients come to us after they have already done chemotherapy, and it didn't work. Or they had radiation, didn't work. So they come to us with the hope, now you can give us a solution.

But in most of these cases, the immune system has been destroyed, so in those cases micro-nutrients are only able to have a limited effect. So what we understand is that in order for having a maximum chance of fighting and overcoming cancer, we need an intact immune system.

And that too, makes the current approach of chemotherapy so unethical. It destroys, the chemotherapy, the first organ that is effected, actually the target organ, is the bone marrow. The destruction of the generation of defense cells, and leukocytes, etc. are built in the bone marrow. So from the very onset, from the very planning of chemotherapy, from the very scientific approach, it is a deception. It is an unethical deceptive business that creates illusion for millions of people.

And everyone, every scientist involved in it, I'm not blaming the doctors, because they sometimes don't have the education to go at that length on it. But every scientist knows that it is a huge fraud. And those who say they don't, they should quit the job of being a scientist.

Dr. Niedzwiecki: And education is the key for patients, for doctors, for everybody. And this is why we put the big, we emphasize the importance of knowing, importance of education in the area of natural approaches to health. This is why we make all our materials, publications, education materials, free, available to everyone.

And if somebody wants to know more details about our scientific work, they should go to our research website, www.drrathresearch.org, where we have, we give access to all scientific work that we publish in the area of cancer, and, of course, in other areas as well.

Dr. Rath: An interesting story that shows the transitional time that we are living in. One of our first patients, that's now almost 20 years ago, who went on the program here in Europe, he had lung cancer. And he was given half a year to live and put his affairs in order. And he decided to go on this program, and I think six, seven months later, he came back, and an X-ray was taken, there was no more tumor. So the doctor apologized, he said, "You know, sorry. You have to come back a week later. We need to repair our machine. It is apparently kaput," as they say in German.

And so the gentleman said, "Sure, I understand. I'll come back in a week." And they redid the X-ray, it was the same picture. And then the doctor started to try to find other excuses, because, this was a female doctor, she had not seen anything like that. But our patient, he said, "Well, I don't think I need to come back. I know what I've been doing."

And I'm not telling that to add an episode to this conversation. I'm telling it to underline the transformational time, that it is inconceivable for health professionals, for doctors, educated people, that cancer can disappear in a natural way.

Dr. Niedzwiecki: Mm-hmm.

Dr. Rath: Just go away. Again, we're not promising that to anyone for sure. But these things that we developed is, scientifically speaking, the most direct way to have a chance to see that happening.

Dr. Niedzwiecki: Yeah, and we confirmed it in so many different models, not only in vitro studies, but also in vivo studies, and we look at different aspects of it, using the same methods, the same tools that pharmaceutical industry is using in testing, developing their drugs.

So we are not using any magic testing systems, no. And our studies are approved in peer review journals. But yes, it's a change of perception, that natural substances can be effective in controlling many diseases, many pathologies, and it's a mindset change that is, has to occur not only in patients but also in medical profession as well.

And I think that we see, especially in the US, that there are more and more doctors who are open into learning more, and also applying natural approaches. So it's a good step, but still, there is a lot of work to be done when it comes to education, and also when it comes to science, supporting the power of natural substances. Because there is scientific proof.

Dr. Rath: The fact is, example that I just mentioned with this lung cancer that disappeared, and that couldn't be understood by doctors. Our research shows—we now understand what happened. Because micro-nutrients give, in layman's terms now, give the cancer cell two options. Either you think about how you operate properly and become a healthy cell again, or you die, you commit suicide.

And this is this process that Dr. Niedzwiecki said, apoptosis. And that happens at a genetic level, and we understand quite a bit about the regulation, how micro-nutrients got directed to the core of a cancer cell, to the DNA, and challenges the very, the inner sanctum of this cell into this process.

Of course, it's not an intellectual deliberation, it is a forced biological interception. Either you function properly or you commit suicide. And that's really powerful. That is something that no chemical chemotherapy drug, or no synthetic drug can do. And of course, again, this is a sign for the real power of natural health.

These regulatory processes, they didn't appear in a reagent lens, or a petri dish in a laboratory of the pharmaceutical industry 20 years ago, or five years ago. These were processes that nature developed over millennia, and this is why they function so distinctly.

And we're just about to learn how they work, and what substance we need. And that is another aspect that we like to emphasize. There are those among our friends in the natural health field that educate, mega-doses of vitamins that you just take one vitamin, for example, vitamin C, and you give it in dosages of 100 or 200 grams a day, etc.

What our research shows, is that we, in order to have a maximum effect, as Dr. Niedzwiecki already indicated, we need to understand how these micro-nutrients work together. Like the artist of an orchestra. And when the music plays, that's when we have the maximum effect. And that's what we call synergy, and that's an essential part of cellular medicine.

Dr. Niedzwiecki: Yeah, and in this aspect, the vitamin C mega-doses—we also compared in our study the high dose of vitamin C, with vitamin C used in much lower dose, within this nutrient synergy complex. And the synergy works better, not mentioning with using multiple nutrients, we can address several mechanisms of cancer at once, so the final effect is much, much better and wider, more pronounced.

Ty: So could you kind of reiterate these micro-nutrients that cause cancer, they stop cancer cell growth, they stop the spreading, they stop the blood vessels, the growth of new blood vessels, the angiogenesis, and that also cause the apoptosis, the programmed cell death? What are these nutrients that have the synergistic effect, the orchestra? What are the components of this?

Dr. Niedzwiecki: Yeah. This is vitamin C, for simple reasons, since we are targeting the stability and integrity of connective tissue. Without vitamin C, connective tissue cannot be produced. The other compounds of this synergy, a very powerful component, is the amino acid Lysine.

Lysine is an inhibitor of those collagen digestive enzymes, but also Lysine is a component of collagen. One third of amino acids in collagen are Lysine and Proline. So it is important that they are included. And Lysine, similarly to vitamin C, is not produced in our body. It only comes from the diet.

We are also having other components like N-Acetylcystine. We are having trace elements including copper, selenium. And we are having the active component from green tea, called apigallocatechin gallate, or EGCG for short. And quercetin. So this is the mixture of several components. You can find the information on our website.

And this is what we tested them, we tested individual compounds and also we combined them in the synergy. So they are components acting on different mechanisms in our body, including, what we see they also have an anti-inflammatory effect. And what we know from one side, inflammation is associated with cancer, and also long-lasting inflammation is the triggering factor for developing cancer. And these micro-nutrients are also effective in addressing this important aspect. So this is this pleiotropic effect of micro-nutrient synergy that we are working with.

Dr. Rath: When we had the first proof of the concept that actually micro-nutrients are the solution to the cancer epidemic, we were thinking about how to present this to the public at large, and we decided to go into USA Today, in 2002, in March. And the largest circulation newspaper at the time.

And they didn't want to publish, so we said, "Well, but we just presented this information at the Breast Cancer Conference in Miami, Florida, so why shouldn't you publish things that are there in the scientific community?" So finally they did. It was a whole page, "Breakthrough in the Natural Control of Cancer," and listing some of the micro-nutrients, vitamin C, Lysine, Proline, and showing some of the research, all in layman's terms.

That did it. It triggered the war against this breakthrough that I just mentioned before, with more than 100 lawsuits, mostly focusing on cancer. The American Medical Association gave a media alert about Dr. Rath and his research institute, that no media should be publishing anything about our results. I thought, how could you deal with such an unethical approach?

And we took out another page in the newspaper, US newspaper, and I wrote an open letter to the President of the American Medical Association saying, "Well, you are heading an organization that is supposed to do good to the people of America. Here is some advanced research that can actually help benefit millions of people, and you are opposing it. Why is this?"

And I printed his email address at the bottom, and encouraged the readers to send their comments to the President of the AMA. We've never heard anything about them, so we assume that he got a lot of mails. I'm telling this not to brag about this battle and some lines episodes.

It tells again, that it is extremely important to state the truth, to fight for the truth, and this is why we appreciate you coming to us and interviewing us at length on this process. Because it is a courageous thing that you are doing, Ty, and not just with us, but with opening up this curtain of deception and lies about cancer and for a lot of diseases, and giving the people of America and the world a chance to see through that maze of deception, and make their own choice. I think you must be complimented. I'm complimenting you for that.

Ty: Thank you.

Dr. Niedzwiecki: Yeah. Because now, I think it's even more difficult in fighting for scientific proof, truth, because in old days, before pharmaceutical industry was created, it was more convincing others to accept the concept. So this was mostly fighting somebody's egos, and careers. But now, we are challenging the most powerful industry on Earth.

So this is not accepting science, and we see from our other contexts, that many doctors, scientists, agree with what we are doing and what we are publishing. But there is an economic aspect, and economic pressure, which is very difficult to overcome. And it is only by education, by spreading information and knowledge to people, this is how we can change it.

Ty: Yeah, that's with our group, *The Truth About Cancer*, that's our goal, to educate. Which, I appreciate everything that you've shared today, because it's very educational. It's to eradicate cancer, which, I think that using approaches like this, that's possible. But it's also to expose. That's the three E's.

And so we want to expose this beast, and it really seems to me that the real war is actually being fought against people that are offering natural treatments for cancer. I don't think there's a war against cancer, I think it's a war against natural treatments.

Dr. Rath: It's very true. And there's a reason for that. We talked about concentration camps. They are surrounded by a fence. If someone tries to escape the fences of the modern concentration camp, the ones that confine the cancer patient within the parameter of conventional thinking, of chemotherapy thinking, they are being hunted.

How many court cases have been filed around the world for withdrawing custody of parents who went into natural health as opposed to staying within the confines, within the fences, of conventional chemotherapy treatments? It's nothing else. The dimension of a child dying in a concentration camp, or dying from leukemia, that is being intoxicated by chemotherapy, as opposed to choosing natural paths, are the same.

The parents are losing a child. The family is losing their future. And that's the deeper dimension of what you're talking about, that the same interest groups that have proven again and again in the past, namely the pharmaceutical investment business, how ruthless they are, are still around trying to fool us, trying to tell us, "Well, believe us."

Why should we? If we don't have the courage to liberate ourselves, then we will not make progress. And this is why this is important, this series that you are doing, Ty. It's being kept alive, and I just can encourage everyone who's seeing this show, that you spread it and help Ty to get his message around the world, and not only tame this beast, but eliminate it. Not by violence, but by education, by becoming aware about the three E's that you mentioned.

Dr. Niedzwiecki: Yeah. We need to recognize that fear is being used in controlling patients, in controlling society. Fear is a very powerful weapon, and fear of cancer is being used in manipulating people. And so by educating, by bringing this knowledge to people, explaining both the basis of the problem, but also showing about possibility of new solutions to it, this fear is being alleviated.

Dr. Rath: Elaborating on that, Alex, among all diseases, the one disease that the status quo, meaning the pharmaceutical investment, needs most to continue its business, to stabilize, to cement its system, is cancer. They can afford to allow, let's say, advances in osteoporosis, that decrease the number of bone fractures, without major damage to its future existence.

They can allow progress in this and that disease to kind of mask their principle business. But they cannot allow, they cannot allow cancer to disappear, being identified as a disease that can be regulated or prevented. So long ago, they have initiated what Dr. Niedzwiecki mentioned, the fact of fear.

In fact, it's more than that. It's a psychological warfare on humanity that the pharmaceutical industry is leading with the tool cancer. Keeping cancer as a death verdict is the platform, is a precondition for this entire investment industry to continue.

Ty: Wow.

Dr. Niedzwiecki: It's strong, yeah?

Ty: It is.

Dr. Niedzwiecki: Yep.

Ty: Really amazing information that you've shared. I'd like to stop, but I'd like to ask one more question, because that would be a perfect ending for the interview. But there's one more question I want to ask you, because you just mentioned children.

Children are being taken from their parents. I've had the opportunity to interview several parents that have had their children literally taken from them because they refused chemotherapy. Why do you see—why have we seen over these last couple decades, this huge increase of children with cancer?

Dr. Rath: Well, I would start, but one of the answers is that during the phase of growth of the human body, cancer cells divide naturally. They multiply, otherwise we don't grow. Bones do, our skeleton expands.

And that's why we have already, by natural means, the risk that certain cancers are developing in the juvenile age, for example, osteosarcoma, a typical form of juvenile cancer, develops during the phase of bone growth in the epiphysis, the growth zone of the bone.

And then we have this effect, that chemotherapy is offered as a solution, and actually makes our cancer really explode. We have the fact that by now, 42 percent of all prescription drugs currently offered and sold in the United States, and for that matter, in the Western World, are potentially carcinogenic, according to US statistics.

And so we have, by the very means of reacting to the problem of cancer, by the way they do it, by the methods that are being used, we have a very strong reason why there is this explosion. Plus, we have lots of environmental factors and nutritional factors, etc.

Dr. Niedzwiecki: Pollutions. Yeah. So the same factors that Dr. Rath said, that children are vulnerable because their cells are already in this growing phase, means the enzymes that destroy connective tissue are active. And therefore, if there is exposure to carcinogenic compounds, the cells can reprogram and start digesting this connective tissue indefinitely and then other changes occur. So it's a combination of different factors.

Ty: Well, Dr. Rath, Dr. Niedzwiecki, thank you for helping us today to engage in our mission to educate, to expose, and to eradicate cancer. I know that this has been a very informative interview for the viewers, and so I just really thank you for the fact that you're providing science-based natural medicine that most medical doctors say, "I want to see the scientific evidence." They've got it with these treatments that you're currently using with these micro-nutrients. So I thank you for what you're doing, and just keep up the good work. It's great to be on your team.

Dr. Niedzwiecki: Thank you.

Dr. Rath: Thanks, Ty.

Ty: Appreciate it. Thank you so much.

[end of transcript]

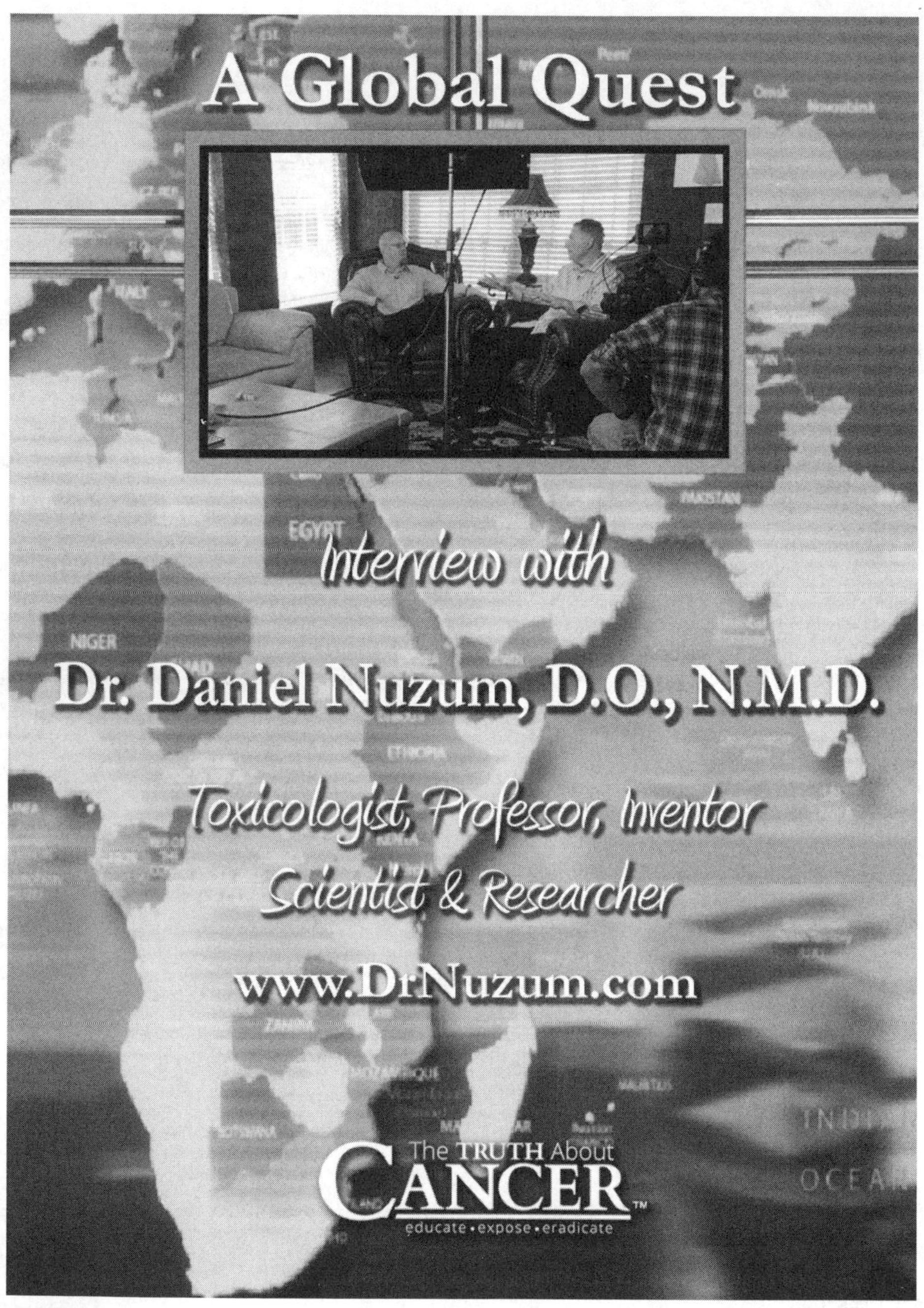
A Global Quest
Interview with
Dr. Daniel Nuzum, D.O., N.M.D.
Toxicologist, Professor, Inventor
Scientist & Researcher
www.DrNuzum.com
The TRUTH About CANCER
educate • expose • eradicate

Ty: Doc, I wanted to get you to sit down with us today and share a little bit more about detoxification. Because, as you know, being on the *The Quest For The Cures Continues* last year, we sat down and we talked detox. But we had such a huge response to that interview and so many people have come up to me and have emailed me and have contacted us and said, "We got to get more of Doc Nuzum. We want to know some details about this detoxification thing."

So, let's grab a seat here. I want to get some details from you on detoxification, if you could.

Dr. Nuzum: Well, you know, 80 percent of the problems people would normally deal with involve toxicity in some way, shape, or form. If you can minimize the amount of waste the body is carrying you're going to minimize inflammation, all the irritation that happens via the waste product build-up in the system, you're going to have reduced inflammation, reduced swelling, you're probably going to lose weight because you're reducing swelling. Girth is going to change.

Ty: Let's do this. Let me direct this a little bit more specific. These are the questions that we're getting. We're getting, "Doc convinced us that we need to detox. Doc told us the example of the fact that you've got a stadium full of people and you only got two exits. You got to clear the exits." What they're asking is this, "how do I do it? How do I detox?"

Let say that somebody is full of toxicity. They are full of toxins. They got 30 days to detox. Give us Doc Nuzum's 30-day detox program. And I know this is kind of spur of the moment thing but give me some products that you would recommend that they can detoxify their colon, their liver, their kidneys, whatever it might be.

Dr. Nuzum: Well, the way to do this would be like the stadium. You got a hundred thousand people in the stadium and there's a fire. You got to get them out right now. If you only have one exit open, you are just going to make a mess. So, if we can open up multiple exits and clear them, we can get everybody out safe.

Ty: Right. So how do you do that?

Dr. Nuzum: First off, the garbage chute. We got to take the garbage out. Clean the colon. We got to clean the colon.

Ty: Clean the colon. How do we clean it?

Dr. Nuzum: We could use coffee enemas, we can use colon hydrotherapy. My preference is usually with herbal supplements using herbal cleanses.

Ty: Like psyllium.

Dr. Nuzum: Psyllium, cascara sagrada, bentonite, slippery elm bark, buckthorn, very, very good. Those are good, good herbs. Humic acid, excellent for the entire digestive tract.

You've got to clear the exits, you've got to clear one exit to clear the next. Your colon would be number one. The next best exit to go to would be the urinary tract, the kidneys, the bladder, clear that urinary tract system.

Ty: How do we do that?

Dr. Nuzum: Parsley, asparagus. Your marshmallow root. Those types are very good here.

Ty: Lots of water?

Dr. Nuzum: Lots of water, yes.

Ty: Which you would want to go back in your colon if you're taking psyllium husk. You have to be drinking lots of water.

Dr. Nuzum: Right. That's going to swell up and take up space so if you don't want to bloat, you have to keep it moist so it moves easy. Once the urinary tract is cleared, your best bet would be to the liver. Follow that with the liver. Clean the liver, clear the liver.

Ty: And coffee enemas as Dr. Nick Gonzalez shared with us last time. One of the best ways to clean the liver.

Dr. Nuzum: The best ways. Your turmeric, milk thistle. Virtually all of your root vegetables, beets, ginger, burdock, all of those things are very, very good at cleaning the liver.

Ty: You're recommending that people to eat those or do they take extracts?

Dr. Nuzum: If you want to clean it quick, extracts. You need the concentration. They need to be concentrated.

Here's the thing, you have two kidneys, one liver, you have a hundred lymph nodes. If you don't clean out those lymph nodes, there's no way to then drain the tissues. So if we clean the colon, clean the kidneys, clean the liver, lymph nodes will be the last thing to focus on.

Ty: And how do you do that?

Dr. Nuzum: You need things like cat's claw, pau d'arco, burdock root. The essiac formula [is] excellent for cleaning out lymph nodes and draining those lymph nodes, getting the lymph fluid drained up.

Ty: Would you use that in conjunction with a daily rebounding to stimulate the lymphatic system?

Dr. Nuzum: Rebounding would be excellent especially if you're trying to drain it. The lymphatic fluid is what's called a thixotropic fluid. Thixotropic fluid is like butter, the warmer it gets, the softer it gets, the more fluid it gets. The colder it gets, the harder it gets.

Ty: So, as you heat your body up it's going to flow better.

Dr. Nuzum: As you heat your body up, you get moving, bounce on a trampoline, do those types of things, you get it moving. You raise your temperature a little bit, it liquefies the lymphatic fluid, it flows easier. If you can do that while you're doing things to clean the lymph nodes, they'll clean much faster, more efficient, and probably with fewer hiccups. The detox effect, minimize.

Ty: Is that last?

Dr. Nuzum: That would be last. Yes.

Ty: You've really basically—just in the last five to ten minutes—you've gone over step-by-step the order by which you would detox.

Dr. Nuzum: You've got to open the exits. Things drain south. So they have to drain down so you open up the drains.

Ty: These specifics that you just went over, these herbs, these roots, that's what people are asking for.

Dr. Nuzum: That's what they need.

Ty: You just gave some practical advice. You need to develop some supplements. Do you already have them developed, are you developing them?

Dr. Nuzum: We have formulas. We need to implement.

Ty: Do you have the formulas that you—I know that you're in to the fulvic acid. Are some of these formulas that you have for cleaning out the kidneys, liver, colon, or whatever are they based on fulvic acid as well?

Dr. Nuzum: We would definitely incorporate the fulvic acid and humic acid in particular. Humic acid does a lot for detoxifying, de-parasitizing, de-bugging the gut. So in dealing with anything in the gut and the liver in particular, the humic acid would be really important.

Fulvic acid detox is always useful with any type of detoxing. You need that delivery system and you need a good garbage man.

Ty: By the time this airs it is going to be October. You're going to get inundated with people wanting to know how to detox or where they can get these some of this stuff. So maybe by October this year, you are going to have some of this stuff.

Dr. Nuzum: We'll have it. Yes, sir.

Ty: If you're interested, don't contact me.

Dr. Nuzum: We'll put something together.

Ty: Contact Dr. Nuzum. I really appreciate you spending time with us again because as I mentioned, you were in the last quest. We were inundated with people saying, "Get Doc back on there and get us some specifics." So you shared that with us. I think it's really practical knowledge and it's going to help people to where they know how to detox. They know they *should*. You've just shared the *how*.

Dr. Nuzum: *How*. That's important. If you don't have *how*, you never get to your destination.

Ty: I'm glad that you shared *how* because if you didn't share *how*, I was going to have to do some muay thai on you. And actually, I'm just joking about that because he's like eight-black-belt or something.

Dr. Nuzum: I'm six. Only six.

Ty: Six black belts. He'd knock me down in two hits. So we would be over and people would say, "What happened to Ty?" I'm glad we didn't have to do that, Doc.

Dr. Nuzum: Thank you, sir.

Ty: We had a blast, my friend. Thank you for helping us.

Dr. Nuzum: Thank you.

[end of transcript]

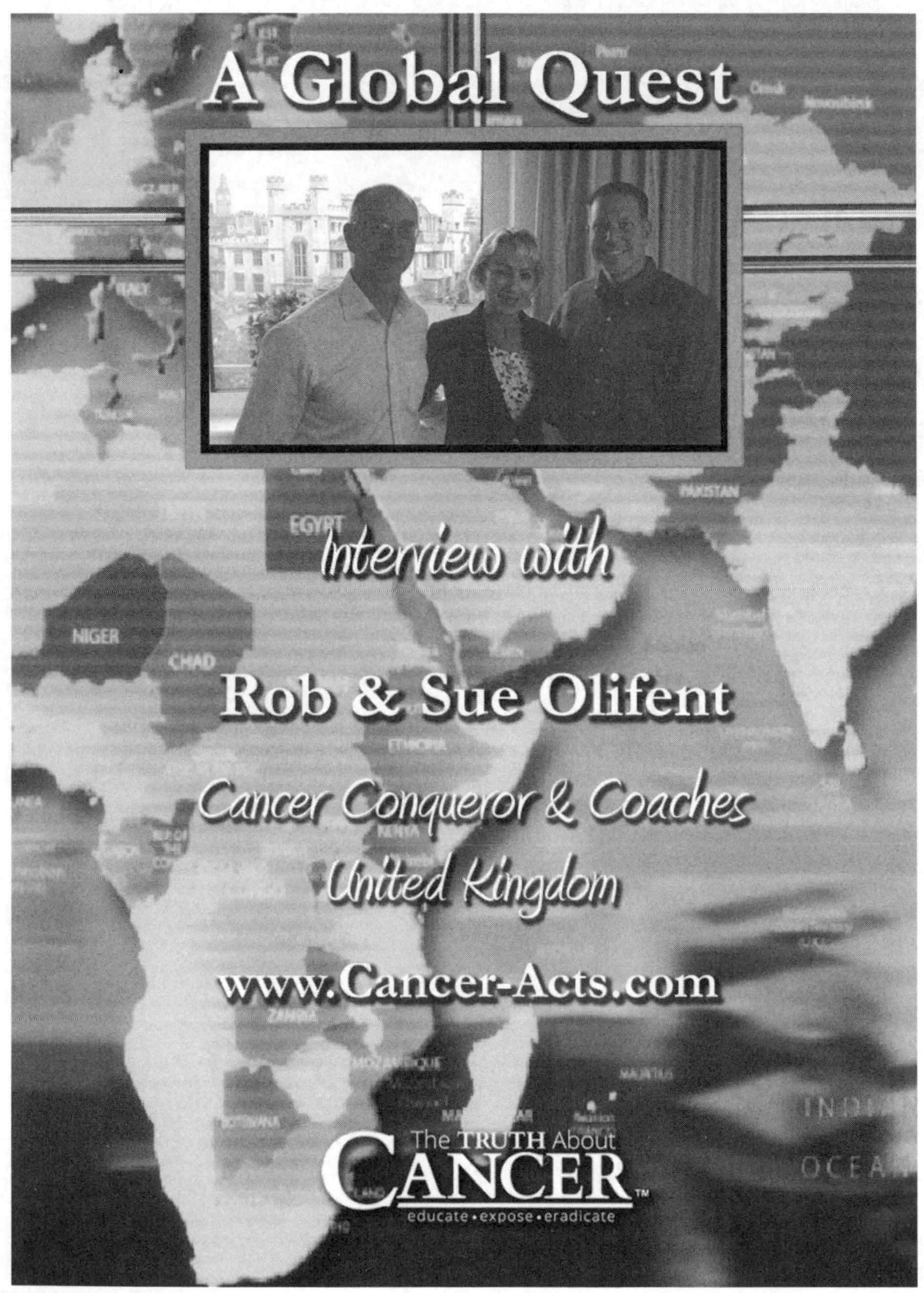
A Global Quest
Interview with
Rob & Sue Olifent
Cancer Conqueror & Coaches
United Kingdom
www.Cancer-Acts.com
The TRUTH About CANCER
educate • expose • eradicate
EGYPT
NIGER
CHAD
PAKISTAN
ETHIOPIA
KENYA
MOZAMBIQUE
INDIAN
OCEAN

Ty: I'm excited to be here in London, England today, with Robert and Sue Olifent. Robert and Sue, thank you for being here with us today.

Robert: Pleasure.

Ty: Your story begins back in 2008, Robert, with your parents being diagnosed with cancer. Can you tell the viewers about that story?

Robert: Both of them, they got cancer at the same time and they died within three weeks of each other, which was quite a horrendous time.

Ty: What kind of cancer did your parents have, Robert?

Robert: My father had a brain tumor. My mother had it everywhere, pretty much everywhere. So I witnessed quite a few things that I was really uncomfortable with in the medical paradigm, and it just got me asking questions, and I went into researching quite a lot. And Sue wasn't on board at all.

Sue: I thought he was crazy.

Robert: And I researched for two and a half years.

Sue: Video after video, after DVD, after all...

Robert: And reading stuff, all that.

Sue: Yeah, just constantly researching. I didn't see him at all, really. He was always upstairs.

Robert: I don't think I was all that bad, but then maybe, maybe I was.

Ty: So Robert, what did you find in your research on cancer?

Robert: Well, I wondered why one in two people are going to get cancer in their lifetime and yet, the media was saying, "Well, we're winning the war on cancer. Just give us more money and we can beat cancer." Yet, I researched that there were natural protocols that were going to basically stack the odds in the person's favor who has cancer, to deal with the root causation, to deal with toxicity issues.

And all these seem to be being ignored by the medical foundations that, you know—when I think back on it now, the things that they fed my parents when they were in hospital, things like root vegetables. I mean, there's nothing wrong with root vegetables as such. But if you have cancer, an overload on these—their starch turn immediately to sugar and sugar feeds cancer. So these were principles that I learned. And I wondered why they had chocolate bar dispensers on every oncology ward. I wondered why they had coke machines, fizzy drink machines containing sugar on all these wards, and why they gave my dad and mom, and uncle, who later died of cancer, apple pie and ice cream.

And—just didn't make sense. So I did all this research, but then, two and a half years down the line, Sue got very poorly. And she lost a stone and a half in weight, and every time she ate, she had tremendous stabbing pains in the stomach. And she couldn't eat particularly acidic foods. And she had a scan and they found a two and a half inch tumor in the liver, where the tubes are coming out, and it was strangulating the tubes. So that's the position that we're in. She'd also got three smaller growths on the pancreas and we basically had to throw everything in, because the doctor said, "I'm so very sorry. I've never seen a cancer of this type in a woman of your age."

And we were left in a position where he said, "There's nothing we can do. They can't do anything. It's such a sensitive area." And Sue went out and bought 25 pounds worth of goodbye cards and it was quite a horrendous time.

Ty: So Sue, how did it feel when you were told by the oncologist that, "I'm sorry,"—you know, from an emotional perspective, he told you, "There's no hope." Tell me how that felt.

Sue: I was on my own when I was diagnosed. But I didn't want to—at the time Rob himself was quite ill. After losing his parents, he was struggling. He had to be off work so, I didn't want to put any more pressure on him. He really wasn't well at the time. So I decided to go—I had a feeling it was going to be bad news when I went, because of the way the receptionist spoke to me on the phone the night before, when I rung up.

So when I did go in, it was off just slightly, it was numb, it was like it was a haze, like it wasn't happening and I just kept thinking, "I can't tell Rob, it will make him ill." I didn't know what to do. I just got on a bus and went into town, in this daze, and then found myself in the card shop. But then I realized I had to tell him in the end, because when he walked in the door I was shaking from head to toe. I thought I'd hold it together, but I couldn't stop crying. The thought of telling my 16 year old son, you know—I just—my head was all over the place. It was really hard.

Robert: But, we had an advantage, because I've done quite a lot of research involving this and, because we had nowhere else to go basically, those—they said there was no hope by medical standards.

We threw everything into what we'd learned, what I'd learned, and we started instigating an anti-cancer protocol. We're quite strict on the diet. Sue was climbing the walls occasionally, more than occasionally, because you know, what can they—I can't have this and I can't have this.

Sue: It's just getting used to that change, isn't it? All the things that you used to think were good for you, you're learning that they're actually not. It's hard to totally change your whole lifestyle, with choices and that, it's...

Robert: Yeah.

Sue: We were brought up thinking that milk, cheese, bread, white bread, pork, it was all good for you, in my family.

Ty: So basically, what you had to do Robert and Sue, you had to unlearn everything that you grew up thinking was true, is that correct?

Sue: Yeah, yeah.

Robert: Yeah, yeah. Because these are staples, aren't they? They're a staple diet. Bread, cheese, milk, and you know, sometimes people think you're absolutely crazy. "You don't have what? You don't have bread, and you don't have cheese, and you don't have milk? What?" Yeah.

Sue: The foods that we eat now are just full of color, herbs and spices, and salads—it's not just salads that we, we do still eat casseroles, soups, lots of healthy foods.

Robert: Curries, plenty curries.

Sue: But we're always having fresh, live foods with whatever main meal we have, lots of green juices and spices in the green juices, constantly herbs and spices daily.

Robert: Apple teas, pineapple tea.

Sue: Just so, it was a case of packing everything—what goodness you possibly could into the body, because you know it was sick and I suddenly start believing in what I was doing, that I got more of the, well—once I got my positivity back after that I really got stuck into the diet and I enjoyed it instead of suffering.

Robert: I think there was a time which I remember in the kitchen and it was a really positive time where we were discussing all what we were doing and so we decided to go on the apricot kernels. When we were discussing those and I've got my arms around Sue and I said, "We're going to really do this. This is going to be okay." And I felt really positive at that time and I think that was a change around for Sue as well and I think you saw the apricot kernels.

There's no silver bullet as such, because the cancer is a holistic thing and you have to deal with everything, emotional, and psychological, and nutritional, hydration, detoxification. But that was a moment which was a step forward.

Sue: I think to me, each time I put them in my mouth, I was feeling they were the medicine, they were what was going to break this cancer down. Something switched on with me with that that I didn't mind taking thirty a day. It didn't bother me because people were trying to scare me off from taking them, but I had faith in them. And I chose to—I mean we watched films on them. Lots of different books.

Robert: We've got a lot of information about them and knew how it worked, and the theory behind it. We just went for it and it's crazy that cancer organizations actually state that if you have these products, these apricot kernels, that you have a long list of things that happen to you. You get nauseous, you vomit all over the place, you get hives, you get headaches, you'll get migraines, and then ending in death. I've read the cancer research UK website and this is what it says. Well, it's not my experience and I've had thousands of them. It's not Sue's experience. She's still alive without cancer. I know various other people that have taken these things and they're still alive without cancer.

We shout this from the rooftops, all about the information that we have gained and we put on meetings, and we set up a little support group. It's just me and Sue and we put on meetings every month and explain to people the principles of what we chose to do. We don't give advice, but we give information and that is where—our strength is in that, if not protection, because with us not giving advice we're not breaching any laws. We are seeing people that don't have cancer anymore—some people that have been written off by the cancer industry, societies that literally—they don't have the cancer anymore.

Sue: We've been watching them every month getting better and better and better. Especially Bernie Walsh and the Collins'. But from being so sick and then seeing them starting to do a bit of exercise and just seeing them start to put the weight back on and then finally to be told they're not terminal anymore.

Robert: Yeah, those tumors are getting smaller and smaller.

Sue: We share it with so many people, don't we? All the different stories we get. And we asked her when she came to our meeting what she got from it and she just said "Hope," because she's been told she was terminal. You know, there was nothing more they could do and she suddenly realized, "Hang on a minute. Maybe I can do something here," and she's okay knowing that she had lung cancer. It was in her neck, in her bones.

Robert: It wrapped itself around an abscess in her lungs. She broke all the ribs down one side through excessive coughing, this lady, and she could barely get out of the steps the first meeting last May. And now she's jogging four miles a day. It's just amazing.

Ty: Talk about the changes that you made in your diet after this cancer diagnosis.

Robert: Well, what we chose to do was to detox. Find the body starting with the colon. We did magnesium oxide for ten days, taking a small teaspoonful of magnesium oxide in a glass of warm water. Most people that we say this to—it's, like, very gentle. But some people said, "You know that gentle stuff that you told us was gentle?"

Sue: It wasn't that at all, it wasn't. For me, anyway.

Robert: It wasn't bad. Then we went on to the liver cleanse and we started having lemons first thing in the morning. Juicing green leafy vegetables, maybe include an apple in there, sweeten it up a little bit, a little bit of ginger, celery, cucumber, things to liven the taste up, because sometimes when you have green juices on their own, they leave a little bit to be desired on the taste factor front.

So we included other things in them—like apples are great because they are low in sugar, low glycemic, and they just lift the flavor that little bit. So we got organic veg box delivered every week. We made sure that what was coming inside us was pure. It didn't have toxicity of all these things that are going into mass farm production today, which are pesticides and fungicides and the rest of it. These are part of the protocols. We took out milk, dairy products. We still did have bread, but we didn't have white bread. We've since learnt—because it's a progression of learning and there's better things like the ancient grained bread—which is far better for you—that isn't prone toward commercialized farming techniques and the toxicity that goes with that. So it's going to serve your body rather than tax your body. And other protocols—what else did we do?

Sue: Lots of water.

Robert: Yeah, we got water filters to make sure that the water was clean and pure as much as we were able. Because we weren't wealthy or anything like that, we just got a Britta water filter, carbon filter, and that served its purpose. And they are all parts of the armory.

Sue: Really, the more alkaline diet I had the less pains I was having and I think within three months the pains were gone from being on that type of diet. It didn't happen straight away obviously, but it started being easier and easier to eat. I mean, there were times I was forcing myself to eat because I knew I needed it, but I was still getting the pain.

Robert: I think what was quite incredible, because we were doing this diet and then we'd got another scan, an MRI scan due, and we were looking—because we read Phillip Day's book *Cancer: Why We're Still Dying To Know The Truth*. Read quite a few of the books. But we were looking to see some notable change in the two messiahs, that's what we were really aiming for. It was scar tissue, this two and a half inch long—which is, you know, no small size. It was strangulating the tubes. It was just scar tissue.

Not that it wasn't there. It was scar tissue, so there was clearly something there and Sue actually saw her on the computer monitor screen at the doctors. There it is. It's strangulating the tubes, two and a half inches, and he's pointing it out to you. So there's no mistaking that and she'd also got the three on the pancreas as well. Now, she still had the three on the pancreas, which was a worry. We wouldn't let them biopsy because what we knew about biopsies—and it was Sue's decision at the end of the day.

Sue: He wasn't very happy at all, was he? He was cross with us, but in my view I wanted to see—as I could feel I was getting better, I didn't want them going in and starting something that—it might not have been cancerous or might not have been active and if they had gone in, it could have start and made it spread and cause metastasis.

Ty: So this risk of metastasis or spreading, is this the reason you avoided the biopsy?

Robert: Pretty much.

Sue: On the pancreas definitely. Because within three months of the pains going—I believe that's where the pains were actually coming from rather than the liver—that's what the oncologist was saying in the hospital. But because the pains were gone, I just believe that that was okay in that area now and there was no need to investigate. And he was really not happy with it, was he?

Robert: The second oncologist was a little bit pleasanter. He was accepting, "Well, if you don't want us to biopsy, then we'll just monitor the situation and come back if you have any further problems." And we've not had any further problems. Sue's been good. You've put on a little bit more weight.

Ty: What was the oncologist's reaction when you told him what you were doing to treat your cancer?

Robert: Well, we only went to see him the two times and we've not been back.

Sue: We just said, "Oh. Well, it's scar tissue."

Robert: Yeah, come back if you find that these things aren't going anywhere.

Sue: We walked away thinking about it, didn't we? What did he just say? We just couldn't believe it, because it was so quickly changed from being a two and a half inch tumor to nothing.

Robert: We explained that we were taking apricot kernels and I think he wrote it down as apple seeds, which is B17 basically.

Sue: They didn't have a problem with that, though, which was good because sometimes they try to frighten people into not using them.

Robert: But he wasn't on board in terms of—he wasn't happy. The first oncologist was quite obstinate really, whereas the second one—he was okay. He was alright.

Sue: I think as soon as we'd gotten the belief in what we were doing to be the right thing—because I was getting a lot better and I realized I was getting better—we've never been back since, because I feel once you start on that conveyor belt of them checking you out for the—and I know some people might think it's a risk to not have this examined to see if it is anything to worry about, but I just feel from the way we're eating, I'm not going to be ill.

Robert: And it's personal choice, isn't it? We still, at the moment, have personal choice as to whether we have biopsies or have radiotherapy or chemotherapy. That's our choice, but I think people would do well to arm themselves with knowledge to make a balanced judgment and balanced assessment of what's right for them. Some people that come to the meetings that we put on, they still want to do the medical realm, but see the importance of doing this. And if that's right for them, then that's what they want to do. We don't really tell them not to do anything or to do anything. We just give them information to make their own choices and we always suggest that they actually check out everything that we say. Check out everything that the medical people say because there's a lot of untruths or things that are not explained to the people by the medical oncologists.

And I heard it put like this: it's a little bit like going into a Chinese takeaway and asking for a king prawn Rogan Josh. Well, that's Indian food. You're not going to get it because they don't make it and they don't know how to make it. And the same applies with the medical realm, they don't really know anything about the nutritional side of things. Otherwise, they wouldn't have all these chocolate bars on oncology wards and they wouldn't feed them foods—like they've fed to my family—that are going to feed the cancer. They wouldn't do that. They have no idea. In fact, we've got information and booklets from prestigious hospitals that actually tell people to consume sugar, and donuts, and ice cream, and apple pie.

Sue: That's a diet for children as well with cancer and they say in it not to bulk up on fruits and vegetables and to microwave food—and this is a quite local hospital.

Robert: We won't say the name of the hospital, probably for legal reasons, but it's in their booklets I mean, so it's public knowledge, it's public domain material. All we do is to bring this information to people. If this is the case, if cancer works on the system called glycolysis, which is the metabolism of sugar, then why would you increase the sugar load in the body? That's just crazy.

Ty: That makes no sense at all, does it?

Robert: Makes no sense.

Sue: This is also—we didn't mention the processed food, the amount of chemicals.

Robert: And sugars.

Sue: And the labels and the hidden sugars and the salts, but particularly the chemicals. You know, when we read a loaf of bread—I mean most people in England they'll go and buy a loaf of—I was going to say a name then and I'm not allowed to. But if you look at the labels, there's probably about 20, 25 ingredients in that one loaf of bread and you think, "It's crazy, there should only be about three or four ingredients in bread."

Robert: Half of the things you can't pronounce and there are these long-winded chemical things so…

Sue: And in supermarkets, you look at people's trolleys and there is no color in the trolleys. It's all light beige. There's no greens, and oranges, and yellows. It's all very bland.

Robert: All packaged nice and neatly and plastic and, you know—some people say, "I eat healthy. I read all the labels." If you're eating healthy, what are you doing reading labels? Is my sort of thoughts.

Ty: That's right. Healthy food does not have labels.

Robert: Absolutely, it's God's foods,—what I would class as God's foods—and it's plucked straight from the ground, fresh, local, organic if you can have it, or responsibly produced on your back garden or your neighbor's allotment. These are foods that are going to give you the nutrients to help your body to heal your body and your body knows perfectly well how to heal your body if you give it the right nutrients, is my thoughts.

And so, it takes the confusion out of things as well, because some people say, "Well, there's so much information at the meetings. Do I have this, do I have that?" Hang on a minute, stop. You just have to think, how was it produced? Has man had his finger in the pie, so to speak? Has he had his finger in the pie of manipulating that food by genetic modification or by processing? And if he has, that's not going to be a food that's going to serve you well. It really simplifies things, I think.

Ty: When did the meetings begin?

Robert: How long—

Sue: It must have been nearly two years now, probably. We used to do about two a month because it was so popular, but now we're on one a month. We often get some really good speakers to come talk for us as well, like Dr. Patrick Kingsley and there's been a few others.

Robert: Yeah, we saw a nutritionist one time. Again, we were in a bit of a financial pickle at the time, and we could only afford to see the nutritionist once. But she was a great lady, and she gave balance to what we were doing, a little bit, because we were quite strict. We got her to come along and do a talk, and it was interesting to see what she had to say about her thoughts towards us. And she said she couldn't get a word in edgewise with—it was mainly me doing the talking, wasn't it, at that time?

Sue: We also do meetings in a hyperbaric oxygen chamber center, so that when people come to the meetings they can go inside the chambers and see what they're all about. Because where we live, we were very fortunate. There's one that's quite easily available to people that doesn't charge very much and it's very affordable.

We're finding people that use it with cancer are doing really well with it, with helping them heal scar tissue, and radiotherapy bones. And one of the ladies using it got her eyesight back from it. She doesn't need her glasses anymore, so that was amazing.

Robert: I don't know how that works, but she said she came out of there and she said she could see! Yeah, Jenny—she's great.

Sue: I suppose what we're trying to do is, like, sign poster people, trying to create a network around us, not just locally but—

Robert: People are coming from further afield now, I think.

Sue: Yeah, yeah. And then Emma Collins and her husband, he's healed now of his cancers. He'd got it in the kidneys and then in the lungs. And she's been totally on board with this diet. Now she's sort of spreading the wings, and she's writing a book, and she's telling other people what she's done. It's just getting shared out, isn't it, amongst everybody?

Robert: Yeah, the husband had no choice in the matter. He was doing it.

Sue: She is formidable. What she's normally—

Robert: Yeah, she's great. She's passionate. And sometimes it's about the positivity that's actually given to people, inspired into people, because they come to the meetings and often they've been told, "There is no hope. There's nothing we can do for you. Go home and die," pretty much. And yet they come to the meetings and this gives that air of confidence and positivity, that actually there is something to do.

And it empowers people. And yes, they have to take personal responsibility. Often, people they see on this hand a pill, a red pill, a blue pill, whatever, and they don't have to do anything, they don't have to change their lifestyle. On this hand, they see exercise. They see changing the diet to things that they don't normally eat and it's hard work. All this getting stuff together. So the pill or all this hard work?

We'll go for this because there's no responsibility with that. And yet, the people that take the responsibility inspire themselves with confidence, and they tend to do well, whereas the people that go down the traditional route of poison and burn— that's basically going to give the cancer every condition that it needs to thrive by acidifying the body, by chemotherapy, or poisoning the body, which is taxing the body, depleting the immune system. Why would you do that? You're just pandering to the cancer's needs.

And then it might get rid of the cancer initially, but then it comes back. Because the very nature of what they are—if you read the MSDS sheet, the Material Safety Data Sheet of the chemicals, then they tell you that they're Category 1 and Category 2 carcinogens, which means that they cause cancer in themselves. It's just—we had one guy come to our meeting. And we were talking about one specific drug, and he said, "I'm on that drug and I don't believe you."

And I had the actual Material Safety Data Sheet with me, and I said, "Well, what part of this don't you believe? Because it's here. I didn't write it. It's from the manufacturers. You can download it. You can get it. And it tells you that it's Category 1 carcinogenic." And he was quite cross about it and he said—what was happening, because his family was so prone to cancer—that they'd actually gotten his daughters on this drug as a preventative.

Ty: That's absurd. They're doing chemo as a preventative.

Robert: We just couldn't believe what we were hearing. And then a lady shot up from the front and her husband was an oncologist. And she was a medical lady, and she said, "Yes, but it doesn't happen for five years. It doesn't cause cancer for five years." What? Are you listening to what you're saying?

Sue: I hope he went home, though, and thought about that. And after being with us for three hours, I hope that we planted some seeds in there that would help him change his mind with that.

Ty: Robert and Sue, what is your message to someone that might have recently been diagnosed with cancer?

Robert: I think, to understand that cancer requires certain things to flourish. And if you understand the basic principles of it requiring three things—I mean, there's a lot of other things surrounding this—but it requires deoxygenation, so a lack of oxygen. It requires acidity, so if you alkalize the body, that's going to go away from acidity. And if you introduce sugar into that environment, then you've got fermentation, respiration of the cells, rather than oxygen respiration.

So we know three things there—from Dr. Otto Warburg who got the Nobel Prize for knowing all these in 1932—that we can fight the cancer with. We can oxygenate the body. We can alkalize the body. And it's like two sides of the same coin, though. If you've got an alkalized body, your body, on a cellular basis, is able to absorb more oxygen. And then you take out sugar.

Now, wow, that's incredibly stacking the odds in people's favor. And you start adding into all this thing detoxification and apricot kernels or whatever you choose. Cannabis oil. We didn't go down the cannabis oil route. But you start adding in these things and it's all stacking the odds in your favor. And to have the positive mindset that you're not in the hands of the man in the white coat, that there's something in your hands that you can actually do, is empowering. There's so much that people can do, yet they're not told this.

And it's criminal. It's absolutely criminal that people aren't being told these things and they're just being given foods that are actually causing cancer in themselves. Certainly, you wouldn't class them as healthy foods, even for a healthy person, so why would you give them to a sick person? But understanding this, getting basic information, is the key to actually stacking the odds in your favor, is what I would say.

Ty: Is there hope for someone that's been given that terminal diagnosis?

Sue: Oh, gosh. Yes. We've met them. So many. It certainly was for me.

Robert: I think there's always hope, isn't there? Because a common thing that we're told, and I hate it when people say this, is that, "You can't give people false hope, can you?" What are you talking about? Hope is hope. Hope is positive. And hope is inspirational.

So you're saying that you're going to tell someone that they're going to die in three months time? You prefer to do that? It just doesn't make sense, because it's almost like they're cursing people to death. I think I heard that on one of your documentaries. Yeah, the power of the spoken word over people—when someone says you've got three months to live, people live that out or die that out.

We had one gentleman that we were asked—he was a good friend of some friends of ours—and we were asked to speak to him. We explained some things to him and he was given three months, or—I think it was three months—and he says, "Ah, you don't understand." Because we'd explained that Sue was actually written off, nothing we could do. And he says, "You don't understand. The doctors have said that I've got three months to live."

And I said, "Yes, but if you do these things, you'll greatly stack the odds in your favor, potentially." And, "No, you don't understand. The doctors have said I have no chance. That's it." And he wouldn't listen. It was like a brick wall that came up like this, and there was nothing getting past that wall. And that was sad. And he died almost the three months later.

Sue: I think we're finding a lot of people are so depressed after they come away from the oncologist as well—that seem to go into a depression, don't they, where they've got no life left in them. They're just sitting around all day waiting to die. We know of somebody who hung himself a few months ago after a diagnosis.

He couldn't cope with the word "terminal," and it just breaks your heart that this is happening, that there's no positivity around cancer. It's such a scary thing for everybody. It should be—I don't know why they can't create a bit more hope around it rather than it being such a dire illness to have.

Ty: How can people get in touch with you and attend those meetings that you offer?

Robert: Well, we've got a website, and that's www.cancer-acts.com. We've also written a book, which we'll let you have a copy of. It just details all what we did, and it's called *Do You Want to Know What We Did to Beat Cancer?* Simple, it says it as it is on the tin. That's what it is. We've been having such a lot of positive feedback from that. It just looks—the reasons why I started researching, where we were, where we are now, and the principles and protocols of how we got there. So it's a fairly simple book, 158 pages, and it's—

Sue: We also do lifestyle coaching that we don't charge for, locally. Two days a week. And we meet up with people, anyone that wants to have a one-on-one with us, just to talk through what they think is a difficult diet and make them realize it's not so difficult once they learn to give up a few things that they're used to having.

Robert: And the meetings are free. We don't charge for the meetings. We don't charge for speaking with people. It's just become our passion, hasn't it? It's what we do. It's who we are.

Ty: Robert and Sue, thank you for spending this time with us today, travelling all the way down here to London to share your inspiring story. I'm inspired. I know the people that are watching are inspired, so thank you very much.

Sue: Pleasure to meet you too.

Robert: Thank you for all you're doing as well, Ty.

Sue: We wouldn't have—

Robert: Yeah, it's quite inspirational. It's great stuff.

Sue: We wonder how you get away with it.

Ty: The inspiration goes both ways here. I really admire what you're doing.

Sue: Thank you.

Robert: Yeah, it's all good.

[end of transcript]

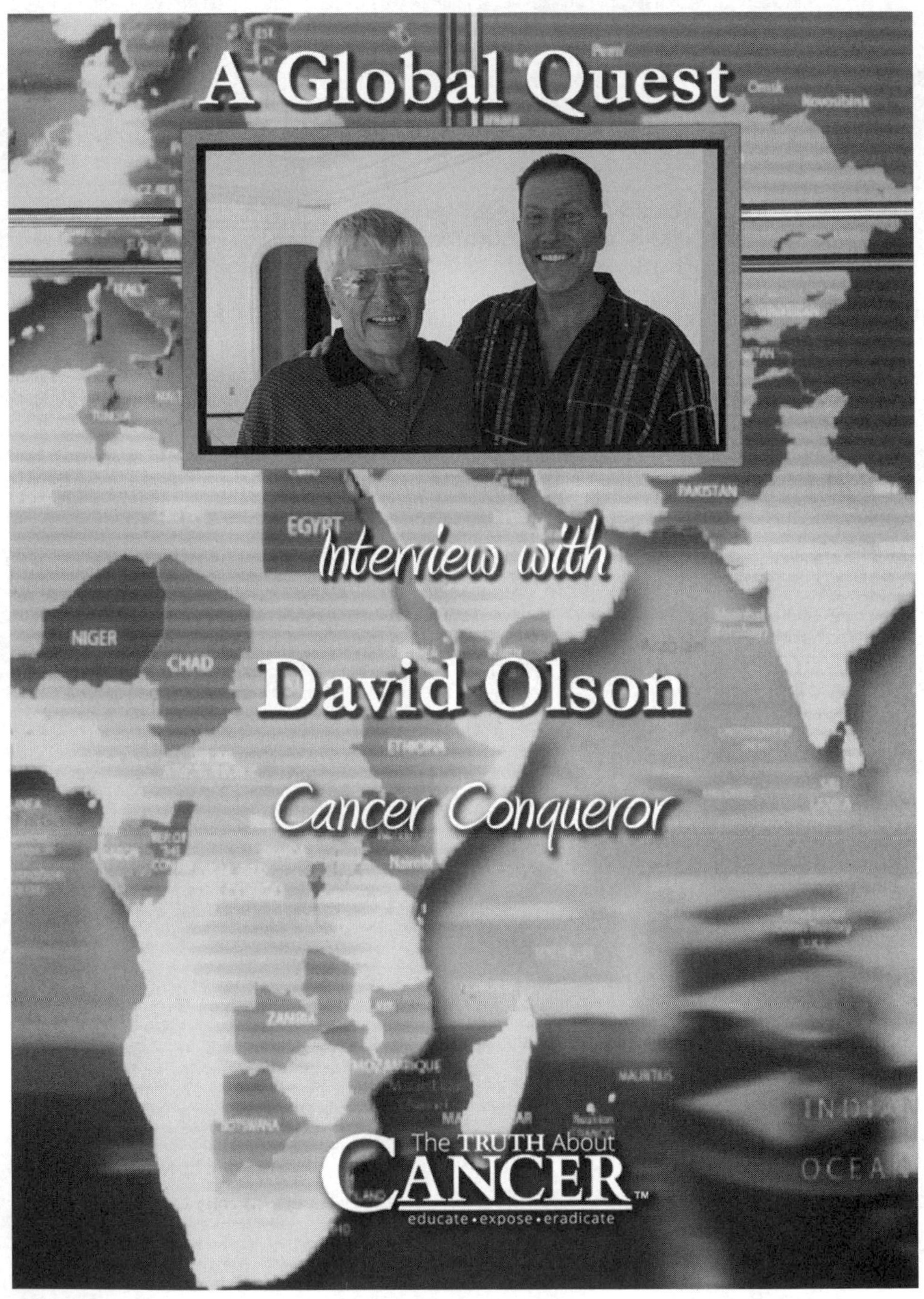
A Global Quest
Interview with
David Olson
Cancer Conqueror
The TRUTH About
CANCER
educate • expose • eradicate

Ty: David Olsen, so glad to be with you here today at the Bio Medical Center in Tijuana.

David: Yes.

Ty: Formally known as the Hoxsey Center. I've shared this story with others. I wanted to get my dad here when he was diagnosed, but he died in 25 days. But this was the place we wanted to bring him. Now, eight years ago, you'd been told a lot of things about your cancer. So let's walk back eight years and tell us your story.

David: Well, experts at Mayo Clinic started—I had 13 doctors here diagnose me. And at first, they didn't know I had cancer. From the blood test, they could not tell me I had cancer. And then a couple of days later they said, "Yes, you've got the easiest kind of cancer to take care of." And then a couple of days later, "Nah, you've got the worst kind of cancer there is to take care of." It went from bad to worse in just a couple of days. After they finally got it totally diagnosed after about three weeks—roughly from middle of August of 06' until 12th of September. So about three weeks of all their tests and whatever, whatever, whatever and then they had to take the marrow from my bones and it was in the bones, so I had it in the esophagus, the liver, the kidney, the lymph nodes all over, especially under the arm and the groin.

Ty: It was everywhere.

David: I had a tumor bigger than a volleyball in the stomach and then in the bone, stage four, and all of the doctors kissed me goodbye. And that was the 13 at Mayo, then I went to the University of Minnesota and then at Fairview Hospital in Minneapolis and then the Masonic Cancer Center and everyone gave me a really rare diagnosis. If you had the best stuff they could give you, I might make three months. Might. And one of the doctors there he says, the last guy we treated like you, made it three days. Three days is not a very good forecast, but anyway I could not lay down—from that I time I could not lay down and use a bed for three months. I had to sit up. And if I was leaning back this much I could not stand the pain.

Ty: But was it the volleyball sized tumor in your—

David: It was something else.

Ty: I can't believe that they could not detect cancer with a tumor that big.

David: Well, it took them two weeks to detect it. Then they finally had it. It took two and a half weeks actually and they didn't know I had it in the bones yet and they took this test, this test, this test. I was literally tested out of everything imaginable. Anyway, they finally discovered—and I had it in the bones so they told me that. It was at two o'clock one day and I'd already made a flight to get down here. I had to be in Minneapolis— from Rochester, Minneapolis, about an hour and a half, in time to get everything done and up in the tenth floor of the [Inaudible 00:02:26] building—get way down the bottom and then on the subway, get over the parking ramp, way up the eighth floor of the parking ramp and on the park ramp, eight different floors, get out of there, making the airport—made it to the airport in 13 minutes to get the flight down here.

Ty: Really?

David: And the next morning I found out at two o'clock in Rochester I had cancer in my bones and at two o'clock from then till I was here the next morning at 7:30.

Ty: What was it about the clinic that made you get here so quickly?

David: I'd already had the flight coming down here, but I didn't tell the doctors that— they'd told me—I want my reports, my third year reports with me and I better have— as soon as you got— coming down the parking ramp and I waited in the airport and she starts crying and I say, "You haven't got time to cry. Look out for cops. We're on our way." They hit it and made about 13 minutes to get on the plane to get down here.

Ty: Wow.

David: And I wanted to get here and I knew other people had been here and I had other friends that'd been down here before and that sent other people down here before and... Anyway, for three months I could not use a bed and I had to sleep sitting straight up. I had to get on an airplane—neck pillows would blow up and just—they applied that and if I would wake up for instance after—I didn't go to bed till about two o'clock in the morning and I'd sleep from two till—maybe for an hour or two and then I'd—if I woke up, just wiggle and wake up and I'd call this faith healer and he would pray for me for 30 seconds to two minutes and then I'd make another hour of sleep, might not and five o'clock, ready to go again for the day and I never missed a day at work. But I could not sit down or lay down or use a bed. Could not stand the pain. And oxycodone, for instance, didn't even phase the pain, just like sugar pills. Nothing. But come down here and they got the diet—on the diet on there and took about three months for the pain to start going away and one night I could lay down for about two or three minutes and the next day for ten minutes, next day for an hour and after that I haven't looked back since.

Ty: Really?

David: Really.

Ty: Remarkable recovery. Almost miraculous.

David: Right and then in March of 07' Mayo could not find my cancer.

Ty: Eight months from the diagnosis they said they—

David: They could not find it.

Ty: —that soon—couldn't find the cancer. Well, they couldn't find it to start with either, could they?

David: No, they couldn't. But I'll tell you, it was there.

Ty: Yes.

David: It was there and that tumor was right down in here and no radiation, no chemo—did not get cut and it came and it went and I had six alternatives and one was biomedical of course at Hoxsey Clinic here.

Ty: Right.

David: Now it's—it was a very interesting six, eight months.

Ty: I bet it was. Now you're—you know, eight years later here, are you still taking the Hoxsey tonic?

David: I still take it because I—every place that I've talked about there's no side effect for taking it. And I've talked to different doctors here and they have no side effect for taking the tonic from here on. So if I'm not on a trip—I'm on quite a few trips. I'm gone a lot, and if I'm gone for a month at a time I don't take it.

Ty: Okay.

David: I still take my—I take vitamins and the only prescription I take is for an aspirin, because I had a stroke back in Budapest a year and a half or almost two years ago now, but that's my only prescription medicine, is an aspirin a day, a full aspirin, but other than that, vitamins, a bunch of vitamins.

Ty: Okay.

David: I'll be—a lot of them every day. Maybe 80 a day.

Ty: Okay.

David: Vitamins and the tonic and so forth and I was taking four teaspoons four times a day of the tonic, which I think is the most powerful dose I've ever heard anybody take so far. And I know a lot of people take a half of teaspoon four times a day, but I was taking four teaspoons four times a day and I'd take probably three—about three times a day instead of four times. And I just—with a forecast of three days to three months, how does a year fit in that schedule as far as—and even—I like to come here every six months for a checkup, and I was here last Thanksgiving—the day before Thanksgiving for my check up and I usually make it every six months, but they said I could wait for a year and could be off the tonic for at least six months at a time, but I haven't got guts enough to.

Ty: You want to stay monitored?

David: I want to stay on it and I've—with no side effect, no known side effect whatsoever yet—and I haven't seen any side effect of it and it doesn't bother my stomach, it never did—and one of the side effects of having the tonic, it makes your nose run. Well, I've been from Minnesota in Olsen. My nose ran for 60 years before and it still runs, so I don't know if it had any effect on that. So it still runs and that's sinuses. My sinuses aren't near as bad in Arizona as they are in Minnesota. Nothing like the dry heat.

Ty: You're in Arizona most of the year now?

David: Eight months. I've been an Arizona residence for going on six years.

Ty: Well, it's been quite a transformation and your wife is—from a point of—she's in tears—I can only imagine with a diagnosis that's that grim, the effect that had on your family, and you have a son as well—

David: Yes, I've got two sons and three grandsons.

Ty: Okay.

David: And one of my grandsons who's with me today—which is a challenge to get his folks to let him come to this place called Mexico. But I told them it's a piece a cake, even though he only has a driver's permit—he's 16, just got his permit, and his folks are very concerned about getting him across the border, but I've seen numerous people in the 18 trips down here so far—19th today—that have had just a driver's license to get back across. You don't need a passport, it's better to have a passport, and it takes like ten seconds for a driver's license only. A driver's license and a birth certificate takes about six seconds and a passport takes two seconds.

Ty: It's easy.

David: And I know some people here that—a dentist that came down the first time with me—I took him down—rode down with him, he has had people back with no ID whatsoever and it still got them back to the states, which is a challenge but it can be done. And the medical line—I didn't get out of the medical line—piece of cake and I've never waited more than 20 minutes to get out of here yet.

Ty: So it's easy back and forth.

David: Oh, very easy. It's embarrassingly easy. It's easier here than Canada.

Ty: I'm laughing because we went up to Canada and I thought we weren't going to get in.

David: I'm not surprised and I have a story from a friend that had driven a truck up there, a 3M truck for 20 something years, three times a week and then he went fishing summer—the spring, summer, and fall, three times a year for 20 something years, fishing up there, no problem. A year ago, right now he went up for a spring trip and they turned him down. They wouldn't let him in and the records—he did something in California 44 years ago and finally the computers and the records caught up with him and they wouldn't let him in.

Ty: Wow.

David: He had to maybe pay $2000.00 to see if he could get through the red tape to get in again, or maybe he can't get in. And he's not in yet. It's been over a year ago already.

Ty: You've got your two grandsons then, right?

David: Three.

Ty: Three grandsons.

David: One is here and two more are in St. Louis.

Ty: How old are they?

David: 16—16, 15 and 13.

Ty: Okay, so at the time of your diagnosis they were like five, six, eight, something like that. So you would have never even seen them growing up.

David: No, not at all and it's—the one that's here with me now comes to Minnesota every—he's from Denver, comes to Minnesota about three weeks every summer and he was down to Arizona with me for about a week and his spring break this year. And we brought the Jeeps and he went up one hill, and he said he—you can't get up that hill. Well, he drove. We went up it, but…

If he would've had a four wheel drive we wouldn't have made it, but we have all wheel drive, so it's a big difference. Anyway, we do a lot of things together, everything from four wheelers, shooting, chainsaws, tractors, skid loaders. We do a lot of things. He's had a lot of education I would have never been able to give him. He's a city boy as such and a city boys don't get the stuff the farm boys get, if that makes any sense.

Ty: Oh it does. It does.

David: Anyway, he's a very good kid and does a lot of things and he's had a lot of experiences in the last eight years he would've never had.

Ty: He would have never had them.

David: No, and I would have never been able to have been with him at all.

Ty: If—Harry Hoxsey was a man that wanted his Hoxsey tonic to be available for everyone and I can't remember when it was that Hoxsey died, but it was several decades ago, but what would you tell him if he were here?

David: What would I tell him—Harry?

Ty: What would you tell Harry?

David: Thank you for having this available and on the wall down there. If you saw the stars on the wall—I've known a number of people who would—I've sent down that didn't have any money and it used to be able to just say you didn't have any money because Harry didn't want to have this treatment—he wanted to have this treatment available to anybody and not be denied because of lack of money and you just had to tell somebody—tell the office—tell them you didn't have any money and they'd give it to you for free or a little bit. Now you've got to bring a 10-40 with you, so you can still get here for reduced and I sent one guy down from Minnesota—matter of fact he lives ten miles from the Mayo Clinic and he came down here and his family got him a ticket to fly down and he gave the clinic a hundred bucks and that was paid in full and they're not chasing him.

Ty: Really?

David: Really.

Ty: A hundred bucks, full treatment.

David: Full treatment, because he didn't have anything and that's what Harry wanted and that's what Harry has achieved numerous times and all the stars on the wall are the benefactors of the people who have given money or donated money to the foundation so that these people can get free treatment or a real low cost treatment. So they don't have to be deprived, because I know a number of people have been down in Mexico for treatment and I know one clinic down here that I know a number of people have gone to—not here—that cost $17,000 for 12 days. They come down on a Sunday, so it's Monday to Friday for five. Then they stay the weekend for two more and then five more the next week. So that 12 days costs 17,000 bucks. My first four years here, I spent just under $5,000.00 and our insurance at our store—we had a two thousand year deductible. Two thousand times four is eight thousand. I only spent five, so with the deductible—no, it wasn't, but they didn't make the deductible and now they have an insurance program since, that they take 15 percent. So if you have a $1000.00 bill for instance, you would pay $150 and the insurance will pay $850. So you're still 85 percent covered.

Ty: That's very, very affordable.

David: Extremely affordable and if you have nothing, it can be free. And how much cheaper can you get than free? And going across the border with a driver's license, easier than Canada.

Ty: Yes, and you got people like yourself that are alive years and years later.

David: Nothing like this. Being living is great.

Ty: I'll tell you what, each day is great. What was it you told me downstairs?

David: Living is great, but everyone thinks that life is—what did I tell you?

Ty: Each day is blessing, something like that.

David: Each day is a gift. Even a stroke that get debilitated in Budapest on there. The four doctors in Budapest and the 14 at Banner Baywood in Phoenix and they said I should be a vegetable. They said I shouldn't be able to walk. I should be in a wheelchair and I should never ride a bicycle again. Can't ride a cycle. I ride a motorcycle. I've got a Gold Wing in Arizona, a Gold Wing in Minnesota and I ride cycles a lot and scooters and bicycles and basically no effect.

Ty: Well, that makes two major inconsistencies in their predictions.

David: Every day is a good day.

Ty: They told you that you'd be dead within a few months and you weren't. They said you'd be debilitated from the stroke and you weren't.

David: That's right.

Ty: Every day's a good day. David, thanks for sharing with us today. I really appreciate it.. Loved getting your story.

David: I loved being able to give it, and I've given, like I said, nine and a half seminars to over a thousand people.

Ty: Well, you keep up the good work and stay healthy so you can get back to your Jeeps.

David: Right.

[end of transcript]

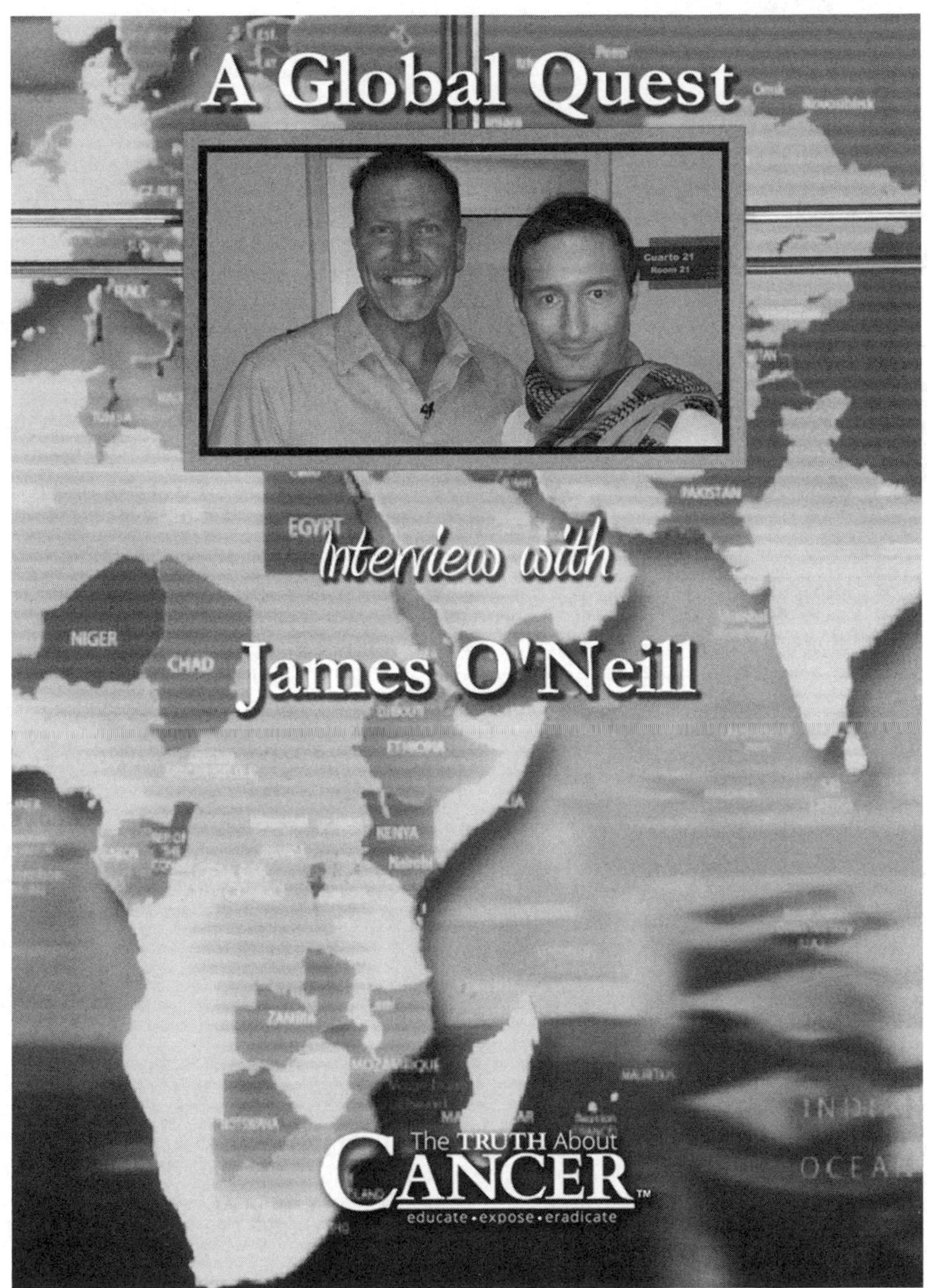
A Global Quest
Cuarto 21
Room 21
EGYPT
PAKISTAN
NIGER
CHAD
ETHIOPIA
KENYA
ZAMBIA
MOZAMBIQUE
Interview with
James O'Neill
The TRUTH About
CANCER
educate • expose • eradicate
INDIA
OCEA

Ty: Wow, James, thanks for joining me today.

James: My pleasure. Thank you.

Ty: We're here at Hope for Cancer. We were just on a little patient roundtable with Dr. Jimenez.

James: That was great.

Ty: I got a little bit of your story then and we've gotten a little bit of your story off the air. Now we're going to get it for the people who are watching this video, this documentary miniseries— your cancer experience and your experience here at Hope for Cancer.

James: I was diagnosed last October, but the first lymph node that popped up about 10 months prior to that. My doctor wasn't too concerned and told me to come back in a couple of months. I did. Then he sent me to get a biopsy. They biopsied my thyroid by mistake actually. I went back to get it right to biopsy the lymph node.

The blood test said that it expired so another couple of months had to go by. We had to get a fresh blood test and it kept getting pushed back. About six months in we finally got a fine-needle biopsy, and it came up negative. So they did more blood tests, and they said, "No cancer. You're fine." I had another lymph node that popped up and then my tonsil popped up. They still kept saying, "No, you're cancer free. The fine-needle biopsy found a few irregular cells so we're a little concerned, but we don't think you have cancer."

Needless to say, about 10 months in, I just felt like something was wrong. I checked myself into Cedars-Sinai Hospital. They rushed me to get a CAT scan. They said you have a three-centimeter by a 10-centimeter tumor in the base of your tongue. So then they did a fine-needle biopsy of my tonsil, and they were able to diagnose and find squamous-cell carcinoma HPV-related throat cancer cells.

Ty: Wow.

James: So, that is when I got the first diagnosis.

Ty: Seems like a long time to go with them supposedly trying to find cancer to finally find it.

James: An extremely long time, and this is top notch. I had Beverly Hills Insurance, Beverly Hills doctors, Cedars-Sinai Hospital to the stars. They finally got it, but I—10 months in, that was 10 months of incredible stress.

Ty: I bet it was. So finally you're diagnosed when? What was the month?

James: It was about October 24th of 2014.

Ty: Okay. So at that point, what's your options according to the docs?

James: The option was, one year of hard-core chemo and radiation. I was just begging them—I'm like—do I have time to think about it? Do I have a month, do I have two weeks? The doctor said, "I've already made an appointment with you tomorrow to go to Beverly Hills Radiological Center with a radiologist oncologist." I'm like—whoa … it just—literally my whole world just swept, spun around in circles.

Ty: To me that's just crazy. They screwed up for 10 months, didn't diagnose it and now they got the diagnosis and you have two days to think about.

James: I've no time whatsoever.

Ty: Wow.

James: So I actually called up and cancelled those appointments and I just knew, I have a month. I have to be able to think about this, process it, I'm in shock. What am I going to do?

Ty: So at that point you started doing some research, I learned earlier. You're a researcher.

James: Right. So, I'm just eating, living and breathing online research, books, Amazon. I didn't know anyone with cancer. I didn't know anyone with experience in any of this. I was a fish out of water, but very good at online research.

Ty: Where did your research lead you to?

James: Research led me to a lot of different websites and I kept tripping over Hope for Cancer as a clinic. They weren't the only place. I called quite a few places. It was a place that sounded the most professional, with the most therapies under one roof, and I'm still researching. I'm still talking to a lot of people, but I was getting phone calls back faster from Hope for Cancer. They're calling me, the way they're speaking to me is personable, and I just developed enough of a rapport to where my girlfriend and I decided, "Well, let's drive down there and look at it." I'm still not—I don't know if I want to be in a clinic. I don't know if I want to be around people with cancer.

So I come down here and even walking through the doors, I'm scared, I'm nervous, I'm still in shock from a fresh diagnosis. So I didn't make any immediate decisions. It wasn't until after interviewing with the staff, talking to some of the patients and talking to Tony that a lot of my apprehension really started to settle and I started to feel like, well, out of everything I've researched, I'm going to give this a try. I still—there was a part of me that was still terrified and scared and wanted to run out the door and just pretend nothing was happening.

Ty: Right. But you didn't because you're here.

James: I didn't.

Ty: You pulled the trigger, right?

James: I pulled the trigger and it was the best thing I've ever done because it just—like a domino effect. It's set so many things in motion. Being able to be around other patients too, I can't stress how amazing that was for me, because a lot of these patients have been dealing with it a lot longer than I had before they came to the clinic as well. So they were braver than me, tougher than me, stronger than me, more resilient than me. I felt like here I was, just nervous, shivering, cowering, completely still in shock, and I was able to just be at ease seeing their bravery, their courage, their ability to stand up, was my motivation. Then on top of that, Dr. Tony, actually finding a doctor that I could trust. He would shake my hand, then hug me, and then talk to me. He wanted to know how the diagnosis is affecting me emotionally, what our plans are for the future. Those were things I wasn't hearing. I was getting very sterile, cold answers from the doctors. If I ask a question, like, well, do I have another couple of months to think about it? "Do you want to live?" was the only answer I got back. "You have to do this now." I know that they cared. I'm really not saying anything bad. That's their schooling. It's what they know. But in my heart of hearts, I just wasn't going to just jump because they told me to jump.

Ty: Right. I'm glad you didn't. You're here four weeks into it? Five weeks into the treatment?

James: Yes. I am four weeks in. I have two more weeks.

Ty: What treatments are you using here?

James: Here I'm using M-formula, which is brand new. That's one great thing about Tony, he's open-minded to brand-new things. Basically it's IV-therapy, DMSO-based formula with a proprietary blend of anti-cancer agents. I'll let him or other people talk more about the technicalities of it, but it's an IV and so mixed with all of the other therapies, it's a personal therapy just for me. I think there are three patients total doing that therapy also with IPT, which is a low-dose chemotherapy that they do by reducing your insulin. It's very targeted. When I spoke to them, I don't lose my hair, I don't lose my saliva glands, I don't lose my teeth, I can eat food for the rest of my life. I don't have to have liquid or anything like that. And we're having phenomenal results.

Ty: You are? Good. Good. That was my next question. What are the tests looking like—the markers—how are we doing?

James: Right now, the last MRI I had, my main tumor in the base of my tongue, which was three centimeters by 10 centimeters, they didn't even see it on the MRI, they had to look again. They're like,"Oh, yeah, we do still see it a little bit."It's at least 80/90 percent down. The tumor of origin. The tonsil and around in my mouth area is at least 70/80 percent down and I can eat an apple without pain now. For the first time since this whole journey began I see light at the end of the tunnel. It's a brand-new world for me.

Ty: Wow. That's so awesome, man. I'm really happy for you. You look great. You look like you're thriving here.

James: Thank you. I didn't—I was not looking this good when I first got here. I put on a little weight and I've got a lot more energy.

Ty: And you have a great mental attitude. That's important isn't it? Your mental attitude.

James: It is. It is. They stress that here, but they also let you—whatever you're into because I was doing a lot of things—they support all of the other—no matter how crazy or wild the other things I was doing—if it can be incorporated here, they're like—do it and they'll help you support it. They'll let you know if it integrates well with what they're doing or if it doesn't. So far, all the wild, crazy stuff I had been doing, they've been really okay with. Dr. Tony wants to hear about that stuff too, which I love. He always wants to learn new things and he's always really supportive and that trust/patient/doctor bond that I have with him is—we're like family at this point.

Ty: That's great, man. And it's so different than many clinics where they're like, "Okay, this is our regime, x, y, z, period." You don't do anything different and so Tony—he lets you incorporate anything as long as it's not going to contra-indicate something that you're taking.

James: In fact, I was quite surprised of his curiosity for some of the things that I do, whether it's crazy meditation stuff or whether it's something I found on YouTube. He's cool with hearing about it. If I'm gung-ho about it, he gets that's important to me. He's going to show some enthusiasm for it. If it's logical, I guess.

Ty: You know what man? James, thanks for sharing your crazy, whacky story with us.

James: I appreciate it.

Ty: You didn't share all of the details, but man, it's really awesome to meet you.

James: My pleasure.

Ty: Your enthusiasm and your zest for life is contagious.

James: I appreciate it.

Ty: I know you help people out here—they're watching.

James: All right. Thank you. ***[end of transcript]***

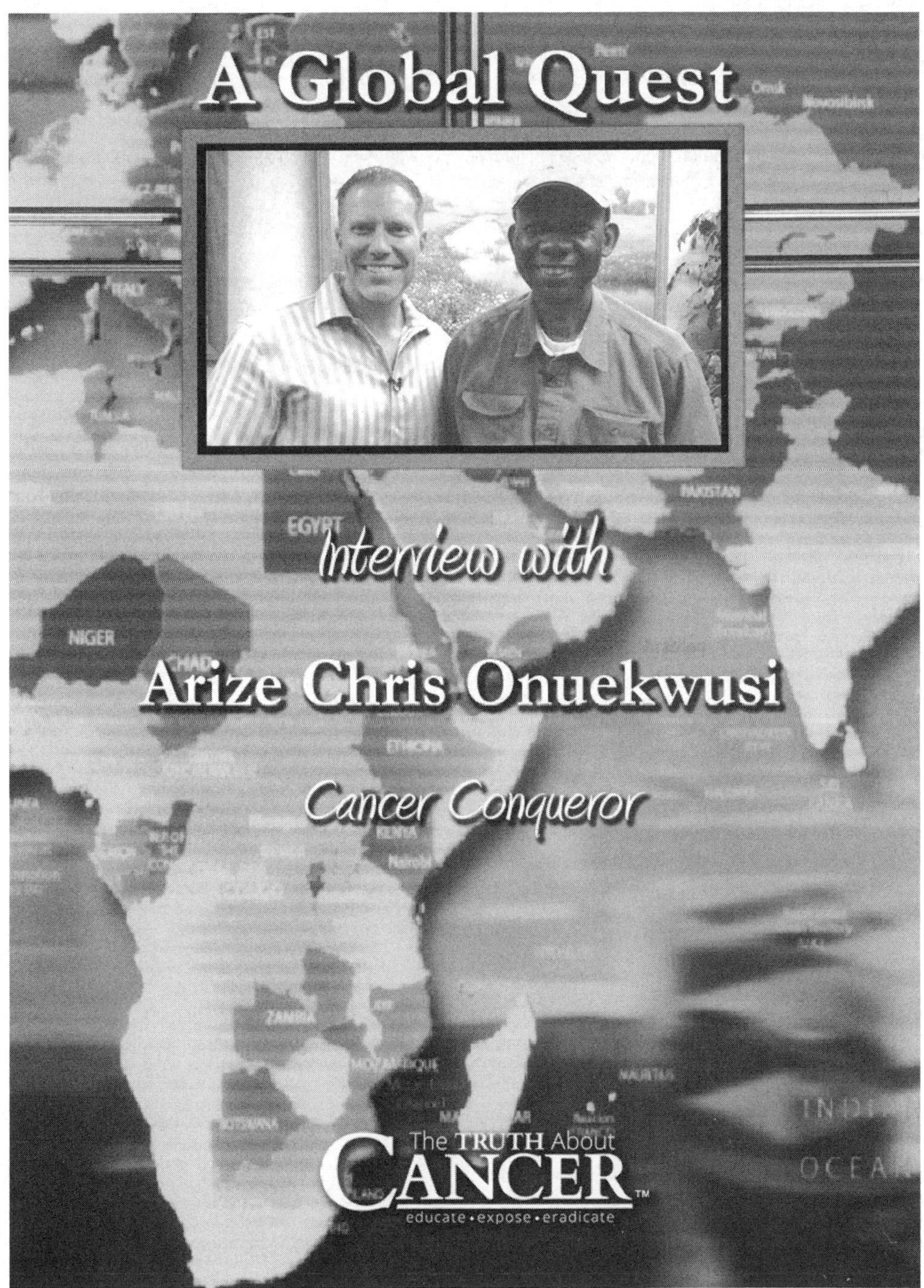
A Global Quest
Interview with
Arize Chris Onuekwusi
Cancer Conqueror
The TRUTH About
CANCER
educate • expose • eradicate

Ty: I am here at the Burzynski Clinic, in Houston, Texas. I'm sitting with Chris. Just met you Chris.

Chris: Nice to meet you.

Ty: Yes, nice to meet you, too. And I'm really thankful that you're willing to share your story, your success story, with the Burzynski treatment method. Tell us a little bit about eight years ago when you were diagnosed with cancer.

Chris: This is such an impromptu, we'll call it, interview, or whatever. I wasn't prepared, but I don't need a script anyway. I just have my story.

Ty: Tell us your story.

Chris: As much as I can remember. And forgive me because I have a porous memory. So what little I have retained in my brain, that's what I'm going to tell you. I was diagnosed with colon cancer back in May of 2008. I was diagnosed with colon cancer. That was at Memorial Hermann Hospital in Houston, Southwest Freeway. My doctor said there was going to be surgery and nothing else. There was going to be surgery, there was no alternative.

And I didn't buy that. I went to discuss things with the surgeon and he said he would cut off my colon this long, and I said, "How long?" He said, "I don't know. I'll know when I get to the theater." And that raised a red flag. I said, "Hm…hm…hm." This guy is going to cut my colon, he's going to do whatever he wants, and I was living by myself. So I went back to my doctor and said, "You know what? I want a second opinion." My doctor didn't really like it. And he said, "Whether there is a fourth opinion, or a fifth opinion, or whatever opinion, there is going to be surgery." So I went to MD Anderson anyway, and lo and behold, it was going to be surgery, too. And I was scared of surgery.

Ty: You didn't like the idea of them putting you out.

Chris: I did not like it, not one bit. And I didn't like the idea of chemo either, or radiation, or whatever. So I went on the Internet. I had to look for alternatives to the surgery because I couldn't figure out—the problem was when I come back home who is going to take care of me? That was really one of the deciding factors.

So I went on the Internet and I started looking around and searching all over Germany, New Mexico, Mexico, and I ran into Burzynski Clinic. But there were so many negative articles about Dr. Burzynski. He was treating with urine, he was a quack, ***Ty:*** I am here at the Burzynski Clinic, in Houston, Texas. I'm sitting with Chris. Just met you Chris.

Chris: Nice to meet you.

Ty: Yes, nice to meet you, too. And I'm really thankful that you're willing to share your story, your success story, with the Burzynski treatment method. Tell us a little bit about eight years ago when you were diagnosed with cancer.

Chris: This is such an impromptu, we'll call it, interview, or whatever. I wasn't prepared, but I don't need a script anyway. I just have my story.

Ty: Tell us your story.

Chris: As much as I can remember. And forgive me because I have a porous memory. So what little I have retained in my brain, that's what I'm going to tell you. I was diagnosed with colon cancer back in May of 2008. I was diagnosed with colon cancer. That was at Memorial Hermann Hospital in Houston, Southwest Freeway. My doctor said there was going to be surgery and nothing else. There was going to be surgery, there was no alternative.

And I didn't buy that. I went to discuss things with the surgeon and he said he would cut off my colon this long, and I said, "How long?" He said, "I don't know. I'll know when I get to the theater."

And that raised a red flag. I said, "Hm…hm…hm." This guy is going to cut my colon, he's going to do whatever he wants, and I was living by myself. So I went back to my doctor and said, "You know what? I want a second opinion." My doctor didn't really like it. And he said, "Whether there is a fourth opinion, or a fifth opinion, or whatever opinion, there is going to be surgery." So I went to MD Anderson anyway, and lo and behold, it was going to be surgery, too. And I was scared of surgery.

Ty: You didn't like the idea of them putting you out.

Chris: I did not like it, not one bit. And I didn't like the idea of chemo either, or radiation, or whatever. So I went on the Internet. I had to look for alternatives to the surgery because I couldn't figure out—the problem was when I come back home who is going to take care of me? That was really one of the deciding factors.

So I went on the Internet and I started looking around and searching all over Germany, New Mexico, Mexico, and I ran into Burzynski Clinic. But there were so many negative articles about Dr. Burzynski. He was treating with urine, he was a quack, it was all that—blah, blah, blah. And that kind of really, really discouraged me.

But he was living here in Houston, and I was desperate because once you are diagnosed with cancer your perspective on life changes—I mean, like that—and you see life in a different way. And I have relatives here in Houston and everybody was saying, "What are you waiting for? Go for surgery. Go get your surgery, and then you can talk about the Burzynski Clinic later on, but you need to do the surgery. That's what the doctor says."

My older brother is a doctor, his friends are doctors, and they just—the pressure was too much. But you know what? I was a little bit stubborn. So, finally, when I cooled down a little bit and I started thinking about the chances I had and the alternatives, and this Burzynski Clinic kept on coming and coming. And I started reading about the patient stories, and the lawsuits, and the reasons behind the lawsuits, and on and on and on.

I said to myself, "I don't really care, I just want to get cured. Whether he treats with urine, or he treats with tomato juice, I don't care."

Ty: You just want to be healed, right?

Chris: Yes, I just want to be healed. And then when I looked at all the accusations and all that, for me, from a patient's standpoint, that's really none of my business. There are people that this guy has treated, and they are there, and they are witnessing, and they are part of the group. So, I said, "You know what? I'm going with him. If that's where it's going to end, that's where it's going to end, but I'm not going to do surgery. I'm not going to do radiation and all that stuff."

So I called him up and he said, "Well, have you done surgery?" And I said, "No, I haven't done surgery." "What kind of treatment have you received?" I said, "None so far." He said, "Come on down, maybe we can help you." They didn't say, "We'll cure you." They didn't tell me that. I have to be honest with you. They said, "Maybe we can help you."

So, I came on down here and they took me through what they were going to do, their treatment protocol, and they laid it out for me. And they said they had to do blood work and mark my genes, I don't remember what—mark my genes and then see what kind of treatment would be best for me. Which is—and I really liked that, you know?

Ty: Individualized treatment.

Chris: Yes, individualized. That's really one of the things that made me say, "Hm, this guy is different." And I said, "Okay, I'm going ahead with it." So they took my blood and then marked my genes—whatever they did. And they put me on some chemo tablets. I was hoping I would go on the antineoplaston, but then I don't think the FDA allowed them to use that kind of treatment for people like me.

Ty: But you said that you did do some oral antineoplaston. Sure.

Chris: Yes, he gave me oral, in combination, with little tablets. You stay for two weeks, and he will up the amount of medication once you get to a certain threshold. And then he sends you away for two weeks to go back to your doctor, and he will be sending periodic results of your monitoring. That's the way I understood it back then, I don't know how he does it now.

So I was there for two weeks and they took my blood and marked it, whatever they had to do. And then put me on oral medication, a bunch of—maybe one, two, maybe three different chemo tablets, maybe two or three, some of that stuff I was taking. And then I started taking it and within three months—I don't want to go into too many details because there are some instances I don't remember.

Within three months—first of all, I had to go for a baseline PET scan. And then from there you can monitor how much progress you are making. And so I went for the baseline PET scan. Of course, the cancer was there. And so, after three months I went for a checkup. I had a PET scan checkup. That was on a Friday. The result came back—the tumor was gone. Can you believe it?

Ty: The tumor was gone.

Chris: The tumor was gone. The tumor was gone. If I had gone for surgery—because my tumor was right at the junction of the small and large intestine, and there is a valve there called the cecum valve that regulates the flow of nutrients from your small intestine to your large intestine, and that could have been taken out during surgery. And so I would have been a candidate for—what is that bag—colonoscopy? What do they call that bag?

Ty: Yes, the ileostomy?

Chris: No, this bag that people wear?

Ty: Yes, I know what you're talking about.

Chris: Colostomy bag.

Ty: Colostomy bag, yes.

Chris: Colostomy bag. So I would have been carrying colostomy bag and I wouldn't have met you because I would be dead by now. You know?

Ty: So this treatment saved your life.

Chris: It did. And plus, so much other stuff. And so after three months the tumor was gone. I was shocked, my brothers were shocked. Everybody was—people got stunned, you know? And was it easy for me? No. Chemo is chemo, I don't care whether it is in tablet form, or in liquid form, or whatever. It is tough, no picnic, I tell you.

But what I liked about the clinic was, when I came here he had a full-time dietitian that I had to see that guided me as to what to eat to help me with my treatment. I came to realize later that nutrition is a key component of your treatment. Because the chemo itself—whether it is in tablet form—it destroys a lot of your body. Your fat-growing cells, your blood, and on and on and on.

And you need something to replenish that. So if you don't emphasize the proper nutrition you are going to get in trouble.

Ty: So that was a big part of your protocol, was the nutrition?

Chris: Yes, the nutrition was, personally. Because after I met with the nutritionist, I realized that was a key part of the treatment. Maybe nutrition was—so I started reading about nutrition and looking at alternatives. That's where I ran into all these alternative cancer treatment and I said, "Wow." So I became—you know Whole Food Market?

Ty: Whole Foods, yes, I shop there all the time.

Chris: I got sold on that one.

Ty: We just ate there yesterday.

Chris: Okay, so I said to them, "I realized that if you give your body what it needs, you know, plus the chemo, and then your body will do—you can take care of yourself." And that's exactly what—plus the medication I was taking and they were monitoring me regularly. I was coming here for blood work on a very regular basis.

So after three months the tumor was gone, but they said, "No, you cannot stop your treatment, because the fact that the tumor is gone doesn't mean that your cancer is gone." It may be somewhere else. So I had to go on with the treatment for some time and then gradually they tapered down the dosage. And gradually, gradually, gradually—eventually I was no longer taking all the chemo tablets. And I stayed on that and they kept on monitoring me and since then I feel great.

Ty: Yes, you look great.

Chris: I feel great.

Ty: Yes, you look healthy.

Chris: Yes, I'm healthy. When I hear about all this, whatever, lawsuits, I feel bad for the cancer patients. If there is anything I can do for a cancer patient I would do it, because they are the ones that get caught in the middle. The insurance company will not help you, as far as this clinic is concerned.

Because I had a bunch of, "Oh no, not approved, not approved, not approved," some of the medications that I was taking, and they are pretty expensive. And that really scares a lot of people away from a place like this. And maybe other clinics, too, because the insurance company will not pick up their tab.

Ty: Because Dr. Burzynski is doing treatments that are not approved.

Chris: Exactly. So they get hung up on that, and that's it. But look at the number of people he has taken care of. Compare that to the number of—percentage-wise, he gets the worst of the worst.

Ty: Yes, and you said, "Look at the number of people he has taken care of." Right over here behind me, this wall, all these people that are alive because of his treatment.

Chris: And most of those are people who have gone through the system and they are told, "There is nothing we can do for you." And they come here and somehow he gets some of them okay. And those people have been written off by the system. And then, if people like me who haven't gone through the system come here, the success rate would be much, much higher.

Ty: Yes, success rates are very good if you haven't been experimented on.

Chris: Exactly. But when you have been fried, and barbecued, and minced, and all that, and you come over here, you have to keep your fingers crossed. But people are expecting miracles to happen. And when somebody dies, or one or two, they say, "Oh, he's a quack, he's killed someone."

I understand it's painful to lose somebody, but you have to be fair when judging people. It has to be on an even playing field. But in this case, everything is stacked against him. You can see I am biased toward Burzynski. Right? You can tell.

Ty: Well, there's no reason that you shouldn't be biased toward him, because if it weren't for him you wouldn't be here.

Chris: I wouldn't be here. And I've met so many other people, so many other people I've met here. Unbelievable stories, you know, brain tumors and all that, and on and on and on and on. Unfortunately, a lot of people don't know that there is a place like this or there are alternatives—natural alternatives, that can get you wherever you are going. If you get the food that mother nature gave you and your body can take care of itself. I believe that 100 percent.

Ty: I do too.

Chris: I don't care what it is. And I experimented with myself over the years and I kept on tweaking my diet, tweaking my diet, tweaking my diet. To the point now, to be honest with you, I have made a list.

Ty: Of things that you eat.

Chris: That I give to people.

Ty: Oh, so the things they should be eating.

Chris: Yes. And I have some cancer patients that have been through the system, my cousins, and I say, "You know what? If you believe me, do this." And I wrote it out. One of them, she has had cancer for two years now. And she hasn't been walking, and I gave it to her about three months ago.

Ty: She's getting better.

Chris: Not getting better, she is about to walk.

Ty: She's about to walk?

Chris: Yes. And there are so many other things. So food, nutrition, there is no substitute.

Ty: I agree. So you're not only a cancer conqueror, you're a cancer coach now for other people.

Chris: Yes, I am. And that's my goal. And I don't charge anybody money, but you've got to eat, baby, you've got to eat.

Ty: Eat clean foods, right?

Chris: Yes, you've got to eat real food and you'll be okay.

Ty: Yes. I like your quote, "If you eat what mother nature gave, you're going to be on the right track."

Chris: Eventually, we will all die, don't get me wrong. But eat, baby, eat. Eat the right foods.

Ty: The first doctor that you visited, Chris, did he have any kind of a nutritional plan over at MD Anderson?

Chris: No. No, no, no, no. They never talked about nutrition. The first doctor that I went for a colonoscopy, right? All he said was surgery, so he didn't say anything about nutrition or anything else. He said it didn't matter what opinion I got he was going to do surgery anyway. So I went to MD Anderson and they told me the same, and as a matter of fact they scheduled surgery about three days after I met them.

Ty: Really, they were going to rush to do surgery?

Chris: And I hadn't even told my family that I had cancer, and here you've already schedule me for surgery. I've got to go home and tell my family first. So there was nothing about nutrition whatsoever, until I went back in and I started reading. And I started going on the Internet and I started reading a lot of people that were advocates of nutrition, and on and on and on—The Cancer Tutor and Dr. Ross and there's a Dr. Ross.

Ty: The Cancer Tutor, yes.

Chris: And Dr. Ross—what's his name? Dr. Ross. He blew the whistle on one of the hospitals and they fired him. So I started reading a lot about it and I came across a lot of people.

Ty: Yes. What was the original prognosis when you were told you had colon cancer? Was it advanced? Did they give you any kind of a timeline? You were going to either do this or you were going to die? What was the stage?

Chris: No. My doctor—I gave him credit, and I called him back to tell him that my tumor was gone he never returned my call to today.

Ty: He never called?

Chris: No. I called so many times, and nobody.

Ty: So you called him to tell him that your tumor was gone and he never returned it?

Chris: He never called me until today, when I'm talking to you, so you know?

Ty: Seven years.

Chris: I refused the surgery, and maybe he got upset, or whatever. But I am still grateful to him, though, because he is the one that found out my cancer. But the prognosis was—it wasn't like I was going to die tomorrow, or whatever, he didn't say anything like that. But one guy who looked at—I wish I—If I knew the interview would be today I would have brought my colonoscopy photographs, before and after.

Ty: I can get you to send them to me. I'll get you my email.

Chris: And it was like night and day. It was like night and day. And I did the second one on my own. Burzynski didn't even know. I said I wanted to make sure this guy was not a quack like they said he was. So, I went on my own, independently, and did a colonoscopy after about a year or two years, and it was just—you know? And I don't know what to say. I don't know what to say. I just wish everybody well, but that's life.

Ty: So, if somebody is diagnosed with cancer you would whole-heartedly recommend that they see this clinic?

Chris: Right away. Not even go anywhere, because going to there from other places will not be as good as what you get from here. Here is the thing. And I read a lot. When you get cancer—when the FDA approves drugs, from what I am reading, and I'm just a layman. But when the FDA approves drugs—a new drug comes on the market—maybe it helps only 20 people out of a hundred. But it is better than whatever you have out there.

So you have 100 people go to the hospital and they give them that drug. Only 20 people will be helped, the other 80 people (inaudible - 17:15). So you go in there and keep on getting this drug over and over and over, and eventually you go home because it didn't work for you. So there should be a system where you can do like allergy tests to find out what kind of foods you are allergic to and you eliminate those that you know you are allergic to, right?

And that will increase your chances of symptom—that's what they call—what do they call it? They have a name for it, I'll remember in a minute. And so you don't—but you don't have—that's what Burzynski does, because he takes your blood, marks your genes, or whatever, and then picks out which medications are best for you.

Ty: It is an individualized approach.

Chris: An individualized approach. I don't know if they do it in other hospitals or not but that's the way it should go because it increases your chances of getting better. If anyone has cancer, if you have the money—unfortunately, it is expensive, and insurance will not pick up the tab, but if you have the money, come on here.

Ty: Well, Chris, you keep on keeping on, and keep on coaching people, and keep on sharing your story.

Chris: I'm blessed, so, whatever you guys have, I know the odds are against you, but it's not like that. It's going to start changing.

Ty: Well, it's changing now, and it's going to keep changing because of people like you.

Chris: It's going to keep changing. They may try to—people say, "Oh, why didn't I believe that before?" But it's going to come. It's going to come.

Ty: It is. Well, you keep up the good work and thanks for sharing your story, brother.

Chris: Nice to meet you, man.

Ty: Appreciate it. God bless you.

[end of transcript]

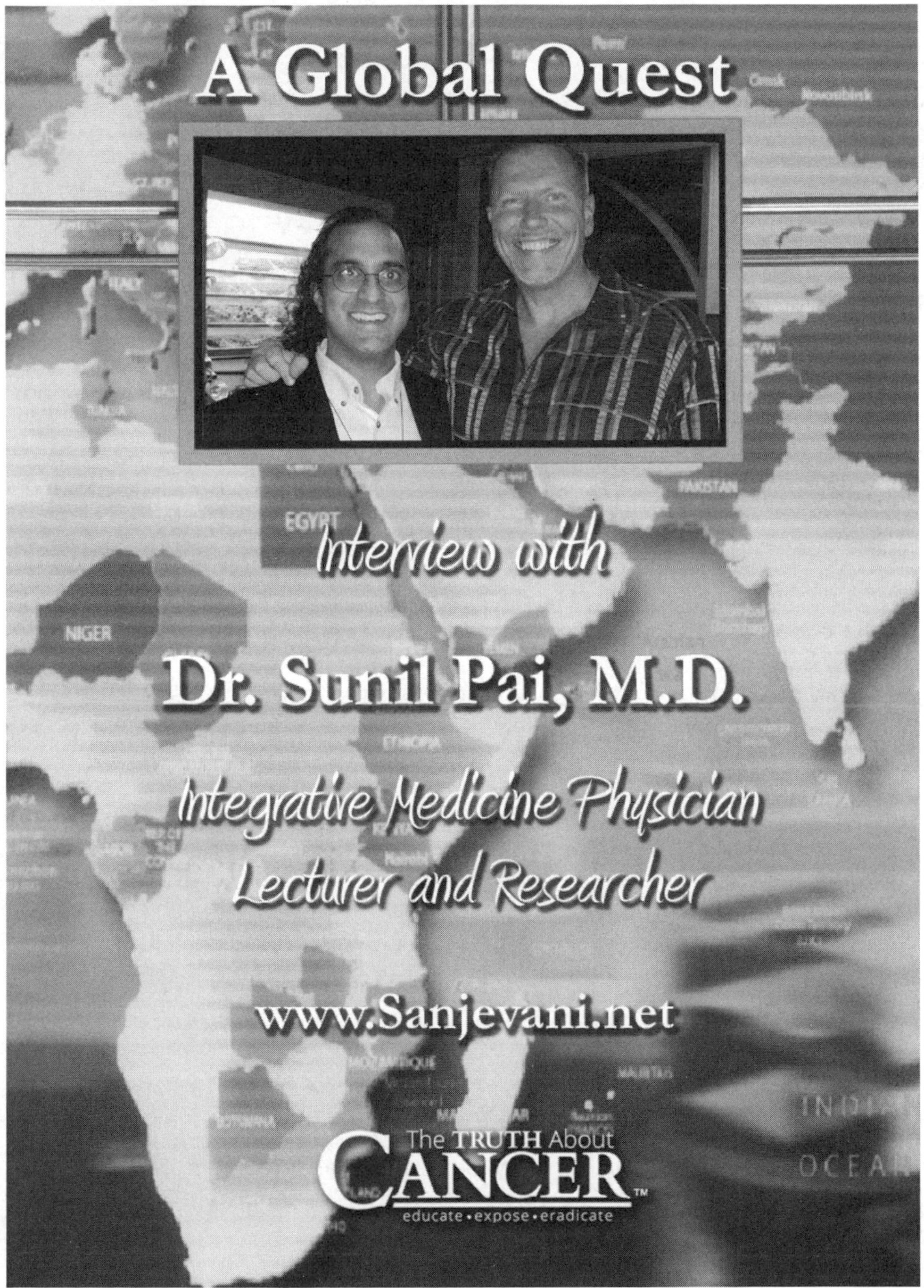
A Global Quest
Interview with
Dr. Sunil Pai, M.D.
Integrative Medicine Physician
Lecturer and Researcher
www.Sanjevani.net
The TRUTH About
CANCER
educate • expose • eradicate

Ty: Dr. Pai, the first thing I want to talk to you about is the money involved with, not only cancer, but just most medical treatments today. You said something last time in the "Quest for the Cures" that resonated with people. You said, "Follow the money."

Dr. Pai: Right.

Ty: And you got a lot of response from the viewers that said, "I've always thought money was a big driving force in a lot of these decisions that are being made." Talk about following the money trail, and how that could apply to the cancer treatments that are available today.

Dr. Pai: There are a few aspects that money does play a role, and cancer is a big business. It is over 127 billion dollars that is being spent on cancer care. The majority of that is in the pharmaceutical drug costs of the care. The average patient, now, according to a study that came out by Kaiser Health, last year, was that they spend between 10,000 dollars a month and 30,000 dollars a month, so that's 10,000 to 30,000 dollars just for the chemotherapy agents that they are using.

And this price keeps on going up higher and higher, so that the average person has, say, three to four months of treatment. Some people have continuously ongoing treatment, so they kind of suppress the cancer, but we're not curing the cancer, for example, and that can go up to 12 months or more, unless they keep coming back for tune-ups, they would say.

So most people don't realize that in cancer treatments, that the facility, or more importantly, the physician that has been prescribing some of these medications, say if that person is a Medicare patient, the government allows the physician to charge the cost of the drug plus a percentage. So Medicare, for example, gives six percent on the cost of the drug, as a reimbursement for de facto aspects of overhead costs, whatever it was.

So what happens is, if I was [sic] a physician and I was in that system, for example, I would prescribe a 100-dollar drug, I would get six dollars back. Now, if I prescribe a 10,000-dollar drug, I get 600 dollars back.

Ty: Wow. In other realms that would be called a kickback, but in this realm, since it is legal—

Dr. Pai: It's reimbursement.

Ty: It's a reimbursement.

Dr. Pai: The thing is, this is the only field, in oncological care that gets that type of reimbursement. And what the studies are showing is that it drives the cost of care higher because now we have a financial incentive, meaning the health care practitioners or hospital systems, to bill for higher, more expensive, costs of drugs or therapies.

And, so, for example, if you had a sore throat, for example, and you come to me, and I have a choice, I could either give you natural therapies, which we have a lot of, that would help your strep throat, or say, amoxicillin. So you say, "Hey, you know what? I want to take amoxicillin." What I do as a physician is make sure you don't have an allergy, and I look at, okay, what is the cheapest generic of that and let me prescribe that. But I don't get a reimbursement from the maker of the amoxicillin company.

So, if I treat your diabetes, your hypertension, your blood pressure, whatever it is, if I use a prescription drug, I don't get reimbursed for any of that cost. I am prescribing it as a provider because I'm trying to give you the best evidence-based medicine, medical practice, and what is the risk/benefit of taking this medication or intervention, for example, of helping manage, and hopefully resolving—what we do is resolving your disease by lifestyle changes. But in oncological care it is almost the opposite.

Ty: So you are talking, specifically, in cancer care, oncological care—

Dr. Pai: Right.

Ty: That this is really the only branch of medicine that the doctors receive reimbursements for prescribing drugs.

Dr. Pai: According to this study, yes. And what the study was showing is that over the last couple of years is that the hospital systems are purchasing what we call physician practices. So you usually, say, if you were to go see an oncologist and they have a little office, the cost of the overhead was very low—the doctor, the nurse, some staff, a small reception room, a couple of treatment rooms. That's kind of the standard practice.

And, so, people would go in, and in the study that was a Kaiser Health study, in which they're showing—Kaiser Health is saying that patients would come and get, say, Herceptin. They actually gave an example, so I'm going to quote the example. The patient was saying, "Oh, I came in and I was being charged 5000 dollars a month for my treatment, for the drug. And I spent a certain amount of time with the doctor, the nurse, in the treatment center."

And then what happens is that the hospital systems are now buying out the oncology practices of physicians. Now what happens is the doctor still works in the same office, they have the same staff, nothing has changed, but the billing of that drug and that treatment now is considered an outpatient hospital center. And the studies will now show that that increase in cost, now that they can bill, is between 50 percent and 184 percent.

Ty: Whoa.

Dr. Pai: So that 5,000 dollars that patient was charged just a week before, or a month before, now can be up to 16,000 dollars, for the same doctor, the same treatment, the same amount of time, in the same room.

Ty: So how did—

Dr. Pai: So the problem is, and that's where some insurance companies, rightfully so, are looking at, well, some companies make money on all of this because it is vertically integrated, right? So the insurance company might own the doctor's group, they might own the pharmacy, they have the financial interest in the laboratory. So the more that they bill, the higher they bill, the better, because they can raise their premiums on all the members.

Some insurance companies that have to take a variety of members, that is, they maybe see more universal coverage, they are trying to look at how they can control the costs. Because I don't want to be paying for a 10,000-dollar drug and 600 dollars to a physician, for example, as an insurance company, to someone that might get a treatment that is half that cost and may be just as effective, or even safer. But there is a dichotomy because it all depends on who and what is the insurance company, which hospital, and what the relationships are.

Ty: Right. Well, you know what is sounds like—I've heard the phrase that there are more people making a living on cancer than are even dying from it. Cancer is a big business.

Dr. Pai: It's a very big business.

Ty: How did it get to this situation? It wasn't this way 50, 60 years ago.

Dr. Pai: No, and in fact, what has always worried me is before, 50 years ago, even 20 years ago—I'm a product of the '80s and watching television, for example. And we would never see cancer on television. It was really taboo. Even mentioning or speaking about cancer was kind of taboo. Even on television it was kind of like the bad C-word.

And now we see commercials on television. I always tell people, you can watch television this weekend and one commercial will be going to a beach in the Bahamas and swim with the dolphins and the next exact commercial will be, "Come to this cancer center for your treatment." And it's becoming very, very common. The problem is, making it so common, not due to its prevalence that more people are getting it, but it just makes it that it is common that we expect to get it. So it should be alarming, that why are they advertising me to go and check in at this place?

And they are competing. Every hospital is competing, the one in Texas competing with the one in Arizona, and the one in Florida, and the one in Chicago. And they are really spending a lot of marketing dollars to get your admission—I call it the "health care amusement parks" or "Disneyland" for example. They want you to come and spend your vacation, but instead of taking your vacation you're actually being treated.

Ty: But if you sit in a nice comfortable lounge chair with a view of the golf course while you're getting chemotherapy dripped into you...

Dr. Pai: Yes. That's not the ride I want to be on.

Ty: No, me either. I interviewed Courtney Campbell and her husband, Kevin, last year for the "Quest for the Cures," and they mentioned that exact thing, that when she was diagnosed with, I think she had non-Hodgkin's lymphoma, they went into this huge cancer-care clinic in Atlanta and they got the tour.

Dr. Pai: Right.

Ty: They got the tour of the beautiful paintings and those huge lounge chairs and the high-def TVs and all these things. And they said the ironic thing was that there were skeletons in the chairs that were being poisoned with chemotherapy and these other drugs. They were being sold a bill of goods to come there and spend their money. And, as you said, this is—we are expecting now to get cancer. It's not, can we prevent cancer anymore, it's, "You're going to get cancer, let's go find the most exciting, nicest, state-of-the-art facility to be treated."

Dr. Pai: Sure.

Ty: When you get it.

Dr. Pai: Right. And sometimes what we have to look at is that people get the tour, it's like going to a showroom of a house, they go, "Wow, that house is beautiful." It's filled with everything, and then when you get your home, though, that is the same model home, it's empty. [laughs] Right? It has no furniture. You're like, "It doesn't look the same; it doesn't feel the same."

Ty: Yes.

Dr. Pai: And, unfortunately, then, what happens, people get sometimes the tour from the hospital, but then they get shifted to that outpatient center, which was the doctor's clinic that they have been seeing all the time, but they are being charged at the higher-end cost of the outpatient hospital billing.

Ty: So these treatments that are standard today, that are the standard of care, the conventional oncologist is pretty much hamstrung. They have to use these if they are going to follow the standard of care.

Dr. Pai: Right.

Ty: How effective are they? How effective are the chemo and radiation?

Dr. Pai: Well, there is a lot of—it all depends on how you want to spin the statistics.

Ty: How about you unspin the statistics?

Dr. Pai: Well, there is a couple of articles that have been published in the conservative journals about the wonders of modern medicine. I think that was in the title of the article, actually. And we're looking at certain anti-cancer drugs—we call them TNF-alpha blockers, or biologics, we call them. They are kind of one of the mainstays now of blocking inflammation in certain treatments of cancers. Except the cost of that being now—some of those are 10,000 to 40,000 dollars for the treatment.

The survival rate of those patients, particularly when they are end-stage, Stage III, Stage IV—more people are coming in to get chemotherapy by the time they are diagnosed, the cost again, as I mentioned before, can be up to 10,000 to 40,000 dollars, but the survival rate of that patient is anywhere from 15 days up to three months more. So, is that a cost benefit? If this patient lives for a year getting treatment then those costs, again, can go up to 250,000 dollars to what they call quality-of-life years, up to 1.3 million. And I mentioned that before when we interviewed.

And the reason is that, what does that cost? Can we spend any of this money, in terms of telling someone to change their diet, change their lifestyle? Can we use natural therapies? And we know that 95 percent of cancer is preventable. In my lecture yesterday—30 percent is related to tobacco, another 30 to 35 percent, or 40 percent, is related just to diet, about 20 percent is related to obesity, another 10 to 15 percent is related to environmental toxins, another 10 to 15 percent is also related to chronic infections that also cause inflammation, and less than 5 percent is genetically related. And we're so worried about the genes, even spending a lot of money on genetic testing, but we know that 90 to 95 percent, there are things that right now, that your viewers, rightfully so, can start doing to change and prevent the risk of having cancer, and even if they have cancer, to improve the outcomes, at least.

Ty: So then why are we not focusing on that? Not you and I, and the group of people that are really trying to get the word out about natural treatments for cancer, or integrative medicine, however you want to put it, because there are some good integrative techniques. As you mentioned last night, we want to do whatever we can to give the patient better outcomes.

Dr. Pai: Right.

Ty: But why are traditional doctors not focusing on this? Why are they stuck in the rut of these treatments that really are very, very expensive, and most of the time don't really work all that well?

Dr. Pai: It first comes from the training and education of the physician. So, we haven't been trained in nutrition; we haven't been trained in natural therapies. So that's why I always recommend people to go seek a formally trained integrative medicine physician, because we need to have knowledge of conventional training, understanding chemotherapy drugs, or radiation therapies, or surgeries, and other medications, but understanding what are the natural therapies? What would they be doing in India, or China, or South America, or France right now, for the same outcome?

And how can we improve our outcomes? We are ranking now 46 out of 48 industrial nations in terms of outcomes of all health care parameters. So there are 46 other countries that are ahead of us in terms of doing better at everything. So we have to look at—in an integrative approach we look at what other things we can be doing and just integrate them. We're not saying, "Don't do this, don't do that." How can we always improve the outcome?

And we are able to, now, with conventional therapies, with natural therapies, like I mentioned at the conference here, the Bosmeric SR—the curcumin, the boswellia, the ginger, the black pepper. There is a lot of data that will show that with the top-15 chemotherapy agents, we can help sensitize a tumor, meaning it takes a toxic agent and makes it more targeted, and it also has a protective effect of, say, oral mucosa damage, heart damage, kidney damage, lung damage, so we are protecting the healthy tissues.

Sometimes, most people, as we talked about yesterday, most people are going to be getting conventional care. Most people are already in the treatment right now. What can we do to help improve their outcome? And now the data will show that if you have a physician who actually did some studies, or if you told your oncologist to go on PubMed and look up curcumin and these other chemotherapy agents, you will see how the data will support using it in conjunction will have a better outcome than just using chemotherapy alone.

Ty: So, Dr. Pai, we always hear that we need to use evidence-based medicine. What you are telling me is, this combination of these different herbs that you are telling me about—the Bosmeric—and I want you to go into details about it—this *is* evidence-based.

Dr. Pai: It *is* evidence-based.

Ty: You're saying, you do research—and I appreciate what you said. Many people that are watching this, they've already undergone chemotherapy.

Dr. Pai: Sure.

Ty: So we want to give—our message is that there is hope, and there is hope for you if you've done chemotherapy.

Dr. Pai: Absolutely!

Ty: It's never too late, you're not in over your head now because you did chemo and now you just found out...

Dr. Pai: And there should never be guilt or fear. Everybody has decisions to make, and sometimes they were forced decisions, or decisions in an untimely manner that were pressing, that they had to do. I never fault anybody for making their decisions.

Ty: And we don't either.

Dr. Pai: But the decision that they have to do is, from today, is changing and making better decisions in terms of making more informed decisions.

Ty: Right. And so this combination of these herbs—go into, real quickly, the details—the Bosmeric, that you are saying, can help people that have undergone chemo, or they are going to continue undergoing chemo, because you're in the system, your doctor is going to keep you on chemo, and if that's your choice, there are things that they can do to help it become more targeted.

Dr. Pai: Right. We always want to—the fear of chemotherapy is the side effects. People lose weight, they have cachexia, diarrhea, hair loss—all these other—the fear of the chemo.

Ty: The *direct* effects of chemo.

Dr. Pai: The direct effects of chemo. The *common* effects of chemo. And so everybody is uniquely different when they get chemo. Some people can get chemo and not have much problems, and some people, they don't survive even the treatment. So we want to improve everybody's outcome. And so what the studies will show, again, when we take things like Bosmeric, which has a curcumin C3 complex, it has Boswellin PS, ginger, and black pepper, in a special delivery form.

During the treatment, in fact, people will do better, and, in fact, with our patients we always improve outcomes. So a lot of people will call us and say, "I'm already in my sixth round, and they are expecting me to do another six more. What can I do?" And so we are looking at giving natural anti-inflammatories. These all work on the same pathways, but they also work on preventative and protective pathways, so some of these ingredients like curcumin will increase genetic expression of what we want to turn cancer cells off. So we're not just talking about suppression of cancer growth; we're looking at turning on your own immune system, the inherent ability for the body to heal itself, which is there.

Ty: Is that also considered part of epigenetics?

Dr. Pai: Absolutely.

Ty: Turning on as well as turning off the gene expression?

Dr. Pai: Yes. In Western medicine you have only ways to turn it off. And that is why when we give some of these agents, they are very good at doing what they are doing—they are turning off certain cells, like cancer cells. But the side effect is that they also turn off a lot of normal cells. And through that process there is also damage that some of those cells can become more resistant to chemotherapy over time, and they can also genetically change where they start creating more cancer, or secondary cancers, or other chronic conditions down the line. So we have to be careful; we want to give that targeted, to toxic, to targeted effect and reduce the side effects by improving the outcomes.

Ty: That makes a lot of sense to me because a lot of times people that are undergoing chemo, or have undergone chemo, sometimes we almost give up on them, and say, "You went conventional, your immune system is shot, there is nothing you can do now." That's not true.

Dr. Pai: That's not true.

Ty: The fact of the matter is, there is a lot that they can do. This is one combination of herbs that you use. Name some other products that you are using.

Dr. Pai: We always want to recommend probiotics because the gut microbiome is one of the most important things to our health. And what people don't realize is, they understand that when they take an antibiotic it lowers the good bacteria in my [sic] gut, but chemotherapy we would consider a hundred times stronger than an antibiotic. And that's why people lose weight, they have diarrhea, they have malabsorption, because when you give chemotherapy it also knocks out the good bacteria in the gut. By doing that then they have malabsorption problems, and then their nutrition is poor. So no matter what they are eating, it goes right through them, and then they lose weight, they don't have enough strength, their immune system is down, and then sometimes they die from the therapy. So we have to look at strengthening the GI tract.

So a lot a lot of times when we work with patients, looking at, how do we keep your immune system up? How do we decrease swelling post-chemo, or from the radiation? How do we decrease a burn, for example? Or the tumor is dying off, rightfully so, there is still going to be swelling around that tissue. What natural agents, like proteolytic enzyme formulas? Or if they have a hormone-sensitive cancer, how can we help the excretion of the hormones, through the liver, for example?

So we have certain drugs that block it. I mentioned here in the conference, Tamoxifen, and all these other type of drugs. Okay, they block it, but it's still in the body, circulating. How can we help the body augment that excretion, even through diet? We can increase fiber, for example. People who eat a plant-based diet get about 40 grams a day. Studies show that women who had estrogen-positive breast cancer who had three bowel movements a day had the lowest recurrence rate because their body is able to, once the hormones go through the liver, it goes into the—the gallbladder takes it out with the bile, it goes into the small intestine, and fiber binds that and excretes it.

But if you don't have enough fiber in the diet, something as simple as fiber—I'm talking fiber from vegetables, not fiber supplements, because you want all the other nutrients—when the fiber is in the body then it binds to the hormones and excretes it. But if we don't have enough fiber, then it is called enterohepatic circulation—it just recirculates. The average American has seven to 12 grams of fiber a day, and we need about 40 or more. And so when you look at other countries, there are other people in the studies who are surviving the most, meaning the least reoccurrence, they're having more bowel movements, they're eating more fiber, and it is flushing the body.

So when we're talking about detoxification it is very, very important. But the average American right now is usually on the constipated side—bowel movement every two days, three days. In certain states I won't mention, but up to 10 days, 12 days—people are horribly constipated. So if you go to the store you can see all these stool softeners and bowel movement stimulants. And then people don't realize that that is a dysfunction of the body. So probiotics, vitamin D, increasing the immune system, we use a lot of mushroom extracts that increase your natural killer cells.

So it's always getting the person's body's own innate ability to heal itself and its innate immune system to participate. Because when we shut everything off with certain drugs like chemotherapy or biologics, for example, the patient is at risk of getting higher secondary infections. So a lot of times you will hear people say, "Oh, my mother went to go get her chemotherapy and in the hospital she got pneumonia." And sometimes they die from the pneumonia, not the chemotherapy, or the cancer.

Ty: I actually just talked to someone last night that told me that. I think it was their daughter that had undergone several rounds of chemotherapy and died of pneumonia.

Dr. Pai: Right.

Ty: The exact same thing.

Dr. Pai: So, what we want to do is, we want to improve that outcome by saying, "Okay, let's get your soldier cells, your immune system, stronger while it's being beaten down on the other end."

Ty: Right. And the immune system is the key, isn't it?

Dr. Pai: The immune system is the key. So lowering the inflammation, increasing the immune system, eating a plant-based diet. You need all the phytonutrients, you need all the antioxidants, you need the fiber, and the protein.

Ty: And I appreciate what you said about eating the whole foods.

Dr. Pai: Right.

Ty: Because there is a synergy between the active ingredients in the herbs, and plants, and foods, that you don't get when you extract one particular component.

Dr. Pai: Right. For example, when we give the Bosmeric, we are giving four ingredients for a reason, because these four are more potent and efficacious than just giving one. So if somebody says, "Oh, I take tons and tons of curcumin," then they're kind of overloading one pathway. And, actually, sometimes that can also have a detriment effect, or burnout effect, because the body becomes tolerant to it. When we look at synergistic formulas, they can take it for longer periods of time without developing the tolerance. So we can actually balance a potential side effect and also maintain efficacy for a long period of time.

Ty: Great advice. Let me ask you this. What would you recommend to someone that has just been diagnosed with cancer? What is the first thing you would recommend that someone do that has just been diagnosed?

Dr. Pai: Well, first thing, no fear, no guilt, second opinion, find an integrative doctor to get on your team. It doesn't mean that you are going to run from conventional care, but you need to have all the educational options and make a truly informed consent of what those options are. Most cancers, as I mention in my lecture, most cancers, that once we find it, there are very rare cancers—very few cancers, about five percent of cancer, is very aggressive, like you need to do something now, you need to have it taken out right now. Sometimes by the time the patient actually gets diagnosed, unfortunately, it is very late, so we have to rush them to surgery.

But most cancer growth is very slow-growing. And, in fact, by the time we see it on a mammogram, or a biopsy, or an ultrasound or CT scan, it can to 10 to 20 years in the making. So another week for most people is not going to be a big difference, unless it's an emergency. But everybody is treated as if it is an emergency. And the reason why is that if we give a patient more than about three days or four days to think about it, they might get a second opinion.

Now, what the conventional system is worried about is not an opinion from an integrative or holistical alternative; they're afraid of someone contacting the other cancer hospital that is also advertising on television. So they're competing against—so they want you to as soon—as quick as possible make this decision because otherwise you might go to a different center and then they lose all that revenue.

Ty: So, in other words, this is the same logic that is used for Internet marketing, or for any kind of marketing. It is sales.

Dr. Pai: It is sales.

Ty: You convince somebody of the urgency, they need to act now, because if not—anyone that does any kind of sales knows you got to close the sale.

Dr. Pai: Right. I was on the Internet the other day and I clicked on some advertisement and a little clock came up and it was like, "Well, you purchased this, but if you do this in the next two minutes," and then I go, "Oh my God, should I get it?"

Ty: "Should I get it, should I get it?"

Dr. Pai: And I clicked it again and another thing came up. And so it's almost like that. They put on pressure. But this is not buying a skin care product or something—

Ty: Or a Vegematic.

Dr. Pai: Yes, or something like that. This is your life that we're talking about.

Ty: Yes, that's true. This is serious.

Dr. Pai: But it is easier to persuade someone in that life-and-death situation to do something now. And the intention, for everybody, even the family members that are putting on a lot of pressure, is because they do want their loved ones to have a better outcome. So it's not coming from a bad place, but it's coming from a place of not understanding what all the full options are.

Ty: Yes. Do you think that most of the oncologists that are prescribing these pills for everybody, all these chemotherapies, do they know that they're not really working too well? I mean, how in the know are they, really? Because I've seen statistics that most oncologists won't do chemo if they were diagnosed. But it seems like they know this isn't good.

Dr. Pai: But that has become the standard of care. So they're not held to any higher or lower standard. So if the standard of care is that we give these drugs, and then these are the outcomes, then they're doing a good job per the standard of care. But I always, like I mentioned yesterday in the conference, I said, well, you know, hopefully I won't have a legal aspect problem with this, but McDonald's was the official restaurant of the Olympics.

Ty: Yes.

Dr. Pai: Now, if you use the word "restaurant" and "McDonald's" in the same sentence, I may disagree with that definition.

Dr. Pai: Even for the Olympics. And they're making it official. And they're a sponsor. So the idea is that we have to look at what is that standard of care? So if someone says, "Well, that is a great kind of food establishment," well, that's their decision. Then that means people eating at that restaurant should be getting healthier, or should be an Olympic athlete, but we don't really see that. We see the rest of what's happening with America being "supersized," for example. So same thing when it comes down to these aspects of what are we looking at, how we're selling it. We have to be very careful of getting caught into the marketing aspect.

And I don't think that the oncologists are coming from a place of ill intent, or mal intent; I think they're just doing the job that they've been told to do. But we need to have more oncologists step outside the box saying, "You know what? I'm going to practice more on my consciousness, and my ethical and moral value, than what the group, or the hospital, or the insurance company is saying, this is what you must do." I mean, many people follow the "I'm just following orders" attitude, which has gone through history for a long period of time, but I don't think physicians can no longer do that anymore.

Ty: I'm with you. I mean, that was the common response at the Nuremberg trials. "We were just following orders when we put them in the gas chambers."

Dr. Pai: Right. And you know, when you look at interesting things, how to roundabout this conversation, how we first discovered chemotherapy, the first chemotherapy agents in the early 1940s, was because in Italy, when they dropped nitrogen mustard gas on these missions, and they were doing the post-mortem autopsies on the bodies, the lymphocytes of these patients dropped down. And then some of these doctors got an idea, "Well, gosh, someone has leukemia, or lymphoma, where these lymphocytes are producing too much, it was suppressing these people that were dropped with mustard gas. So the chemotherapy agent comes from the history of actually making

Ty: Mustard gas.

Dr. Pai: You said it.

Ty: Wow, I did. And you've told us a lot of information today that is very valuable, Dr. Pai. I really appreciate this second interview.

Dr. Pai: Thank you very much; I appreciate it. I hope best of health for everyone.

Ty: I appreciate what you're doing.

Dr. Pai: Yes, I appreciate what you're doing, too.

Ty: All right.

Dr. Pai: Thanks.

[end transcript]

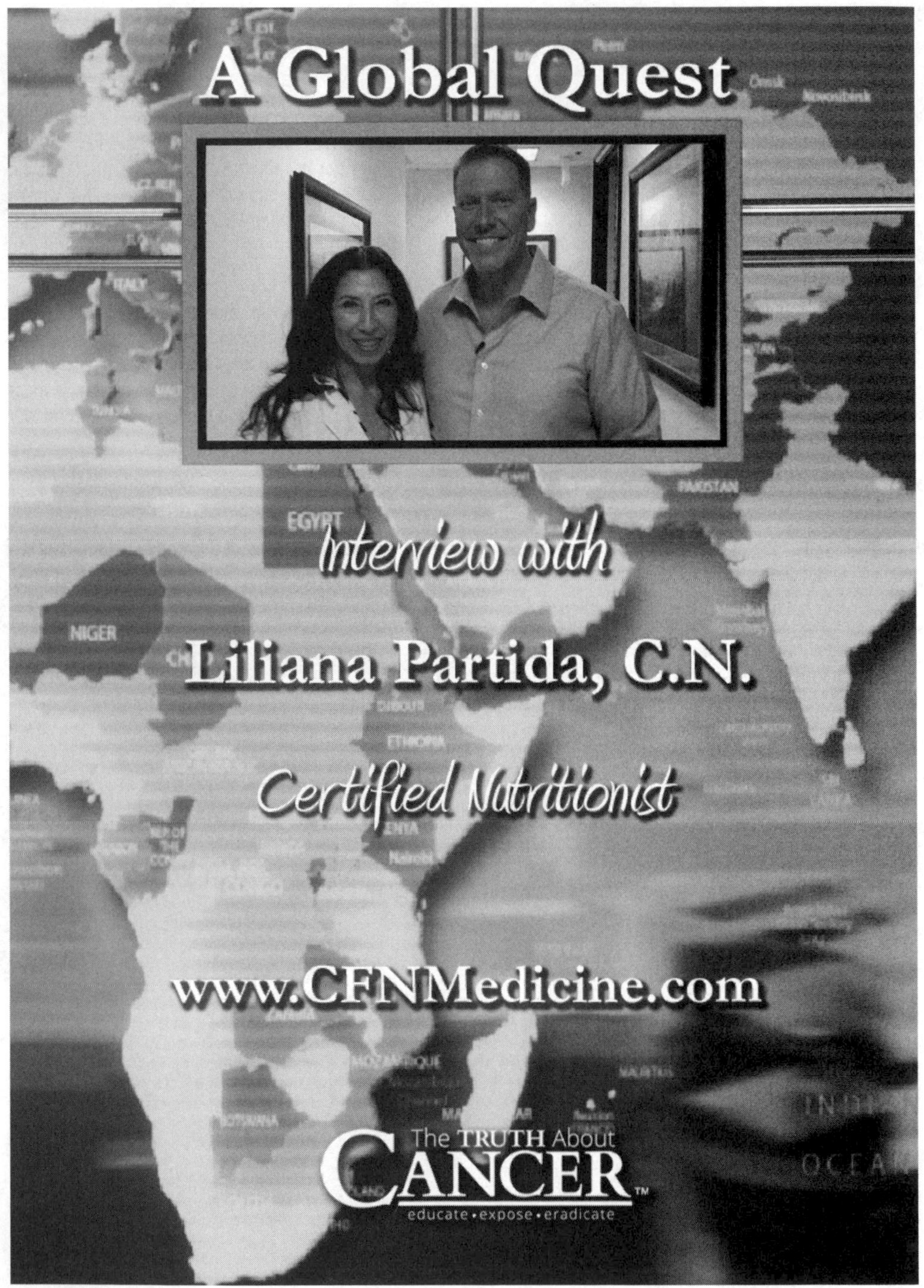
A Global Quest
Interview with
Liliana Partida, C.N.
Certified Nutritionist
www.CFNMedicine.com
The TRUTH About
CANCER™
educate • expose • eradicate

Ty: So I'm here with Liliana Partida, a clinical nutritionist here. Dr. Connealy's medical center here in Irvine. Thank you for joining us, and I want you to explain the Evox machine.

Liliana: Okay. Well, I compare the Evox to what I would consider emotional acupuncture. So it's pretty amazing because it's done with bio feedback and so what it's doing it's picking up voice recognition. So we use a cradle and it works on galvanic response. A patient will have a microphone on and then I just ask them to speak their name so that I can just pick up the patterning.

Then it will come put with a little mandala, it will have what we call PIs, perception indexes from one to twelve. So each area is associated with an organ and also with an emotion. So often times the patient doesn't know what's really running their lives and potentially even running their health in regards to their crisis that they're experiencing.

So what's really fascinating about it is the patient doesn't even really have to tell me about it. The feedback actually comes up with the areas of stagnation or what we call extreme energy, or let's say, even if you were thinking in terms of acupuncture where there would be extreme excess in a specific organ.

So through that determination the program is equipped to send specific frequencies to unlock those emotional stagnation. So it's pretty amazing. So each time we do a recording we do about five recordings that we can actually see the unlocking of those emotions. And that is kind of like an onion, each voice recording goes deeper and deeper in regards to what potentially is the underlying of even that emotional stagnation.

Ty: So kind of peeling off the layers off the onion?

Liliana: Exactly.

Ty: And then eventually you get to the real root cause.

Liliana: Eventually we get to the root cause which is really pretty amazing for the patient because often times they'll have an "aha" moment. They'll be potentially experiencing a lot of depression and really what we're looking at as we go deeper and deeper, the depression is based potentially on unworthiness or repetitive thinking. And I always ask them, "How does that show up for you in your life?"

So we try to get some feedback, and they say "actually, you know, I just churn things until they turn into butter, you know, I can't let go of thing when they happen to me." So when a patient is really able to identify what they actually do, they can begin to actually recognize, oh I'm doing it again, this is a stuck pattern. And just even that begins to unravel those energies that are stuck.

Ty: So this can be really beneficial for cancer patients because of the emotional link that we've seen to cancer. Here we have so many cancer patients that have this emotional trauma, these things that have happened in the past that they can't let go of, this baggage, whatever you want to call it. This allows them to help release that, doesn't it?

Liliana: Absolutely. I'm definitely a believer in Hamer's work in regards to every disease has an emotional component, whether it's a sore throat or cancer. And so it's pretty exciting that we have this information so that we can really look at, potentially, is it the emotion that's causing the problem? Or is it the actual organ function that's causing the emotion, you know. Which is really pretty cool.

The sister machine to this is the LSA, the Limbic Stress Assessment. So what I love doing is I love checking the organ function. So, for example, they might show that they have a deficiency, for example, in the liver and it'll show up here that they have a lot of anger. And then I might run Bach flower remedies to support them and then we might do affirmations.

So then really can go home with the full package in regards to trying to balance out their emotions through creating beliefs, re-imprinting their beliefs by giving them affirmations. Or with the Bach flower remedy and then also working with the organ itself.

Ty: So I can just see this as being a huge adjunct to other therapies that are being used. Many doctors aren't addressing the emotions. So if you're not hitting cancer from all these different areas, especially from the emotional area, you're missing a big piece of the puzzle.

Liliana: Oh absolutely. I mean so many patients have fear as their underlying issue. And even when they have been treated and are in remission, it's like the Boogie Man is going to come back at some point. So they have this kind of underlying fear. And so if we can just really look at it, stare it in the face. I always say kind of like an opera singer when she hits the right note, she can shatter a glass.

Well, the same thing with the Evox. When it really finds those areas of stagnation it sends the frequency and it can shatter it so that we can begin to release some of these emotions.

Ty: That's a great analogy. I love that.

Liliana: This is Perception Index, a patient has given us a basic voice transitioning. And then what happens is it comes up with this area of depression versus inner peace. So I would ask the patient does she associate with that at all. And then you know, obviously they're going to say, “Yeah, I really feel depressed” and this and that. And I said, “Do you want to continue experiencing that?” Because the patient has to want to get well.

When we start working with our patient, we can actually work trans-generational. We can work on the mother, the father, we'll actually look to see who did you pattern after most emotionally, who did you take stuff from? And they can always just say, “Oh my God, everybody always said I'm just like my father.” And so it's pretty amazing that we can actually go deeper and not just working on themselves but trans-generationally all the way to the grand parents or to a significant other, like their spouse, and so it's pretty amazing.

Ty: I bet it is. And I bet it's rewarding to see the changes.

Liliana: Oh yeah, it is so awesome. I mean I get chills all the time when I'm in here and the people are going, “Oh my gosh, I've never told anybody that before.” I said, “Well, I'm not telling you, your body is telling me, it's speaking.” So I said, “The body never lies.”

Ty: Well, you guys keep on shattering that glass of ill health that's being caused by ill emotions and thank you for sharing this today.

Liliana: Oh, thank you very, very much for having us to share with you.

Ty: Yeah, this is great information. I appreciate it.

[end of transcript]

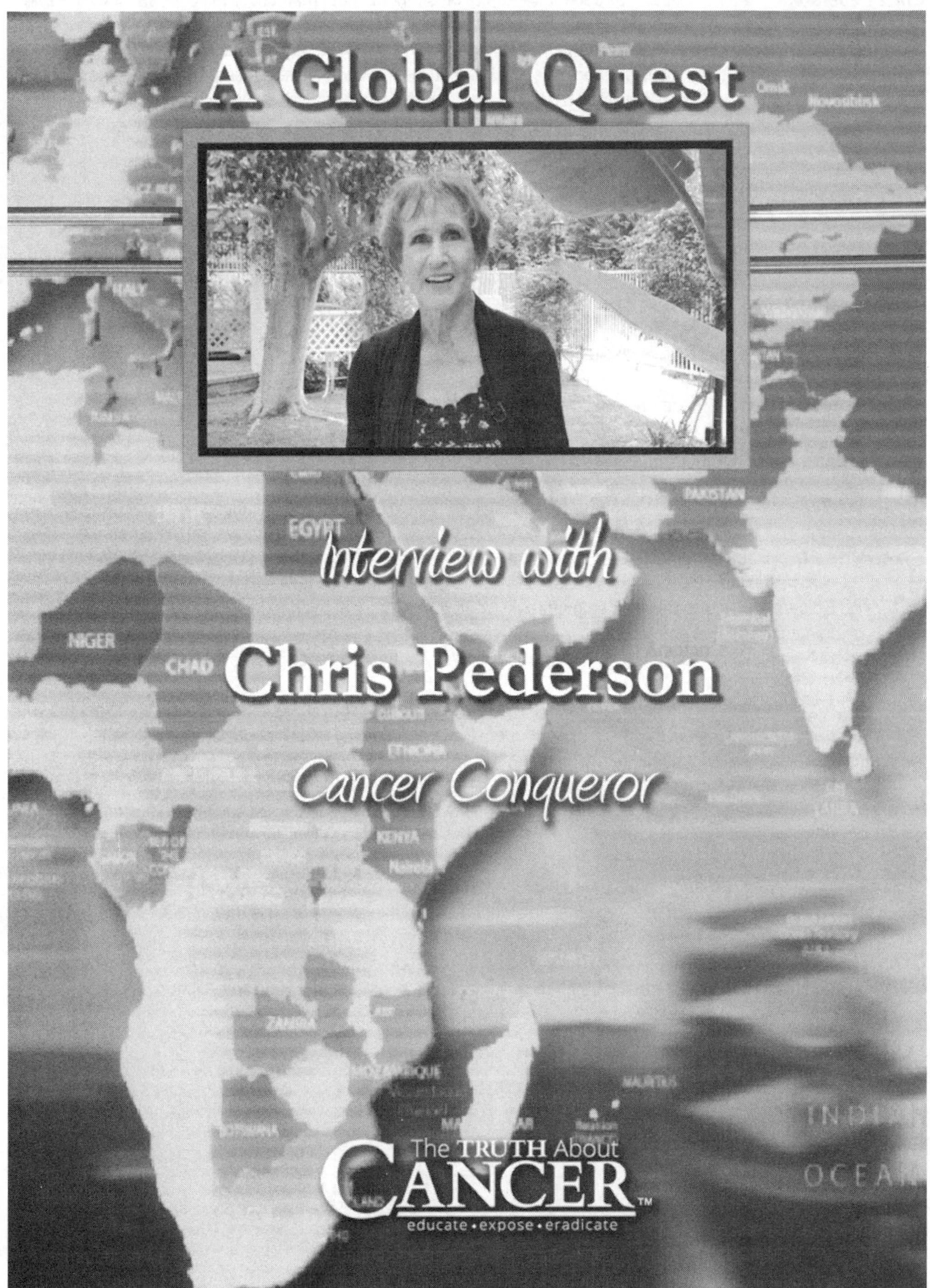
A Global Quest
Interview with
Chris Pederson
Cancer Conqueror
The TRUTH About
CANCER
educate • expose • eradicate

Chris Pederson: March 2009, my husband brought home a book that I read cover to cover and it was Verne Verona's *Nature's Cancer Fighting Foods*, and I embraced everything in that book. The next day, after I had my cry-pity-party, "I can't do this," I changed my diet the next day. I'm very disciplined, I got that from my dad. I'm very disciplined, so I stuck with it, just all kinds of vegetables. I'd cut up vegetables and I'd make my own dressing. I didn't even have lettuce in it either. I would just cut up a variety of vegetables and eat those and that was my main meal, my main thing. Then I would juice and blend those, and do all different things.

Ty: You were getting serious nutrition.

Chris Pederson: I was getting serious nutrition. I also added some, very few, but a few supplements and an herbal combination. B17 I took that. So, I took these things and then went through those, still removing the polyps. About a year onto my whole diet, big regimen change, I had zero polyps.

Ty: Wow. That's amazing. How did that make you feel?

Chris Pederson: That made me feel great. It was really a blessing.

Ty: The fruits of your one year labor of being so disciplined and strict eating paid off quickly.

Chris Pederson: Very much. I was ready to shout it from the mountain tops because I had beat genetic cancer. To be honest, when I started out, I wasn't sure, but I had been doing tons of research on my gene to figure out what it was and what it was all about. It had only been discovered in 2002. I wasn't really sure what the effect would be, but I started looking into this new science called Epigenetics. Epigenetics simply said it's being affected by your environment to change your genes. Well, the first thing that you can control about your environment is what you put in your body, and so I was doing that. I started feeling like, "Okay, this can probably work." When it did work, I was just thrilled.

Now, the interesting thing is the doctor who did that colonoscopy, I thought he would be, "What did you do? Tell me all about it," because I told them that I was doing a diet. I was really making big changes there. He walked in, handed my husband the pictures of my colon, he just said, "You're clear," and walked out the room. That's the only words he said, and I was still reeling from the anesthesia, but I wanted to scream at him, "Don't you want to know about what I do so you can share that with your other patients?"

Ty: What's your message to cancer patients that may have been told they have some kind of a genetic cancer? What is your message that you want them to take away from this interview?

Chris Pederson: Well, I tell friends of mine who complain about, "Well, you know, the genes in my family," and I just shake them off and say, "Look at me. Look what I did and you can do it, too. You just have to make some changes in your life."

[end of transcript]

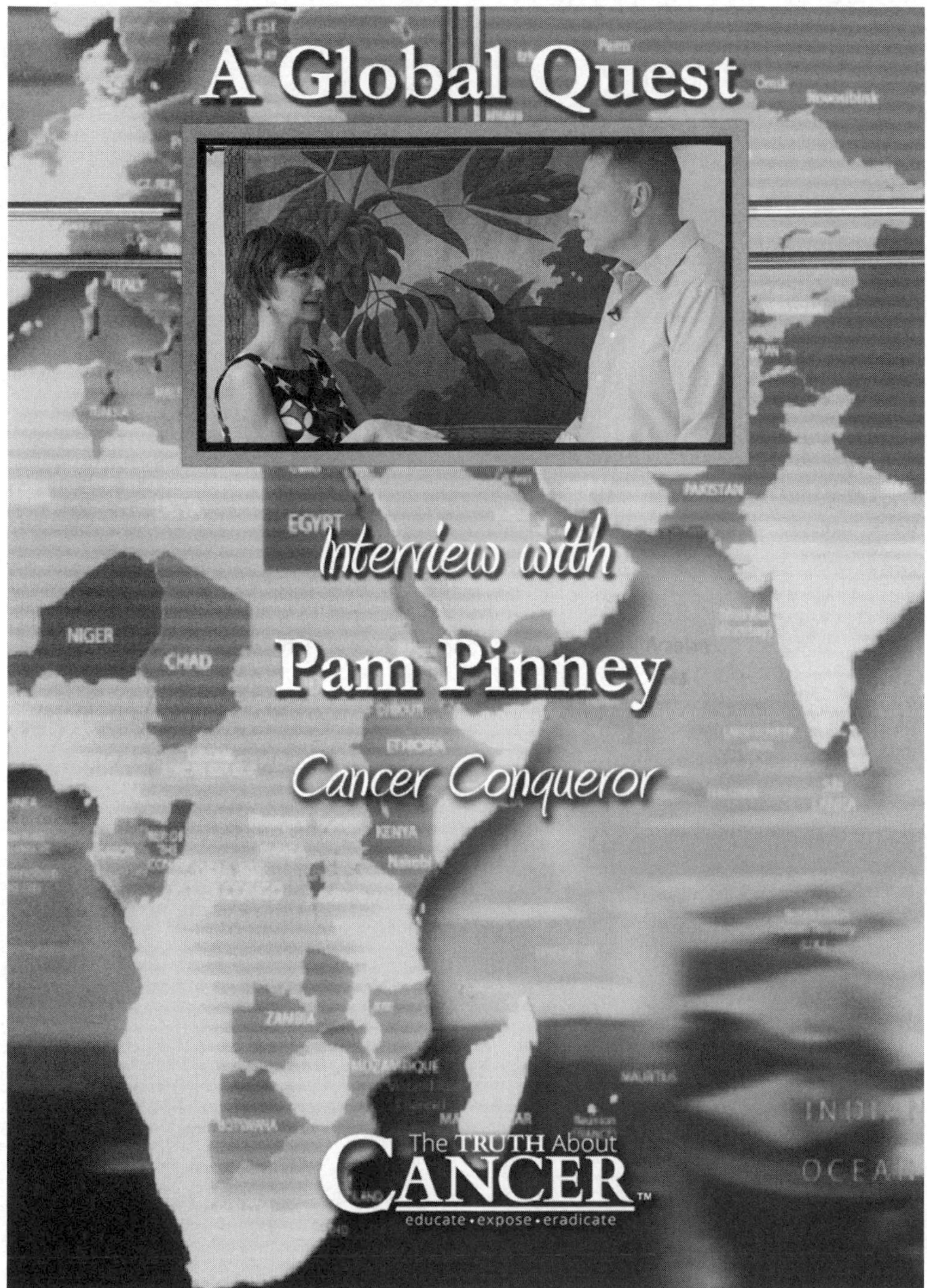
A Global Quest
Interview with
Pam Pinney
Cancer Conqueror
The TRUTH About
CANCER
educate • expose • eradicate

Ty: Pam so good to be here with you today.

Pam: It's so good to be here, Ty.

Ty: Yes, we're here at the Hope4Cancer Institute and we were just on a little round table with a bunch of other patients and I got the chance to hear a little bit about your story but I want to hear some more now, and learn about how you got here, and what you are doing with your cancer. Very inspiring story, what I've heard so far, so what was yours?

Pam: Well, when I was a little girl, I don't if I was 10 or 12, I went into the hospital. I was doubled over in stomach pain. They checked my appendix, said it's not that, and they diagnosed me with an old-fashioned stomach ache.

When I left the hospital I was crooked, my spine was crooked. My mom noticed I was walking funny. Well, years later I was diagnosed with scoliosis. We progress, and in 2007 my husband and I, Harry, we did a 40-day fast and I lost 25 pounds. And so, I was lying in bed one day and I laid my hand on my chest and I noticed this pea-like thing in my chest. I was like, "Huh, that's interesting."

One physician said if I hadn't lost the weight with the fast I would have never known, never seen it, never felt it. So I caught it stage one. I went in, they did testing, a biopsy. Said it was stage one invasive ductal carcinoma. So I had surgery. There was this urgency—have surgery, have chemo, have radiation. I quickly did the surgery out of fear.

Ty: And they removed the little pea-sized lump.

Pam: Removed the lump, had a lumpectomy. And they said, "You need to have chemo and radiation." Actually, there was mixed—some days they said, "We don't know what to do with you." Other days, "You're going to die if you don't have it." So I prayed about what to do and I felt the Lord said, "Every good and perfect gift comes from above." And he said, "Chemo causes cancer, why would you do that?" And so, I thought, "I'm just not going to do it."

Well, announcing that to the family was not—it didn't go well. Everybody—it's not just you in fear, the whole family gets in fear. So I didn't do chemo or radiation. We began making lifestyle changes. I started reading books like crazy.

Ty: What year is this?

Pam: This is 2007 still. So 2008, 2009, and 2010 we're reading. My husband and I both have medical backgrounds. He is a speech pathologist and I was an occupational therapist. So we had a medical background and we started researching. Four years later, the tumor grows back in the same exact spot and when they did the testing they said, "Wow, it looks exactly the same as four years ago, same size." They said, "It's a little more aggressive."

My genetic testing, my oncotype, was a 14. Low risk of it ever coming back, they did that the first time. My genetic testing with 23andMe—it's a great testing. It said my risk of cancer was lower than the average person.

So I began praying even more so, "Lord, what are the roots to this cancer?" I got a phone call, asked to come speak at a chiropractor's office, Dr. Aaron Rose, a "Maximized Living" doc. And the lady said, "He heard you're fighting cancer different and he wants you to come give your testimony."

So I went and gave my testimony. And he said, "I think you're supposed to see me." And I said, "I think I am, too," because I'm doing four of the five "Maximized Living" things. I'm not doing the one, and that's getting my spine adjusted. I had had scoliosis my whole life and no one had ever said they could fix it other than rods and surgery.

So he looks at my spine—I was running 5Ks at the time—and he said, "You need to stop running, and I can straighten your spine." It was a 30-something degree curve. He said, "I can get it down to two degrees," and I'm like, "You're kidding me." Because I was 50 years old at the time.

Ty: That's a huge improvement.

Pam: And my parents were like, "Nobody ever thought they could straighten it." So he starts adjusting me, and my thyroid hadn't been working, hadn't taken any medicine—the doctor kept trying to get me to. Two months after adjustments my thyroid starts working, and it was verified with the blood. And he's like, "Wow, your thyroid's working better." And so I told him, "I'm getting adjustments."

So as my spine began to get straightened, I was praying and a naturopathic friend of a friend called. She said, "Can I look at your blood work?" I said, "Absolutely." So she looks at it and she says, "Will you do a colon cleanse?" And I said, "I've done colon cleanses." And she said, "No, will you do a colon cleanse called Blessed Herbs?" We were financially so broke I said, "I can't afford it." We'd been fighting this for—it had been five years or something. She said, "I'll buy it for you, and I'll bring it to you." And I'm like, "Wow." She said, "But you have to promise you'll do it."

So I did it. And when I did it I got deathly sick. I spent one night thinking, "Am I going to die tonight, am I going to go to the hospital? What should I do?" But I was throwing up and just very, very ill, as this old stuff started coming out of my colon. And I looked like this, I weighed 120-something. It wasn't like I looked like I had parasites.

So as I did this colon cleanse and it started coming out. Over the next few weeks as that stuff came out, then I began seeing lots of parasites. And it was what the naturopath had suspected. Nothing on my blood work had shown it, the numbers hadn't indicated it, but she had a revelation of what was wrong. I mean, nothing was showing that was what was wrong. I know Hulda Clark had said every person with cancer has liver flukes.

Ty: Yes, parasites in the liver.

Pam: And I've been tested by Dr. D'Angelo with ParaWellness, and he said that every person with cancer that sent their samples to him had parasites. So I feel like that's probably my message that God has for me to give to people, because I see some people overcoming but I see many people not. And I think parasites is a missing link, definitely. Because there was no sign, I had run three 5Ks right before I found out I was infested.

Ty: What was in this Blessed Herbs that you used to cleanse, because it was a parasite cleanse, as well, apparently?

Pam: No, it was just a colon cleanse.

Ty: It was just for the colon, but the parasites came out?

Pam: Exactly. What happened was as the mucoid plaque came out I began to notice that as I went to the bathroom the parasites were trying to hide in my stool. And I thought, "Wow, they've been hiding in that mucoid plaque." And I had taken parasite medicine eight years ago when I first got diagnosed. We saw Dr. Simon Yu in St. Louis. Dr. Tony actually went to a presentation he did on parasites. He gave me parasite medicine back then. It did nothing, but I think it was because they were hiding in that mucoid plaque. So as it came out I would use a spaghetti strainer and go in and watch and see what was there. And I just began to see, the photos will show you, tons and tons of parasites.

So, my naturopathic doctor followed me every day. She would write me, and we would call and talk, and she said, "You should be free by now." It was six months later and I had done the parasite thing with Dr. D'Angelo at ParaWellness. He tested me and found several. And she said, "You should be free by now." So I kept battling, kept battling.

Some changes with the tumor. We felt like we were winning, but we thought, "We need some extra help." And that's when my chiropractor bought me your book, *Cancer: Step Outside the Box*, and we watched your series, saw Dr. Tony on episode two. So, we knew that was probably—I felt like I needed to come and get my blood cleansed.

In your book you have a chart about how there is an order to cleansing. I have preached that to so many people, and I'm still preaching it every day, because I did it out of order and it really cost us time, money—it can cost you your life if don't get this toxic stuff out fast enough.

Ty: In the right order.

Pam: Yes. So I had done six gallbladder liver cleanses with no results. And I would feel yucky when I did them. After I did the Blessed Herbs colon cleanse, my husband said, "We need to do the gallbladder liver cleanse again." And I said, "No way, I've done six of these." So we do it and I have thousands of stones come out.

So in your book you had listed colon, parasite, kidney, gallbladder, liver, blood. Well, I was feeling like my blood really needed a cleanse from killing parasites for two years so we came here. And for three weeks here, I did nothing for parasites while I was here but my eosinophil number now was showing the parasites in my system—it was 8.7 or something.

And when I left here, just with the cancer-killing things here, my number was 3.0. So it significantly reduced the load of parasites. I had ZYTO testing when I came. I showed him a picture of a parasite and I said, "What is this?" And he did ZYTO testing, turns the screen around, and it was a picture of what I've just shown you. And he said, "That's taenia"-something. And I was like, "Thank you, God, I'm finally getting answers."

And I had 31 types of parasites. And I'm still battling some of the last ones. I'm still battling, but the load is definitely decreasing. My teeth grinding at night is improving, my hair and my nails, and my energy—everything is getting better. And it is interesting, because I'm not really concerned about the cancer and the tumor, my concern is the parasites because I know that's what led to this.

Ty: That's the cause.

Pam: It broke down my immune system.

Ty: So Pam, you've been at Hope4Cancer how many months now? Or at least, originally, when did you come here?

Pam: In October we saw your docuseries, October 31st we got here. I mean, my husband really got on it. We were here for three weeks. The third week of November we went back home and started doing all the daily—I stay busy with my home program every day just like you do here. That's the really nice thing, you're not just waiting on a doctor to do something to you, you are empowered to take back your own health. And we had looked for someone like Dr. Tony for seven years. Seven years we had looked for someone, so it was an answer to prayer, and we are just so grateful.

Ty: That's a great story. And you're doing well?

Pam: Doing well, doing well. Still battling the parasites. I go through seasons where I know certain kinds are causing certain problems. But I have no doubt that I'm going to be running my next 5K in the next, maybe, couple of months. We ran through the airport on the way here and I said, "I can run a 5K, we ran through the Chicago airport."

Ty: Where are you from?

Pam: We're from Missouri. From Columbia, Missouri.

Ty: What kind of substances are you taking for the parasites?

Pam: A variety. Definitely, we battle them with food—God's food—garlic and onions and pomegranates, and carrot juice. There are just so many foods that are potent—oregano, the list goes on and on. So food, especially. Essential oils. Dr. D'Angelo with ParaWellness—his wife is really into essential oils. She says, "It is the lifeblood of the plant." Together they make these concoctions of formulas.

Parasites are like cancer, in my opinion. They figure out what you're doing and then they adapt to it. And so when he first sent me the first formula and I started taking it, they started running from my colon. And I began to have asthma attacks. My husband said, "I've never seen you have an asthma attack."

So the naturopath sent over an essential oil for me to breathe. I was like, "Sure, this isn't going to work." I start breathing in this oil and my asthma quit. I was like, "That's incredible," because as a kid I had to have an inhaler or treatment. So when I got them out of my lungs they went to my head and behind my eyes, and I began having extreme eye pain and headaches. I remember I would sit in the bathtub throwing up, asking Harry, "Call anybody to pray. Call anybody to pray." I went to the eye doctor because the eye pain was tremendous. He said, "Your eyes are beautiful, nothing is wrong with your eyes."

And so, I've just noticed they go wherever in your body—they're opportunistic, and they just go in your body wherever they can try to thrive. So the problem right now is in my triceps in this arm, in my lymph, is the one that I'm overcoming right now. Yes, it's been quite a journey.

Ty: Well, keep up the good work. I'm sure that in the end you will overcome.

Pam: Yes, I am overcoming. It's manna fasting.

Ty: You will eventually be the ultimate overcomer.

Pam: Exactly.

Ty: Pam, thanks for sharing. I want to see some of these pictures here in a second.

Pam: Absolutely.

Ty: Awesome. Thanks for sharing with us.

Pam: Sure. Thank you, Ty. God bless you.

Ty: God bless you, too.

[end of transcript]

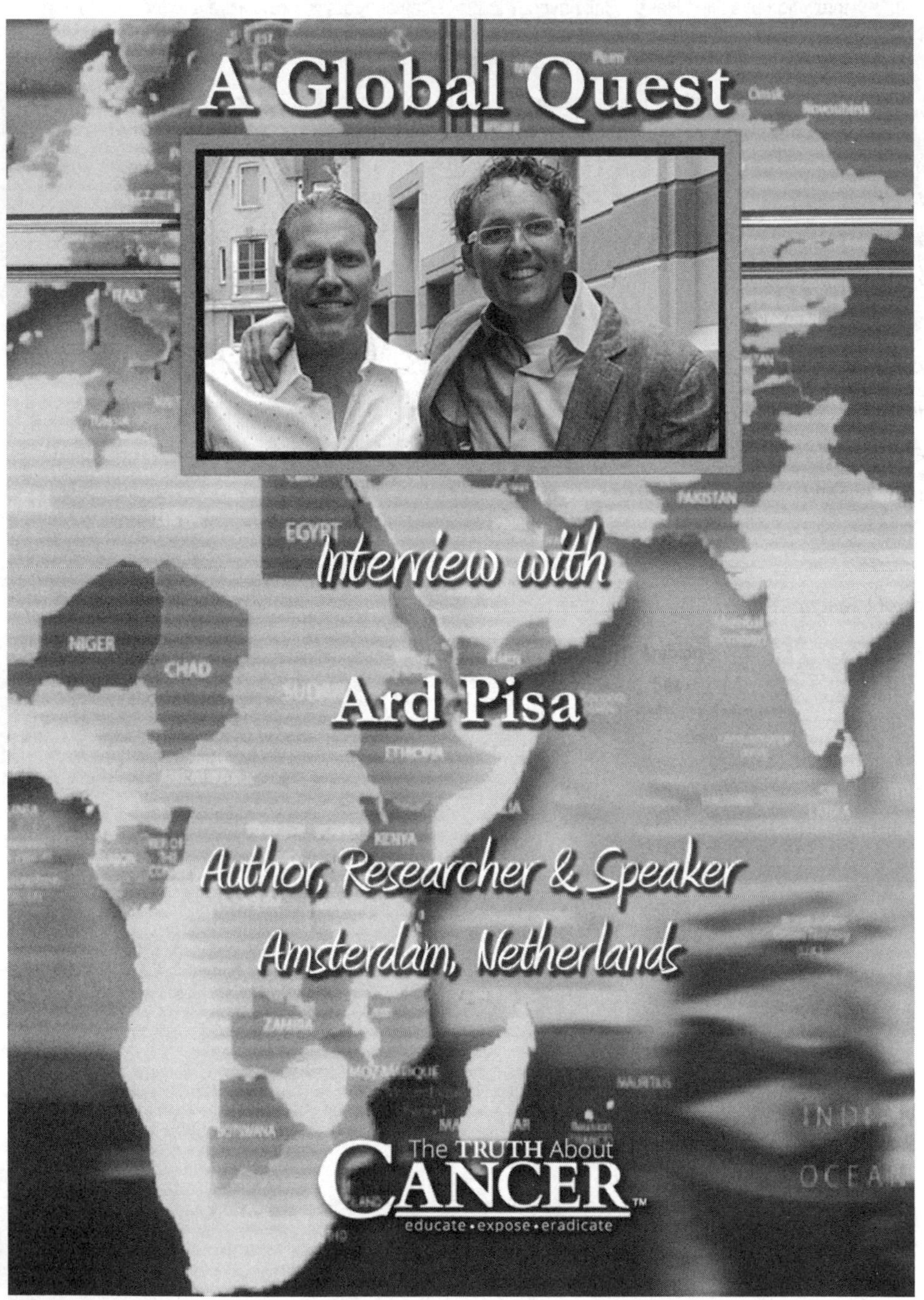
A Global Quest
Interview with
Ard Pisa
Author, Researcher & Speaker
Amsterdam, Netherlands
The TRUTH About
CANCER
educate • expose • eradicate

Ty: I'm really excited to be here in Amsterdam with Ard Pisa.

Ard: Hi Ty.

Ty: Thank you for joining me. It's really good to meet you finally. You're holding in your hand there a book. Can you hold it up to the camera and tell everybody what's the title in Dutch and then tell us what it means in English.

Ard: It is [Dutch title], *What Angelina Didn't Know about Cancer But Should Have Known*; that's the title in English.

Ty: It's a great title. So tell us what should she have known?

Ard: Okay, I will tell you about myself first because I'm a common guy like you. I'm not a doctor, I have no white jacket, I use my common sense. When you take a look in Holland about health care, there is no health care in Holland. We have only sick care because we have 5.3 million people, patients who have chronic disease. And if you look at cancer we have 650,000 people with cancer. And every year we have 100,000 new patients. Unbelievable!

So I ask myself a lot of questions. What's cancer? Is there a way for prevention? And if I have cancer what can I do? Are there also natural treatments? If we have to solve our health problems we have to understand nature. And that's my mission to tell people what is nature, how does this body work, what is cancer and what can we do for prevention. And if we get sick what can we do in a natural way. I tell people about this. That's my job; that's our mission.

Ty: We have the same mission.

Ard: Yes, I know. You have four children and we have four children. You have written a book, I have written a book. You have lovely wife and I have also a lovely wife.

Ty: We have a lot in common.

Ard: Yes.

Ty: So you just asked a question, what is cancer? What is cancer?

Ard: Cancer is an immune disease, a disease from the immune system.

Ty: Immune System.

Ard: It's an immune system disease, nothing else. If you look at the way nature works we need four things to live and everybody knows. We need sunlight. We need nutrition – minerals, vitamins, proteins, fatty acids. We need water, two liters of water every day for the transportation of minerals and vitamins. And we need oxygen. I read a book five years ago about Dr. Otto Heinrich Warburg. You know Otto Warburg? He discovered the main cause of cancer in 1926. The main cause of cancer is short of oxygen in our cells, a lack of oxygen in our cells.

And because our metabolism needs 100 percent oxygen and if our cells did not get enough oxygen you went to Plan B. And in Plan B we use sugar to make energy. That is cancer because there is a lack of oxygen. And then a tumor grows, an excessive tumor and that is cancer. But nobody knows this story, but it was discovered in 1926 by Dr. Warburg. He got in 1931 the Noble Price for this great discovery and historic discovery. But who knows?

Ty: Let me ask you a question then, Ard. Is cancer a result of a lack of chemotherapy in someone's body?

Ard: We don't need chemo. There are natural treatments. Chemo breaks down our immune system. That's what chemo does because we have to stop several things if we have cancer. We have to build up our system and not to break it down. And chemo breaks it down.

Ty: So with cancer being a disease of the immune system that's broken down, why do you think we have this explosion of cancer over these last several decades? Why so much cancer?

Ard: Why so much cancer? There's only one answer. It is related to our lifestyle. It's a lifestyle problem. All the chronic diseases are related to lifestyle. Alzheimer's, cardiovascular diseases, diabetes. It's all related to our immune system and our lifestyle. Look at this world and we can get in every corner, also in Amsterdam here, unhealthy food. If you want healthy food you have to search for it.

Ty: What does healthy food look like?

Ard: It's organic food, not from an industry. You go to a farmer and you get his food without pesticides. That's organic food and that is nutrition. We have to feed our system not only with nutrition but also with emotional well-being. There's a lot of stress. Look at Amsterdam. What a speed in Amsterdam, it's fast 24/7 and so much stress. And look at the people you see their mouth frowning and not happy. They are surviving instead of living. We have to live and we have to be emotionally in balance. We need nutrition, we need exercise and we need a healthy environment. That's what we need. And that's when we can reactivate our immune system and that's what we have to do.

Ty: You mentioned stress. Does stress play a big part in cancer?

Ard: I think the most important factor is stress because we are energetic. People are not only with a skin and material but inside we have energy, we are more energetic persons than material persons. So our emotions have a lot of influence on our health and our sickness. We have too much stress. Yes, we have to deal with it but that's not only stress, we have also a lot of anger. We have a lot of sadness, frustration, and as well sexual frustration, which is a big issue. We see that every time at home where Helen treats her patients on a holistic energetic way, a lot of sexual frustrations and traumatic issues. So stress is most important. You know Dr. Howard, also the German? He talks always about our emotions and problems related to cancer.

Ty: So you've not only got to get oxygen to the cells, you not only have got to feed your body with nutrition, you've got to get rid of the stress as well.

Ard: Yes, also, because a stressful body needs more oxygen. And if we do not [have] a lot of exercise it's not good for our immune system. We should have a lot of oxygen and we have to transport it into our cells. I tell the story of Dr. Warburg in my book. Oxygen needs a transportation, blood or water. But we need a third transport and that is fatty acids. Fatty acid transports from the vessels inside the cells because there are inner spaces in our body that we have to transport the oxygen from the vessels. What the vessels stops not in the cells. They are stopped in the inner spaces.

Ty: So fatty acids are important to transport the oxygen. So it doesn't make sense when we have these low-fat diets, does it? That's not a healthy diet, is it?

Ard: No. We need these fatty acids.

Ty: Where do you get the good fatty acids? What foods would provide you with good fatty acids?

Ard: What we need is marine phytoplankton, the whole food of this world. Do you know marine phytoplankton is the whole food of this world and is full of fatty acids? And not only fatty acids but also minerals, vitamins, and proteins. So it is called the whole food. The super food. We need marine phytoplankton.

Ty: And so it contains all the fatty acids that you need?

Ard: Yes. Like we eat fish, but fish eats phytoplankton, so that makes sense. That's nutrition. So we have to learn about nature that most people do not understand this or haven't learned this.

Ty: What do you think it is that most people or even most doctors don't understand about nature?

Ard: Because it's not in their education. They learn about medicine but they don't learn about nutrition and what is good nutrition. A lot of doctors do not know this even here in Holland. Even here in Holland most doctors haven't learned about good nutrition, minerals, and vitamins.

Ty: Why is that? Why do you think that doctors are generally not taught about nutrition as they are preparing to become a doctor?

Ard: That's a good question. I don't know. It's not in the program.

Ty: It seems like it should be, doesn't it?

Ard: Yes, it should be in the program. But it's not, at a stretch, and that is very strange. So we have to do our mission.

Ty: To get the word out to everyone.

Ard: Yes.

Ty: You think it might be the reason it's not in the program the fact that there's a big influence of the pharmaceutical companies on the medical schools?

Ard: Yes, there's a big influence. It is by law arranged in Holland that a doctor must give chemo, radiation and surgery, but no natural treatments; it's not allowed in Holland.

Ty: Oh, natural treatments are not allowed?

Ard: No. You are going tomorrow to Cologne to Professor Dr. Gorter at the Medical Center Cologne. You can't open the doors of a Medical Center in Holland like that. It isn't allowed in Holland.

Ty: Well, I guess at least people in Holland have access to go to the clinic in Germany, it's close.

Ard: Yeah, it's close. But you have to pay for it yourself. And that's a big problem.

Ty: Insurance doesn't cover it?

Ard: Exactly. Here in Holland they pay insurance for chemo – 50,000 Euros. But for 30,000 Euros for a natural treatment in Germany and they won't pay it. It's crazy. It's the world upside down. So we have to do our work. Let's continue our work.

Ty: Yeah, I agree. You know, an interesting thing we were talking to a fellow yesterday in Latvia, before we left Latvia. He said in Latvia the oncologists are now being called Chemotherapists because that's all they use which is chemotherapy, but it doesn't work. So what would your advice be, after all the research that you've done and written this book on cancer, *What Angelina Should Have Known*, what would your advice be to someone that's been recently diagnosed with cancer? What should they do?

Ard: Stop doing things. You have to change your lifestyle. Begin to throw away all your food you have in your home and buy natural, efficient, organic foods. The first one is drink two liters of water. Eat marine phytoplankton. Exercise a little bit. Reduce your stress; that's the first things you can do.

And no sugar, sugar is fuel for cancer. Everyone should know this but it's never told in our hospitals. There's no doctor who tells you, "stop with sugar." Okay, we need the essential sugars from the vegetables and the fruits, but no sugars from industry.

Ty: No processed sugars?

Ard: No processed sugars.

Ty: So what if you're diagnosed and your doctor says you are advanced and you need to hurry and begin chemotherapy treatment and the doctor also tells you, "don't worry about what you eat it has nothing to do with your illness?" What kind of advice is that?

Ard: Do your own research. Everyone who is sick, do your own research. Look at your videos, take a book, and do your own research. Call someone who has experienced this before. I speak to so many patients who did it another way and live today. And the doctors they say, "it's impossible." But they did it and I have talks with these people.

Ty: You know they say, "you shouldn't be alive, but you are." So our last question, you wrote a book called *What Angelina Should Have Known and Didn't Know*. So what should she have known?

Ard: I feel very sorry for her because she has removed healthy breasts. Can you imagine Ty if you removed your manhood, your healthy manhood because of fear. It's crazy. But she thought that it's the only way for prevention. But there's another way for prevention because she should have known that our genes do not control life. You can activate genes and deactivate. And if we deactivate our genes with our healthy lifestyle we do not get cancer. That's what she should have known.

Ty: So that's what you're talking about, it's the science of epigenetics.

Ard: Yes, that's what I'm talking about in my book. And it's in simple language in my book for the common people. Everyone has the human right and this is not some tour against cancer, but it is about the human rights to know what is cancer, what is the best prevention and what can I do in a natural way to treat my cancer? That's what we are doing and that's our mission – human rights.

Ty: And as Ard just said, if you've been diagnosed with cancer and if you're watching this series right now, we want you to know what Angelina didn't know. And that's the fact that let's say the doctor just told you that your genetic predisposition is that you're going to get cancer. It does not have to be so.

As Ard just described there's a science called epigenetics and these lifestyle choices that we make can affect the expression of our genes. So don't listen to them if they say, "you've got bad genes, you've got bad luck, you're going to die of cancer." Don't listen to a doctor who says that, right, because there's always hope. That's our mission to get there, right?

Ard: There's always hope. Yes, there's always hope. Our mission is that there is hope always and we can change that today.

Ty: Keep up the good work.

Ard: Okay, keep on the good work.

Ty: Alright my friend.

[end of transcript]

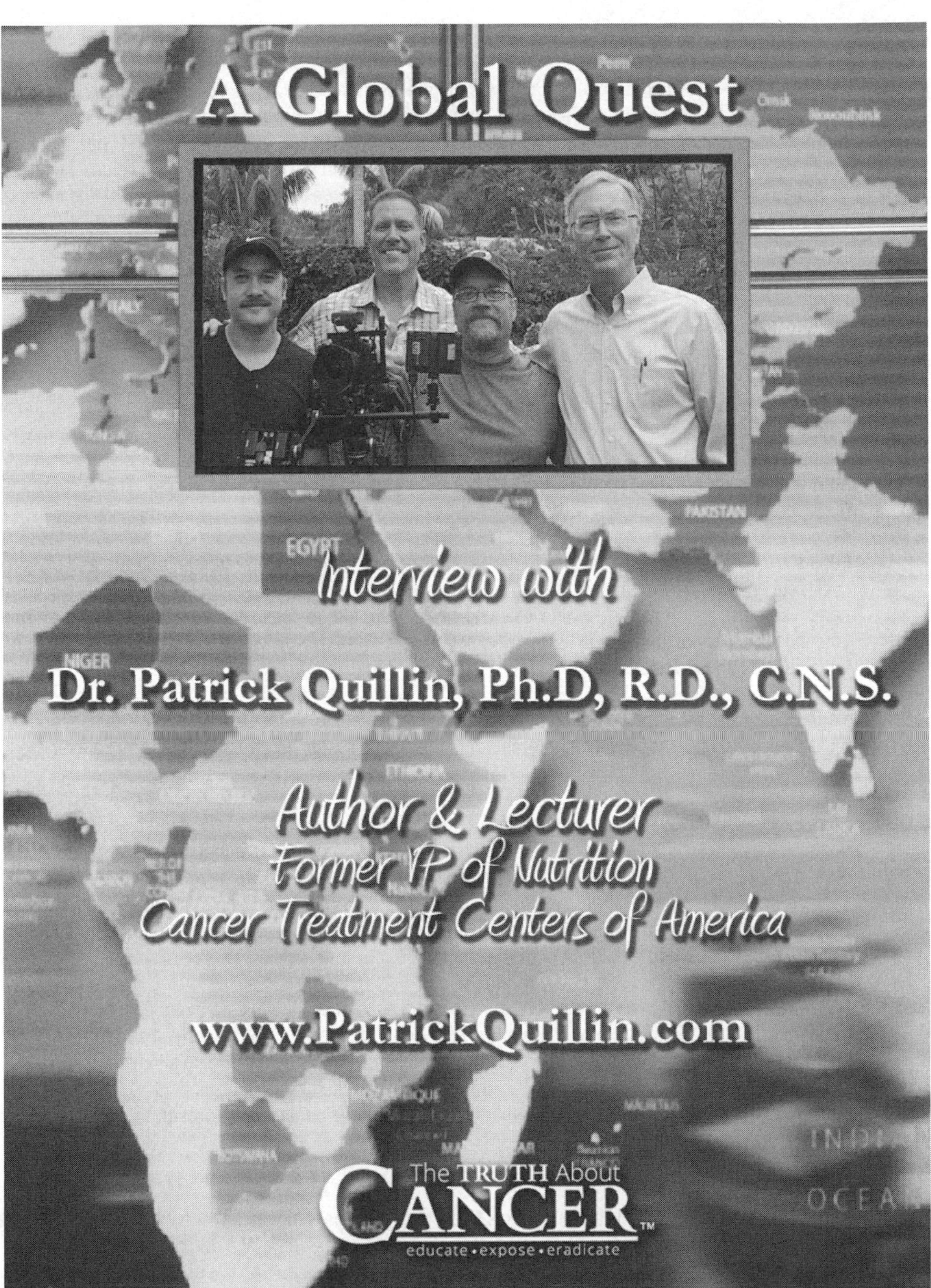
A Global Quest
Interview with
Dr. Patrick Quillin, Ph.D, R.D., C.N.S.
Author & Lecturer
Former VP of Nutrition
Cancer Treatment Centers of America
www.PatrickQuillin.com
The TRUTH About CANCER
educate • expose • eradicate

Ty: So really excited to be back here in Carlsbad, California, with Dr. Patrick Quillin.

Dr. Quillin: Ty, thanks for coming back.

Ty: You bet. Yeah, so you know last year you were in the *Quest for the Cures*. You were literally one of the favorites, if not the favorite. People loved your explanations, your really down-to-earth explanations of nutrition, the different phytonutrients, as we went through the yard for a few minutes last year. But I said, "You know what will be better this year? We're going to do the whole interview outside." I want you to go plant the plant here in your yard, and describe what we might do, what we might find in these berries, these fruits, that would fight cancer.

Dr. Quillin: Perfect. Welcome to my pharmacy. This is where we start talking about—people think that modern medicine has to be controlling, invasive, disabling, expensive and dangerous, and that's what most modern medicine is. In fact, real medicine is phytonutrients that nourish the body. They're antioxidants. They regulate abnormal growths. They stimulate apoptosis, or program cell death.

We're going to start with one of my 60 fruit trees, black raspberries. What we have here, Ty, is arguably one of the most impressive medicines that you can find, anthocyanins, antioxidants, ORACs, so oxygen radical absorbable capacity off the charts. Add in ellagic acid, which stimulates cancer cells to commit suicide. What you have is, this feeds the brain, the lens of the eye, it prevents cancer. This is real medicine. We move on.

Let's show ourselves around a mulberry tree right over here. The mulberry tree is near the end of its cycle, but once again we have—let's see if we can find any fruits doing very well. The mulberry fruit, again, is high in pigments. And what we're looking for is go for the color. And so in those dark pigments, you find accessory pigments that help in photosynthesis. Here, I know we've got some green figs here. Let's go back and look at fisetin.

Ty: Yeah, you know, last year we did—we were here a little bit earlier in the season and we did get some mulberries. And I remember tasting them, one of them, and it was the sweetest mulberry I'd ever tasted.

Dr. Quillin: Oh, they're just delightful. You can see these figs, and we'll see if we can find something that's ripe, because it's the early part of the harvest. There we go. Ty, you get to taste that. So, longue verde means green, but inside, they're purple. If you'd show the camera what we have inside there. And so, fisetin is one of the more important phytochemicals in figs, and again, proven to stimulate apoptosis, or program cell death in cancer cells. Delicious. And if you think of all the ingredients, one of the things you're looking for here is prebiotics.

Plant food, fruits, vegetables, grains, legumes, contain substances that we cannot digest, but our hundred trillion cells in the gut are using it for food. And if we feed our gut properly, it's called the microbiota, what we end up is we're making vitamin biotin, vitamin K. We're also stimulating the immune system. What they find now is two-thirds of the immune system surrounds the gut, and by things we cannot digest—that prebiotics—are going to improve our immune system.

Ty: Incredible.

Dr. Quillin: This is dark, this is Black Mission figs. This one's not quite ripe, but you can see we're going to have a great harvest here. And you know, people will think, "Yeah you're some rich doctor in California. I can't afford that." Sixty-two percent of Americans own their own home. You don't need much land. About 20 years ago, Sierra Club put out a book called *Edible Landscaping*, in which they talked about, if you're going to spend time on it, if you're going to water it, make it something you'd eat.

And two-thirds of Americans could do the same thing. And if you don't have land, there's a lot of cities where they're taking land that's unused, downtown Detroit and other places, and they say, "This is a community garden." Put some fruit trees in. It might be a couple of years before you get a harvest, but a garden, you're going to get it in a couple of months.

Ty: Grow gardens, not grass. Right?

Dr. Quillin: Exactly. And I live in a desert, you know. Southern California's a desert. We're in the worst drought in history. Why would you water something unless you can eat it? And here's an interesting point. We are good to Mother Earth, and it nourishes us. And so there's this symbiotic relationship. I feed the soil, and then the plant feeds me. And the same thing for you folks.

Ty: I mean, you know, by the way, Patrick, that fig that I just ate. That's the sweetest fig I've ever tasted.

Dr. Quillin: Isn't it delicious?

Ty: That's incredible.

Dr. Quillin: I'll tell you what. One of the things that I do, I add Epsom salts to the soil. Epsom salt is magnesium sulfate. If you look at green plants, what you have here is green chlorophyll, and chlorophyll takes the energy of the sun combined with water and carbon dioxide, to make sugar.

And then from that it makes proteins, and all these exotic phytochemicals that protect us from disease. Well, the beauty of this whole business of that the middle of that chlorophyll molecule is magnesium. If the plant doesn't get enough magnesium, it doesn't make enough chlorophyll. It doesn't get enough chlorophyll, it won't make enough sugar, it's not going to get sweet enough, and all the other chemicals that it makes. So, I put like a handful of Epsom salts in a gallon of water, and dissolve it at the base of the tree about three times a year. Delicious fruit.

Ty: That's a great tip for people that are growing their own food.

Dr. Quillin: Do you see any bugs or anything on that?

Ty: No.

Dr. Quillin: This is all biodynamic, organic, and I'm not fighting any bugs. Essentially, the plant has its own immune system. Just like you and I do, just like you people do. If you're nourishing yourself, you have a good immune system, vaccinations it's a whole other subject. Move on here.

Ty: Okay. So basically, if you nourish the plant, you won't have the issue with the bugs.

Dr. Quillin: That's right. These are Surinam cherries. And fascinating. Surinam cherries, I get three harvests a year out of this.

Ty: And by the way, you guys are missing out. You have to be behind the camera. I'm getting to eat these. This is incredible.

Dr. Quillin: The hard part is to eat and talk at the same time. I find I salivate so much that I can't talk well, which is...

Ty: I'll let you do most of the talking, I'll do most of the eating.

Dr. Quillin: Perfect.

Ty: We'll be happy here.

Dr. Quillin: Think about this. What you have is these beautiful, dark cherries, and they're sweet, aren't they?

Ty: Delicious.

Dr. Quillin: And what nature is saying is, "Alright. What I've got is some sugar here, and the fungus living around us in the trillions wants to eat this." And so the plant has to create its own protection. It creates a substance called phytoalexins, and that is, one of those is resveratrol.

People have heard about it in red grapes. Grapes are another thing. So the sweet thing in the grape has to protect itself. So if a fungus lands on this, and it eats that phytoalexin, it dies. It's sort of its own, it's a pre-drug, essentially. The drug companies can't duplicate this stuff.

And that's the beauty of what we've got here, is that you cannot patent a natural substance. And that's why the 280 billion dollar a year drug industry can't come up with something as effective as this. Phytoalexins, in red and green fruits and vegetables, have been shown to be anti-cancer the same way that they protect the plant against fungus.

Moving on here, we've got another. This is another Surinam cherry of a different color.

This is mangoes. These are green and small right now, but they're going to get to be the size of a baseball or bigger. And what you have is, there's at least 8,000 different carotenoids, at least 20,000 different bioflavonoids, in fruits and vegetables.

And they find that these things are extraordinary as anti-aging, antioxidant, anti-inflammatory. There's what? Twelve million Americans who are on the Vioxx, Celebrex drugs. They have chronic inflammation, chronic pain. Eat more fruits and vegetables.

As a matter of fact, there's a group, if you look them up, NORI, on the web. Nutrition Oncology Research Institute. They recommend nothing but fruit to cure cancer, a whole-fruit diet. Now I'm not sure that I go on that enthusiastic, but I am clearly on board with them when you talk about the biochemical, scientific reasons why fruit and vegetables are going to slow down cancer.

These are Golden Dorsett apples. Apples, if you look at it and do a little analysis of it, you find not much vitamin C and yet, the ORAC score is higher than vitamin C, because it's a combination of all of these substances that are in the apple.

Moving on over here. Here we go. Mulberries. These are Oscar mulberries.

Ty: Now this one wasn't ripe last year.

Dr. Quillin: You're right. You came at a different time of the year. So dark purple is going to have this rich mixture of phytochemicals, bioflavonoids, carotenoids. The medicinal value is beyond argument.

Ty: Oh my goodness. That's ridiculously sweet.

Dr. Quillin: Delicious. And this is why I'm saying, we're not denying ourselves, people. People think, "If I can't have my Twinkies and Coke every day." No, this stuff is delicious, and once you develop an appetite for it, what's fascinating is, the human tongue has got four sensors - sour, sweet, salt and bitter.

That sweet is for fruit. The earliest food of humans was fruit, eggs and insects. I'm not telling you you have to eat insects, but eggs and fruit are good, and the sweetness is to make fruit taste good and feel good in our body.

And then what the food manufacturers have done is said, "We're going to create all of these substitute sugars," which are not good for you, and now we're eating 140 pounds per year of refined white sugar, which is killing us. Obesity, diabetes, depression, heart disease, cancer, among other diseases that come with refined sugar.

This is a different sugar. What you find is, if you take the fructose and other natural sugars that are in the matrix. Matrix means mother in Latin. And literally, here's this sugar sitting in the middle of this cell membrane, and it's got all these phytochemicals around it, and fiber, and it works.

And if you take a different sugar, and take all the matrix away, which is white sugar, corn syrup, now it's killing people instead of healing people.

Ty: I'm glad you picked that, because I was about to pick another one. Ridiculously sweet.

Dr. Quillin: Moving on here. Apricots. We're at the end of the apricot season, but we've got, hopefully—I've got a few silent partners that work with me, the birds. And what I sort of give them, I tithe to them.

I give them 10 percent. They eat the insects. And everybody's happy. So this is the tail-end of my apricot season, and apparently we're not going to be able to eat any of those. I did a great harvest the other day. Blood orange, here we go, Ty. Blood orange.

What we have is—you want to use your strong Texas hands just to rip the thing open. Basically, oranges are good for you. Citrus has got everything from bioflavonoids, rutin, hesperidin, vitamin C, fiber, all those things that I mentioned.

But blood orange goes a step further, and it develops these red pigments that we were talking about, not unlike the mulberry and the deep inside of the fig. And so this is going to look a little bit like a beet inside.

Ty: Yeah, it's darker.

Dr. Quillin: And so, the ORAC score, once again, Oxygen Radical Absorbent Capacity, is just phenomenal.

Ty: Pop this thing open here.

Dr. Quillin: There you go.

Ty: So you can see.

Dr. Quillin: Pop it open.

Ty: Don't want to get it too close to this white shirt, because it is dark as you can see. I've never seen orange juice that red. Look at that.

Dr. Quillin: So, blood orange is another one of these things, if you grow, if you live in a reasonably warm climate, you can eat this thing, and it's...

Ty: It's really sweet.

Dr. Quillin: ...off the charts for all the phytochemicals that are going to protect you against heart disease, cancer, aging, inflammations. It's phenomenal. We've got avocados up here.

Ty: You know, Patrick, it almost looks like in the interior of this blood orange, it looks like the little seeds that you have inside pomegranates. See that?

Dr. Quillin: That's true, you're right. Good point. And I've got a pomegranate tree over here we're going to go to. This is avocados. These are small ones, they're only the size of a marble. They're going to get to be the size of a baseball. But avocados have become the darling of the health food industry, because they have fat, but it's a healthy fat.

It's a mono-unsaturated fat, not unlike olive oil. Very high in natural vitamin Es. And it's interesting, there's been a couple of scientific studies that said that vitamin E was unhealthy. One meta-analysis said that vitamin E shortened lifespan. Another one said it caused prostate cancer.

Two bizarre studies, when in fact, what they're doing is, there's four different vitamin Es: alpha, beta, lambda, delta, and there's four different tocopherols, tocotrienols and tocopherols. They're in natural foods, such as wheat germ and avocado.

They're not in these vitamins, and what they usually do, is they take a mirror image of the natural molecule. It doesn't fit anywhere, it actually is probably counter-productive. So some of the supplements, unless they're naturally-based, are counter-productive.

Ty: So they didn't do the study on the real thing?

Dr. Quillin: Well, if you think about the difference between a man and a woman, is literally one hydroxyl group. If you take a molecule of cholesterol and amplify it, and turn it into androgen or testosterone, there's one hydroxyl group on this giant molecule that's different, and that becomes estrogen, and now you've got a man or a woman. Is it Vin Diesel, or Miss September?

And there's tiny changes in a molecule that make a huge difference in its chemical structure and its activity in the body. Vitamin E, androgen, testosterone, same with these molecules in the foods. Mother Nature knows how to make it. Francis Bacon was the founder of the modern scientific principle. In 1600 he said, "Nature, to be commanded, must be obeyed."

And what we're doing in modern medicine is saying, "We don't care about the rules. We're going to change the rules. We know that you need vitamin D in sunshine, but we're going to say we can't patent that, so we're going to try and come up with a drug that bypasses all of those pathways." Nature, to be commanded, must be obeyed.

Ty: I love that quote.

Dr. Quillin: Moving up here.

Ty: I'm going to tithe to the birds.

Dr. Quillin: Pixie tangerines. These things are unbelievable. More citrus, and more food, that tastes absolutely delicious, if you want to peel that rascal.

Ty: I love these, the kids would love these.

Dr. Quillin: Yeah. And there are no seeds in these. And so, we're looking at more blood orange, and basically, I wanted a third of an acre. This is not a mansion. I'm very blessed to have this, but essentially, you can take a tiny yard, put in a few fruit trees. With literally about a 30 by 30 foot plot, you can feed you and your family with vegetables. If you don't have a yard, your community probably has some land that they're willing to have serve as a communal farm, a group property.

Ty: Let's see. You know what I'm going to do?

Dr. Quillin: Pixie tangerine.

Ty: I'm going to taste it, but then, these guys are working hard. You're all going to get a taste too. I see Zack there with his hand out. Allan there's yours. Travis, you got it. Incredible. Is that good? They can't see you but tell us, is it good?

Speaker: Yeah, it's great.

Ty: Okay. Incredible.

Dr. Quillin: Now Zack just had his Cheetos in the car as he was coming out here. So he's got your standard young guy's taste buds. No, I'm just kidding Zack. But the fact is, you're not giving anything up with these foods.

Ty: No, it's incredible. This tangerine here, the mulberry that I ate earlier, the Greek mulberry, is that what it is?

Dr. Quillin: That was Oscar mulberry.

Ty: Okay, the Oscar mulberry. I don't know where I got Greek. But it's, that is sweeter than any sweet you will buy in the store.

Dr. Quillin: What it gives you is a sweet and sour taste too.

Ty: Yeah, it's really hearty.

Dr. Quillin: There's something unusual about it that just says it's delicious. Moving our way on down here to grapefruit.

Ty: Pretty incredible.

Dr. Quillin: This is a grapefruit tree, and we may not have any fruit on this one. We have some up front. Here we go. Here's some of the tiny stuff right here, size of a marble, it's going to be of course a grapefruit the size of a softball before it's through. I find grapefruit a fascinating subject, Ty, because every pharmacist, every medical doctor, tells all their patients, "Don't touch grapefruit."

And what happens is, grapefruit accelerates a detoxification enzyme in the liver, which changes the pharmaco-kinetics of drugs. So if you take a drug, it will have different activity if you're on grapefruit than If you're not. And so they tell you, "Don't eat grapefruit if you're on drugs." And I agree. I'm not against that. I've got another idea. Get healthy and start eating the grapefruit. Because it improves the function of your liver in detoxification pathways. So you know, while everybody says, "Don't eat grapefruit," get healthy, and then start eating grapefruit.

Ty: Get healthy so you can get off the drugs.

Dr. Quillin: Exactly.

Ty: And then eat the grapefruit.

Dr. Quillin: Exactly.

Ty: Makes sense.

Dr. Quillin: We've got orange, Valencia orange here. This was an incredible tree that I, you know, when I went to the fruit nursery, I picked out a lot of fruit. I had no idea what it was. This is a pink guava.

Ty: Guava.

Dr. Quillin: So this is it right now. It's small, it's going to be about the size of a baseball. It's going to be about, it's going to turn a light yellow, and inside, it's just got this delicious fruit. This thing produced, maybe, if you look at this tree, it's not that big, maybe 10 feet tall, it produced at least 40 pounds of fruit last year. And you can see that I don't have some huge area here. It's just right up against a fence.

Ty: You've just chosen to grow fruit trees instead of bushes.

Dr. Quillin: Exactly. So ornamentals, fine, if that's what you want. If you want to play baseball and football on the lawn, that's fine, have fun. But I thought, if you live in a desert, and you're going to water it, you've got to be able to eat it, and it should nourish you. So nourish the soil.

You mentioned pomegranates.I've got them right over here. These are small fruits, and they're going to ripen into a nice red thing eventually.

Ty: Yeah, kids love pomegranates.

Dr. Quillin: Wood pile. Valencia oranges. And we could go on and on. Basically in a third of an acre, I put in 60 fruit trees, and it's a year-round harvest. And so you folks who live up north, there are some things you can grow that I can't grow. Cherries and apples, and many different types of fruit need a good hard frost before they can lay down fruit.

And admittedly, this is a delayed gratification thing. You know, what you're looking at in health care right now, Ty, is that we know what to eat, but there are some people who ignore it, and they say, "I like the taste of this sack of potato chips," and sitting in front of the TV and having a six-pack of beer.

And they know the repercussions from it. And so medicine is more than willing to sit by and say, "We'll provide medication to palliate the symptoms you're going to get from that unhealthy lifestyle." There's what they call delayed gratification and immediate gratification.

Delayed gratification says, "You know I know eating a quart of ice cream might taste good right now, but I'm probably not going to feel good tomorrow. And eventually I might look pretty obese." And so plant some fruit trees. It will take a couple years before you're getting a harvest. Put in some garden.

I've got some vegetable garden over here. It will take a couple of months before you get a harvest. But the same thing with your health, if you're willing to delay your gratification: exercise, eat right, maybe you can put off going to the doctors and the hospital.

We could go out front, Ty, but I think we've given the essence of it, is modern medicine has this confused notion that the human body is a fragile, frail vehicle that is prone to breakdown, when in fact, we are built wondrously. This is a moving miracle.

They tell us the human body has maybe 20 trillion cells, maybe 100 trillion cells in the gut, 60,000 miles of blood vessels. And here is the sound bite I hope our viewers can take home: A healthy human body is self-regulating and self-repairing. It will protect itself from infections.

It will slow down the aging process. If it finds any cancer, it will eliminate them. It will keep the blood vessels open. Why don't you and I have a headache right now? Some people have a headache, why don't you and I? Because the body is self-regulating and self-repairing. It takes in these various minerals. It regulates blood pressure. And this miraculous process occurs because we feed the body properly. And much of that comes from fruits and vegetables.

Ty: And I feel even better than I did when I got here, because of all the fruits I've just eaten.

Dr. Quillin: Well, you're looking good.

Ty: Fantastic. Well, thank you. One thing I don't see here in the yard is hemp. But in California, it is legal to grow.

Dr. Quillin: That's true.

Ty: Under certain parameters.

Dr. Quillin: That's true.

Ty: Talk real quickly, if you will, about the medicinal effects of the hemp plant, or cannabis.

Dr. Quillin: Hemp, cannabis, is arguably the most useful plant on earth. If you do a history of it, you look at canvas, which is what our ancestors used for Conestoga wagons and for the clothing. Canvas comes from the word cannabis, because cannabis was the material that they used to make all of their clothing and canvas.

It lasts longer than cotton or polyester. If you go back and look at your history, it was around 1937 when DuPont got its patent for polyester, and that was the beginning of the witch hunt to get rid of cannabis. Because it was competition. You look at, you can use it for paper pulp, for clothing.

You can eat it, the food, the seeds are high in omega-3 fats, high in protein. The oils, from hemp oil, is delicious, nutty tasting, and high in omega-3s. And then there's the medicinal parts, the cannabinoids. And the THC, tetrahydracannabinoid, and CBD, are two different fractions.

The government has had this illogical approach to cannabis, because you think. It's a category-1 drug, meaning they think it's more dangerous than cocaine, schedule-1. Schedule-1 means that it's addictive, dangerous, and has no therapeutic value, which is ridiculous. I mean, there are many studies that have been done. One of them, for instance, the DEA, Department of...

Ty: Drug Enforcement Agency.

Dr. Quillin: Drug Enforcement Agency, decided they want to prove how unhealthy marijuana was. And so they went to a major researcher at UCLA, University of California at Los Angeles, and said, "We want you to prove that smoking marijuana causes lung cancer." He said, "Shouldn't be a problem." They did a huge study, prospective, randomized trial, and he said, "Not only it doesn't cause it, it actually helps to prevent it."

THC has an anti-cancer property. I'm not telling people you should smoke marijuana. I'm telling you that we need to have a rational discussion on marijuana, hemp, cannabis, because there's an abundance of data now that says that it's non-toxic and has therapeutic benefits.

The CBD, cannabinoids, apparently there are cannabinoid receptors in the human body, and it's almost as if nature designed, "Here's lock and key. And this fits in, and it improves." It's an adaptogen, not unlike ginseng, or garlic, or substances that just make everything work a little bit better.

We need to have an adult discussion on it. If you compare it to tobacco and alcohol, the risk to benefit, the cost ratio of cannabis is in favor of legalizing it, regulating it, and taxing it.

Ty: One thing. And thank you for sharing all that about hemp, cannabis, because that's kind of a little bit of our hidden history. People don't realize that. They think, they hear the word marijuana, which is actually a slang for the hemp, or the cannabis, plant, and they think, "Oh. You must be a pothead."

Dr. Quillin: No.

Ty: Right? They don't realize the thousands of medicinal and therapeutic uses for this plant. And so I think that's really important for people that are watching to know that this is a medicinal plant. And so, thank you for sharing in those details.

Dr. Quillin: It's an industrial plant. I mean, instead of—one of the beauties of hemp is you don't have to, there's no insect that will eat the plant, and so you don't have to spray it. And so, instead of cutting down trees to make paper, we could grow hemp and use that to make paper. You can use it to make materials, canvas, clothing, it's an industrial material. It's a nutritive material, and it's a medicinal substance.

Ty: And you mentioned the DEA study at UCLA. The first study that I'm aware of was back in the early 70s. Also at the behest of the DEA and the National Institute of Health. And they found that it cured other types of cancers as well, mitigated other types of cancers. So it's really fascinating that we have this plant that people think if you smoke it you're going to get cancer, but really it protects against cancer.

Dr. Quillin: It's not a gateway to more drugs, it's a gateway to health. And I'm not, you know, I'm not smoking it, I'm not using it. I think it should be legalized and available, and taxed and regulated, so that we have standardized concentrations of it.

If you compare it to the 280 billion dollar a year drug industry, and according to an article in the *Journal of the American Medical Association*, at least 100,000 Americans die each year from the on label use of prescription drugs. Find me the deaths from cannabis.

Ty: They're not there.

Dr. Quillin: They aren't there. No.

Ty: And when you look at, on the flipside of the coin, people that have been healed from cannabis. We were just over in the UK and London. We interviewed a man that was diagnosed with terminal cancer, and he used cannabis. Unfortunately, there it had to be illegally black market, because that's illegal in London as well. And he...

Dr. Quillin: I thought they changed it from Schedule-1 to Schedule-3?

Ty: It's still—I don't think it's as big of a prison sentence.

Dr. Quillin: Probation type thing?

Ty: If you get caught. It's lower. It's like a misdemeanor. But it's still against the law.

Dr. Quillin: Well on that subject, Ty, if you think about it. America has more incarcerated people than any other county on Earth. We've got 315 million people, and 2.2 million in prison. And half of those people are in prison for non-violent drug offenders, and 17,000 are in there for marijuana use. That's ridiculous.

Ty: It is.

Dr. Quillin: We pay $55,000 a year to keep somebody in jail for this? That makes no sense.

Ty: For growing or smoking a plant.

Dr. Quillin: So, I'm hoping that rational thought comes to modern medicine, that the government officials employ rational thought as part of regulations, and that Americans get healthier. And the best ideas, you don't have to go to the doctor or hospital if you take care of yourself. And that's what this "Welcome to my pharmacy" is all about.

Ty: I love it, Patrick. Well thank you for sharing with us today. This is fascinating. I mean, I know that this, I'm going to get a flood of emails after this airs saying, "We want more of Patrick Quillin."

Dr. Quillin: It's a pleasure. Thanks for being here.

Ty: Thank you.

Dr. Quillin: Thank you, Ty.

[end of transcript]

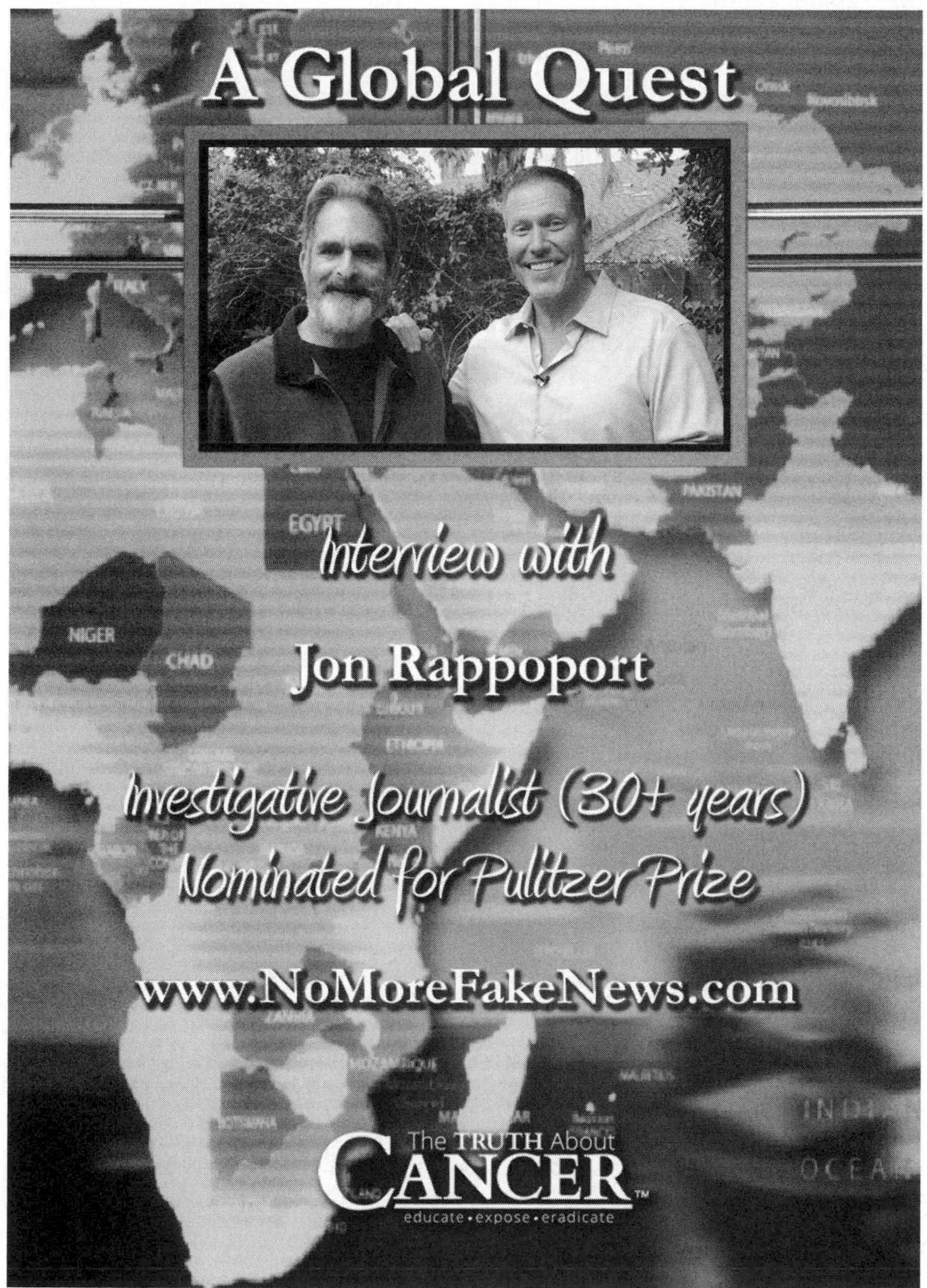
A Global Quest
Interview with
Jon Rappoport
Investigative Journalist (30+ years)
Nominated for Pulitzer Prize
www.NoMoreFakeNews.com
The TRUTH About
CANCER
educate • expose • eradicate

Ty: So we're pumped to be here in Southern California just north of San Diego with Jon Rappaport.

Jon: Glad to be here.

Ty: Thank you for inviting us here to your house.

Jon: Thank you for coming.

Ty: We really want to get your take today on several issues relating to health. The main one being vaccines. I know that you and Robert Scott Bell have put together a—there's like a DVD or CD series called *Armed and Dangerous*.

Jon: Yeah, that was lots of hours about vaccines.

Ty: Lots of research on vaccines. So, one of the things that we try to focus on with *The Truth About Cancer* is there's certain things you can do to prevent cancer. One of my opinions is that if you don't get vaccines, you've got a better chance of not getting cancer because they've got so many carcinogens.

Give us your take on vaccines. Are they a modern medical miracle or not?

Jon: You know, I think that people have to look at vaccines from the ground up. I mean, let's take away all of the propaganda and so forth. You've got a needle and you're injecting it into babies, into adults even, into children of all ages. What's in the syringe?

You've got many different chemicals, some of which are obviously carcinogenic, like formaldehyde, for example. You've got aluminium which is extremely toxic. You've got other heavy metals.

You've got unknown elements in vaccines, germs that were not intended to be there, but are there. Partial genetic sequences of things that were either put there on purpose or not. And it's all right there in the syringe and these toxic chemicals and these germs and the whole soup.

You are basically saying to a mother, "Look, this is what we want to do to your baby, okay? I'm going to take this needle with a syringe full of this stuff that I just explained and I want to shoot it into your baby who doesn't really have any immune system at all—except derived from you, the mother—and this will be a good thing." And if that is really what you've said, then the mothers are going to respond, "Wait a minute. Where's the fairy tale? Where's the promise? Where's all this?"

And that's where I start with people, "Let's understand what we are doing here." And even in people with developed immune systems—when you're injecting anything into the body, you're intentionally bypassing a lot of portals of immune defense that would normally be active and working because you want this to penetrate deep into the body. Well, that's the idea of vaccination.

So, beginning from there, I say, fundamentally, yes, vaccines can cause cancer. No question about it. Vaccines are not safe. They are not effective. They don't do what they are supposed to be doing. They are not responsible for the major declines in infectious or contagious diseases in the West. That was done by revolutionizing society, better sanitation, better nutrition, less overcrowding, development of the middle class, etc, etc. The fundamental environmental things that you would do in order to improve life for people. That's why those diseases basically went away.

Ty: Right.

Jon: And when they returned, it's basically because those factors have diminished again, which we are now seeing especially when it comes to nutrition. It has gotten a lot worse over the past few decades. So, the whole thing, to me, is a gigantic hoax and I make no bones about it.

I mean, there are people who argue this issue on both sides from different angles, and I can appreciate that. But for me, I start with—I don't accept it as being legitimate at all. And that's not just some faith-based conviction on my part, that's from my investigation into vaccines, interviewing many, many people who have lived without ever getting vaccination who have lived well, who've remained disease-free, strong, alert, able to enjoy life.

Ty: And you're an investigative journalist, right? Describe a little bit of your background.

Jon: Thirty years plus of investigative journalism. I have written for a number of publications in the US and Europe. Magazines, newspapers, *CBS Health Watch, LA Weekly, In These Times, Spin Magazine*. But then I stopped most of that in the late 80s and eventually I went online to write my own material because I wanted to have freedom from censorship.

But most—I would say half of what I have researched over the last 30 years has had medical connotations. Medical research fraud, deep laboratory research fraud having to do with viruses, toxic pharmaceuticals, major investigations into all aspects of what I call "the medical cartel."

Ty: And why do you call it "the medical cartel?"

Jon: Because it aims to be a monopoly. Because it aims to control the entire field of health by substituting itself for what other people would choose to do on their own. It wants to eventually—and I'm talking the combination of medical schools, public health agencies in the US, for example like the FDA and the Centers for Disease Control, doctors themselves, medical bureaucrats at universities, pharmaceutical companies, of course.

All of these together form a kind of a cartel because they work together. They collaborate and they cooperate in order to bring more drugs to the market, more medical procedures to the market, more diagnoses of conditions—in many cases that don't even exist—to the market and to cut out competition, which would be natural health practitioners, people who want to live their lives naturally and are not interested in being reliant on medical care their whole lives.

So, that's a medical cartel. And I've studied that medical cartel from all angles for 30 years to see—what are these people doing? How are they bamboozling the public? And it isn't just about money. Money is there for sure—profits, yes, yes, yes. But it isn't just about money. It's about power and control and monopoly.

Ty: You mentioned research fraud. I've read many instances of research fraud, but name a couple of instances of research fraud for, maybe, drugs that people would be aware of.

Jon: Well, any drug that is on the market, available through prescription that has serious widespread adverse effects, as they say, was previously declared safe and effective by the FDA. That's the only reason that drug reached the market.

So if, after approval, it suddenly has opposite effects—very dangerous—that's fraud. Fraud at the level of the FDA for not investigating the drug properly or concealing the truth because the FDA's clients are the drug companies, not really the public as it is supposed to be.

So take a drug like Prozac for depression, as they say, you know. This was really the first blockbuster depression drug called SSRI. It had to do with serotonin levels in the body. And this drug was perpetrated on the public through studies that were falsified. In other words, the manufacturer really knew in advance that this drug could have very serious problems, could cause dangerous effects in people and yet they managed to wriggle their way to FDA approval of the drug as safe and effective.

And then, early on, when people started killing other people—people who were on Prozac started killing other people. Some lawsuits against—really were piling up in the courts and the famous case called

Fentress was laid on about a worker who went back—disgruntled employee—and shot lots of people. I think this happened in Kentucky. Joseph Wesbecker.

Well, Peter Breggin, a psychiatrist, was an expert witness at that trial. It was a lawsuit against—mounted by the families of the people who were killed—against Eli Lilly. And essentially, what happened was—Lilly, of course, tried to defend itself and say, "Hey look, our drug had nothing to do with the reason this guy went in and shot all these people," and so on and so forth.

But behind the scenes, Lilly was making a deal with the lawyer for the plaintiffs on the other side to pass what had to be enormous amounts of money under the table so that the case would be won by Lilly, but the money would go to the people who were suing Lilly.

Well, that's a felony. You can't do that, you know. Lilly won the case, which forestalled, and put off all those other suits that were piling up in courts for people who'd killed people, committed suicide on Prozac, you know, who were about to come down on Lilly. That gave everybody pause for thought. "Wow! If Lilly won this case, we better back off."

Well, the judge in the case, Potter, sniffed out what happened and he called the lawyers and he said, "I have a feeling that what's happened here—and I'm not just blowing smoke—that money has changed hands here." That a felony has been committed. And he sent the case on to a higher court.

And it just kept on swinging back and forth and eventually just sort of dissolved in the air. But the truth was there. A verdict was bought in the case. The drug was a fraud. The drug causes multiple serious problems in children and adults and everybody and it can cause suicide and homicide. That's what I call an instance of research fraud.

Ty: And it's true or isn't it true that many of the mass shootings over the last couple of decades—the shooters are always on Prozac?

Jon: Yeah, or Zoloft or Paxil or any of the other so called—

Ty: One of the SSRIs?

Jon: —one of the SSRI anti-depressants, right? So, this drug is supposed to lift people up while they're feeling chronically sad and then the person ends up killing somebody else? That's the solution to feeling sad? I mean, this is really dangerous stuff.

And the way I look at it, these drugs—it's like an evil Jonny Appleseed. Psychiatrists—they are seeding the population and not just in America. In England, Australia, Canada, other countries around the world where these drugs have really caught on in huge quantities. Walking away, as it were, from it, you turn around and you see a story of somebody who just killed 13 people. Over here, somebody killed his parents. What happened? Over here somebody walked into school, opened fire, and killing 20 children, you know.

This is spreading the seeds of destruction, pharmaceutically. The cops want to have nothing to do—I tell you—with investigating this aspect of things. They don't want to get close to it. Neither do the prosecutors, neither do courts, judges, anybody. They don't want to hear about this. Occasionally, they are forced to, but, most part, they don't want to get close to this. But this is eating society out from within.

Ty: Right. I guess then it shouldn't surprise us in a lot of these factual stories— when we look back at the history of chemotherapy to the mustard gases and all these destructive chemicals in the world wars—that that's the origins. But we still believe that they are safe and effective. They are used on a cancer patient to cure them, but they were used to kill people 78 years ago. So is that cognitive dissonance at its finest?

Jon: Yeah, I would say so. It is cognitive dissonance at its finest.

People want to believe. They want to have faith in something. And so, the guy in the white coat becomes a priest. Wearing a stethoscope around his neck. He's got an office and he's in the hospital and says, "Listen, this is the way it is. We're going to give you the best care possible." Person's sick, feels horrible, family's in chaos, diagnosed with serious cancer—they are going to go for the faith in the doctor. "You sure the drug's okay?" "Absolutely."

And now, poison, poison, poison, poison, poison. Death. This is really the height of what medical practice can achieve, you know? And then, you look at the people who have been suppressed. The independent researchers over the years. Not just suppressed and shoved to the sidelines, but careers destroyed, prosecuted in court. "We're going to do a study, finally, on your experimental compound, Dr. So-and-So, and we'll see if it really works," and then they do a study and they twist the protocol all up to ensure that the study is going to fail.

Ty: Which they did with Linus Pauling and vitamin C.

Jon: Which they did with Stan Burzynski, doctor in Houston. Which they did with Nick Gonzales, another doctor in New York. You know, this is typical kind of behavior. And these people were on the road to really knowing something about how to treat cancer. And you would think that in a profession like medicine—where first, "Do no harm." Obviously trying to help people get better—they would show some interest in this instead of saying, "Well, if it hasn't been studied and published in a peer reviewed journal, then we don't have anything to do with it. And you're a fraud. You're a quack," and so forth. And you're keeping people from getting real help. Being real poison. Now, that's evil.

It's not just disinterest or professional arrogance. It's evil.

Ty: People are dying from lack of access to these treatments.

Jon: People are dying.

Ty: It's like—it's almost like a medical holocaust in my opinion.

Jon: It is. It is a medical holocaust. There is no question about it. I've often cited this study and—I mean, this would include cancer patients, who include all American patients, you know—but the so-called *Starfield Report*, July 26, 2000 American journal—*Journal of the American Medical Association* and her review is called "Is US Health Really the Best in the World?" And the conclusion was the US medical system kills, directly, every year, in the US, 225,000 people.

And she told me in an interview, she said, "That's a conservative estimate." So, that would mean that the US medical system is killing 2.25 million people every decade. Wow! I mean, this is not a mystery. Journal of the American Medical Association. She was working at the Johns Hopkins School of Public Health. MD; doctor; public health expert; revered public health expert.

Ty: Not exactly a quack?

Jon: Yeah. I mean, just right up their alley. Right up the old mainstream—meticulous credentials—everything. And here's the conclusion. So I said to her, "Did the federal government ever come to you since the year 2000 when you published your study to ask you for any advice or help or consultation on remedying this holocaust?" And this was an email interview. And she writes back—capital "N", capital "O." NO. I said, "To your knowledge, has the federal government ever tried to do anything to remedy this horrendous situation?" NO.

So, they know what they are doing. They know—the medical cartel knows the effects of what they are doing. This is no mystery. And yet, they just keep doing it. I mean, I call it murder. I don't think there is any other word for it. It's not just indifference. You know this is happening. You know that you're participating in it and you do nothing about it.

Ty: It is sad when you think of the fact that it's not just adults that are dying. It's children that are dying as well. We recently did an interview up in Seattle with a man who's trying to use the Burzynski treatment, but the FDA won't let them and kids are dying. It's sad.

Jon: Right. Oh man, as far as I know they are still saying that in order to get help from Burzynski, you have to have exhausted every other possible conventional treatment and then there are other conditions and so forth.

Ty: Which is why people are dying. They are dying from the treatments.

Jon: Exactly. They don't even get that far.

Ty: Jon, this is a fast interview and I appreciate you spending your time with us today. But last question, we call ourselves *The Truth About Cancer,* but if there is one truth that you wanted people to know, that has been hidden from them—not necessarily even about cancer—but just one truth, what would it be?

Jon: Boy, if I have to narrow it down to one...

Ty: A couple is fine.

Jon: Living a healthy life is not really a medical proposition. That's what we've been led to believe especially in recent years. If you watch television, if you're aware of media, you're led to believe that there's no possible way that a human being can go from cradle to grave without constantly relying on medical doctors. That's the message.

And people don't seem to realize that's a fairly new message, you know. That's 30, 40, 50 years, maybe, of huge long history in which suddenly this is pounded on day and night. People have to wake up and remember, "Wait a minute. It wasn't always like this and I am capable of living my full complete life without thinking of myself as a medical patient primarily. Without having to rely and rely and rely and rely on doctors all the time." That would be, in a nutshell, what I'd leave people with.

Ty: So, as Robert says, at the end of each show, "The power to heal is yours."

Jon: "The power to heal is yours." Yeah, exactly.

Ty: Thank you, Jon. Appreciate it.

Jon: Thank you, son.

[end of transcript]

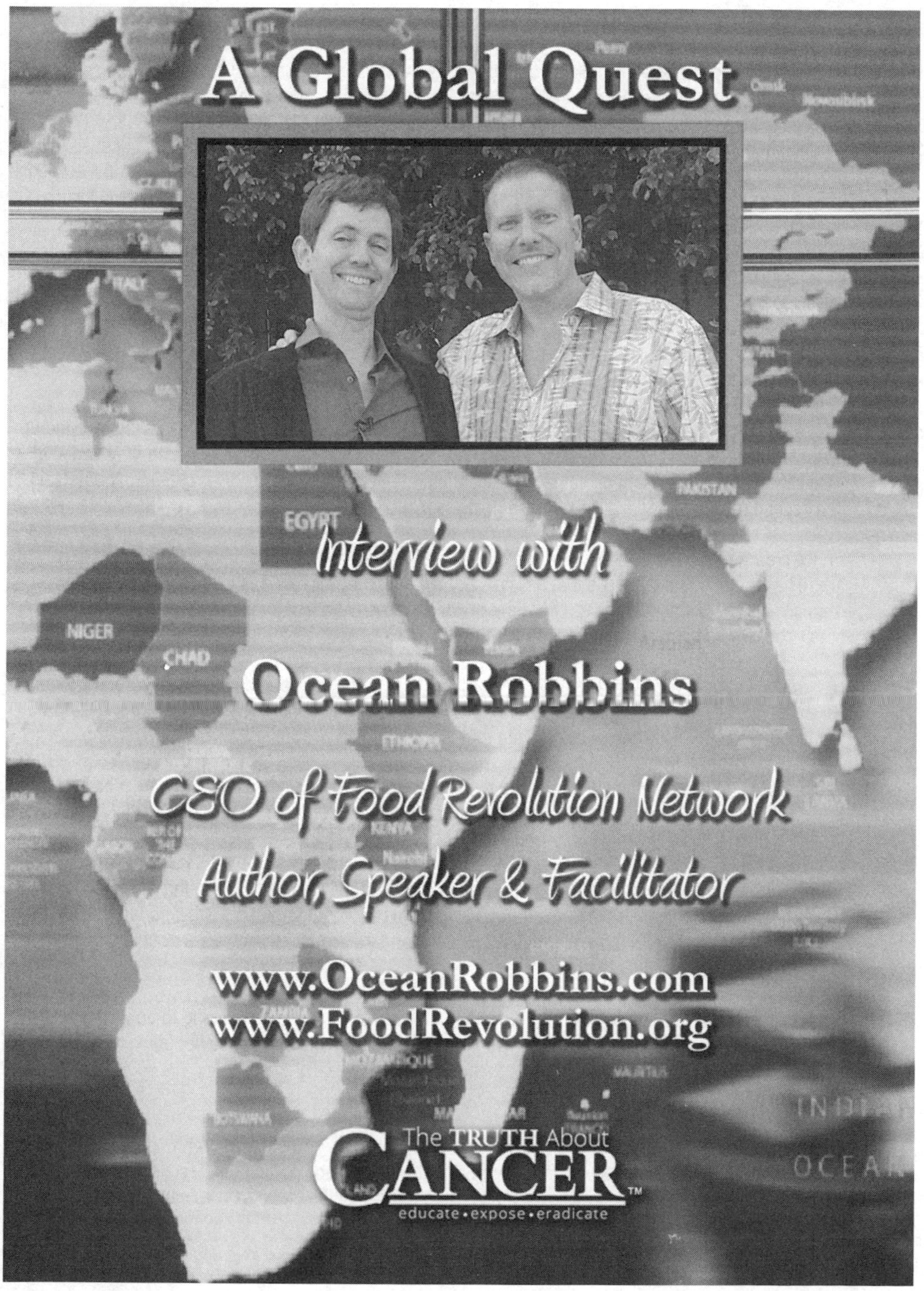
A Global Quest
Interview with
Ocean Robbins
CEO of Food Revolution Network
Author, Speaker & Facilitator
www.OceanRobbins.com
www.FoodRevolution.org
The TRUTH About CANCER
educate • expose • eradicate

Ty: Ocean, thank you for hanging out with us today. I know you had to come a ways to get to this interview.

Ocean: It's my privilege.

Ty: I'm really excited to be able to talk to you today to get you to share some of your knowledge specifically about food. For the viewers out there, could you tell us a little bit about yourself?

Ocean: Alright. My name is Ocean Robbins. My last name may sound familiar to some viewers because my grandfather founded an ice cream company. It's called Baskin Robbins. So he came up with the notion of 31 flavors of ice cream. My dad grew up with an ice cream cone shaped swimming pool in the backyard and 31 flavors of temptation in the freezer at all times.

He was groomed from early childhood to one day join in running the family company, and it was fully expected that he would. But when he was in his early 20s his uncle Burt Baskin, my grandpa's partner in the business, and brother-in-law—

Ty: That's where the Baskin came from.

Ocean: That's where the Baskin came from. Burt Baskin came down with serious heart disease that wound up taking his life. My dad's uncle Burt was a big man. He ate a lot of the family product and my dad said, "you know what, there might be some connection here." He started doing some research and he said, "I can't spend my life selling a product that's going to make people sick."

An ice cream cone isn't going to kill anybody, right? But the more ice cream you eat the more likely you are to have a lot of the diseases that are prevalent in our times. So my dad followed his own rocky road. He walked away from the family company and then any access to the family wealth to go on in time to become a best-selling author on food and health issues.

He wrote *Diet for a New America* in 1987 which inspired millions of people to look at our food choices as an opportunity to make a difference for our health and for our world. We received about a hundred thousand letters from readers thanking him for his work and I was inspired by my dad's example.

I said, "I want to do something to reach out to my generation with this message." Because he had taken this stand for integrity. He had walked away from an ice cream fortune and now he was helping people to walk a different path towards greater health.

Remarkably enough, my grandfather Irvine Robbins wound up in his early 70s being diagnosed with a whole host of serious health problems that you would expect for a man of his age who ate the diet that he had eaten in his life. Which was pretty much the standard American diet plus a double scoop of ice cream on top.

So his doctors told him, "you've only got a couple of years to live and you're going to be taking a serious amount of medications for those two years and we're afraid that you're not going to be too happy." They said, "unless you want to get serious and make real changes." And his doctor hands him a copy of my dad's book.

So my grandpa winds up reading it, making changes in his diet, giving up ice cream, giving up junk food and processed food, moving towards a more plant strong diet, and getting real results. His golf game improved seven strokes. He lost thirty pounds. He got off all of the diabetes medications that he was taking.

He wound up living fifteen more vibrant healthy years. I have this vivid memory of my dad and I, we were marathon runners, and we would run in these marathons. We would run by my grandpa who was out taking his hour-long morning walk and he's cheering and waving us on as we're going. That's the kind of thing that's possible when you're willing to make changes.

You can have radical transformations. So my whole life since then has been dedicated to helping people have the kind of radical breakthroughs that my own grandpa got to have, that his brother-in-law never tragically got to have, but that everyone deserves.

Ty: Ocean, to me that's really admirable on many levels. The first of which is that here in the United States everybody is in search of the all mighty dollar. So you've got a father, even a grandfather eventually that made changes that actually affected their wealth. They made changes that actually diminished what we look at wealth here, but really health is true wealth, isn't it?

Ocean: I mean well it is. If you don't have your health, what good is money? Right? I don't think anybody in the world would be willing to take unlimited money and give up their health and be in misery and suffering and pain and then death. Yet the reality is that when you actually look at what's happening, as you say, we have made money and economic opportunity in some ways a greater priority than our own physical well-being.

When it comes to food, Food 1.0 was about survival. If you could get enough calories to survive another day that was success. Food 2.0, which is dominant today in most of the modern world, the developed world at least, is about commerce.

We've got this huge variety of flavors and textures and tastes and cuisines and opportunities, incredible opportunities, but it's morally bankrupt. We've got a food system that is full of flavorings, and additives, and chemicals, and colors, and genetically modified organisms, and pesticides, and hormones, and antibiotics.

All of these things together are creating this toxic soup. The tragedy, Ty, is that this toxic soup is killing us. It's killing our kids. It's leading to two-thirds of our population suffering from obesity. A third of our kids expected to get diabetes in their lifetimes. Massive epidemics of cancer, as you know, and so much of that could be prevented. We can do so much better which is why I'm calling for Food 3.0. which means we make health the central organizing principle of our food system.

Ty: I like that idea. I like Food 3.0. Let's talk about Food Revolution Network. You're CEO of Food Revolution Network. A hundred and fifty thousand plus people that are mobilizing for healthy living, right? So Ocean, tell us a little bit about the Food Revolution Network.

Ocean: We're standing up for healthy, sustainable, humane, and delicious food for everybody. People ask me, "is 'revolution' kind of strong word?" I say, "yeah it's a strong word." We got some strong problems and we need some strong solutions. We can do so much better.

I think it's not an exaggeration to say that in a society where toxic food is normal, and where illness and suffering and feeling like crap are increasingly considered normal, it's time for a serious change. So we're standing for our revolution and we do that through education, through the Food Revolution Summit, through mobilizing with resources and information and knowledge. We want to empower people to put the food revolution into action.

Now the beautiful thing about the food revolution is that you don't have to wait for Monsanto or McDonald's, or Coca-Cola, or the U.S. government to be able to make changes. You can be an everyday food revolutionary in your own life and when you do that you actually change the system.

We are actually creating a demand for a whole new food economy. Even companies as big as McDonald's and Coca-Cola are feeling the effects and are realizing that what made them food giants in the 20th century is going to make them dinosaurs in the 21st century if they don't make some big changes.

Consumers are sick of being sick. We're tired of being tired. We're fed up with toxic food. We're hungry for a change and we're demanding it. That's why we're seeing this massive change in sales of organic food, certified non-GMO food, natural food, local food, farmers markets have tripled in the last decade.

Ty: It's real food, right?

Ocean: Real food.

Ty: We shouldn't even have to call it organic. Should we or shouldn't we? Food by nature should be organic. They should have to call their food "pesticide laden food" and ours should just be called "food." It's kind of flipped, what we call organic, but that's what we're after. We're after clean foods. So Ocean tell us, what does a clean diet look like to you?

Ocean: I'm excited about diets that are based around real, whole, organic, natural foods that are full of lots of plants. I want to see us eating a lot more vegetables and fruits. I think the medical research is so clear. There's just about no nutritionist out there that doesn't agree that we need to eat a heck of a lot more vegetables.

I think that whole grains make a great contribution to a healthy diet. I think legumes make a great contribution to a healthy diet. I think if people are going to eat animal products they should come from animals that were treated humanely and that were raised without a bunch of chemicals and junk.

That's a personal choice people need to make for themselves. On the whole, I think we need to eat less meat, collectively, for the survival of our planet. Fifteen percent of our global warming impact is coming from our livestock production. A huge amount of our water is going to livestock production. It takes about eighteen hundred gallons of water to produce one pound of grain-fed beef in a factory farm.

Ty: I can attest to the water. We've got horses on our property and man, those big animals drink a lot of water. Let me ask you a question about that. I've got a quote here. Somebody I heard recently said that, "a trillion GMO meals have been served and not a single case of GMO-induced illness has ever turned up." What do you say to that statement?

Ocean: Well how would we know because we are all participants in a mass experiment. Pretty much unless you've been living in a cave somewhere or growing all your own food, you have consumed some GMOs at some point. They're only in five major food crops but those food crops are so wide spread.

We're talking corn, soy, canola, sugar beets, and then of course cotton which ends up in cottonseed oil. But all of our restaurants virtually contain genetically modified organisms in their ingredient supply. So unless you never eat out at restaurants you're probably being exposed to them.

So the reality then is we have to say that we don't have any placebo, and we don't have any control group in this experiment. We are all in on it. So we wouldn't know. Unless they caused immediate death, right? We have very little way of knowing.

Ty: Which they don't because as we saw three years ago in the Seralini Study, it took them two years to kill the mice. So they didn't cause immediate death. As Jeffrey Smith shared with us last year, that testing that was done by Monsanto on these GMO crops, they always stopped the test at 90 days before the rats got the tumors and before they became sterile, and before they had premature deaths.

Ocean: So what I find rather terrifying is that we do see some trends since GMOs have come into our food supply. In the same 25 years that we've been adding more and more GMOs into our food supply, we have seen a rapid increase in rates of autism, digestive problems, diabetes, obesity, a whole host of health problems. Now correlation isn't causation.

The Chinese economy follows a very similar trajectory, right? But when you see a correlation this strong, I think it bears a deeper examination. We do have quite a few scientists that have come out saying that GMOs seem to be completely safe.

The reality is that most of those scientists have been funded by the biotech industry that has a direct interest in those results being what people conclude. So when you look at independent scientists, they're much more divided on the issue.

When you look at the studies that have been done by scientists who are not on the payroll of the biotech industry, you find about a third of those studies find serious problems. So I don't think that this is like, "case closed, we know for sure what the impact is." I'd say the case should be opened, in a serious way. In the meanwhile we as consumers should have the right to make informed choices.

Ty: We should also have the right to know what's in the food, right?

Ocean: We should, we should. Absolutely. And I'll tell you what else we do know with certainty, that genetically modified organisms are leading to vastly increased use of Roundup, glyphosate, which has just been declared by the World Health Organization to be a likely carcinogen.

We do know that they are leading to vastly increased use of 2, 4-D, which is one of the two ingredients in Agent Orange which has been linked to a host of metabolic and health and neurological dysfunction and birth defects in large numbers.

We do know that when we spray these chemicals on our croplands we wind up eating crops that have literally absorbed herbicide. Which is unprecedented in human history because before if you sprayed them on your crops, the crops would die.

Ty: That would be a resistant crop.

Ocean: Right. We have resistant crops so they're absorbing herbicide so we're consuming the herbicide. So what is the impact on human beings of consuming large amounts of glyphosate and 2, 4-D, and other toxic herbicides? I think it's pretty alarming.

Ty: The experiment is still underway.

Ocean: It's underway. But we do know that the rapid increase in digestive problems and food allergies that we're seeing, which is dramatic in the United States today, tripling in the last fifteen years by the way, could very well be linked to this because we know that glyphosate has also been patented by Monsanto as an antibiotic.

So there is the possibility that these chemicals could be interfering with our gut bacteria, with our digestive process. If that's the case, then obviously that would help to explain why we're seeing this rapid increase in allergic reaction.

Ty: How important is the gut bacteria in health?

Ocean: It's fundamental to everything. What you digest is what you become. What you eat is important of course, but what you digest of it is equally important. Your body's ability to make use of the vital nutrients that it takes in is essential to your survival and well-being.

That's why gut bacteria is absolutely paramount. That's why if you take antibiotics it's highly advisable, because they do tend to wipe out a lot of good bacteria, to take some probiotics thereafter to help get your system back in balance.

Ty: What are some foods that you coul eat that would have that natural probiotic effect?

Ocean: I love to make fermented foods from sauerkraut to homemade kefir. I make soy yogurt, some people make regular yogurt. I don't like the stuff with all the sugar in it. The actual fermentation process, getting all the good culture going is great for our bodies.

Ty: So that's kind of a natural probiotic.

Ocean: Exactly. Coconut kefirs are really good. There are a lot of ways to enjoy fermented foods, misos, that can really provide some of that beneficial bacteria. But here's the other thing, if you don't kill it, it'll naturally proliferate.

We all have a lot of bacteria in our bodies and we want to encourage the good stuff and take out the bad stuff. Ultimately, eating good healthy food turns out to be one of the best things you can do for encouraging good stuff.

Ty: You seem to be very, very well educated on food. The thing that's ironic to me—and this is something that I was informed of in many, many interviews last year, with many medical doctors—is that after asking them about their education when they were in medical school on food and nutrition, they got numb. Medical doctors today aren't educated on food and nutrition.

Ocean: Out of all the medical schools in the United States, less than a third of them have a single required course on nutrition. So it's possible for a doctor to go through six years of medical school, plus all their residency, and never have a single course in nutrition.

Ty: Like my good buddy Dr. Irving Sahni who was in *Quest For the Cures Continues* last year, he had a course on nutrition. It was a one day course and it was a two hour, literally two hours, course and they just talked about the effects of vitamins on the body. It was about the chemical effect, more from a chemistry effect, not from a nutritional effect, and not from, "what can this do for your health." So it's really not even beneficial, some of the courses that are even offered.

Ocean: It's not. I mean, we've got a food industry that pays no attention to health and we've got a health industry that pays no attention to food. And yet food is the foundation of health. We all know intellectually that an ounce of prevention is worth a pound of cure. Yet functionally the way we're living is the complete opposite of that and that's not by accident.

We have a lot of money being made by the food industry for selling whatever it can sell for the lowest possible price. We got a lot of money being made by the medical industry that's now 19 percent of gross domestic product in the United States. Most of that money is being made off treating the symptoms of disease. Disease that we know how to prevent, but there's not money to be made in that.

I'm not accusing every individual doctor of being out just to make a buck. I'm saying that we've got a system in place that systematically causes us to be sick.

Ty: We have a system that's broken. I would completely agree with that and we actually have a medical school system that's actually been hijacked. We covered that last year, over 100 years ago the way that big business aligned itself with the medical schools to push drugs.

As a result we got a pill for every ill, but people are sicker than ever and the doctors don't know how to fix it because they've never been educated.

Ocean: I'll tell you what else, even the Academy of Nutrition and Dietetics, which is the major group for the dieticians of the United States. They have their annual meetings and some of their sponsors are companies like McDonald's and Coca-Cola.

They literally give away Coca-Cola to everyone at those meetings for free. They will sponsor meetings, sponsor sessions, discussion groups on topics. It will literally say in the program, "Sponsored by McDonald's,", "Sponsored by Coca-Cola."

How objective do you think that information is going to be and how revolutionary do you think it's going to be? When you actually look at the data and what is the impact of these companies on the health of our kids. On the health of our population. Then this isn't just funny, it's also scandalous.

That nutritionists and dieticians whose job it is to look out for the public well-being and to help individuals to get on a path of health, are being bought off, functionally speaking, by industries that are polluting the health of the people these folks are supposed to be serving.

Ty: It is. It's sad. It borders on criminal. You mention McDonald's sponsoring these meetings. One of the things that I brought up last year was the fact that, I think it was in 2009, one of the sponsors for breast cancer awareness month was Kentucky Fried Chicken.

So you have foods that are very well causing cancer, companies that are producing these foods are sponsoring breast cancer awareness month. It makes no sense whatsoever.

Ocean: And they have their whole "pink bucket campaign" where you could buy your chicken in a pink bucket and they would donate money to help fund research on cancer. Research on how to cure the diseases they're causing.

Now we can do better. That's what your work's all about, that's what my work's all about. Saying we can do better and because we can do better, we've got to do better. What thrills me, honestly, is that we have the opportunity, right here and now. We know everything we need to know to radically improve the health outcomes for millions and millions of people.

We can lose weight, we can have more energy, we can have better sleep, we can prevent cancer, we can prevent heart disease. We can recover from diseases we already have, we can even reduce Alzheimer's Disease by up to two-thirds with improved nutrition and lifestyle.

Ty: The interviews that I've gotten of people that are on this quest, the Global Quest for the Cures that we're doing here, to a tee the people that are recovering and are healing, they all radically changed their diet. They all got rid of eating the junk and the things that were causing disease and they went to organic and vegetarian, clean meats, those that eat meats, clean, clean dairies.

They got away from the genetically modified organisms, stopped eating processed foods, stopped going out. They all have that in common. So it's not just a coincidence. This is one of the fundamentals, Ocean, of regaining your health, preventing disease, overcoming cancer and other diseases, it is that you must change your nutrition because that's your fuel for your body.

Ocean: It's true. We look at genetics and the role of genetics, obviously they're fascinating and important. We also know that where people come from—when you look at international migration patterns and human beings, where they come from is not nearly as important as where they go to.

People in Japan have very low rates of a lot of diseases that when they come to the US and eat our western styled diet they suddenly start getting all those diseases just as much as the rest of us do. So genetics are significant but I think the modern research on cancer is showing that probably about 10 percent is genetically caused, and about 90 percent is lifestyle and environment caused.

Ty: The modern research too that we have now is on the five to ten percent that the American Cancer Society mentions is genetically linked. They have the studies on epigenetics. Things that you can do now to prevent that gene expression. A diet of organic foods and all these things that we've been talking about is one of the main ways that you can take that epigenetic control of your genes and you can keep them from expressing.

So even if you have these genes that are supposedly causing cancer, if you eat a clean organic diet, avoid GMOs and processed foods, and pesticides, and all these things that we've talked about, and exercise, and keep the lymphatic system flowing, on, and on, and on. They may never express themselves.

Ocean: There are two parts to a healthy diet I think. One is avoiding the bad stuff and the other is taking advantage of the good stuff. Avoiding the bad stuff is things like pesticides, and hormones, and chemicals, and antibiotics, and all those sorts of things, and processed foods, additives, flavorings, and colorings, and the list goes on.

Taking advantage of the good stuff is getting all the phytonutrients and all the flavonoids and all the beautiful things that fruits and vegetables and a balanced varied diet provides to us. We need the fiber to help clean our colon out. We need the phytonutrients to give us that vitality and that energy, and that ability to fight off cancer.

It's incredible what can happen when you don't just eat a little less bad, when you actually make your food an expression of what you love. Your body is more vital and more alive, and you have more bounce in your step, and you have more clarity in your mind.

That's what I love getting to see happen in the work that I do. Every day I'm interacting with people whose lives are transforming. We're getting to see their smiles brighter, and their work more productive, and their energy stronger, and their lives longer as times goes by. And it's thrilling.

Ty: It's evident just from your aura that you love what you're doing. It's evident that you're practicing what you're preaching. I think you've been getting plenty of phytonutrients because you got that vitality going on. I think that what you're doing with Food Revolution Network is amazing and I'm really happy to be working with you on this mutual mission that we have to get the world healthier, to prevent disease, and just to help all humanity to live better lives, to live better quality lives.

So I'm really thankful that you've traveled down here today to interview with us. Thank you for the information that you shared. And I just wish you all the best in the future. I look forward to working with you on this mutual mission.

Ocean: Likewise, Ty. Thank you.

Ty: Alright. God bless you.

[end of transcript]

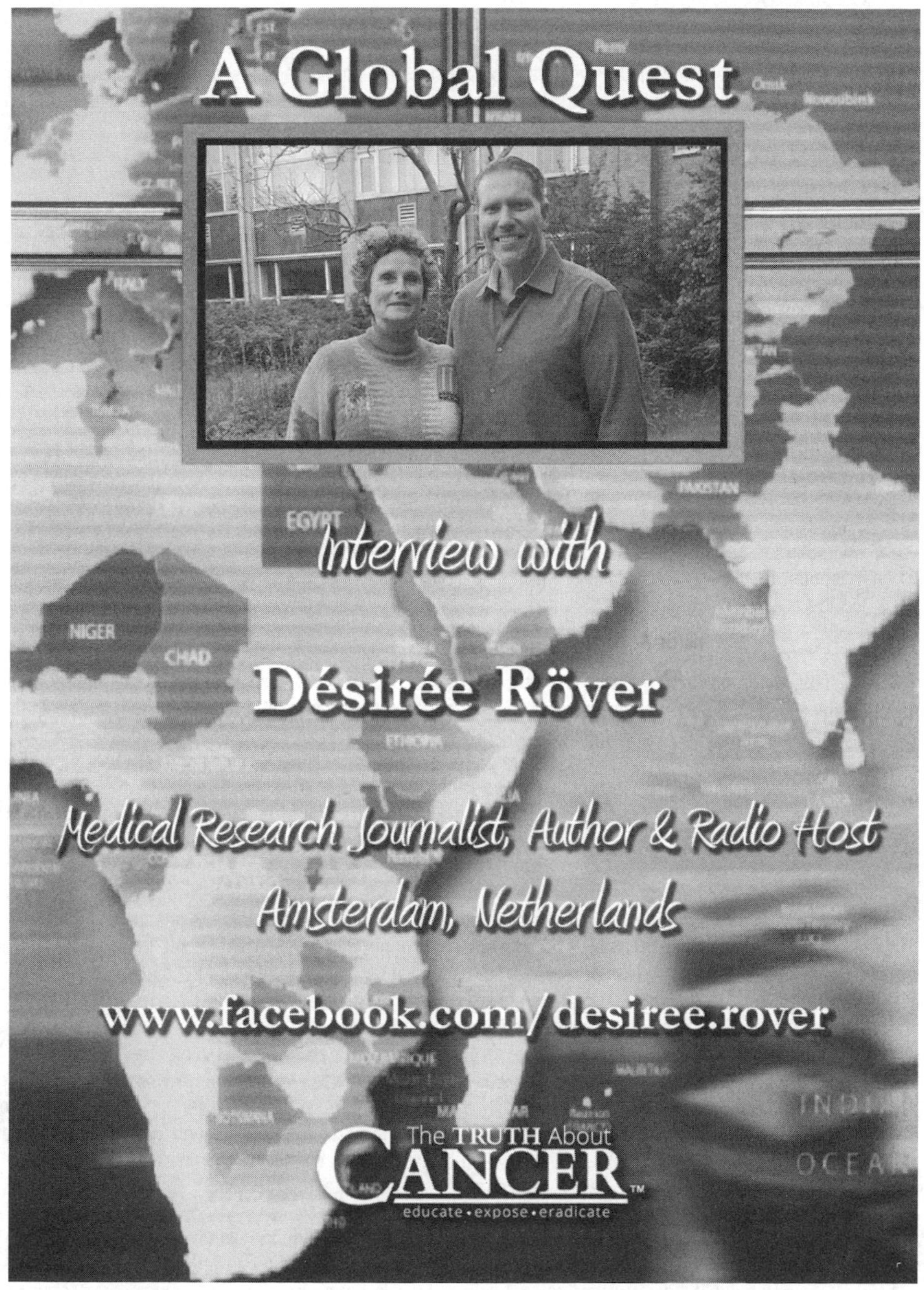
A Global Quest
Interview with
Désirée Röver
Medical Research Journalist, Author & Radio Host
Amsterdam, Netherlands
www.facebook.com/desiree.rover
The TRUTH About CANCER
educate • expose • eradicate

Ty: I'm here with Desiree Rover. It's a pleasure to finally meet you.

Desiree: Yes, same here.

Ty: Well, you interviewed me a few years back on your radio show. And here with John Consemulder tonight. Did not even know you were going to be here, but I'm so glad that you're here.

Desiree: Was it a nice surprise?

Ty: It is a great surprise because I want to ask you a couple of questions. The first question is being about vaccines. I know you're an expert and you've been looking at vaccines for 25 years. We hear they're safe and effective. We hear they don't cause cancer. We hear that they prevented all these diseases. What's the truth?

Desiree: The opposite; that's the short answer. It's totally the opposite. I wrote a book in 2009 on the HPV vaccines, Cervarix and Gardasil. And then for that book I delved even deeper into the history of vaccination. To my big, big surprise I found out that Edward Jenner had a folk myth. That if you had had cowpox you were supposedly protected against smallpox. But these are two viral entities. So it's a nonsense story. What he did, he was the first guy who introduced proteins and DNA and RNA from animals, from other species, into humans. It was called inoculation or variolation. They made a scratch and then they put in the smallpox pus. That's how it originally started. And Jenner did a variation on that and he put in the cowpox pus or the goatpox or the pigpox or whatever, all sorts of crap. He did that with his son and the son of his gardener. And both boys never got older than 20 or 21 years old because they died of tuberculosis, which is an illness related to cows. And then that's the one faulty leg underneath vaccination.

The other one is Louis Pasteur. His rabies vaccines and what he did with that is he created havoc in the health of the people who got rabies. These days they have rabies vaccines and they play around with rabies in the laboratories. Now you can get rabies from something that's going around in the air. In the States they have been dropping bait packages with rabies in it for the wildlife to vaccinate them. Rabies and cannibalism is a connection. So there are all sorts of crazy things happening and it has often to do with rabies. With vaccination, whether you do it the way Jenner did it with his scratch and putting material into the wound or you do it by a syringe like we do now, you introduce foreign material into the human body. So you change the genetic information and you introduce a lot of toxic chemicals.

What I often do when I speak to parents is I say, "Well, see this beautiful green apple I have here, now I'm going to inject into that formaldehyde, aluminum hydroxide, polysorbate 80, phenoxyethanol, this that and the other." So then these parents say, "No I'm not going to feed that apple to my kids." And then I say, "Well, have you ever realized that when you have your kid vaccinated that you have these materials introduced into the blood stream of your child. And what do you think is happening in the body of your child when these toxins are there?" And then, they scratch their heads. And even then because the emotional blackmail is very strong, even then sometimes parents still do vaccinate because everybody does it. And the doctor said it was safe and effective. Well, doctors do what they know. And their course in vaccination at the university was one sentence, "vaccines are safe and effective, period." And in studies that they read about what vaccines do, they read the headline and they read the abstract and the conclusion maybe. And at the bottom of the article there's always the disclaimer either that more studies are needed or well, we can't say for sure that they are not safe.

Ty: So Desiree, one of the things that you just mentioned is the fact that they are really not proven to be safe and effective. One of the comments that I got last year when I interviewed Dr. Sherri Tenpenny—Dr. Tenpenny said that vaccines are not being tested for carcinogenicity. In other words, they have not been tested if they cause cancer. Could this be one of the reasons we are seeing this huge spike in childhood cancers?

Desiree: I'm absolutely sure for two reasons. One, I have many old books written by doctors in the beginning of 1900s and after that, stating that vaccination causes cancer. There is a Dr. Clarke from Indianapolis who wrote in 1906 that he had seen 200 cases of cancer. And he had never seen cancer in a non-vaccinated person. The second reason why I know that there is a connection between vaccines and cancer is because Dr. Vera Shivener in Australia is a very dear close personal friend of mine. She told me that the cancer that my second son got in 1981 when he was two years old was caused by the SV40 in the polio vaccine. My son died three weeks before his fourth birthday, after his 17th chemotherapy treatment. And that is what killed him, not the cancer. With any cancer patient as you know, no doubt, it's the treatment that will kill you, not the cancer.

Ty: I'm sorry for that, I did not know that.

Desiree: Yeah, but the reason that he has been in my life is that I do what I do today. That I do with all my heart knowing where I'm coming from and being authentic in it. I have studied for years in this subject to know what I'm talking about.

Ty: Just so that somebody doesn't watch this and say, "that's just anecdotal," many vaccines contain formaldehyde. Formaldehyde is a known carcinogen.

Desiree: Yeah, how can they say that? It's only a tiny, tiny bit Ty, that's why. Apparently they have never heard about homeopathy.

Ty: Right, that's a good connection.

Desiree: Yeah. Also vaccines have never been tested teratogenicity. How do you say that?

Ty: Carcinogenicity?

Desiree: No, it's that you get birth defects. Teratogenicity or whatever, it's a difficult word. And also vaccines are not tested for sterility. If you ask me the HPV vaccines, Gardasil and Cervarix are a covert sterilization agenda. Everything that I wrote in my book as a question, "is this going to happen, this awful effect of these vaccines?" It has all come true. I'm sorry to say it. I would have loved to be wrong about it, but yeah.

Ty: You mentioned Gardasil, the vaccine to prevent cervical cancer. Is it true that it can also cause cancer?

Desiree: Oh, you bet, of course. Have you seen the crap that's in it?

Ty: Have you seen the package insert, right?

Desiree: Yeah, I've read them all. On my website I have taken apart every vaccine in the Dutch Vaccination Program. I've taken it apart from the product inserts for the doctors, not for the patients.

Ty: Desiree, you mentioned the package inserts. Are they the same for patients as for doctors?

Desiree: No, not at all. For patients it's a soft story and it's more like public relations. It's good and it's going to do this and that and the other and maybe you get a red spot and maybe a little bit of this or that, but it's very mild. When you read the product inserts for the doctors, then you have a whole list of stuff that can seldom happen or less rare or often, and they have a whole thing. And then there is something very important because the studies that have been done with vaccines, that's been paid by the manufacturers. But the FDA in America and the ADVM here in Holland, for adding it to their program, they go with these studies. So it's the fox is guarding the hen house.

Ty: So Desiree, this is the last question for you. Every oncologist knows that radiation causes cancer.

Desiree: Exactly, as do chemicals.

Ty: They know this, right? Should we be concerned about the radiation that began spilling from Fukushima four years ago?

Desiree: Yeah, definitely, absolutely. Even Chernobyl has created havoc. Because people don't know but the radiation fallout is not some spread, like it's an even spread in an area, but you have pockets where there is extra radiation. And that has happened with Chernobyl, which is in Ukraine, which is quite nearby here relatively speaking. But Fukushima, after 4 years I can tell you has taken out all the life in tide pools at the west coast of America, Alaska, and Canada.

Ty: I've seen reports and I've seen documentaries on this.

Desiree: Dana Durnford has been working with a zodiac and a camera and Testsoft and everything. He has a beautiful website, thenuclearproctologist.org. You see every picture he took. And from the 5,000 species that were there in the tide pools he finds maybe 50 now. Yes, it's quite dramatic. It is very dramatic. They have stopped fishing for sardines because there are none. They're gone.

Ty: So in light of this really shocking information, what can we do? What can the viewer do to protect themselves against this radiation?

Desiree: Taking extra potassium iodide and extra vitamin C. Don't eat dairy and don't drink cow's milk. Have your own garden under a shade, that's more for the chemtrails also. But basically there is no place to flee to anymore. It's everywhere.

Ty: So when you mentioned, "don't drink milk," is that because the radiation accumulates in the grass and then the cow eats it?

Desiree: Exactly. You added bio accumulation in the cow, in the milk, and that sort of a thing.

Ty: So one of the things you can do practically is to take iodine.

Desiree: You know what a very interesting thing is Sonoma County in California, the health department said to doctors, "don't give your patients iodine."

Ty: Really. One of the few things that will protect us they are not supposed to give.

Desiree: Exactly.

Ty: Surprised.

Desiree: I haven't done it today but with iodine you can do a fun thing. There is a product called Lugol. You can paint it on your arm. I paint little hearts with it on my arm. And then I see how fast it disappears. When it's disappearing within 24 hours, you can take a lot more iodine because iodine has many different functions in the body, not only for your thyroid, but many other places iodine has a role to play. And they took it out of the bread and they changed it for bromine. We are being poisoned by the authorities. It's amazing. They love people getting cancer. They love people dying and that sort of a thing. Listen to Bill Gates and you'll know where they are coming from.

Ty: Well, we've got to keep fighting, don't we?

Desiree: Yeah, we should do that.

Ty: Well Desiree, thanks for sharing. We really appreciate your input.

Desiree: I'm sorry it wasn't nice news, but people need to know this.

Ty: The truth is not always nice. ***[end of transcript]***

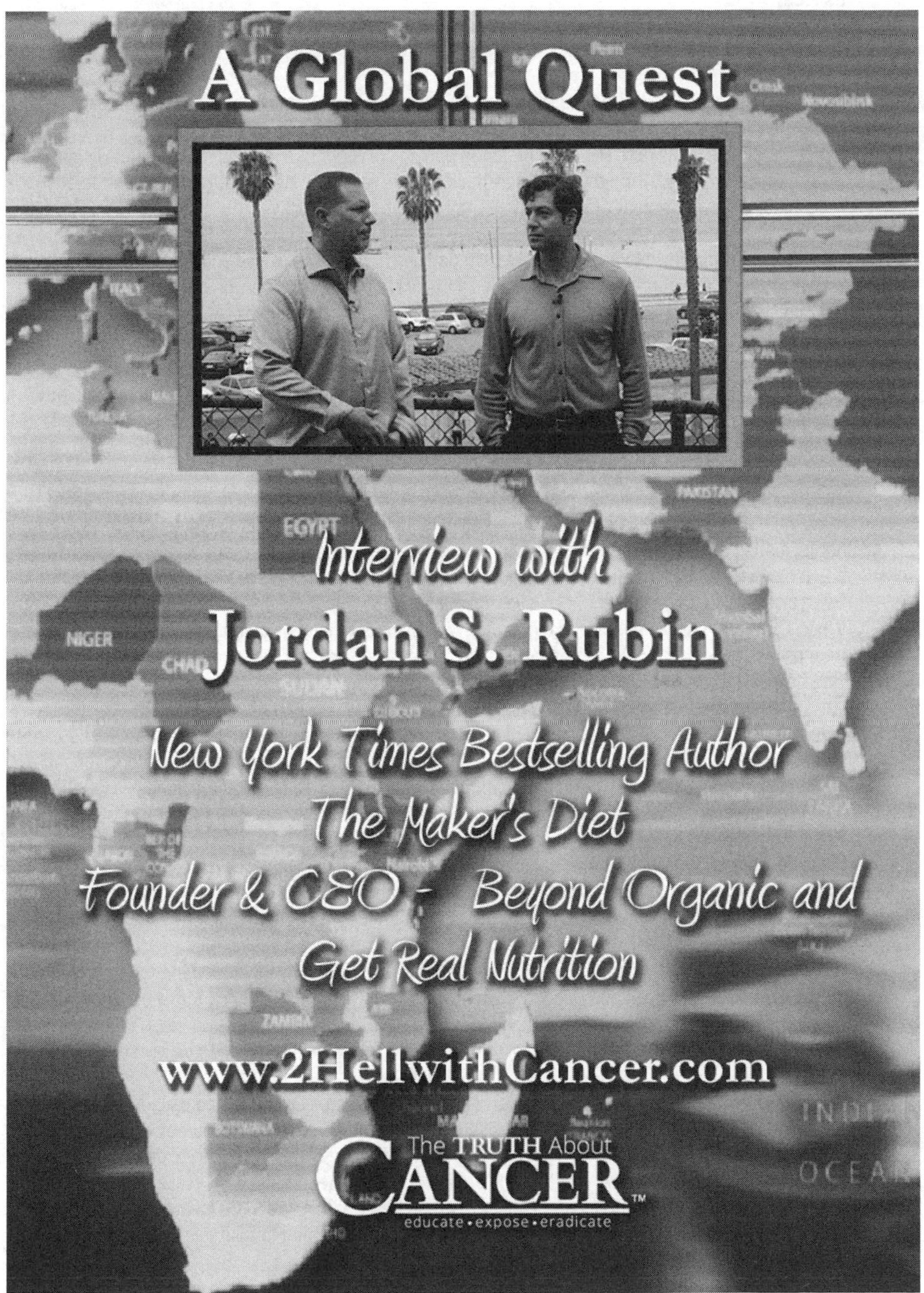
A Global Quest
Interview with
Jordan S. Rubin
New York Times Bestselling Author
The Maker's Diet
Founder & CEO - Beyond Organic and
Get Real Nutrition
www.2HellwithCancer.com
The TRUTH About
CANCER
educate • expose • eradicate

Ty: So excited to be here at Muscle Beach, Venice Beach, California with Jordan Rubin. Thanks for joining us today.

Jordan: Great to be here.

Ty: I'm really looking forward to your interview today and getting your story. I remember years ago when I first got into what we call "natural health" and beginning to take some of your products. I read a couple of your books, *The Maker's Diet*, and I learned about your story of overcoming a lot of really bad health issues a long time ago. Would you walk us back to some of those issues that got you interested in natural health and eventually led you on the path that you're on today?

Jordan: I started in my journey into natural health from day one. I was born at Naturopathic University. My father was a naturopathic student at the National College of Naturopathic Medicine outside of Portland, Oregon. I like to say I was born with a silver sprout in my mouth. So in the 1970s, eating healthy, cleansing, detoxification, chiropractic was not commonplace. However, my parents were non-conformists. I guess you could call them hippie-health nuts in the 70s. They started in Kansas and then moved to Oregon to follow the school and my dad was all about natural health. I think for fun, they would all take activated charcoal and measure each other's transit times. You know what I'm talking about. This was way before anything was accepted. It was definitely outside of the norm so to speak.

I was born in a naturopathic university, wasn't vaccinated, was really ushered into the natural health movement. But as a child, I only thought about what I couldn't do—what my restrictions were. The health foods back in the day were very limited. I think we had seaweed, there was wheat germ, brewer's yeast and all manner of soy products. Nothing like today. No big health food stores. Everything was small and niche. However, growing up, having a healthy constitution was part of my life. When I was 15 years of age, I was threatened by my school that if I was not vaccinated for measles, mumps, and rubella, I would be suspended. My father said take the suspension, it's not worth it. One little needle and a second of time may have contributed to my diagnosis of Crohn's colitis three years later. It was in the midst of a very fun and successful college career that I was blindsided by these digestive and immune system issues. I went from 185 lbs. at nearly 6'1," college athlete, just on fire for God, on fire for life, to being bed ridden, suffering for two years with now 18 medical conditions. I had diabetes, I had symptoms of rheumatoid arthritis, parasites, fungal infection, bacterial—a lot of what is now implicated in the disease that we collectively call cancer.

I was devastated. I visited 69 medical experts, conventional medicine failed, natural cures—I went to Mexican clinics, mostly treating cancer, but also some autoimmune conditions, to Germany, several of the places that you visited recently—nothing helped. One day, I came to this really apex of faith and I was reading my Bible, and I read a verse that I had read before, but this scripture now spoke to me differently. It was Hebrews 11:1. It said, "Faith is the substance of things hoped for, the evidence of things not seen." So here I am, bedridden, in a wheelchair, looking like skin and bones, emaciated, a failure for all things that we consider important in life. Yet, I felt God was asking me to take a step of faith. I took eight steps from my bedroom that I had now inhabited that used to be my sister's room.

When I left to college, my parents downsized and pretty much came home and caused major challenges in the family. I was sleeping in this bedroom, and I'd have to walk about eight steps to the bathroom, which I visited all too frequently as is common with inflammatory bowel disease. I stood up in boxer shorts and nothing else, 111 lbs. and I said, "Mom you need to take my picture." She said, "Jordan, I can barely stand to look at you, it breaks my heart. Can't we wait until you're better? And she said, "Why do you insist I take your picture?" I said, "Mom, you need to take this picture because the world is not going to believe what God's about to do in my life."

Ty, this was in the midst of my illness, no doctor could help me, no natural health method or integrated medicine, but I knew that God was in control and I had my mom take that photograph and it's now been seen by millions of people. I didn't get well right away. It took weeks and months.

Nearly a year later, I met a man who taught me how to eat and live like the Bible says. It's really the Bible meets history, meets modern science. Out of that experience of 40 days, just living and eating the way that our ancestors, the way that my ancestors did, I overcame my diseases in just 40 days of what I had later called the "Maker's Diet-40 day Health Experience," I not only got well, but I had a new mission in life.

I went from having a certain path to knowing that my life was going to be about helping others, either overcome disease or better yet, avoid it. Out of that, I started a company called Garden of Life, where we manufactured whole food nutritional supplements. Later, I would write 25 books on health and wellness. And recently, Ibecame an organic farmer, and now I'm really on a similar quest to you. I'd love to see this disease, this group of challenges and a tax on our body that we call cancer be ameliorated and I believe it can. I believe out of personal experience that the way we approach cancer from the onset can determine our success or our failure.

Ty: I've seen the picture, along with millions of others of you. Let me go back to when you were 15. So you're saying that you did have the MMR?

Jordan: I did.

Ty: Okay. I thought that's what you were saying.

Jordan: It was my only vaccination. I was not immunized as a child. I took MMR and obviously, we know that there certainly is in our mind valid research and evidence that this vaccine can lead to pervasive developmental disorders and inflammatory bowel disease. I can't say it was the cause, but it certainly set my immune system I believe into a cascade that was in the wrong direction.

Ty: Say, Jordan, it sounds like we really share the same purpose. Our goal with the "The Truth About Cancer" is to educate and to eventually eradicate this cancer epidemic. So share some of the things that you learned with what you call the "Maker's Diet" about how we can get our bodies healthy and stop cancer.

Jordan: When it came to the "Maker's Diet" I was someone who had experienced digestive illnesses—autoimmune disease, if you believe that IBD is an autoimmune disease. But I definitely dealt with all of the—let's call it toxins the microorganism and bacterial, viral fungal invaders, etc. I learned about eating whole nutritious foods. I believe in a mixed—I would call it conscious—omnivorous diet. I really focused on every single thing I put into my mouth—fermented foods, raw foods were a big part of what I did to overcome Crohn's disease and those other conditions and it's still part of what I do today. But nothing prepared me for the shock in 2008 that I received.

Now, I had written books, not only *The Maker's Diet*, but an entire series on specific health issues and diseases, including *The Great Physician's Rx For Cancer*. I helped my own grandmother have a great result with cancer. I've coached thousands of people over the years. In 2008, due to a surgery that I should have had at birth—at least my parents should have considered it—I was led into something in 2008, that once again changed my life forever and it was a cancer diagnosis. Ty, I was really at a crossroads, because here I was helping—in my mind, be part of the solution and all of a sudden, I was not only dealt the blow of a cancer diagnosis, but I had to deal with so many others, the waiting game of, have we gotten it all? Has it spread?

I had what they call an exploratory surgical procedure in my pelvic cavity, thinking it was a hernia, and it ultimately was an advanced form of embryonal testicular cancer. Another reason being for me is I had an undescended testicle that was never operated on, that lodged in my pelvis, not knowing there was a thousand fold increase in cancer risk. And here I am, thinking it was a surgical procedure for an inguinal hernia, or what they call a sports hernia and instead, I was given a cancer diagnosis. I'm writing books on health, I'm helping coach thousands of people, developing products that have been used by millions and now I'm dealing with what many people fear greater than anything.

Ty: So this is a real shocker to you?

Jordan: An understatement.

Ty: Yeah, understatement of the year. You've written all of these books and you've coached hundreds of thousands of people to their health and then you're diagnosed with cancer. What's the first thing that goes through your mind at that point?

Jordan: I wish that I could tell you that I had some great epiphany—that I thought long and hard what would happen if I was ever diagnosed with cancer. But you know what I did, Ty? And it's something that I've done probably seven times in my life and I believe it made all of the difference. I am a man of deep faith. God saved me, God healed me. And in that instant, when I was in the doctor's office and I was getting some of the staples removed and I was sitting in an examination room and I knew that the physician was going to come tell me what stage or what level of metastatic condition I was in—instead, he came through and I said, "So doc, what are the results?" And he said, "We have more to discuss." I knew that wasn't good.

So he left the exam room and a nurse walked me into his office. I told my wife to stand against the door and block the door, and I did something very powerful. I got on my hands and knees—this is in a doctor's office—put my face on the ground and I quoted a Bible verse that I have quoted probably seven times in the past. And I call it Job's Prayer. Job was a man in the Bible who was righteous in all of his ways, lost his kids, lost his finances and lost his health. In Job 1:21, when he lost his children, he put his face on the ground, clothed himself in sack cloth—I wasn't anywhere where I could get some black goat hair to cover myself, but I put my face on the ground in a submissive or humble position and I said, "Naked I came into this earth and naked I shall return. It is the Lord who gives and the Lord who takes away, blessed be the name of the Lord."

What I meant by that, Ty, is this is bigger than me. This is a God-sized attack and it's going to require a God-sized miracle. My first inclination was to show where I stood and where I needed God to be. I did that, the doctor walked back in, my wife and I were sitting there and he said, "You have a fast growing form of cancer," and he said there are treatments now that can help you. Years ago, this cancer killed everyone who was diagnosed with this progressive state. I said, "Doc, God's gonna heal me, and I need time. I need time to attack this." And he said, "I was afraid you would say that. I looked you up online, I know who you are." And he said something I won't say on camera, but he said, "Don't blank around with this. If you wait for conventional treatment, you'll be dead within three months—100 percent chance."

Now, I'm sitting here partially thinking, could it be 97, like, can you throw me a bone here? But then I realized, this is set up for a testimony. We've all heard about life expectancies within the five year mark—68 percent at Stage Two die within five years or 42 percent but 100 percent. And he said, "If it were prostate cancer," and he listed a bunch of other cancers, "I would give you time, but you either need to get to Indiana"—that's where Lance Armstrong went—"or you need to go the Harvard Medical System in Boston—Brigham and Women's Dana-Farber Cancer Institute to see Dr. Jerome Richie, who wrote the latest textbook on this cancer." He said, "You've got to get there within the week. I'm an experienced surgeon in the surgery you're likely to require, but you need someone who does this week in and week out."

I wanted to put it off and I immediately began a program that involved spiritual, mental and physical health. And I want to be very clear, spiritual was first. I did end up really attacking my diet. For the first few weeks, I was on an all raw diet, I postponed the Boston trip. I did go—I wanted to be responsible. I didn't want to make natural health an idol and I think this is very important, Ty. So many of us who are in the natural health movement, we're physicians, we're practitioners we're authors. Those of us who are considered natural health experts, oftentimes make these natural health methods our diet, our idol.

I first said, "Look, Lord, I am going to do whatever it takes to get well." I've got a wonderful wife, and I just had adopted or was in the process of adopting two children in addition to our biological son. I was going to have three kids, two infants, I needed to be here.

Ty: Right.

Jordan: I would never imagine myself undergoing chemotherapy or a surgical procedure which would slice my body up and remove lymph nodes, which I knew I needed. But what I did was—I said to my wife, who is completely onboard with all of what I teach and even as much or more so as me—I said "Honey, just 40 days. Let's do this for 40 days, God did it before, he'll do it again, I'm going to go to Boston."

I had a friend, who was a cardiologist at the Harvard Medical System at Brigham and Women's Hospital. He met us there, went to see Dr. Richie. And I have to tell you, the signs were clear. I was walking down the halls of the most celebrated, educational institution maybe in the world, arguably in the world, and all I felt was darkness. I had tested various markers in the blood that would indicate cancer activity and I was going to do another blood test. I had a number, let's call it 278 in the beginning and the number that needed to be was 1 or less to be normal. I was already on a raw diet for three weeks.

I consulted with Dr. Richie—his first thing he said to me, Ty, and I'm sure a lot of people who are seeking natural health and talking to their doctors about to get this—he said, "Oh, you write books on natural health, don't you?" I said, "Yes." He said, "I've heard of you. Now that you've had this diagnosis what are your readers going to think now?" I'm thinking, every question I asked him, my digestive tract had been rocked with IBD years ago, how will the chemotherapy you're recommending affect me? He didn't really want to answer anything—everything was sarcasm. I got a blood test. I was believing it was going to be good.

On my way out, I picked up what was a little slip—it looked like a receipt from a store. Now mind you, Ty, those of us that have been diagnosed with cancer, this waiting game of an answer, this understanding from checkup to checkup of where we are—it's horrible. Just seeing a little slip of paper that was going to determine my future. So the slip comes out—I'm expecting a number to go down, it goes up. But instead of my heart sinking I did something that was, again, I think a reflex. I said, "I curse this number in the name of Jesus."

Now I know I'm getting spiritual here, but you know what? When it's your life, you call on the strength that you have and my strength has and is in God. I knew He was in control and I said, "I don't care what this number says, I'm going to move forward." My wife and I did not feel peace about proceeding with treatment from Dr. Richie, not chemotherapy, not surgery 40 days. My good friend, Dr. Joe Brasco, who is another co-author of mine—I said, "Dr. Brasco, here's what I've got going on." He said, "Jordan, I love you. I'm into integrated medicine as you know. I can't recommend you avoid conventional treatment." I said, "Listen, just order me the scans, I want to go to the same radiology center. I will do everything in the exact fashion of my diagnosis. Give me 40 days and if I don't see a regression and if I'm not cancer free, I will consider the next step."

Now, mind you, during this time we were investigating IPT. We were investigating a laparoscopic procedure that was being pioneered to avoid the—my opinion—was an archaic surgical procedure to remove my lymph nodes and other things I wanted inside my body. I always said, "I'm doing research, but this isn't for me. I'm healed. I know that God's already paid the price for me. I'm going to walk it out and work, work, work on nutrition and detoxification, but I'm looking for somebody else. This isn't for me." I kept that in mind, but we did some research on integrative cancer treatments, which would be much preferred over the conventional barbaric treatments.

So 40 days. I went to my team at Garden of Life and I told them what had happened to me. They were freaked out. I said "Listen, God has already paid the price for me. I am healed, you're going to see it. But I need to step away from work, six weeks you won't hear from me, no emails, no texts." For me, Ty, that's a miracle if I can go 30 minutes without that much less six weeks. I did the opposite of what most cancer patients do. Cancer patients go and basically submit themselves to the convention. And it's easy. "What do you mean it's easy? You have side effects and hair loss." No, it's easy because you let someone else tell you what to do. You let somebody else tell you how your side effects are going to go. What's going to happen—what your outcome is going to be, what your prognosis is. They can do radiation, chemotherapy, and surgery, but they're doing it. You don't have to think for yourself. There is no individuality. You're just a number.

But I said, "You know what, I'm doing this. I'm going to go after it in every way, 12 to 14 hours a day," Ty, spiritual, emotional, healing, nutrition and detoxification—I started with spiritual. I had written a prayer that really was a combination of scripture and some great teachers and I quoted it three times a day, out loud. And I honestly felt like the demons in hell were holding their ears like a dog whistle to a dog. I was storming the gates of hell to get well here.

Some people will say, "But Jordan, I don't share the same faith as you." All I can tell you is, if you're desperate enough, you will find God on your knees, because I believe in essence, cancer is a spiritual disease. I have a theory on this, from observation, but when you experience this, I've seen people with amyotrophic lateral sclerosis, or Lou Gehrig's Disease, multiple sclerosis. I've seen people with Hashimoto's, I've seen people with rheumatoid arthritis, very disfigured, systemic lupus. I've seen people with all manner of digestive and skin disorders and I've seen them get better. But cancer is different. Cancer attacks the spirit like nothing else.

I'll give you an example. You go in for a physical and you're told you have terminal cancer. You walk out of there different. You literally—it's like your body and your spirit have been hijacked. When you have a headache after a cancer diagnosis, it's not a headache, it's spread to the brain. If your elbow hurts, you don't have a bruise or a broken bone, it's cancer—it's spreading. You wake up every morning like you're looking behind your back—over your shoulder—when is this disease going to kill me? I believe, Ty, that people who are diagnosed with cancer they either make up their mind immediately that they're going to conquer or they begin to die that minute.

I've heard years ago, that there was a study done and I believe this is probably a myth, but think about it for a moment. One hundred healthy people go into their annual physical and they're told—every one of them, "I'm sorry, I have terrible news. You have cancer." Lab coats—stethoscope—doctor—small g-god, we elevate doctors in this country and world to God—you're told you have cancer and you have six months to live. I believe that those 100 people without cancer—no pathology here—I believe about 50 of them die within six months. You know why? Because they leave there and they say, "I've got cancer. I've got six months to live." They quote, "get their affairs in order." I am a firm believer now more than ever that out of the overflow of the heart the mouth speaks and the Bible says, "Life and death is in the power of the tongue." So for me, when I was diagnosed, I told a handful of people. People wanted to pray for me, but even going public would have been overwhelming.

Ty: Right.

Jordan: Because every time I talk to somebody, I could feel their pain and they were scared—I trusted. I would talk to friends who were physicians and they would say, "Jordan, I know you have faith that if anyone can beat it, you can." I talked to the head of oncology—and he said, "Don't mess around with this, this is serious."

It was hard for me when I talked to my physician friends about dealing with things. So I told a few people, but I made it a point, Ty—I didn't say the word cancer very much during those 40 days. I didn't call myself a "cancer victim." People go around and say, "My son's autistic, I'm diabetic," and if you're goint to have a title or a label, don't make it that. It's as if you're saying and believing and receiving that. I didn't receive it.

I spent 40 days working my rear end off. I literally was in a sauna, infrared sauna, two hours a day. I was doing amazing raw food cocktails, phytotherapy or herbalism, consuming an all raw omnivorous diet. I went after it. You know what I didn't do? Suffer in misery. I had more joy and more peace during my 40 days of healing than most people have with all of the money and all of the stuff in the world. I was facing a death sentence, 100 percent chance, and I decided to live. I chose it from the beginning. I walked it out. I prayed those three times a day. I went back over every memory that I had in my life. This is work. Starting from two years old and any time anyone hurt me or I had hurt them, I wrote the experience down and I prayed until I felt peace. Ty, I'm talking about when I was ten years old and my baseball coach told me, "If you strike out again, I'm going to do something terrible to you." We actually store cellular memories, emotions and failures or unforgiveness that turned to bitterness and we store it in my mind, like our body grows cancer cells.

I felt like if we fear a malignancy, we should fear unforgiveness and bitterness much more. I dealt with issues. It took me days, but I dealt with everyone. I'm talking about thousands of memories. And people say, "Well, Jordan, what does it have to do with my health that someone turned me down for the prom when I'm 16?" What did it make you feel like? Did you say you were worthless? Did you decide you weren't good enough? There are people out there, Ty, that have had marriages with infidelity, they've had their spouse divorce them, they've had their parents tell them they don't love them. These are serious and we store them in our body like a virus on a hard drive computer and if we don't take care of it, it will eat us away. Taking a pill is easier. Taking an IV cocktail of hydrogen peroxide and ascorbic acid and other vitamins and minerals, that's easy. Forgiveness is hard. We dealt with that in my life—hard core.

And then the nutrition, detoxification—as I said, 12 to 14 hours a day—I was doing essential oil therapy. I was on infrared heating mats, I was trying to exercise the best I could on a mini-trampoline 20 to 30 minutes a day. Everything you can think of, everything that I knew. I put together that program and you know what else I did? I found a doctor, Dr. Emil Shandel, in Fort Lauderdale, Florida. He would give me not only one blood test, but tested three ways every two weeks and then there was the 40 day, CT scan, with contrast. So I could it exactly the same way, same radiologist, although, he didn't realize I wasn't under an oncologist's supervision at the time.

So first two weeks program, hard core. I go, get my blood drawn, I'm praying the whole time—now remember my number was about 278, so to speak, my HCG, which is typically the pregnancy hormone, but in testicular cancer, oftentimes it is elevated. I went 278, told Dr. Shandel, he also recommends nutrition and integrative medicine, but he's got his own laboratory that he would run. I took the blood test, three days later, which was the two week mark, I was going to get my results. I see my phone ring, Dr. Shandel's name comes. I begin to shake. I had a lot of peace and a lot of faith, but man, when you're going to hear those results. Look at what was riding on this.

I answer it and he says, "Jordan," and I said, "Yes?" He said I got your results. I tested three ways, but you said you were in the 260s, 270, I'm getting 32, 20, 26. And I said, "Praise God." And then I told my parents. I told my wife and then I said, "But wait a minute. What if he tested a different way? What if it's not comparable with the methodology?" Doubt began to creep in. But, no time for that, two more weeks of hard core spiritual, emotional mental and physical, nutrition, detoxification, healing, go get my blood drawn again, praying, praying, praying, wanting this to be a positive result. I got a call. It was on a Friday afternoon. I see Dr. Shandel's name on my caller ID, I answer, he says, "Jordan," I said, "Yes," he said, "I have your results." He said, "I'm getting zero, zero, zero."

Ty: Wow.

Jordan: I was elated. Praise God, called my wife, called my parents. And then I said, "Well, wait a minute, what if it wasn't my blood he tested, what if it was somebody else's?" That instant of doubt can just ruin all of this peace, but I moved on.

Two more weeks, talked to Dr. Brasco, my friend who was helping—and just order the diagnostic for me, etc. And he said, "Jordan, I am so thrilled, I would love to see one more result of zero, zero, zero." Two more weeks, I dug in, I was doing more therapy, more detoxification, more emotional healing, spiritual battling than ever before and I went and got my blood tested and in three days, I was going to get my results. Dr. Shandel called again, see his number on my phone, my hand begins to shake. This is it. This is the big moment. This is huge. It's confirmatory and I answer and he said, "Jordan, what's your address again? I want to make sure I have the right blood results?" I said, "C'mon." And he said, "Jordan, it's zero, zero, zero."

Ty: Wow.

Jordan: I was excited. I said, "Praise God." I called my wife, called my parents and then I made a mistake. I looked online. You see I had never gone to WebMD, never looked at any of the PubMed articles. I didn't see what percentage of people who had the cancer diagnosis I did live or die, but I did now. I said "Okay, I have blood results that would be as good or better than around the chemo. I'm normal, but how many people have a normal HCG, but still have enlarged lymph nodes?" I found research and what did disturb me was the 94 percent of people with testicular cancer have a cure, that's a testicular cancer.

I looked at all causes of death and I realized these treatments are not helping people the way that they should be and I knew that. But I also learned that some people who have a zero HCG still do have residual traces of cancer or even enlarged lymph nodes. It got me down a little bit, but no time for that. It was time for celebration. A couple of days later, I had my CAT scan. I went in and I don't know about you, but if you've ever had an enclosed CAT scan or MRI—I guess I'm more claustrophobic than I thought—that was awful. But I prayed the whole time. I don't believe in getting radiation, or contrast fluid or drinking barium or any of that nonsense, but I needed to show the world what God was going to do in my life.

Three days later, I was going to get the results. Dr. Brasco said, "Jordan do you want them to send the results to me or do you want them first?" I said, "Joe, I actually can't handle hearing from you, I need them right away." He said, "Okay, they'll be ready for you at 11:00." I got up in the morning, and this was someone who had faith and peace most of the 40 days. I was sitting at my counter consuming some liquid herbs, holding a glass and I began to think about all the ramifications of the results that were going to come. What happened if I still had the cancer? What would I have to say to the industry? What would I have to say to my family? How would life change for me?

I began to have fear again and my hands shook as the glass fell out, smashed all over the tile floor. And I said, "God, I know I'm going to regret this. I know that I'm going to regret not having faith." I quoted another scripture. "I want to believe, but help me in my unbelief." I said to my wife, Nicki, "You've got to drive me to the radiologist center. I'm too shaky." So she drove me and we approached the doors in the front. Got out of the car, and everything slowed down. This was it. This was the moment of truth. I saw the woman, the receptionist at the front with a manila envelope, walked in, opened the door, and she handed it to me. I said to my wife, "I don't want to open this in here let's go out in the parking lot."

I stood there in the parking lot—opened up this envelope and I pulled out the front page and it listed a bunch of stuff. I don't know if you know a bunch of stuff on a radiology report is not good, so I saw enlarged lymph nodes, I saw all kind of tumor activity and my heart sank. I looked at the top of the page and it said, July 3rd, which was my diagnosis date. They had to stick the diagnosis document in there. Nothing is easy. So I flipped the page real quick and I look and I see, "normal, normal, normal, normal."

Ty: Wow.

Jordan: I drop the packet, I started to weave, I hugged my wife and I couldn't believe it, but yet I believed it. It's like nothing I could ever explain. I was free. This disease that I never claimed was a part of my life was now officially gone. I called 20 or 30 people that I had shared this with and they were the best phone calls I've ever had.

Ty: I bet.

Jordan: To be able to tell them what miracle had happened in my life. Some of them admitted to me that they were really concerned. Some of them were overjoyed and said they knew all along. But it was an awesome day for me. And my son, Joshua, who was four or five years old at the time—I said to my wife, "Hey, can we pick up Joshua from school and take him to ToysRUs and buy him anything in the store?" She said, "Why?" I said, "I can't explain to him what miracle I've just experienced other than telling him you can get any toy you want." Of course, he was excited. He asked me why and I said, "Dad's experienced a great gift. God gave me a great gift to me." From that point on I decided that part of my life was going to be devoted to helping people overcome this dreaded disease.

Ty, as I stand here with you today, I am convinced that what you eat, the supplements you take, IV therapies, hydrotherapies, certainly infrared saunas and various exercises and various machines can make a difference in your health. Can help you build your immune system. I'm convinced that emotional health is critical, but I can tell you something that probably no one else in this series will—cancer starts with a spiritual disease. And if I were to be with somebody for 20 minutes after their diagnosis, I bet I could predict if they're going to live and thrive or suffer and die. Don't own the disease. Cancer is not who you are. I think you've realized after all of these interviews that cancer isn't one disease. How could it affect somebody's blood, another person's bone marrow, someone's colon? How could it be a solid tumor in one person and not in another? And be the same disease? The name cancer is evil, but it's evil for different ways than we think. You decide if you win or lose. I think you're going to find the common denominator in people that are survivors or conquerors as I like better, are those that decide to go after it and win. Don't sit back and let somebody tell you what to do. Make the most important decisions of your life. You know what's crazy, Ty?

Ty: What?

Jordan: If you try natural health with cancer and you die—"they killed you." If you go conventional and you die—"we did the best that we could do."

Ty: Right.

Jordan: How is that possible? We lost loved ones. You've lost loved ones. And you know what, I'm writing a book soon and I think the most appropriate title is, *To Hell With Cancer*. That's where it came from in my opinion. I want to help send it back. I do believe that if somebody—if anybody wants to overcome this dreaded disease, you start by making the decision that cancer will not win. Cancer will not own you. You are not a cancer patient. You are more than a conqueror. And frankly, next time I hear somebody get diagnosed with cancer, my first encouragement is going to be—you say it, "To Hell With Cancer."

We go around and celebrate wearing pink socks and pink ribbons and buying pink lemonade on airlines to contribute to cancer. It sure does. It's ridiculous. I coach youth sports. I won't wear pink. I won't put pink on. I don't believe in that. Why? Because the pharmaceutical intervention, conventional methods are not saving lives. I don't tell people if they should or shouldn't do conventional treatment. But no matter what you choose, conventional or integrative and I far believe in diet, detoxification, integrative medicine—but no matter what course you go on, you must believe cancer starts as a spiritual disease. And if you don't get on your knees and if you don't believe that your healing is available—first spiritually, then emotionally, then physically, your chances are much greater of succumbing to a disease that we've given too much power.

Ty: Wow, Jordan. Thanks for sharing your story. It's incredible what you've just shared with us and it's incredible for several reasons. One of the things that you've mentioned that's so powerful, I believe is when you said you quoted the verse, "I believe, but help my unbelief." It is about belief, isn't it? It is about believing you can conquer and I love the "Cancer Conqueror." You're not a cancer victim, you're a conqueror. So let's—your 40 days. I know that people that have watched this, they're going to want to know in the 40 days you did the spiritual healing, the forgiveness, you got rid of all this baggage potentially. You did the emotional work. You did the physical work. As far as you mentioned rebounding. But I know people are going to say what did you eat?

Jordan: Absolutely.

Ty: What were the oils? You mentioned essential oils. Give us a quick rundown of what you ate and the essential oils that you used over that 40 day period.

Jordan: I did essential oil massage every day while on hot infrared mat. So not only was I perspiring out toxins, but I was getting an essential oil massage. In fact today, I have taken these oil blends that I use—and they're the basic ones, frankincense, myrrh, galbanum, we certainly use lavender, we use citrus oils. So nothing unusual in terms of the oils. I have actually put together a way to apply them and I believe in a way for spiritual healing and I call it BHW or "By His Wounds" and this is a very spiritual message. It takes essential oils and applies them in all of the areas that Jesus bled for our sins.

Look Ty, I am not telling everyone who is watching this to believe exactly the way I believe. What I'm telling them is what I did. I certainly believe the truth is the truth and principles behind my faith and action work. So I apply the essential oils to my feet. I apply them to my forehead and my scalp. I apply them to my side—the rib areas. I apply them sort of close to underarms, sometimes I'll use a carrier oil because underarm area is sensitive and then I have someone apply them to my back 39 times. Jesus took 39 lashes.

If you believe like I do, jump all over this. I did essential oil massage every single day, several hours. I did various lymphatic treatments. I recommend lymphatic massage. There are a lot of things now that I do that are even greater than I did previously. Phytotherapy, herbal therapy is critical, fermented powerful herbs in various combinations is amazing and my diet is all raw, omnivorous, no salt. I believe that certain mineral salts are really good for you, but in this case, all raw.

I did green juices added a little bit of raw coconut cream. I did raw dairy, made these raw butter drinks. I call it a super lipid drink which helps get the combination of botanicals and foods into your system quickly and doesn't taste the best. I consumed raw organic grass fed beef, raw salmon—not only for the omega 3s, but the astaxanthin. Consumed lots of coconut products. I took systemic enzymes, I'm a big believer in systemic enzymes, 60 a day because I believe fully in Dr. Kelly, Dr. Gonzalez' work.

But the *One Answer to Cancer* book is pretty clear. Followed some of those things. There are various other elements that I had. I made sure that my vitamin D levels were high. I either got a lot of sun or took a whole food vitamin D supplement and that was pretty much it. It kept me really busy, but lots of raw fats. My opinion is that raw fats are critical to not only help build the system in the cells, but to help pull waste out. Lots of raw pastured eggs. I did various mineral clays and zeolites along with certain probiotics that I developed and each and every day worked at.

I did things like foot baths. I walked on the beach. But Ty, it isn't simply one food, it's not avoiding something, it's not one detoxification method, it's a total commitment to healing. Here's the best news. I haven't told very many people about my story, but people have come to me and I've seen amazing results that are as miraculous as mine by following similar or the same principles. But it all starts with faith, and confession. You either own this so-called disease or it owns you. There is no in between.

I'm a huge sports fan. We celebrate Olympic gold medalists, Hall of Fame athletes, Most Valuable Players, but you know who I celebrate? Those who pick themselves up by their bootstraps, and go after this Goliath that is cancer. Bottom line, you're David—it's Goliath. But those five smooth stones are in your sling and it's time to get going. I celebrate the heroes who overcome this disease that's taken our loved ones—taken your loved ones and I'm not going to stand idly by anymore. "To Hell With Cancer."

Ty: I love that Jordan, "To Hell With Cancer," and I love the analogy. David and Goliath. But you got him right between the eyes with this 40 day diet plan and the emotional plan, the spiritual plan—all of this wrapped together.

One of the most fascinating things about what you just said to me was about the importance of the fats. There's a lot of fats in many things, but you mentioned the fats. There's so many diets that we hear. Stay away from all of the fats, but it sounds like that was an integral piece of your food that you were eating during that 40 days that helped you to heal.

Jordan: Absolutely. I was easily consuming 12 raw eggs a day, I consumed what would be the equivalent of sticks of raw butter. And mind you, I'm an organic farmer, so I have access to the best of the best. I believe that fats not only nourish the body, but I believe some fats—fats from avocado, fats from eggs—act in a sacrificial way to remove fat soluble toxins like metals and other toxins we've been exposed to and that's really critical.

Most people think of detox as green juice and I drank plenty of it. Drank coconut water—lots of raw cleansing juices. I had a tomato and cucumber drink with unheated honey and all kinds of amazing nutrients added, but fat is absolutely the key and it was for me and I've seen it work for others. Not to say that a juice cleanse or various fasts don't work, but in my case, I feel very strongly about the consumption of raw fats if you're going after this dreaded disease that is beatable called cancer.

Ty: Yes, it's interesting that you did it from the perspective that worked for you. That diet works for you. I think it's important for people that are watching to know that you treat it on an individual basis. But I think that many things—many of the takeaways that you can get from what you just said are number one, you've got to believe—and number two, you've got to not have a victim mentality—to see that you are already a cancer conqueror. I love that term. Do you mind if we use that?

Jordan: Absolutely. Survivor means you're barely hanging on. You're thriving, you're conquering. That's what it takes. This is a big game here. This is the big game. Get ready for it. Gird yourself up. Don't let anyone around you who is going to say, "Oh, but you have cancer, how long do you have to live?" I did not allow anyone in my life to speak death over me. The doctors that spoke death, were no longer my doctors. Relatives who spoke death, temporarily, were no longer my relatives—if you know what I mean.

Ty: Yeah.

Jordan: Get yourself an inner circle that supports you and believes you and go after this thing with gusto. But the universal truths here are, believe, have faith, and get that bitterness out of your body. I don't care if you use oxidative therapies, I don't care if you are using hyperthermia, I don't care if you're going to use all of these different various frequency machines. There are all kinds of good things to do, but you've got to believe, you've got to have faith, you have to speak the truth. You can't accept this diagnosis as your life.

This doctor with a stethoscope and a lab coat does not know your future. He is not God, she is not God. But there is a God and He has already conquered sickness and death and my results prove that in my life and I believe it can in so many others.

Ty: Amen brother and you know what? Cancer Conqueror, this is the last episode and we're going to call it "Cancer Conquerors" now. I love that. I'm giving you credit now.

Jordan: All right.

Ty: I'm ready for that. Thank you so much for sharing brother. Great information. God Bless you too.

[end of transcript]

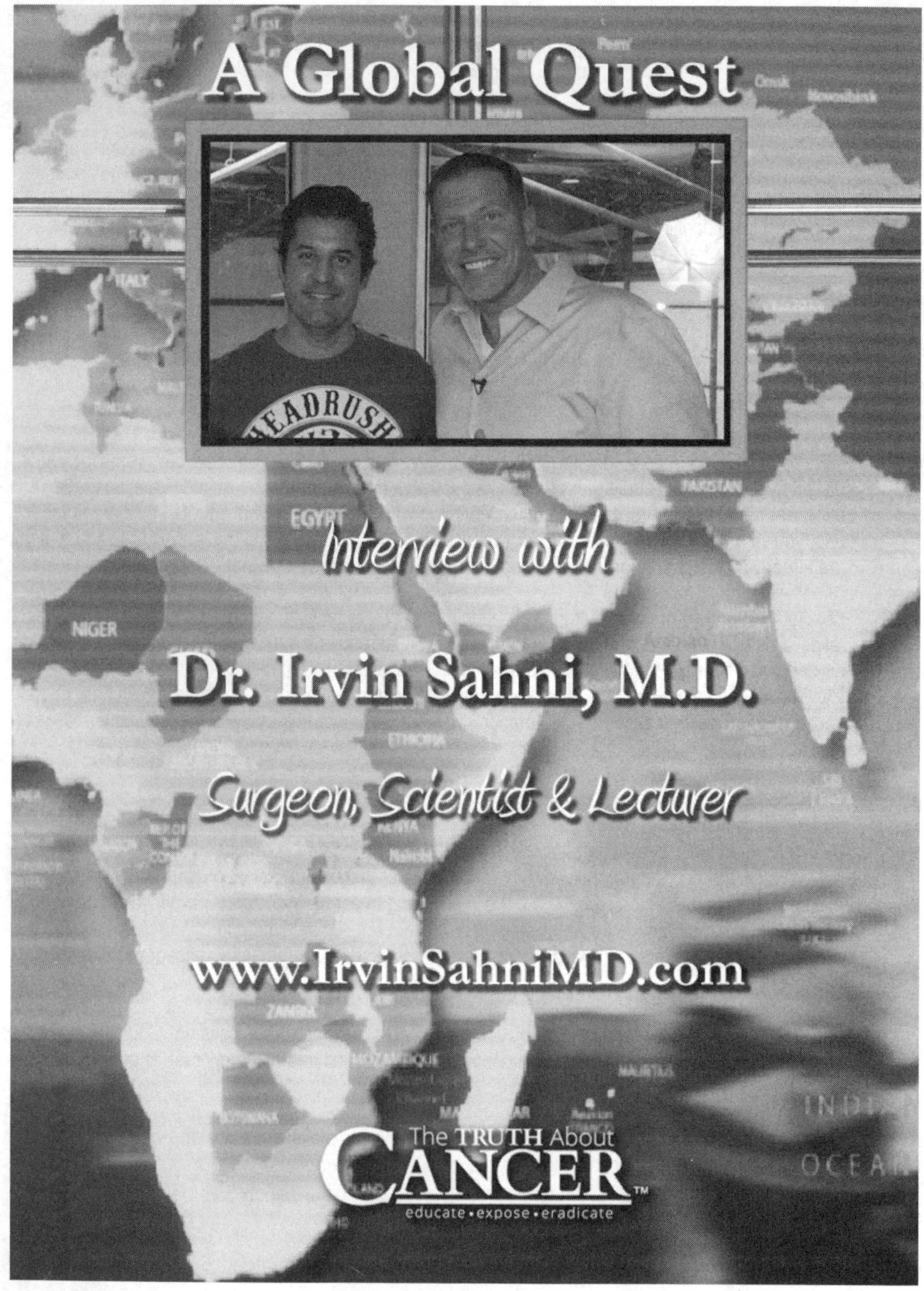
A Global Quest
Interview with
Dr. Irvin Sahni, M.D.
Surgeon, Scientist & Lecturer
www.IrvinSahniMD.com
The TRUTH About CANCER
educate • expose • eradicate

Ty: Well, I'm really happy to be back in Seguin, Texas with my good buddy, Dr. Irvin Sahni. Man, thanks for the invite today.

Dr. Sahni: Glad to have you, bud.

Ty: So last year, you were in both of the documentaries, *The Quest* and *The Quest Continues*. Now, *Global Quest* and I had to get back and get some more information from you. You were one of the very popular ones last year. One of the big comments we got was about your dramatic weight loss. People really liked to see the fact that you had implemented a lot of the things that you had actually learned in the first documentary, and you dropped a bunch of weight.

We wanted to have you back to get your perspective on some other things this time. First thing I wanted to ask you about is, what's been happening in the last year?

Dr. Sahni: What's been happening for me personally?

Ty: Yeah, just personal. What's been happening?

Dr. Sahni: Well, I have been working on growing my practice, and of course, continuing to try provide quality healthcare, and provide good service to my patients. And raising my three kids. My daughter is eight now, and my twin boys are six, and they all go to the Christian Academy together.

In terms of my health, with anybody, it's a constant battle. You've got to keep your eye on the ball, and it's a lot of work. It's not like you just lose weight, and it stays off magically. And certainly, I've tried to continue to learn. And a lot of that has been thanks to you and other friends and sources of information to have access to unbiased information. I haven't watched TV in ten years and I still haven't. I get all of my information mostly through alternative sources.

Ty: So, it's been a good year, living the dream, right?

Dr. Sahni: It's been a good year. Yeah. It's been a great year. Sure.

Ty: Good. Good. Yeah. Well, I'm excited to be back. I wanted to ask you about this case that's in the news here recently. And this is about a doctor in Detroit, Dr. Farid Fata, that was convicted and sentenced to 45 years for prescribing chemotherapy to patients that didn't even have cancer.

Dr. Sahni: This recently came out in the news, and I just became aware of it I think when everybody else did just recently when he was sentenced. Certainly, there's probably information about it before then but I tried to get as much as I could off of the conventional media website.

So my understanding is he was a 52-year-old Lebanese man who became a citizen of the United States, I believe, in 2009, but he was running one of the largest cancer centers in Michigan. I believe it was the largest actually in Michigan. I think he had seven clinics. I read some stuff on it. I lost count, but it's something in the order of six or seven clinics. He billed Medicare, according to the articles that I read, $169 million—Medicare, and Blue Cross, and probably some other insurers. That's a lot of money. That's an unusually high number.

I don't know how many providers there were. Sure, I guess if your network was big enough, maybe that wouldn't be such a large number. But if it's just him and a few other people, that's a pretty insane number.

So obviously, this is probably the most egregious example of Medicare fraud, but to me, that's just the tip of the iceberg. This person, this man, is a monster. He committed one of the most heinous acts, probably the most heinous act I know of in American history at this point.

We're talking about people with cancer, people who when—you're told you have cancer, you're desperate. You're scared to death. You're vulnerable and you're really putting your trust in, in this case, conventional medicine, to help you. And so this guy completely violated that trust and treated people who didn't even have cancer with very expensive cancer treatments, and it's a disaster.

Whatever punishment he gets, it's not enough. He killed people's family members. One person reported that all their teeth fell out. All of the side effects that are associated with receiving chemotherapy, you can imagine. He wasn't just treating—there's 500 people who even didn't have cancer, but he was also over-treating people who had cancer and were in remission. In one case, there was a drug—and again, I don't remember the name of it—but it was a drug that you should only receive 24 treatments, and he gave—one example is he gave a patient 122 treatments. So, the guy was obviously completely driven by money. He is clearly, in my opinion a sociopath, and thank goodness, he has been taken off the streets.

A whistle blower in 2011—she was a nurse—she came to his clinic to apply for a job noted discrepancies, things that were quite unusual to her, and she reported that to the Medical Board. She tried to be a whistleblower, and they basically disregarded her concerns, which is kind of sad because this could have stopped sooner. It wasn't until a couple of years later that this was brought to the attention of another doctor. I believe a patient went for a second opinion. But whatever the circumstances, this other doctor ended up reviewing 25 of these cases and realized that how ridiculous, how completely fraudulent they were. He then became a whistle blower, and that's when this guy, Farid Fata, was investigated and ultimately taken down.

Ty: What is your opinion on the impact that the current system had on this set of crimes? Because for chemotherapy, doctors were able to purchase that at wholesale, and they basically retailed the chemotherapy. They're able to mark it up. So what kind of an impact did that have potentially on this case?

Dr. Sahni: Well, it's extremely ludicrous. This is the reason that people are—for the same reason that people aren't out selling organic spinach, which arguably is very healthy for you and can—eating healthy and having good nutrition can certainly have a very positive impact on your health, but there's no money in it because you can't make billions of dollars selling organic spinach. I mean maybe you can, but not in the same way.

The point is you can't patent that, and the premium that's put on by these drug companies and the—I don't want to say excessive because that's all relative, and this is capitalism. But I mean I think you can argue excessive profits in some cases that are available will ensnare someone like him who is obviously inherently greedy, unethical, and a sociopath. And if those profits weren't there to be made, I would question whether he would have done any of these things. I don't think it would have been either an option for him.

So I'm not blaming the pharmaceutical companies, but certainly, the opportunity was there because of the very lucrative nature of being an oncologist. He had his own imaging centers, if I understand correctly. He also had his own pharmacies, if I understand correctly. And so that added a completely different element than, say, just someone who is an employed oncologist. He was really engaging in the very lucrative business aspects of oncology.

Oncology is an unbelievably lucrative field of medicine, especially if you're in the business side of it. I had been told by an oncologist, and I don't have this confirmed in a periodical or the research, but the average cost of treating a cancer patient is $80,000. I don't know if that's Medicare, or Blue Cross, or where that number comes from, but that's a big number. That's big money. And again, I'm not indicting the pharmaceutical companies, but they made a lot of money off him billing Medicare and Blue Cross $169 million too for unnecessary treatments. They're not going to have to give that money back.

I'm not saying that they should. I'm not trying to get into that area, but I understand that there's a lot of people that made money off that deal besides him—a lot of money. So he's marking up, like you said, the retail aspect of that. He's marking up those drugs and making a lot of money, but those drug companies, and those people who sell those imaging centers, and all the other ancillary revenue that's associated with treating cancer, there was lots of people obviously making money. I think he billed $169 million, but I think he actually collected $93 million. That's a lot of money. I think that was somewhere between 2006 and 2009, so this is a busy, busy clinic.

Ty: Thirty million a year.

Dr. Sahni: Yeah. If those numbers are accurate, that's a busy clinic. That's a lot of fraud. The problem, the thing that is so disgusting to me about this situation—I'm a spine surgeon. I'm an orthopedic surgeon. If someone comes to me, and I'm certain we're not saying that orthopedic surgeons and spine surgeons are immune to fraud, but the big difference here is that if someone comes to me with a broken arm or arthritic knee, they feel the pain. They know there's a problem.

If I tell someone who doesn't have any pain that they need to have a shot in their knee, or need to have their knee replaced, or have their knee scoped, or even go to physical therapy, it's going to be pretty easy for them to clue in on that, that that doesn't make sense. It just doesn't make sense. But you don't necessarily—in fact in most cases, you don't feel cancer. You're told you have cancer, but you don't necessarily feel it. You can. You can certainly have some symptoms.

But in many cases, when you're diagnosed with cancer, there's not symptoms associated with that. So you're taking the word. You're trusting someone to tell you the truth and then to further recommend treatments, which are incredibly toxic, incredibly disabling, fatal in some cases. It's just unbelievable what this guy did. It's sad.

Ty: Yeah, it is. You know, what's bizarre to me is that they—I've seen news reports of people that have said, "This man killed my relative with these chemotherapy treatments," that they died from the treatment. But it's such a double thing. It's such an oxymoron, I guess, for us to be seeing this on the mainstream news that the chemotherapy killed these people that were diagnosed for cancer that really didn't have it, but they died from the treatment. But they refused to believe that the chemotherapy killed someone that did have cancer.

Dr. Sahni: Sure. And if you take that a step further, and again, these are numbers that we need to be confirmed by the individual, but I think in some cases, there are reports or there are statistics that show that if you look at cancer treatment and chemotherapy specifically - and again, I'm not 100 percent sure about but you and I have discussed it before - the overall success rate of treating people with cancer utilizing chemotherapy is somewhere in the neighborhood of three percent. Let's just say it's ten percent.

Ty: Yeah, when you look at five years. Sure.

Dr. Sahni: That even means—I'm not indicting an oncologist who's following normal treatment protocols but that means even if you're doing it right, even if you're an honest oncologist, you're still poisoning 90 percent of the people arguably. Obviously, hindsight is 20/20. When it doesn't work, it doesn't work and they can't predict that, but yeah.

To me, if I had a surgical procedure that only worked three percent of the time, I would never even consider doing that surgical procedure. To me, that would be insane. Unless, of course, it was an emergency, a trauma case, and I guess you could argue that with cancer. The point being that even in the best of cases, when you're delivering chemotherapy appropriately, you're still harming a lot of people without any benefit or at least ultimate benefit. If that's what your point was.

Ty: Yeah, I think it is. To me, it just seems like it's a complete illogical inconsistency to claim that.

Dr. Sahni: When I hear about this guy, you start thinking about Charles Manson. You start thinking about Ted Bundy. You start thinking about Adolf Hitler, or Stalin, or any of the many, many people that have hurt large groups of people—mass murderers, rapists, whatever you want to call them. People that are tyrannical. But this guy in one sense is worse than, say, Adolf Hitler, because at least if you were a victim of Adolf Hitler, you knew when the SS was coming or you knew when Adolf Hitler was coming. You better run.

If you're one African tribe attacking another African tribe, when the guys are coming down the road with machine guns, you know to run. But in this case, you're trusting this person with your life. You're going to him asking for help. And even in cases where people really did have cancer, he was inappropriately continuing to administer chemotherapy to them when they didn't need it. Or just as bad or worse giving chemotherapy to people who simply didn't even have cancer.

To me, that's just unbelievable. It really is mind boggling that someone could be that evil and that greedy.

Ty: One could make the argument that chemotherapy is never needed in a sick body, couldn't they?

Dr. Sahni: Well, yes. And here's where I might diverge from you a little bit, from this line of thinking, and we talked about this before. In my opinion, chemotherapy is very different, depending on the type of cancer. So if you look at, let's say—here's a really interesting comparison. If you look at gonad cancer—

Ty: Testicular, sure.

Dr. Sahni: Yeah, testicular cancer, seminoma, and you compare it to the female version of the gonads, which is the ovaries. If you look at patients who have testicular cancer, their survival rates with chemotherapy are 95 percent. So, I would certainly argue, in the case of seminoma, that particular chemotherapy, although it may be toxic, tends to be very successful. In the case of pancreatic cancer or ovarian cancer, the results are abysmal. And the five-year survival rate is somewhere in the order of a few percentage points. And so in that case, yeah, I completely agree.

But there are some forms of cancer where I do believe chemotherapy is a good option. Now if there were a natural way to treat that cancer, then absolutely. I've always argued in all the Quest Series that they are not necessarily telling people, and I know you're not telling people to abstain or avoid conventional treatments, what you're saying is there's other choices out there. And after reviewing natural means or alternative means and you want to go back and do those conventional treatments, maybe because it's seminoma versus ovarian cancer, then that's exactly what this is all about.

It's about education, information, and being self-empowered in making your own decisions based on the facts, not inserting your bias. But the problem is when you go to see an oncologist, at least as far as I know, they don't offer you those other opportunities. The menu is very short. The menu is typically three things—chemotherapy, radiation, and surgery.

And in fact, if an oncologist wanted to discuss other alternative or natural means of curing your cancer, they would probably be investigated by the medical board and possibly even prosecuted in some cases depending on the situation. Not only are they not incentivized to do it, but I think in a lot of cases, they are probably scared to even bring up some of these truths.

Ty: Actually, we agree on that—the testicular cancer. There's a few rare cancers that the chemo does actually work on. I think my question was that it was really more intended to bring out the fact that people are not sick with cancer because they're shy on chemotherapy. So the reason they're sick is not that they're chemotherapy-deficient. Not that there are certain cancers that chemo doesn't work on, like some non-Hodgkin's lymphoma, testicular cancer, and a few other cancers.

Dr. Sahni: Chemotherapy is not a vitamin. Chemotherapy is not a vitamin D or a vitamin C. If they were to correct their physiology, and they were to give their body the nutrition or abstain from the toxins that cause the cancer, they would actually solve the problem. If someone is exposed to a chemical that is known to cause cancer, they get cancer. They get chemotherapy, and let's say they get lucky, and they're successfully treated with chemotherapy, but then they go back and get exposed to that chemical again.

Well, guess what? They're going to have cancer again. The chemotherapy didn't fix that. The chemotherapy may have placated it, even if it worked, like we just said. And in some cases, only three percent success rate overall. The problem is not a deficiency of chemotherapy. The problem is some other outside factor that's causing them to be sick.

Ty: That's definitely what I was trying to get to is that chemotherapy can be a very effective Band-Aid. Sometimes it can be a huge Band-Aid, and maybe it's a permanent Band-Aid, but it never really corrects that imbalance.

Dr. Sahni: I think a lot of people still believe—because I talk to patients all the time about this—and they really believe that the fact that they're going to get cancer is sort of preordained. It's in their genes. It's nothing they can do about that. They have no control over it.

They don't realize that by cleaning up their body or cleaning up the area in their life that's toxic that they absolutely cannot only prevent themselves from getting cancer but even cure or reverse cancer once they have it. I think that's still part of the big misconception. There's sort of bad luck. What can I do? What can I do but go to the doctor and get chemotherapy, radiation, or surgery.

Ty: One of the things you can do is change your diet to stay healthy. Diet has a big impact on it. One of the quotes that you gave us last year for the Quest was—I said how much education did you get in medical school on nutrition? You said pretty much none.

Dr. Sahni: Pretty much none. You know, let's expound upon that. I don't know how it is now. You would hope it would be better, but I'm not so sure that it is. This all goes back to, I think, something you did talk about in one of the episodes, the Flexner report, and basically how corporate America, once again, intervened, limited people's choice, controlled the narrative, and basically influenced on what kind of medical education the doctors get with the current medical education.

And I went to one of the best medical schools in the country, Baylor College of Medicine. It's an outstanding school, but this is what they taught. We spent an inordinate amount of time in basic science—there's basic science and there's clinical. Basic science is the first portion of medical school where you learn out of a book, basically sit in a classroom. And we went on, and on, and on about all kinds of different pharmaceutical drugs.

We did have a nutrition course, and basically, here's vitamin D, and here's the molecule, and here's the mechanism of vitamin D and then here's how somebody gets rickets, that kind of thing. But not here's how to eat, or you should tell your patients to eat this way, or to eat naturally or synthetic vitamins versus natural vitamins, or anything along those lines. And then that's literally a few days maybe that we cover that kind of stuff. Certainly, vitamin D might come up a couple of times again, but again, we're talking about the molecule and metabolism.

And that's important information, but that's not learning nutrition, and that's not learning practically how to educate someone. It's like they don't teach doctors a thing about business. And then they ultimately come out and a lot of them suffer for that reason trying to run their own business. Who know? Maybe that's by design as well. Anyway, different topic. But certainly, the education that we get concerning nutrition is non-existent. It was non-existent. Pretty much none is probably an overstatement.

Ty: Pretty much none.

Dr. Sahni: Yeah, pretty much none is too much. I didn't really understand practical nutrition, if you will, until after med school, until after being in practice.

Ty: So you learned that after school, after you got out of medical school.

Dr. Sahni: Which is very normal as a doctor. There's a lot of surgical procedures that I've learned because we don't go back to residency every time a new procedure comes out. We have to be able to reeducate ourselves. But the person has to be willing to endeavor in that reeducation. I told you the story. We'll talk about it again.

When I was in the midst of losing weight, I was juicing. So many different ways to do it and there's so many different healthy ways to do it. I chose intermittent fasting, and I chose juicing, and I was going green and raw and trying to stay away from processed foods and so forth.

I ran into a doctor in the doctor's lounge in the hospital here locally. We talked about this, and I said, "Hey, you know, if you lose weight, if you get off diet," just talked about the benefits. He goes, "Well, why would you do that?" He goes, "I'm just going to eat my cheese nachos and take my cholesterol medicine." I don't know if he's messing with me a little bit, probably. Kind of sent me through the roof. I was like, "really?" "And by the way, if we did that, we wouldn't have a job." Again, probably messing with me to some degree, but this is how these guys think.

I could tell you right now that if every doctor thought more like me and really pushed—let's not say it that way. If every doctor really pushed nutrition and really, really generally pushed nutrition, it would be generations—it would be never really before all of us would be out of a job. There's always going to be a job. There's going to be a use for pharmaceutical medications. I'm not anti-pharmaceutical medication, I'm anti crutch. Some people use drugs as a crutch and then make zero effort to improve their health, and take personal responsibility for their health.

We've talked about this before 50 percent, and some people even say 75 percent. It depends on what you look at, but certainly, it's true. At least 50 percent, as you get older, of the medications you're taking are going to counteract the side effects of the first 50 percent of the medications that you're taking.

A lot of medications are taken because you're having side effects from the first one. So it's this sort of downward spiral of taking more and more medications. I sort of have this alert in my mind. My computer screen, I think we have maybe a 15-inch monitor—I'm not sure—a 13-inch monitor.

But on my EMR when the list of the medications the patient is taking can't be seen on the page—it's cut off at the top and the bottom—I'm just like, "Wow, this is a sick patient." I usually do have lot of stuff going on, but that just blows my mind. I even wondered, I say, "How do you fit these in your stomach? How's there enough room in your—what do you eat? Where's the room in your stomach?" It's unbelievable how many pills some people take. I've seen people come off that. I've seen people make the efforts to come off that. I'm not saying all doctors are that way but certainly the prevailing attitude that I've seen is that doctors don't really—they don't get paid, first of all. If you look at the way we get paid—and we've talked about that in a previous segment or in the previous series. They don't get paid to educate people. They get paid to write the prescriptions. And you can imagine the drug lobbying—they make sure that's the case.

And so, I make the same amount of money writing a new prescription for a patient spending 15 seconds with them, that's a certain code, as I do spending 45 minutes with them talking about nutrition. I can speak to them for 45 minutes, and talk about all the stuff we are talking about, and get the same a hundred bucks for Medicare, or I can just give them a new prescription, change a prescription or do a procedure on them, and it qualifies for that same code. So you can imagine if the doctor is trying to pay his bills, is he going to see ten patients an hour and give them all new drugs or is he going to spend 45 minutes with each person and really try to make them healthy? The system is literally designed to get people on medication in my opinion.

Ty: So the system is flawed at its roots?

Dr. Sahni: Yeah. And the changes that have occurred in recent years, they've only—in my experience, attitude of bureaucracy. There's more paperwork. There's more regulation. I think of it in terms of minutes spent looking patients in the eyes, not trying to force myself to do that, but as time is time going on, I spend so much more time and just think of meaningful use.

I mean the intentions are good with these things, but it's bureaucrats and computer programmers, who don't ever see patients, trying to come up with ways that seem really neat in a think tank or sitting around a table. But in a real world, they create excessive regulation, documentation that doesn't really add to the quality of the care.

And what it really, really detracts from and destroys, in my opinion, is the doctor-patient relationship and communication, because you're spending so much time staring at a computer screen, making sure that all your little things are put in there, and end up spending very little time actually looking at a patient in the eyes. Looking a patient in the eyes is important, because you learn a lot, not from even what they say, what they're telling you, in their physical exam, but how they look back at you, and their facial expressions. That's important. I think you miss out on a lot of stuff by spending your time looking at a computer screen. So, I do think medicine needs an overhaul. I do think medicine is broken, but I don't think—I haven't seen a lot of cases in history where increased government involvement in regulation has resulted in an improvement in any industry, and I think we can all probably see some truth in that.

Ty: Yeah. Let's shift gears here to diet. Your heritage is Indian?

Dr. Sahni: Yeah.

Ty: Right? And so the Indians use a lot of spices in their foods.

Dr. Sahni: Yeah. So there's a type of medicine, which by the way, the kind of medicine we're talking about, cholesterol medicine and blood pressure medication has been around for about a hundred years. That's not a very long time when you think how long the Earth's been around and people have been around. Ayurvedic medicine, which is an Indian form of medicine—it's sort of the analog to Chinese traditional medicine—has been around for 5000 years.

People probably don't do something for 5000 years unless there's a little bit to it, I would imagine. So am I an Indian cook? I'm half-Indian. My father's Indian. My mother's Caucasian. And so, "Am I an Indian cook? Certainly not." I mean I definitely cook some Indian food. I think I've cooked some good Indian food.

Ty: Yeah, I've had some of it.

Dr. Sahni: Yeah. And I cook actual Indian food, but what I like to do, and I really encourage people to play with—because Indian spices are just amazing—is just cook what you normally cook. My kids will get up in the morning and say, "Dad, I want some of your healthy eggs." Because I talk to them about the difference between eating Froot Loops, which occasionally, they do have some sugar cereals, but I love it when they get up in the morning and say, "I want your healthy eggs."

And this is a matter of maybe taking some cumin. The components in Indian spices, you can Google it. We'll talk about how they're anti-inflammatory and they're anti-cancer, and there's a lot of them. But they're also just amazingly delicious, and so I usually—and I have an Indian—my dad actually and even my mother-in-law have said to me, "Oh, no, Indian food is not healthy." Well, I mean it depends on what your perception—how people think butter's bad for you and cream's bad for you. And I talked about this. Maybe butter and cream aren't so bad for you after all.

There's probably some greasy Indian food, but I've altered mine a little bit, so I'll cook with coconut oil, and I'll brown some cumin seeds and throw some turmeric or some curry. All these are amazing spices, and I'll just cook some onions and some peppers, maybe some mushrooms with some eggs. Sometimes I'll throw meat in there, sometimes I don't, but this is super healthy. We already know the benefits of coconut oil versus other types of oils. It's probably the best oil to cook with or at least one of the top two, coconut oil and grape-seed oil, and it's just so easy.

You can whip these things up, and these things are good for inflammation. These things can be good for people who have arthritis or other types of inflammatory ailments, so yeah, I think that Indian spices are not only delicious, but can absolutely benefit your health, and there's so much information out there on this, and it's really easy, and it's fun.

Ty: Yeah, especially the cumin and then the curry powder, right?

Dr. Sahni: The turmeric.

Ty: Yeah, the curry is really the equivalent of turmeric, isn't it? Or is it different? I mean I know the turmeric—

Dr. Sahni: Like I said, I'm no Indian cook. I'd have to go back—to, me they're two different spices that I use when I cook.

Ty: Are they?

Dr. Sahni: Yeah, they may somehow come from the same family—

Ty: I think they come from the same root. I think it's the turmeric comes from the—I think curcumin is the active ingredient in the turmeric root. And then I think from the curcumin, you get the curry powder. But I'm not sure the way they all work. I have seen them different. I've seen some curry powder. I've seen turmeric powder. I honestly don't know the difference.

Dr. Sahni: You know, the bottom line is I just throw it in there, and it's delicious, and my kids love, and it really is a fun way to cook. And Ayurvedic medicine I encourage people to take a look at that and see what type of options are available, the different spices they can cook with. It's delicious. It's something you're not shortcutting it. It tastes way better than Froot Loops.

Ty: Yeah, me too. And if you do get the Froot Loops, you've got to get the organic ones they'll eat. Nature's Path actually it's a good brand. They're non-GMO. They're very low levels of glyphosate, and other contaminants, and lead. But they make a Froot Loop knockoff. Because we get it for the kids sometimes too. They're kids. Occasionally, they'll get that. Talk about the many instances where we've have lately that children have been taking their parents and forced into chemotherapy.

Dr. Sahni: Yeah. And again, I know what I've seen in the media but again, horrendous. So there was this recent case of this, and I believe you've interviewed Cassandra. What do I think about that personally? I mean you're talking to a guy who's got an eight-year-old daughter and twin boys. I'm not even going to say on camera what I would do to a person who basically abducted my children and then injected poison into their body. But I don't think that even needs to be said.

I think everyone agrees how they would feel if that were done to their kid. I think the thing to talk about is that it's absolutely ridiculous to me that these bureaucrats—these people with very little qualification—are given that level of power. How could someone, with a phone call, have the police come to your house—I'm sure at gunpoint or some other forceful way—

Ty: Yeah, there was the police.

Dr. Sahni: —take your child, and in my opinion, kidnap them, abduct them, whatever. Take them away. And then take them to a hospital, and 12 people hold them down, and force them to have a needle or an IV, or a port, or whatever the method was to enter your intravascular system, and then literally inject poison into your body. That's a complete violation of your constitutional rights.

Now the fact that this young lady ultimately turned out not even to have cancer to begin with, that just takes the whole thing over the top. But even if she did, it's inappropriate. We're getting into political things now. These are decisions the parents make for their children. This isn't something that the government or the federal or state government should be making for our kids. I find it just absolutely unbelievable. Unbelievable that that could happen. I think most Americans would feel that way.

Ty: What's your take on the new law that was recently passed in California with the SB-277, forced vaccines for kids in school?

Dr. Sahni: Well, again, vaccination is extremely controversial. Even my wife and I don't even agree on all of those issues, okay. And I don't feel maybe as strongly as some do, say, Robert Scott Bell. But again, the point is that it's my constitutional right as a parent to make those decisions for my children. And certainly, other people should not be making those decisions for my children. If I want to make the decision not to receive a vaccine or have my children receive a vaccine, that's not the government's business. It's just simply not the government's business.

An example, I believe in some vaccines. I think some vaccines are important. I think the flu vaccine—and there's lots of them I don't believe in, but the flu vaccine is a good example—is worthless. The strain that you're getting vaccinated for is basically a guessing game. There's so many strains that you could get, and the government or whoever is preparing the vaccine is just making a best guess. I'm not going to have anyone inject mercury into my body, or even if it didn't have mercury, mercury-free vaccine, that's essentially going to have no effect.

I don't take the flu vaccine. I'm a doctor. I'm exposed to sick patients all the time. I haven't been—actually, I got a little bit sick here lately, but that was the first time I had some GI stuff going on, more than usual, but before that, I literally hadn't been sick in a long time, years, 15 years really. Knock on wood, right? But I believe that eating right and taking care of yourself—personally, I use colloidal silver and have had a very good experience with that. Maybe that's anecdotal, but it's been good for me. I'm a big believer in colloidal silver, been around for a long time.

And so I think it's the individual's right to determine, and as a parent, the parent's right, to determine whether their child receives a vaccine or not.

Ty: It really is a matter of personal choice and the individual freedom that we should be upheld. We're granted it by the Creator this liberty. The constitution, the bylaws enumerate that. They don't give it to us, but it should be something that's protected by those that are in power.

Dr. Sahni: It makes it very difficult—it's hard enough to be healthy. It really is. It's a challenge, but the environment makes it even more difficult. I always—the doctor's lounge, I go into the doctor's lounge. We've talked about that before.

I've given you pictures in the doctor's lounge. These are the people again telling me I should just take my cholesterol medicine and eat my cheese nachos. These are the people that are supposedly educating their patients on real health, and the doctor's lounge is just unbelievable. It's all Cheetos, Fritos, Pop Tarts. It's garbage. There's one little bowl of fruit, and I'm sure it's also soaked in pesticides. I don't know, maybe, maybe not. But there's one little bowl of fruit in the middle of the table. It's always full by the way. I don't know that anyone has touched the fruit.

Ty: It's been there for about six months.

Dr. Sahni: Yeah. So they got a Starbucks machine in there that they had had—I do drink the coffee. I think a little coffee is actually good for you. It's ridiculous. And then there's a big giant Coke machine with full of diet Cokes. This is not at the hospital I'm at now, but the old hospital.

The new hospital and the hospital that I know work at—Resolute Health, in New Braunfels—that's a really, really—it's a glimmer of hope. And I was actually talking to Dr. [Bitar] about this. It's a pilot program for the whole country. So who knows if it's going to work out? I certainly hope it does. But it's owned by Tenet and founded about 80 hospitals nationwide.

Ty: I used to work for them.

Dr. Sahni: Tenet Health has a hospital in New Braunfels, Texas that's essentially a pilot program that was started to be completely different than any other hospital. They truly preach and believe in and promote preventative health. They don't use Sysco for their food services. They have a cook that cooks for the patients. All of the food is grown locally by farmers. The majority of the food is brought in by local farmers. I've never seen a hospital do this or even try to do this. I'm not sure if they're always successful, because obviously, crops don't always come up the way they should.

But their doctor's lounge, it's got a few bags of chips, but other than that, it's a completely scenario. It's extremely healthy. They aren't allowed sodas in the hospital. That's Tenet taking a stand against Coca-Cola. I think that's inspiring. I don't know what the end result will be. It's been open for about a year. But it makes me hopeful that someone is sort of listening to what the rest of us want. Really, it made me excited to go and to work there because they're for true health.

If you look at hospital food, it's pretty unbelievable what we feed patients after we do surgery on them or if they're sick. It's really toxic stuff. Sysco, I'm not picking on them. I'm sure anybody who does that sort of corporate preservative, hormone, antibiotic laden type foods, it's not going to be very healthy. You've seen hospital food. It's pretty unbelievable. And the doctors aren't eating anything better. If you go up the doctor's room, their lounge, they're eating really healthy food. No, they're not. They're eating garbage.

In fact, I was speaking to one of the people who work in our cafeteria at the old hospital that I used to work at, and I said, "Why do we always have this greasy bacon and these biscuits and gravy, just that kind of nasty stuff?" And she said, "You know, we actually tried to bring healthier food in, and the doctors complained."

Ty: They complained about healthy food?

Dr. Sahni: They were furious. They wanted their bacon, and their sausage, and their biscuits. They complained. They said, "We actually try to bring in healthier stuff for breakfast." They put breakfast in the doctor's lounge. The doctors were upset. They didn't want that. I guess you like what you grow up eating, right?

Ty: Yeah.

Dr. Sahni: And you could have taken your cholesterol medicine, right?

Ty: And to be fair to them, they weren't educated about it in medical school.

Dr. Sahni: But when I try to bring some of these issues up, I've tried to talk to a lot of—I mean I'm viewed as crazy. I'm viewed as the conspiracy theorist guy or the nut-job. The nut-job who lost 50 pounds.

Ty: When you try to talk about the importance of nutrition, and obviously, it worked for you, you're crazy?

Dr. Sahni: I'm crazy. I mean it was taken—it was actually taken to a level much—this isn't something I hadn't planned on talking about, but I think I will. I was actually called before a group of doctors and questioned whether I had cancer or not because I had lost 50 pounds. Now first of all, people saw me drinking green smoothies and knew that I was working out aggressively. No one ever came up and said, "Wow, I'm so impressed. How do you do that? Can you teach me because I want to get in better shape," or, "can you teach me because I want to help my patients?"

But what they did do was sit me in front a group of doctors saying, "We think you're on drugs. We think that you're an alcoholic. We wonder—" They literally asked me these questions. "Are you an alcoholic?" I have to answer this in front of a group of doctors now. "Are you on drugs?" Because people are like, "You lost so much weight, we can't believe it." I mean it's that unbelievable to a group of doctors, and that's one reason I left the hospital because you can imagine how mind-numbing that is when you've—and I said, "Well, actually—"

And I was pretty unhappy with the line of question. I wasn't really friendly about my answers. I said, "Actually, I can tell you that I drink less alcohol than everyone in this room. I don't drink any alcohol." At that point, I quit drinking altogether. I had a few glass of wine now and a little bit of drinking here and there, very little. And I happen to know for fact that everyone in that room drinks alcohol, eats Cheetos, abuses their body, and they see someone who's healthy, and now they're going to question that person. They're going to try to tear me down and ask me if I have a psychological illness. Am I seeing a psychiatrist? Are you on drugs? Are you an alcoholic? I mean I guess these are the questions they felt they had to ask, but literally because I have lost weight.

Ty: And they also thought you might have cancer.

Dr. Sahni: And they asked me, specifically, "Do you have cancer?" I said, "You think I have cancer because—" To me, that's just unbelievable. It's like somebody coming home with a gold medal. And the first thing winning the Olympics and say, "Oh, were you on steroids?" And it's thinking the worst.

Ty: I think it shows the fundamental lack of understanding of the importance of nutrition from their perspective.

Dr. Sahni: They couldn't believe that I could be in that good of shape by just eating right. By just eating. And I told them. I said, "Look, not only do I not take drugs, not only do I—I'm not on alcohol. I also don't take testosterone," because I happen to know a couple of them who are on testosterone—fat guys with big bellies on testosterone. I said, "Yeah, I actually raised my testosterone level naturally."

Ty: We know that testosterone is important. Having adequate levels of testosterone is important, especially when we see the estrogen sensitive cancers. So one of the things that you've done recently is you've been able to boost your levels of testosterone naturally. Could you tell us how you did that?

Dr. Sahni: Yeah. In fact, I think, maybe going back to the beginning of my story there. I'll try to keep it short. God, what year was that? It was a few years ago. I went to a natural—this is after interacting with you and I was heavy, and I felt like I probably had low T. I wasn't experiencing early morning, expected type of things you expect early morning when you wake up. And I didn't have energy. I felt fatigue.

And I went to a naturopathic doctor in Austin. Great guy. Dr. Manzanero, I think, was his name. And he was a really short guy actually. And was shocked that after he did some lab on me, he recommended testosterone because I wasn't expecting to be given some plants or something [chuckles]. I was expecting some sort of natural medication. I was sort of shocked that I ended up with—you know, it makes sense.

My testosterone level was 187, so it's extremely low. It was very, very low. A lot of it had to do with being fat. As you understand, when you are have especially belly fat, you have an enzyme called aromatase, and aromatase converts enzymes to estrogen. So even if your testicles are producing inadequate amount of testosterone, the belly fat or overall body fat will convert that testosterone, and that's where you can get male breasts and all that kind of stuff. So, it doesn't necessarily mean your testicles aren't working just because your T is low. There's a lot of different ways that can happen.

Anyway, he put me on testosterone, and I started taking testosterone, and it just didn't settle well with me. I'm sure I probably could have taken it a little differently and done better. I was taking a ten-day cycle, and what would happen is I would inject some testosterone, and I would actually feel really good in the beginning. By day seven or eight—somewhere in there—the tail end of before my next dose, I just get headaches. It was horrible. It was so bad that I said, "I'd rather have low T than do this for the rest of my life." I probably could have gone back to him, and he probably could have changed things up. But I decided I did not—I went to him because in my mind I was trying to not go the pharmaceutical route, and so I just started doing a little research.

And there were studies that show that something called interval training where you basically, the way I do it is I work out for 40 seconds. I'll do a set—like a set of five, say, push-ups, as many push-ups as I can do, as hard as I can—and then rest for 20 seconds and then immediately go back to 40 seconds. In 30 minutes, you can do six different exercises, five reps—because five times six is 30—and you basically take no rest except the 20 seconds. So that's been shown to naturally raise your testosterone. It also raises your metabolism much better than, say, getting on an elliptical for an hour, not that that's bad. You can mix those together, but I wouldn't just do an elliptical. You're going to gain the weight right back. So anyway, I was able to raise my testosterone from 187 to almost 600 doing interval training, which is pretty impressive.

Ty: Wow.

Dr. Sahni: Yeah. And I've got the labs to prove it, so I'm not getting much—

Ty: So doing interval training, which is basically 40 seconds on, 20 second rest, 40 seconds exercise, 20 seconds rest.

Dr. Sahni: Yeah.

Ty: For 30 minutes.

Dr. Sahni: For 30 minutes. I do 30 minute work out. I do a lot of jump rope, and I start mixing other things in. And let's be clear, I also changed my diet dramatically, so there's a lot of things going on there. Who knows what all the factors were, but I do believe the interval training was a big part of it. It helped me lose the weight, and I cleaned up my diet, but the bottom line is, you know— and I would say, I spoke to a urologist at the same hospital and he seemed relatively unimpressed, "Oh yeah, that's great."

That's what a lot of people have experienced. He wasn't my doctor. They go to a doctor, and their doctor tells them or sees that they need to lose weight or get off their diabetes medication. They come back, and they've lost a ton of weight or they've completely changed their health situation and their doctor is not interested because their doctor wasn't the one that did it. That doesn't empower the doctor. For you to be able to go and do that on your own is almost a threat to them. It's a threat to their business. Now I'm speculating here a little bit, but that's my impression.

And so I think when I went to my doctor, for instance, "Guys, this is amazing." Let me tell you these are fat guys that need to exercise. They're in terrible shape. They're eating the Cheetos. They're eating the Pop Tarts. They're eating the garbage. And they could have clearly benefited from this. They didn't even want to hear what I had to say. Probably didn't even believe me. Although looking at me, I was 50 pounds lighter. They have to know something—oh, that's right, I was on drugs or maybe I had cancer, but I was able to naturally raise my testosterone.

Ty: You know that reaction is not uncommon when it comes to—this specifically you are talking about losing weight—but I don't know, what guys, a dozen people that we've talked to in these interviews have told us that they have treated cancer naturally, and went into remission, and their markers are all down. They go back to the oncologist, and they don't want to know what they did. They didn't care.

Dr. Sahni: And you'd think they would be like, "Wow, how did you do that? That's amazing." You know I would as a doctor when someone does something I always say, "Well how did you do it?" I want to know. I'm curious you know. Or some product they bought off that television. Well, if it worked for them, I want to know what it is, but a lot of doctors aren't that way. And since I didn't get the testosterone shots from that doctor, he's probably thinking, "Shut up." Don't talk about that. Everybody will start doing that, and I'll be out of business. But that's not—if I can raise my testosterone level without injecting drugs into my body, that's how I'd rather do it. I mean, who wouldn't?

Ty: Well, the bottom line is—I'm trying to think who told me this. It was Dr. Pai, Dr. Sunil Pai. We interviewed him for the *Quest*, and he said, "Our job as physicians is to get the patient better however we can, period." He said, "Our only desire should be to have the best patient outcome, and if it is through conventional treatments, then we should use them. If it's through natural, then we should use them. If it's through integrated, we should use them." But he said, "The only thing that should be at the forefront of our mind is that we want the patient to get better no matter what we have to do, as long as we don't hurt them in the process."

Dr. Sahni: Yeah, I couldn't agree more. I tell patients this all the time. I'm a spine surgeon. Spine surgery is a very drastic thing. Nobody should want spine surgery. So when people ask me, "Can I go to a chiropractor?" which, by the way, I don't have a problem with chiropractors. I'm not discounting chiropractors. But what I say to them is, "You know what? If jumping up and down on one foot and slapping yourself in the head makes your back pain better and you can avoid surgery, do it." In other words, try anything first.

Now, if you're doing a treatment and it's not working, I don't think you should just keep—you know, I don't like that. When I see some people sucked into paying medicine clinics or chiropractor clinics, and they just sort of keep them in their systems as much as they can, whether they're getting better or not—that's where I have a problem with that.

I encourage people to try anything before having their body cut open to have their problem fixed. Sometimes that has to be done sooner than later, but I wouldn't be upset with someone because they bought the new back machine off of Amazon, and it made them better. They didn't have to have surgery. I'd be very happy for them. In fact, I'd probably want to know a little bit more about it to see if maybe it could help some of my other patients. So I completely agree with that philosophy. Whatever it takes to get people better the right way.

And the funny thing is, is when I really started becoming more interested in alternative medicine—I guess you might call it—and really almost got ridiculous, almost obnoxious about really talking people out of surgery, and I'm a spine surgeon that's always talking people out of surgery. I felt my practice blew up. We got busier and busier because this is what people want. They want honesty. They want somebody who's really looking out for their welfare and not just want—I've seen some horrible examples of the kind of surgeries that people got that in my opinion probably would have been better off avoiding the surgery altogether.

So surgery is definitely a last resort and one that should always be saved for very extreme cases. You always want people to get better by any means, whether it's chiropractic, whether it's acupuncture, whether it's Chinese medicine, whether it's herbal medicine, or whether it's conventional medicine, whether it's epidural steroid injections, and facet blocks, and any sort of allopathic medicine that we do routinely.

Ty: Yeah, so I think that would cause a lot of the friction that exists today between conventional and natural medicine would go away if at the forefront of every physician's mind was just let's get the patient better.

Dr. Sahni: There's plenty of business. There's a shortage of doctors. A lot of patients, I think, don't go to the doctor because they just feel like the doctor's not really going to do anything for them. And if they really felt like maybe the doctor in a particular situation is really looking out for their best interest, they might come out of there—I mean I hear people all the time saying, "I never want to the doctor." Like I believed when the guy told me, "Well, if you start preaching health, we're going to be out of business [chuckles]. We're going to out of business." It's going to be 1,000 years before out of business. There's always going to be a need.

When your product is a dinosaur, you need to find a new product. You need to evolve. If what you're doing to treat patients is no longer effective or archaic, then you need to evolve and come up with a new way to treat patients or be open minded to new types of treatments. A lot of people just get stuck in that rut. And when you have a hammer, everything's a nail.

And that's the problem I see a lot of times with medicine. If you're a spine surgeon, that's all you do, because we do a lot in a clinic beside spine surgery. In fact, spine surgery is probably one of the least things I do now. But when you're a spine surgeon and all you do is spine surgery, guess what? You're not going to make your rent payment that month, the mortgage payment if somebody don't get spine surgery. If I'm a mechanic, and all I can do is fix alternators, and I can't fix any other part of the car, all there's going to be some alternators. If you're missing alternators—

Ty: You got to find some alternator problems.

Dr. Sahni: —I'd better find some alternator problems or my kids aren't going to go to college. So I have a problem with that. That's a sort of philosophy, this tunnel vision philosophy where medicine's gone. You put that in the hands of an unscrupulous—hands of a sociopath, like Farid Fata and look at the results. And this happens whether it's spine surgery, or ENT, or family practice, or oncology, and that's unfortunate.

Ty: It is.

Well, Dr. Sahni, as usual, thanks for the interview. I appreciate your input. I appreciate your honesty. It's nice to be able to get kind of some behind the scenes of what goes on in the doctor's lounge, and you know, thanks for sharing your story about being called before a group of doctors, because you'd actually had the audacity to lose weight and get healthy. I guess if you've been on the weight loss drugs they we we're trying to get you, that would have been okay.

Dr. Sahni: Were there always financial motivation behind these? And this had to do with me, honestly doing procedures in my office and not using their facility. And that's really, again, speculation. But I know that's what it is.

Ty: It's all money motivated.

Dr. Sahni: It's all money motivated. We don't need to get into that. That's not the point of this series, but I'm happy to share those things with you. It is the reality of not just the politics of medicine, but the politics in any business. The good news is that I'm actually doing much better after getting away from those sort of negative people. They did me a favor by making me not want to be around them anymore.

Ty: Cool, man. Let's end this interview and go and make some of those good eggs [chuckles].

Dr. Sahni: All right, buddy.

Ty: All right, buddy.

[end of transcript]

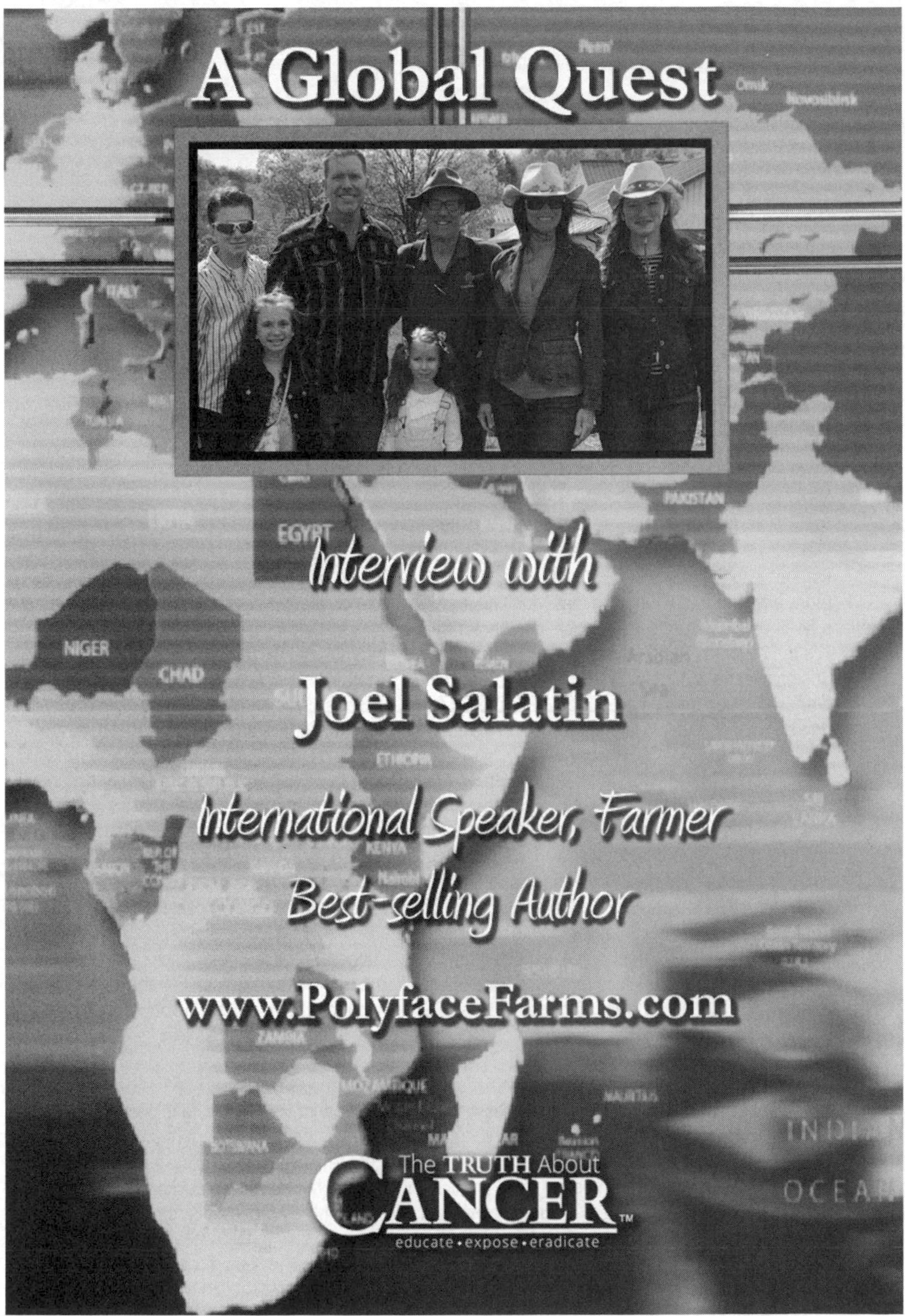
A Global Quest
Interview with
Joel Salatin
International Speaker, Farmer
Best-selling Author
www.PolyfaceFarms.com
The TRUTH About
CANCER
educate • expose • eradicate

Ty: I'm here today at Polyface Farms in Virginia with Joel Salatin. Thanks for joining me today.

Joel: Alright, Ty. It's great to have you.

Ty: What does Polyface mean?

Joel: Polyface is the farm of many faces. We're not just two-faced, we're many-faced.

Ty: Not just two-faced. So many faces as far as many…

Joel: Different livestock, different kinds of animals, plants, diversified landscape. It's about multi-speciation, multi-enterprises, and lots of people.

Ty: And lots of faces of your family as well, right? You've got a lot of your family that lives here with you?

Joel: Yes.

Ty: Joel, one of the things—I've seen a meme, out there on the internet of you and it says, you think organic is expensive, eating organic is expensive. Have you priced cancer lately? Let's talk about that, because one of the things that I hear a lot is—I can't afford to eat organic food. I know I should, but I can't afford it. So what's your response to someone who says that?

Joel: Sure. Well, there are several answers. One is that if you buy in volume you can save a lot of money. Get a freezer. We're in the animal business, so I'm thinking frozen beef, chicken and whatever. But you can get a huge price break if you buy in volume. Number two, look in the mirror and ask yourself, "Is there anything that I'm buying that I don't need?" Whenever anybody says that, I want to grab them and say, "Okay, take me to your house, and here's what we're not going to find, I'm sure at your house. We're not going to find—soda, we're not going to find lottery tickets, we're not going to find $100 designer jeans with holes already in the knees, coffee, alcohol, hot pockets, frozen microwavable dinners, French fries." You can go down the list and the truth is, there aren't very many households that don't have those things in them and none of that is actually nutritious. None of it.

I went to New York City's Union Square Green Market, arguably the most expensive farmer's market in the world. I asked my hostess, could she take me to the most expensive potato in the New York City's Union Square Green Market? She said, "Yes, I know just the guy." She elbows her way through and we go up and we get to this potato guy. He's got about 30 potatoes out there. There are red ones and white ones, blue ones and green ones and orange ones, fat ones and long ones and skinny ones, and all of this stuff. I look through all of the little boxes there, and I find the most expensive one. It's an heirloom Peruvian blue fingerling potato, and it's $1.99 a pound. That whole market is surrounded by supermarkets with 100 feet of fluorescent-lighted, handicapped-accessed, retail floor space, selling French fries and potato chips for $3 a pound. All right? The point is that you can buy the most expensive potato in the world and use the sophisticated techno-glitzy gadgetry in your kitchen. We've never remodeled and gadgetized our kitchens with so many things and been so lost as where the kitchen is.

So getting in your kitchen, buying unprocessed, and then preparing it, processing it, packaging, and preserving in your own kitchen ultimately, you cannot have an integrity food system until it becomes home-centric. Home-centricity is the foundation of an accountable integrity food system and when you do that, you're able to save massive amounts of money. When you buy single packages—highly expensively packaged, actually—single-serving material that's highly processed, ready to eat, that is expensive stuff. It's very expensive and you can buy—especially bulk, unprocessed local, highest quality you know, I call it royalty food. You can buy royalty food for way less money. It means that you're going to have to participate. You have to come down off the bleachers and you're going to have to stop whining and being a victim, put down your Netflix and actually get in the game of visceral participation in your body's energy field.

Ty: It's really a choice. It's really, "What do you put your priority on?"

Joel: Absolutely.

Ty: It's a choice. And when we compare it to cancer, the average cancer patient is going to bring anywhere to three quarters of a million to $1.5 million to the cancer industry. So it's not even a fair comparison when we look at the disease that can be created if you don't eat healthy. It reminds me, I was speaking up in Kentucky a couple of weeks ago. We were at a store and there's a little girl that wants an apple and her mom is in front of her and she's got cigarettes, and a coke and a lottery ticket, which reminded me of that when you said the lottery ticket. The little girl wants the apple, it's $1 an apple. The mom says, "We can't afford that."

Joel: Can't afford the apple.

Ty: But she bought cigarettes, a coke and a lottery ticket. Do we need to say any more? It's really a choice isn't it?

Joel: It absolutely is a choice and as far as time is concerned, do you know that right now the average American male between 25 and 35 years old, spends 20 hours—25 to 35 years old—American male spends 20 hours a week playing video games? That's enough time to get a second job, enough time to cook all your own food and eat leftovers. You don't need to eat out.

Ty: No. And that's another place that people can cut back, isn't it? Eating out.

Joel: Absolutely. There's no reason to eat out. When I was working off the farm, I took my lunch. There's a thing called a thermos. There's a thing called a brown bag.

Ty: Paper sacks.

Joel: Paper sacks. I've decided that now the litmus test of a person who gets this food thing is the person who eats leftovers because leftovers are a fundamental outgrowth of familial personal home-centric food prep—leftovers. That should be the badge of honor. I eat leftovers. Yes.

Ty: That makes me feel good, Joel, because I've got four kids and sometimes I'll eat leftovers from all of them, You can't tell. So, Joel, what you said makes a lot of sense. One of the things that's interesting to me—last year I toured across the United States and I spoke to numerous, dozens, of doctors and I asked them, "How much education did you get on nutrition when you were in medical school?" None of them got any education. So there's this disconnect between what we're eating and our health. So what you're sharing makes a lot of sense. We're sick because we're eating foods as you mentioned you can't even pronounce—50 different ingredients and 49 of them are manmade chemicals. So we're sick because we're ingesting foods that our bodies don't even see as food, right?

Joel: I go with Michael Pollan's idea that we really shouldn't eat anything that wasn't available before 1900. That's kind of the cutoff, 1900, beginning of the industrial era, and we can be really thankful that hot dogs were introduced in the 1890 World's Fair. They had 10 years to spare—they just sort of slipped in right there.

Ty: One of the things about hot dogs—people hear hot dogs and they're terrible for you. Not necessary as long as you know what's in them? Right? It's not about the food. It's about what's in the food.

Joel: That's right.

Ty: Right? So you can eat a hot dog that you get at the supermarket that's full of nitrates and nitrites and all of these processing and it's terrible for you.

Joel: Especially a salvage operation.

Ty: Right. But okay, so talk about your hot dogs.

Joel: Our hot dogs are essentially 60 percent beef and 40 percent pork and the beef that we use is the same stuff that would go into ground beef, for example, or chuck roast.

Ty: And it's from grass-fed cows.

Joel: Grass fed-animals, grass-finished animals. Of course the pork, the pigs are out running around and also pastured pork—and so the pork is actually rose-colored. It's not white. When the industry says, pork the other white meat, what that means is the other white, tasteless whatever—slovenly…

Ty: Denatured.

Joel: Denatured, devitamined, whatever. Good, good food should have color. A garden club lady doesn't get the first prize for a pale rose. You want a rich one. Our children, you can tell they're sick when their cheeks are off-color. You kind of turn white. So this whole paleness thing,it is symptomatic of a lack of keratins of the salad bar in the diet. So having the animals out on a salad bar where we move the animals every day on to a fresh salad bar to stimulate the ingestion of all of this salad bar green material, that's where the vitamins and minerals are. That fundamentally changes the omega 3, omega 6 ratio. It changes the conjugated linoleic acid. We participated with *Mother Earth News* magazine a couple of years ago on an egg test with 11 other pastured egg producers in the country and, I'll just pick out one of the 11 nutrients they tested for was folic acid, which of course is really important for pregnant women. The USDA generic nutritional statement for eggs is like 48 micrograms per egg, and our eggs average 1,038 micrograms. The differences in this food are not like five and 10 percent deviations …

Ty: That's 20 times better.

Joel: Yeah. It's just off the charts.

Ty: You mentioned salad bar beef, you mentioned the omega 3 and omega 6, the CLA—this is all important stuff because there's going to be people who watch this and they say, "Look we shouldn't be eating meat at all." If you choose to be vegetarian or vegan that's your choice and God bless you for it, but if you want to eat meat, which we eat meat, you have to make sure it's a high-quality meat. So what I'm hearing you say—and this is very important for people to understand—is that if you're going to eat meat, you want to get it from pigs that are out there expressing their pigness. From cows that are being fed and finished with grass.

Joel: That's right.

Ty: You go to a factory farm where they're raising 200 cows in a little barn. They're cooped up, they're treated very inhumanely, we've all seen the videos—

Joel: Right.

Ty: Not only that are they treated inhumanely, which you don't and we'll see that later—but they're being fed grains instead of grass and the grains are genetically modified and you are what you eat, right? Even a child knows this.

Joel: Beyond that you are what you eat eats.

Ty: That's where I'm going.

Joel: I would take it back—you are what you eat eats.

Ty: So the cows are what they eat, so talk about that.

Joel: Sir Albert Howard, said, and he's of course the godfather of modern scientific aerobic composting. And his iconic book *The Agricultural Testament* in 1943, he said, "When we feed the soil with artificials,"—that's what he calls chemical fertilizer, artificials He said, "When we feed the soil with artificials, it creates artificial plants, which make artificial animals, which make artificial people who can only be kept alive with artificials."

Ty: Wow.

Joel: That was 1943.

Ty: He knew something didn't he?

Joel: That was so prescient that you can't improve on it. He was obviously looking into the future. We're fundamentally interested in creating a habitat and a diet that appreciates and honors the full the glory of that animal. It's phenotypical expression. And so just like we would want to honor the tomato-ness of the tomato, we want to honor the pig-ness of the pig, the chicken-ness of the chicken. And for those who think, "C'mon, haven't we gotten beyond meat? C'mon and aren't we achieving some sort of cosmic nirvana as we sail off into this non-murderous route." Let me tell you something. Everything is eating and being eaten. And if you don't believe it, go lie naked in your flowerbed for three days and see what gets eaten.

Ty: That would be you.

Joel: Yes. The fact is that the beautiful cycle of life, of life, death, decomposition—which is digestion—regeneration, through excrement, through waste, through the energy stream—life, death, decomposition, regeneration, life death, decomposition, that beautiful mystical circle goes on and on. You cannot have life without death and decomposition. A compost pile is all about, life, death, decomposition. It's bacterial, microbial, but it's about communities living and dying and eating each other. The way the plant community works in the soil, is the grass takes in solar energy and trades carbohydrates to the microbes, which then bring the minerals from the soil into the plant, and it's all an animal-plant community. Of course, now we know the plants are talking in pheromones and strange languages and they're responding to each other. The plants are responding and the animals are responding and there's a lot of communication going on out here in this amazing world of beings.

Ty: What we do—in all of our wisdom—being sarcastic here.

Joel: Sure.

Ty: Is we've got these—our bodies are trillions of microbes. We're—

Joel: We're only actually 85—we're actually only 15 percent human, we're 85 percent non-human, according to MIT.

Ty: Because of the bacteria and the microbes. So what we do, we spray things on the plants that kill the bacteria, that kill the microbes and it not only kills it on the plants it kills it in us.

Joel: They all end in "cide", which is the Greek suffix for death. Why would we be spraying all of our life with death? What we want it do is have life right up to intake.

Ty: Yes.

Joel: That's what we want. And when that life is right up to intake, then that's when it can bestow the greatest amount of life force, energy, in our bodies. The fact is that most people are actually more informed and interested in the latest dysfunction in the Kardashian household than what's going to become flesh of their flesh and bone of their bones at six o'clock.

Ty: Right. And that's why we're sick. That's why we're sick. That's sick enough in and of itself.

Joel: Sure it is.

Ty: Right?

Joel: Sure it is. Yeah. Friends shouldn't let their friends read *People* magazine, but anyway, that we eat with such little conscious effort, that we, as a culture, have so profoundly abdicated our responsibility, our visceral role in our body's fuel, is indicative not of a new Star Trek nirvana future, it's indicative of a profound devolution I would say, a de-volution into a diss-appreciation from what are actually the most important things.

Ty: Right. Because what we eat become us. It becomes every cell of our body.

Joel: Sure it does.

Ty: We are not paying attention to the foods that we eat. We can't be healthy because it's not going to happen by eating the standard American diet, right? We look at the ingredients in your typical processed—you mentioned earlier processed foods, but you were talking about the way the foods are processed, but if we look at processed foods, on the shelf…

Joel: Yes.

Ty: That will last for billions of years and never deteriorate. You have all of these chemicals and then add the preservatives. That can't be good for us and that has to somehow contribute to our ill health today.

Joel: Again, life gives life.

Ty: Right.

Joel: And if it won't decompose, it won't digest.

Ty: And look at all of the incidents in colon cancer.

Joel: Sure. And all of your ultra-pasteurized milk. Milk is not supposed to sit shelf-stable for six months without deteriorating. I mean a nut or a bolt will, or a copper fitting or a piece of PVC pipe, but we don't consider that food and so we've essentially plastic—

Ty: Plasticized…

Joel: Essentially mechanized and inanimitized our food to where it's just in our stuff.

Ty: I heard Dr. Tim O'Shea, refer to pasteurized homogenized milk as liquid Formica.

Joel: That's right. That's right. So what we want is stuff that will actually decompose.

Ty: Raw milk. You look at a few years ago, I'm sure you're familiar with the raid in California of the Rawesome Foods where they—raw milk—and one of the charges against them was that they had mislabeled cheese. And so then they sent in a SWAT Team—

Joel: Guns drawn.

Ty: Yeah.

Joel: There is an overwhelming orthodox in our culture today. And this orthodoxy, which permeates all of the developed countries—what we call the first world nations, right? That orthodoxy is pretty simple. One is that safe food has to be sterile and that's how we've come to... Coca Cola and Mountain Dew are safe, but raw milk is unsafe. Another orthodoxy is that people are too dumb to choose their food so some bureaucrat or a government agency has to choose and sanction what's acceptable for food. Another one is that we do anything to have cheap food, that you shouldn't have to pay for food. Food should be cheaper so you can afford more Las Vegas time, Hollywood time and Caribbean cruises and get to the soccer game.

And then another orthodoxy is that we want a fundamentally segregated food system rather than being hyper-integrated like it used to be. We have a fundamentally segregated where the food is growing over here, the people go over here, the food is processed over here, it's sold over here and none of these things meet, so we have massive waste streams, massive spoilage. At no time in human history has half of all human edible food been thrown away. That's never happened. The biggest lie of our time is that we're short of food. How are we going to feed all of these people? Right now we're throwing away enough food to feed the whole planet a second time.

Ty: Wow.

Joel: That's never happened in human history, and it's happened because of the inefficiencies in the industrial food system and the global food system where we have so much waste and spoilage, sell-by dates, dented, bent, crashed—whatever—that's what's creating that.

Ty: One of the popular things that you hear about genetically modified foods is that we have food, genetically modified foods so we can feed the world.

Joel: Absolutely.

Ty: So what you just shared, that kind of flies in the fact of that.

Joel: No, absolutely and in fact, that has completely been debunked now with lots of studies coming out showing that there is no increase in production with genetically modified foods

Ty: Is there actually a decrease?

Joel: Sometimes there is a decrease.

Ty: Yeah.

Joel: And so the data now,GMOs—It took 14 years from the development of DDT until we finally connected the dots that it really is making infertile frogs, three-legged salamanders and eagle eggs that won't hatch. It took 14 years. Well, GMOs have only been out for 15. We're finally now really beginning to connect these dots with infertility, with some studies are showing autistic results. Of course, the thing is, the science, science is pretty subjective. It depends on who you want to believe as to which scientist you believe, how they set up the ...

Ty: You can rig a study.

Joel: You can rig a study as easy as pie.

Ty: One of the things we learned last year with, you know who Jeffrey Smith is, right?

Joel: Oh, yeah.

Ty: So he shared with us that the fact that the GMOs—all of the studies from the scientists that are performing real studies, objective studies that they're causing cancer, they're causing tumors. You mentioned a link to autism, you mentioned a link to sterility. We're the guinea pigs.

Joel: All of this has not been done before and of course, the people that say. "O, c'mon! GMOs, they're just an extension of plant selection and animal breeding that we've been doing for centuries." Mendel's peas were peas on peas. They weren't peas on watermelons on pigs. They were peas on peas. Let me tell you what. When the sexual plumbing doesn't match up, it ain't right.

Ty: Okay.

Joel: It's like God put barriers in here. Barriers are good. Cell walls are really functional. They protect what's supposed to be in, in and keep out what's supposed to be out, out and so actually there is reason to have barriers, to have ence around your yard so your toddler can't fall into the street. These barriers are actually very protective things. There is only one that we've been able to naturally go over in nature. That's the donkey and a horse and it makes a mule, but a mule is sterile. It's almost like God says, "All right, you can do this, but this is a far as I'll let you go." And so the truth is that we are forcing something that nature actually has a lot of protections to make sure can't happen. Nobody has looked down on their garden and seen a squash plant impregnating a potato plant. All right? That doesn't happen. You have to overrun a whole bunch of natural barriers and hurdles to make that run. I believe that those barriers are actually templates of truth that are to keep genetic purity the way it's supposed to be and not have just complete mass confusion. There is an order, and the order needs to be honored and appreciated. When the USDA—I call it the US"duh"—for 30 years, it took farmers like me to a free steak dinner to teach us this new scientific method of feeding dead cows to cows. We didn't buy into that. They accused us of being anti-progressive—

Ty: Anti-science—

Joel: Anti-science—yeah, yeah, yeah. That wasn't it at all. We looked around the planet and we said, where is an herbivore eating carrion? When a lion kills a wildebeest, you don't see a bunch of wildebeest come around and start eating the liver out of the wildebeest. You don't see it. Omnivores do. A chicken dies in the yard, the chickens they'll get around there. They don't bury their sister, they eat her. That's the way chickens do, and pigs the same way. But herbivores, no, they don't eat that. And so we didn't buy into it not because we hated science or innovation. We didn't buy into it because we said, "You know what, there's an order here. There's an order and there's a template, There's a template of function. We don't understand all of the nuances of it. But we come to nature assuming nature is fundamentally well, and it's well because it's designed to function correctly and if it's sick, if it's broken, then I probably broke it. And then 30 years later there is this world wide oops, maybe we shouldn't have done that—with the mad cow disease, bovine spongiform encephalopathy.

Ty: Sure.

Joel: Who was right? The dumb peasant Luddite was right. And so my dad used to say that we're pretty clever. We've got this big brain and opposing thumbs, monkeys can't do that. We have this amazing mechanical intellectual ability and we're so smart that we can innovate things that we can't physically, spiritually, mentally or physically metabolize. Or emotionally metabolize.

Ty: Right.

Joel: And so what happens is we invent things that cause problems, and then we spend generations trying to remediate the very things that we thought were clever and innovative. Like Velveeta, like cheese that ...

Ty: Like plastic cheese.

Joel: Like plastic cheese. Like ultra-pasteurized milk, like medicated chicken, like apples that don't turn brown when you cut into them.

Ty: Grapples. We have grapples now. Grapes and apples. What you shared Joel, this makes a lot of sense because nature seems to have it right. Specifically, with the genetically modified issue here, one of the things you said was really profound. We've overridden that one time with a horse and a donkey, and that gives rise to a mule that's sterile.

Joel: That's right.

Ty: That picture is I believe exactly what's going on with these genetically modified foods.

Joel: Yes.

Ty: They may look good at first, and there may be all of these really altruistic reasons for us doing this, but in the end the sterility is one of the results when we eat them.

Joel: That's right. It's funny how sure we are of things and one of the things we were sure of... Remember when the human genome matching project was started?

Ty: Yeah.

Joel: And it was budgeted and it was allocated three years and mathematically the mathematicians and the scientists deduced that they were going to find a 100,000 pairs and that's what the whole project was budgeted and scheduled for. Was for find these 100,000 pairs of genetic variances, right?

Ty: Yeah.

Joel: Well, that's probably the first government program that ever came in under budget and sooner instead of later. And the reason is because they only found what 24,000 ...

Ty: Yeah, a little over 24,000.

Joel: Twenty-four thousand , , and they said that's mathematically impossible. We know this can't be and of course, it was. So then the question was, well, what's responsible for all of the hanky panky going on up and down the DNA strand? That then created another whole new field called epigenetics.

Ty: Epigenetics.

Joel: This is brand new and so there's a lot more going on here. We think we're really smart. We can fly to the moon, we have smartphones, we've got clever cool stuff. But boy when it comes to life we are profoundly ignorant without the nuances and the connectiveness, the connective elements of the microbes in the soil, to the microbes in my digestive tract, to the microbes in the food that you're ready to eat.

Ty: Which leads me to an interesting observation. Across the world we have tribes that live remotely that eat diets like this.

Joel: Sure.

Ty: They eat clean meats and vegetables that they grow and they're not exposed to all of these sides that we talked about that cause death.

Joel: Uh huh.

Ty: And they live—they're centenarians, a lot of them. They have very little incidence of any diseases, but when those people move to the United States or the other civilized, industrialized part of the world and they begin to eat what we eat—

Joel: The Westernized diet.

Ty: The Western diet, they get sick.

Joel: They fall apart really fast. Of course, this was documented by Dr. Weston A. Price, in his degenerative studies and it just shows that ultimately you can't get health out of a bottle. Trust me, if you're sick it's not because you're pharmaceutically disadvantaged. It's probably because there's some underlying thing. Now it might not be food, it might be stress, it might be something else. And certainly, there are genetic propensities, but what we've now learned already through epigenetics is that we can actually move our diet to a profoundly elevated nutritional plane enough to actually override our genetic propensity and through epigenetics, realign in a healthy fashion those genetic propensities and start over. Now whether you can say you can start over completely, we could argue, but at least you can give yourself a new shot at it. You're not just inevitably programmed for whatever Mom had or whatever. We can absolutely change that epigenetic code through care and attention to our body's fuel.

Ty: Yeah. I think that's a great subject to address at this point, and to actually end on with this interview, is this epigenetic issue because our message to people who are watching this documentary is that you may have been told by your oncologist that you've been diagnosed with cancer, that you've got bad genes and there's nothing you can do about it. Our message is a message of hope, and what you just shared is completely accurate. People don't need to despair if they've been diagnosed with cancer or another disease. There is always hope because of the fact that we're now discovering this epigenetic link that the food that you eat, if we eat a diet that we're describing here today, we're letting the animals be animals. We're eating these vegetables that don't have any of the sides on them. You start fueling your body with that kind of nutrition, maybe those genes won't express, right? Is that what I'm hearing you say?

Joel: Yes, that's correct and I think it's important because there are naysayers. I can hear people in a room as a family watching this and there will be a naysayer there that says, "Oh, c'mon. We debunked the whole—people still die." That's true. Like you said, one in 80 had cancer even in 1900. But we're talking about averages. We're not saying, and I know you're not saying, that if you eat right you'll never die.

Ty: No.

Joel: No. Okay.

Ty: We're all going to die.

Joel: Exactly. That is appointed. All right? But what we're talking about is quality of life and your chances of aging gracefully rather than aging pharmaceutically or dying extremely young, and it's the averages. Sure, I could walk out in front of a freight train tomorrow. I get that. Whether I eat industrial chicken or pastured chicken is not going to save me if I walk in front of a freight train tomorrow. So there are no guarantees here. What we're talking about risk and percentages. Metadata. What are your chances? What's the way to bet? And the way to bet is, that if you eat things you can pronounce and you eat things—the plants and animals from sources that honor the distinctives, the glory of those beings, the chances are it will honor your place and your glory as well.

Ty: Wow. That's a great way to end the interview. I've not heard it said that way, but I think that's going to resonate with people because that's the message, isn't it, Joel?

Joel: It is indeed.

Ty: Wow. Thanks for sharing that. This has been awesome.

Joel: Great.

Ty: I really enjoyed it.

Joel: Thanks for coming. ***[end of transcript]***

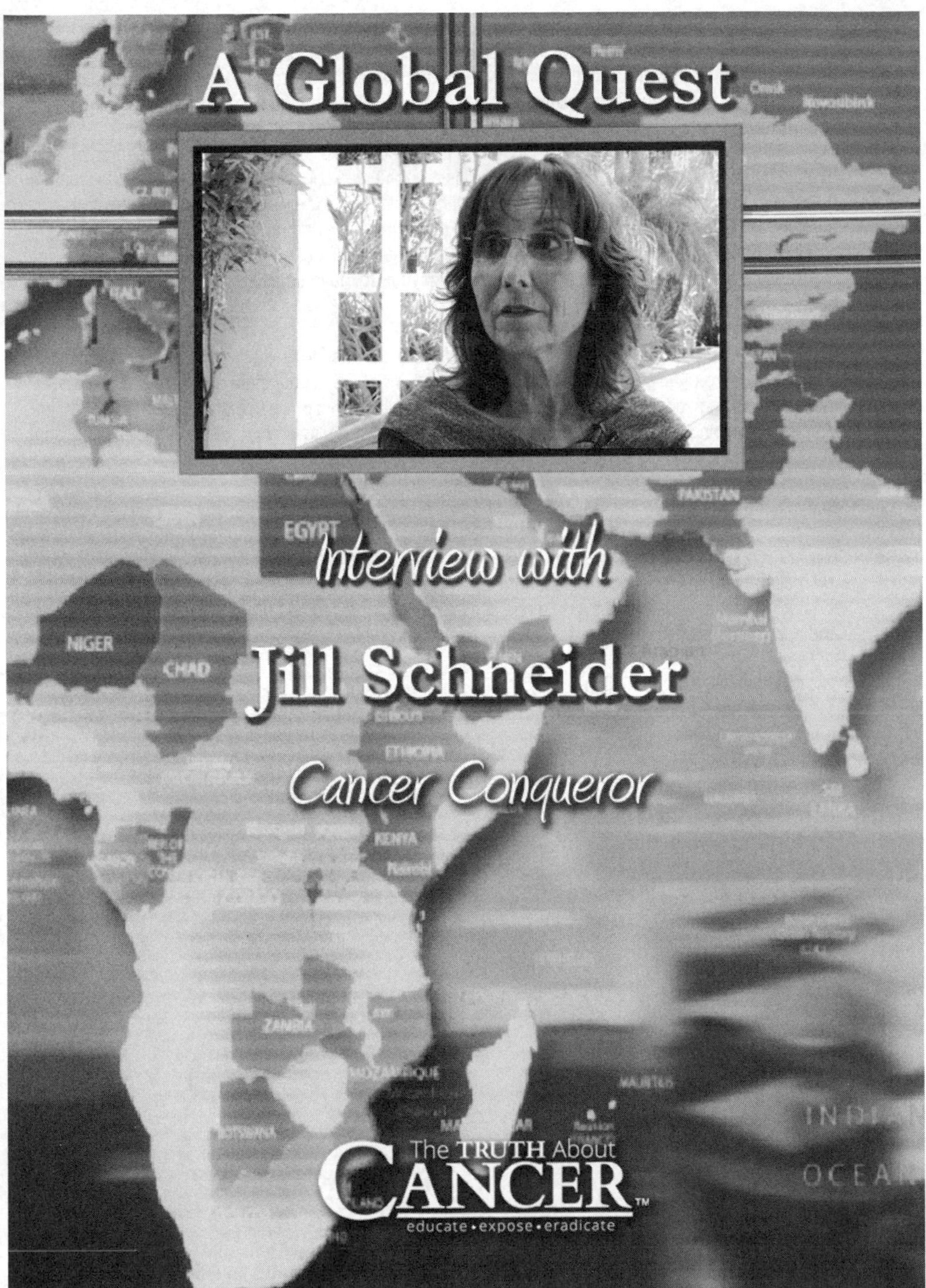
A Global Quest
Interview with
Jill Schneider
Cancer Conqueror
The TRUTH About
CANCER
educate • expose • eradicate

Jill Schneider: In 975 I went to have a PAP test with my OBGYN. Maybe it had been a couple of years since I had had one. And the doctor said that it was a classification 5 PAP test and he wanted to take another test. After they did that, they called me in and said that you have cervical cancer which is very severe and we want you in the hospital next week.

I just looked at the doctor and I said, "I think this is something that I need to do some research on and begin a program of nutrition." He looked at me as though I was completely off the wall and he slammed the door in my face. I just walked out of the doctor's office, and I knew I never wanted to see that person again. That evening, I had to perform – I'm a singer/songwriter/guitarist – on a radio station. From the time I had the appointment, I found out that I had malignant cervical cancer, until I sang that night because I knew I couldn't sing if I had fear, I gave it up, gave up all the fear. What point would it have in my life at that moment?

Shortly after that, I quit a job that was very stressful. I knew I had to leave the country just to have the time to take care of myself. So, a month later – after a month of acupuncture and herbs – I had another test, it had already gone to a number three. I said, "I'm clear. This is a piece of cake. I'm off to South America. I'm going to hang out in the jungle for a while and then go down to Peru and do some hiking, Machu Picchu, 1975."

Ty: So, you already saw progress within a month, and then you left.

Jill Schneider: Yeah. Then I left to go and really have a real health vacation. I went to hot springs, I hiked in the mountains, I ate their food, I lived. Immediately, as soon as I got home, I was responsible. I went to the doctor, and it went from a five to a one in five months, and two and a half years later, I had a child, and now I'm a grandmother of two little girls.

Ty: Wow. Congratulations!

[end of transcript]

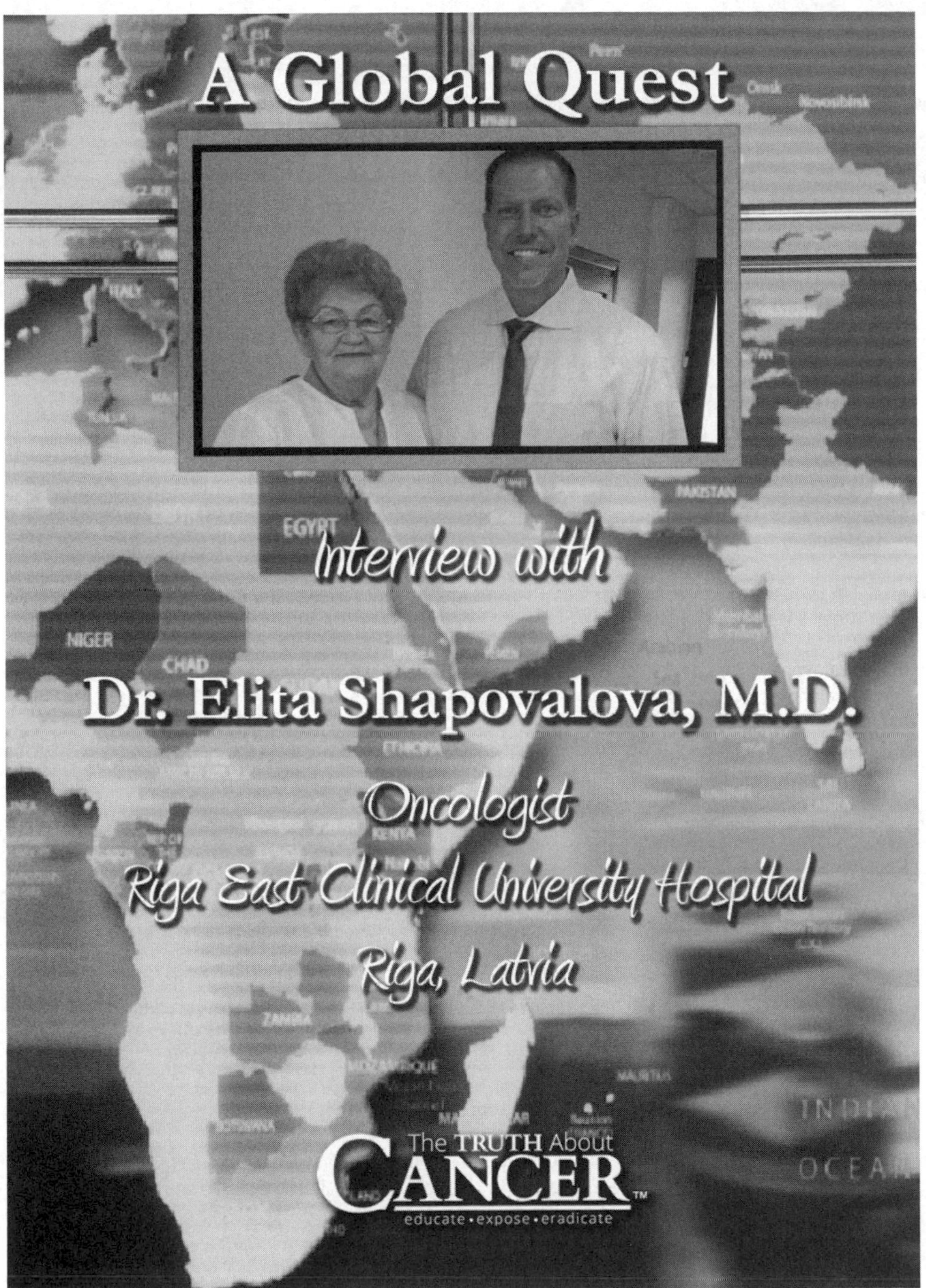
A Global Quest
Interview with
Dr. Elita Shapovalova, M.D.
Oncologist
Riga East Clinical University Hospital
Riga, Latvia
The TRUTH About
CANCER™
educate • expose • eradicate

Ty: I am honored to be here today at the Latvian Oncology [Center] with Dr. Elita Shapovalova. Thank you for joining me today.

Dr. Shapovalova: And great to see you here.

Ty: Dr. Elita, could you share with the viewing audience your experience, your education in medicine and specifically oncology?

Dr. Shapovalova: [Translated 00:29 - 1:00] I have graduated from the university in 1963 and after that I have worked for three years as a surgeon. And then I had also continued my education for two years. And then starting from 1971, I am working here in this center.

Ty: So you have been working in this place for over 40 years.

Dr. Shapovalova: [Translated 1:30 - 2:13] Starting from '71 to '84, it was located on the other bank of the river on the other side of the city. But from '84, thanks to the donations of people, it got moved to this place and it got united. And after 1984, it's been located here and it's always been held here at these premises.

Ty: So you have been an oncologist for how many total years?

Dr. Shapovalova: [Translated 2:46 - 2:52] Starting from 1969. [Translated 2:56 - 3:05] Since the 6th of January, 1967. In Oncology.

Ty: In Oncology. Can you describe the treatments that you have used over the years as an oncologist and their success?

Dr. Shapovalova: [Translated 3:25 - 4:15] I have experienced all the oncology history in Latvia throughout my life, throughout my working experience. And 15 years ago, there were patients that we could not help when they contacted us, but today we can help these people. And this is also thanks to the diagnosis, the technical things that we use to monitor the disease, to find out about the disease, and to help all the aspects of the disease.

Ty: What were the standard treatments for cancer 40 years ago when you began?

Dr. Shapovalova: [Translated 4:52 - 5:53] We were working according to all union standards, the USSR union standards. And the oncology developed mostly thanks to the very popular people in the field of oncology, for example, Professor Stradins. And in 1977, we were also cooperating with the USA researchers and we were researching melanoma disease.

[Translated 6:26 - 6:57] We had to study the specific bacteria in melanoma patients and, for this, we needed young people and that's why we cooperated with the USA and other USSR institutes to research it in the young and strong people.

Ty: You were one of the first oncologists that were involved with Rigvir.

Dr. Shapovalova: [Translated 7:26 - 8:08] Actually, I was not the very first. Most of the first specialists were Dr. Priedite who was heading the Republican Oncologist Center at that time so she had the most difficult job to do in the beginning. And Dr. [inaudible - 08:27] also, the chief, the leading oncologist.

Ty: How is Rigvir different than the other treatments that you used previously to treat melanoma?

Dr. Shapovalova: [Translated 8:39 - 10:30] Rigvir firstly affects the humoral factors in the blood and also it has the immunomodulating ability, when we talk about differences. And as we also can monitor, when patients receive Rigvir, their quality of life is also getting much better.

For example, we have statistics and percentages. When there's a surgery for stomach cancer and people who receive Rigvir, after this, 42 percent of patients survive and have better results. But without Rigvir only 20 percent. For example, also with melanoma patients, people receiving Rigvir they have much higher standard of quality of life. And our country's small so it's hard nowadays to divide into groups and to study. We take into consideration the studies that were held previously some years ago where the statistic data was bigger. So in melanoma cases, at earlier stages when patients receive Rigvir, the percentage survived is 92 percent. And, at later stages, for example, if they receive Rigvir, it's 60 percent. And if they don't receive it, it's only nine percent at later stages.

Ty: How effective is Rigvir compared to chemotherapy and radiation for treating melanoma?

Dr. Shapovalova: [Translated 12:03 - 12:49] Those treatments cannot be compared because, until date, there is no chemotherapy medicine that can treat melanoma if it's not found. And in the beginning, we were using virotherapy, but then it even got rejected so we cannot use it because it heals the immune system, it's very hard to fight this melanoma disease. [Translated 13:16 - 13:37] If we come back to chemotherapy, the medicine in chemotherapy, it's not found to cure melanoma. And the second negative is that it has the side effects, which simply destroy the immune system, which lowers the quality of life of the patient. It simply changes the whole life of the patient by these side effects.

Ty: So does Rigvir have negative side effects like chemotherapy or radiation?

Dr. Shapovalova: [Translated 14:07 - 14:49] During this age, most of the oncology patients they have gone through our department and usually—not usually , but in most of the cases, almost always, patients had only little a slightly [inaudible - 15:04] temperature of 37 degrees. There were no feelings of sickness. There was no vomiting as the ones that we can see in chemotherapy and radiotherapy.

Ty: Can you explain simply, if possible, to those that are watching how Rigvir works to fight cancer?

Dr. Shapovalova: [Translated 15:31 - 16:05] If there is an echovirus, and it's trained to find the cancer cells and when it gets to the cancer, the tumor, it simply gets to the cancer cells and kills it. And the second option is that it boosts the immune system and helps the body to fight as the immune system is boosted.

Ty: So would it be fair to say that Rigvir is selectively toxic to cancer cells without harming normal cells?

Dr. Shapovalova: [Translated 16:40 - 17:05] Yes, we can say it because usually, on average, a patient receives the therapy during three years and patients don't feel any side effects. They feel very good.

[Translated 17:19 - 17:29] And in case if a surgery is needed, those who receive the Rigvir before the surgery, even those don't feel any side effects. They feel good also.

Ty: And Dr. Elita, I want to thank you for joining us today for the interview. I'm confident that any patient that comes here to the center that has you as their oncologist is in good hands. So thank you for joining us today.

Dr. Shapovalova: [Translated 17:58 - 18:42] First, I also want to thank you for the warm words. We have many patients and Virotherapy Center also has many patients and I hope and believe that this therapy, this medicine, will leave a very long, good, and never-ending life.

And from my side, I have also experienced two very legendary, historic events, moments in medicine. First, it was when the heart was transplanted in Cape Town in 1969 by Dr. Barnard and the second is the whole work, which was done by Professor Aina Muceniece by discovering this medicine.

Ty: Thank you.

Dr. Shapovalova: Thank you. **[end of transcript]**

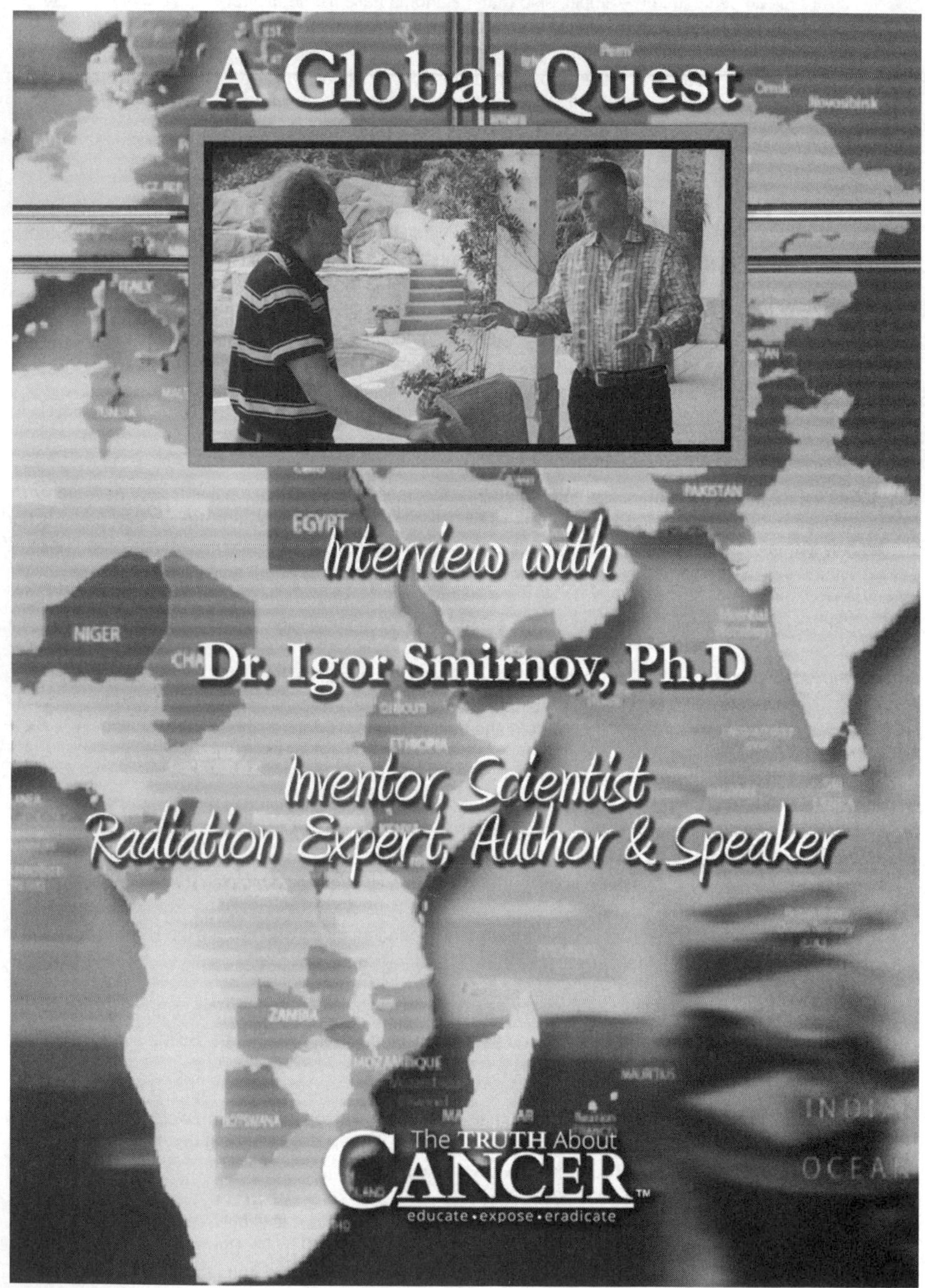
A Global Quest
Interview with
Dr. Igor Smirnov, Ph.D
Inventor, Scientist
Radiation Expert, Author & Speaker
The TRUTH About
CANCER
educate • expose • eradicate

Ty: I'm here today in normally sunny Southern California, today it's a little bit overcast, with Dr. Igor Smirnov. Thank you for inviting us to your home. And I look forward to talking to you today.

You've got some information that you can share with us that is unique, it's revolutionary, and it's regarding activated water and also other ways that we can mitigate radiation.

Dr. Smirnov: Right. So, basically the development of activated water. I mean I was involved in some scientific research back in [the] 1980s.

Ty: Where did you initially grow up and were educated?

Dr. Smirnov: I was educated in Russia in St. Petersburg. I graduated from a naval academy and University in St. Petersburg. I was involved in this in 1980s in research related to the effect of radiation on human subjects after the 1986 Chernobyl fall out. And by chance they found that in some areas the groups of people suffering from radiation were placed in different resorts. And in some areas their rehabilitation was much better compared with other groups. And by accident they found it was because of the spring mineral water.

So we got samples, we did some studies. Within a couple of years we actually found that it's not because of the mineral content of the water, but because of the unique molecular structure of the water. And then it took me probably another 10 years to develop a technology—how to recreate the same type of water in your kitchen.

Basically it's a unique equipment and it's actually treat[ing] water with extremely low intensity, low frequency electromagnetic isolation, which kind of resembles the earth's magnetic field intensity. And we did a lot of research in regards to how this water can affect human physiology and we found it has a very profound effect. There were a lot of studies done in Europe, in United States, and in Russia in regards to how this activated water, MRET activated water, can affect humans.

Ty: What does MRET stands for?

Dr. Smirnov: It stands for Molecular Resonance Effect Technology. Basically this very extremely low intensity and weak signals, electromagnetic signals, they change molecular structure of water. In 1995, two American scientists they got a Nobel Prize for discovery of so called aquaporin channels. Aquaporin it means—they named this aquaporin—in other words how human cells, how they receive water inside the cell.

Ty: Okay. Could you spell that?

Dr. Smirnov: A-Q-U-A-P-O-R-E, I guess. That's right. The main reason for proper hydration of cells is aquaporin channels. And what they found [is] that actually the water molecules go inside these channels one by one with the speed of several billions per second. This is how it works.

In other words, it's very important for the human body when you drink water to reorganize water in so called single linear structure. In this case it can easily go inside the cells. If the water has a different type of structure, then it requires a lot of energy for the human body to create the proper structure. So called intra-cellular structure of the water. After doing research for MRET water we found that the structure of this water quite closely resembles the structure of the intra-cellular water. For this reason, when we ran the so called bioimpedance testing for water, we found that after the MRET treatment, water goes inside the cells three times faster compared with regular water.

It obviously improves hydration of the body and we know that hydration of the body is very important. Because for ten thousands molecules of water in the human body, there is only one molecule of the protein.

The hydration of the body is number one mechanism which supports the whole homeostasis in the body. So, then we conducted a lot of research in regards to how this water can affect, for example, different forms of cancer.

This research was conducted at the Kiev State University in Ukraine in collaboration with [an] oncology centre. And they used mice. It was done in vivo. They used 500 mice. Which means it's very good statistics. And what they found is that if you just treat mice with regular average water, that inhibition of the tumor growth is about 60 to 50 percent compared with control groups. When they were just consuming the regular water. The lifespan of the mice in the group which was treated with MRET water was about 70 percent higher.

Ty: Seventy percent longer.

Dr. Smirnov: Longer. So they live longer.

Ty: So you have mice that were treated with the—the only thing that was different with the two groups was they drank the MRET water?

Dr. Smirnov: That's it. Everything else was exactly the same, like in control group.

Ty: Fifty percent less cancer, 70 percent longer life.

Dr. Smirnov: Longer life, yeah.

Ty: And there's no placebo effect with mice.

Dr. Smirnov: There's no placebo effect with mice, obviously. Because we did a lot of so called in vitro tests on cancer cells with this water. For example, in AltheaDx, it's a San Diego based biotech company, they just treated the cell media with MRET equipment, because cell media is about 90 percent water. And then they placed the HeLa cancer cells and regular human cells in this media. And obviously there was a control cells group.

So what they found, number one, that on the regular cell human cell there is no effect of MRET water. It's completely safe, low effect, it doesn't inhibit, it doesn't enhance growth of these cells. It's just normal. But on the HeLa cancer cells the inhibition was 52 percent.

Ty: So the MRET water it gets into the cells faster. It hydrates better, but it doesn't have any kind of detrimental effects on a normal cell.

Dr. Smirnov: Absolutely. For normal cells.

Ty: But the cancer cells it does.

Dr. Smirnov: But the cancer cells it just inhibits their growth. This is what we found in vitro and in vivo in animal models.

Ty: Dr. Smirnov, this MRET water, you helped to develop this machine that will create the water that's very similar to the water that helped the radiation victims of Chernobyl. And that some of these victims were healing faster.

Dr. Smirnov: Quite closely resembles this water, but of course it's a different technology. It was natural water. This is man-made technology.

Ty: But it resembles the water that helped to mitigate the negative effects of radiation.

Dr. Smirnov: Exactly.

Ty: It also has effects on the cancer cells as well. Selectively toxic to the cancer cells. It inhibits their growth.

Dr. Smirnov: It inhibits the growth. And this is what we found. We run a lot of experiments with cancer cells. As I said, for example, with AltheaDx a biotech company in San Diego, they run tests on HeLa cancer cells. And they run tests on normal human cells. So what they found that MRET water has no effect on normal human cells, which means it's safe for consumption. And there is significant 52 percent inhibition of HeLa cancer cells.

Ty: So it stops them from growing.

Dr. Smirnov: Exactly. Right.

Ty: That's fascinating. So you have water. What do you call it? Activated water?

Dr. Smirnov: It's activated. MRET activated water, yes.

Ty: So it has this effect on radiation as well as cancer cells.

Dr. Smirnov: Exactly, because the result of any radiation effect is cancers. Mostly is cancers.

Ty: So is this water something that, let's say—this documentary is specifically focusing on cancer. Many people that are watching may already be undergoing chemotherapy or radiation treatments. Is this water something that they could take to help lessen the side effects?

Dr. Smirnov: Exactly. We were actually very much surprised. When we did a lot of biological tests for this water, including the effect on harmful bacteria. It inhibits growth of harmful bacteria. And it actually, in general, improved the homeostasis of the body.

So, it's kind of like an immune boost. And the main point is it has a proper molecular structure which quite closely resembles intra-cellular water. Basically when you drink this water, your body doesn't need to spend energy to restructure water, because regular water is supposed to be restructured inside the body.

Obviously this energy and this input of the MRET water just helps the body to function properly and to develop to boost immune system, to resist different type of harmful bacteria including growth of the cancer cells.

Ty: And apparently it helps with healthy growth as well, because right over there behind you is a lemon tree – a lime tree actually. And I noticed over there before we started the interview that these limes are bigger than any lime I've ever seen in my life. And you're telling me that you're feeding the tree MRET water.

Dr. Smirnov: That's right. We're doing this private experiment with my wife. But obviously we did serious lab research, how the water affects...

Ty: Some of it is sitting here. So this isn't something that's just fly-by-night. This is very heavily researched technology.

Dr. Smirnov: Exactly. And this research was actually published with the World Scientific Publishers in Singapore. It's one of the largest scientific publishers. And it includes all this research in regards to how this water affects different type of cancer.

We conducted this test on two different type of cancer. It's carcinoma and sarcoma. And tests were done in animal models.

Ty: So as you can see here we got a book, *Introduction to the Biophysics of Activated Water*. We got a ton of research here. And this is just the tip of the iceberg. This is very heavily researched science, isn't it? That's why I wanted to share. There's some anecdotal cases of different types of illnesses that the activated water...

Dr. Smirnov: Right. Because the water is very important for the human body. For example, we have some anecdotal cases in regards to how the MRET water if you have different types of problems like for example, eczema or psoriasis.

This case as you can see this is the original and after two moths of consumption MRET water. So it's almost gone. This is another case with psoriasis.

Ty: That's unbelievable.

Dr. Smirnov: So this gentleman was suffering like 18 years from this heavy problem. And this is after 20 days.

Ty: That's unbelievable.

Dr. Smirnov: Unbelievable. This is another case in China. This is Singapore. This is China case. How clean the body is cleaning. Detoxing. This is the cancer case. This gentleman was diagnosed with the nose cancer so called.

Ty: Nose cancer, lymphoma, bone cancer, and liver cancer.

Dr. Smirnov: Liver cancer. Right. So he was taking MRET water for one year. So this is later, that's his letter of a clean [bill of health]. No cancer cells. And this is just one of the many anecdotal cases we have in our records.

Ty: That's really interesting that water can have that profound an effect on your health. So this MRET water, there is machines that you have invented that will create this water?

Dr. Smirnov: Right. Exactly.

Ty: They are called MRET machine?

Dr. Smirnov: MRET activator. MRET machine, yes.

Ty: So as you can see here on my phone I've got a little device here. And this is called an MRET device?

Dr. Smirnov: It's an MRET-Nylon device.

Ty: What does this do because I've got it on my phone because we know about the dangers of cell phone radiation? I've had this on my phone ever since I learned about this technology over a year ago. So what is this and how does it work?

Dr. Smirnov: It basically works [the] same way like a MRET water machine, because it's based on these so called generation of the low frequency, low intensity, so called noise field, magnetic field, which quite closely resemble natural geomagnetic field.

So in other words, for million of years of evolution the human body was developed when around us was just natural earth magnetic fields. And after probably within the last 150 years there is a lot of distortion of these electromagnetic fields because we developed a lot of man-made electromagnetic pollution around.

In order to protect the human body we have to recreate the same natural noise field to protect the human cells. Because how the human cells react to the man-made electromagnetic field, it immediately shut downs their membranes, so called channels. It's called hardening of the cellular membrane.

So when man-made electromagnetic field effect the cells they shut down their membrane, so called hardening of these cells membranes mechanism. And it's designed – it's a natural mechanism. The same way cells behave when kind of like a chemical poison can be introduced to the cells.

So the only difference is that you can easily remove because of the flush and human body activity, the chemicals can easily be removed out of the body. But when you expose to the electromagnetic – you cannot remove it. You cannot stop it. You're continuously exposed to this pollution, especially after introduction of Wi-Fi.

Ty: And the cell phone towers.

Dr. Smirnov: Right. Towers.

Ty: So this recreates the noise field that we're used to for our bodies. So how does it protect us?

Dr. Smirnov: So when it generates this noise field, extremely low intensity noise field, the noise field can be superimposed on the micro-wave signals, man-made electricity. It's kind of like it's a piggyback. It carries these noise field frequencies. The microwave signals carry these noise field frequencies.

So in other words when it hits the cells, the noise field is kind of like a mask. The microwave signal. So cells cannot recognize microwave signals and they don't shut down their membrane.

Ty: So basically it makes it invisible. You're tricking them. So this thing is generating the healthy noise field that we're used to for ourselves and then – so let's say when it rings or whatever, is that when the microwave radiation comes in and then it piggybacks it and it makes it invisible to the body so you don't have a reaction to it?

Dr. Smirnov: There is no reaction. Cells don't shut down their membranes.

Ty: That's what causes the problems. Is when the cell membrane shuts down. So is this something that once it's placed on the phone like I don't need to recharge this thing, it just continually does that?

Dr. Smirnov: No. It's just the material. It's a polymer material. And when you expose this polymer material to electromagnetic microwave radiation, it's kind of like creates excitation in the molecular structure of the polymer. This is how the polymer generates low frequency.

Ty: I understand how this works better than I ever had now. I didn't understand how it worked. I trusted that it worked because I've read some of the writings on the research on it. I know it works, but that's a really great explanation.

Dr. Smirnov: Because this is a side product of the MRET water machine. Because inside the water machine we used same type of polymer. So in other words how we create the noise field to treat water. We use same type of the polymer material. We activate this polymer material.

And polymer material generates this noise field which actually treats water and restructures the molecular structure of water. But because we know that this water actually has an extremely profound effect on the human physiology, this is exactly the same mechanism.

Ty: Same mechanism. So if I'm carrying this thing, so the cell phone towers and everything around me, is this protecting my whole body or just...?

Dr. Smirnov: It's protecting the whole body because the microwave signal is carrying this noise field, depending on the power of microwave signal. If let's say it's covered 10 feet, so you're protecting 10 feet around you. If it has intensity to cover one mile, you're protecting one mile. But we already developed a new product based on this technology which can actually cover like 30 feet around. You can place it in your office.

Ty: Put it in your home.

Dr. Smirnov: You turn on this machine. This is a passive mechanism because it requires a microwave signal to generate the noise field. This is a new machine which our company is introducing into the market.

It actually has electronics inside. And it stimulates the polymer material any time. It doesn't matter if there's any microwave signal, no microwave signal. So you just push the button and 30 feet around everybody is protected.

Ty: So you if had two or three of those for a big home you could protect the whole house.

Dr. Smirnov: You can cover the house and we actually developed in kind of like a portable one, because you can carry it on your flight in the plane. Because there is a lot of effective radiation. If you go on YouTube you just check when your flight radiation effect, it's about maybe 20-90 times increase of radiation when you fly at 13 [thousand] feet or higher.

Ty: So it's good. But the thing I guess then if you're flying, would this [*indicating the cellphone MRET-Nylon*] protect you in flight or would you need another to protect you in flight?

Dr. Smirnov: It's better to have kind of like a portable one.

Ty: The active one.

Dr. Smirnov: The active one.

Ty: Okay. Got it. Well, that's really fascinating because I know that's really a big topic today is we got all the cell phone towers, all the Wi-Fi, do we turn the Wi-Fi off at night for the family so we get less exposure. These devices that you've invented for your house could protect you at all times.

Dr. Smirnov: Exactly. Yeah.

Ty: That's great information. Well, Dr. Igor, this is great information for our audience. This is something that no one else has covered. But it really makes me more hopeful that we can actually protect ourselves in this toxic world, especially with all this electro-smog that's going on. So thank you for your research. Thank for you time.

Dr. Smirnov: Thank you.

[end of transcript]

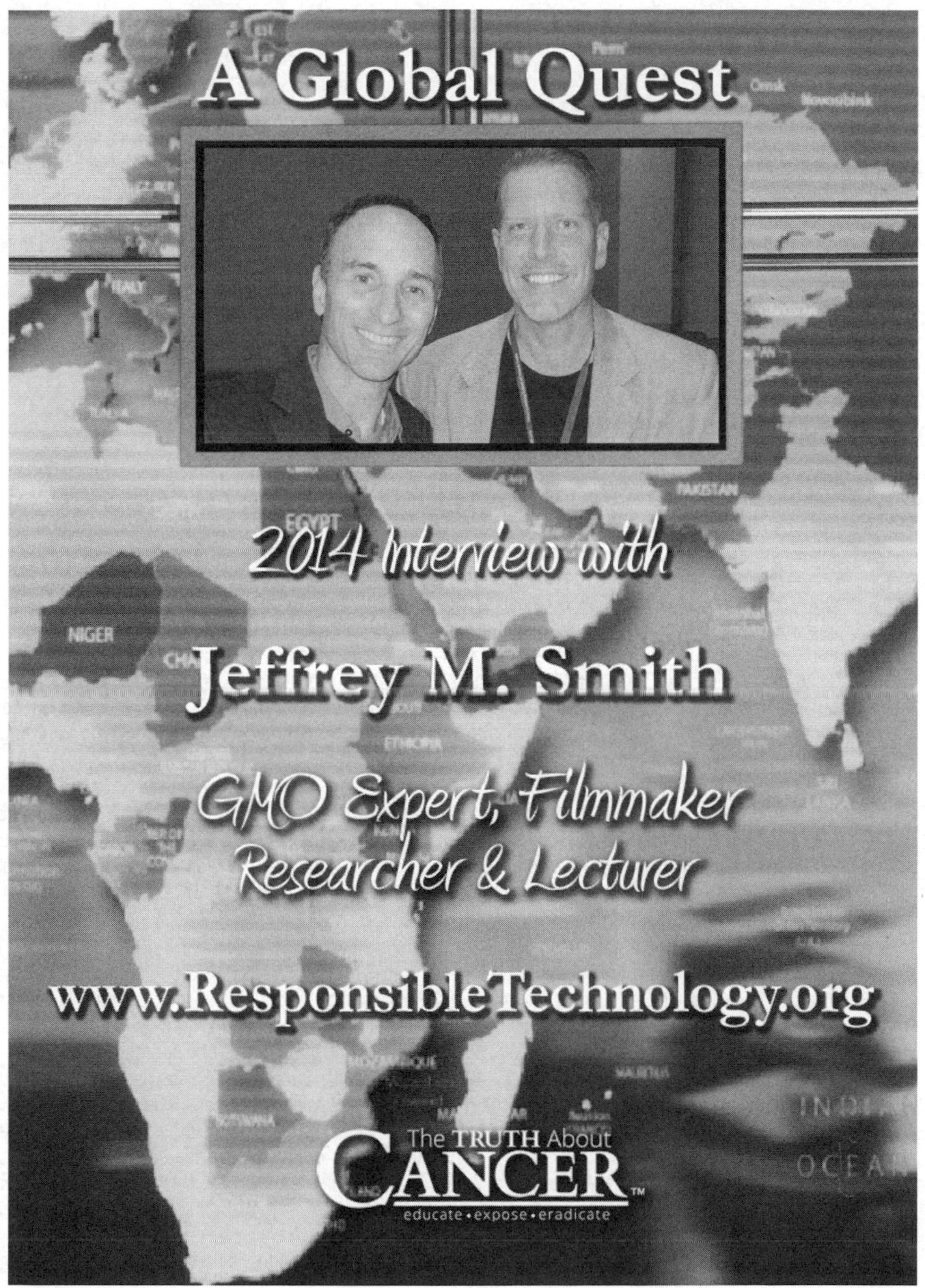
A Global Quest
2014 Interview with
Jeffrey M. Smith
GMO Expert, Filmmaker
Researcher & Lecturer
www.ResponsibleTechnology.org
The TRUTH About
CANCER
educate • expose • eradicate

Ty: So I'm here today with Jeffrey Smith. We're here in Las Vegas, Nevada. And first of all, I just want to thank you for being with us today and taking the time to share some of your knowledge with our viewers.

Jeffrey: Happy to be here, Ty.

Ty: So tell us, Jeffrey, about your background, your education, anything you want people to know about you.

Jeffrey: Well, I just talk about one thing, GMOs, genetically modified organisms. I've been interviewing scientists and translating the science into English for over 18 years. And I've traveled to about 40 countries and I founded the Institute for Responsible Technology. We explain to people why to avoid GMOs and how. And we have a shopping guide, a nonGMOshoppingguide.com and a free iPhone application, Shop No GMO.

Ty: When you were a kid you probably didn't dream that you'd be a GMO research and advocate.

Jeffrey: When I was a kid I never heard of GMOs. They hadn't existed yet. So no, you're right.

Ty: So what got you into this kind of research, this line of research?

Jeffrey: I went to a lecture from a genetic engineer and he was absolutely adamant that it was completely inexcusable to use that technology for food because the technology was prone to side effects. It would be absolutely unpredictable. And not only that, but even those that could be tested were not being evaluated properly and they were able to be planted. This was in 1996 when I went to the lecture. And, moreover, once they were produced and released into the environment they would cross-pollinate, seeds would travel, and they would become part of the gene pool, a self-propagating pollution of the gene pool that would last forever. So the only thing that lasted longer than genetic pollution, not global warming, not nuclear waste, is extinction. So when they realized the profound implications of this technology for all living things and all future generations, I figured, this guy needs a little help and he needs to get the word out in a way that'd be effective and to wake people up. And I wasn't expecting it to take this long, but now we're actually seeing a big wake-up in the United States. People are rejecting GMOs in very large numbers and we see it coming to a tipping point very, very soon.

Ty: Yeah. And you know, I want to thank you personally. You are probably the most vocal, the most well known, anti-GMO researcher person that's getting the word out about GMOs, waking people up on that. You were the reason that I've learned about GMOs. So I just want to thank you for that because I know that you're impacting the world and making it a better place, waking people up. Let's take a step back though. What are GMOs?

Jeffrey: Genetically modified organisms—you take genes from one species and force it into the DNA of other species. Now the GMO crops on the market, there's nine of them, and the primary traits are either herbicide tolerance or pesticide production. So herbicide tolerance, Roundup Ready is the most popular. Roundup Ready soy, corn, cotton, canola, sugar beets and alfalfa. They're engineered with genes from bacteria and pieces of virus, etc. not to die, the plant doesn't die when it's sprayed with Roundup herbicide, which normally kills plants. So it makes weeding easier for farmers. They can simply spray over the crops and kill all the weeds but not the Roundup Ready crops. And the other genetically modified trait that's popular is pesticide production. They take a gene from bacteria in the soil called the bacillus thuringiensis, or BT for short. And take that gene which produces a known insecticide and put it into corn and cotton. So when a bug, certain types of bugs, eat or try to bite the plant the toxin gets released and then it breaks open little holes in their stomach walls and they die. So now we eat that insecticide and we also eat the Roundup laden crops. So we're eating two types of poisons in these GM crops.

Ty: So what are the effects on humans of eating BT toxin and Roundup pesticide?

Jeffrey: Well, it was promised to us up and down that BT toxin was safe because it only affected certain insects. That turned out to be not true. The BT toxin in its natural form, which is used as a spray or even organic agriculture has been linked to inflammation, immune problems, and also tissue damage in mice, but immune problems in humans. The toxin that's produced in the corn is thousands of times more concentrated. It's designed to be more toxic. And it was found to poke holes in human cells. So it pokes holes in insect cells. BT toxin pokes holes in the cell walls of insects and breaks open their stomach to kill them. It's now found to poke holes in human cells. So this means that it might create leaky gut or holes in the walls of our intestines that allow undigested food proteins, chemicals and bacteria directly into the bloodstream. And this is linked to cancer. It's also linked to autism, autoimmune disease, food allergies, inflammation in general, Alzheimer's, Parkinson's, a whole host of diseases and disorders.

Ty: So in light of the fact that the research has shown that this does cause leaky gut, which is…

Jeffrey: No. The research has shown that BT toxin in a laboratory setting can poke holes in human cells. I would say it's preliminary to say that the research has shown that it causes leaky gut in humans. We just know that it has—the entire apparatus is there. It's a hole-poking toxin. It also can promote immune responses in humans. So we're eating corn that can possibly create immune responses, food allergies, not just to the corn but to other things, possibly poke holes in human cells that can possibly cause autoimmune disease. All of these things we say possibly because there's hardly any research conducted from independent scientists on the dangers of GMOs. And when scientists do discover problems they're often fired, threatened, gagged, attacked, they're just treated terribly so that no one else wants to weigh in on the issue. And so there's really very, very few scientists willing to risk their jobs and their reputations by doing GMO research.

Ty: So you have these—this BT toxin, Roundup, these potentially dangerous substance being sprayed on food. They've not been proven to be safe. We think that they may be potentially extremely harmful. How is it that they are—that the companies are allowed to make these and spray them on our food and we're ingesting them without being warned about the potential dangers?

Jeffrey: The companies are in charge of determining if their genetically modified foods are safe. The FDA does not require a single safety study on GMOs. Now this was determined in a policy in 1992 that was overseen by Michael Taylor. Michael Taylor is the former attorney to Monsanto. And he was given a position that was designed for him by the FDA when the agency was told by the White House to promote GMOs. And Taylor's policy falsely claimed that the agency wasn't aware of information showing that GMOs were significantly different, therefore, no testing or labeling was necessary. Companies like Monsanto could determine on their own if their GMOs are safe. And Monsanto told us that agent orange and PCBs and DDT were safe and got that wrong, maybe they'll get it right with GMO's is the thinking by the FDA. Taylor then became Monsanto's vice president and chief lobbyist, now he's back at the FDA as the "US food safety czar."

Ty: It's almost like you have the fox guarding the hen house.

Jeffrey: It's more than almost. We have a situation where the claims in the policy, they weren't aware of information showing that GMOs were different, was a complete lie. It was a total fabrication. The lawsuit forced 44,000 secret FDA memos into the public domain and it showed that the overwhelming consensus among the scientists working at the FDA was exactly the opposite. They said GMOs might create allergens, toxins, new diseases, and nutritional problems, urged their superiors to require testing, complained about the draft of the policy and their concerns were ignored and even denied.

Ty: Now when you say that they are not significant, or at least Monsanto said they are not significantly different than what

Jeffrey: Think the normal foods.

Ty: The normal foods…

Jeffrey: Right.

Ty: Oh, so since they're not significantly different than normal food it doesn't—they don't need to tell us that they're doing this to us.

Jeffrey: They don't need to tell us, they don't need to test it. They can just put it on the market and assume that it's safe. And if they want to do tests they can do tests. And if they don't want to—and the tests that they do, tobacco science, completely rigged to avoid finding problems. We catch them red-handed.

Ty: So the only testing that is required are self tests that they submit and then, of course, it's going to—

Jeffrey: They can submit them if they want and they usually—if they do submit just summaries they will never give a reviewer enough information to determine safety. The tests typically on animals end in 90 days. So you feed an animal, a rat, for example, let's say 33 percent of its diet is a genetically modified corn for 90 days. And if it looks good after 90 days you feed it to humans for their entire lives. Now a research team headed by Dr. Seralini decided to extend the study of 90 days to two years, the approximate lifespan of a rat. Now Seralini had been reviewing the submissions to France and to the European union by Monsanto and saw that Roundup Ready corn fed to rats showed more than 50 different statistically significant changes in the animals compared to the control. And Monsanto said, "Oh, there's no problem." And Seralini says, "What do you mean there's no problem? This is very serious." He published it, showing that there was very significant signs of toxicity. So he secretly extended the study using the same type of rats, the same control group size, but many, many more parameters that they tested for and starting after the 90 days in the next month the first rat started to get tumors. And by the end up to 80 percent of the female rats had tumors, almost all of them mammary gland tumors, up to 50 percent of male rats had tumors compared to far less in the controls.

Now it's interesting that the tumors came from the rats that ate the Roundup Ready corn that had been sprayed with Roundup. But they also came from rats that ate the Roundup Ready that had never been sprayed with Roundup. Now this was never done because if you plant Roundup Ready corn you do it in order to spray Roundup. But he wanted to see what was the cause of any problem that was encountered. So he had a group of rats that ate the Roundup Ready corn that had never been sprayed with Roundup, a group that ate the Roundup corn that had been sprayed with Roundup, and a group that ate the Roundup with no Roundup Ready corn, just the Roundup. All of them got massive multiple tumors as large as 25 percent of their body weight. They also died earlier and had damaged their liver, kidneys, and pituitary.

Ty: So what is—how do you summarize the three different groups? What is the significance of the group that ate just the Roundup, just the corn, and the corn that had been sprayed with Roundup? What exactly does that mean?

Jeffrey: It means that there's something in the corn and there's something in the Roundup that appears to promote tumor growth. And Roundup we know more about. There's more studies on Roundup than on the GMOs. Roundup can promote cancer in many, many ways. First of all, it's an antibiotic and it kills off beneficial gut bacteria, causing overgrowth of the bad gut bacteria. Now this overgrowth of negative gut bacteria is linked to certain cancers—colorectal cancer, for example. The overgrowth of negative gut bacteria can produce Zonulin, which can create leaky gut. It opens the gaps of the cell walls on the intestines. And leaky gut is linked to cancer. Roundup also damages a set of enzymes called the CYP enzymes which are part of the detoxification process and CYP enzymes are linked to cancer. And so it's interesting, and they're linked in different ways but if you're damaging the CYP enzymes. You may be promoting cancer, and no one is looking. The CYP enzymes also should help the body detoxify chemotherapy. There's a certain one that will help the liver detoxify. And one of the problems with Roundup is it can disable some of those enzymes that are involved with detoxification. So any toxic influence from the environment can be much more toxic when you're also exposed to Roundup, or its active ingredient, glyphosate. So even the chemotherapy taken for the cancer which may have been promoted by Roundup may actually not get out of the body as easily and be much worse.

Roundup also chelates or binds with certain trace minerals like zinc and zinc would become more deficient in the presence of Roundup. It'll still be there but it can't be assimilated because it's locked in and bound with the glyphosate molecule. And zinc deficiency is linked to certain cancers, and it's been tested as a possible adjunct or supplement for cancer therapy. In addition, Roundup specifically can promote enhanced breast cell growth and in tiny, tiny amounts, in parts per trillion. So this is the amount of Roundup that's already in our air and in our rain water and in our drinking water because of the overuse of Roundup because of the Roundup Ready crops. So Roundup has all these different ways. It also can promote inflammation through the gut bacteria. Through the gut bacteria overgrowth it can promote inflammation in the gut. And inflammation is also linked to cancer. So Roundup has all these different ways, like a perfect storm. Now there are certain tissues that are the target tissues for Roundup and they—it accumulates in those tissues and those are the cancers that are on the rise in the US population, for example—thyroid cancer, liver cancer, and kidney cancer. So there's a lot of indications out there that Roundup and its active ingredient glyphosate may be promoting the growth of cancer in the United States.

Ty: Wow! So it sounds to me like we're going to have millions of people who are watching this. I guarantee there's tens of thousands of cancer patients watching this. To me it sounds like one of the most important things they should avoid in their diet is anything that contains Roundup or has been sprayed with Roundup because of all of these factors, all of the linkage to cancer but also the fact that it inhibits the CYP enzyme from detoxing the chemo because many of the people are probably taking chemotherapy.

Jeffrey: Yeah. zit used to be just important to avoid the GMOs, the Roundup Ready soy and corn which are in practically everything. And they contain higher levels of Roundup. The cottonseed oil, the canola oil, sugar beets, sugar, which is mostly sugar from sugar beets. But actually it's worse now because Roundup is used as a ripening agent on all sorts of grains and beans and fruits and vegetables. So it's used for sugarcane. So you'll find it in molasses and what not. You'll find it sprayed on wheat. It's sprayed on barley and rice and lentils and potatoes and sweet potatoes and berries and citrus groves. So the way to go really to avoid Roundup, I mean you can find the 160 types of fruits, vegetables and plants that have been approved for high levels of Roundup residue by the EPA but it's just easier to go all organic. And that would be anyone who has a diagnosis of cancer might want to do that to prevent exposure to glyphosate and some other nasty chemicals that are found on conventional foods. Now the BT toxin produced by the corn, because it promotes allergic reactions or immune system reactions, in humans and animals, can create inflammation. And again, inflammation is linked to cancer. Now the BT toxin, it's interesting, they found the BT toxin and Roundup in the blood of pregnant women tested in Canada. In fact, 93 percent of the pregnant women had BT toxin in their blood and so too did 80 percent of their unborn fetuses. Now the BT toxin may have gotten into the blood through the leaky gut that it itself created by poking holes in the cell walls. If it gets in the blood it can be cytotoxic, damaging the red blood cells, and this was found in the case of a mouse study where BT toxin damaged the red blood cells. The fetus doesn't have blood brain barriers well developed so it might end up in the brains of the fetuses. So you have a hole poking toxin in the brains of the next generation in North America.

Now what's interesting is 93 percent of the pregnant women tested had the BT toxin in their blood, but BT toxin washes out quickly. So they must have had a frequent intake of BT toxin, but it wasn't Mexico, where they eat corn tortillas every day. It was Canada and most of the corn they're eating is already devoid of BT toxin, high fructose corn syrup has no BT toxin left in it, corn oil doesn't. So the authors of the study guessed that the source of the BT toxin was probably the milk and meat of animals that do eat BT toxin as part of their daily regimen. And so for some reason they were saying that the BT toxin survived digestion in the animals and then survived digestion in humans and then maybe poked holes in the walls of the intestines and then got into the blood. I think a more plausible explanation comes from a 2004 study, which the only human feeding study is ever done on commercialized GMOs. They found—and this was with soybeans, Roundup Ready soybeans—they found that the Roundup Ready genes that were inserted into the soybeans to allow the soybeans not to die when sprayed with Roundup those genes, part of them, transferred into the DNA of bacteria living inside our intestines. And that bacteria was unkillable with Roundup, suggesting but not proving that once the gene transferred the gut bacteria it might still function. And to function means it might produce proteins. So we may have these Roundup Ready proteins produced continuously 24/7 inside our digestive tract.

Now as soon as the pro-GMO UK government who was funding this study, found out, they pulled the plug on any additional funding. So they never found out if eating a corn chip from genetically modified BT toxin corn also transfers to the DNA of gut bacteria. If the BT gene transfers to gut bacteria and continues to function it can convert our intestinal flora into living pesticide factories producing BT toxin 24/7 which might poke holes along the cell walls causing inflammation and all sorts of gastrointestinal disorders, possibly creating leaky gut, which is also linked to cancer. And that might explain this production of the BT toxin, why 93 percent of the pregnant women tested in Canada had it in their blood because they are producing it in their gut.

Ty: Wow! This is pretty disturbing.

Jeffrey: Yeah, it doesn't get much more disturbing than that.

Ty: It's pretty disturbing because you may be very cognizant of the foods that have genetically modified organisms, the BT toxin, and avoid them, but what you're saying is it's possible…

Jeffrey: Like six months ago before you knew about GMOs you might have colonized your gut bacteria. Now people ask me all the time what to do about it. The good news is this. Actually it's terrific news. People when they stop eating GMOs, they get better from all sorts of diseases and disorders. And we interview them and we hear about it all the time. When I speak to a room full of say, 500 people, you know, dozens and dozens of people will say, "Yes, I feel better and got better, symptoms went away when I switched to non-GMO foods." And it's completely predictable which categories of diseases and disorders get better. The one that is far greater than anything else is gastrointestinal. And you have things like immune system problems like allergies and asthma and autoimmune disease, skin conditions, headaches including migraine headaches, people lose weight when they stop eating GMOs, people who couldn't lose weight before, many of them. We have mental problems like brain fog, depression, aggression, and we understand why that may be the case. We understand why, for example, consuming Roundup might cause mental problems because the gut bacteria normally produces tryptophan and tryptophan is a precursor to serotonin which is important for mood and the tryptophan-producing metabolic pathways dismantle with Roundup. So if you're cut short on serotonin you might have problems with depression. You also might not feel full when you eat. When you get to a certain point it's this tryptophan that kicks in that says, I've eaten enough. Without that you can just continue to eat. It's also a precursor to melatonin and so you may have problems with sleep as well. So the gastrointestinal problems, immune system problems, reproductive disorders, organ damage, all these things that people are talking about getting better from when they get rid of GMOs those are the same categories of diseases and disorders that afflict the lab animals fed GMOs. And it's described in the review study by the American Academy of Environmental Medicine, that said these animals are causally being—creating these disorders from eating GMOs and every doctor should prescribe non-GMO diets to their patients. Thousands of doctors are telling their patients don't eat GMOs and many are telling us that the patients are getting better from these same disorders and diseases.

Now when a human gets rid of GMOs they have to do a strategy, because it's not labeled in the United States, so they'll have to switch to organic or reduce-processed foods to avoid the soy and corn derivatives. And so there's competing cofactors that might explain why a person feels better and why their symptoms disappear. But when livestock are taken off of GMOs there's no competing cofactors. It's just switching from GM corn to non-GM corn, from GM soy to non-GM soy. And the animals get better from the same problems that the humans are getting better from. And this is reported by the farmers and by veterinarians. And now we're hearing from pet owners, cats and dogs taken off of GMOs are getting better from gastrointestinal disorders, immune problems, fur issues, things like that. And we see this all the time.

Ty: I hate to interject this, but I was just speaking with a lady last week and she had had a pet, a dog, that was having all kinds of issues. She took the dog off the of the GMO feed, got organic feed and the dog's doing well.

Jeffrey: I have heard so many stories like that. In fact, I'm putting together a little film with many veterinarians and pet owners saying the exact same thing. You see, in my situation, Ty, I hear more testimonials than anyone on the planet from people who get rid of GMOs for their dogs or cats. Because that's what people tell me. And in fact, I ask audiences to tell so that other people can hear. So to me it's so absolutely predictable. And I originally was skeptical even though I was talking about the dangers of GMOs from a scientific perspective for more than a decade. People come up to me and say,"I react to GMOs." And my skeptics say, "Well, how do you know?" I didn't say that. You don't know if it's from GMOs or not because there's no easy way to do it. And I didn't really get a sense that it would be so blatant, except for very, very sensitive individuals. Then I went to the American Academy of Environmental Medicine for the fourth time. I had been speaking to their group for four years—three years—and people started to prescribe non-GMO diets and I wasn't aware of them. I started interviewing them and they said, "Oh yeah. My patients react more to GMOs and the allergic reactions get worse and I take people off of GMOs. They all get better and GMOs cause inflammation." They weren't speaking like the scientists. The scientists are like, "GMOs might...and it appears...and it could be...and it suggests." These doctors are saying, "Oh no, GMOs are doing this to our patients." And it occurred to me that they treat thousands of patients. And they're experimenting on us. So when they say get rid of GMOs they get to see, and they get to see, well. If I don't tell them to get rid of GMOs, then sometimes the treatment is not working, so well. So GMOs are linked to gluten-related disorders according to research that we've done and others. And one doctor says, "When you get rid of gluten, I say to the patients, get rid of GMOs at the same time because the recovery is quicker and more complete."

Ty: That's encouraging. It's encouraging to see that removing the GMOs from the diet actually shows promising benefits. I like the good news after the devastating, there's the good news, I like that, that we can recover. And that you don't necessarily—can keep the BT toxin in forever or at least the effects of the BT toxin.

Jeffrey: As far as the gut bacteria, I mean, it is now a huge source, a huge topic of study. Everyone's into the microbio now. It's like it's the new tofu. Everyone's into the microbio. And so we have a situation where as the devastation of Roundup becomes bigger and bigger the more they realize this, because it is a potent antibiotic, but it is selective. It kills the lactobacillus and the bifidobacteria, the stuff that's good for us.

Ty: The ones that you want in yogurt.

Jeffrey: The stuff that you're buying and paying for and then you wash it down with something with Roundup in it and you just kill everything you've just put in there plus more. And it allows the overgrowth of salmonella or botulism or e.Coli, the negative stuff.

Ty: Let me ask you this. So you've talked about the Roundup Ready corn and the soy potentially that's sprayed with Roundup. Do they use Roundup or glyphosate on other non-organic vegetables as well or is it just the corn and soy?

Jeffrey: No, no, it's used as a ripening agent. They spray it on wheat, on barley, on rye, on lentils, on sweet potatoes, on sugar cane—there's a 160 or so different fruits, vegetables, grains, beans, etc. that are allowed high residues because of this now practice of using it as what's called a desiccant or ripening agent. Not every farmer uses it but it's hard to tell where it is and where it isn't because it's not labeled. So that's why buying organic is much safer.

Ty: I'm sure that on your website that you have a food guide that we can look at.

Jeffrey: We have nonGMOshoppingguide.com. Now we don't list which foods contain sprays of glyphosate or not because there's an extensive list. We just say in order to avoid glyphosate and Roundup, buy organic. In order to avoid GMOs we have close to 17,000 products in our shopping guide.

Ty: This a huge warning for people I think. And this is a reaffirmation to me. My family tries to only eat organic and stay away from the GMOs, the BT toxins. This is just a reaffirmation to me to be extremely vigilant to not ingest GMOs, and the BT toxin, the Roundup Ready foods.

Jeffrey: And it may get worse because they have now up for approval, we call it Agent Orange crops, crops that are tolerant to be sprayed by 24D which was half the component of Agent Orange, which can create dioxins tjat are linked to cancer. And so it's expected if that gets approved the use of 24D will increase in the United States by as much as 20-fold, and so it'll be in the food, it'll also in the air, because it can vaporize and then move and then land and kill other crops and hurt other people and livestock. So it's an absolute disaster. Now we hope to stop GMOs soon. We actually have seen a tipping point of consumer rejection. We expect to end GMOs soon. And it's because consumers are becoming awake to the dangers. So in Europe because of a high-profile food scandal related to GMOs most people decided they didn't want to eat them. In very short time, huge headlines, hundreds and hundreds of articles, the food companies said, okay, we won't use them. Then bovine growth hormone was kicked out of Wal-Mart and Starbucks and Yoplait and Dannon in most American dairies because of its link to cancer. And that became popular and people didn't want to eat it. And so it had a tipping point. There's now a tipping point against GMOs in the natural products industry, and we expect a tipping point in the conventional food industry any time.

Ty: And recently we had legislation in Vermont.

Jeffrey: Vermont passed a labeling law, yes. It was very, very exciting. So this was passed this year and it'll go into effect on July 1, 2016. They expect to be sued by Monsanto and the biotech industry. It's possible the FDA will come in and preempt it. They're up still against some potential obstacles but it's the first state to pass a labeling law that will go into effect immediately as soon as the date hits. Two other states have a requirement of other states also passing similar laws before theirs become enacted. And most states actually have introduced labeling legislation that has not yet passed.

Ty: That is encouraging news. To me it's ironic that Monsanto says that the GMO crops are safe but they're fighting labeling the crops. So if they're safe why do they care if they're labeled?

Jeffrey: Well, there's a schizophrenia in Monsanto that's rather deep. I mean, they tell the FDA there's no difference. They tell the patent office it's completely different and patentable, you know. They say to consumers it's completely safe and it'll produce better crops, but we don't want you to know that it's in your food. Well, they told us that Agent Orange was safe and PCBs were safe and DDT was safe and got that wrong. And they are really—they're voted every year as the most hated corporation on earth with stiff competition. And I think they have deserved that award every year. Now they also introduced bovine growth hormone. RBGH, recombinant bovine growth hormone, is a genetically engineered drug injected into cows to increase milk supply. And it does a lot of things to the milk. There's more pus, more antibiotics, more bovine growth hormone in the milk but there's also more IGF1 which promotes cell growth and it promotes cancer growth.

Ty: What does IGF stand for?

Jeffrey: Insulin-like growth factor-1. Now the IGF1 increase in the milk was the primary reason why it's been banned in the European Union, Canada, Australia, New Zealand, Japan. And a former Monsanto scientist told me that three of his colleagues found so much IGF1 in the milk from treated cows, and they were doing the safety studies in the milk, that Monsanto's own scientists, the three of them, refused to drink milk thereafter unless it was organic. One bought his own cow.

Ty: Wow!

Jeffrey: So they wouldn't even drink the milk from treated cows but they promised it was safe to everyone else. Now soon after the bovine growth hormone was approved someone went in and did some research and found out that milk duct tissue cancer went up in parallel with the introduction and expansion of the RBGH in dairy by about 60 percent. And it's also possible in many other cancers, slower growing cancers, less aggressive, are also on the rise because of RBGH. And there was a study done in 2006 that linked the use of RBGH in the United States with also higher levels of fraternal twins because in addition to promoting cell growth it also promotes the multiple eggs and also fraternal twins.

Ty: Wow! Now concerning RBGH, I noticed that if you buy milk on the label you'll see no RBGH or RBGH-free. Can we trust those labels?

Jeffrey: With RBGH there's no assay or test to apply to the milk to see if RBGH was used with the cow. So it's done in an affidavit basis. So farmers will sign an affidavit to their bottler that they don't use it. That's as good as we have right now.

Ty: But it's better to buy that because everybody buys milk and so your recommendation I'm guessing would be if you're going to buy the milk buy organic and RBGH-free?

Jeffrey: Organic—there's three levels. There's organic at the top. They're not allowed to use RBGH and they don't feed the animals GMOs. Then there's non-organic but no RBST or no RBGH, same thing. They will feed the animals GMOs but they won't inject them with bovine growth hormone. So that's a second mess. Then there's conventional which is the worst of the three.

Ty: Okay. But it seems to me though the middle category where they might not inject them with RBGH but they still feed them the GMO crops, they cows are what they eat. You might as well go organic.

Jeffrey: Oh well, if you have the choice it's kind of a no-brainer.

Ty: Right

Jeffrey: Because they found that even feeding the animals GMOs versus non-GMOs changes the milk content. And that was found back in 1996 in the same study that Monsanto claims shows that there was no difference between Roundup Ready soybeans and conventional soybeans. The fat content was different in the milk from the cows that ate one versus the other. But they just ignored it as being not important.

Ty: Let me ask you this. One of the common arguments that you get from those that are producing the GMO crops is that we need this to feed the world.

Jeffrey: No, no, they need it to pay their salaries. GMOs are so inept at feeding the world that the biggest paper in the world, the biggest study, more than 400 scientists, sponsored by the UN and signed on by more than 58 countries concluded that the current generation of GMOs has nothing to offer feeding the hungry world, eradicating poverty or creating sustainable agriculture. That's the ISTAD report. In fact, the Union of Concerned Scientists study showed that it actually doesn't increase yields and the USDA recent study verified that GMOs do not increase yields, and in many cases, reduce yields. Now not only do they not increase yields but they concentrate the ownership of agriculture. They bind farmers in a cycle of dependence on agricultural inputs like Roundup. They also disallow farmers from saving seeds year after year. And by spraying the Roundup on the Roundup Ready crops it kills all the other plant biodiversity. We call it weeds in this country. They call it food in the developing country because they eat a lot of those greens as part of their biodiversity so it's not designed properly for feeding the hungry world. And it's really an accident-prone, very dangerous technology, which we think by its very nature is linked to diseases.

The process of genetic engineering—you take a gene from one species. You make millions of copies, put it into a gene gun, shoot that gun into a plate of millions of cells and clone the cell into a plant. So now every single cell of that plant has that gene in it but also its caused massive collateral damage, two to four percent of the DNA is mostly mutated. So you could have hundreds or thousands of mutations up and down the DNA. Now that means that you can turn on genes, shut off genes, or change the levels of gene expression. Now that can be extremely dangerous for diseases and disorders, allergens, etc., because you can have toxins go up, allergens go up, Monsanto's corn has a gene that was switched on that produces an allergen. Monsanto's soy has as much as seven times the amount of a known soy allergen. You can end up switching on an oncogene causing a carcinogen to flourish or an increased level of a cancer-causing compound. You can also change all of the secondary metabolites or the natural products by the plant which we're now discovering today can fight cancer. But we know like just a handful of them. But even before we understand them and catalog them we're changing all that with genetic engineering because when you change it at the DNA level you change all these different expressions at that higher level.

So one study, for example, this was done in the UK, they fed potatoes that were genetically engineered to a group of rats. It was engineered to produce an insecticide. Another group was fed non-GMO potatoes. A third group was fed non-GM potatoes but their meal was spiked with an insecticide, the same one that the GM potatoes produced in the same amount. Only the group that ate the GM potato got sick. Those that ate the non-GM potato spiked with the insecticide did not. So it wasn't the insecticide that was being produced by the GM potato that caused the problem. It was the massive collateral damage, the side effects that result from the process of genetic engineering that cause the problem. And one of the problems was potentially pre-cancerous cell growth in the digestive tract. So they didn't find tumors in these rats but within 10 days their stomach lining was increased by double and this proliferative cell growth is a precursor to cancer in some cases. They also had smaller brains, livers, and testicles, partial atrophy of the liver, and a damaged immune system. And it was not because of the gene, the specific gene, that was put in. It was because of the process of genetic engineering, the same generic process that's used on the food that we eat. That potato was never commercialized but the soy and the corn that we do eat is produced from the same process that resulted in potentially pre-cancerous cell growth in the digestive tract of rats in 10 days.

Ty: It sure seems to me that if you want to avoid cancer or you have cancer GMOs are something that should be number on your list to stay away from.

Jeffrey: Well, you can choose your disorder you want to avoid at this point. I mean you can be avoiding cancer, you can be avoiding Crohn's and colitis and acid reflux, and migraines, so many things we've heard people describe getting better when they get rid of GMOs. But absolutely, there's so many ways that GMOs—and I have to be careful I have to say maybe promoting cancer. You know, I have to make friends with my inner attorney.

Ty: Gotcha! Now let's say we're in Kentucky. Iowa's the better state, but for my knowledge we've got Farmer Hatfield and Farmer McCoy in Kentucky and they're both growing corn. Now Farmer Hatfield is growing GMO corn. Farmer McCoy is trying not to. What's to stop the cross pollination if their farms are close to each other?

Jeffrey: Well, first of all, I just want you to know that if you're a farmer growing GM corn you're now at higher risk of getting the spray into your own body. There was a study done, just an epidemiological evaluation, finding 300 percent higher cancer rates in areas where they were using Roundup in Argentina and 400 percent increase in birth defects. In an entire area, in one little hospital area, there was 70 times the amount of birth defects with a high exposure to Roundup. So the farmers themselves are at risk. Those in farm communities are more at risk. The US geological survey found Roundup residues in 60 to 100 percent of the air samples and rain samples in the Midwest. Now when you plant GMOs and non-GMOs in side-by-side fields if you're planting the non-GMO you want to hope that the wind is blowing in the other direction especially during the time of pollination. So the pollen can transfer. Seeds can be moved by births. They can be moved by rain. The cross contamination is a very real situation and it has been so pervasive that even organic products and products that are labeled non-GMO you can't guarantee a 100 percent purity even with non-GMO project verified label. It still has a 0.9 percent, threshold and that's because of the contamination that's already out there as part of the background. So that's the bad news. If we do switch to a non-GMO world we can't with current technology eliminate all of this contamination. We can make it a tiny amount. If all you're doing is adding more non-GMO seeds and the amount of GMOs that's in the gene pool will get less and less when we have no technology to clean it up completely today.

Ty: Talk real quickly if you would about—I've read about terminator technology where the seeds don't reproduce or you can't use the seeds for next year's crop. Could you address that?

Jeffrey: There's a technology developed in part by the USDA which allows a crop to produce sterile seeds. Now it hasn't yet been commercialized. The uproar of the international family was immediate and intense because the purpose of terminator technology was to target the 1.4 billion farmers who save seeds every year. Now the saving of the seeds provides an increase in the quality of that crop that's customized for the geography and weather. And so you have incredible diversity. The biodiversity, because of seed saving, is millions upon millions of different types of seeds. The biotech industry wants to eliminate all that biodiversity and force farmers to buy seeds from the catalogs. So they're betting the food security of the plant which is based on this biodiversity at a time of global climate change in order to drive more profits into their pockets. So they want to introduce terminator technology. Right now they have farmers sign contracts that they won't replace the genetically modified seeds. And they'll go after farmers even if they suspect that the farmer is saving seeds. They'll sue or threaten and there's been some horrific stories about that.

Ty: So Jeffrey, you just said the key word here in Las Vegas—"betting."

Jeffrey: Oh, yeah, yeah.

***Ty*:** One of your blockbuster documentaries is "Genetic Roulette: The Gamble of Our Lives." Talk about that and making that documentary. It's a movie that I have seen and has really influenced my family's choices. So if you would talk to us about that.

Jeffrey: Well, first of all, I've been very happy with the impact of "Genetic Roulette: The Gamble of Our Lives." It won movie of the year. It won transformational film of the year. And when I go to lectures now and I ask, "How many people have removed GMOs and noticed some big improvement in their health?" so many people say, "Yeah, I saw your film and stopped eating GMOs the next day." It's the number one tool that we have found to be most convincing to change people's diet the quickest. And people can watch it at GeneticRoulettemovie.com. It shows scientists and doctors and veterinarians and farmers and people all describing the problems that we have found with GMOs, and the cover-up by the biotech industry, and all the takeover, the political machinations by the very powerful biotech lobby, etc. So it lays it all out there. But most importantly it's driving more and more people to avoid eating GMOs. It was seen by millions of people and we are now seeing a tipping point under way. Let me explain the dynamics. In 2013 in March the president of Whole Foods said, "When a product becomes non-GMO project verified it increases sales by 15 to 30 percent." Everyone in the natural products industry heard that and it became clear that using GMOs in the natural food industry was a liability.

So there's 20,000 products that are either verified or on their way to be verified this year, most of them in the natural products industry. But there are a few big ones in the conventional food industry like the original Cheerios, the original Grape Nuts, soon Smart Balance, soon Ben & Jerry's completely, etc. Now when they start selling more than their competitors in places like Wal-Mart and Safeway, it'll inform the rest of the food industry that they can't afford to wait until their competitor declares non-GMO first in their product category. So it becomes—they're like the test hanging, out there especially Grape Nuts, which is in the front of the package, non-GMO project verified as opposed to Cheerios which sort of hides it on the side. So if those move the needle in sales we may see a tipping point this year or next. And so it's interesting, Ty, that when you look about—look at protecting the genetic integrity of all living beings and all future generations it may come down in historical context that the most important thing was sales of Grape Nuts at Wal-Mart. And that that moved the whole needle.

Ty: Yeah.

Jeffrey: So we think that it's going to be moved this year or next and we think that the animal feed will be moved within five years, and that we want to ask people to help us.

Ty: And so how can people help you?

Jeffrey: At responsibletechnology.org we have a website. People can sign up for our newsletter and share the pieces that we send out. Sometimes we have petitions, etc., sometimes actions. And we would like to invite people to make donations. We have a master plan to end GMOs within five years, food and feed. We've helped engineer the tipping points that we've currently seen against bovine growth hormone and against GMOs in the natural products industry. We know exactly what to say. We know who to say it to. We know how to say it. Its simply a matter of funding the staff time and the production time to make this a reality. So we need about $5 million a year for five years, which turns out to be not that much. More than two million people came out to protest in the march against Monsanto. If even 50,000 people gave $100 a year that's $5 million. That's less than $10 a month. So in order to protect all who eat and all living beings and all future generations it's pretty easy. And so we also have an opportunity for people to be involved. We have the tipping point network where close to 10,000 people are involved in over a hundred organizations. Let me say that again. We have an opportunity for people to help get the word out in their local communities through the tipping point network. We have a speaker training program. We've trained close to 1,000 people. We have a lot of information. So we would like to invite people to go to our website, responsibletechnology.org, and connect with others and connect with the information and become a click-and-send non-GMO revolutionary from here on in.

Ty: Well, Jeffrey, you are changing the world and you're making it a better place with your information. And so I just want to thank you for your time that you've spent with us today sharing your knowledge about GMOs. I know it's benefitted our viewers quite a bit. So thank you so much.

Jeffrey: You're welcome Ty. And I want to say I've had mothers come up to me and when they meet me they burst into tears. And they say that we saved their kids lives or turned their family around. It's very real. It's very real. You know, it used to be more theoretical for me. It's like I wanted to get rid of GMOs but I wasn't paying so much attention to the individuals. A few years ago that all changed. And now I am listening to the stories and I have this pressure. I want to share this with the world because I don't want to be the only one that knows this. And I'm not. Right now GMOs have become a very popular topic. So I want to thank you because I have the pressure to get what I know out to the world. So thank you for that.

Ty: Thank you Jeffrey.

[end of transcript]

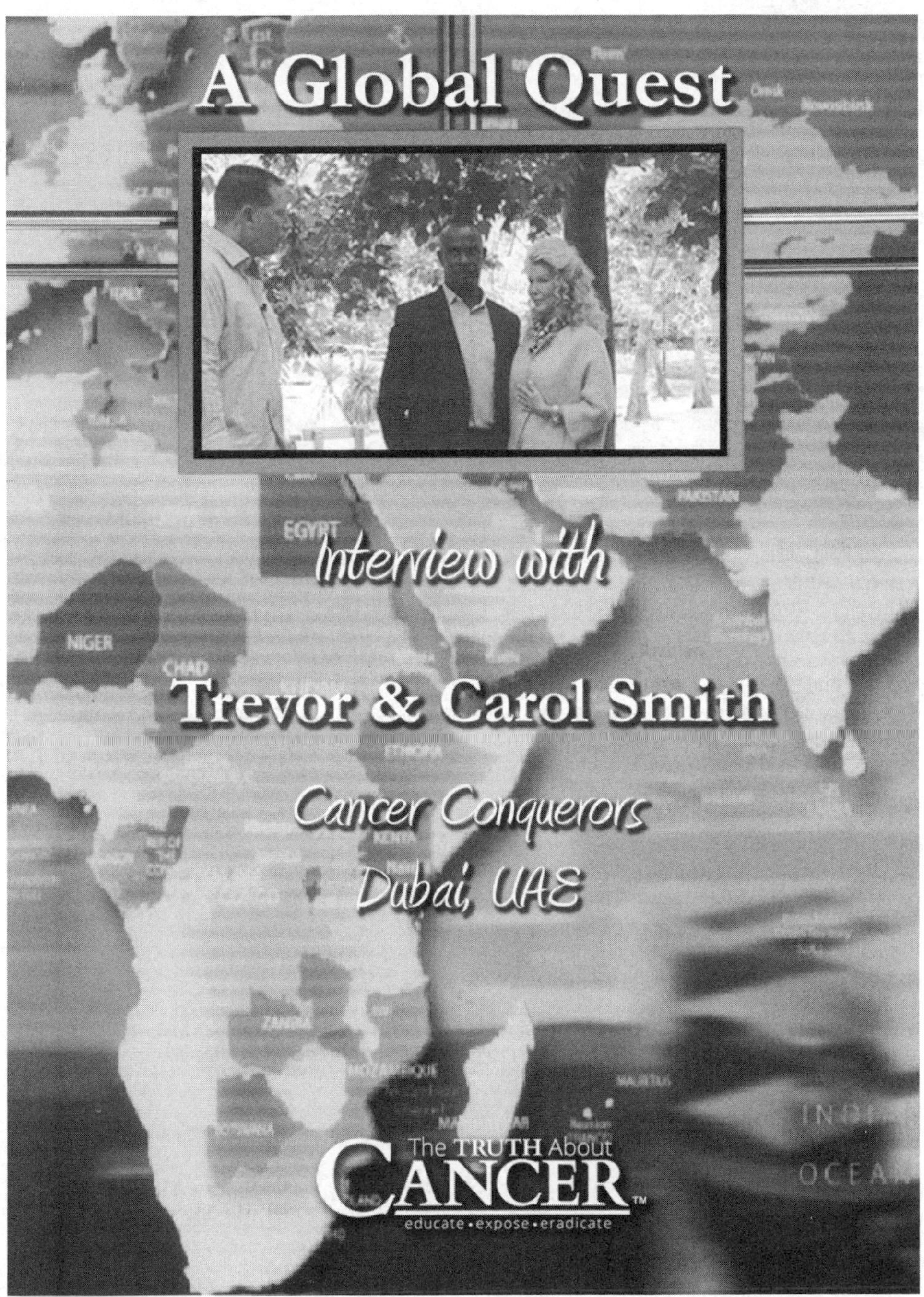
A Global Quest
Interview with
Trevor & Carol Smith
Cancer Conquerors
Dubai, UAE
The TRUTH About
CANCER
educate • expose • eradicate

Ty: So, I'm here with Carol and Trevor Smith. Thank you for travelling to breezy, sunny, rainy, foggy London—

Carol: You're welcome. You're very welcome.

Ty: —from Dubai. It's a little bit chillier here than you're used to, right?

Trevor: I'd say yes. Yeah. A bit dark as well.

Ty: Yeah, we just had a little encounter with a bird.

Trevor: That's why I'm looking up.

Ty: Before the interview, a bird attacked me. Not really, but kind of used me as his toilet but…

Carol: Better you than me.

Ty: It's better me than you. That's right. I'm glad that you're here. I've followed your story over the last couple of years. I've corresponded with you via email but it's really a pleasure to meet you.

Carol: And you.

Ty: Well, thank you. Thank you. Let's walk back in time to the diagnosis. Trevor was diagnosed with cancer.

Carol: Yeah.

Ty: And I want you to share your story just the way that you were just sharing it with me before the camera started rolling about the way that you were feeling and the things that happened. One of the things that you said—and we'll go back from this —is you said that after the diagnosis, one of the doctors—you overheard a doctor say, "It sounds like she is running the show. We're not going to get them to do surgery now," right?

Carol: Yes, yes.

Ty: Isn't that the way it should be? Shouldn't the patient have the choice of what they do and it's not the doctors'?

Carol: Being in control of your health, you know.

Trevor: I think we were really adamant in that interview with the doctor. We were not listening to him and we were going to do things differently. So, I tip my hat off to my wife who took the initiative and found another way to go about and cure me.

Ty: So, talk about the diagnosis. When was it and what kind of cancer did Trevor have?

Carol: In 2012, in June, he started with a backache and then we flew home back to Dubai because we was on vacation in England. We flew home and we thought that he got a kidney stone. But the doctor did say, "If it's a tumor, we'll be able to tell you right away."

Then he went under anesthetic. I was waiting outside the operating room and a surgeon came. He had blood still on his gown. He came to the door and he said, "I couldn't see because there was too much blood. It was like a massive jellied blood" and I said, "But you told me that you'd be able to tell us if it was cancer." And he said, "It is cancer, and it's a very aggressive form of cancer."

I can't tell my husband because he needs to recover from his operation until they got a plan of action to give to him so that he would feel better about it.

Trevor: So all this time I was under anesthetic and I came through.

Carol: And it brought me into my knees because I just learned my husband has got cancer and I can't even tell him. So, I spent four days in the hospital in his room and not being able to tell him that he got cancer and he just thought he's got to wait for the biopsy to come back

Trevor: Back for the results.

Carol: But I knew he'd got cancer. That was the hardest time.

Ty: I bet it it was, from an emotional perspective. That probably just tore you up, didn't it?

Trevor: The emotional part was when I came out of surgery—the way she kissed me, I knew there was something, but I couldn't put my finger on it.

Ty: You knew it was more serious than just kidney stones or gallstones.

Trevor: I guess so, yeah and she tried to keep it to herself until the last minute. I knew something was going on.

Carol: And then we flew to England to get a second opinion within a week and the second opinion gave us a worse prognosis: that he had to have six weeks of chemo and radiotherapy then remove his bladder and his prostate and his intestines to build another bladder.

Trevor: But they weren't forward in telling you that in the initial findings.

Carol: And the doctor had it in his diary to do the operation within six weeks and told us that we didn't have time to mess around. We could go back to Dubai for four weeks at the most before he needed to start chemo, before it spread all over his body.

And when he knew we weren't going to have the operation or he thought we weren't going to take the operation, he went into graphic detail about how it would spread and he'd get cancer all over his lower region.

Trevor: All of this. Your fear tactic, mostly.

Carol: And it would be a very painful, slow death.

Ty: So, they scared you?

Trevor: Yeah.

Carol: Yeah.

Ty: They instilled fear. What type of cancer did he have?

Carol: Bladder cancer.

Ty: Bladder? But you said the doctor said he also needed to remove his intestines?

Carol: To build another bladder. They were going to remove the bladder, remove the prostate. But he didn't tell us he would be impotent, he'd be incontinent for up to a year while they built a new bladder.

He is at the height of his career. He's got an amazing job and he just didn't want to go down that route and so we asked how long if we didn't do the operation and we were told 18 months to 2 years at the most.

Trevor: It was 18 months. It was less than that.

Ty: 18 months—so you better act now.

Carol: Yeah.

Ty: Okay, so they instill a sense of urgency to undergo their protocol.

Trevor: But the one thing about it is we have somewhere to go. Instead of staying in England—

Carol: Where all the family were pushing us to go for chemo, get the bladder out, especially Trevor's family. "No, he needs to have chemo, he needs to do what the doctors say."

Trevor: So, we've taken a step back. We were able to go back home and take some time, away from everybody—

Ty: Back to Dubai?

Carol: Yes.

Trevor: —and make some decisions. Even there, the doctors there—

Carol: First we spoke to our sons and we told them our decision to take the 18 months. We started giving away money to our sons.

Ty: Did you?

Carol: Yeah. We were going to live our life—I was going to go with him. I was going to take some time—

Ty: Tell me that story.

Trevor: What I said was take the 18 months and celebrate, live life to the full, do things that we always said we wanted to do. For me, I was going to walk straight into the desert if it got to a point where it was painful or something that I couldn't do. I was going to walk straight into the desert, not bother anybody and that's the way I was going to do it.

But my wife decided, "No, I'm coming with you. Not mainly straight into the desert but I don't want to be left around without you." So, that made it even worse. But your mind plays tricks on you in these decisions you make. Under duress, can't say—nobody likes to use the word or is able to mention the word. I wasn't able to say the word 'cancer' when I find out that I had it.

Carol was the one who was able to talk to people and actually talk for me.

Carol: I just got to work and then I started meeting people who have killed their own cancer online. My computer saved his life. It wasn't me. It was the computer, it was the Internet—

Trevor: It was the Internet. It was the big one.

Carol: —the Facebook pages. Many, many pages.

Ty: You minimize your importance too much. It was the operator of the computer that was doing the work.

Carol: And I never stopped operating that computer. I never stopped.

Trevor: It's the same as when you're trying to get information. If you wrote a letter and sent to say, Australia, how long would it take to get back?

Ty: True.

Trevor: So, the Internet, the researching—people have got recorded a win-win thing or being cured. That did it.

Carol: And all the time I was keeping a journal because I was emailing my family and they were all talking between themselves and getting the story mixed up so I kept a journal, basically for emails for my family and then when I realized what was happening to him—he lost 19kgs in weight. He never was sick for one day and he got better and better and he looked—he got fitter and fitter. He was playing 11-a-side football.

Ty: What did you decide to do?

Carol: We changed his diet, first off, completely. We cut-out all processed foods. He only ate organic, chicken, fish, vegetables, salads, fruits. We juiced every day. He drank smoothies, nuts, and dried fruits.

Trevor: Basically, what I was not eating—I changed my whole diet.

Carol: We got a naturopathic doctor on board and she did the test and found out it was completely—

Trevor: That was the big turning, the big turning point.

Carol: Yeah, he was completely depleted with vitamin D, weren't you?

Trevor: We went through a point where—so, it was all blood tests of everything. It covered all different spectrums and they found out what was depleted. So the high doses came in to vitamin C or—

Carol: We didn't know what we were doing. We were just taking it off the Internet.

Trevor: Right.

Carol: If I'd had your import, I would have known exactly what to do. I found all the sources and—

Ty: And so you got your blood analyzed and found out you were deficient in vitamin D.

Carol: Yeah, completely depleted.

Ty: Okay.

Carol: And most dark skinned people are depleted in vitamin D.

Trevor: And we don't know about it.

Carol: We since found out most cancer patients have low vitamin D.

Ty: That's right because the darker complexion actually does not absorb the sunlight as well and they produce—

Carol: Yeah, even though we lived in a hot and sunny climate. But if we weren't quiet, I wouldn't have been able to do all that. Like ten months afterwards, I came across cannabis oil.

Ty: Cannabis oil?

Carol: Cannabis oil.

Trevor: But you know what, that's not quite true because we went past it.

Carol: It was ten months.

Trevor: We came across it—

Carol: After six months—

Trevor: And we went home and went past it.

Carol: —we came across it and I was trying to figure out how to get it. And I sourced somebody in Spain and I was trying to figure out how could I get it? I wasn't going to take it to Dubai. How could I get it to the UK?

Ty: Right.

Carol: So, I was going to break the law and fetch the cannabis oil myself. But then, he was getting better so we didn't need to do it then.

Trevor: But there was one thing that was said to you if—

Carol: Yes, one guy said to me, "I can bring it to you, but if I'm not prepared to risk imprisonment for—if you're not prepared to risk imprisonment for somebody you love, then why should I?"

That made me realize I need to risk it, you know?

Ty: Wow.

Carol: But I knew if I went to prison in England, I'd get out. I'd have a slap on the wrist and I'd get out. But I knew if I tried to do it to Dubai, then there's no chance I would get out of prison from there.

Ty: So, you risked it? Did you do treatment here then?

Carol: We flew home to England and took the treatment. I won't say how we got it to England but—

Trevor: I stayed there for three months and went through the whole part of doing the oil.

Carol: But you know, there's so many people saying cannabis oil killed their cancer but nobody actually said how hard it is to take. It was really, really hard. It was the hardest part of our journey.

Ty: Did you make it yourself?

Carol: No.

Ty: No? Okay.

Carol: It was made by a legal cannabis oil maker and she also wrote the foreword—because eventually, I'd publish my journal that I was keeping for emails for my family and I self-published it because I knew that we were onto something and people needed to know what we'd done and how we'd done it when the doctor said there was no other way.

Ty: What is the name of the book that you published?

Carol: The book is called *Taking Control* by Alyssia Sade. Alyssia and Sade are my two beautiful granddaughters. I wanted to do it in their names, first of all, because we lived in Dubai and he took cannabis oil and it's all in the book on how he took it, and secondly, to leave something behind in their names.

Ty: Right. It's really impressive to me that you decided to say, "Doctor, I'm not listening to what you have to say. I don't believe that I will be gone in 18 months," and you went in a different direction.

Trevor: Yeah.

Carol: Trevor is an engineer and he said to the doctor…

Trevor: I said to him, "There has to be a different way, another way to do things." And he said, "Nope, this is the way," but I'm going to do it my way and that was the driver. Everybody believes somebody in the white coat has the answer but it is not necessarily so. For me, I think if you feel there's a doubt, don't go with it.

Carol: And my intuition—it was screaming at me to tell me that I was on to something. And I knew—all the way through my journal, I say that I know that I'm part of something, far bigger than Trevor's illness. I was onto something and so are many, many others. The world was waking up to there being another way to kill cancer.

Trevor: But you know that there's so many people out there. People in Australia, Norway, Holland.

Carol: Everywhere. All over the world people are waking up.

Trevor: We Skyped in. We spoke to people.

Carol: I've got so many Facebook friends now that are on the same path or have been on the same path. And I had to surround myself with people like that otherwise I wouldn't have been able to do what I did.

Trevor: Yeah.

Ty: We just interviewed yesterday a man from England here that used cannabis oil for his cancer as well. He was told he was terminal and there was nothing he could do. And he said, "I've got a 5-year-old little boy and I couldn't let him be alone and I have to say alive," and went to cannabis oil. He had to break the law here in the UK to take it.

Carol: Yeah, and we did.

Ty: But I told him, I asked him isn't it a shame that you had to break the law to use a natural substance that actually can cure your cancer?

Carol: Yeah.

Ty: Did you use that temporarily or do you still use it?

Trevor: No.

Carol: He doesn't use it now.

Trevor: After three months, 90 days—

Carol: He used it three months and then we had to go back to Dubai so we're keeping him well just with his diet change, exercise, spiritual. We also did a lot of spiritual healing and he got rid of some past hurt that he had. Trevor's mother died when he was eight and he was holding onto some real deep hurt issues. And he did some work called *The Journey* work by Brandon Bays.

Ty: Emotional healing.

Carol: Emotional healing, yeah.

Ty: That's a big part of it. Talking about emotional healing, that is a big part of the equation, isn't it?

Carol: Mind, body and spirit.

Trevor: Yeah. In that process, searching for a cure, so to say, we came across *The Journey* work. I'd try anything and I was into doing anything.

Carol: But you didn't believe it would work, but then after one session you came out and you said I think my cancer is gone.

Trevor: No, I'm not skeptical because I never needed to look for something like that.

Carol: But the lady who did the journey work, she said that she'd wished she'd used Trevor like a—

Ty: Test case.

Carol: —Like a test case but she hadn't documented it. She said she'd never had anybody go under, like, hypnotism so fast for so long.

Trevor: I got a great result, but you do start bawling and crying like a baby or trying to…

Carol: And Trevor never cries, but he cried for three hours and he released a lot of pent-up emotions.

Ty: I'm sure that was a big help as well on your healing journey as well.

Trevor: Yes.

Carol: Yeah.

Ty: To get rid of that.

Carol: You know, the second worst part of the journey, when we came back after the cannabis oil—we'd pinned so much hope on this. And we left for England and he had three small tumors in his bladder.

Trevor: When we came over.

Carol: When we came back, we were expecting the tumors to be gone. He was in the surgery and I was in the doctor's surgery and so they go through the penis and into the bladder. And so he's on cameras so I can see on the television screen. There was 23 or more tumors after cannabis oil.

Trevor: Yeah.

Carol: And the doctor thought it was in his prostate now so we thought, "All this and it's not worked." It was the hardest thing that we'd both done and so we had to wait for an MRI the next day—same day—and then to be read by the doctor the next day.

I broke down in there, in the surgery, thinking that was it. It has spread now and he's going to die.

Trevor: And what it was—

Carol: That was the year after.

Trevor: Somehow the cancer was trying to get out of my system, but it had nowhere to go.

Carol: But then—

Trevor: —because it had closed into the bladder. So, when the cameras went in through the penis into the bladder and looked in there, it was full of cancerous cells.

Ty: There was no place to go.

Trevor: Nowhere to go. No.

Carol: So, the next day when the MRI was read, the doctors saw that it was the tumor hanging down onto the prostate and it hadn't actually spread. And he saw all the tumors were superficial. They weren't aggressive, they weren't muscle invasive. So he said we can laser those off.

He lasered them off and they never came back. So the cannabis oil worked in a different way to what we expected. We were expecting it to be gone, but then that's when Trevor had a breakdown.

Trevor: I really don't know what role the cannabis oil plays but there is—

Carol: We don't know what's worked.

Trevor: —but there's a place for it—

Carol: It's everything. It's like cannabis oil was a piece of the jigsaw.

Ty: There's no magic bullet, right? You hit it from different directions and that's what you did.

Trevor: Yeah.

Carol: Yeah.

Ty: And you're still hitting it from the nutritional direction.

Carol: He'll never go back to his diet.

Ty: What does the typical diet or a typical day look like for you?

Carol: He has porridge oats.

Trevor: It is always porridge.

Carol: Yeah, with goats' milk.

Trevor: Yeah, organic.

Carol: So he doesn't have dairy.

Trevor: It's camel or goat's milk.

Ty: Camel or goat's milk? Only in Dubai, right?

Carol: And smoothies.

Trevor: I'll not say it's a bonbon but you can get it from the store.

Carol: And always a green smoothie or juice, carrot juice. Lots of carrot juice.

Trevor: Initially, it was always green but now, I vary it.

Carol: He has no processed foods.

Ty: No processed foods?

Carol: No. No cakes, no biscuits, no white flour, no sugar.

Ty: That is key right there in and of itself.

Carol: And it's two years now, cancer-free.

Ty: Yeah, you look really healthy.

Carol: He does.

Trevor: My weight initially, it was just under 100kg.

Carol: You know, he started looking younger and younger and I started looking older with the stress.

Trevor: Not at all. The drawback on this journey initially when I watched Carol go through, talking to people and everything, I always had this worry that she'd never step off it, off that train that we were riding. It's like the story where a man goes to save his dog on the ice and he goes to save the dog and the dog climbs out and he falls in through the ice. And that is how Carol would be. I get well and Carol may get sick.

Carol: Yeah, because stress is also a factor in cancer and I was in a lot of stress.

Ty: Yeah. Well, you don't look stressed now.

Carol: Thank you.

Trevor: She came out of the cyclone quite well; I mean, both of us have. I have my doubts when I have this three monthly, four monthly—

Carol: Yeah, it's hard every three months but—

Trevor: Few days before I don't quite—

Carol: It's getting easier. This last test was the easiest. Now I feel that we've cured him. I've not said cured yet because I'm waiting for that 5 year mark. And I self-published the book when he was 6 months cancer-free because I needed to get the word out. But now I'll write again when he's 5 years and continue the book I'm writing and update it.

Trevor: We'll share it with whoever wants to know about it. It's virtually free, isn't it?

Carol: I spend my days—my time is spent on a page called Alyssia Sade on Facebook. And I helped many people with cancer and put them in the right direction and I always share all your posts and yeah.

Ty: Well, thank you for what you're doing. Let's talk about your diet before. You said you changed your diet. What were you eating before? Did you have any habits that might have contributed to the cancer as well?

Trevor: I would always go for the biggest steak.

Carol: He always asked in the restaurant, how big is the steak or how big are these spare ribs because he wanted a big meal.

Trevor: Well, I had this phobia because I travelled a lot. I would never go for salads or greens or anything unless they were washed at home or made by my wife. So I always went straight for the meat, nothing green, no salads. I think that was part of it.

Carol: And 30 cigarettes a day.

Trevor: Yeah, there were these cigarettes as well.

Ty: So like a pack of cigarettes?

Carol: A pack and a half.

Trevor: My wife would say I smoked some strong cigarettes from the age of 14.

Carol: And then to quit with no help from 30 to none in one day.

Ty: So you've been smoking since you were 14?

Trevor: Yes.

Ty: Okay. And then how old were you when you quit?

Carol: 52, when he got cancer.

Trevor: On the day we were flying back I picked up the cigarettes and put them on the side of the fence with the lighter and I never smoked since.

Carol: Do you know they say that—in the research that I have done—that cancer craves sugar—I knew Trevor was sick before he got the diagnosis. He kept craving sugar. And he never used to eat sugar.

Trevor: Lemon tarts.

Carol: So he would go and buy two of these big huge lemon cakes and things.

Trevor: I would sit there wanting to bake and eat them.

Carol: So he was craving sugar.

Ty: So here's a question. So the research shows that sugar is more addictive than cocaine. What was more difficult, getting off all the sugar or getting off the cigarettes?

Trevor: The sugar I think because the cigarettes—when I found that I had cancer I would be a hypocrite to keep on smoking if I wanted to get myself better. So to this day I'm really angry because I packed up smoking just like that. There were no patches, there was no anything like that. It was just a straightforward, cold turkey, stopped. I stopped and walked away from it.

Carol: But still now he's craving sugar, but he goes for dried apricots or raisins or fruit or a smoothie if he wants sugar.

Ty: Well, there's a big difference between natural sugars and processed sugars as well.

Trevor: Yeah.

Carol: Yeah.

Trevor: I don't crave for the processed sugar.

Carol: Chocolate cake or biscuits. It's me that's got to get off that now. It's less for me. My diet has completely changed. But I still have the odd biscuit or cake.

Trevor: In fact you changed because I don't take any dairy and my tea is black tea and very little coffee, maybe one or two but definitely no fizzy drinks or pops.

Carol: We don't buy sodas or have anything like that in the house.

Trevor: Our fridge is completely different from what it used to be years ago.

Carol: It's like a pharmacy in the fridge.

Ty: Isn't that good advice? And I like that, pharmacy in the fridge. I like that phrase. Isn't that good advice to someone who wants to change their diet? If you want to eat more healthy don't buy things that are unhealthy because if you have them around you will eat them.

Trevor: You will.

Carol: Do you know if we go into the supermarket now we are in the vegetable isle and then out.

Trevor: Yeah, packed of all that.

Carol: All those rows of...

Ty: You never hit the middle isles, do you?

Trevor: No, we don't. Well, I sometimes ask for one or two things.

Ty: We've got a 23 year old still at home, but he was more healthy than we were. He wouldn't eat red meat or fats, dairy, and now he is saying there's nothing in the fridge to eat because there's nothing prepared. We cook all the time, don't we?

Trevor: Blending or juicing or something.

Ty: But you are preparing it yourself.

Carol: Yeah, always.

Trevor: One thing I find difficult now is when I travel and I go to hotels, they don't quite cater.

Carol: The first thing he looks for is a juice bar to get somebody to make his juices for him.

Trevor: So I buy nuts, definitely raw nuts, and untreated nuts and just pick up fruit. If I'm on an airplane I just have an apple that I carry on the plane with me. And that's how I go through the flight instead of having the airplane food. Because there's not much choices in that dish. I really try to be healthy as much as I can.

Ty: What would your advice be to someone that may have been recently diagnosed with terminal cancer?

Carol: Completely change your diet. Cut out all sugars, all processed foods. Cut out dairy. Go and visit a naturopath, get your blood works done. Find out what your body is deficient in because your body can heal itself. Given the right nutrients it can heal itself.

Trevor: As much as it might cost, the initial blood grouping tests to find out what you're deficient in—that will save a lot of time.

Carol: Even your normal doctor will do a free vitamin D test. And even if you don't get your tests done, change your diet. Completely cut out sugar and dairy. They are the main things I think.

Ty: So that's your number one advice, which is to change your diet?

Trevor: For me I think you do have some time when you're diagnosed with it. You don't have to rush around in fear.

Ty: Don't give into the fear, the fearmongers.

Trevor: You do have some time. I'm not saying how much time you do have; it's not going to happen. If you went through your life and you only just found out that day, you do have some time.

Ty: So even if you've been diagnosed as terminal there's hope, isn't there?

Trevor: Yeah, there is.

Carol: There is hope.

Trevor: There are so many people who recorded... success.

Carol: And Trevor was never sick for one day. He was in cancer and out the other end without being sick for one day. And now he looks 10 years younger.

Trevor: Yeah, but you're fighting fear. And it takes you in different ways.

Carol: I think he lost confidence, didn't you? He's just getting that back now.

Trevor: You go silent. You don't want to talk to anybody. You don't know what to say. But you, (inaudible - 00:25:34) you really do.

Carol: And also if you're taking Cannabis oil make sure that you do some research on it because it's not easy to take. It's very hard.

Ty: Hard to do it properly.

Carol: Yeah.

Trevor: Yeah, because there was never any guidance.

Carol: There was no guidance. That's why I also wrote a chapter called *The Dark Months*. It was May and June when he took it. I thought that that could help a lot of people that decided to go that route.

He stopped from one gram a day to none. It really had a profound effect on his personality. It was hard. And you are supposed to come off it slowly. Like, you build up to one gram a day and you're supposed to come off it slowly as well.

And then you're supposed to take a maintenance dose. But Trevor couldn't because he was in Dubai. Well, I'm glad we are recording it all because perhaps you don't need to take that maintenance dose you know.

Trevor: But I want to put emphasis on the oil because—B17.

Ty: Did you take apricot pills or apple seeds?

Carol: No, B17 capsules. And high doses of vitamin C, 20,000 mg of vitamin D a day.

Ty: We just had our vitamin D here for breakfast. So the combination of changing the diet, the vitamin C, the vitamin D, the hemp oil, the vitamin B17, all of that in combination and keeping a positive mental attitude.

Carol: And I think lots of love and support.

Trevor: Support.

Ty: Ah, I can see that's evident.

Trevor: It's big and it's key, yeah.

Ty: Well, you guys are awesome. I mean your story is very encouraging. Like I said, I followed you for a good long while now. And it's an honor for me to be able to meet you. I know that this is going to encourage people that are watching the show today.

Carol: And it's an honor for us to meet you because you're doing everything that I'd love to be doing. And that's why I self-publish.

Ty: You are doing it. So you keep up the good work.

Carol: I will. Once you're into this and you realize— you can't stop though. It's like a life calling.

Ty: It's a mission, isn't it?

Carol: It's a mission, yeah.

Ty: Well, thanks for being part of the mission.

Carol: Thank you.

Ty: Alright, I appreciate it.

Trevor: Thank you Ty.

Ty: God bless both of you.

[end of transcript]

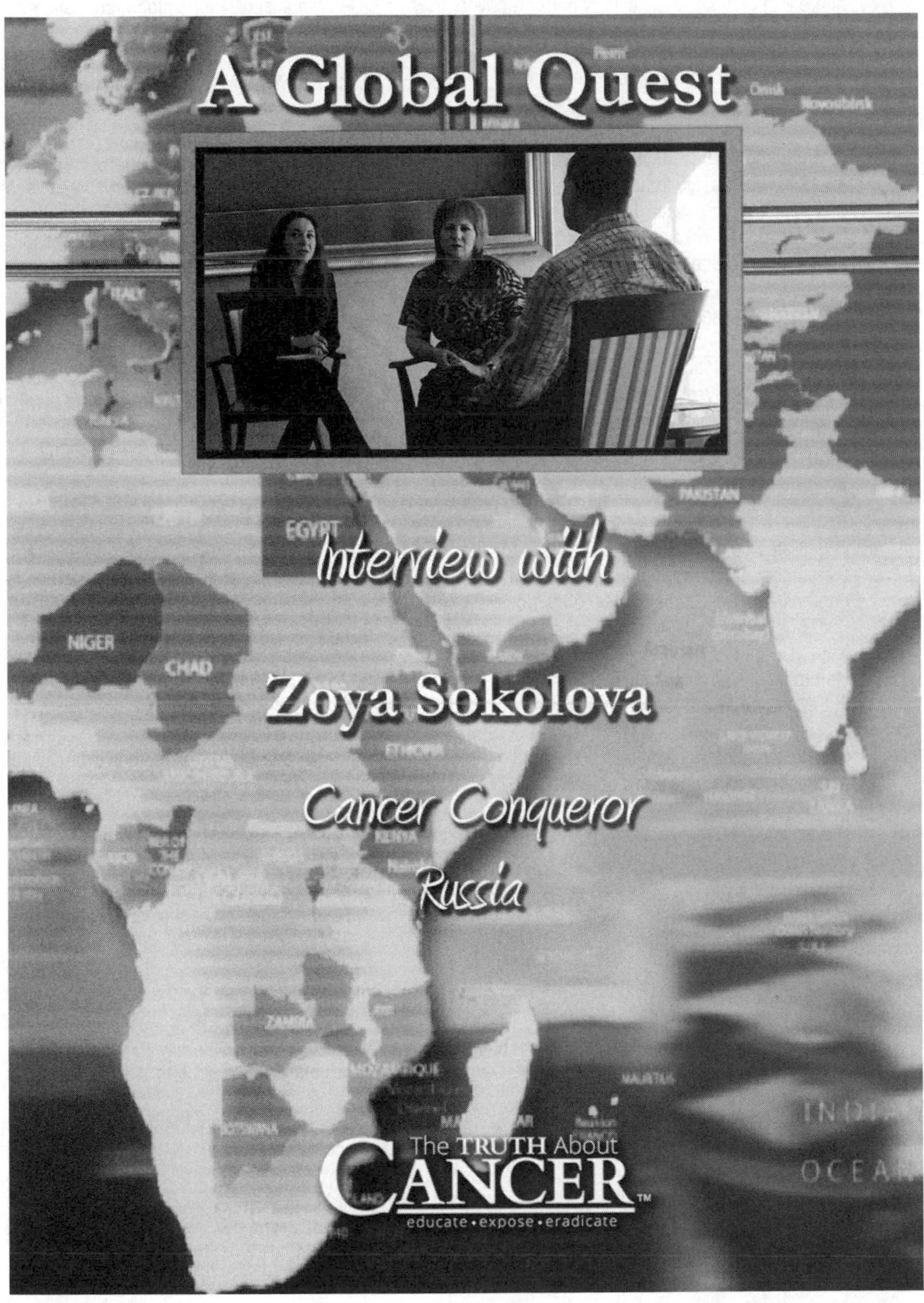
A Global Quest
Interview with
Zoya Sokolova
Cancer Conqueror
Russia
The TRUTH About
CANCER
educate • expose • eradicate

Ty: I'm real excited to be here at the Latvian Virotherapy Center with Zoja this morning. And she's going to share with us an incredible story of her recovery from so called terminal cancer, a stage four cancer, weeks to live. So thank you for joining us today.

So tell us, Zoja, where are you from? Where do you live? And then we're going to walk backwards about four years to your cancer diagnosis.

Zoja: [Translated 00:43 to 00:59] I came from Russia from St. Petersburg, and I want to share my experience about the second life that the specialists of the center have given me. The second life that I wasn't even dreaming of. [Translated 1:13 to 00:01:24] I wanted to say sorry that it is very hard for me to remember this story because I was already a bed patient. I couldn't stand and couldn't work, so it's very hard for me to remember, and I'm being very emotional.

Ty: Tell her that's okay. It's no problem.

Zoja: [Translated 00:01:43 to 00:01:48] I'm sorry beforehand even though there will be a tear or something. I will try to hold myself together. [Translated 00:01:55 to 00:02:13] It was bad news that was very sudden for me. It was after a very strong stressful period, and then after a month and a half I was diagnosed with third stage cancer. [Translated 00:02:27 to 00:02:29] I'm sorry, and I also had surgery already.

Ty: Okay, so stage three cancer, already had surgery. What year was this?

Zoja: [Translated 00:02:38 to 00:02:42] It was the summer of 2011. [Translated 00:02:46 to 00:02:49] After the surgery, I had my chemotherapy. [Translated 00:02:54 to 00:02:55] Then they assigned another six chemotherapies. [Translated 00:03:03 to 00:03:05] And the full course of radiotherapy. [Translated 00:03:09 to 00:03:19] My condition allowed only for the chemotherapy to be handled, and after the fourth I wasn't able to stand up from the bed. I became a bed patient. [Translated 00:03:29 to 00:03:48] Before these courses of chemotherapy I was told about the center, about this treatment, but I believed in this, in our doctors and their treatment methods so I decided to follow that path.

Ty: The doctors who treated you in Russia, did they give you hope that eventually the chemotherapy would cure your cancer, and you'd be able to walk again?

Zoja: [Translated 00:04:23 to 00:04:34] It seemed that they wanted to be so, for me to be treated but they couldn't give a warranty, they couldn't say for sure that they could treat this disease. [Translated 00:04:47 to 00:05:07] And at that moment when I couldn't stand up from the bed on my own completely, I was so weak, my relatives, they decided to take a van to make the bed for me and simply drive me to Riga to the center.

[Translated 00:05:23 to 00:05:31] Before coming to Riga, I had the blood test and the complete observation for the doctors here to have the full picture of my condition. [Translated 00:05:41 to 00:05:53] When the doctor saw my blood test, she was really astonished because the other blood test was lower than that for a live person. She was astonished how I managed to get here staying alive.

Ty: Wow. Just so I understand this properly, your blood work was almost equivalent to that of a dead person. They were amazed that you were still alive at that point.

Zoja: [Translated 00:06:28 to 00:06:30] This was exactly what I heard from them showing my blood test. [Translated 00:06:33 to 00:06:40] The doctor said exactly, "I'm not asking how you got here. I'm asking how you are still alive with this blood test." [Translated 00:06:47 to 00:07:01] From my feelings at that moment, I realized that I would not survive, and I felt how my body is fading from day to day.

Ty: Did you have—I suppose it was your family from Russia who drove you here. Who came with you?

Zoja: [Translated 00:07:22 to 00:07:38] It was my husband who took me here, and I realized that it probably could be my last route, my last route and I was feeling that my body is already dying. [Translated 00:07:54 to 00:08:20] The doctors recommend me to take certain measures, to take certain indications, even before taking Rigvir, to simply boost my immune system to renovate, to repair my immune system, my body so I could be ready for Rigvir. And after a couple of weeks I started to take Rigvir.

Ty: Did you have at that point, did you have the full support of your husband and other family members? They thought this was a good decision?

Zoja: [Translated 00:08:54 to 00:09:09] It was really my family who made the decision because, as for me, I was so weak, I was so down that I simply took this and I was ready to say goodbye to the life and simply—my family made the decision.

[Translated 00:09:27 to 00:09:35] I simply accepted their decision and I thought, "What shall be, this shall be." Simply I followed them.

Ty: I don't know your family, but I'd say you've got an incredible family to make this decision for you.

Zoja: [Translated 00:09:53] Thank you.

[Translated 00:09:55 to 00:10:09] After following the indication of the doctors for boosting my body, my immune system, after two weeks I was able to stand up and walk, sit down on the bed and walk around the house and move, so I was feeling better.

[Translated 00:10:28 to 00:10:48] After a month of already taking Rigvir blood therapy my condition changed entirely. I was now even able to walk around, stand up from the bed. I was even able to drive myself to Riga to receive the therapy.

Ty: So after you began only a month of treatment with the Rigvir therapy, did you ever contact those patients that you used to know in Russia when you were being treated with chemotherapy? I'm sure that you had contact with other cancer patients. Did you ever contact them again and let them know that you found this place?

Zoja: [Translated 00:11:35 to 00:12:07] I can say more that when I got my surgeries I had them with the same women in the same room and so we met. We were performing the same pattern, we met on the same days for chemotherapy, and when I started Rigvir, even though I had only fourth chemotherapy, not the full course, they continued this course. And I was getting better with Rigvir, they on chemotherapy, they were starting to feel worse and worse.

Ty: Have you ever contacted them today to see how they're doing?

Zoja: [Translated 00:12:45 to 00:13:07] I can say again, I can say more but because when I started to receive therapy, very quickly I became a very healthy person. I started to travel, I started to feel full of energy, and they called me and I recommend that they start this treatment. But for some reason they refused them. Now they are all gone.

[Translated 00:13:29 to 00:13:59] It's a pity that a lot of great people are gone now, but I'm happy, I'm healthy, and I can't say that at the beginning I trusted this method. I didn't know, and I was so weak. But currently I don't have any more disability category. I'm completely a healthy person and I'm so thankful to these people who helped me here.

Ty: Similar question that I just asked. Have you ever contacted the oncologist back in St. Petersburg, Russia, and let them know how healthy you are? Because apparently you had a very bleak prognosis. Have you ever talked to them since you've been on Rigvir ?

Zoja: [Translated 00:14:50 to 00:15:15] Yes I go to this clinic because I have to do blood tests and I have to be observed to send this blood test analysis to Riga for my doctors here, Those doctors in Russia, they are surprised that I am looking great, that I am feeling healthy. But then I'm hiding that I'm receiving my treatment here in Riga.

Ty: Do they want to know more about the treatment here so perhaps they can implement it in Russia?

Zoja: [Translated 00:15:47 to 00:16:07] I am trying to give them information. I am showing the materials. I'm providing all kinds of information. But these doctors they are thinking that they also have made some good impact on my condition with their treatment.

Ty: Okay. I don't mean to laugh but you left there on—you were carried out of their hospital on a stretcher and needed to have somebody to drive you to Latvia, and they thought that they helped your improvement? Okay. It just seems absurd to me.

Zoja: [Translated 00:16:56 to 00:17:01] What is, that is.

Ty: I don't think I even need to ask you how you are doing. It is obvious that you are doing very well. You walked here and sat down in the chair, so you are much improved since you have been using Rigvir?

Zoja: [Translated 00:17:40 to 00:17:41] For sure. [Translated 00:17:42 to 00:17:44] Thanks for complimenting me. [Translated 00:17:47 to 00:18:00] I'm receiving these compliments that I'm healthy, that I'm looking great, doing great all the time from all my relatives and friends, and they simply are astonished how I could make it from this negative condition to the way that I am now.

[Translated 00:18:19 to 00:18:44] Now I'm a completely healthy person. I can travel from country to country. I can drive on my own for many hours. I'm taking care of the house. I have two beautiful grandchildren, and I'm normal. I'm like everybody. I couldn't believe that I could be like this.

[Translated 00:19:01 to 00:19:25] Good people gave information to me, to my family about the center. And when I came here it was almost like we can say that it was the last minute, but I came here right on time. I really want for more people to find information about this center, to find their way through this situation.

[Translated 00:19:47 to 00:19:57] I think that God gave me this chance for a second life and I think that it was the reason for Him that I should also give information and chance for other people for their second life.

Ty: I would have to agree with you. I think that God gave you a second chance so that you can share this information and because of your willingness to share today, millions of people are going to be able to be aware of this treatment, and they'll know that despite a bad prognosis from cancer, even weeks to live, that there is always hope. So thank you for joining me in this today.

Zoja: [Translated 00:20:45 to 00:20:51] Now I believe there is a hope and there should be a hope for every person.

Ty: Thank you.

Zoja: [Translated 00:20:56 to 00:21:01] And I believe that with your help, more people will find about it.

Ty: Thank you for contributing to this.

Zoja: [Translated 00:21:09 to 00:21:12] Thank you.

[end of transcript]

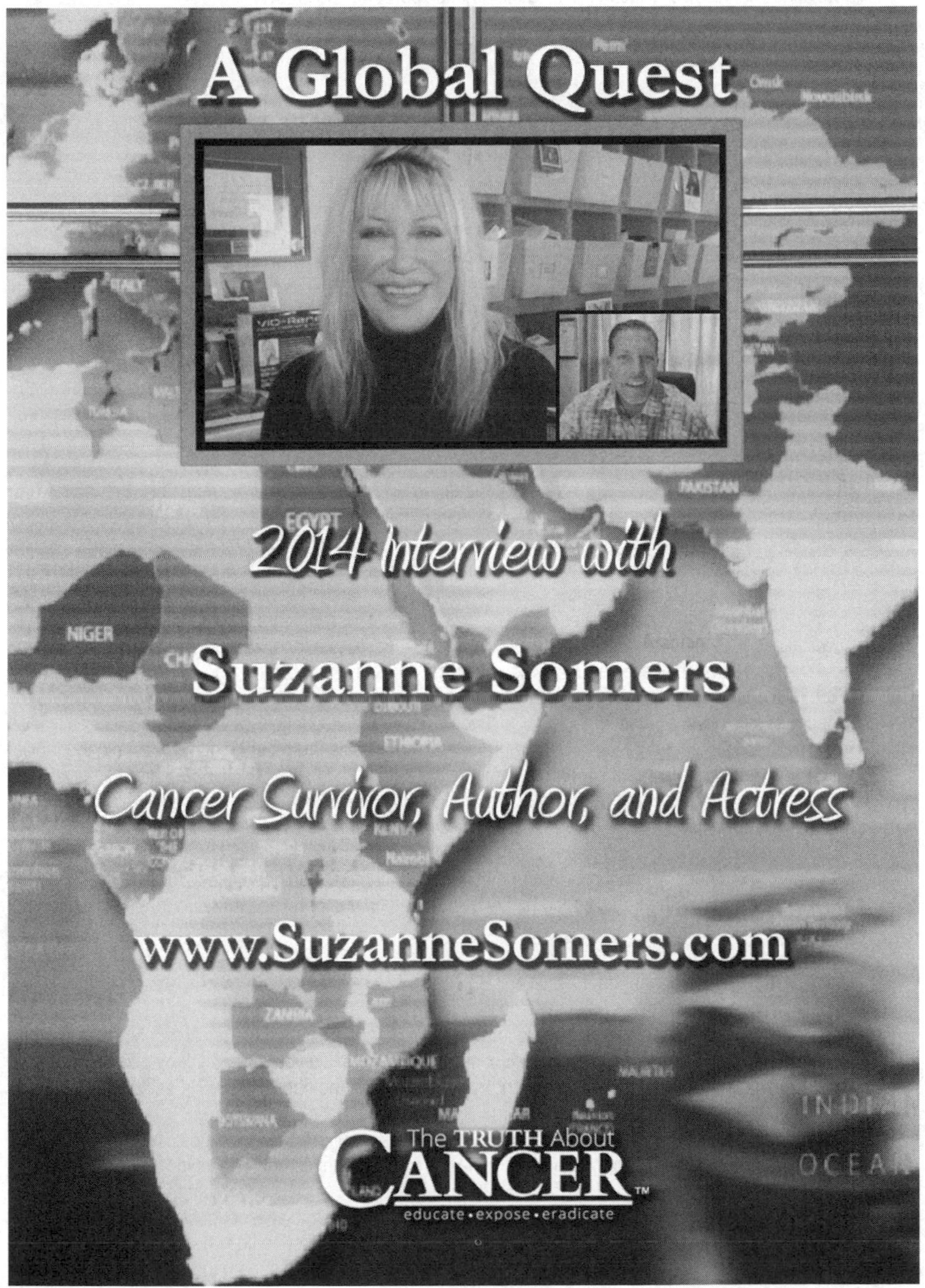
A Global Quest
2014 Interview with
Suzanne Somers
Cancer Survivor, Author, and Actress
www.SuzanneSomers.com
The TRUTH About CANCER
educate • expose • eradicate

Ty: Well, today I am here with Suzanne Somers—one of America's most beloved personalities. Suzanne, thank you so much for taking the time to spend with us today.

Suzanne Somers: My pleasure. This is my passion. I love talking about the things you and I are going to talk about today.

Ty: Awesome. Well, Suzanne, if you could, just let's go back about ten years, actually 14 years now, in time and tell us about your bout with breast cancer and what you did to treat it.

Suzanne Somers: You know, when I look back 14 years, what I am so glad about is what I did not do. I remember that I got the recipe right away; we will do surgery, radiation, chemotherapy and aftercare drug of Tamoxifen. And even at that time, because all of us in the alternative world, from year to year, you know so much more. I cannot do that. The idea of putting chemical poison into my body to cure me just does not make sense. And he said, you will die if you don't. And I said, I think I'll die if I do what you want me to do. So I did end up doing radiation because a doctor I respected very much, who is an alternative doctor, said, well, you have to do radiation. And I said, "Really? You would do it, too?" And she said, "Absolutely."I think today, knowing what I know about radiation and knowing what I know about a nutritional approach to cancer, I really do not think I would have done a radiation. Because any problem I have health wise is as a result of radiation. So, I have a whole different feeling about it. But, you know, we do the best that we can with the information we have at the time. And that is what I knew at that time. So I was looking around at that time for what could I do. And I read some books about Rudolph Steiner. And back in the 1920s, he was doing something call anthroposophic medicine. And one of the medicines that jumped out at me was Iscador. It was said that it builds up your immune system to be so strong that nothing can invade or attack, and that kind of made sense, because clearly I had cancer because there was some flaw in my immune system. So I injected Iscador for—I started to do it for two years. I got it from Weleda in Switzerland. It is legal to bring it into this country. But they, at that time, at least, they were not selling it in America. Maybe they are now. And then I kept on taking it. I took it for—I took it up until the time that, and I am sure we will get there—I ended up in the hospital again, being diagnosed with cancer, which was a misdiagnosis. You know that movie, Genetic Roulette, that was really eye opening, Food Inc., really eye opening.I ran into Laurie David the other night, who just did the movie, "Fed Up." And I said, "First of all, I have name envy." I said, "I am always looking for great titles and 'Fed Up' is an incredible title." And I said, "I wish you had interviewed me for that movie." She said, "Well, you're mentioned in the movie." I said, "Okay." But there are people of influence and substance out there starting to alert the general public that our food has been hijacked. Our food has been degraded to the point where it no longer holds nutrition that a human body needs for support. And nutrition is the fuel of the body, so the higher quality of food you put in the more your body will operate at max, all kind of simple.

Ty: It makes too much sense, doesn't it?

Suzanne Somers: Right. But I was doing a radio interview the other day and they are talking about the obesity epidemic with children. And I said, "Let's just stop for a minute. Do you really think by giving kids smaller sodas and less French fries that that's going to tackle the obesity issue?" I said, "No one wants to call it what it is. The kids are eating chemicals, processed foods, packaged foods." And, you know, chemicals, like I remember when I was interviewing Dr. Russell Blaylock, he said, "They design chemicals to taste scrumptious. And so if that is the first food the kid get," he said, "You have to bribe them to get a floret of broccoli in them and a piece of chicken so that they can have the foods they really love." And that is what needs to happen in schools, is education about, there are no safe levels of chemicals for any human body. That needs to just be known. And I do not believe in our lifetimes or our children's or children's children's lifetime we can clean up the planet. It is such a mess. So that is why a show like yours, books like mine, just keep educating people who are starting to go, hey, what is happening. Or they get cancer, you know, which turns out for me was a gift to get cancer, because it changed my whole life. It changed the thrust of my career.And you can control little world. And then if you have a louder voice, like you do and I do, then you can preach to the choir. And those who are ready to hear will hear. And those who are not, will remain deaf. And you just hope that they get their hearing back before it is too late.

Ty: Hmm, that is true. You mentioned Dr. Blaylock. An interesting statistic that I have heard him quote, and it is regarding breast cancer and mammograms, that mammograms actually increase the risk of breast cancer with each one you get. And then, I have heard you talk about that. Could you expound on that?

Suzanne Somers: Well, I no longer get mammograms. It was Dr. Blaylock who said, "If you start off at age 40 with no breast cancer and you have the prescribed yearly mammogram, by the time you are 50, you will have increased your chances of getting breast cancer from radiation exposure by 331⁄3 percent." He said, "And if you carry the BRCA gene, every time you have a mammogram, you increase your chances 15 percent with each mammogram." And he said, "And most people with the BRCA gene get two, maybe three mammograms a year. So they are actually ensuring that they will get breast cancer."You know, ever since I met Nick Gonzalez, he makes so much sense. I do his protocol preventatively. I do not ever want cancer again and by doing his protocol, I am not afraid of cancer anymore. And I think cancer is one of the motivating fears that most people have tucked away inside them. You know Nick and how altruistic he is and how he is not in it for the money and this is a good guy. And the flack he has taken for having the audacity to treat serious cancers with pancreatic enzymes, coffee enemas, and nutritional supplementation, and a designed diet for their genetic code. But when I wrote Knock Out, I interviewed 17 of his patients. I said, "I'd just like to talk to Stage IVs."And I remember there were these two older women. You know, when I interviewed them, I thought they were older but they are sort of close to what my age is now. Isn't it funny how time flies? And they were both in their 70s. And one had Stage IV breast. One had Stage IV ovarian, only been treated by Nick. One had Stage IV ovarian for 17 years, the other Stage IV breast, at that time for 12 years. I haven't asked Nick recently, but as of last year they were both still alive and thriving. And Devil's advocate. I said, "Really? You're going to do coffee enemas every day?" And they started joking and the older one said, "Yeah, I particularly like French Roast." She said, "It gets me kind of all juiced up." You know, I said, "Okay, whatever."But it makes sense that if you keep cleaning out the liver and a coffee enema goes back to Egyptian, you know, early Egyptian, you know, Cleopatra era. Cleaning out the liver of toxins in a time in the world where our livers are groaning from intoxication, it almost—you wonder how anybody can be alive without doing regular liver cleanse. And then the idea of the pancreatic enzymes, and I always have to do everything visually. So, what I see with his enzymes is, you take them in between meals, and it is a lot of them. I think, I take, and this is where I get ridiculed, but I take about 80 a day because I had cancer and I had a big tumor. So I am not worried about getting it back, but I have to do everything I can in my power to make sure. But, so I visualize the little enzymes. And in between meals they are eating all the debris and what better debris to munch on than cancer? And when you keep yourself cleaned out, then there is no reason for the cancer to grow anew self. So, I believe in him. But also, I think my belief is a big part of why I am so well. You know, if you believe it, you manifest it, and I believe it.

Ty: Yeah, it is obvious that you do by the passion that you speak with. And that does make sense, doesn't it, with the pancreatic enzymes, the way that they digest the proteins. Because the proteins and the cancer cells have a protein lining, so they are attracted to those cancer cells.

Suzanne Somers: Right.

Ty: It makes perfect sense. It makes just too much sense, doesn't it? The fact that if you use pancreatic enzymes to digest cancer cells. You actually eat clean, organic, raw foods to fuel your body and stimulate your immune system. It almost makes too much sense.

Suzanne Somers: Well, you know, it's a Happy Meal for the little bad guys. Now, in my particular genetic coding, I am not a raw food person. I am a moderate vegetarian. So I am allowed to have chicken a few times a week. I can have a steak once a week. And for me, I love the way I eat. People see me eating a steak.

And they will go, "You're eating steak?" And I go, "Yes, yum. I'm feeding my brain. I'm feeding my GI tract."I have another visualization that I do with the GI tract, because what most people have is an imbalance of the GI microflora. And the bad pathogens have overtaken from the toxins because of a lack of people understanding the necessity for probiotics. Anybody who has ever had antibiotics probably needs to replace probiotics for life. You know, anti takes away, pro puts back. This makes sense to me. It is all simple.So, now, how do I—how do I control strong desires to have sugar and carbs, because don't we all like them. They are good. I envision the little bad guys in my gut that would like to overtake the good guys and create havoc. I do not have icky gut right now. I know what it feels like because I have had it. And interestingly, I had it before cancer. So let's connect those dots.When I get tempted, because I have this ice cream shop down the corner that I—I love ice cream. I love ice cream and cake.

Ty: Who doesn't?

Suzanne Somers: Who doesn't? I then envision the little bad guys in my GI tract going, "Come on, you can have some. Come on, give me some." Because all they want is sugar. The need sugar. They thrive on sugar. They have to have sugar. And I say to them, "No. I am going to starve you to death. My job is to stamp you out so I'm never giving you your Happy Meal. In fact, I'm going to flood you with fats, which eventually you'll just have to die and go away." And that is how I have chosen to get rid of my bacterial overgrowth. And it works.

Ty: I love it.

Suzanne Somers: Yeah, yeah.

Ty: I love it. It's a great technique and I have heard that from many medical doctors on this journey. That if you hate your cancer, starve it don't give it the sugar—

Suzanne Somers: Starve it.

Ty: —that it needs to thrive.

Suzanne Somers: But how can the oncologist's office, and I have seen it where you go into their office and they have candy bowls with candy there. Because cancer patients on chemotherapy are so weak and they need a little pick-me-up. And I have looked at that different times in an oncologist's office going, "What are you thinking?"

Ty: Yeah.

Suzanne Somers: Right, right.

Ty: It makes no sense whatsoever. Your diet, actually, Suzanne, sounds very similar to ours. We do the same. We live here in Texas on five acres and we have about 25 laying hens, so we eat—we have fresh eggs every day.

Suzanne Somers: Mmmmmm.

Ty: We eat a lot of pastured hens and then grass-fed steak.

Suzanne Somers: Yep.

Ty: People do not understand that steak is okay as long as you are eating meat that was cow that was eating grass, and not injected with antibiotics, and no hormones and so forth. The cows, the animals are what they eat, as well. And so if you are eating a cow or another animal that was eating a clean diet, you are going to get good meat.

Suzanne Somers: Right.

Ty: Yeah.

Suzanne Somers: You know, it is a, let me just get rid of something here. It is interesting—you have to also think about what was your mother's eco balance in her GI tract and what was your father's? Now, I am at an age where no one would have ever known. But in realizing that the good or bad eco balance of microflora in the pregnant mother's stomach, then gets passed on to the child, only worse. And then that child bears a child who has had digestive problems all their life. And the child that that one has has GI problems, only worse. But right now, there is an epidemic of ADD, ADHD, OCD, autism, schizophrenia, bipolar, asthma, eczema, dyslexia, dysphrasia. And it is the dirty little secret nobody wants to talk about. Because if you get to the bottom of what that is, it is all chemically induced, all the shredded GI tract lining, creating generations. It is not genetic. It is generations of poor health in the GI tract, which then it gets exacerbated by all the chemicals. And now our children are really suffering. Our children are... their brains are under attack.At my grandchildren's schools, I would say half the kids that I am aware of are on mood stabilizing drugs, Vyvanse, Ritalin, Concerta, Adderall. And this is only going to aggravate the problem more. And what the kids need is to be put on the diet that you—what you and I eat. What is so wrong with you and I eat? I love—eggs, fresh eggs, great steak.

Ty: Yeah.

Suzanne Somers: You can put a pat of butter on your steak, if you want. You can have vegetables tossed in butter, all of what, I mean—

Ty: Yeah.

Suzanne Somers: I love the way I eat.

Ty: It is great.

Suzanne Somers: True nutrition, and true nutrition is not a smaller diet soda.

Ty: Right, exactly. Less toxic chemicals to eat holes in your brain.

Suzanne Somers: Right.

Ty: Now, Suzanne—

Suzanne Somers: Uh-huh, yes.

Ty: No, yeah, go ahead. Finish your thought and I will ask you—

Suzanne Somers: Well, what you are describing is the foods we all grew up on.I'm a baby boomer, so I grew up on—there was no organic food, because it never entered anybody's mind to put chemicals and poisons on our—you did not say give me the one without the poison. I always say, in a grocery store, if in the vegetable section they put up poison food and non-poison food. Well, it would be a no-brainer what you bought. But because they cannot label GMO foods, although there are two counties in Oregon in the last month that have voted on labeling GMO food.

Ty: Right.

Suzanne Somers: That is the beginning of a turnaround. That will be really important to do.

Ty: It is huge, huge, in Vermont, as well.

Suzanne Somers: Vermont, too? Okay, I didn't know about—

Ty: Vermont and then, as you know, out there in California, you guys have turned down a couple of propositions. But I think it will pass there one day soon.

Suzanne Somers: Yeah, well, I wonder—I mean, they are deep pockets of big business. And they can outspend. And I cannot tell you when that was up, I started a campaign my own Facebook and Twitter. I cannot tell you how many people said, "Yeah, but it is going to make food more expensive." I said, "That is a crock."

Ty: Yeah.

Suzanne Somers: A penny, a penny at most, if at all.

Ty: Fractions of a penny.

Suzanne Somers: Yeah, fractions of a penny, or go watch Genetic Roulette and look at the little insecticide factory in your intestines then go make your decision.

Ty: Exactly. And then, as Joel Salatin likes to say, "Have you priced cancer lately?"

Suzanne Somers: People are so ill and the chemical treatments, chemical poisoning. I don't even like to call it chemotherapy, so that people will really get a sense of oh, I didn't know I was taking chemical poison. Yeah, that is what chemotherapy is.

Ty: That is exactly right.

Suzanne Somers: It doesn't really work. It, you know—

Ty: Well, it is not—cancer is not a deficiency of chemotherapy. So you cannot really give a long-term cure for it by treating with chemotherapy, especially in light of what we talked about today, with the immune system being so key. If the immune system failure is one of the reasons that you are diagnosed, then why are you going to be treated with chemicals that will destroy the immune system further?

Suzanne Somers: Further, right. And on the other hand, why don't you make a concerted effort to rebuild your immune system. And you can do that through probiotics and healthy fats, and no chemicals. Even when your GI tract is shredded like a tire on a freeway, even high fiber vegetables at that point can turn toxic on you until you get things healed. So you have to even be careful about the amount of—the kinds of vegetables that you take in during that time. And eventually, you can go back to all vegetables. But kale, and cabbage, and those gaseous kinds of vegetables, while you have GI distress, is going to aggravate the situation for a while.

Ty: Yeah, sorry I am laughing. Because we—one of the dishes that we love, we cook up kale, cabbage—

Suzanne Somers: Love it.

Ty: —onions and we put a lot of coconut oil and shook them up. And we did that last night, but it does cause some indigestion, if you are not ready for it.

Suzanne Somers: Yes. You have to be really comfortable with your spouse. Because it's a sort of noisy evening.

Ty: Yeah, absolutely.

Suzanne Somers: But it is good. I probably have four spoons of coconut oil, just on its own, during the day because that is so appealing to the intestines. And then I use it in my cooking. Coconut oil is incredible. In my Suzanne Organic Skincare Line, we have coconut oil in so many of the products. My products are certified toxic-free. I don't know of anybody else who has that, organic, and so certified toxic-free means it has to be grown organically, extracted organically and nothing upwind or downwind of the product can be toxic to contaminate it. And I am developing a nice little business of people who want high quality cosmetics and skincare, and makeup, and do not want any chemicals. You know, I think about how much lead have taken in through lipstick over the years. I make lead-free lipstick.

Ty: Oh, it is phenomenal. Yeah, it is phenomenal the amount of lead of that people have been taking. And I was going to say, my wife is looking for this, so you have another customer.

Suzanne Somers: Oh, go to my website and it is honestly, you know, it sounds self-serving, but it was developed because this is what I wanted. I have never used a line of makeup or skincare as good as this. It is just wonderful. And my skin has gone to a new place, so how nice, coconut oil.

Ty: Awesome, yeah, coconut oil is great.

Suzanne Somers: Over the years, I do not know why, I had been keeping a file of doctors who were curing cancer without drugs. Nick Gonzalez was in there. Stan Burzynski was there. Julian Whitaker, because he is integrative and I assemble this coterie of doctors and because of—because of my being poisoned and writing that book, so many people have had access to these other kinds of doctors.

Ty: Yeah.

Suzanne Somers: And, you know, I look at the people walking into the chemo world and I think, what makes you think it is going to work for you? It doesn't work for anybody else, unless you're lucky and you have childhood leukemia, or even adult leukemia, testicular cancer and non-Hodgkin's lymphoma. After that, zip. And those chemos for those cancers do not work all the time. When I look at Nick Gonzalez and Stan Burzynski and Whitaker, and Forsythe and the other doctors in that book, Taguchi, I think open—if you are diagnosed. It is so devastating and so heavy to be diagnosed. Open your mind. Look at all the options. They get you with fear on the day of your diagnosis. Like the doctor said, "What we can do is start you on chemotherapy today." And most people would be so afraid that they go, "Okay, alright, I'll do it." Cancer is not fast growing. You have time. You have time to think about it and look at another way. And because of what I have learned, because of that incident it has taken away my fear of cancer. And it doesn't mean I may never get it again. It would be hard to get it with my body. It is so clean and so cleaned out and toxic-free, but were it ever to find its way in there—

Ty: Right.

Suzanne Somers: I know exactly what I would do. I would go to Nick and I would have him up the ante.

Ty: Right. Well, you know, it is all about the knowledge, isn't it?

Suzanne Somers: Yeah.

Ty: And that is why your book, your Knockout book has been so powerful and so useful to tens of thousands, and potentially more, hundreds of thousands of people—

Suzanne Somers: What a privilege, what a privilege, yeah. And people from all over the world go to these doctors. And I feel that this is probably why I am famous. I didn't go after fame in the early years. I really, I was a teenage mother and I needed money, and I started as an extra in movies. And one thing led to another and it is a long story. But sitting on the Tonight Show one night, and the man who was running ABC was looking for a Chrissy Snow. And that unbelievable visibility at that time, the number one show in the country, when there were only three choices, gave me a fame beyond anything that people can accomplish on network television anymore. If you really know how to work the internet globally, you can do it a few of those international stars. But I always wondered, when you are not seeking fame why does it come? And why, then, why did I get fired at the height of my success, because I asked to be paid what the men were being paid? It all makes sense to me now. I needed that kind of visibility, that kind of fame, to have a louder voice, to use it for the better good, to write these books, to lecture to these groups so that others can find another way. So, I feel like I am doing what I am supposed to do.

Ty: You definitely are, Suzanne. That has to be reason for the fame is so that you could do something like this, that is really important, that is helping people.

Suzanne Somers: Yep. Very satisfying work and passionate, compassionate.

Ty: Yeah, you clearly are. You know, it is very encouraging to hear your story. It is really amazing the number of people that are now waking up to this line of treatment, these natural treatments that can help the body be healed. And I just want to say thank you for spending the time with us today to share with us your story, your success story, about beating cancer naturally. And then, the things that have happened in your life since then that now you are impacting so many people with just—you have become one of the most outspoken voices for alternative medicine and for natural healing. And so, it is a real privilege to interview you for this series. And I want to say thank you for spending the time with us today to tell about it.

Suzanne Somers: Thank you very much. It is very nice to talk to a like-minded person, who eats steak, too.

Ty: Well, Suzanne, you take care. Thank you so much.

Suzanne Somers: Thanks a lot, Ty, bye-bye.

[end of transcript]

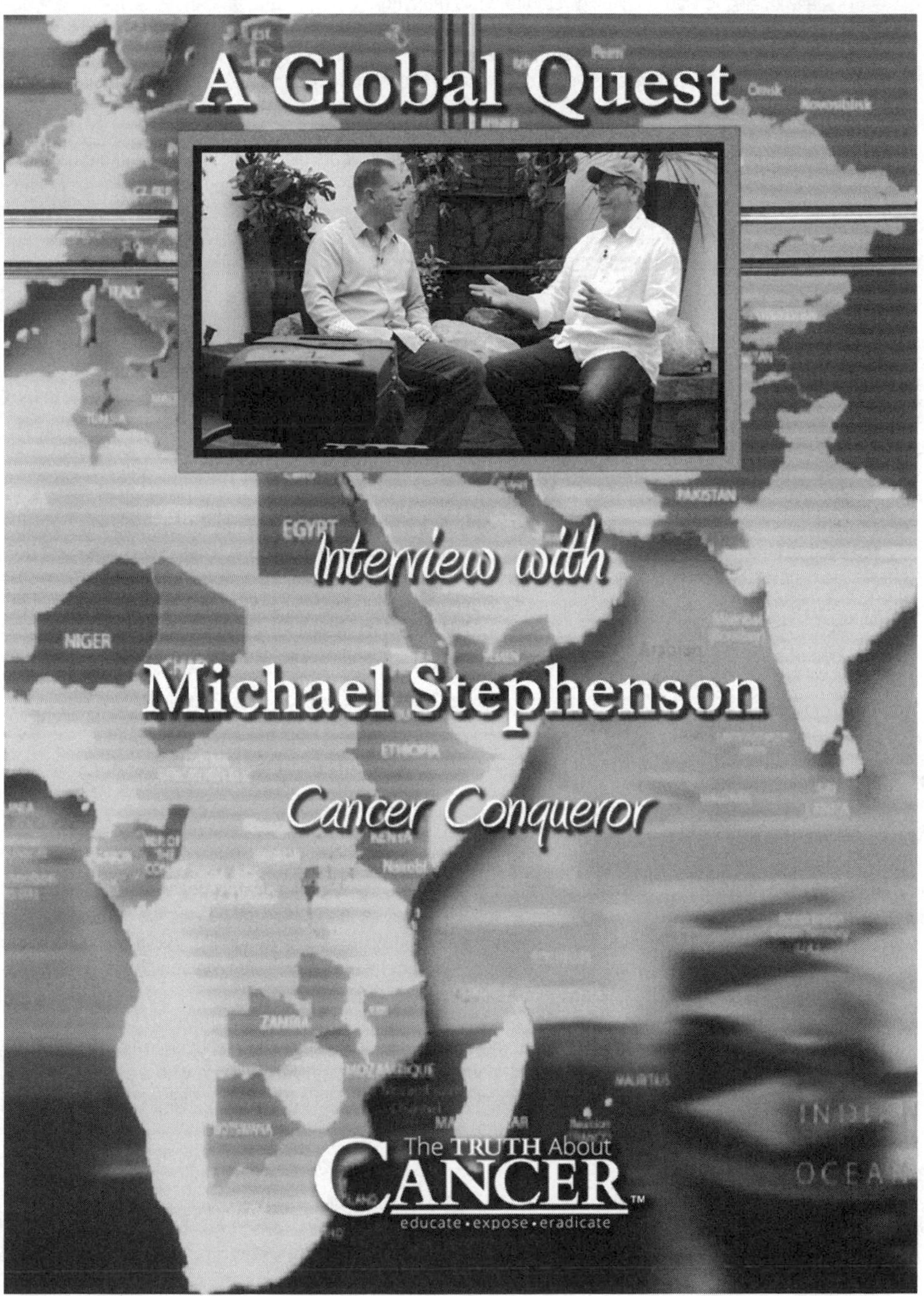
A Global Quest
Interview with
Michael Stephenson
Cancer Conqueror
The TRUTH About CANCER™
educate • expose • eradicate

Ty: I'm here in Tijuana, Mexico with Michael and we're at the Hope For Cancer Clinic, Dr. Tony Jimenez. Really looking forward to getting your story this morning.

Before we got on camera here, you were telling your story beginning about four years ago in Oakland, California, with Cisco Systems and a diagnosis of cancer. So tell us a little bit about yourself and let's walk through your story.

Michael: Well, like you said, I'm Michael Stephenson, and I was 55 years old, feeling great, found the love my life, just gotten married, had a little boy, five months old. The long short of it, I had a really fluky thing happen, as I was telling you. My wife had a doctor's appointment that she couldn't make, so I went. I show up to the doctor's appointment and, lo and behold, I get this news of, "We need to do some more testing because your prostate's a little swollen, or larger or whatever. So let's just send you to urologist," I think that's who it was. "Yeah, okay." And that's when my life changed.

I went. They said, "We're going to take biopsies." Went through that, 17. I was in a meeting at Cisco, and looked down at my watch, "Well, I've got to go back and get the results from my test." But you know, I'm healthy, life is good. We get into the urologist's office, and this is one of the things you don't think about. It's kind of comical. So I got to tell you. We're looking around at all these magazines and it's about prostate cancer, prostate cancer, prostate cancer. I didn't even think, "Well, look where you are." None of this can apply to me. So he walks in. Super guy, and his delivery was quick.

He says, "Michael, your biopsies are back and all 17 are malignant. You have an aggressive cancer." At that time you want to look around and go, "Are you talking to somebody behind me? This can't be happening." When you hear you have cancer—as I told you earlier, my sister died at age 45 from cancer—you're devastated for a moment. But he started to draw pictures, this is what it means. I just had to put my hand up. "I've got to stop you. This is all I can take today." So I want to keep my composure. The long walk down the hallway out of the hospital, was a long walk. We made it to the car …

Ty: Broke down.

Michael: Broke down.

Ty: Your wife with you?

Michael: So, I think that's pretty normal. If you don't break down, there's something wrong with you. But even now I get emotional because it brings back such fierce fear about how fragile your life is. So we went home, we held our little baby. Pretty much cried all night, and the next morning, we wiped those tears away and we said, "What are we going to do? I cannot die. Not now." Well, we don't have any control over it, but we wanted to have some more than we were given.

However, the thing that shocked me the most was—now that I know more about it, is how—I won't say lie because lying is a harsh word. But the counsel that we were given by those who are trained in the profession, I think that's where it really comes down. You put so much faith in their education, their knowledge that you trust, the trust is—it's not even earned, it's just implied.

Ty: It's blind.

Michael: It's blind trust. As I was telling you earlier, he said, "Yours is aggressive." I was 55 years old. "And with prostate cancer, normally, we really don't get too excited about it. It's slow growing, you're going to die from something else probably 70-80 percent of the time, except in your case. You're in that 15-20 percent that we're very concerned about and you need to make some pretty hard decisions very quick."

Ty: What were their recommendations for you?

Michael: Absolute surgery, because he's a surgeon. I did have a choice. I could either use robotics, or I could let him do it. He still does that the old-fashioned way, but that is the only salvation. There is nothing else. "Well, you could do radiation, but with your medical history, radiation wouldn't be a viable option at this point in time." Well, all you can hear is "You've got to make a decision very fast and I know what I'm doing. I've been doing it for 20 years. I've got this success rate. Robotics or this."

So he said "Well, let's talk to a robotics guy. What about this?" "Well, I can …." "Okay." Then he said—the thing that shocked me the most was because I thought "Okay, in the next month or two, I'll have the surgery." He goes, "I have a patient scheduled for Monday morning." It's now Thursday or Friday of the next day, and he told me, he says, "I can put him off, his isn't as critical as yours. We need to get you into surgery."

Ty: So how did that feel? At that point he's telling you it's so critical you need to be operated on within three or four days. What's coming over you at that point?

Michael: It elevates the fear, the lack of knowledge that I'm going to die factor, so high. I don't think you can really think. I think you are so overwhelmed with the fear of dying. And I go, I never feared dying, and I guess that's true with most people until you're faced with it, and so short. And all I could think of is "I'm going to do whatever it takes to be around my little boy. Well, let's schedule it."

I have two older children. My daughter flew back home and as we were walking in the hospital that morning, I'm going "Let me just jump. I'm going to skip and jump because in a few hours I'm not going to be able to walk." That freaks me out. I feel great, and I know when I leave here I'm not. But this is what the best minds are telling me I need to do and I want to follow that.

Went into surgery, came out, it was a great surgery. Complete success, and these words that I've now come to smile at, "We have clear margins. Got it all. Couldn't be better. You're going to be great." Went, "Okay." So you go home and start the recovery process. Mine was a little longer than they expected. Then when I went back in, my PSA was—I have to stop and say this. Why would I even have a PSA if I don't have a prostate anymore? A prostate-specific antigen should be eliminated with the prostate.

Yeah, shouldn't have any, and I was still showing some. So then they were even more concerned. "Well, we thought we got it all, and we had clear margins. What we want to do now is radiation." Let me just tell you a side story here. At this point in time, my wife was working—and I won't tell the name of them—was working for a large health care organization in Northern California, and her specific job at that time was she was helping them create a prostate cancer database of outcomes and going back through history to records, and current. So she was deep into oncology, and it ended up that she did not last at that job very long.

The reason why, she came to her own determination that this wasn't about curing cancer, it was about making money. How can we offer more services, provide more care and generate more revenue? That was disheartening. So she decided this is not the line of work or the organization that I want to associate with, and so she quit and her career has gone another direction. Taken off and life is great.

Ty: Good. Well, good for her to act on her convictions.

Michael: Exactly.

Ty: I mean, how many people out there that know what she knows and learned and don't do anything about it because they're making good money.

Michael: And you become part of the problem.

Ty: Yeah.

Michael: And you perpetuate it. And I'm proud of it, and like I said, one of the things that happens too, is—and this was kind of a back story. Once I did have the diagnosis and I went back to my company, we had a network set up that if anyone who has cancer and wants to join, it's all confidential, you can go into a database online and say, "This is my name, Michael Stephenson. I was just diagnosed with this type of cancer. Anybody has anything, let me know."

It goes out and within 30 minutes of logging in—they were the world's largest network provider, so it's all over the globe—I get a message from a young lady in Israel, and she is the person who turned me on to alternative medicine. Said "You must read this book. It changed my life. I'm alive. There is another way." Fortunately, I've always been open, so I wasn't shut down to it. I bought the book, I read it, and I think I even took one of the what I call concoctions. You could order online and take – didn't really see it doing anything. But at least it got me on the path, and that's what I'm the most grateful for. At least I now know there is another path whereas before I wouldn't have.

In the course of this my wife's sister had a doctor that lived next door and her dad was going through some cancer and he said, "You ought to go to Germany." "Why?" His answer was "They have a great success rate with treating cancer and they don't use …" It was a small amount of the same chemo, radiation. "They use heat, and light, and all kinds of alternatives, and that's their course of treatment."

Ty: With no side effects.

Michael: No side effects, and I'm then going, "Wow!" Okay, so I go online and I look up German clinics for cancer. I find them, they look like these castles. I want to go there just to stay in the castle and get treated. It was kind of awesome. And it's almost like the university is taking care of you because as I was looking online at all these beautiful places in Germany, I thought I read we have a sister clinic in Mexico. I went, "Mexico." I'm in the West Coast, it's closer. So I log onto this Hope For Cancer. Turns out it wasn't a sister clinic, it was just another advertisement on the Internet that I misread, thank goodness. It has been the only fluke I think you can make that's awesome in your life.

Ty: That's good.

Michael: So I called Dr. Tony. I was—again, from the first moment—stunned that I got him on the phone, and I found that to be incredible. I was actually talking to the head of the clinic. We chatted. It was at least 45 minutes, probably an hour, went through everything that I had and he told me, he says, "Well, Michael, first thing if you would just send me all of your information, I'll review it." And I thought, again, it's incredible. You're offering a service. You're not asking about insurance and cost. None of that's mentioned at all. "I'm just here to tell you this is what I do."

When I told him what I had and the diagnosis, one of the things he said is, "I don't ever tell people that I can cure cancer. But I will tell you based on what you've told me here in this interview, is that if you come into my clinic, you're not going to die from cancer. You're still going to die at some point in time, but it won't be from cancer." Wow, that's pretty powerful statement to me, and I went "Okay." Now, that was in 2010. So I got to tell you the truth.

I came here August of 2011. And so, when people ask, "Well, what took you so long?" Again, this is alternative medicine. You've got Stanford University down the street, you've got people telling you this is the way you ought to go, and it's not covered by insurance. It's a pretty substantial amount of money, but to save your life, you're going to come up with whatever you have to do.

Ty: Right.

Michael: I stayed on my vegan track that I had started, but it wasn't until I went back again, I went and circled back to this urologist and I had another PSA, the last one I've ever taken. He says "It's elevated and we're suggesting radiation. I want you to meet with a radiation oncologist, and we've made a lot of headway with radiation today." And I said, "Well, I just have one question. What are you going to radiate?"

Ty: Good question. Prostate's gone.

Michael: The prostate's gone. He says, "We're just going to shoot in the general prostate area." And I went "So, you're not going specifically for … you're just going to start shooting anywhere?" "Yeah, we're going to shoot quite a bit, so we'll catch whatever's there." And that is the last time I ever saw him. No thank you.

Ty: I think that was a good decision on your part. It's almost like he's throwing Jell-O at the wall to see if it sticks.

Michael: Yeah, I hadn't thought about it that way, but that's a great analogy. It is like throwing Jell-O against the wall, but fortunately, I was no longer a wall willing to be thrown anything at. I had knowledge now. I had had time to read and I think the thing that really helps out is knowledge is power. It gives you confidence that you're making a decision based in, in not something that's false, but there is hope, and when I saw Hope For Cancer, what a great tag line. You guys got great marketing that's for sure.

But I think the other thing is one of the things I do believe when it comes to medicine in United States is if it wasn't for doctors and hospitals, my little boy wouldn't be here because of the birth. That's what we need doctors for. But when it comes for cancer, I have a totally different attitude. I think with the billions and billions of dollars that's already been invested, if we wanted to find—well, I think they have found a cure. I just think we don't know about it. I may be wrong. I may be just making all that up, but that's what my gut tells me, that if we wanted to solve this problem, it would've been solved by now.

Look at what it has done with AIDS. AIDS is solved for all intents and purposes. People are living longer. It's no longer a death sentence. Cancer still is, and I believe—and I know you know more than I probably do—but out of 2,000 cancers that are in existence, there are only a treatment for 15 or so, a handful, and then out of that 15, all the statistics on these four or five that are really focused on. Well, unfortunately, I think that's a sad commentary on medicine.

Ty: Unfortunately, you were telling me earlier that one of your colleagues, a young lady that you worked with was also diagnosed, and you tried to share some information with her. Kind of relay that story and then I want to get to some of the treatments that you used here at Hope For Cancer.

Michael: Yeah, fortunately, I've always been open to talking about it, and as I was telling you, as soon as I was diagnosed I didn't hide it from anyone at work, personal. I was pretty surprised to find out how many people aren't that open about it, especially at work, because they're afraid they're going to lose their job. And not to be joking about it, but I go, "You're going to lose your job or your life? Really doesn't make sense to me, but I have to honor however you feel and the choices that you want to make."

So through this network, I would get calls at least once a month or sometimes more often from people who had been diagnosed with cancer and had heard about my story and had seen me. Ty, I tell you what floored me when I came back from here and I went back to work, I was meeting people in the cafeteria that hadn't seen me in a while and they would walk up to me and go "You look great. Wow!" And I'd say, "So, let me ask you this. If I was bald-headed and pale and looked like I'm going to die, would that validate that I have cancer more?" And they were like, "Yeah," cause that's the view of cancer.

Ty: That's the stereotype.

Michael: That's the stereotype, and I go, "No, this is the new face of cancer." Healthy. Survival. Beating it. This is what you can do. I also think I'm incredibly blessed, incredibly lucky, fortunate, all those things too. But all that doesn't just happen. You have to do your part, and my part was coming to Hope For Cancer. I'll go back and answer your question now. This young lady was at Stanford, never been sick a day in her life. Just had a baby about an almost two-year-old, 18-month old baby was told, "You have a rare stomach cancer, there's no hope. You're going to die in two or three months." That's it.

Ty: Death sentence.

Michael: Death sentence. You're 30 years old. Your family, your life is just starting. Devastated. "But we're going to give you some treatment anyway." So they started chemo on her. They made her so sick, they had to stop chemo and she stayed in the hospital for three weeks being treated to get over the chemo treatment. Still telling her there's no hope.

Ty: Three weeks to get over the treatment, or to take the treatment, to mitigate the treatment.

Michael: Exactly. Is that confusing?

Ty: Wow.

Michael: On something that there's no hope for. So if there's no hope, why give me anything. It's like she said, "I feel like I'm just a guinea pig and they're testing this stuff and it's killing me." Well, yes, it is. But first of all, the thing that hit her was standing right in front of me they're saying, "There's no hope for this person. This is not going to work. We're going to try this, but it probably won't work." "Hello, I'm a human being. I'm here."

So when I talked to her, and I would tell this to anyone that I meet. "I've just been diagnosed with cancer, and I'm scared. I'm trying this treatment. I'm going to do that. What would you do?" Well, the first thing that any of us really have to do is just accept it is what it is. Yep, you may die. We're all going to die at some point. You've just been given a look into how much sooner it may be. But all we have is today.

That's the philosophy I think hit me pretty quick. All I have is today. So whatever I have left, I want to use it. And I want to live it, and I don't want to go out the way I've seen other people go out. Unfortunately, it took her a few weeks to make the decision. We did get her down here to Hope For Cancer and she did have a rare and terrible cancer, but she was so debilitated physically by the chemo and the cancer that by the time they got here, Dr. Tony said, "We need to get you to the hospital because I can't treat you until your body's strong enough to even be treated." I was with her in Oakland, and her husband, when she passed. And you want to give hope, and what doctors told her at Stanford is, "We don't want to give you false hope." I came to her and said, "There's no such thing. You either have hope or you don't."

Ty: There's no such thing as false hope.

Michael: There's no such thing. So, that's what I just want to make sure is that you have all the hope that you can muster up, and don't let them take that away from you. It is a reality. And unfortunately I've seen and had a few other friends who weren't as fortunate as me. A gentleman that I work with, exact same cancer, prostate, exact same Gleason scores, and by then I think I'd matured in my cancer knowledge, in my soapbox and I said, "If you ever want me to tell you what I've done and what's worked for me and what I believe, all you got to do is ask. But I don't want to impose it on you."

But he already knew my story that I'd come to Mexico and I had treatment, and he never asked. And I got a call about six months ago that he had passed away. I was sad because the very treatment that he was given is the one treatment that Dr. Tony told me here was the worst thing you can possibly do for prostate cancer. And we did the exact opposite of that here, which—this is going to sound crazy, but made common sense. If you look at prostate cancer and you look at what it does, you don't give estrogen, you give testosterone. And I went, "Why does that just make sense right when I hear it?" Because it's true.

Ty: Truth resonates.

Michael: It just resonates with you. So I came down—long story short—I had made it down to Hope For Cancer and I have to say this. When Jesus, who picked us up at the airport, my wife, little boy and I, we drove down the street—and I just had the same flashback as we were coming today—turned the corner, we're driving down and I'm seeing a pretty grim sight for a ... I'd been to Mexico a lot, but this cannot be a world-renowned cancer center this street.

He pulls up and he stops and I go, "Jesus, where's the clinic?" and he points, it was right here. And my thought was "Oh, my god. What have I done?" Literally, I went, "Okay. You got to go with it." I walked through the doors. It was 7:30 in the morning, nobody was here. Jesus says, "You just go back there and sit on the sofa and somebody will be out there sometime." My wife is looking around, and we're thinking this isn't professional and there's nobody here. And I see a gentleman walking down the hall. He has an IV. I came to know him, Rick from Sacramento. He says, "You're new here, huh?" I'm like, "Yeah." He goes, "Just relax. Best decision you've ever made."

Ty: Really. Confirmed you the first day.

Michael: It was over. He says, "And remember you're in Mexico. You'll get your treatment when you get your treatment, and it'll be fine, but this is the right place to be." And from that moment, that little bit of encouragement that you're not stupid, that you haven't made a bad decision, that all your research is right, came to fruition. When the doctors took me in for my first evaluation, they go through it and the gentleman that was the lead doctor at the time spoke pretty broken English, but he had my medical records, and there were a couple of nurses and another doctor. They go through it, they ask me. I say,"Yep, yep. Yep. That all sounds correct. You got a good handle on it." He says, "Do you have any questions for us?" I went, "Yeah. When do I pay? Nobody's asked me for insurance, or credit card, or that check." He goes, "Well, they'll get to that. We just care about treating you."

Ty: Really?

Michael: Wow.

Ty: They're focused on the right thing.

Michael: "Wow. You care about treating me? Not that you're going to get not paid." Dr. Tony, later when I was chatting with him about it, he just laughed. He goes, "That's the least of our worries around here." People don't come here who don't pay us. We never have any problem, so we don't have to worry about that. We can focus on medicine and the treatments that we know are working and give you the best service we can. And then we started into the treatments and the first—I'd never been in the sweatbox, is what they call it. And there was a lady here from back East, a Vietnamese woman, a little older and spoke broken English. And I was getting ready to go in for my first 45-minute treatment, and I asked her, "How was it?" She goes "Pig cooker."

Ty: Pig cooker.

Michael: Pig cooker. And I went, "Oh, pig cooker." I'm from North Carolina, so I know what a pig cooker is like. So I get in, they put me in, they heat it up and within like two minutes I go, "I will never make 45 minutes in here. Are you kidding me? I'm going to fry." And all I could think about was this little lady out in the foyer. And I went, "If she can do, I can do it," and I toughed through it.

I get back out and I go up to her and I say "Wow, I did 45 minutes." She goes, "Huh. Ten minutes." She only made it 10 minutes the first time. I went, "I'm glad you didn't tell me that." And that's how I think life is. When you think you can do something, you can do it. Had she told me 10 minutes, I might have made 20 or 30 and thought it was good, but I made it the whole time.

And then when you're first introduced to a coffee enema—I've read about them, so I knew this was sane and there are doctors in New York using them. This is not weird, but I never had one. Coffee. So you think, "Okay, we're going to do that." But I think the other thing, too, that happens to you especially where my cancer was, you have to get very comfortable really quick with being served. And none of these doctors and nurses here, they're not just probing. They are trying to cure your cancer. And they're looking at you from that standpoint, and it's humbling. Very humbling.

I had to go in, had the enema. Wow! I was just—I felt comfortable in their hands. They were kind. They were efficient. They did a great job. They didn't make me feel uncomfortable at all. Whatever I needed to do, they were very gracious about it, and we got it all done. So what I look at is this, I go, since I've left the center—and then when I had to do the serum, that was another "aha" moment for me. Dr. Tony says "We need to collect a gallon of urine from you by the end of the day and we're going to extract some PSA. We're going to make what we call anti-venom, and you're going to give yourself five shots of these." And I go, "I'm going to give myself a shot. Didn't know that. And it's going to come from my urine. Okay."

So you really do start to think this is alternative medicine, but as he explained it you go, again, "Why does that resonate so instantly? Why does it make sense?" First time I had to do my shot, I was like, "I know I'm going to hurt doing this." We had to train my wife so she could do it. And we went, "Oh, not bad. Not bad." Did that. Got through those. You took it home and you did it at home. You're doing everything that you had to do and they ask you to do that you didn't think was possible, you did.

Ty: And they let you know that you could do it. They gave you the confidence that you could.

Michael: Yeah. You really—just watching how they operate here, and I keep going back to it. I told Dr. Tony, I said, "There were no God complexes." There was no, "We're just here to check you off number 601 patient." So it's Michael. Called you by your name. Oh my gosh, how does that feel?

Ty: That's a novel concept.

Michael: So I think all those things and Dr. Tony, you've met him and people who meet him, wow. You just go, "If you told me to just start cutting my wrist, I'd probably start doing that too because the confidence level is there must be a sound reason for it." That's kind of a weird graphic thing that you can cut out of this film if you want to. But if he had asked you to do something that you hesitated for a moment, it would just be for a moment. Now, if I go back to American medicine and they say—and this would be how I would sum it up too: "Should the cancer come back one day, it comes back, what's the first thing you're going to do?" "I'm headed to Mexico."

Ty: Headed to Mexico.

Michael: I'm calling up Dr. Tony, "I'm headed in, make a bed or a pallet or something, I'm headed to Mexico." And it will work because the alternatives don't. It's that simple. And when people go, "Well, we've made such great strides in radiation and chemo and we're doing ..."

I had some friends—a well-known biotech company, I won't call it by name. Their mother got sick with cancer, and I went over to talk with them and this young lady's a scientist there. She thought I was a lunatic. And yet, I go,"But here's the thing. I'm not forcing people to come to Hope For Cancer." All I can do is just say, "If you want to be treated and..." What's that Hippocratic Oath thing?

Ty: First do no harm.

Michael: "Do no harm, then you're going to go here. If you want to go bald, if you want to get sick." I watched my sister go through this, and she was at a well-known cancer clinic in Houston, Texas. And a night or two before she died, I asked her, I said, "If I ever get cancer, what should I do?" She goes, "Never let them stick a needle in your arm."

Ty: Really? You heeded her advice, didn't you?

Michael: Oh, yeah.

Ty: Yeah. Four years later, from 2011, you're here, healthy. The only thing that's missing is your son. Where's your son?

Michael: Well, now he's six, so he's this big and he just graduated from the first grade last Thursday, and one of his graduation presents—my wife had to come down for a conference in San Diego anyway. So the timing of this was awesome. Again, the universe is just lined up the stars for Dr. Tony and my family and everyone.

But had a choice to go here to Dr. Tony's, where he's been before, or LEGOLAND. And that's just not a fair choice when you're six years old. And I couldn't force him to come. I'd love to, but one thing I can tell you is I was the manager of his little league baseball team this year. To watch him go from he can't even catch a ball—and not T-ball—we're talking coach pitch to catching a fly hit by another team.

Ty: Yeah. That's huge.

Michael: That's life.

Ty: And you wouldn't have been able to do that without Hope prevention.

Michael: You know I think about that all the time, how blessed I am, and when I hear others have chosen a different path, and even with Dr. Tony, if they choose a different path, his heart is, "I hope it works. I hope whatever anybody's doing out there works, but I know what the path that I'm on and the treatments I give do no harm and can work and they do work."

I asked him in my interview with him, I said, "So, again, what's your success rate, Dr. Tony?" He was so humble. He goes, "Well, Michael, you have to understand most of the people that I see have been sent home to die. They have been chemo-ed and radiated and told there's no hope. And then they come to me. And so, I'm going to say I have about a 30 percent success rate, even at that." I thought, "You're kidding."

Ty: That's awesome.

Michael: I was looking for like a two to five percent. Thirty percent. Even 20, 10, and double digits, it was incredible. And the fact that I go, "Wow, I got down here..." And it was like he was smiling. He's going, "You know how few people never had chemo, never had radiation. You've been a vegan, your immune system's strong. We're going to just supercharge you." And then some of the probes, the heating probes. That was interesting. Again humbling and interesting. But you go, "What's the purpose of it? It all makes sense."

And I will tell you this. When my sister died—we're from North Carolina. She was a hardcore Southern Baptist. So being buried is part of her religion, and she chose to be cremated. My grandmother was just beside herself, but I knew why. And it came into my mind, here in the treatment because they use heat and light to kill cancer. She says, "This cancer may kill me, but I'm going to have the last laugh because cancer can't live in heat and I'm going to burn it to death."

Ty: And that's one of the things they do here, but they keep you alive.

Michael: It keeps you alive. So it resonated that she knew it can't live in heat. Wow! That's what they're telling me.

Ty: Yeah. And these far infrared saunas that they use here are amazing.

Michael: Yeah, and then I went home, built my own in my garage, heat that sucker up to 140 degrees. Dr. Tony was up in San Francisco for alternative health conference. Called me up, I went. I got probably one of the greatest pleasures in my life to introduce him at the conference. And after that, meeting people at the conference, and I met five or six people from my own company who were there. Incredible stories and other people and this infrared came up and there had just being a doctor talking about near or far infrared and how far infrared was better than near infrared.

Again, Dr. Tony doesn't flinch, and he is gracious. He gets up and he says, "Well, my colleague here, distinguished has just quoted this, but I have to professionally disagree and I've talked to Dr.—and he called the doctor by name—, who's written what I think is the definitive book on it, and I think near infrared is the way to go." And I'm going, "And that's what I have in my home." There's a gentleman in Maine who makes kits you can buy, put them together. It's not something that you invite people over to have a sauna with. But it works. And that's what I was looking for, something that I can continue that and the devices that I got from here to take home with me.

I did that for about two years and then I just waned off of it and I go—every now and then, I'll go—well, not this in-house sauna because now my wife, my daughter, they go—when you have cancer—this is some of the—sweating it from the inside out and then going in exercising, it all works. We don't think it's alternative anymore. That's what's so funny. We think this is normal.

So even my daughter, who thought I was a little crazy for coming down here, coffee enemas, feels, "Yeah, that makes sense." She done some reading on it. There are some people who take a little longer to get on the path, and that's been probably my biggest growth is to allow people to walk the path that they need to walk, and be there whenever they're ready and open. And I'm here today.

Ty: Well, thanks for being here today with us, and thanks for being there for people when they need you.

Michael: It's an awesome pleasure.

Ty: Yeah, and tell your son hello and your wife hello from us. Wish we could've met them.

Michael: I will. Thank you so much.

Ty: Yeah, thank you.

Michael: Thank you.

[end of transcript]

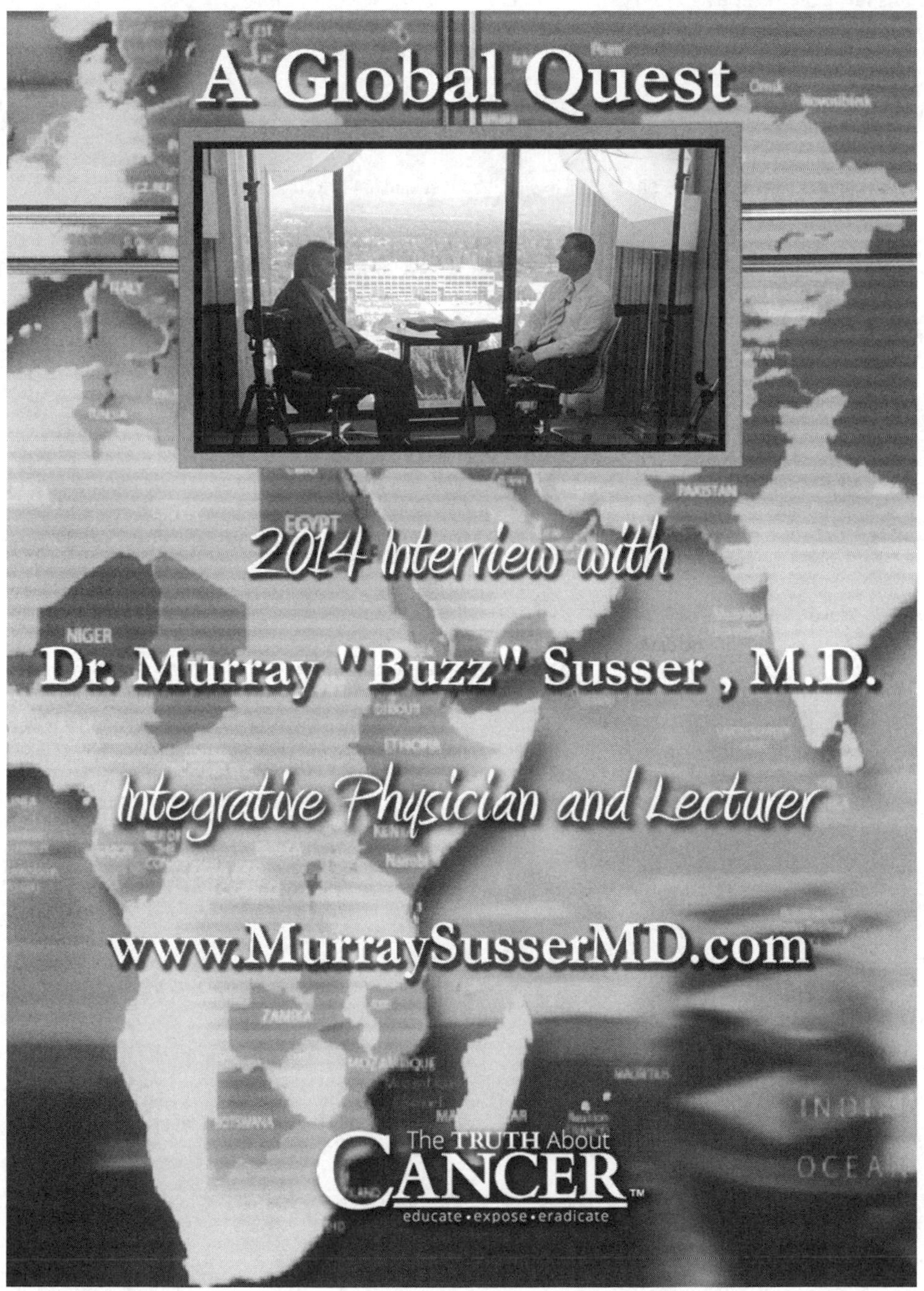
A Global Quest
2014 Interview with
Dr. Murray "Buzz" Susser , M.D.
Integrative Physician and Lecturer
www.MurraySusserMD.com
The TRUTH About CANCER
educate • expose • eradicate

Ty: I am honored to be here today with Dr. Murray Susser. Dr. Susser, thank you for being with us today.

***Dr. Susser*:** Oh, it's my pleasure, Ty.

Ty: I'm going to pick your brain about cancer if you allow me today.

***Dr. Susser*:** I don't have any cancer in my brain, I hope. But you could—yeah, you're welcome to do all the picking you like.

***Ty*:** I hope you don't have any but tell us about your education. How did you get involved with cancer research?

Dr. Susser: Well, I got involved with nutrition first. I got my MD degree from the University of Pittsburgh in 1966. That's hard to imagine that long ago. I was already a fighter pilot, by the way. So I was late—I was the oldest guy in my medical school class at the University of Pittsburgh. And when I graduated at the University of Pittsburgh in 1966, I thought, now I'm a doctor, and I really know a lot, right? Wrong. I found that it was very hard for me to lie to myself. I couldn't feel somebody's belly and look for the spleen and look for the liver and get really skimpy information, and then make some definitive decision out of that on what to do for that patient. And that's—and then treating the people was the same kind of thing. I felt that a lot of it was lies to myself. And I just really couldn't do that. It just went against my grain. So within a year of finishing my internship in 1967 I was looking for alternatives. And the alternatives include looking for alternatives to cancer treatment. And so it was—it's been a real odyssey. I think I'm going to write my memoir but I don't like my name. I was going to call my memoir, My Mother Never Called Me Murray.

Ty: Okay. That's a good title.

Dr. Susser: Is it? And so, I still may do that because my nickname is Buzz. So that's all I knew when I got to school. But the point of alternatives is that everything is an alternative, including chemotherapy and radiation and surgery. They are alternatives. And the alternatives that I like do not include those most of the time. I like alternatives with the dozens of different cancer things that have come up as alternatives over the years, and you could find it on the internet, every time we go to a conference like Cancer Control Society, where we met. But there's tremendous information there and a lot of fantastic cases. I started to talk about a patient I had who had lung cancer, who had a bone metastasis from breast cancer. And I treated her with the Reardon technique of threshold vitamin C, high dose, getting her blood level up to 400 mg percent of vitamin C, which is about a hundred times the amount you can possibly get by taking it orally.

***Ty*:** Right, it would really upset your stomach, wouldn't it?

Dr. Susser: Yeah, it would. Yeah, it would blow everything apart.

***Ty*:** Yeah.

***Dr. Susser*:** But she had bone metastases, which were painful. They got better when I gave her the Reardon technique, which is the 400 mg percentage of venous vitamin C.

Ty: Right, which was the same technique that Dr. Pauling espoused, correct?

***Dr. Susser*:** No, no, he was oral.

Ty: Oral, okay.

Dr. Susser: He was oral vitamin C. But the thing about it that was interesting is, she suddenly developed bone pain one day after being treated for months successfully. And she got this pain in her shoulder. And I said, uh—oh, this treatment's failing. I said, let's get a bone scan and a CAT scan, and have her checked out. And it was arthritis.

Ty: Okay.

Dr. Susser: And it really had nothing to do with her cancer. And she had kind of sprained the shoulder. It was scary. But she did very well, as many people do using the Reardon technique.

Ty: I like what you said about the options, the alternatives. So you've got everything as an alternative. Everything—basically a synonym for alternative is an option. Everything is an option. So chemo and radiation are just as much an alternative as the other alternative treatments.

Dr. Susser: Yeah, which—and they're getting better. You know, when I first starting doing this, 35 years ago or so, chemotherapy was horrible. I mean it wasn't even close to decent. It was totally indecent. And now there's some really good chemotherapy.

Ty: Now what do you think about the IPT, the IPTLD, the targeted low dose?

Dr. Susser: I think IPT is a good option.

Ty: Okay.

Dr. Susser: I've seen people who had exhausted everything in conventional medicine and conventional chemotherapy, conventional everything, and they always give that little phrase, go home and get your things in order.

Ty: Sure.

Dr. Susser: You know that's a real doctor thing.

Ty: Yeah.

Dr. Susser: And with the IPT, a lot of these people instead of getting their things in order took IPT and got a lot of good results and a good quality of life. IPT is insulin-potentiation therapy. Now they're calling it low dose chemotherapy.

Ty: IPTLD, sure. Can you kind of describe what IPTLD is, what is the low dose IPT?

Dr. Susser: Well, the low dose IPT, the low dose therapy, has to do with getting the cancer cells, fooling the cancer cells. Cancer cells eat sugar at about 19 times the speed of healthy cells. And cancer cells are voracious for sugar, which, you should say, that's one of the good management aspects of treating cancer patients, is take them off every drop of sugar, not a spec. But with IPT, what you do is, you give insulin, and insulin lowers the blood sugar. And you just get the right amount of insulin, and you give it, and you lower the blood sugar below its normal range of about 90 or 100 mg percent. And when it gets down to 40 range, you get really sick. I mean you get—you feel sick. It's not dangerous but it feels terrible. It gets dangerous when you get down to around 20 or 10 or zero. But at 40, it's not dangerous but it's quite unpleasant. And what's happening is, it's unpleasant for the cancer cells. It's more because they're starving. And cancer cells are really good at selecting out chemotherapy. They won't take chemotherapy but they will take sugar. And when you take away all the sugar, then the cancer cells will take anything. That's kind of like someone dying of thirst on the ocean in an ocean raft and they drink salt water. They know it's not good for them and it kills them. But the cancer cells then will take the chemotherapy instead because they can't get sugar.

Ty: Okay.

Dr. Susser: And that gives a tremendous benefit, therapeutically. And the numbers are really fantastic on that, because the IPT gives you 200 percent, 200 or 300 percent, therapy with 10 percent of the toxicity. You give a tiny dose of chemotherapy at the therapeutic moment when the blood sugar reaches 40. And you give the IV chemotherapy.

Ty: And so that's more of a selectivity toxic treatment towards the cancer cells than just blasting the whole body with chemo.

***Dr. Susser*:** Very—exactly, that's exactly the way to put it.

Ty: So then you can use a smaller dose, you can lessen the side effects because you're using, what you said, one-tenth of a dose of normal chemo, and get better results.

Dr. Susser: You use 10 percent of the dose.

Ty: Okay.

Dr. Susser: And these are people, many of them, most of the perhaps, have already failed at all the conventional methods. And so, there's nothing left. But the conventional methods are growing now and they—and some of these people wind up getting deeper and deeper radiation. So it's really frying them and they need larger and larger doses of chemo. So that's frying them.

Ty: Sure. Invades things that you can't cut out.

***Ty*:** Right. I have heard—I can't remember who it was, said that IPTLD turns chemo, it changes chemo from a shot gun into a rifle, so.

Dr. Susser: A sniper rifle.

Ty: A sniper rifle, there you go.

Dr. Susser: And I watch the military channel.

Ty: Okay. There you go, so. We got a sniper rifle chemotherapy treatment with IPTLD that's able to...

Dr. Susser: Yeah. And I used to fire missiles and rockets from fighter planes.

Ty: Did you?

Dr. Susser: Yeah. That was my Disneyland stuff.

Ty: That was pre-med school days.

Dr. Susser: Pre-med school, yeah. I was a trained killer.

Ty: Were you? And now you're a trained healer.

Dr. Susser: Yeah.

Ty: You're on the other side of the coin.

***Dr. Susser*:** Yeah. I'd rather do healing than killing.

Ty: I love your accent because my wife's from the Pittsburgh area. So the folks from the Pittsburgh area have a distinctive Pittsburghian tone. And so I knew the first time I had met you a couple years ago, I was like, he's from Pittsburgh.

Dr. Susser: I got rid of that accent for a while but then when the Steelers won four championships I got it back.

Ty: The Steelers.

***Dr. Susser*:** Yeah, the Steelers.

Ty: The Steelers, because when we lived up in Pittsburgh for a while...

***Dr. Susser*:** Pittsburgh...

Ty: Yeah, "the Burg"... There's not a crazier city in the United States that I've been to on a Sunday than Pittsburgh getting ready for a football game.

Dr. Susser: Oh yeah, yeah.

Ty: It's nuts. Now let me ask you this. We'll get off the football and back onto cancer.

Dr. Susser: Just one thing, they got Frank Lloyd Wright to look at the city when they wanted to redesign it. And they went around the city and said, okay, what are your recommendations? He said, abandon it.

Ty: Abandon it. Well, you know, the perception—we'll keep talking about it for a second because the perception is that Pittsburgh is this dirty, old town from many people across the country, but it's one of the most beautiful cities in the country now.

Dr. Susser: No, it is.

Ty: They have redone that whole downtown area.

Dr. Susser: When I grew up we were still using bituminous coal in our furnaces, and I walk across the street and my shirt had already had a black collar just walking across the street.

Ty: Yeah. It's not like that anymore.

Dr. Susser: No, it's not.

Ty: It's a beautiful city.

Dr. Susser: Yeah. But...

Ty: So they cleaned up Pittsburgh. How do you clean up your body? If you have a detox, if you have this toxic burden in your body, you've got these environmental toxicities, these things that we're exposed to that have compromised the immune system, what effect does the immune system play in the cancer equation and is detox a good idea?

Dr. Susser: Well, I think the immune plays a pivotal role in cancer. It may be the reason we get cancer, when the immune system fails for whatever reason. And what is the reason for failure, as you mentioned, toxicity and what kind of toxicity you have. Well, we all have too much toxic metals in our body. We all have too much lead, cadmium, mercury. And Walter Bloomer, have you heard of Walter Bloomer from Switzerland?

Ty: Yes.

Dr. Susser: He did a study where he gave—I forget the exact numbers. 50 some people got chelation every month. Chelation means metal binding. It's a process of putting a substance like EDTA in the body. It hooks onto the metal, and floats it out the kidney. And that's a major detoxifier for heavy metal. Sweating is good too. In Finland, they did a study with saunas and sweating and they found you could sweat more lead in an hour than you could pee out in 24 hours.

Ty: Wow!

Dr. Susser: So sweating is good but it's still not enough in most cases to get rid of the lead toxicity. And Walter Bloomer gave—said that there was a 90 percent decrease in cancer in patients who got the chelation.

Ty: Wow!

Dr. Susser: And 90 percent decrease, he had 59 patients who got treated, one of them got cancer over an 18-year period of 117 patients or so who didn't—who were the controls in a sense. They didn't get the chelation. And that group had 17 cancers.

Ty: Okay. So you have 1/17th of the cancer.

Dr. Susser: Yeah, we had 1/11th of the cancer. It came to 10 percent.

Ty: That's pretty effective.

Dr. Susser: You know, the study was not a perfect study, but it was a very good study and it was approved by the Swiss government.

Ty: Okay. So you've got the heavy metals, one of the toxic burdens that compromise the immunity.

Dr. Susser: Heavy metals is a biggie.

Ty: Okay.

Dr. Susser: And then there's bio films and toxic infections, Lyme disease probably, many other infections, chronic viral infections like chronic herpes. And all these things—by the way, the talk I gave today was on vitamin C and cancer. Vitamin C is a great detoxifier for these vicious things like chronic herpes. Chronic Lyme disease is another one. I treat a lot of Lyme disease.

Ty: With vitamin C.

Dr. Susser: With vitamin C, with peroxide, sometimes with antibiotics, and you notice we're talking about using unnatural things. We're using scientific unnatural things. And I went through a phase in my career. I said, I don't want to use any unnatural things. So I would only use natural things. Well, there aren't any totally natural things. And those that are, are not near as natural as we think they are.

Ty: Sure.

Dr. Susser: And so the...

Ty: So really maybe a better term would be not something that's totally natural or unnatural, but looking for something that is less toxic on the system, is what we should aim to do.

Dr. Susser: Yeah. And you have to fight fire with fire. If you have a patient who—and you want to play shaman and give them tree bark and leaves and stuff like that, that's all well and good if it works. But if you have something like chelation therapy and you have detoxifying vitamins like vitamin C and glutathione. There's a lot of nutritional treatments that detoxify.

Ty: Right.

Dr. Susser: And so I think—I use those things. I try to. Once I went three months without writing a prescription for a pharmacologic drug.

Ty: Awesome.

Dr. Susser: Because I said, I can do everything with nutrition, and I can do everything natural, and people were not getting better. Now I gave each person the choice to be—I didn't just force this on them, or trick them into it. I said this is a possibility. I could give you the antibiotic for your bronchitis. I can give you lots of vitamin C and vitamin A and vitamin D, and duh, duh, duh. And I'll give you a choice. And everyone for three months chose what I wanted them to choose. There was a little bit of coercion there.

Ty: I gotcha!

Dr. Susser: But mostly they were pretty eager to try. And what I found was it wasn't fair to them. Instead of getting over a cold or bronchitis in two or three days, it might take two or three weeks. They got better, and in the long run maybe it was better. But...

Ty: So you're more in favor of an integrative approach.

Dr. Susser: That's right. The blending of east and west.

Ty: Got it.

Dr. Susser: You know I call myself on the cutting edge of ancient medicine.

Ty: On the cutting edge of ancient medicine, I like it. Let me ask you this, cancer versus stem cells. We've got treatments that focus on killing cancer cells but not necessarily the stem cells. What's your take on the importance of targeting stem cells?

Dr. Susser: Well, I think stem cells in general are a really good idea. I don't know if we've perfected them enough to use them cavalierly. I've had fetal stem cells from Eastern Europe as a treatment. I had a miraculous result with it. My wife had a miraculous result. It lasted about 11 or 12 years. But now, we've lost that result. But it was phenomenal. I injured my back when I was in the Air Force in 19—I was 22 years-old so in 1956, I guess. And I really—and it was a hyperextension football injury. And it bugged me for 40 years. And I went to Jesse Wright and Henry Manchon [ph], and Albert Ferguson, and these top orthopedist people, and nobody could help my back. Then there was a chiropractor named George Rambacher [ph]. And we weren't allowed to talk to chiropractors. I don't know if you knew that.

Ty: Uh-uh.

Dr. Susser: It was in the AMA dictum that we weren't allowed to socialize with cultists.

Ty: Really? So medical doctors were not allowed to talk to chiropractors.

Dr. Susser: Now allowed to even talk to them in the hall.

Ty: According to the AMA.

Dr. Susser: Yeah, according to AMA.

Ty: Wow! So you broke the rule.

Dr. Susser: I've done that before. Rambacher helped my back, got rid of about 50 percent of the pain. And he was a cigar chewing, jeans and Braganza, and flannel shirt, and suspenders. He was an old time redneck looking guy.

Ty: He was a character.

Dr. Susser: But he was a great chiropractor and he was a great guy. And he was my first chiropractor. I've had about 50 or 60 since then. But Rambacher helped my back. He was the first one who helped when all these famous orthopedists couldn't help it. And then in 1998, I got the stem cells accidentally. My wife had atrophic purpura. Her arteries were bruising and shredding and had a terrible, and nobody could help that. So we went to probably 30 or 40 doctors over a long period of time, and she—over a period of six years. And she didn't get any better with anything we found from some of the best doctors anywhere. And when she got the stem cells, her arms got all better in two months. And my back, which had bothered me for 40 years I did—I got the stem cells just because I believed they would increase my longevity. And I didn't even think anything could help my back at this point. And two months after I got the stem cells I woke up one morning and everything was different. That's strange. What's missing? Oh, my back doesn't hurt. And so it got all better for about 12 years and now it's starting to bother me again, so I'm looking at the next option.

Ty: Well, let us know what it is.

Dr. Susser: Yeah. I think I'm going to see if I can arrange—if I can afford another set of stem cells, so. But stem cells and cancer, remember there's a telomer issue, and telomerase. Telomer is a little blip at the end of the DNA molecule and every time the cell divides, and we have to have cell division to have rejuvenation and revitalization. And stem cells, well all cells, have this DNA blip called the telomer. And every time the cell divides and you create a new set of tissue, a piece of the telomer snips off. And presently the natural state of things, we can only have about 60 telomer divisions in a lifetime then the cells won't divide anymore. And they're working with an enzyme called telomerase, which was discovered about 15 years ago, I guess. But they don't know exactly what to do with it. They haven't found any good solution with it. And telomerase is an issue in cancer cells because cancer cells have telomerase and their ability to divide never ends. They can—they're immortal in that way.

Ty: Right.

Dr. Susser: So stem cells and cancer, the jury is way out on this one. But I think there's a lot of problems there. Somebody's going to come up with a little manipulation to switch the telomer, the telomerase so it's purely good instead of good or evil.

Ty: Instead of carrying that same cancer propensity when they divide.

Dr. Susser: Yeah. We don't want to carry the endless division of this cell.

Ty: Let me ask, you think then, Dr. Susser, you treat cancer with vitamin C, one of the things that you use.

Dr. Susser: Absolutely!

Ty: So...

Dr. Susser: I don't treat cancer. I treat cancer patients.

Ty: Gotcha! You treat cancer patients.

Dr. Susser: We're not allowed to treat cancer with anything but the radiation and chemotherapy and surgery.

Ty: And what you're doing with the vitamin is definitely impacting the immune system.

Dr. Susser: I'd definitely have to say that. Definitely!

Ty: So what are other treatments other than the vitamin C that you might use to treat cancer patients to help them with that immunocompromised....

Dr. Susser: I have—there's so many possibilities. One of the treatments I like is the tea from Canada. I can't think of the name right now. But there was a tea developed in Canada, which for some reason or another will stop the growth of cancer in some people.

Ty: Are you talking about Essiac tea?

Dr. Susser: Essiac, thank you.

Ty: Yeah, okay, Essiac tea, great, yeah, what was the name of it? The Ojibwa Indians in Canada used to use for hundreds of years and they gave it to nurse Renee Caisse.

Dr. Susser: And her name backwards is Essiac.

Ty: Yeah. So you've seen good results with Essiac tea.

Dr. Susser: Yeah. I've seen some really excellent results with that.

Ty: My grandmother who died of cancer in 98 was diagnosed in the late 80s, and she was supposedly terminal. And she used Essiac tea for 10 years and it made her—it gave her another decade.

Dr. Susser: Yeah. I had a patient who had bowel obstruction and they opened it up and he had a cancer of the cecum where his appendix was. And they cut it out but he had—it had already spread to his liver. And so, he was kind of doomed by conventional things. And instead of taking chemotherapy, he took Essiac tea. And he went for years under my care and the tumor never came back.

Ty: Awesome. So you've seen good results with Essiac. Anything else that you're using currently when you're treating cancer patients?

Dr. Susser: Well, there's a lot of possibilities. Sometimes mega doses of things like vitamin A. Ramsberger in Germany used vitamin A in giant doses. Vitamin A is considered toxic above 25 thousand units a day. He, just for experimental sake, went up to half a million units a day of vitamin A. His skin kind of fell off, but as soon as he stopped taking the vitamin A he got all better. But sometimes mega doses of things like A, vitamin C mega doses, vitamin D now has been shown to have value.

Ty: Lots of vitamin D out today.

Dr. Susser: Vitamin D...

Ty: Let me ask you this, as far as nutrition is concerned, what's a good diet that you would recommend to your patients that may be compromised because they've been eating crap their whole life?

Dr. Susser: I'd say no sugar and then the other thing is no sugar, and then the other thing is no sugar.

Ty: Okay.

Dr. Susser: What we said before, the vitamins that—the cancer cells consume sugar about 19 times as fast as healthy cells. So then the question is, no junk, eat wholesome foods. You can eat animal foods. I don't believe in the vegetarian diet. Some people do. I've seen people who really seem to waste away on vegetarian diets. I think you could do a low meat diet but you got to have enough protein to rebuild your cells.

Ty: Sure.

Dr. Susser: And so you need some animal foods I believe. You could probably do—well, there's a diet for a small planet where if you bled—remember that book, Diet for a Small Planet?

Ty: Uh-uh.

Dr. Susser: That was one of the first nutritional books about cancer and about nutrition, in general, that if you combined beans and grains you can get a complete protein because vegetarian proteins never have all the amino acids that you need. But if you combine beans and grains then you can have both. So if you're going to try to do something low animal food, read Diet for a Small Planet and be sure that you get enough of the broad spectrum of amino acids. There are 20 or 22, depending on who you believe, amino acids that are essential to our body. Now all but about eight of them we can make ourselves, and so eight or arguably 10 depending on who you believe.

Ty: The jury's out on that still.

Dr. Susser: Yeah, which you wouldn't think in this day and age it would be.

Ty: Right.

Dr. Susser: But just say you need 10 amino acids that are considered to be essential because we can't make them. We have to eat them. And so, if we have a complete list of them, a complete diet of amino acids, all the good fatty acids, the omega-3, omega-6, and omega-9 in the right proportion, and of course, good starches. And the good starches—one of the best foods is watercress.

Ty: Watercress.

Dr. Susser: Yeah, it's high in sulforaphane. Sulforaphanes are plant enzymes that are plant hormones, actually, that fight infection that fight damage. So when you crush a plant it release sulforaphane. So sulfur is one of the best ways to fight invaders like cancer or infection.

Ty: Gotcha! Watercress....

Dr. Susser: Watercress is like arugula, those are the cruciferous vegetables. And so, I like those. And you can overdo those also because then they start binding iodine and your thyroid gets depleted. Iodine, by the way, is another important item that we're very neglectful of.

Ty: You know, I just interviewed yesterday Dr. David Brownstein about iodine in Detroit.

Dr. Susser: In Detroit.

Ty: Yes and he talked about the importance of iodine.

Dr. Susser: Yeah, I use it. I treat almost every one of my patients with iodine. The recommended daily allowance of iodine is a 160 mcg. I have a product that has 20 mg per drop SSKI.

Ty: Okay. Yeah. That's what Dr. Brownstein said was anywhere from 12 to 25 mg a day of iodine. Well, let me ask you this final question. If you were diagnosed with cancer, what direction would you head?

Dr. Susser: I think it would depend on the cancer. But I would certainly do the basic stuff and really clean up my act.

Ty: And no sugar, no sugar, no sugar...

Dr. Susser: No sugar, no sugar, no sugar....

Ty: I like it.

Dr. Susser: And I would get into a lot of good green vegetables like arugula and watercress. I do that now anyway to some extent, but I could do better.

Ty: So a good cancer treatment is a good cancer prevention then.

Dr. Susser: Absolutely! And that's one of the things that's true about healthcare in general. When you're doing natural things, the cure is also the maintenance and prevention, whereas in conventional medicine with drugs and surgery, the cure—if you get a cure it's not the natural thing to do continuously.

Ty: Yeah. Absolutely! Well, Dr. Susser, thank you so much for your time today. I really appreciate it. That's some enlightening information.

Dr. Susser: Well, it's good. That's my job.

[end of transcript]

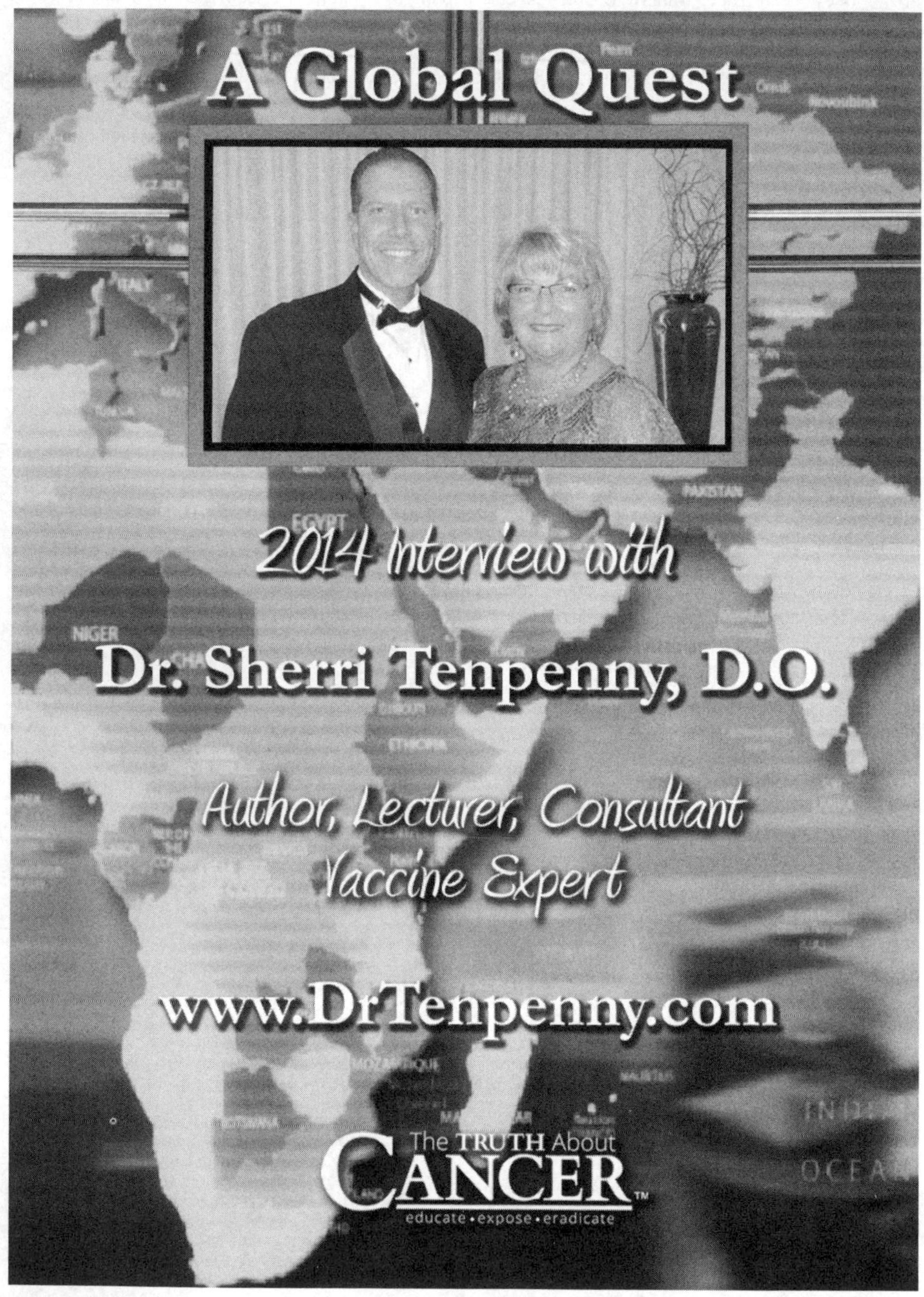
A Global Quest
2014 Interview with
Dr. Sherri Tenpenny, D.O.
Author, Lecturer, Consultant
Vaccine Expert
www.DrTenpenny.com
The TRUTH About
CANCER
educate • expose • eradicate

Ty: I am here in Cambridge, Maryland, and I am sitting here with Dr. Sherri Tenpenny. I am so happy to be able to talk to you today.

Dr. Tenpenny: Thank you so much. Thanks for the invitation.

Ty: Oh, thank you for being willing to do the interview.

Dr. Tenpenny: Sure.

Ty: I'm really looking forward to getting your take on, of course, vaccines. And as you know this series, the Truth About Cancer. And so we're going to kind of see what we can do to connect the dots between vaccines and cancer. But, first of all, let me kind of read a couple of things that I made notes of. About a year ago you were attacked by UNICEF regarding your stance against vaccines. It seems that the United Nations doesn't believe that we can actually read packed inserts on our own.

Dr. Tenpenny: Absolutely!

Ty: So can you talk about that? What happened with you being attacked by UNICEF?

Dr. Tenpenny: Well, I don't know that I was actually attacked but I think it was interesting that of all of the anti-vaccine, if you want to qualify it that way, I do not really think of myself as anti-vaccine. I think of myself as more pro information and pro education. And once you understand what is in the vaccines, how they work, and how they do not work, then you become one who says no thank you. And I think that is a very different position than just being anti-something just for the sake of being against it. So with all of the people out there these days who are now talking about problems associated with vaccines, I would say I have probably one of the biggest audiences for that. And so UNICEF was going out and looking at Facebook pages and decided that I was one of the biggest terrorists in terms of vaccine information.

Ty: A domestic terrorist…

Dr. Tenpenny: A domestic terrorist, that is right, probably global terrorist because my Facebook page goes out to about 12 million people globally. And so they decided that I was one of the people that needed to be brought to attention to say that this is one of those people we really need to keep an eye on.

Ty: Now you are a medical doctor.

Dr. Tenpenny: I am. I'm an osteopathic medical doctor, which is a D.O., which is in my opinion better than an M.D. because we not only get trained to do everything that an M.D. can do but we also have been trained in osteopathic manipulation, which is kind of like being a chiropractor or maybe a little level above. And so I am an osteopathic medical doctor. I was board certified in three medical specialties, emergency medicine, osteopathic, manual medicine, and holistic, and integrative medicine. I was the director of an ER for 12 years before I started my own clinic in Cleveland, Ohio in 1996. I used to be in charge of a three county EMS system that was involved with the sheriff's department, the police department, and the state highway patrol. So I have done all of the conventional stuff. And so I think that I am capable of reading package inserts, medical literature, CDC documents, and interpreting them in light of the way all physicians should be doing it, not just people who spend their time, their evenings, and their weekends, reading about all of these things.

Ty: Right, right. So speaking of CDC, recently you had this big CDC whistleblower story that broke.

Dr. Tenpenny: Yeah. I think that that's still an evolving story. We do not know exactly what those documents look like. We are waiting for this person to come out and really show his face in the light of day. I have heard rumors through several different sources that there are four or five other whistle blowers who may be interested in coming forth with information about various vaccines. And I really hope that this will be the start of a motion, of a movement. I don't know if you have ever seen that video of the crazy dancing guy, how to create a movement. It has got, I don't know, three or four million views on YouTube. That one person starts and then you have got the brave follower. And then the first thing you know you have got hundreds if not thousands of people following behind. And I am really hoping that perhaps there is starting to be some cracks in the dam to where we will get to the bottom of how vaccines are not safe, they are not effective, they do not protect you, and they definitely do harm.

Ty: Now, you mentioned that one of your goals is just to educate, and that is our goal as well. So educate the viewers here. How are vaccines dangerous? How are they doing harm? How are they not effective? Because if you listen to most conventional medical doctors they will say, oh of course, you need to get vaccinated. You are going to do your child if you do not. So how is that?

Dr. Tenpenny: Well, it is just amazing to me how we think we can inject something that has never been tested for carcinogenicity, never been tested to see if it's mutagenic, which means changes your DNA, never know whether or not it can cause any autoimmune disease, but we can perfectly say that it is safe and effective and causes no harm. If somebody died and made me health czar tomorrow what I would do is I would round up all the medical doctors, all of them, and I would put them in a big football stadium, and have them read all of the package inserts particularly the package—particularly the pediatricians. Read their reports from the vaccine adverse event reporting system, and then take an entire test, a written test, on immunology to prove that they know something about the human body. And then have them with good conscience say that what we are injecting into human beings is harmless.

Ty: They probably could not do it.

Dr. Tenpenny: It would be impossible but that would change everything overnight, wouldn't it, if suddenly we forced physicians to look at the truth about these injectables because all we are really doing with these things is trying to prevent diseases that are a fever, a cough, a rash, and some diarrhea. Really, for what kind of harm that we are causing?

Ty: Well, you know, look at the HPV vaccine. One the package insert it says it may cause other kinds of cancers.

Dr. Tenpenny: Yes. And we have already known that it has through the VAERS report that there have been many girls who have been fully vaccinated with the HPV vaccine that within three months to about two years that are diagnosed with cervical cancer, massive cases of venereal warts. We know that less than four percent of the women in the United States have actually ever been exposed to the two viruses that are in the vaccine. So if the vaccine did anything, which it does not, and it can cause a lot of harm, there are at least eight strains of HPV, human papillomavirus that are supposed to be associated with or known to be associated with cancer. But the vaccine only covers two of them. So it gives this false sense of security to moms who think they are protecting their girls to think they will not get cancer. And that will say to the girls, well, I do not need to get a pap test because I have been protected. But there are other strains that can cause the cancer. And that brings up another point. Does the virus cause the cancer or is the cervix, which is an exposed organ, have a nutritional deficiency, the organ starts to break down and deteriorate, and then the virus gets embedded into that decaying and sick organ. And the medical community says that the HPV caused the cancer when I actuality I believe that a lot of cervical dysfunction and cervical dysplasia are nutritional deficiency diseases. And we have treated many of them in our office with vitamin A, vitamin D, vitamin C, natural progesterone, and other types of—get them to stop smoking, get off the birth control pill, and it clears up and goes away in more than 90 percent of people that we have kept track of.

Ty: So when you give the body what it needs to run properly it runs properly.

Dr. Tenpenny: Imagine that.

Ty: Wow!

Dr. Tenpenny: Yeah.

Ty: And one of the things you said earlier about that most vaccines or all vaccines have not been tested for carcinogenicity.

Dr. Tenpenny: Very good.

Ty: Yeah. I have only got it right once. That is all I can say about it today. That is shocking in light of the fact that you are saying that they have not been tested. The ingredients in the vaccines have not been tested to see if they could cause cancer especially in light of the fact that you look at the ingredients in some of these vaccines today, and I mean it is a virtual who-is who of poisons.

Dr. Tenpenny: It is. There are several things that really, really continue—well, all of it concerns me, but to your point. Formaldehyde is used in the DPT vaccines and in the polio vaccines. And we have said or known for years that formaldehyde can cause all sorts of health problems and that the amount of formaldehyde exposure, either through ambient air that you come in contact with, or that you breathe in very, very small particulate amounts have been known to cause lots of different problems, including cancer. And it was only about, what, two or three years ago now that they formally said, yes, formaldehyde will be added to the list of known carcinogens but yet we continue to have known carcinogens in the vaccines and have them not be removed. And they have been injected for 50 years or more.

Ty: Wow! So it is worse than, they have not been tested for carcinogenicity—I got it right— but they have been tested and the formaldehyde...

Dr. Tenpenny: At least some of the ingredients...

Ty: ...has been shown...

Dr. Tenpenny: ...have shown to be known carcinogens.

Ty: Wow!

Dr. Tenpenny: There is also stray viruses that end up in these vaccines and they end up in the vaccines because a virus in order to replicate needs to be embedded into a living cell. And so they use these cells to grow these large quantities of viruses for which, then they harvest, and run them through a long line of chemicals to weaken them to put them into the vaccines. Well, the polio vaccine has been known for many, many years to have a virus in it called SV40, which stands for simian virus-40 because those polio vaccines are made from monkey kidney cells. And so simian virus is a monkey virus. And in 2002, the Lancet published a paper that said it was suspected that more than half of the 55 thousand cases of non-Hodgkin's lymphoma that were out there with a very high probability could be associated with the SV40 vaccine from the polio, the SV40 virus from the polio vaccine. So that is something in the published literature that was in the Lancet. And that came out in 2002. There are two other stray viruses that end up in there from avian cells, which are all the vaccines that are made from eggs because they are passed down through the chickens and they get into their eggs. And there are two different cells, two different viruses that are known to be associated with breast cancer. And I have written a couple of articles about that because we are now pushing flu vaccines on everybody including starting at six months of age in children. We are giving it to pregnant women. We are giving it to everyone. And I just read an article just today that said that the flu shot was less than 50 percent effective. It was 50 percent effective in pregnant women. Well, that is no better than the toss of a coin. And so could those women have done better while they were pregnant by taking high doses of vitamin and high doses of vitamin D and washed their hands more frequently?

Ty: Right. Yeah, just basic common sense things, right.

Dr. Tenpenny: Yeah. Well, I have often said that someday I'm going to start a whole company and I am going to have one product. And there is going to be a bumper sticker and t-shirt, two products, that says common sense ain't so common.

Ty: What people think…

Dr. Tenpenny: Exactly!

Ty: Well, the ingredients that you mentioned in eggs, is that ALV, is that what you were talking about that has been linked to leukemia?

Dr. Tenpenny: Avian leucosis virus, yes, it can be linked to leukemia, but that is also one that can turn on some of the genes that can cause breast cancer.

Ty: Okay. Great! You are doing great stuff here. [Informal background]

Ty: We are probably just going to go a couple more questions here. So you talked SV40, you talked about that. You are hitting all of these.

Dr. Tenpenny: And we could talk a little bit more about some of the animal cells. I think that is really important.

Ty: Okay.

Dr. Tenpenny: I think one of the more concerning things that comes from vaccines is coming from the cells for which the vaccines are manufactured in. That was a clunky sentence, wasn't it?

Ty: But I understood it. [Laughter]

Dr. Tenpenny: The vaccines, or the viruses, are manufactured in cells. Some of the cells are bovine cells. They are cow cells. And bovine serum has been known to have bovine diarrhea virus in it that has been passed into children that causes chronic diarrhea and maybe other types of issues. But the bovine cells, and then we have avian cells from chickens, and we have monkey cells, and we have dog kidney cells, now, that are now being used for some of the flu shots, and caterpillar egg cells, and all of this DNA ends up in the cells that gets transmitted into humans. There is a process called transcession, which is an old term that comes from the 1970s, which means that DNA of one animal or of one entity gets incorporated into the DNA of another entity. And I have a lot of concerns about these stray viruses and about the DNA matter from these cells being incorporated into the DNA of our children. And we cannot even find it necessarily because it has been actively incorporated into the DNA so we cannot—they say, well, it is not there. Well, how do you know? Just because you didn't find it does not mean it is not there. We also have human cells. There are two different cell, three different cell lines that are made from cells of aborted fetal tissue. So we have other human DNA and we have albumen that is many of the vaccines. Well, albumen is human protein. So if you inject protein into the bloodstream it acts as a pro-inflammatory molecule and it is also foreign so our immune system turns on immediately and starts to attack this human albumen. We create an antibody to that albumen which nobody is testing for. Could it very well be that that antibody then turns on genes to cause cancer, turns on genes to cause autoimmune diseases, attacks joints for inflammation, for all this autoimmune stuff that's going on? All of these things are starting from childhood. We are, in my opinion, one generation away of having very few humans left on the planet who have non-contaminated DNA to propagate our species.

Ty: Wow! And so not just the genetically modified foods that are getting into our DNA but the vaccines because of the fact the albumen mounting this immune response…

Dr. Tenpenny: Autoimmune response…

Ty: Wow!

Dr. Tenpenny: And I think that a lot of people will say, well, how can you just say it is the vaccines? Why is it not genetically modified food, or fluoride, or mercury, like dental fillings? It is all of it.

Ty: All of the above.

Dr. Tenpenny: And when I assess a patient in my office I sort of picture them visually as having a pie diagram sitting on the front of their chest. And each of the little slices of the pie represent different things, one is genetics and family history, one is chemical pesticide exposure, one is vaccines, one is chemicals; I mean a whole list of things. And in each individual person that slice of the pie will be a different size. And in some people that have been vaccinated the slice of that pie might be one or two percent risk. It might be more of something, the genetically modified food. It depends on how much high fructose corn syrup they eat, right.

Ty: Yeah.

Dr. Tenpenny: But in some people the slice of that pie might be 75 percent. But as long as you have been vaccinated the risk is never zero. And if your parents and your grandparents have been vaccinated, because that means that you are still at risk even if your children are not, because now we have seen some of these viruses pass through generationally from parent to child, or from grandparent to child. And we know that happens in the animal world, and now we're seeing it in the human world.

Ty: But didn't vaccines wipe out all the communicable disease, the diphtheria, the pertussis, the polio, weren't vaccines responsible for that?

Dr. Tenpenny: You know, it's interesting because every time someone is new to this topic it always starts from, well, what about smallpox, what about polio? Well, I do an hour and a half talk on that so I can maybe give you two sentences that say the answer is no, that less than 10 percent of the global population was actually vaccinated for the smallpox vaccine. And it was a virus that was dying out and becoming weaker over time. And when we introduced hygiene and refrigeration that is when the smallpox started to go away. And then, of course, it morphed into this other type of virus called monkey pox, and so smallpox is still around. It is just given a different name. The same thing, polio, the epidemic of polio in this country was well on its way out before 1954 when FDR released the polio vaccine. And we have seen nothing but travesty about that ever since. And the only places in the world that still report any polio are places that are using the oral polio vaccine, which is a live virus. The other thing is that polio is not a synonym for paralysis and that the vast majority of people don't understand that 98 percent of people who actually were exposed to the polio virus and maybe even contracted the infection that caused polio, it was nothing more than looking like a stomach flu. It was some diarrhea. It was maybe a little bit of fever, and it just passed through that you maybe thought you had food poisoning and then you had lifetime immunity to this gastrointestinal virus. But we have done such an amazingly good job impregnating multi-generationally into people's brains about iron lungs and little children with braces and people with deformed limbs but that happens so infrequently in the big picture but yet we have this horrifying terror of polio when we really should not. I mean we have spent billions of dollars around the world to eliminate that virus. What if we would have spent those billions of dollars on potable water and refrigeration and better hygiene? What could we have done with that?

Ty: Yeah, good question. Well, that leads into my last question. You talked about better hygiene, potable water. So health is not—health is an inside out phenomenon.

Dr. Tenpenny: That is my phrase.

Ty: Right.

Dr. Tenpenny: It is what I say all the time.

Ty: That is where I got it from.

Dr. Tenpenny: Oh.

Ty: I read some of your lectures.

Dr. Tenpenny: That's good.

Ty: So health is an inside out phenomenon, which I have heard you say. So could you explain what you mean by that? Is bad health a result of a lack of needles?

Dr. Tenpenny: No. And on the opposite side of that is health does not come through a needle. It just cannot. We just cannot in anyway think that we are going to inject something into a little baby or an adult that in any way is going to positively impact their health. So health is an inside out phenomenon. You have an intact immune system, good nutrition, adequate detox, organs of detoxification, liver, kidney, colon, and skin, all of those things come out easily. You have got all of the appropriate nutrients in there, your B vitamins, vitamin D, vitamin C, all the appropriate things that you need that you could be swimming in bugs. In fact, sitting in this room right here, how many bugs do you think are in the air in this massive hotel, and the carpeting, and if you live on a farm and you're going out and petting animals and all of that, you are not succumbing to all of these viruses and bacteria that are around you. If you are healthy from the inside out and your immune system does what God intended it to do, and what we were humanly designed to be.

Ty: Well, Dr. Tenpenny, what you say makes a lot sense. It is just common sense. And I think that I understand why they are honoring you tonight. You are the sacred—what is it called?

Ty: Well, Dr. Tenpenny, what you say makes too much sense. I can see why they are honoring you at the Sacred Fire Liberty Gala tonight. Thank you so much for spending time with us today.

Dr. Tenpenny: Oh, you are so welcome. Thanks for having me.

Ty Bollinger: Awesome! **[end of transcript]**

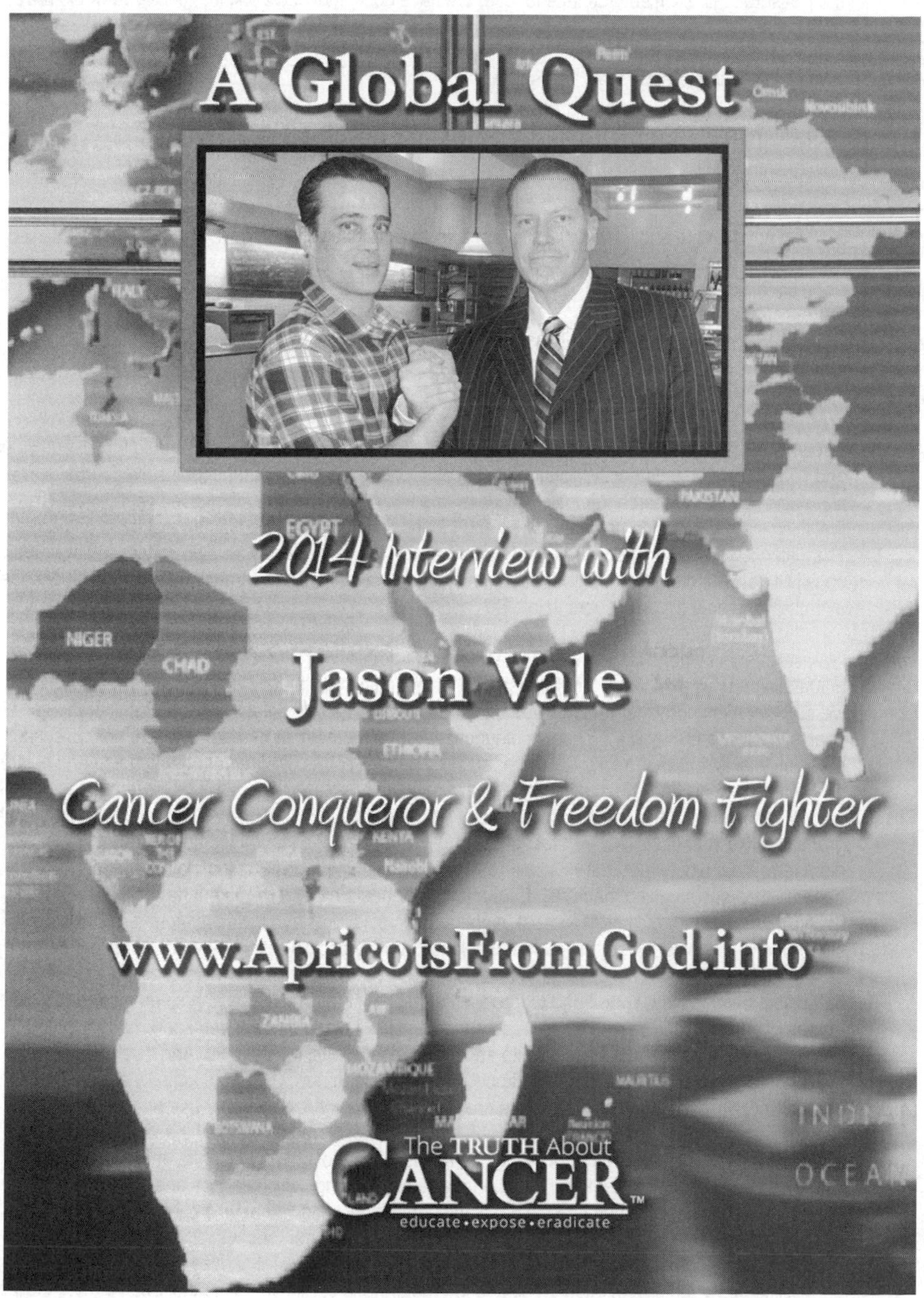
A Global Quest
2014 Interview with
Jason Vale
Cancer Conqueror & Freedom Fighter
www.ApricotsFromGod.info
The TRUTH About CANCER
educate • expose • eradicate

Ty: All right, so we are in New York City at Marjio Organics Restaurant with my friend Jason Vale. Jason, it is a pleasure to finally meet you face to face. We have done interviews online. I think you would have beaten me with the arm wrestle.

Jason: We just have to meet like that, that is good.

Ty: The arm wrestling champion here.

Jason: That is good.

Ty: But I am not going to arm wrestle you because you will probably flip me over.

Jason: You are blushing.

Ty: Yeah, I am embarrassed man, because you would probably knock me off.

Jason: No, no.

Ty: But anyway, Jason and I have never met before, but we have interviewed on the radio for several times and I am so excited to interview you tonight because this is the reason that I got involved with alternative cancer research almost 20 years ago when my Dad was diagnosed with cancer. The first thing that I did was do some research and I found Jason's video. He was on a show called Extra. They interviewed him on the show about the protocol you used to cure your own cancer. What I want to do is just get your story tonight. Talk about being diagnosed and the treatments that you used, and then eventually the time that you spent in jail. So Jason, take it away my friend.

Jason: Please, interject whenever you want to keep me on track or whatever. But when I was 18 years old, actually, when I was 15 years old, honest truth, I felt a pain in my back. Later on, when we did research, we saw that everybody that had my type of cancer, which was called the Askin's tumor, it started at 15 years old. There is only like 15 people diagnosed. At 15 I remember, I had smoked pot, excuse me, but this is in New York, up there at the handball courts. I remember going home and being real sensitive to my body. I felt something in my back, and I actually said, I will never forget, the Lord, I said, "Lord, if this is a tumor please do not let it come out now because my life..." You know at 15, ninth grade, it is like your life is like, you feel great, you are the best. Then, nothing happened.At 18 years old, I remember when I got really sick at 18 years old; actually I was in a lot of pain. I was playing handball that was my thing, handball. Every day, eight hours a day, six hours a day, excuse me. And hitting that ball and I came home at night and I could not lay down anymore. I had to actually sit up when I was sleeping, or my mother would just rub my back. That was the only thing gave me any relief. We did not know what it was and I was coughing some. I went to camp, actually had to leave camp from upstate New York. I had to leave in the middle of the, you know, the sleep away camp. I had an x-ray done and they said, "You have pneumonia." Now I do not know if you know, but when you have pneumonia your whole lung is white and that is what it was, it was white. And if you have a tumor in your lung, a tumor is white. So they did not see this huge tumor, which was actually a grapefruit size.So about two months later I still have pneumonia and my, the doctor, my personal doctor, Mr. Ribinowitz said, "Listen, I am going to put him in for exploratory surgery because this is not going away." I went in for exploratory surgery because they thought I might have an empyema. Empyema is like a pus pocket that is on the outside of your lung, which causes pneumonia to stay a couple extra months, and they have to go in and get that out. And you have a chest tube and all that stuff. Anyway, they operated on me and I woke up eight hours later, because it was not a normal operation, they actually, when they went in, they found a tumor the size of a grapefruit, a connecting tumor the size of a lemon next to it. When I woke up, they told me that and I did not realize the seriousness of it, because I just did not realize anything. My mother and father, they know they have to get a pathology report, and we are going to know in a week or two if it is cancer or not. I was not even thinking along those lines yet. So it turns out, I am still in the hospital and they came back with the diagnoses that it was cancer. It was a very, very rare cancer. It was a very deadly cancer. Everybody had died from it in one year.

Ty: Less than 20 people in the world with that type of cancer.

Jason: Yes. That had it diagnosed and right. There is probably much more than that but not on the books. So we are in the hospital and they were really nervous. My mother and my father, like I said on the Inside Edition of the Extra show, they were at the foot of the bed and they were like, just about crying. I felt very confident and I was brought up, not that I was brought up so much in the church, which I was, but I really had a deep relationship. I was praying every day. At Halloween, we did not go trick or treating, we actually had a 24 hour prayer meeting at night, with the kids. So I just told them, "Listen, there is a reason for this." I told my mother and my father, "and I believed it is going to be okay."Over that year, after I got out of the hospital at 18, my father took me to the medical library. It is a good thing he did because we saw that everybody that had this type of tumor did either chemo or radiation, never did chemo and radiation, but did either chemo or radiation and they still died within six months. One person lived eight years. Other than that, everyone had died right away. And they all had the tumor, originally 15 or 16 is when it came out originally. Now there is more cases of it. But back then, that was all that was there. So I said, we are not going to do chemo and radiation, there is no way I am going to do this, because everybody died. So I just went right back, got my hockey equipment out, and just went back to playing hockey again. Literally twelve months later, to the day about, I was in tremendous pain again and went and got a CAT scan. By that time, I knew how to read the CAT scans. Not that I knew how to read it so much, except that in this spot if there is any white, you have a tumor.

Ty: That is not good.

Jason: I knew that, right. I went in the other room after they did the CAT scan and learned that they do not let you, the technicians do not let you, they do not give you any diagnosis. They are not allowed to, they get in trouble. They do not even really let you look at the stuff. But they let me look. I begged them. I said, "Listen, please, this is my life, my body, and I want to know before I get a call." Who wants to get a call from the hospital saying we have news? So anyway, it was there. I saw it. Same thing tumor, same as the other time, it was just as big already.

Ty: Within a year.

Jason: Within a year. It was big, it was huge, a very aggressive, it was not like just starting out or anything.

Ty: By this time, you are 18 or so?

Jason: I am 19.

Ty: Nineteen, okay.

Jason: Already had it once, they did the thoracotomy on me, they took it out, and now it came back now. This time I remember I was getting pretty sick, I was at home, I was actually laying on my mother and father's bed. They were sleeping on the couch. I could not walk. I did not know it, but the tumor had a tumor. Then, remember before, I said there was a lemon piece? Well, it was a tumor, then there was this trail that went over to my spine and ate on my spine and was just about to eat my spinal column.

Ty: Wow.

Jason: I could not really walk, I was having a hard time, actually, I was stepping before I hit the ground. My mother said, "Don't worry, we have an appointment next week." My father immediately called the hospital and said, "We have to come in now." So because of my father I can walk. My mother was listening to what they said, my father just steamrolled right over and said, "We have to get him to the hospital now." So that is what we did. We went to the hospital and they said, we are not going to do it now, because it is twelve o'clock at night, whatever, we are going to have a fresh team in the morning and we are going to operate on you in the morning. So morning comes, and all I remember from that day is, that they laid me down on the bed, Dr. Cosgrove, Dr. Batey, this was Sloan Kettering, and Dr. Berglund, he was the nerve doctor that was going to take over when they got to the cancer that was near the spine. Dr. Batey was the chest doctor; he was going to take it out from there. Dr. Cosgrove turned out to be a friend to this day and a good friend. He was like an intern at the time. A resident or whatever, you know. So they told me count back from ten and by the time you get to one, you are going to be asleep. So I remember saying I was going to play a trick on them, I will never forget this. I said, "Ten, nine, eight, [snoring noise]." I went like this and the whole team; you hear them starting to get their stuff together, getting on. Three seconds later I went, "Just kidding." To this day, they all say that that really brightened the whole attitude of the operating room. Another second I was out cold.

Ty: Okay.

Jason: It was really afterwards that that really gave them a new outlook. They do not like seeing an 18-year-old kid with a deadly incurable cancer in his body. Anyway, they did an amazing operation, and so forth, and that time I said to them, I did not know better, and I still do not know until this day what did what. But I do know that I said to them, if I am going to do this chemo and radiation, everyone did chemo and everybody did radiation. I was strong; I felt I was strong as an ox, even though I had the cancer the year before. I said, let me do a chemo and the radiation. So they gave me the most poison you can possibly take in the world without dying. I almost did die. I remember like four months into the treatment my blood was down to, I think it was a four. Your hemoglobin is like a 14, when it goes below nine or eight you get a transfusion.

Ty: You had a four?

Jason: It was like really super low. I thought it was a one, but it could not have been a one. Anyway, it was really super low and that is when I stopped, I think I went for a transfusion, I am not sure, that is when I stopped doing the chemo. I did four rounds of chemo, did the radiation. We waited two or three weeks and I could not walk again. They tell me know, something was going on in the spine. A couple of things happened. I remember I went out one day and a bouncer ran by me and hit into me. I fell on the floor. When I saw the CAT scan, I had a scan after that, it was a big, and the whole thing was white. Turn out it was just pus and fluid from getting hit, but we thought the cancer was back. We were already talking about bone marrow transplants, and that would have been it. There was something wrong with my spine again and we went for radiation treatments just on my spine. It was not cancer, I think it was just fluid, I am not 100 percent sure, but my mother tells me that it was just fluid. Anyway, so everything changed from that day. My taste buds changed, I did not like Kentucky, McDonalds, Chinese food. There were certain foods; I remember that I detested them at that point. Even until this day, I really cannot eat them anymore, except for Kentucky once in a while. I really got grossed out by certain foods. My mother started making chicken soup. I started eating sunflower seeds. I knew nothing about the apricot seeds yet, nothing about them. For four years, five years, nothing happened. I do not know, for those four years, what did it? I was not taking any drugs; I was not taking any painkillers then. I had stopped the painkillers. So I do not know if it was my immune system, it was prayer. Because we had in our church a 24 hour prayer chain. Everybody would sign up. You would sign up, like from 12 o'clock until 12:30, you would sign up from 12:30 until 1 o'clock, 1 o'clock until 1:30, 1:30 until 2 o'clock and all the rest, pretend there is a million people here, from 2 o'clock until 2:30. Anyway, everybody throughout the night was waking up and saying a prayer. No one had lived through this thing. Five years later, actually once or twice they thought they saw something, turned out it was nothing. It was a big scare, you know. But five years later they found something, maybe six years, they found something in my kidney. I think the size of it was 3.5, when they found it originally. I think I was going for a scan every year or so. First it was every six months, then it was every year, and then they found something that was 3.5 centimeters in my kidney. They said it parallels renal cell carcinoma. I said I did not want to get a biopsy because you get a biopsy if you are going to, who knows.

Ty: Spread it.

Jason: Spread it. Doctors say that, or other people say that. Biopsy.

Ty: Many doctors that we have interviewed say the same thing.

Jason: Good, because the needle aspiration, they pull the needle out, it can pull, I do not know. Some doctors believe that, some doctors actually do not believe that. At this point it was that I found out about the apricot seeds. This is when I found out, the man's name is Sal Calapano, this has nothing to do with the seeds. This is someone who gave me a typhoid vaccine, which was going to build the immune system. He was working with AIDs patients that had their T-cell counts were maybe like 100 or 200, and they are supposed to be higher, whatever, I do not know, 900, 800. My T-cells were kind of low, 400 or 500. He gave me the vaccine, which at the same time, doing the apricot seeds. This is why I am not sure which was doing what, because I did the vaccine for a while and my tumor got under control. Then I stopped the vaccine, continued with the seeds, and it seemed like the tumor kept shrinking. Every time we went to the doctor's we saw it. The first time I went it only down from 3.5 to 3.2, and I was discouraged, but kidney cancers can be very slow growing, slow shrinking also. I did not let it discourage me much, but every time I went, it was going down a little bit more. Three point five, 2.8, 2.5, 2.0.

Ty: All the while, you are eating apricot seeds?

Jason: I am eating seeds, yes. I actually stopped doing the vaccine. But the vaccine could have built the immune system, I do not know, because as I am finding out now the seeds are amazing for certain cancers and especially amazing for metastasis, stopping things from growing other places. Certain people tell me for kidney cancer it is not that great. So I am not 100 percent sure about my cancer and about, I mean kidney cancer is known to be something that your immune system is number one. Really all cancers are, but when it comes to kidney cancer it is, they are more emphatic about it. Saying that it is your immune system that has to take over with that one.

Ty: Jason, here let's talk about, once you successfully used the apricot seeds and your cancer was under control, talk about apricots from God and what happened with your website and then the FDA issue that followed.

Jason: Okay. Well at about, I was like 26 or 27, I was arm wrestling and I was starting to become the New York State Champion, and you know, I was U.S. champion at one point, I was the World Champion at one point. But before I was the World Champion, the show Extra from Inside Edition, they are not connected. I am not sure. I have been saying that for years though, so anyway. The show Extra they called me up and they wanted to do an interview. I said sure, I will do an interview because they saw that this guy with can... That this very good arm wrestler also had cancer had beat the worst cancer.

Ty: Yeah, that is good fodder for TV.

Jason: Right. So they came over, we did the interview, and the next thing I know they were calling me up and saying, "Listen, Jason, we have hundreds and hundreds of people calling the show. They want to know your phone number; they want to know how they can get in touch with, to talk to you. Is it okay if we give your phone number out?" I said sure, give my phone number out. Immediately people started calling me and I put together a business package. I found a way to get the seeds, which I could only find like a place that had five or ten pounds at a time. Like the video says, "Well without cancer," about this whole thing.

Ty: I still remember it was a video tape about cancer.

Jason: Oh, you ordered it.

Ty: Yeah.

Jason: All the people, who know the health food stores in the past, the FDA would break the windows, shut the stores down, because they had these seeds. So until this day a lot of health food stores, or until that day, when I was talking about. I was 26, I am 46 now. They did not carry them. I could not find them anywhere. If I did find them somewhere, it was like an underground Chinese health food store in the city that had like five pounds in the back somewhere.

Ty: Right.

Jason: So anyway, I got the seeds and I made some, I got a duplicating machine and I put the seeds, for like 50 dollars I sold the seeds and the DVD. It was probably cheaper than that because the seeds were only like 15 dollars. Anyway, I put it together and I got a credit card account and put up a quick website. I just started selling tons of these things. I would tell each person, "Now, listen, I do not want to be, if this is not true, I don't want to be touting something that is not true. Call me back if there are any success stories." I started getting calls immediately. People saying, look I had a tumor in my skin, it shrunk down. Or I had a tumor in my arm and it got bigger, swelled up and then shrunk down. It started itching, or something. I got every story in the book and I asked the people, can I put your phone number at the website? Can I put your email at the website, because people do not believe this? So they said okay, and then I learned how to spam. Which I do not know if you know what spamming is. Spamming is bulk marketing. Back then, it was easy to do. I would buy like 30 million email addresses and I set up a program, which turns out to be a fellow arm wrestler writes these programs. Amazing coincidence, we found out. I put the emails in, I put my thing, and The Answer to Cancer is Laetrile. If you want to know more go to this website, and I pressed the button. It was just like you see like there was a drop all over the United States. Millions and millions and millions of emails, it was four hundred, I remember the highest was about five hundred thousand an hour were being dropped around the United States. At the website, I had a counter at the bottom, which would say like, say it started at 5000, I would click it like ten seconds later and it was 5100. I was getting 100 hits an hour; no excuse me every ten, fifteen minutes, maybe less than that. It was just so many hits I was getting at that website. Then the next day the phone calls started coming in. Some people saying, "Don't spam me," some people saying, "Is this true what you are saying," some people ready to order right away. So I immediately called some kids from church and said come on over. We have to answer calls. We need to take orders. I got a phone system where I could take six calls at once. I started selling the seeds more, a lot more than the gorilla marketing way.

Ty: So how did you get sideways with the FDA, what happened?

Jason: At that point, I was learning about, you know all these like, they say you do not have to pay your taxes because of income things. This amendment was never ratified. They are really like extremists out there. One of these extremists taught me, like, if your name is on something, your commercial name, I do not know if you have heard of this, the CC.

Ty: The UCC, sure.

Jason: The UCC thing and all that, which, please, I went through it to the end and it does not work. But anyway, the FTC sends me a letter, and they spelled my name wrong. So should have stuck with them, but I said, listen, I do not know who you are talking about, there is no this name at this address, so we went back and forth. They sent the letter saying we have proof of this happening and proof and showing the proof.

Ty: So they are saying you are making unapproved claims for curing or what was it?

Jason: They kicked it over to the FDA and the FDA started saying that. So at that point they had my right name and right address, I just had a lawyer, Mr. Dillon [PH], and I do not know if he is alive to this day, but Mr. Dillon was in the middle of this fight forty years ago when this whole thing was going on. He told me, "Listen we just have to change the labelling." Which I did, then the FDA said no good, then we changed it again. They kept saying no good. To everything we did, they kept saying no good. Then I realized that there is nothing we can do to make this work.

Ty: It is a stacked deck.

Jason: It sure was. That is when they got a temporary injunction against me and the injunction was not to sell, the whole crux of it was they said we cannot sell seeds. At first, they said, you cannot sell them as a cure. You cannot sell them according to FDA law. Which only means I cannot sell them as a cure. Does not mean I cannot sell them period, because then I cannot own a grocery store.

Ty: You just cannot say that they cure anything.

Jason: Right. In the end of them adjusting and marking things out and redacting things from the injunction, it read a lot more to say, you cannot sell seeds, period. This is when I said, "You cannot tell me I cannot sell seeds." You cannot tell me I cannot sell apples because it has the same thing in it. They stuck to that and the judge, it was a stacked trial, they actually had, then they had a permanent injunction against me. They said I violated both, but I would say, listen, you have to prove that I sold them as a cure. Which I stopped, I did not do that anymore. I told people that, I gave the FDA warning at the bottom. I also told people it was third party information. I just said, I never told people it was going to cure you. I would never say that to people, even if it does. So I had a trial basically. At one point I actually ran away when I was going to the initial, whatever that is, not arraignment.

Ty: Hearing?

Jason: Yeah, the initial hearing. I left. I was on my way with a bunch of friends, all dressed up and I just, I am not kidding, this sound weird, but a flock of birds, like as I am heading this way a flock of birds came right over the car going this way. I was like, I am sorry, I am not superstitious like that but I was like, I am not going. This has got to be a sign. I am not going. Anyway, I left. I went to my other apartment for three months. They were looking for me, I was talking to the marshals, and finally I turned myself in. There was a million dollar bail they gave me.

Ty: A million dollars.

Jason: Eight hundred eighty three thousand dollars.

Ty: You could have raped children and killed them and not gotten that kind of bail.

Jason: Right. Exactly. But you know, I think it is a little pretense. You are, you know, defrauding older people, so you are killing older people. If it is called, to them though it is like you have killed thousands of people by defrauding them. So in that sense.

Ty: So in the trial they acquitted you, right?

Jason: I almost won the trial. My lawyer, who was telling me, I will get you eight years. What do you mean you will get me eight years? This is a, this is contempt of court. Contempt of court is like a six-month thing the most if you are guilty. I was not even guilty and they were saying. So it was a trial but there was no statutory maximum and no minimum. So it was a very, they would say he could get 20 years. I said, listen, if I am going to go to prison, it is going to be, I am doing my own trial then. So I kicked them out and the judge would not let them completely get off. The judge made them sit at the table. I will never forget the one question that I asked that the lawyer jumped up on my side and said, "Don't answer that question." I was going to ask, the FDA agent was up at the, he was on the witness stand, and I was redirecting. I was doing my cross examination, excuse me, and the question was, I was going to say, "Did you have like 40 or 50 complaints about me?" The lawyer got up and said, "Hold on, wait, time out." He told him, do not answer that question. I said, listen, I am asking this question, because I was going to come down to the end saying, "Did you ever get a complaint against me?" So I made him sit down I said did you have 30 or 40 complaints. He said no. Did you have 20 or 30, did you have 10 or 5. Did you ever have one complaint about me with the seeds, about me defrauding people? And he had to say no. I have those transcripts at the website actually. Where he had to actually admit no.So who, why was I on trial. That is the point. Nobody was injured. There has to be an injured party for there to be a trial. This should not have even been a civil thing. Anyway, it was a big kangaroo court. It was a big farce. The jury is over here, the place is immaculate. The prosecutor is over here, and I am over there, the defense is over there, so the prosecutor, anything that they wanted to enter into evidence, they could whisper over here. But we cannot say that they did this and they did that. They could hear everything. It was just completely, you can completely brainwash the jury by being in the spot where the prosecution was. It was just unfair. The one argument that I had was that the injunction was ambiguous. It did not say that I could not sell seeds. It said according to the FDA law, and that is what I am saying. And the judge actually stopped me from saying and said, "You cannot argue that." That is my defense, what do you mean? He says, "You can take it up on appeal. You cannot argue that." I am like, what are you talking about. Anyway.

Ty: The whole claim was that you violated an injunction, but he would not let you talk about the injunction.

Jason: He would not let me talk about that aspect of the injunction. I was sick to my stomach. That was my whole argument. My whole defense is that. Actually, there were four charges. One of the charges was, the charges were I broke the preliminary injunction, the second one. I broke the primary injunction. One of them was that I defrauded the people by selling these B17 seeds against FDA law. They dropped that charge. I refused to let that charge be dropped. I said listen, I don't want, I want you to try me on that charge. The judge says, "No, I am not going to let you do anything that can injure you." I said, no I want that charge in there. They would not allow that charge to be dropped. And that was the whole crux of the case that I wanted to prove, and they would not allow it. The judge just wanted the people to think I was not allowed to sell seeds period. Which is not really it. The injunction, if you read it in the original form, it says, "You cannot sell it against FDA law." Which of course is how it is. They cannot tell a person you cannot sell apples. They just cannot do it. But they did and it was not fair.

Ty: So in the end you got a sentence of how long?

Jason: In the end, well, almost at the end, someone from my family put out these fliers on the outside that said, "Your right to the freedom of speech." There was a case in England where, I think it was some type, it was a freedom of speech case but the king wanted a guilty charge and the jury stayed in the room and said, "We have the power." And the king said, "You stay in thisroom until you come up with guilty." They said, "No we are not, period." A week later, they won. And this paper had that, the paper I had had that stuff on it. Like the jury has the power. You do not have to listen to this judge; you do not have to listen to what they are saying. When the prosecutor came in the morning of the trial that day, he came in waving these flyers."We found these on the car, and he is the only one that could have done this." Out of all the cases that were going on in the place. The judge looked at me and I could not lie, I said, "I think it was one of my friends, maybe." At that point, he said right away, you are in contempt, you have to show me why you should not be held in contempt by the end of this day or else they were going to detain me anyway that day. I was guilty that day, and that was it, they held me from that day. I did not come out for five years from that day.

Ty: Five years.

Jason: Five years. Four years eleven months.

Ty: County jail? Where did you go?

Jason: I went to MDC, not county. This was federal.

Ty: Federal prison.

Jason: Oh yeah. County is a whole other world. I am glad I was not in county. Yeah. I had a blast. A lot of the time, I had a good time. Actually, the judge, on sentencing day the judge actually could not help laughing. I said, "Can I go to Florida?" I had heard good things about the Florida thing. I did not know better.

Ty: Talk about real quick for the five years that you were in prison; you told me a story a few years ago about when your mother would come to visit you and she brought you mixed nuts. Tell us that story.

Jason: She could get arrested. I do not want to say that. She would sneak stuff in for me. She would sneak apricot seeds in all the time for me. Every week she would bring seeds. Meanwhile the tumor is growing in me a little bit. She would sneak apricot seeds in. She would go up to the vending machine and buy some nuts. The seeds exactly like almonds, and put them in there, that was it. If she ever got caught with them, she could just say, huh.

Ty: It is almonds.

Jason: No one knows. Even if they are seeds, no one knows that that is what I am in there for. Even though the inmates did. They called me Johnny Appleseed and stuff like that. I learned how to laugh at myself in prison.

Ty: So you did five years and you got out, what was it 2008 when you got out of prison?

Jason: 2008, yeah. Five years.

Ty: Well, to me it is amazing that you actually spent five years in jail for that, but I am glad you made it out and now you are back to. What is your website so people can get to you?

Jason: Christianbrothers.net or apricotsfromgod.com.

Ty: apricotsfromgod.com.

Jason: Goes to the same place.

Ty: Okay, same as you had before.

Jason: Yes.

Ty: Well, Jason, I want to thank you for sharing your story with us tonight. And I just want to thank you personally. This miniseries The Truth About Cancer would not be happening if it were not for you.

Jason: Thanks, Ty.

Ty: Because you are the first person that woke me up to natural cancer treatments back in 1996. A long time ago. So it was 18 years ago.

Jason: 1986?

Ty: It was 96 that I saw it.

Jason: I think it was 94.

Ty: Ninety four is maybe when you filmed the show. Ninety six is when my dad died and that is when I first saw the video. So I just want to thank you personally. This would not have been happening without you.

Jason: Ty, everybody mentions you. So many people that called up my company, they all say, "Ty." I wish there was a way I could have, I mean I owe you a lot too. There is a lot of people; they owe you a lot, too. A lot of people read your book the way you market it. A lot of people read it and they got better. Or they lived an extra five, ten years, which all counts.

Ty: With quality of life. We are all in the same fight. We are all here to spread the truth and to spread knowledge about this so it was my honor to interview tonight, man.

Jason: Thank you.

Ty: And we will arm wrestle in a second, but off camera.

Jason: Yeah, sure.

[end of transcript]

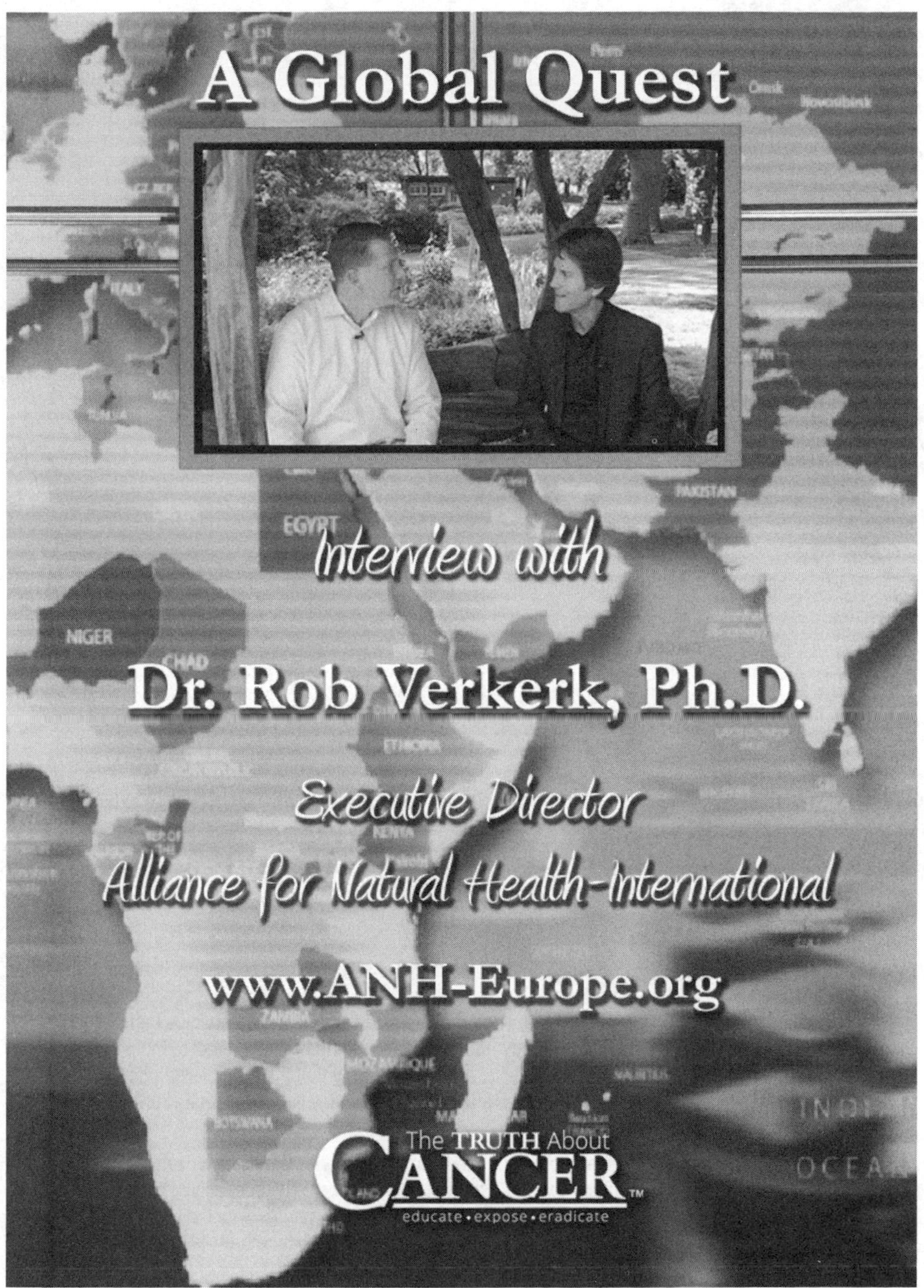
A Global Quest
Interview with
Dr. Rob Verkerk, Ph.D.
Executive Director
Alliance for Natural Health-International
www.ANH-Europe.org
The TRUTH About
CANCER
educate • expose • eradicate

Ty: So, I am honored today to be sitting next to my friend, Dr. Rob Verkerk. This is our second interview in as many years.

Dr. Verkerk: Absolutely.

Ty: Only now, we're in your hometown.

Dr. Verkerk: Absolutely, we're in London.

Ty: London, England.

Dr. Verkerk: We've got beautiful London weather.

Ty: We do.

Dr. Verkerk: Bit of rain, bit of sunshine.

Ty: We've had it all day long; every half hour it changes.

Dr. Verkerk: Exactly.

Ty: Anyway, thanks for sitting here and joining me today.

Dr. Verkerk: Amazing to see you again, Ty. Love what you're doing. Getting such an important word out.

Ty: Thank you. I really appreciate it. Tell the viewers a little bit about what you do here with the Alliance for Natural Health.

Dr. Verkerk: Well, Ty, we're a research information communication organization that is about creating a sea change in health care. We're an alliance because we have many different sectors within the community from the consumer, through to practitioners, through to the companies that support the practitioners. Looking at the food industry and of course looking at the healthcare industry with its gamuts of different professions. We believe very passionately that the model—the dominant health care model—is broken. There are many aspects of it particularly when you look at chronic diseases that isn't [sic] working.

We've seen a major shift in the science over the last decade or so that shows us that what we might loosely term as natural health or working with, if you like, biologically compatible health care that's about nutrition and about lifestyle change, using products from nature in such a way that you are not interfering—you're not working against nature; you are working with nature—is the way to resolve many of the world's problems. But, at the same time, we've got some major challenges and these challenges are negative media that is often influenced by pharmaceutical interests or parts of the medical establishment that themselves are very impacted by the dominant role of pharmaceuticals in health care. We've also got a lot of regulatory challenges that also it's a little bit like putting a noose around the system that you don't want to exist. So we're really looking at fundamental rights and freedoms to try and create a scientific and legal framework that allows natural health to really flourish.

Ty: So aside from these things that you've just mentioned, what are the biggest threats that we currently see on—not just here in UK, but on a global scale—that might inhibit our ability to have freedom of choice when it comes to our own health?

Dr. Verkerk: There are so many different ways of looking at that. If you look at the part of the environment that we're most intimately exposed to, it's food. We really face such a major issue with the globalization of the food supply with essentially what is unwitting adulteration of the food supply. So there are people out there who know that they need to eat more fruit and veg, or high-quality protein, or fat sources, but a lot of it is not what it says on the tin, as it were. It's certainly at odds with what we've co-evolved with over millennia. And the kind of food that we eat is so deficient. It is fascinating that when we choose to then supplement our food with dietary supplements or food supplements, barring very, very few exceptions, and an obvious one would be a requirement for vitamin D, but the question is how much? Another one is folic acid and neural tube defects. Governments out there don't want people to know about supplements and they treat them much as they would want to treat medicines and basically as soon as you have a supplement, especially in Europe, that has a therapeutic effect, it's automatically illegal. Because, by definition under the medicinal code of Europe that was evolved in 1965 to protect people from thalidomide, it basically said any substance that has a pharmacological effect should be termed a medicine.

So that leaves foods as this thing that you can consume to provide energy, but not something you can use therapeutically. So food cannot be medicine, which of course is contrary to what our dear friend, Hippocrates, supposedly said many hundreds of years ago. Yes, we have major challenges with the food supply and also ingesting concentrated source of nutrients. On another side, we have a major problem with the way in which we view the science. Science has become the—if you like—the lens through which we determine if something is good for us or bad for us. And evidence-based medicine has become the guardian of decision making, yet itself it's being twisted and manipulated in such a way that it works well. If you have a drug and you're using a randomized controlled trial to measure the specific therapeutic effect of a drug, it doesn't work well at all within a natural health care framework, which is often about using multi-modalities. It's not using a single pill. It's often about changing someone's emotional attitude. It's about changing the environment, their sleep hygiene, their relationship with others, the food they're eating, the addition of concentrated nutrients. It may also be about some body work. And we don't have a framework that looks at these multi-modality inputs that a lot of, if you like, so-called complementary and alternative medicine practitioners are working with that are giving people really positive outcomes. But there's nowhere that we can actually find studies or epidemiological evidence that shows how this works.

That's one of the reasons you have so many millions of people out there demanding to have access to complementary and alternative medicine or integrative medicine. And yet the mainstream medical profession keeps turning around and saying, "Through our lens of evidence-based medicine, we see no evidence of it working." There's this complete discontinuity...

Ty: But they already have a presupposition that they're working with, don't they?

Dr. Verkerk: Well, exactly. The irony is, even if you use their lens of EBM and look at the 3,000 or so interventions that have been studied through BMJ clinical evidence, they find that only 11 percent of conventional treatments have been proven to be beneficial, 50 percent—a staggering 50 percent—of unknown effectiveness. Yet the average person still believes when they go to their doctor, they're only going to be given an intervention that has been proven to work. And they don't realize that, say, even a lot of the drugs that have been prescribed are prescribed off label for purposes that no one really has any idea of exactly what the outcome is going to be. It's actually clinical practice that informs those decisions.

Ty: Right, and as Casey Prachi mentioned last year, they don't do studies on the interaction of drugs together. They do the studies on the separate prescription of the drugs, but no studies are done on this drug with that drug with that drug with that drug. It's impossible to predict the clinical outcome of drugs prescribed concurrently.

Dr. Verkerk: And that's exactly the same model that is of course used with industrial chemicals or food additives. Each is studied individually and a decision is made about what a so-called safe threshold is. Of course, in the real world we're exposed to 20,000 or so different industrial chemicals every day if we live in the city and the expression of that is all around, of course. One of the fascinating things is as the science of gene sequencing has evolved since 2003 when the human genome project was unraveled—the human genome, we now understand so much more about how that environment interacts with our genes and how they're expressed. Epigenetics and nutrigenomics and nutrigenetics are now branches of science—if you like, mainstream science—that give real credence for why nutrition and lifestyle medicine should actually be the dominant paradigm in health care, yet it stills pushes the margins.

Ty: Talk about—you mentioned epigenetics. Can you explain exactly what that is for the viewers and how might that be something that could encourage, let's say, a cancer patient? That mama or grandmama had breast cancer and then so, "I'm going to get breast cancer. I got the gene." How can that encourage them?

Dr. Verkerk: Epigenetics is looking at the level above. That's what "epi-" means from the Greek, "above the genetics." So we all have a particular genetic code and the way in which the environment interacts with our genes creates changes. So our genetic makeup as we age changes all the time, through process of DNA methylation and histone modification. And, as a result of those changes, we can actually pass those changes on to our children. And one of the major problems that we have in terms of our old understanding of genetics is that people believed if they were born, say, as a woman with a BRCA gene that might increase their [sic] risk of breast cancer, they have not been told and certainly wouldn't expect to hear from their doctor that the way they live their life will alter the expression of those genes and their risk of cancer. And that applies to pretty much all conditions. I've had many of my genes sequenced. I have a real propensity towards obesity, type 2 diabetes, insulin resistance. If I don't look after how I live my life, I'd become very overweight very, very easily.

Ty: Couldn't tell it, because you're living your life the way that would prevent it.

Dr. Verkerk: A few years back, I was still eating a lot of organic food, but I wasn't intermittent fasting. As you age, your metabolism changes. When I hit 50, for me things started going a bit off course in terms of my own health and I was noticing...

Ty: I have to interrupt you here. You're over 50?

Dr. Verkerk: I'm 55. I just had my 55th birthday.

Ty: I would have never guessed.

Dr. Verkerk: I was gaining a lot of weight. I was still eating very good quality food, but the timing of that food, I was—my fat-burning capacity is not great. I really have to move to a process where two meals a day suit me much better than three.

Ty: So what's your window? You eat in the six-hour window?

Dr. Verkerk: Yeah. I've got to always leave at least five or six hours between meals. It's also how you exercise in relation to that activity, and realizing that we should really often be exerting a lot of activity *before* we eat, rather than *after* we eat. Just changing certain parameters in terms of how we can shift our body to being better at fat burning.

Ty: Intermittent fasting.

Dr. Verkerk: Yeah, intermittent fasting, caloric restriction, combined with enhancing your antioxidation fat-burning pathways, so you can actually burn fat in your sleep, which is great. And these are messages that many of us know about, many of us are putting into practice, some alternative docs are putting it into practice, but, unfortunately, that science hasn't found its way into mainstream medicine, where pills are still being prescribed as a rule—as a generality, I should say.

Ty: You're absolutely right. On the walk over here, you were mentioning to me the story of Sarah, who is a conventional medical doctor here in the UK, and her breast cancer story. Share that with the audience.

Dr. Verkerk: You know, what's really interesting is that there are people out there—I was just working the weekend before last with a leading academic who was trained as a medical doctor—Professor Sarah Stewart-Brown—and she is one of the leading researchers in complementary and alternative medicine in the UK. But, for her, she saw at an early stage that there were some issues with the allopathic model. What's really powerful is when you understand that kind of issue, and then you are faced with a major health challenge as she was with cancer, she didn't revert back to the allopathic model. She stayed with a kind of biocompatible, natural health care model and has resolved the cancer. I think that kind of—to have the power of your convictions to stick with it, and I'm a great believer in integrative medicine. There are sometimes really important times when allopathic medicine has a place. But then at the same time the basis of how you manage that and how you reduce the side effects is about integration with natural therapies. As a society, we've got a very long way to go to stop this war that exists between two divergent factions. And I should also say that sometimes it is the guys on the so-called alternative side that are as much the offenders, throwing rotten eggs at the guys in the allopathic camp. And when you have that kind of rivalry what it tends to do is just further entrench each of the camps and you don't get to this kind of nirvana place where you get the best of both worlds.

Ty: Right, sure. Many of the physicians that we have interviewed in the past and that we are interviewing this year for the Global Quest, they're integrative physicians. They use whatever they can. In other words, I think—Dr. Sunil Pai is an integrative physician, and he said, "My job is to do whatever I can to get my patient well. Whether it's conventional, whether it's alternative, whether it's a mix of the two, my only concern is, get them well and don't harm them."

Dr. Verkerk: Ty, this is absolutely spot on. One of the big issues we have is language. We use language that creates separation and really what we're all talking about is the best medicine when people have debates about complementary and alternative medicine versus allopathic medicine. What I often say is that, the bit I like about that is the word "medicine." Let's not lose that word. Medicine is a useful term, but we just want the best medicine and sometimes it's going to come out of ultra-modern high-tech allopathic side. Other times it might come out of ancient traditions, and what it has to be, nearly all, is holistic. It has to look at the whole system probably from an ecological context because we are essentially of—a living organism that has co-evolved with the natural environment. And it is no great surprise that as a result we function really well when that environment is in tune with our bodies, and the 10-fold more microbes that are within our bodies. And it also works really well when we eat very healthy food that is grown in very healthy soils that are in hugely limited supply these days as agriculture continues to damage the natural.

Ty: It only makes sense, doesn't it?

Dr. Verkerk: It's logical, but when you've got nine billion people that need to be supported by the year 2050, you can understand that in agriculture, as in health care, you actually have very similar debates. How can we manage the burden of either looking after the sick, or aged, or people with dementia, and also supply enough food for the world? When you start to break it down, you see that there are some commonalities with the problem. A lot of the business model that is working on either side of this is looking at how it can protect its own business interest. There have been so many studies looking at GMOs. There's very little science that suggests that, at the moment, there's any evidence that GMOs can play a realistic part in resolving world hunger. Yet governments and the biotech industry is [sic] saying this is going to be the savior. Just as in the pharmaceutical side, the next drug is going to be the savior. We should learn from our history. Apart from very limited times in history have drugs been absolutely vital. Most of the real solutions have been about cultural, biological, ecological approaches that are in tune with our bodies. And that's what we're losing sight of as we start to think of the human body more as a machine than as a part of nature.

Ty: Sure. I agree completely. And whether we look at the GMOs, whether we look at the drugs—follow the money. It doesn't matter if you're in UK, in America, South America, wherever we're at—follow the money. And that's what's guiding a lot of these decisions, isn't it?

Dr. Verkerk: Exactly. And there's a really unhealthy interplay sometimes between some of these industry sectors, the media, and governments, and the public is made to feel disempowered. And one of the great messages about what you're doing and what we're doing, too, is actually empowering people to say, "Guys, if you choose what kind of health care you want and if you choose what kind of food you want to put in your bodies, you can actually collapse that system. It's only there because you keep buying into it. If you stop buying into it, it'll fall apart."

Ty: Exercise your rights.—

Dr. Verkerk: Exactly.

Ty: —to choose. I think a lot of people don't even realize what a privilege it is for us to have the choices that we have today and they can't imagine that it would ever be taken. They just can't fathom having government should make all these choices for you, but if we don't continue to stand up for all these rights—it's not a privilege, I say it's a privilege; these rights of ours—then we may lose them.

Dr. Verkerk: Exactly, and it has always been like that. These rights have always been under threat and it's always taken people to have to stand up to those rights, and it's, again, it's another system that is trying to find an equilibrium, to every action there's an equal and opposite reaction. The reason that we're sitting here right now is because there is a system that has some imbalance in it, and we're trying to bring that balance back.

Ty: Everyone has probably heard of Codex in one context or another. Is Codex still a threat on a global scale?

Dr. Verkerk: Codex is always a threat in terms of how food production, the entire system of international food trade and regulation of that food trade as long as we buy into it. So Codex really affects the type of products that are turning up in our supermarkets. So if you want to buy those products, yes, Codex has a big ramification. One of the—if I can say this—few positive things would be that if you have an intolerance to gluten, which one in five westerners do or more, at least Codex has put in a requirement to make sure that to be gluten-free you have to be less than 20 parts per million. It used to be about 100 parts per million...

Ty: So there are some good parts of it.

Dr. Verkerk: There are some good parts of it. Where it is really problematic is that it develops standards of practice and safety that are good for international food trade, which is all about kind of moving—growing food that is of very low quality in one part of the world, moving it to another part of the world, agreeing what level of pesticides or food additives can be in that, all of it having been studied independently with often relying on data that's now very old and with no real idea how it interacts with our bodies. So Codex kind of agrees these standards, these guidelines, these recommendations, and then the food trade lives on it. Now if you want to live outside of that system and buy from the farm gate or buy sustainably produced organic food, well, it's getting harder and harder because that system is starting to have tentacles that influence the way in which food production generally is offered.

And, of course, now Codex has also moved slightly into the world of dietary supplements by looking at vitamin and mineral food supplements. It's using as its template, because Codex is really built out of a European model—the EU European Food Supplements Directive. It's also been building a system for scientific substantiation of health claims that is fundamentally being used as the basis for an EU law on health claims that has had a dramatic impact on the ability of any commercial producer saying anything positive about food. From the tens of thousands of ingredients that exists [sic] in our food or in our supplements, just over 250 have been authorized health claims, which—and over 2000 commonly used health plans around the EU have been banned. So, presently, if you look at the nine essential amino acids, there is not one authorized health claim. We are not allowed to say, "If you're selling amino acid..." even though they are essential to life...

Ty: You can't say anything about them.

Dr. Verkerk: You can't say anything positive about them. You can't say anything positive about glucosamine, and that's because, again, the scientific lens that's being built in Codex, which requires proof of a causal effect, which is very, very difficult to do. I mean you remember how hard it was to prove that tobacco or cigarette smoking causes lung cancer. It took over 30 years to do that. So trying to prove that particular foods have specific effects in healthy people. So glucosamine didn't get a claim because all the evidence was based on people who had knee and hip osteoarthritis. So European foods safety authorities said, "Sorry guys. Can't look at those trials because they're based on a diseased population. We're in food so we don't deal with the diseased population. Anything with diseased population is restricted to drug use." So it's a way, again, of carving out whole sectors that we've been used to dealing with in relation to foods that get left as a future playground for the drug companies that they want to move into that area.

Ty: So it could potentially really hamstring our ability to get good supplements in the future. Is that correct?

Dr. Verkerk: Yeah. I mean, if it's allowed to develop. My sense is that the savior now is the change in the way in which science is looking at our interaction with natural products and natural foods. So it's no longer tenable to say, as EU law does, that actually you can't have a food that's therapeutic. You're telling me that if I have 500 calories worth of broccoli, that that has the same impact on my body as eating 500 calories of ice cream.

Ty: That's what oncologists tell you.

Dr. Verkerk: Yeah. Exactly.

Ty: It's interesting...

Dr. Verkerk: The way in which our metabolic pathways and the way our genes change their expression depending on how you consume those two foods are dramatically different. And food *is* medicine. It is one of the most fundamental medicines, but it's incredibly complex.

Ty: According to the medical director for Codex though, it's not.

Dr. Verkerk: It's because they come out of this paradigm that anything to do with a therapeutic relationship has got to be reserved only for medicines. And, again, historically, we look at Germany as being the origin of this. It was back in the 1930s that some of the precursors to IG Farben, the company that made the Zyklon B that was used in the gas chambers during the Holocaust, were actually some of the pioneers in terms of vitamin research. And they were doing vitamin research as the next health care solution. As the importance of the individual vitamins being found, we then had the Second World War. As we emerged from the Second World War, organic chemistry was really flourishing and once you had organic chemistry you had the ability to take natural molecules and alter them so you could develop patents. And so, after the war, we saw this massive evolution both in terms of agrochemicals and pharmaceuticals of patented models that became the business model. So all the vitamin research was left, and, frankly, it was your brethren, it was the US companies in the '60s, the flower-power generation in America that picked up that science and said, "Hey, we can create health foods. We can take these healthy ingredients. We can work with nature, not against it." And, of course, in 1994, in the States, as the people's interest in this started to grow, you had the risk of supplements being medicalized as well, and it was only because of such a huge public uprising against it that DSHEA carved out a segment for dietary supplements that were a category of food...

Ty: DSHEA standing for?

Dr. Verkerk: Dietary Supplement Health and Education Act in the United States, so more people responded to Congress on the Hill on that issue than they did against the Vietnam War. So Americans have always felt very, very strongly about being told what they can and can't put into their mouths. So that freedom is really essential to their nature. In Europe, I always feel the reason why Europeans have been less rebellious against the system when it is trying to interfere with their freedoms is because we've had two major world wars in recent history. Many Europeans have lived in occupied territories. I'm doing a lot of work in Scandinavia at the moment where the regulators are literally pulling products off health store shelves. And then finally we've got a group of companies to come together who are going to stand up for this. But they just sit there and say, "Oh, the regulators must be right." And we've had to explain to them that these guys are acting beyond their legal jurisdiction, and they must be stopped, and they must be educated about what they can do. And, if need be, we need to go into court with these issues and sort it out in court.

Ty: Yeah, you're absolutely right on the Scandinavia. I've got friends up in that area that we'll actually be interviewing in a few weeks and because of one claim over one product, it's forbidden to be imported in the country now from the United States.

Dr. Verkerk: Exactly. So you take something—an herb that is vital for liver health. Been used for years and years—milk thistle. The Swedes have made it a medicine only. I mean this is something that has an anti-oxidant effect on the body. It works as a food, if you like. Okay, it has particular specificity in the liver, some in the kidney as well, but it is essentially a food that is found in milk thistle and because it has such a clear battery of clinical evidence for how good it is in terms of managing toxicity in the liver, it's only a medicine and, of course, it then requires people to license it as a medicine. The drug companies don't want to spend their money licensing it as a medicine. You now have some very inferior forms that are licensed using a European fast-track medicinal licensing system, but if you want good old natural milk thistle from seed and leaf together as a food supplement, it is now illegal.

Ty: Can't get it. Yeah. You know, Rob, what you're doing is so important because you're standing up for our freedom. You're fighting for our freedom, for our food freedom, freedom for our supplements—choices in supplements—freedom for our overall health, choices in our health. And so, I'm really grateful for what you're doing. People need to understand that are watching this series that what you're doing is so important because if this is incrementally taken from us—our right to choose what foods we put in our body, the right to take the certain supplements we need for our health, the access to those supplements—that is an integral part of treatments for people that are doing—that have cancer that are trying to heal. If they don't have access to good foods, to clean foods, to clean supplements, then they don't have access to the best treatments for cancer. So what you're doing is vitally important for cancer patients, but not only for that, but for everyone because we all—our health will deteriorate if we lose access to these supplements, to these natural foods that you're fighting for us to have access to every day. So you're a hero of mine for what you're doing. Thank you for doing what you're doing.

Dr. Verkerk: Well, vice versa. We have a mutual-appreciation society, getting the word out. We had Ralph Moss over a few weeks ago to London at a think-tank event that we organized looking at some of the issues of how the, if you like, the alternative side of medicine can feed into the mainstream, and, of course, Ralph has been involved in helping people in the cancer world for many, many years. I think one of the things we're all in common agreement that the science is now so fundamentally shifted that it becomes irrational to block the door. If you look at someone who has cancer, you've had for a long time in Europe this notion that if you're using a natural approach you run the risk as a doctor of having your license revoked. If you're a non-medical practitioner, you can be basically put into jail as the Cancer Act of 1939 in the UK to deal with you. This is utterly wrong because an individual that has cancer is just another individual whose body needs nourishment and support—more than a person who is healthy. And yet, to have that denied to those individuals is a real loss of fundamental rights of freedoms, and that needs to be changed.

Ty: It's a crime.

Dr. Verkerk: It is a crime. Indeed.

Ty: Keep fighting against the criminals and keep doing what you're doing.

Dr. Verkerk: Thank you, Ty. It's been a real pleasure.

[End of Transcript]

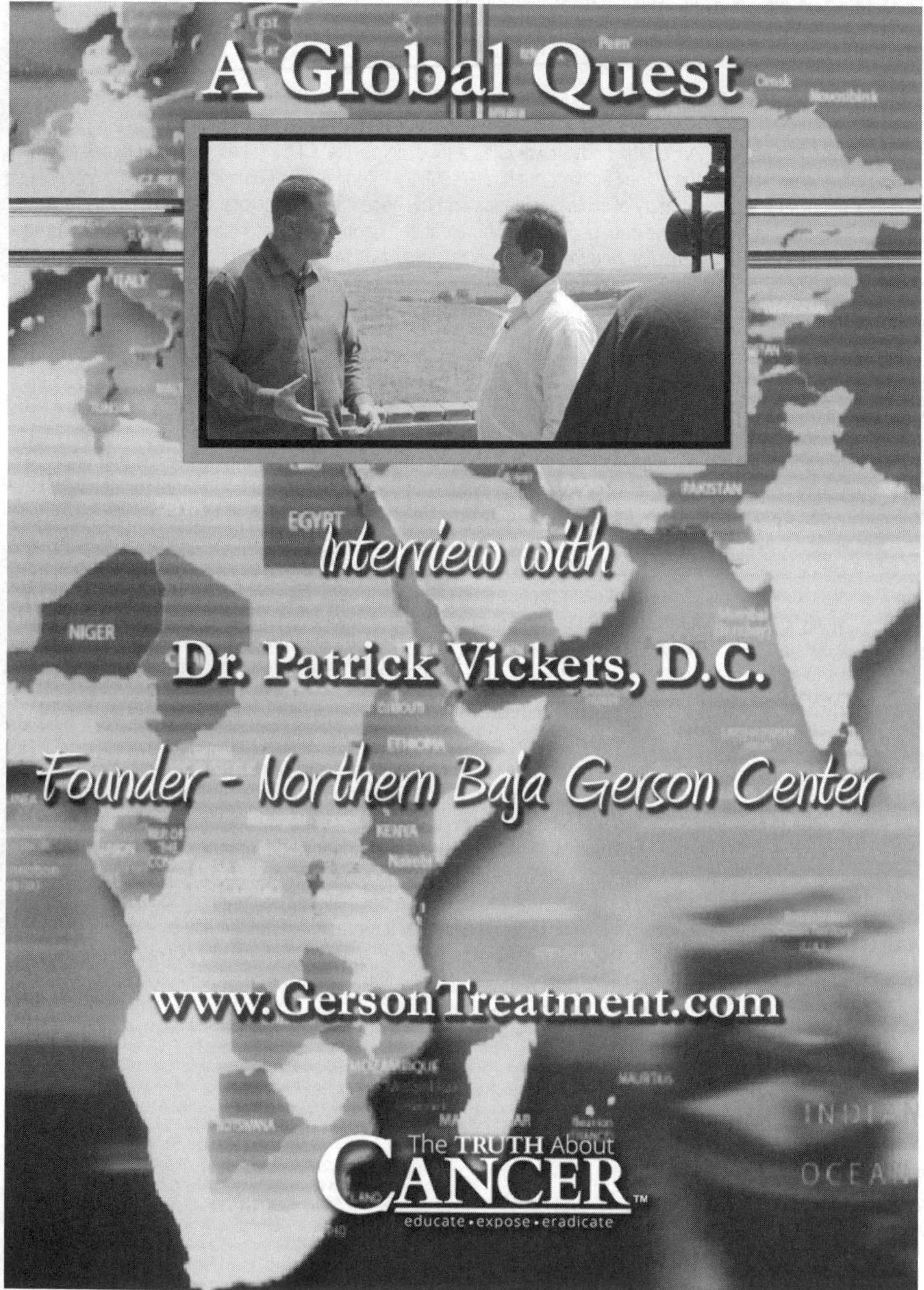
A Global Quest
Interview with
Dr. Patrick Vickers, D.C.
Founder - Northern Baja Gerson Center
www.GersonTreatment.com
The TRUTH About CANCER
educate • expose • eradicate

Ty: I'm really happy to be here at the Gerson Clinic in Northern Baja, Mexico with Dr. Patrick Vickers.

Dr. Vickers: Hi.

Ty: Thank you so much for the invitation out here to your clinic.

Dr. Vickers: My pleasure. Thanks for coming.

Ty: Looking forward to getting you to explain us the Gerson Therapy and really hitting nutrition hard today. Because I know that's the focus of the treatment.

Dr. Vickers: Absolutely.

Ty: But before we do that, if you could tell us your education. Where did you go to school? Tell us your history. How did you get involved with medicine and healing?

Dr. Vickers: Well, absolutely. I wanted to be a chiropractor ever since I was 11 years old. And my last year in chiropractic school, one year away from graduating, Charlotte Gerson, Dr. Gerson's last living daughter, who is now 94 years old, she came and spoke at our school. That was nearly 20 years ago.

And the moment she opened her mouth, I knew that's exactly what I would be doing. I just felt it was the higher calling. Chiropractic is a wonderful profession but being involved with one of the most renowned natural therapies in the history of natural medicine, it just seemed like the higher calling to me. As soon as I graduated from chiropractic school I lived with Charlotte Gerson for two months at her home at San Diego where in her garage, she has boxes of her father's handwritten files of all his active patients, up until 1910 to 1959 when he died. And I'm one of maybe a dozen people who have ever had the opportunity to go through those handwritten files. That's really how my love for the therapy and my passion for the therapy was born.

I graduated from the University of Wisconsin at Madison, a Big Ten School, back in 1992 with a degree in pre-med and in international economics, believe it or not. And then, I went on to New York Chiropractic College where I got my degree as a chiropractor and graduated from there in 1997.

Ty: Did you learn much about nutrition while you were in chiropractic school? Because I know that medical doctors don't learn much of anything about nutrition. Did you in chiropractic school?

Dr. Vickers: Absolutely, yes. Medical doctors, they get 10 hours of nutrition in their entire eight years of education and it's just crazy. How can you be a doctor and you get 10 hours of nutrition, and that's where healing lies. In Chiropractic school, we got some 160 hours of nutrition while we were in school. And I studied nutrition like crazy outside of my classes.

And you know, it's funny because we studied so much nutrition in school and I was studying outside of class and you almost learn nutrition and supplementation in a medical model. You take this for that and that for this. And next thing you know, your patient is walking out $2,500 worth of supplements which ultimately don't heal. It was when I came across the Gerson Therapy that everything became so simple and so finely packaged. Because Dr. Gerson was such a finely-packaged genius. In fact, Nobel Peace Prize winner Dr. Albert Schweitzer, he called Dr. Gerson the "greatest genius in medical history."

And all of a sudden, when I came across Gerson Therapy, I put all the nutritional journals down because they weren't teaching the proper model of nutrition. They were teaching more a medical-based paradigm on how to supplement the body but supplements are just that. They are to be supplemented with proper diet and proper detoxification. So again, when I came across Gerson Therapy, it simplified everything and put it into a finely made package that truly benefits a majority of patients that we are dealing with.

Ty: Great. So as a chiropractor—we were talking about this at breakfast this morning and I wanted you to share this—you're a quack since you are a chiropractor. Until 1989, was it?

Dr. Vickers: 1987.

Ty: Tell me about the ruling. Because we went back in *The Truth about Cancer* last year and we got the history of why chiropractors and homeopaths, naturopaths, all these natural doctors are considered to be quacks and it goes back to the AMA. But talk about that in relating to this 1987 ruling.

Dr. Vickers: That is exactly right. In 1987, four chiropractors from Illinois, particularly Chester Wilk, he was the head chiropractor that took the AMA to court, they actually took the entire American Medical Association to court. Accusing them of having a branch within their organization designed to eliminate chiropractic as a profession, a licensed profession they were trying to eliminate through the use of propaganda. Well, a federal district court judge in Illinois, Susan Getzendanner in 1987, found the AMA guilty of conspiracy. That was the judgment. So if anybody tells you when you are talking about these things, "You're just a conspiracy theorist." You can lead them straight to the Wilk versus the AMA court ruling of 1987. And the judgement was "guilty of conspiracy."

What they did was they ended up violating the Sherman anti-trust act which kept organizations and companies from monopolizing industries and that was the basis of that judgment. So to this day, if you go to a medical doctor and they tell you—you tell them you don't want to have surgery on your back, you want to try something less invasive like chiropractic and they tell you, "No, don't go to a chiropractor, they are quacks." Well, based on this judgment, they can lose their license and go to jail.

Ty: It is a conspiracy but it is a fact.

Dr. Vickers: It's a total fact.

Ty: It's a total fact, it's not a theory anymore.

Dr. Vickers: It's no longer a theory, it's a judgment.

Ty: Right. And we talked about this earlier too. Dr. Jonathan Wright reiterated this for us in Seattle. But in 1953, the US Senate determined that there was a conspiracy to suppress natural cancer treatments in the US. So it is no longer a conspiracy theory, it's a fact.

Dr. Vickers: That is a fact. It's an absolute fact.

Ty: Yes, very interesting.

Dr. Vickers: And you know, medical doctors from the day they enter school, literally, in their first semester of school, they are given a book that is called *Quackery in America* and what do you think that book is comprised of? It's compromised of all natural therapies, including the Gerson Therapy.

That is in those books, programming these medical doctors' minds from the very beginning of their education to believe that these therapies that we utilize are quackery. When the reality is, when you break it down to its hard core science, it doesn't get any more scientific than what we are doing on a cellular level.

Ty: Right. So, explain to me what are you doing on a cellular level? What is the Gerson Therapy? Most people have heard of it and they think it is a juicing and coffee enemas. Elaborate a little bit on that, please.

Dr. Vickers: That is the foundation, juicing and coffee enemas but it's a lot more than that, it's not that simple. What Gerson discovered, really the secret of the Gerson Therapy, is the production of energy on a cellular level. Gerson clearly understood that to rally an immune system, you had increase the production of energy on a cellular level in a form what's called ATP. ATP is Adenosine Triphosphate, it's the energy molecule that the mitochondria produce inside your cells.

When you see someone who is sick and/or dying, what's one of the first things you notice? They are lethargic. Why are they lethargic? They are lethargic because they lost the capacity to produce energy on a cellular level.

You need energy to eat, sleep, drink, walk, talk. You need it to maintain a healthy immune system. You most certainly need it to cure a sick and dying one. And today, that's what we're doing to reverse advanced disease.

So how do you increase the production of energy on a cellular level? There's only one way. There's only one way the human body does that and that's through the consumption of fruit and vegetable sugars and other various supplementation and detoxification procedures that can do that. And the Gerson Therapy—everything we give our patients, rallies around the production of energy.

For example, there's absolutely no sodium on the Gerson Therapy. Gerson quickly found out that sodium was one of the primary causes of all disease, not just heart disease and high-blood pressure but all disease. Why? When you eat a lot of sodium, what else do you have to do? You need to drink a lot of water, right? Well, sodium and water enter the cells and they swell the cell up and the mitochondria cannot function in that environment.

When our patients come in here, not only are we bombarding their body with 20 pounds of organic fruits and vegetables every single day—which is loaded with potassium because potassium is the only way you can get sodium out of the body. Sodium get stored up in our cells and the only way to get it out is through potassium. Because there's an inverse relationship in the human body between potassium and sodium. If you eat too much sodium, the body is going to dump potassium. If you eat too much potassium, the body is going to dump sodium.

So when our patients come in—Gerson created special potassium compound powder and when we give that to our patients in their juices, our patients will literally lose 7 to 15 pounds in a week or two-period in water and sodium weight alone that they are storing up inside their cells. So we have to get that sodium and water out of the cells.

And there are various other things that we're doing. For example, we're giving thyroid glandular because the thyroid is specifically responsible for replicating mitochondrial DNA. Let say in your cells right now, you have a thousand mitochondria in a cell. If we give you thyroid glandular and we give you Lugol's solution which is iodine—we know that the thyroid is dependent on iodine. Well, if we're giving you thyroid glandular, now instead of a thousand mitochondrial in a cell, you now have two thousand mitochondria in a cell.

And mitochondria, they produce energy through sugar and oxygen. Sugar and oxygen is the way the body produces energy. The body can use fat to produce energy but it doesn't want to use fat because it can't do it efficiently. It requires massive amounts of nutrients to take fat and convert it to energy. So the body's natural preference is fruit and vegetables, sugars. So in the presence of oxygen, the mitochondria can convert sugar into energy.

CoQ10 is responsible for the electron transport chain. When sugar enters the mitochondria, it goes through three reactions and it produces molecules, three molecules of something called nicotinc acid dehydrogenase. Those three molecules then get shoveled down something called electron transport chain. And the final production of the electron transport chain is ATP—energy.

And that electron transport chain is completely dependent on Coenzyme Q10. So our patients are getting potassium, Coenzyme Q10, thyroid glandular. All to stimulate the mitochondrial production of ATP. And that's one of the first things our patients always say when they're here for the first week is that their energy levels changed and that's because there's an internal change in the metabolic processes of the body.

Metabolism by definition is the breakdown of food into energy and that's what rallies the immune response. So the underlying principle of what's going on here is we're changing the metabolism of the body. Metabolism by definition is the breakdown of food into energy.

Now, with that said, in my eyes, one of the most irresponsible and dangerous theories out there in regards to cancer treatment, even in natural therapy realms, they are telling people not to eat sugars even fruits and vegetables because they contained too much sugar.

Our patients are getting 20 pounds of organic fruits and vegetables every day. They are getting 4,000 to 4,500 calories per day in juices. And if cancers were feeding—excuse me—if sugars are feeding cancer, there's no way in the history of the Gerson Therapy that we'd be able to reverse one case of cancer. Because our therapy is completely based on fruit and vegetable sugars. So, how is it that we're able to reverse all these diseases, not just cancer. We're reversing virtually every single degenerative disease, whether it is heart disease, diabetes, lupus, MS, rheumatoid-arthritis.

Cancer is what the Gerson Therapy become synonymous with because we have the history of reversing advanced terminal disease. So why are people saying that sugar feeds cancer? Well, the reason why they are saying is this—cancer will be fed by sugar in an acidic body. We hear about alkalinity and acidity all the time. Those two terms, they are thrown around like confetti at a country fair without anybody really explaining what does that mean.

When we're talking about alkalinity and acidity, we're talking about pH, right? PH means potential hydrogen. What acidity is by definition—it's the build-up of massive amounts of hydrogen within the body. Why is that significant? It's significant because in order to run the immune system, you need to be able to properly utilize oxygen. You have to be able to convert sugars into energy and you can only do that with oxygen.

There are two type of sugar breakdown, sugar metabolism, and you know this. There's aerobic glycolysis which is with oxygen and there's anaerobic glycolysis which means lacking oxygen. When oxygen is present, massive amounts of energy by the mitochondria can be produced. When oxygen can't get into the cell, then it goes into anaerobic glycolysis and the foundation of that or the final product of that is lactic acid build-up and tumors and cancers feed on lactic acid.

So, why is it that lactic acid can build up in the body? When you have a build-up of hydrogen or you have an acidic body, the charge at the level of the cell literally repels oxygen away from the cell. So, as oxygen is approaching that cell in an acidic body, the charge at the level of the cell membrane literally repels it away. It's a matter of bio-physics at that point. And if you can't get oxygen into that cell, that sugar is going to form lactic acid. And that is the major cause of disease when we talk about an acidic body causing disease.

So why does this therapy heal? Here's why—when you eat raw fruit, raw vegetables, you're drinking raw juices. Do you know if you tested those juices with litmus paper before they went into your body, they test acidic? They test acidic with litmus paper. But when you drink it, that gets broken down into an alkaline ash called potassium hydroxide.

The hydroxyl molecule literally goes into your body. Now, chemically written, a hydroxyl molecule is (OH-), oxygen, hydrogen negative changed. What's hydrogen? The acidic nature of hydrogen is a positively charged hydrogen ion (H+).

Imagine what happens when that juice gets broken down into hydroxyl ions (OH-) and reacts with the positively charged hydrogen ions. What reaction do you think takes place? You have an (OH-) and an (H+). Two Hs and an O. That reaction forms water. Water is neutral. You neutralize that acidity.

You've now changed the charge at the level of the cell membrane and you've now just allowed your body to properly oxygenate tissues. Making the sugars in these fruits and vegetable juices and of natural fruits and vegetables that they get at our clinic—they can now be easily converted to massive amounts of energy. And that is what ultimately fires up the immune system and that's why we have the storied history of reversing these advanced diseases.

Ty: Is that why you couple the juices with hyperbaric oxygen chamber?

Dr. Vickers: That is exactly right. You know that in 1931, Otto Warburg, he won the Nobel Prize in medicine when he was able to prove that viruses, bacteria in cancer cells could not survive in highly oxygenated environments. That's proof. That cannot be disputed, that's what he won the Nobel Prize in back then. And that's exactly why we utilize oxygen therapy on this protocol. It is an incredible combination of therapy to combat disease.

Ty: So you've got the juices, you've got the hyperbaric oxygen as part of the protocol. There are several other pieces of this protocol I'd like you to share. So continue with the different parts of the Gerson protocol that many people may not be aware of because there were three or four that I didn't even know that you included until yesterday.

Dr. Vickers: That's exactly right. One of the biggest portions of the therapy is the detoxification procedures of the Gerson Therapy. And the Gerson Therapy has made this famous and that's the coffee enema. Now, we were talking about the juicing and how the juicing neutralizes that acidity and forms water. Well, if you're forming massive amounts of water in the body like that, what do you think is happening on a cellular level? The toxins are getting flushed out of the cells into the blood stream and those toxins, they have to get released.

In the beginning of Dr. Gerson's Therapy, he actually lost several of his first few patients. He lost several of his beginning patients. Why? Because he was destroying tumors and cancer so quickly that it was releasing massive amounts of toxicity into the body and he had to come up with something to release that toxicity. And he came up with something absolutely ingenious and it was the coffee enema. Now, people say, "Come on, now I've heard everything. The coffee enema? I prefer to take mine in the morning first thing when I wake up."

Ty: With cream and sugar.

Dr. Vickers: With cream and sugar. But it's ingenius. Let me explain why. There are a lot of reasons why but the main reason is this—your liver produces an enzyme, it is called glutathione transferace. Glutathione transferace is the most potent, detoxifying enzyme in the human body. The liver produces it. What the liver uses is palmitic acid as the chemical base to produce glutathione transferace.

Properly roasted organic coffee, it's lightly, lightly roasted—it's not a drinking coffee. It's a particular bean, it's not a drinking bean and it's also roasted so lightly that you don't de-naturize it like you would in a drinking coffee. But properly roasted coffee is loaded with palmitic acid. And studies on coffee enemas have proven that when you do one coffee enema, the production of glutathione transferace by the body goes up 600-700% greater than normal. And our patients, they are getting five a day. Now, whenever I lecture or whenever I talk about this, people want to do two things—they want the potassium supplement that I mentioned and they want to do the coffee enemas. But here's the problem, when patients are coming to you sick, they are coming to you with severely depleted bodies from the over abuse of processed foods, and stress, and environment toxicity.

These things are depleting the reserve systems of our body are to maintain a healthy immune system. When we stimulate the glutathione transferace system with the coffee enema that requires nutrients, that requires vitamin C, all your B vitamins, iron, potassium, magnesium, zinc. All those things go into firing that system. If you're doing coffee enemas and you're not doing them in conjunction with a massive amount of nutrient intake, you're going to deplete your body further over time.

And so, everything that we do, you can't pick and choose on what you want to do. This is a system that was developed by a medical genius over 50 years of clinical observation. So, the coffee enemas, Dr. Gerson made those famous. And without those, plain and simple, we cannot cure them. They are so absolutely vital to what we do.

That's one of the therapies that we're doing. Some of the other things you mentioned or that you wanted me to mention were Coley's therapy. In 1959, Gerson wrote a book right before he died. And he theorized the direction he wanted to take his therapy in and he mentioned the word, "Coleys." He mentioned William B. Coley.

William B. Coley was a Harvard Oncologist. And back in the late 1800s actually, he discovered that when his patients came down with staph or strep infections, their cancers got better or they reduced or went away completely. But once the infection was gone, they started to come back. So what he did was he began to culture the toxins that staph and strep bacteria make. And he began injecting them into the connective tissue of his patients and he got the same fever response. The patients would break out in fevers and their tumors would reduce and their fever would go away.

So he began to try to get upper hand on the tumors by constantly injecting them with the toxins and produce this fever. He was able to achieve some permanent cures, especially in sarcomas but what Coley failed to recognized was that again, he was artificially stimulating the immune system which requires massive amounts of nutrients.

Gerson knew that if he could do Coley's while doing the Gerson Therapy, he could get exponentially greater results. But he never got the chance to do it because he passed away. Well, we're doing it. And when we give Coley's, we get the same response that William B. Coley got. The only difference is, our patients are getting boosted up immune systems with all these massive amounts of nutrients that they are taking and all these detoxification procedures. So Coley's is probably the greatest addition to the Gerson Therapy since Dr. Gerson passed away.

Other immuno-therapies that we are using—dendritic cell therapy. A very famous therapy out there today. In the States, it's ridiculously expensive to get. Here, where we are in Mexico, it is not expensive at all. What are dendritic cells? They are like generals in your body. They go around your body, seeking out threats to the system and then they present that threat to the white blood cells, to the immune system.

And it's the immune system that rallies the response. So we contract that out. Somebody comes in, they draw your blood, they go back to a laboratory and they separate your dendritic cells from your red blood cells and then they culture your dendritic cells over a three to four day period.

Let's say they took out a million dendritic cells, when they come back, three to four days later, they are now putting five million. And you can imagine what that would do to the immune system, it would put it on high alert. So dendritic cell therapy is becoming a very renowned therapy in the realm of alternative medicine. But it is always exponentially greater when you are doing it in the realm of massive nutritional regime.

Ty: Okay, so dendritic dells. You mentioned the laetrile. Are you also using laetrile?

Dr. Vickers: Yes. Laetrile, that's one of the darling therapies that people come to Mexico for and they've been coming for years. Laetrile is vitamin B17. It comes from apricot kernel, apricot kernel pits. Its active agent is cyanide, ultimately. And it causes immediate cell death of cancer cells. But it really has to be done in conjunction with hyperthermia. Hyperthermia—it's been shown that you do laetrile with hyperthermia, its effects go up nearly 7-10 fold.

There are a lot of people out there, they are eating up apricot kernel seeds and they are taking laetrile supplements, it doesn't work. It simply doesn't work. Not only does it doesn't work, it actually taxes the digestive tract of these patients. For example, we know that the digestive tract is 75 percent of the immune system. So if you are sick and dying, your digestive tract is shot. So it simply cannot take vitamin B17 from an apricot kernel and extract the nutrients out of there and utilize it for proper response that you'd typically would get using an IV.

Ty: So that's why you're using IVs and you're coupling with hyperthermia.

Dr. Vickers: Yes, you have to use IV. Because the patients need six to nine grams of pure laetrile to get a therapeutic response. Do you know how many seeds you would have to eat in order to get six to nine grams of pure vitamin B17? They say anywhere from 12-15,000.

Ty: A small mountain.

Dr. Vickers: It's useless. It really is worthless to be eating the seeds. The supplements that come in 500mg tablets, I guess that would be arguable. You would need 20 of those each day and then your body would have to absorb all of it in order to achieve six to nine grams of laetrile. I don't see that happening.

Ty: So let me ask you this then. For laetrile, and this is just kind of a side note, we're all familiar with Jason Vale.

Dr. Vickers: I'm not. I'm sorry.

Ty: Jason was the first guy who made laetrile famous in the 90's. Actually, there was the Krebs, Dr. Krebs in the 50s. But the first guy since we had TV really publicizing this. He was an arm wrestler from New York City, diagnosed with terminal cancer. And he ate apple seeds and apricot seeds. It totally cured his cancer. So you're saying that's an anomaly?

Dr. Vickers: That has to be an anomaly.

Ty: It shouldn't happen normally that way?

Dr. Vickers: You talked to a lot of people—we have a patient here now. They were eating apricot kernel seeds. They said, after a handful, they were so ill and it wasn't from the laetrile. It was from the body's inability to break down the apricot kernel seeds. Not to mention that the bitterness and just the bitterness of those seeds, they are horrible. That is not good on the digestive tract. You know, there's a lot of anecdotal stories out there. And when you start to break down and you find out more information about these anecdotal stories, you'll hear that they made radical changes in their lifestyles as well. Typically, nutrition. But today—and this is how long ago was that, back in the 50s?

Ty: No, this was in '97.

Dr. Vickers: Ninety seven. Okay. I can tell you today, what we're seeing in our clinics today is nothing like we were seeing 20 years ago. Cancer has become a completely different monster. And these individual therapies like laetrile or IV Vitamin C which we utilize here at the clinic, they are not curing advanced cancer anymore. And even back then, it was few and far between to get a advanced terminal cancer cured using just those modalities. Now, you got to attack it from so many different angles and that's what we're trying to do here at our clinic.

Ty: Sure. What you are doing here is you're treating cancer as—you're treating the tumor as the symptom and not the cancer.

Dr. Vickers: That's exactly right.

Ty: And so, you got these treatments like laetrile or the vitamin C or whatever it might be or even the Coley's toxins. Those are targeting the shrinkage of the tumors but if you don't affect the internal terrain of the body and change it you won't have a long term success.

Dr. Vickers: That is exactly right. Your numbers—

Ty: You're focusing on nutrition.

Dr. Vickers: That's exactly right. It has to be the foundation of everything. Look, Hippocrates to this day, he's still considered the greatest physician who ever lived. You know his famous quote, right?

Ty: What was his second famous quote?

Dr. Vickers: His second famous quote was, "Look to the spine as the cause of disease."

Ty: "Look to the spine."

Dr. Vickers: So when Thomas Edison said, "The doctor of the future will give no medicine but will interest his patients in nutrition and caring for the human spine." He was talking about a chiropractor and a Gerson therapist.

Ty: He was a very smart fellow.

Dr. Vickers: He was.

Ty: Now what's the other way you were telling me about yesterday, P27?

Dr. Vickers: PNC-27. We're using that now at the clinic. It's been around for about five years. It's showing a lot of promise in particular cancers, metastasis, and delivery system because it can be delivered in a variety of ways. It can be delivered through nebulization. So if we have somebody with lung cancer or lung metastasis, it's phenomenal. We've heard some really fantastic stories already coming out of our clinic where people with lung mats or even brain mats have been nebulizing it and their metastasis had been resolved. You can give it as a suppository, either vaginally—in cervical, vaginal or uterine cancer—or we can give it rectally with rectal, prostate and colon cancer.

PNC-27 was discovered by some researchers in upstate New York at SUNY Medical College. Dr. Pincus was his name. It's a protein derived from a moth and a fruit fly and it's specific for cancer cells only. It leaves normal cells completely alone. What this protein does is it envelopes itself around the membrane of the cancer cell and it burrows a hole into the cancer cell and causes immediate implosion or apoptosis, it's called, of cancer cells because of the sudden dramatic change in osmotic pressure when you burrow the hole into the cell membrane.

So we've been using PNC now for about, probably, close to a year and four months and we see success with it. We see some not-successful things going on with it. It's specifically for pancreatic cell line tumors.

Ty: Is that what "P" in PNC stands for? Pancreatic something?

Dr. Vickers: Possibly, I believe so. But PNC-27, it's specific for pancreatic cell lines. That's where it is the most effective but we're finding it very effective in these other delivery systems in cancers that I mentioned earlier.

Ty: Great. Interesting. So really, with the Gerson Therapy that you're using here specifically in this clinic, because there are other Gerson clinics. You're doing it differently here?

Dr. Vickers: Completely.

Ty: So really the foundational principle is you're really forcing all this massive amounts of nutrition into these patients with sick bodies.

Dr. Vickers: That's right.

Ty: You know, to me, it makes a heck lot of sense. You have somebody that is sick, give him nutrition to make him better.

Dr. Vickers: That's right.

Ty: And so, on the flip side, tell us the wisdom or lack thereof of traditional treatment protocol that takes a sick body and poisons them with chemotherapy.

Dr. Vickers: Well, you and I know that the foundations of chemotherapy is, what? Mustard gas, right? World War II ended, they've nothing to do with their Mustard Gas. So they pumped off on the pharmaceutical industry and they're pumping it off on the American and the world public.

You can't heal a sick and dying body with poison. These are bodies that have come to us completely depleted from years of chemical, emotional, environmental abuse. And it's depleted organic systems and weakened them tremendously. You can't rebuild a body with poison. There's only one way you can rebuild a human body and that's pure nutrition and pure detoxification. And then, on top of that, supplementation, proper supplementation.

Ty: So, yesterday, your staff was kind enough to serve us a lot of the juices, the fresh fruits, the vegetables and some really—I had a watermelon steak. If you've never have a watermelon steak, you're missing out on the watermelon steak. Just some incredible food. And so walk us through a day in the life of a Gerson patient.

Dr. Vickers: Absolutely. It's a full time job. I mean, look, if you've abused your body for the last 50-60 years and you've been diagnosed with an advanced disease, for us to be able to reverse and cure your terminal cancer in two year,s which is typically the amount of time a cancer patient has to be on a therapy, that's an absolute miracle. And you're not going to cut corners in order to be cured. It's a full time job for two years straight.

Our patients wake up at seven o'clock in the morning and they get their first enema and they get the first round of supplements. They get a probiotic, a very highly-concentrated probiotic. Why? Because we need to rebuild the digestive tract. So they get their probiotic, they get some enzymes to prepare their stomach for their eight o'clock meal.

So, they do their enema at seven o'clock. At eight o'clock, they're given their breakfast which is typically oatmeal with some stewed dried fruits, organic apricot, organic prunes, organic raisins. They get flax oil. We didn't talk about flax oil but it's absolutely vital to the human body because it literally draws oxygen into the cells. It has an electrical charge that literally attracts oxygen into the cell membrane to be broken down to help break down sugar and energy.

So they're getting two tablespoons of flax oil a day and they can use two to three teaspoons of a natural sweetener, sucanat, honey, maple syrup or blackstrap molasses. So that's their breakfast. And they get fresh-pressed orange juice at eight o'clock.

Nine o'clock, the day begins, the juicing day. They get their green juice at nine. They get a carrot juice at 9:30. They get a carrot-apple juice at ten, and then they're getting carrot and apple and green juices until seven o'clock at night. And in between, every three hours, they are getting a coffee enema. So that's a typical day.

Then, we take them through the adjunctive therapies that we mentioned. They are getting IV vitamin C, IV chelation, IV laetrile. If they choose to get PNC, they get PNC. They're getting their hyperbaric oxygen chamber for an hour.

One thing we forgot to mention is we just included infrared. We just got a full spectrum infrared sauna. Why is that important? The literature that is coming out today is making something very clear, that far infrared light is destroying cancer cells in particular when it's done in conjunction with massive amounts of chlorophyll.

Cancer cells, they suck up the chlorophyll. And chlorophyll because of its nature, it's natural instinct activity with photosynthesis is drawing light to itself. So these cancer cells are sucking up the chlorophyll and then when you hit the body with infrared light, it is immediately destroying cancer cells. They are saying it is as effective as chemotherapy. Obviously, without the side effects of chemotherapy.

So throughout the day, they're getting all their juices, they're doing their enemas and when there's any time in between, they are hopping into the hyperbaric oxygen chamber or they are hoping into the infrared sauna.

Ty: So, it's really a full-time job.

Dr. Vickers: It's a full-time job here. But I'll tell you something. In spite of the trying circumstances that all our patients are going through—obviously, they've been given God knows how many months to live, that's why they are here. They'll be the first to tell you that their three weeks at our clinic, it's a complete transformation on all levels. They say it's one of the greatest experiences that they've ever had in their life because it really is. It's opening up their mind to something they never really knew existed.

And it's giving them something that they didn't have with chemotherapy and radiation because they were sent home to die. And we literally—this isn't some false hope that we're giving people. This is pure science taken to a level of healing that is giving them a real hope. Now, are we going to cure everybody? No, we don't cure everybody. We don't make that claim. Some people come to us—their organic systems, particularly their liver and their kidneys are too far gone to restore. So we can't heal everybody but we heal a lot of people that had been sent home to die. And those that we can't heal, we extend their lives significantly and their quality of life. It's unimaginable compared to chemotherapy and radiation.

Ty: One of the things I noticed and another camera team noticed yesterday as we walked through the clinic is that the people, they were smiling, the patients were happy, that you could see that they have hope in their yes. And I just contrast that to your typical hospital ward, chemotherapy ward and it's depressing. This is completely the opposite of that.

Dr. Vickers: That's right.

Ty: And so I sensed that—one of things that I mentioned to the guys yesterday, several times is, "Wow! This is so different than what you think of a hospital being." This is not a hospital, this is a healing center.

Dr. Vickers: That's exactly right. And when I established this clinic three years ago, two and half years ago, I was adamant that it didn't look like an institutional setting, a hospital setting. Because an institutional setting, it doesn't address on some of the other aspects of healing—rest, relaxation, love, compassion. And when you come to our place, it's beautiful. Take a look at this view. We have a condo down on the ocean, where you have the pleasure of staying in last night.

Ty: It's not a great view, believe me. It's just the Pacific Ocean.

Dr. Vickers: It's stunningly beautiful, no?

Ty: It's beautiful.

Dr. Vickers: It's one of the primest pieces of real estate in all of Mexico. And we have that for our patients to go down and enjoy on the weekends. So I was adamant about creating an environment where they can have fresh air, they can be in an environment that's like more of a home environment than an institutionalized hospital setting. And that's something always that people comment on when they come here, "This doesn't feel like a hospital. This feels like a home." And my staff, they are second to none. The other thing that people say is that they just can't believe how incredible my staff is. And I can't believe that I have the privilege of working with 15 of some of the finest, most loving compassionate and hardworking people that I honestly have ever had the opportunity to work with.

***Ty*:** Awesome staff. Really genuine concern in their eyes. Explain to me—last question here. Explain to me—yesterday, we had a meal. We had some juice, then we had a grilled watermelon with some onions. We had a slice of eggplant that was grilled with some sweet potatoes on it, fresh salad and then we had a fantastic desert that was mango- banana ice cream and a little apple fritter that was made with squash. Everything was just phenomenal.

Dr. Vickers: Unbelievable.

***Ty*:** Why was I so full?

Dr. Vickers: Why were you so full? We have an obesity epidemic in the United States. People eat and eat and eat and they think they're never satiated enough to stop eating. Why? Because they are eating countless dead calories that have absolutely no nutrition in them. So their brain—your body communicates with your brain and it tells it when it's full based on the amount of nutrients that are in that food. So when you come to our clinic, the amount of nutrients that you're getting has—as you said yesterday—a leptic on the brain. The amount of nutrition in the food that you eat communicates with the brain that says, "Okay, I've had enough. I'm satiated. I'm satisfied. I'm full." And it literally turns off the mechanism which tells you that you're hungry. Your staff recognized that as well. They ate and they were full just from one relatively normal plate of food. And that's the reason why, because of the nutrient content.

***Ty*:** And you know, one of the things we were mentioning is—that'll never happen. We were saying—one of the guys, I can't remember who it was, said, "What they should do with these buffets is get rid of all this crappy food they're serving and serve this nutrient dense food and save a lot of money."

Dr. Vickers: It would save them a lot of money.

***Ty*:** Because people don't eat as much.

Dr. Vickers: That is exactly right.

***Ty*:** Because they're getting nutrition.

Dr. Vickers: That's exactly right. They wouldn't eat as much either.

***Ty*:** That's true. Of course I guess we are addicted to the taste.

Dr. Vickers: Addicted to the what?

***Ty*:** Addicted to the junk food taste. Addicted to all of the artificial flavorings and all that mess. I'll tell you what, Dr. Vickers, you have filled up my cup of information today on the Gerson treatment and I really understand it a lot better than I did. I really appreciate you spending time today.

Dr. Vickers: Thank you. It's a pleasure having you.

Ty*:** Thanks. Keep up the good work. ***[end of transcript]

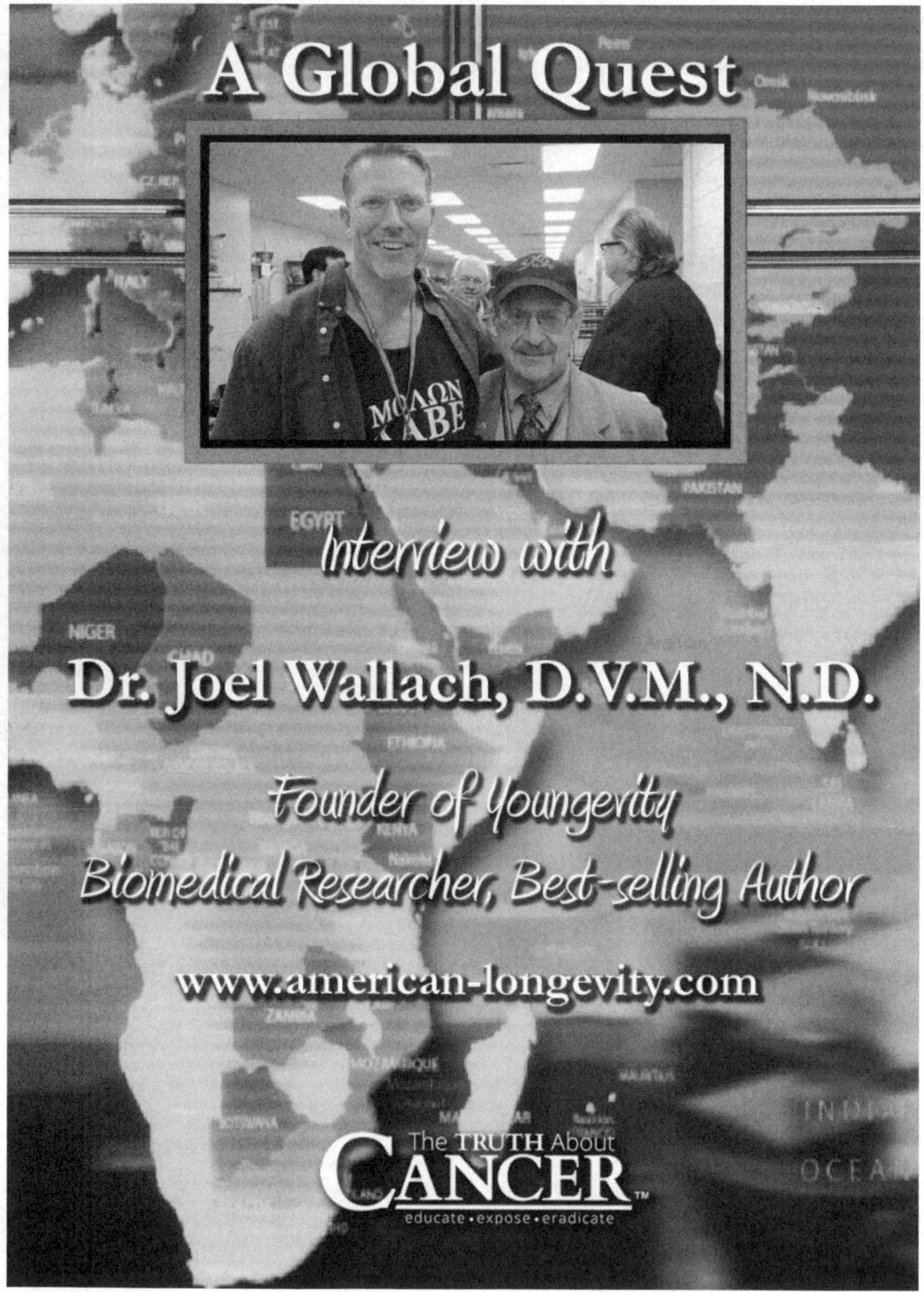
A Global Quest
Interview with
Dr. Joel Wallach, D.V.M., N.D.
Founder of Youngevity
Biomedical Researcher, Best-selling Author
www.american-longevity.com
The TRUTH About CANCER
educate • expose • eradicate

Dr. Wallach: I think probably it's worth a minute to go through what makes me different was that my background was different. I have a degree in Agriculture, I'm a veterinarian. I have a Post-Doctoral Fellowship in Comparative Pathology where I did animal and human autopsies and chemistries. And I've been a primary care physician private practice for 37 years.

It gives me a little bit different perspective because I'm coming at things from four different directions. What I've learned is that cancer, in my experience, is not genetic. It is a self-inflicted disease, totally preventable once you consciously know what the parameters, or what got your family or yourself in trouble.

We can almost always say, "Look, if your doctor says you're at Stage 4 plus or Stage 5 or Stage 6, or whatever. And you have weeks or months to live, we can make your quality of life much better. We can actually extend life considerably longer than the average prediction of a medical doctor."

Many times a diagnosis is incorrect. Sometimes ulcerative colitis will be called colon cancer. Sometimes myelofibrosis, which is a manifestation of osteoporosis, will be called multiple myeloma, which is bone marrow cancer.

Sometimes things that are—cystic disease of the breast will be called breast cancer when it's really just fibrocystic disease of the breast. And I don't know if that's because the doctors need a Mercedes payment, they're doing it on purpose, or if they are just ignorant of all the manifestations of the non-cancer things.

To me, the things you can do to prevent cancer are as useful as the ones that treat it once you have it. And that is you stay away from free radicals. I mean stay away from—don't even go in the same room with them.

For instance, just cooking your meat well done has been well established to show that you can increase a woman's chance of having breast cancer by 462 percent against a control group. If she cooks her meat very well done where the fat is burned, it turns into acrylamides, heterocyclic amines, and Trans fats. Which will not only cause inflammation in the arteries, which plug arteries, but also cause inflammation to glandular and ductile tissues including breast tissue and prostate tissue and results in cancerous changes.

You want to stay away from all fried foods. Don't even keep frying pans in your house because they use the word "fry." Use skillets. If you're going to cook meat, there is nothing wrong with meat, but cook it medium rare as opposed to well done.

Do not eat processed meats with nitrates or nitrites. That means no deli slices, no sandwich meats, no sausage, ham, bacon, bologna, salami, pastrami, pepperoni, jerky, corned beef, Spam. All that stuff has got to go.

No oils. The only good oil is a dead oil. No oils. It means no olive oil, no coconut oil, no margarines, no mayonnaise, no salad dressing, or cooking oils because they turn into Trans fats, heterocyclic amines, and acrylamides all of which are inflammatory.

And I actually wrote papers on this in 1971. After 20,000 autopsies it was very clear that the medical system was actually missing the cause of things. And, of course, every century there are thousands and thousands of failed medical theories. In the 20th century and 21st century there's no difference.

The only difference between a failed medical theory in the 20th and 21st century versus a failed medical theory, including cancer theories, going back say five, six, seven, eight thousand years ago is if a doctor had a failed theory 5,000 years ago, he'd kill 100 people. Today, if a doctor has a failed theory in cancer, he kills a million people.

When people are self-educated, when they know what to do to prevent cancer, what they need to support their body's ability to defend itself against cancer, we're going to get a much better result instead of depending on hospitals and clinics and doctors.

And so my whole thing is train the person individually and let them do what they know to be done and they get a much better result than if they just hand themselves over and say, "Do with me what you will." That doesn't work out very well. They have to be a major player in their own treatment, a major player in their own defense.

Interviewer: So you've seen people turn around, like terminal diagnoses?

Dr. Wallach: Sure.

Interviewer: Have you witnessed that using the protocols you've been teaching and then seeing, "Wow! This person is alive today?"

Dr. Wallach: Every year we see—I'd say honestly anywhere from 15 to 30, 40, 50 people who are given death sentences. They say, "Look, you have less than three months to live."

And we get them off the bad stuff. Which is equally as important as doing the good stuff—no fried foods, no processed meats, no oils, no glutens, got to stay away from burnt foods. And if you do that, you stop the ongoing damage, which is equally important as to supporting the body's ability to repair stuff.

I think this is where people fall short. This is where doctors fall short. They really don't stress enough what they need to do to stop the ongoing damage when it comes to cancer. Because no matter what you do, if you are doing everything right and supporting the immune system and your body is trying to heal itself, but you are still eating deep fried chicken and burnt meat on the barbeque, you're going to have a struggle because you have the good forces fighting the bad forces.

A person has to be obsessive about avoiding the bad stuff and we see people turn around all the time. At the very least, we see them and they have a much better quality of life and they actually—if the doctor says, "You have less than three months to live," we've seen them live five months, six months, two years, five years. This is very common.

Just by staying away from the bad stuff and doing the good stuff. But if you just do the good stuff and and keep doing what you were doing then it will be a struggle.

Interviewer: Yes. That's incredible. Have you seen those total turn-arounds where they've been given a death sentence and then they live like—?

Dr. Wallach: Twice as long. Yes, they'll live twice as long, sometimes five times longer than the doctors will say and their quality of life is way up there. Instead of saying, "Look, I've got this one new experimental drug. Let's try one more round of chemotherapy. " The person should say, "No, absolutely no. Never, never, never." Because they really don't understand life and death if they grasp for that last round of chemotherapy.

Because if the doctor said, "Look. You have six weeks to live if we do nothing. But if this chemotherapy works, you might live eight weeks or twelve weeks. But it also might kill you in three days. This new experimental chemotherapy."

So I'm not big on trying—let them try on somebody else, not my family, not me. And I wouldn't recommend trying the experimental drug because the outcomes usually aren't good.

Interviewer: Yes. That makes sense. Dr. Wallach, most of the time, doctors that are practicing the natural and pursuing that part, they get quite slammed in that. And I'm sure you've gone through that as well.

But isn't it interesting that, for you, you've experienced that in some cases it turns back the other way and you've obviously had that opportunity.

What's happened recently? What has that meant to you? You didn't do it for recognition, I know that. You did it because you wanted to help the people. And now, after all these years, there has finally been a piece of recognition. What was it and what does it mean to you?

Dr. Wallach: The recognition?

Interviewer: Yes.

Dr. Wallach: Well, in August of this year, August 7th, I was given an award from the United Nations as recognition for a lifetime of achievement in natural medicine as well as philanthropy because I don't take any fees for my services. I do all of this for nothing, take nothing.

The only products we will sell to people is at wholesale. We never sell anything retail and nobody that works on my systems, nobody in our organization, takes any fees. We do this all without taking a fee. I think there are very few doctors that do that and we're very, very proud of that.

Our whole goal here is to educate people so that they can take care of themselves. At the very least, we're going to educate their families so their families themselves don't have to go through the things that their loved one went through.

The exciting thing is that people are now beginning to look at this. Where ten, twelve, fifteen years ago, "Well, my doctor said. I better ask my doctor." The one who failed you. The one who said you only had three months to live. You're going to consult with him to see if you're going to try something else?

So they're saying, "Well, I guess you're right. Why would I consult with him? He said I only had a couple of months to live." So people are willing to try things. And we do this in such a manner—there is nothing that is going to harm anybody. And people always say, "Will this interfere with my medication?" I always say, "I wish it would, but it won't. It won't interfere with your medication."

"Well, can I overdose on the vitamins and minerals?" Well, you can, but there are cheaper ways to kill yourself. To overdose with vitamins and minerals you're going to have to take 60 bottles a day. Who is going to take 60 bottles of a supplement a day? It's just insane. Of course, doctors say that so you'll stay on their protocols.

Interviewer: Did you say Obama is sending you patients?

Dr. Wallach: The Affordable Healthcare Act is bringing 10,000 new patients to me every month. This is sort of a surprise. Why am I getting these 10,000 new patients a month? Because when people get moved from being full time status at their workplace to part-time, suddenly now the company doesn't have to cover their health insurance costs.

They can't afford it, so they are without health insurance. So now it seems like $3.00 or $4.00 a day isn't too expensive. Whereas if you're getting free treatment from insurance, $3.00 or $4.00, a day you would say, "Well, I'd rather just have insurance pay it. I don't care if it works or not. I want the insurance to pay for it."

Another thing that has happened is that people, especially kids, have been asking for $15.00 an hour for part-time work during the summer time. And, of course, companies are out there taking pictures of them. And when they apply for a job the next time they tell them, "So you're that guy. I'm sorry, I'm not going to hire you at all."

They are actually getting these big boards inside the fast food places where you put your order in yourself—no cashiers, put your credit card in, and some little retired person comes out and gives you your food instead of a high school kid. And the high school kids aren't getting jobs anymore because they went from making $6.00 or $8.00 an hour now they're wanting $15.00 an hour. Of course, that's not going to happen.

So the Affordable Healthcare Act and all these various things that have to do with availability of insurance or not insurance. Including when the deductible goes up from $100 a month to $3,000—or not a month—$100 deductible for any event versus $3,000 deductible. Suddenly now, "Well, I don't have $3,000 to get the insurance, so I'd just rather pay the $3.00 or $4.00 a day for the supplements and support my immune system and let my own body fend off the cancer and repair itself."

We see miracles all the time. We see miracles, whether it's cancer, or heart disease, or Alzheimer's disease. We see miracles.

Interviewer: What does that mean to you? Truly, you have helped so many people. You have helped influence people that are influencers. You have helped doctors to be able to understand—you've helped patients, you've helped doctors to understand. You've helped lead a field that has saved the lives of precious people and kept families together and all those things that are most important about this whole line of work.

What is it like reflecting on that and looking in the lives of those people that you've touched? What does that mean to you?

Dr. Wallach: Well, it has been, again, very useful that people who are in politics and power, money and power, or billionaires and people who are Ambassadors to the United Nations, people who are Mayors of cities and Governors, movie actors of all kinds, Olympic athletes, Gold Medal winners, professional athletes—these people do great things. They volunteer their services for deaf camps, for sports and for homeless and battered women and families that are broken up and children that are born with birth defects. These are the sorts of things that make it all worthwhile.

Then, of course, I'm a very religious person and I kind of learned these things when I was nine years old. How does a nine year old by himself or herself learn this when you're nine years old? You don't. I realize if you learn it that young, there has got to be some divine guidance there. And that is how I look at it.

As long as I understand that it is divine guidance that sent me this direction, I'm always going to never take a fee for helping these people. Because I believe I'm doing God's work. And so if you're doing God's work—I can't bring myself to take payment for it.

Well, an individual like Ty, he could have just gotten drunk, become a drug addict or hit the streets and gone some place and forgotten about the whole thing. But it tells a lot about the person when he suffers through these terrible events that took his family. And he is putting his energies into helping other people so they never have to suffer the same way. I believe he was inspired by God also because it's a godly thing that he's doing and I cannot thank him enough for everything he is doing to get the word out so people can protect themselves and their loved ones.

I think it helps doctors, too. Even though I have crossed swords with doctors many, many times. I think that they need to hear the truth and see the non-injurious options, the possibilities of other things.

When people say, "I don't want to do that." So instead of saying, "Well, I can't help you." say, "Okay, well here's an option. I don't have a lot of experience with it." But Ty has done such a great job of bringing this to the surface and you'll see so many wonderful things happen, why not?

"If you don't want to do chemotherapy and radiation and surgery, let's try these other things." There have been many, many blessings over and over and over. You've got to respect Ty for bringing all this to the surface.

Interviewer: Do you think he is saving lives?

Dr. Wallach: Absolutely. Saving lives, quality of life—it doesn't get better than that.

Interviewer: That's awesome. And one last one. The epigenetics in cancer, what could you tell us about the important role?

Dr. Wallach: Sure. Again, people have to appreciate that cancer is not genetically transmitted. This is where epigenetics comes in and, of course, my book—I'm fond of it—my new book, *Epigenetics: The Death of the Genetic Theory of Disease Transmission* goes into cancer quite a bit.

Epigenetics, I knew about it back in the 1960s. We're talking 50 years ago. That's because I worked on a big National Institutes of Health project called the Center for the Biology of Natural Systems. I did over 20,000 autopsies, 10 million chemistries, 10 million slides of special stains looking for pollution and genetics as causes of death from natural causes.

To make a long story short, after ten years and all these autopsies and chemistries and slides, the results showed that none of these diseases are genetic and none of them are nutritional. None of them are genetic, certainly none of them are things that pollution—they are, in fact, a nutritional deficiency disease.

The book that came out of it, 1,200 pages, one of these things, is in the Smithsonian Institute as a national treasure because it brought epigenetics to the surface back in the 1960s, 50 years ago. People didn't have a real word for it back then. But when you find all these diseases, that are supposed to be human genetic diseases in crocodiles and hummingbirds and antelope, it didn't fit the genetic picture.

It was quite a relief to know that we're in control of these things. We can prevent them by treating them properly with nutrition and getting rid of the bad stuff. We can have a better quality of life and increase our length of life. Maybe your body is able to totally defend itself and eliminate the disease.

Those are phenomenal, monumental observations. Again, the failed medical theory is that cancer is a genetic thing. No. Absolutely not. So for those of you who are out there that everybody in your family has had breast cancer, don't get your breasts cut off because it's not genetic.

It's epigenetic. Stay away from the bad stuff. No fried foods, no processed meats, no oils, no gluten, and take the good stuff. Take all 90 essential nutrients, 16 minerals, 16 vitamins, 12 amino acids, three fatty acids. Give your body the raw materials it needs to defend itself and God will bless you with a long healthy life.

Interviewer: That's awesome. So then I don't have to live in fear.

Dr. Wallach: Nobody has to live in fear. Nobody has to believe in fear. You believe in yourself, you believe in the good Lord. It doesn't get any better than that. You do not—nobody should live in fear.

Absolutely. Thanks for the opportunity and we'll all work together to keep saving humanity one person at a time. And thank you.

[end of transcript]

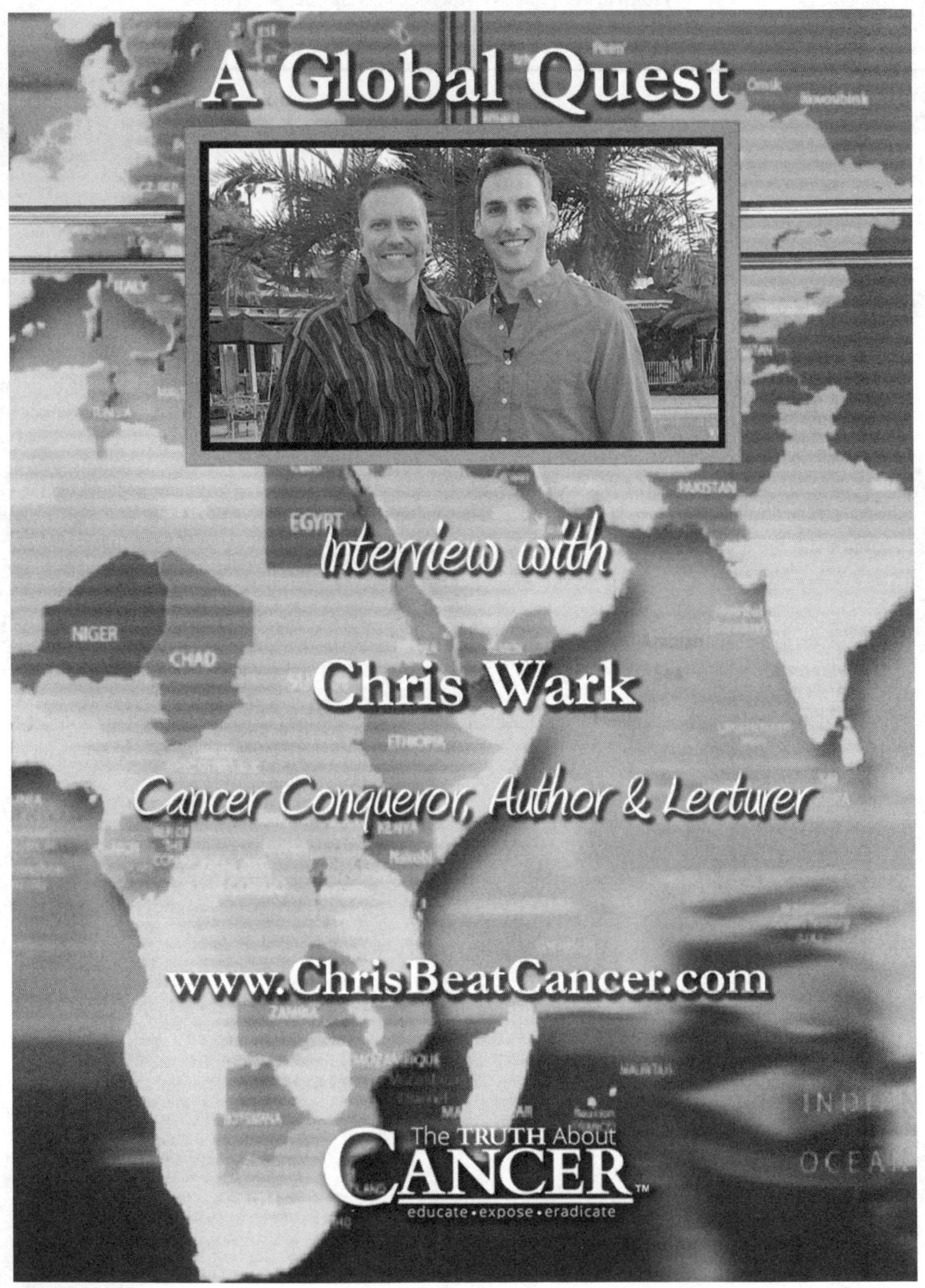
A Global Quest
EGYPT
NIGER
CHAD
Interview with
Chris Wark
Cancer Conqueror, Author & Lecturer
www.ChrisBeatCancer.com
The TRUTH About
CANCER
educate • expose • eradicate

Ty: So I'm here today with Chris Wark and I'm really looking forward to this interview; we're going to get your take on treating your cancer and we're actually going to get your take on what is cancer. We are going to go all across the board today, but first of all just thank you for being with us Chris.

Chris: Thanks Ty. Great to see you again.

Ty: Yeah it's good to see you again too. I'm really excited to have you here today. You're going to be a really beautiful addition to this project. So if you could please tell us your story about diagnosis to start with. Tell us about being diagnosed with cancer. What did that feel like, what was the recommendation from your oncologist? Just go back in time. Put yourself at that place and give us the story from step one.

Chris: Well I was 26. Okay so I was a newlywed, been married two years. I was working in real estate business buying rental property and renovating houses and I've been doing that just a couple years so you know I really just kind of felt like I was just being an adult, you know what I mean? Like out of college a couple years, working, newlywed and I started having abdominal pain.

Ty: And this was what year?

Chris: This was 2003.

Ty: Okay.

Chris: And I thought I had an ulcer. I've never had any illness before, never had any major—you know the flu when I was a kid or something but nothing major. And I thought "I don't know, is this an ulcer; like what's going on?" And I had this pain that would come and go and it was kind of like Groundhog Day, you know because every morning I would wake up and I'd immediately think like "How do I feel?" Like "I feel good, okay no pain." And then I'd go throughout the day but then I would get these twinges of pain you know, most days and I'd be like "Oh, there it is again." And then I'd go to sleep kind of worried about it and then I'd wake up and I'd go, "Well no pain," right and so that kind of went on for many months. And I kept thinking, Maybe my body would get better, because my body had always healed in the past and I believe that the body is designed to heal, and so—but the problem was I didn't make any changes in my life, right? I didn't understand cancer at the time and so I just kept living my life the way I was living it, which was in a very unhealthy way.

And this pain got worse and worse and eventually I went to a doctor and they thought I had an ulcer and gave me some medication that didn't help. And then I through a series of doctor's appointments eventually ended up at a gastroenterologist who did a colonoscopy and found a golf ball size tumor in my large intestine. And you know I came out of the procedure, they put me under and I woke up and you know I was still medicated, you know it was like "Where am I? What's happening?" And the doctor came in and he was—he basically said, "We found this tumor, you might have cancer. We have to send it to the lab" and you know my wife started crying on the nurse's shoulder and I was just like "What? What's going on?" You know I wasn't even—

Ty: You were at that time, how old were you?

Chris: I was 26.

Ty: 26 years old.

Chris: And so at that moment I wasn't even sober, you know what I mean? So it didn't really make sense; it just felt like a dream that I didn't understand. But a couple days later I got the call from the doctor and he said, "Listen you know, the lab report came back and you have colon cancer." And so that was heavy and you know, that's kind of when my life came to a grinding halt and I thought "Well okay, I guess I'm the cancer guy now. What does this even look like," you know? I don't even understand what this means. I'd never had anyone in my family diagnosed with cancer so I had no experience. Never seen anybody go through treatment. I've seen a few people out in the world that were like "Oh that's a cancer patient," and "Whoa they look really bad,," and that's all I knew about cancer. And so I was a very typical patient, clueless. They said—the doctor said, "We got to get you into surgery right away; we got to get this thing out of you before it spreads and kills you." And you know they used fear to manipulate you and motivate you to take immediate action.

Ty: And so I take it that you were scared?

Chris: Of course; yes. Confused, scared, just you know bewildered, you know? Just a total—that time was very, very surreal and I was just kind of in a daze you know? I went into shock I think, mentally and emotionally.

Ty: What I've heard from other patients is that that's supposed to happen to someone else. But when it happens to you it's just the time when mentally it's hard to grasp.

Chris: Yeah and of course at any age it's not great to get diagnosed with a potentially life threatening or terminal illness. When you're 26 it's so far off the radar, I mean it just completely blindsided me so you know the next step was surgery and they said, "We got to get you in surgery right away," and they basically, I was like, "Okay you know I guess this is what I have to do." I didn't really know what else to do. And they—on New Year's Eve they took out a third of my large intestine, a third of my colon. You know, 18 cm or something like that, and I was in the hospital and doped up. My wife was laying in the bed next to me you know, keeping me company, and we were just, I mean, what do you do? You're just sort of trapped. And that's how I felt and the—they came in and said, "You know it's worse than we thought. You have stage three C," which, it had spread to lymph nodes. It was on its way to other organs, my liver or whatever.

Ty: Is that what the C means, spread to the liver?

Chris: Yeah the difference between B and C I really honestly don't know but I mean stage three typically means it's spread to lymph nodes. But then there's stage three A, B, and C, which, you can ask an oncologist. C is obviously worse than B.

Ty: But it's just shy of stage four?

Chris: Yes, yeah it's like one click away. Stage four means it's in another organ, okay, so it had not yet appeared in another organ. It was just in the lymph nodes trying to spread. So you know they took out the tumor, they took out a bunch of lymph nodes, the surgeon said, "Look I took out everything I could see. We got clear margins, but you're going to need 9 to 12 months of chemotherapy." So they brought an oncologist into the—into my hospital room to introduce me to him and I thought, "Okay well this is my life now and I guess I have to—I'm a cancer patient and I have to do what that entails." But there were a few things that happened in the hospital that were very serendipitous that really started the wheels turning. And one of them was the first meal that they served me.

Ty: And this is after you were—after your operation?

Chris: After my operation—

Ty: Where they removed 18 inches—

Chris: Yes they cut out 18 inches of my large intestines—18 cm, a third, right? And the first meal they served me was a sloppy Joe and I'm kind of famous for the sloppy Joe story because it's the most ridiculous food that you could serve a sick person, right? It's the best example of the worst cafeteria food, you know what I mean? What is the worst cafeteria food you can think of? It's a sloppy Joe. And that's what they gave me first meal, after, you know, cutting my abdomen open, removing part of my guts. And they set it in front of me and I was just looking at it going "This doesn't seem like the best thing for me right now."

Ty: Just innately you knew?

Chris: Yeah, right? I wouldn't even eat that—I wouldn't want to eat that any time, okay? I'm never in the mood for a sloppy Joe and so not only was I not really happy about that as a food choice but I just thought like, "This is like a hospital; this is full of sick people. Shouldn't they be feeding them better than this?" Like, "Shouldn't I be eating some applesauce or something?" At that time I really didn't know anything about nutrition but just my instincts you know, the red flag kind of went up. The next thing that happened was the day I was checking out from the hospital the surgeon came in to check on me and I said, "Hey you know is there anything I need to eat or avoid or whatever?" And—because I was a little concerned. I didn't want to go home and like eat something like some Doritos and like screw it up. And he was like "No, just don't lift anything heavier than a beer."

Ty: That was the nutritional advice you got?

Chris: Yep, that was it.

Ty: So where did that leave you mentally? Did you check out?

Chris: Confusing. No, I mean, it's like, wait a minute, really? Like I get it, he's trying to kind of pal around with me, and like hey, you know, but I was really concerned about my health, you know, and it mattered to me. And when—the sloppy Joe and then him saying "Don't lift anything heavier than a beer," no nutritional advice. I was really starting to think "What's wrong here? What is wrong with the medical system when there is such a huge disconnect between nutrition and health care," right? Health care needs to involve nutrition and they just didn't seem to think it mattered. And so I went home and I was thinking about my life, I was thinking about was I going to—how many birthdays was I going to see? Was I going to be able to have kids? I'm an only child; I was thinking about my parents and you know what it would be like to bury their only child. I thought about my wife and what it would be like to bury her husband and person that she's, you know, dated for six years and married to for two; so we've been together for eight years, a third of her life basically with me. Not that I'm super important but it's just, I'm important to a few people, you know? My parents and my wife.

And I thought about chemotherapy and this idea kept coming back to me about the fact that it was poison. And I couldn't understand poisoning my way back to health. Like I couldn't make sense of that and I thought, "I'm sick, why would I want to get sicker to get better," you know I just couldn't make sense of it. Now I understand there's a lot of very sophisticated explanations about why chemotherapy is a good thing but instinctively and intuitively I didn't like it; I didn't like the idea and I didn't want to do it.

Ty: Did you go to the oncologist and tell him why?

Chris: Well, I didn't want to do chemotherapy but I didn't know what else to do. And so it was at that point that my wife and I prayed and we've been praying. It's not the first time we prayed; we've been praying a lot but we prayed specifically together about my next steps. And I basically just said, "God if there is another way, just show me because I don't know what to do," you know I was really conflicted. And I needed an answer, you know and so I just said "If there's another way just show me" and two days later I got a book that was mailed to me from a man in Alaska, all the way to Memphis, Tennessee. I've never met this man to this day, it's been 10 years, but he knew my dad. And he was very bold and he sent me a book that was written by another man who had healed his own colon cancer using nutrition. Tons of raw food and juicing.

And as I started to read this book, turning the pages I was sitting at home on the couch one morning just reading it and I just choked up you know; I knew it was an answer to prayer, tears coming down my face. I was just like, "Thank you God; this is it." I asked for something else, right. I asked for another way and this is what I got. And so I was super excited, right? It's like there's times in life when you ask God for something and you just get a clear answer and it just happens so succinctly, right? Instantaneous, and you just know he's working, you know in your life and I just knew in that moment that he was, and so I called my wife at work and I was trying to tell her about the book and I was really excited and, "I'm not going to do chemo and I'm going to start juicing and start eating raw foods," and she just thought I was nuts you know? She was like "What do you mean you're not doing chemo? Of course you're doing chemo."

And then I started getting calls from family members. "We heard you were thinking about not doing chemo and you know you have to do chemotherapy. You really need to do what the doctors says because this is the best treatment they have and don't you think if they had something better they would be using it?" And when I heard things like that from people around me that made me very, very confused and I started to doubt that this was an answer to prayer and that this was even possible, that it was possible to heal the body. And that was very hard because I had all this pressure, new pressure from people who love me, right? They weren't against me, they love me and they care for me but they wanted me to follow the doctor's advice. And so I reluctantly agreed to go see an oncologist and we go—we're sitting in the clinic and—well first of all the parking lot is packed; couldn't even get a parking place. And the waiting room is packed. I sit down and I'm looking around and there's no one in there even remotely near my age. I'm 26 and I've got long shaggy hair, a handlebar mustache, like rock dude and I'm just kind of checking it out, who else is in the cancer club, it was me and a bunch of seniors—senior citizens, not high school or college seniors.
And I just thought "God I don't belong here." The television was on and out comes Jack Lalanne right as I'm sitting in the cancer clinic couch and he starts going off about nutrition and fruits and vegetables and the reason we're sick is because we're all eating junk food, right? And you need—if man made it, don't eat it. And I was like "Oh man he's just speaking to me through the television right now," like this is exactly—he's reaffirming everything that I just started to understand.

And we go into see the oncologist finally, it's like you wait in a waiting room for an hour, then they put you in a smaller waiting room for another hour and then you get in another little room. Eventually the oncologist comes in and it's just very robotic, you know they see 20 patients, 30 or 40 patients a day and he just comes in, he looked at my chart, I'm sure, for two minutes, "What's this guy got?" Comes in and gives me the standard pitch, he said, "Look you've got stage three colon cancer, you have—with therapies you have a 60 percent chance of living five years." And I thought—

Ty: At the age of 26, what did you think of those odds?

Chris: Yeah I mean I was not impressed by those odds and I thought "Gee that's not much better than a coin toss."

Ty: That's true.

Chris: Not much and I asked him if there were any alternative therapies available and he said, "No, there are none. If you don't do chemotherapy, you're insane."

Ty: He literally said "You're insane?"

Chris: Yeah, yeah. I asked him about the raw food diet and he said, "No, you can't do that, it'll fight the chemo."

Ty: Why would it fight the chemo?

Chris: At the time I was like, "What does that mean?" Well later, I realized I found out that raw food diet is a very aggressive detoxification diet and when you're on a raw food diet your body starts kicking out chemotherapy and it doesn't do what they want it to do. It doesn't destroy your body. And it doesn't do the damage they want it to do. And so they don't want you to go on a raw food diet. The other reason is because chemotherapy is also very destructive on your immune system and bacteria that's normally harmless on an apple let's say could pose a potential problems in your body because your immune system is so weak from chemo. So they won't let you—they don't want you to do raw food.

I was already on the raw food diet; I've been on it for a weak. I was like hard core. I'd just adopted it, right? I was excited about it, I felt going into the clinic, I felt very confident about what I was doing. And everything else he's told me, everything else the oncologist has said to me is really a blur because he really scared me so bad that I kind of shut down. And I walked into the clinic confident and I walked out terrified. And I went to the desk and I made an appointment to get a port put in to start chemotherapy.

And my wife and I walked out into the parking lot and we sat in her car and we held hands and we cried and we prayed and we were just terrified. And I believe that was on a Friday because I had a few days before they were supposed to put this port in; I think it might have been like a Monday or Tuesday or something.

Ty: And when you say a port that's—they're putting in a port so they can—they don't have to inject you with chemo; they can just put it directly into the port each time?

Chris: That's right; they put a port in your chest that's basically a direct line into your arteries or whatever your arteries so they can—it's easier than giving a—

Ty: IV.

Chris: Yeah, it destroys your veins so a port is a better way to do it because chemotherapy is so toxic that it destroys your veins. So yeah I—they just scared me so bad that I agreed to chemotherapy even though I had originally decided not to. And but over that weekend you know I kind of came to my senses again and I thought about my life and I thought about this book and I thought about Jack Lalanne and I thought about the weird stuff the oncologist said to me. One other thing he said, I forgot—he said sort of in the middle of his pitch he said, 'Look man," he said, "I'm not telling you this because I need your business." And I just thought, "Why in the world would you say that? What does business have to do with it, right?" And then I was "Wait, a minute, this is a business. This is his business. He needs patients to make money."

Ty: And this is the same oncologist that told you you were insane if you didn't do chemo?

Chris: That's right, same guy. And it was like a Freudian slip, you know what I mean? Either that or it was the push away, which is a sales technique and where they—you know you kind of give someone like, "I don't really need your business," and then it kind of makes them want to do business with you, you know what I mean? And—but I thought about everything and I thought you know what; nutrition makes more sense to me. I would rather overdose on nutrition and give my body everything that it can use to repair, regenerate and detoxify and heal and trust God to lead me in the process than let someone who doesn't even know me at all, probably has already forgotten my name, poison in me—poison me and experiment on me with a 60 percent chance of living five years.

I found out later that he was lying. When he told me was a—that I had a 60 percent chance of living five years, but that's the average for all cancer patients; so if you take every cancer patient, lump them into one group, and average it out, you get 60 percent of them make it to the five year mark. It doesn't mean they're cancer free in five years, it just means they have a beating heart. Some of them are on life support, right; some of them are knock, knock, knocking on Heaven's door, they are dying. But they still are counted as a success towards five year survival. Well the odds for stage three colon cancer stage three C were about 30 percent make it to five years. And only 16 percent make it 10 years.

Ty: Wow.

Chris: Here I am, 10 years without their therapies.

Ty: Okay so 10 years out and cancer free without—so you decided not to do chemotherapy?

Chris: That's right.

Ty: So before you got the port put in I assume?

Chris: I was a no-show for the port. After that they sent me a certified letter, they were calling my house, they were after me to try to get me to do—to do chemotherapy. And I just was, you know, avoiding their calls and like, "Leave me alone; I've made up my mind, this is what I'm doing."

Ty: Did you ever talk to the oncologist about the phony statistics or the incorrect statistics that he gave you because that was not accurate?

Chris: No, I never went back. And I know why he did it; he did it because he knew the truth was extremely discouraging. If he had come in and said, "Look with the therapies we have available you've got about a 30 percent chance of living five years," I would have been out the door in five seconds.

Ty: Right.

Chris: See ya, you know but he told me 60 percent because he thought, "Well maybe this will sound better; this will be more encouraging. Maybe it will give him more hope," right? It will make the treatment sound more appealing, right? 60 is way better than 30. So that's why I did it, you know? That's why I did it. It's just basic economics, you know? They need a steady supply of patients to make money, and you know doctors aren't bad people, but they're trained—they go to med school and they go to—they have residency and it takes 15 to 20 years for a doctor to go through all the training and actually go through enough practice before they realize that everything they've been trained to do doesn't really work and that most of their patients end up dying.

By that time it's too late to change careers and they're making a high six figure income. The average oncologist makes almost $300,000 a year. And yet in a survey that just came out about a month ago on Med Scape, 52 percent of oncologists reported that they were unsatisfied with their income.

Ty: Wow and they're making—the average makes over—

Chris: $290,000 a year.

Ty: That's a lot of money.

Chris: That's a lot of money to be unsatisfied.

Ty: That's not enough apparently.

Chris: So from there basically it was—I just—I was totally trusting in God to lead me at that point because it's like, "All right, everybody thinks I'm crazy. I'm alone, you know?" I was very much alone.

Ty: So once you made the decision to avoid chemo and to overdose on nutrition as you put it you told your family, what was your reaction like?

Chris: Well they—they weren't comfortable with it you know; they thought I was being stubborn and hard headed and foolish. My mom was a big supporter of me, she's always been—my mom has always been into health food. She's always been sort of a health junkie, and so she was a huge, huge ally for me at that time. And I love my wife, we're still married. We've been together 18 years and she was terrified—

Ty: Congratulations.

Chris: Thank you. She didn't know what to do, she didn't know how to help me and she really thought I was making a mistake and a lot of other people did too. But I had to trust that God was leading me, that he had answered my prayer, and if, so that I could trust that that was the route I—that would lead me ultimately to health. So I had very little support; I was very much alone in the beginning. But what's neat is my mom had a bunch of books about alternative cancer therapy and a bunch of books about health and stuff written by Paul Bragg and all kinds of these just great health books that she had collected over the years for no real reason and as soon as I started reading and researching and found out about different authors and books and health leaders and experts and I would mention them to her she'd say, "Oh I have that book." And I'm like, "You've got this library of books like for me," you know there was no other reason—she was like saving them up for me and I didn't realize it.

Ty: She was collecting them for you over the years and didn't know what the purpose was until now?

Chris: Yeah, yeah and it was stuff—obviously she was interested in them but she'd saved them all and so that was—that was amazing, I just knew God was in control. I knew he was working; so what did my diet look like? It was very simple and I think a hard core nutritional approach to cancer needs to be very simple because there are a lot of options out there, it can get very complicated and a lot of people have—they're seeing so many different directions they don't even know where to go and they get paralyzed.

And so I realized, "Okay, what is the most fundamental foundational part of my healing approach," and that's food. I've got to get as much nutrition in my body as I can from the earth. And so I started juicing and I drank about 64 ounces of vegetable juice every day, mostly carrot juice. I ate giant salads full of perciphorous (ph) and allium vegetables that's broccoli, cauliflower, kale, cabbage, onions, garlic, peppers, right? Just spinach, all that good stuff.

Ty: Sounds good.

Chris: Yeah, I mean the amazing giant salad you can—we shared one at Jason's Deli recently. Yeah, just a giant salad full of like all this really amazing food from the earth, that was put here for us and I ate that twice a day and I would eat fruit smoothies with a fresh coconut and berries, two cups of blueberries, blackberries, raspberries, strawberries; berries are very potent anticancer fruits. And that was it, that was the daily diet and it was every day and I did that for 90 days. It was 100 percent raw food for 90 days. I was working with a naturopath and he checked my blood work and my urine and my hair samples and all kinds of stuff and he helped me modify the diet and he had me on different supplements that he thought would help boost my immune system, help deal with any parasites or help detoxify, just sort of address those things that are common to a lot of cancer patients. Cancer is the product of a sick body. Now you're sick—you have cancer because you're sick, not the other way around.

Ty: So cancer is really the symptom?

Chris: Cancer is the symptom of sick body. And you cannot cut a tumor off or shrink a tumor or poison a tumor and expect to stay well and stay healthy because you're not addressing the real problem here, you're only addressing the symptom. And it's like cutting off your nose to get rid of a cold; it doesn't solve the real underlying problem.

Ty: Yeah I've not heard that before but it makes sense—

Chris: It's cause I made it up.

Ty: You got a runny nose so you cut it off.

Chris: Yeah and the problem is that most people think cancer is a physical problem and they treat it physically, right? With surgery, chemo, and radiation, they're treating a physical symptom, or they even maybe they, nutrition, and they're using nutrition and supplements to treat a physical problem and those are important things. There is a physical component that cancer is a life problem; it's mental, physical, emotional and spiritual. And what I tell cancer patients often is the reason you have cancer is because the way that you're living is killing you; the way you're living is killing you. And the only way to solve that problem is you have to change everything in your life, everything has to change.

Ty: You said cancer is a life problem; as you look back at your own personal story I remember that you mentioned that you had been eating—your diet was full of junk. So that apparently was a big component of your life? That was part of that life issue. What were other issues as you look back in retrospect that may have contributed other than the junk food you were eating what other issues might have been part of that cancer equation for you personally?

Chris: Well, it's hard to know what all caused or contributed, but what we do know from all the science that's been published, from the cancer industry, we know that we live in a world that's full of cancer causing toxins, they're in the environment, they're in the air we breathe, they're in the water we drink, they're sprayed on the food we eat. We're eating a nutrient deficient food that's mostly man made, processed junk food, right? So all of these—all these factors are all physical factors that affect the health of your body and ultimately suppress your immune system and create an environment in where cancer cells can thrive. Everyone has cancer cells in their body; the only permanent cure to cancer is your immune system. And nutrition gives your immune system the fire power it needs to keep you well. So without nutrition you're fighting with no weapons. Without your immune system you're fighting with no army. Chemotherapy destroys your army, destroys your immune system.

Not only that it causes secondary cancers in the body, it makes existing cancer stem cells more aggressive and it causes a host of lifelong, potentially life long damages to the body from brain damage to hearing loss to neuropathy with loss of the use of your hands and feet, to kidney and bladder damage. I mean bone damage, heart damage, lung damage; it's just total collateral damage from chemotherapy and I didn't know that in 2004, but I researched it for 10 years and it's mind blowing how destructive it is and yet we've been conditioned to accept that this is the way you treat cancer. And you have to suffer, right? Cancer is a battle. If we frame it as a battle and use the war analogy, right the war on cancer, it's a cancer battle. You got to fight cancer, right? You got to be a warrior. The reason all that—all of those terms are necessary is because the current model of cancer treatment involves suffering. So if you believe you're fighting then it means it makes suffering necessary. If you believe it's a fight and it's a battle and you're at war, right? And it, cognitively the cancer patient is more likely to accept it if they're told it's a battle, it's a fight and you have to suffer. The truth is you don't have to suffer, and you will not suffer from nutrition. Nutrition will only do you good.

Ty: I like your analogy earlier that—or your statement that cancer is a result of a sick body and not vice versa. So this is a bit rhetorical then so I'm gathering from you that in light of all of the different symptoms, in light of all of the different—let me say that again. From gathering from you in light of all of the different problems that chemotherapy causes in a body that you're not a big fan of that in light of the fact that it makes the body sicker and if cancer is a result of a sick body and we're treating with something that makes the body sicker, there's not a lot of wisdom in that.

Chris: I don't see it; it doesn't make sense to me and I think what's amazing is so many cancer patients when they're diagnosed and they're told they need chemotherapy almost all of them don't want to do it. Instinctively they don't want to do it; they don't want to be poisoned, they don't want to suffer, they don't want to get sicker but everyone tells them they have to and so they reluctantly agree to do it and for most of them it doesn't end well. They get a treatment or series of treatments and there will be a very short window of time where they—the doctors can't find any tumors and so they'll say, "You're in remission, you're cancer free. Yay, right? We see celebrity headlines all the time, "I'm cancer free now after having a tumor cut off," right? But the truth is you're not cancer free, you still have cancer cells in your body. You still have a sick body, you still have a depleted immune system and it's just a matter of time before new tumors form. And it's really sad to watch cancer patients go through this process of, "Oh I'm in remission," and they think everything is great and they go back to normal life. And in a few months later they have another scan and there's a new spot or several or it's migrated from what started as a tiny lump in one breast is now in their brain, in their liver, spots on their bones, in their lungs and we know that's from the chemotherapy. It's causing it to spread, it's making it more aggressive and it's causing secondary cancers in the body—radiation as well.

Ty: Yeah that was my next question is do you think that it's related to the chemotherapy?

Chris: We know it is because of the industry studies. The studies that have come from the cancer industry tell us that chemotherapy is carcinogenic, it causes secondary cancers. It's—there are many chemotherapy drugs that are known carcinogens and listed by the US National Toxicology Board as carcinogens that cause cancer.

Ty: So why don't the doctors tell the patients about the fact that thee chemotherapy agents that are being used could cause further cancers, or do they?

Chris: Most doctors are good people, but you know there's good people and bad people in the world. There's good doctors and bad doctors in the world. Just assuming all doctors are good for the sake of this conversation, they're trapped in a system that pays them very well to do three things, surgery, chemo, and radiation. And they don't have the freedom to use nutrition, right, or what people call alternative therapies, which are really just other non-toxic therapies, right? It's not like they're experimenting on patients with nerve gas, right? But they don't have the freedom to use anything else and if they do they risk losing their license and losing their income and their job. And so I think there's a lot of well-meaning doctors out there that are really hoping that "cure" is developed soon, right? Because in the meantime all they can do is prescribe chemotherapy drugs, watch their patients suffer and eventually most of their patients die. And they have to celebrate these small victories like, "Well, we shrunk a tumor, yay," right? And they have to find some kind of comfort or job satisfaction in their ability to shrink a tumor, you know, it's not in curing cancer and it's—so again I can empathize with oncologists because I feel like they've probably gone into it with very high hopes and good intentions and it takes 20 years to realize, "Oh these treatments don't really work and most of my patients aren't restoring their health and going back to normal lives and they're living cancer free."

Ty: Do you think that—pause one second. Okay, do you think that most oncologists, or even just normal medical doctors, do they have an education in nutrition that they would be able to properly advise someone on how to regain or maintain their health through nutritional advice and through traditional protocols?

Chris: It appears that doctors get almost zero nutritional training. The vast majority of medical schools, the curriculum is really underwritten by the pharmaceutical industry. Doctors are trained on anatomy that they need to understand the human body and then they're trained how to prescribe drugs and memorizing which drugs do what in the body. And then if they become specialists they may be trained in radiotherapy or they may be trained in surgery, obviously, trauma care. By the way trauma care is where medicine is at it's absolute best. If I get a gunshot wound or break a leg, I'm going to the emergency room and that's where doctors do amazing things. But doctors that are involved in chronic disease management like heart disease, diabetes, and cancer, they're really just prescribing drugs that don't work and alleviate symptoms, but they don't heal the body. They don't solve the real problem; they just make you a little more comfortable living with the problem.

Ty: And as you said earlier they might actually cause more symptoms.

Chris: Well we know that there are hundreds, if not thousands, of side effects caused by pharmaceutical drugs. I mean it's too many to even talk about, but any pharmaceutical drug is an unnatural substance, it's a chemical that was never meant to be put in the body and it causes a—an unnatural biochemical reaction in the body that will have unintended side effects. And some of those are cancer; look at—watch television. Actually I don't recommend you watch television, but if you watch television you will see prescription drug ads and at the end of every drug ad you'll hear a disclaimer about all of the side effects it may include and many of them say, “May include cancer,” “May cause cancer." So here's a drug for your restless legs, which by the way can be completely solved with diet change, but it also may give you cancer.

Ty: It's funny you mention that because we don't watch a lot of television but when my kids see a commercial we always watch the drug commercials because of the fact that I've tried to teach them you know, “Listen to what the side effects are,” and it's really mind blowing. As a matter of fact sometimes you'll have a drug that is used to treat X, Y, Z that actually in the list of side effects may cause X, Y, Z.

Chris: Well, yeah, chemotherapy will be one of those. It's true—it's just unfortunate because money is really the driver of medicine. Money is the driver and we live in a world where there are, the industry is trying to promote itself and rebrand itself as science based medicine. And the truth is it's not science based; it's patent based and it's profit based because the only science they're interested in is science that will lead to the development of a patentable highly profitable drug. They ignore the huge body of scientific evidence on nutrition, it's completely ignored. And yet medicine tries to claim that it's science based but again it's ignoring nutritional science and lifestyle medicine. So it's a pretty bogus claim but you'll see—there's people out there with blogs and whatever claiming to be all about science and they use this blog as the platform to promote conventional therapy, surgery, and drugs. And—but they ignore all nutritional science and so you know there's a journal called nutrition and cancer, it's been published since 1979, medical journal. You're not going to see any studies from that published on some of these websites that claim to be all about science.

Ty: So they're very selective.

Chris: Absolutely, and you know that a lot of the science is fraud. A lot of the science is fraud science that has to do with the development of drugs because you look at the number of drug recalls that happen every year. You look at the side effects that happen with drugs and you look at the fact that the FDA panels consist of many conflict of interest researchers that work to develop a drug and then sit on a panel with the FDA that's supposed to be neutral to get that drug approved.

Ty: Isn't that illegal?

Chris: It's not illegal in the US; it should be, it's unethical and there's a huge conflict of interest and they have to disclose their conflict in these drug studies, a lot of the researchers that promote drugs and do studies to show that the drugs work, they're effective. Also have to disclose that they work for the drug company but no one seems to mind. Just like, "Oh that's fine, no problem." I'm sure they wouldn't have any reason to manipulate the data on this study; they're income has nothing to do with the results of this study. So it really is a really—it's mind blowing how much money has influenced medicine and how little real truth is out there in the medical world, it's all built on how can we make the most money off of sick people. What procedures, what drugs make the most money and how can we sell more of them?

Ty: That's sad and disturbing.

Chris: Yeah, and that's why nutrition is never going to be a part of conventional medicine, because there's no money in it. There's no money in broccoli, there's no money in green tea, there's no money in blueberries. They're amazing for you, right? Amazing for your body—they have so many nutritional components, vitamins, minerals, nutrients, enzymes, antioxidants, and thousands of chemicals that exist in plants and fruits and vegetables, beans, nuts, grains that all support your health. You don't even need to understand the studies, you don't even have to read the research if you don't want to. You don't even need to know the science, you just need to know put them in your body, eat them, right? By the way I don't own a grocery store; I'm not selling fruits and vegetables—

Ty: Right, so you can tell the truth?

Chris: Yeah, I've got no financial incentive to tell people to eat fruits and vegetables.

Ty: You mentioned earlier that this is an industry that's based on patents and profits so while we're using iterations tell me a bit about the relationship between sugar and stress and cancer?

Chris: Yeah stress is a major component and we haven't even talked about this in the interview, I'm so glad you brought it up because what are three causes of cancer? If we're looking at the three main causes its pollution, right? Environmental toxins, diet and lifestyle, right? Unhealthy diet and lifestyle choices are going to produce sickness and disease in your body eventually. The smoker who gets cancer, right? Hello, obesity is the number two cause of cancer, smoking is number one. Those are diet and lifestyle choices but the third major cause is stress and stress is a huge topic but what happens is stress comes from negative emotions, it comes from unforgiveness, it comes from bitterness and resentment and all negativity in your mind and in your life, raises your anxiety, it raises your stress which starts in your mind being anxious, but that translates into your body. It raises your stress hormones to cope and that's adrenaline and cortisol and those hormones are immunosuppressant. The cortisol tells your liver to dump sugar into your bloodstream to give you energy, that's what that nervous energy is, stress energy. It's because cortisol is dumping sugar into your bloodstream, but then it cause intense sugar cravings to replenish. This is why there are such—this is why the term "comfort food" was coined because people that are stressed seek high sugar foods because they're living on stress energy, they're depleting their sugar reserves. Glucose, really glycogen, which is glucose, and they need to replenish it with sugar and so in our world the nearest source of sugar is soft drinks and junk food and pizza and ice cream. And so that—the relationship between stress and stress makes you eat crap food. When you're stressed you make bad choices. You make irrational, impulsive and illogical choices not only about the food you eat but just in life in general you make bad choices and fear is a major stress emotion and when cancer patients are afraid and they're stressed they make illogical and irrational decisions and they agree to therapies and treatments that they look back on and say "What was I thinking; why did I let them do that to me?" And I hear that all the time from cancer patients. "I don't know why I would ever let them give me chemo; I never wanted to do it." And now the cancer is back and it's spread and it's worse and the chemo was a total waste, it did nothing for me and pretty sure it made me worse, hear that all the time. And why? Because fear is so powerful and stress is so powerful and it affects the way you think and the decisions you make.

Ty: So and then that's something—that's something that many people don't really get that relationship between stress, between fear that emotional relationship and that's something I've heard consistently over this interview series where people have been diagnosed with cancer from doctors that treat cancer is that there is a big emotional component to cancer and that when you clear that out that's a big step towards recovering. So let me ask you this, last question, what is the typical Chris Wark diet each day because I would ask you what you recommend that people eat because I know that you're eating is the way that you would think people should eat to avoid or to recover from cancer because I know you practice what you preach?

Chris: Yeah and again I do want to acknowledge that something you said is so important; it's not all about diet. Diet is one important component in maintaining health, right? There's three, you got to—if you're working in a chemical factory, eating a healthy diet like Chris Wark, it'll help you but you've got to get out of the chemical factory, you know what I mean? You know if you're living with tons of chronic stress in your life, if you've got—you're in an unhealthy work environment and toxic relationships and you have unresolved emotional conflicts with people in your past those are very powerfully health destructive forces. But the diet is one part of that puzzle and it's very important; so how do I eat now? The diet that I eat today is basically the same diet I've eaten for 10 years; it's 90 to 95 percent plant based. So I eat a little bit of animal protein. Clean, organic, wild or free range or wild caught type animal proteins—that's about three times a week. And the rest of the food I eat is fruits, vegetables, beans, grains, food from the earth.

Ty: And those sloppy Joes—

Chris: I haven't had a sloppy Joe since the hospital in December 2003.

Ty: So that's the diet basically you started out eating when you wanted to overdose on nutrition and treat your cancers that you're continuing to eat today?

Chris: Absolutely. Now I don't juice as hardcore today as I did then, I'm not drinking 64 ounces of vegetable juice a day; that's a medicinal food, right? I don't think that health requires juicing 64 ounces a day for the rest of your life; I don't think that's necessary. But I love to juice and I love to drink fresh juice and I make smoothies, and I eat oatmeal and I eat cooked veggies and I eat raw veggies and I eat you know lots of fruit. So anything from the earth, I eat rice and beans, I eat sweet potatoes; if it comes from the earth, yes I'll eat it as long as it's non GMO and it's organic then that passes my sniff test.

Ty: I've heard it if God made it's good; if man made it, it's madness.

Chris: I like that.

Ty: Whatever you're doing Chris it's working; you look like you're the picture of health and I really appreciate you taking the time to talk to us today; your story has been inspiring to me and I know it's going to encourage people that are watching.

Chris: Thank you Ty.

[end of transcript]

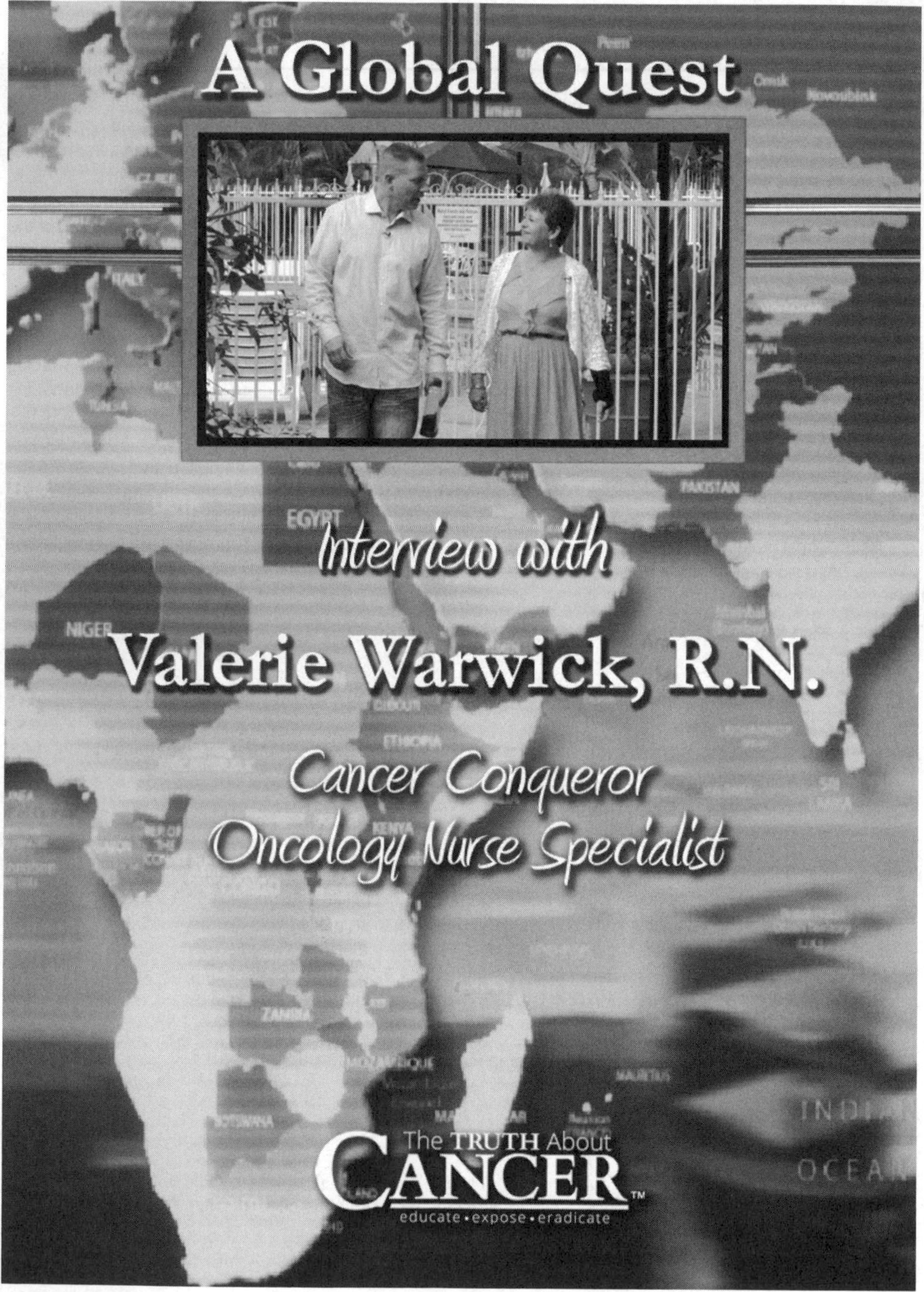
A Global Quest
Interview with
Valerie Warwick, R.N.
Cancer Conqueror
Oncology Nurse Specialist
The TRUTH About
CANCER
educate • expose • eradicate

Valerie: There's been some so-called progress, but really mortality and morbidity have not changed at all, and have not improved. With all the money that we're pouring into Relay for Life and Komen, really it hasn't helped change things for the patients.

Ty: And so you saw that first-hand as an oncology nurse for 17 years.

Valerie: I did.

Ty: So what was it? Was it like a trigger that eventually you said, "I've had enough of this, this is not working. There's got to be a better way." Did anything happen in your life that triggered that or was it kind of a slow progression?

Valerie: It was somewhat of a slow progression. I started to change my diet and improve my health just by shopping at the farmer's market and I saw how it totally changed my health. And I started looking at the patients differently, and seen that they needed nutrition. When my best friend from childhood was diagnosed with cancer, I started searching for answers for her because I knew that the chemotherapy was toxic and that she was going to suffer greatly and that it would not, it would not cure her. It was not going to cure her. It would just make her sick. So that was really the pivoting point when I changed my focus and really started to search for other answers.

Ty: You mentioned nutrition, they needed nutrition. Is that something that they didn't get from the doctors that you noticed?

Valerie: No, they didn't get any nutrition. They were fed really nutrient-depleted foods that were really unhealthy. Because cancer cells have so many more glucose receptors, they're sugar-obligate feeders. They're hungry for sugar and they were just eating way too many carbs and sugars, and processed foods. They were really low in nutrition, and actually in traditional oncology, they tell patients don't eat rough fruits and vegetables. So they really kind of discourage them from eating vegetables.

Ty: Because of the fallacy that you shouldn't take any oxidants, right? One of the reasons.

Valerie: You're right. And they're worried about the microbes because the chemotherapy totally wipes out your immune system. So they're worried about the microbes that might be on the vegetables and fruits, and getting infections.

Ty: Let's talk about the wisdom, or the lack thereof, in that kind of approach to cancer. Don't eat vegetables that are healthy because the microbes might harm you because we just — what did they just do with the chemo to your immune system? What does chemo do to your immune system?

Valerie: Yeah, they just destroy your immune system, and really the key to overcoming cancer and getting your health back is in your gut and your immune system. And if you destroy your immune system, that's the very thing that you need to heal. So you may kill the cancer cells in your body with the chemo because, yes, it's going to kill those, it's going to kill everything. It's like dropping an A-bomb on your body and then expecting health to rebound when really when you know in a garden, when you fill it with pesticides, all you're going to get back is weeds. So you need to rebuild your immune system and support your body in healing itself because it knows how to do that.

Ty: Could that be one of the reasons, inevitably, when people get on chemotherapy that six, 12, 18 months later, the cancer comes back because of the fact that the chemo destroyed the immune system.

Valerie: Exactly. Cancer wants to survive. It's part of your body. It wants to survive, and it'll make adjustments to do that. So it gets smart. It'll put up markers and different pathways so that it can continue to grow.

Ty: But the doctors typically, in your experience, 17 years as a nurse in the oncology department, the doctors don't talk about nutrition. Chiefly — well, they don't know about nutrition, number one. In the

Quest for the Cures Continues last year, we talked about the fact that doctors don't get educated on nutrition when they're in medical school. But also, when we look at it from a financial perspective, is it more lucrative for them to go natural or to go toxic?

Valerie: Oh, right because they're getting kickbacks from the drug companies when they use their products.

Ty: So the doctors get kickbacks using …?

Valerie: That's primarily where their income comes from is making money on the chemotherapies.

Ty: So they literally get kickbacks on the chemo. So they're very incentivized, then, to prescribe it because they make money on it.

Valerie: Right. And it's really, legally, their only option because that's all they can do. They're limited in their practice to only prescribe those pharmaceuticals. And it's really …

Ty: They're hamstrung.

Valerie: It's not their decision.

Ty: They're hamstrung.

Valerie: Yeah. It's not even a creative medical art where the doctor individually treats each person. They're going by a recipe that's already prescribed for you according to what you're diagnosed with, and each individual, each cancer is different, each person is different. And the cause of the cancer may be different from each person. Someone might have toxic metals in their mouth, infections, viral infections.

So each person is different, and the art of medicine has been taken away from physicians, and they are restricted in their practice anymore by just prescribing this drug for that problem. It doesn't matter who you are or what's going on with you, they don't even have to see your face. They just hear two seconds and they're already, "Okay, that's what you're going to get."

Ty: And so, I guess that's one of the reasons that we don't see a very good success rate with the chemotherapy and the radiation and those type of treatments because, in essence, they've not really corrected any kind of a root problem. They've really treated a symptom.

Valerie: Right. They're not correcting the root problem, and they're treating from the top down, so really they just want to suppress your symptoms. We're going to suppress your symptoms. We're going to give you toxic drugs to kill all the cancer cells, right. But really if you don't correct the root problem and deal with the whole environment of the body, you're not going to heal. And then you destroy the immune system on top of that.

Ty: Right. And really from what I've learned over the past couple of years interviewing doctors and in my own research, the compromised immune system, oftentimes, is the primary cause for the cancer. Your immune system's compromise allows the cancer to get a foothold. So what can we do? Let's say if somebody's watching this that is undergoing chemotherapy — because a lot of people just don't know. They're learning about this for the first time now. What can people do to rebuild that immune system after they've undergone chemotherapy?

Valerie: There are immune therapies that — well, first of all, lab testing. So you want to get lab testing to measure, to see if you have circulating cancer stem cells for one. That's very important because you need to then get some immune therapy to reboot your immune system, whether it's medicinal mushrooms, or the GcMAF or Bravo probiotics. You want to make sure your vitamin D level is up between 70 and 100. That's very important because low vitamin D levels virtually shut down your immune system.

Ty: Now you just mentioned two things I want to touch on. Probiotics, very important from what I've learned because your immune system, 70 percent generated in your gut, you destroy that floor with vaccines, GMO foods, antibiotics, also with chemotherapy. You got to rebuild it, so that's a great suggestion. You mentioned GcMAF. Talk about GcMAF that stands for macrophage activating factor, and you mentioned to me before we sat down here that there was a European clinic that recently got raided.

Valerie: Yeah, the GcMAF clinic is over in Europe, and their version of the FDA came into their lab and took all their product, all their medicine, and took all their lab equipment, seized all their bank accounts and virtually shut them down. They were helping thousands of patients reboot their immune system. They were helping kids with autism. They were an answer to cancer, and they shut them down.

Ty: That was something that Dr. Connelly, last year in *Quest for the Cures* mentioned GcMAF, that's one of the treatments that she uses, and I believe that the place that she was getting her product from is the lab that they raided.

Valerie: Right.

Ty: So now we don't have access to this. Macrophage activating factor, this is a natural substance. There were no known side effects.

Valerie: No.

Ty: What was the supposed cause that they raided the lab because I heard about that happening here in the United States, but this happened over in Europe? What was the supposed reason to shut them down?

Valerie: Well, they said that their product was contaminated, but they used the same testing facilities that the pharmaceutical drug companies used to test their products, and they went through nine tests before it ever got to the public. And they were all A-1. Never had any contamination issues. So it was just a made-up story.

Ty: It sounds like they were trying to get rid of some competition.

Valerie: Yeah. They don't want anybody treating cancer and curing cancer.

Ty: Well, it cuts into the revenue stream, and that's another common thread that I learned last year from a lot of medical doctors, even, that were saying, "Follow the money. Follow the money. You'll find out why we're making these decisions."

And you mentioned sunlight. Very great for the immune system. Studies have shown sunlight, the vitamin D that's generated from the cholesterol in your skin mixed in with the UV rays produces the vitamin D3. Great at protecting against cancer. So let's talk about that because you hear today, "Stay out of the sun. Sun's your enemy." In reality, why do we have so much skin cancer?

Valerie: Oh, yeah, because we're low on vitamin D, which puts us at horrible risk, and we're low in vitamin C. So, being in the sun in really important. You don't, of course, want to fry in the sun, but you need to get out in the sun. We're always indoors, and we're seeing the majority of people are super low in their vitamin D. They're about 30, some are 20. This is scary because it puts you at risk for disease. So you really need to make sure your vitamin D level is up.

Ty: And you've got the sunscreens. Can you talk about some of the chemicals that are in the sunscreens that are actually carcinogenic?

Valerie: Yeah. Yep, that's right. They are carcinogenic.

Ty: I think there's one chemical called OMC. I can't think of what it — it's a long medical name for this chemical, but it's a known carcinogen. We know that it causes cancer, and I believe that OMC is in over 90 percent of the sunscreens. So we are just lathering on sunscreen to protect us from something that could cure cancer, and absorbing through our skin carcinogenic chemicals that cause cancer. No wonder we have such high rates of skin cancer today. I've interviewed folks that said the reason that the skin cancer rates are so high is because of the sunscreens.

Valerie: Right, right. They're totally toxic chemicals. They're overburdenning the body and harming the immune system. So there we go again, putting toxins on our body and really hurting our immune system. When we think we're protecting ourselves, we're not. We're not.

Ty: Right. Right. Can you talk about some early detection methods for cancer because we're going to hear in October, "Go get your mammograms." You got all these detection methods that are really harmful, but there's a lot of natural ways that we can detect cancer that are — non-toxic ways that we can detect cancer.

Valerie: Right. So in allopathic medicine, their early detection is like a colonoscopy, a mammogram, maybe some tumor markers, MRIs, PET scans. But they really only detect cancer when it's fairly advanced. So you want to do early — true early detection comes with lab work, getting — there are labs available today that your doctor probably isn't aware of that aren't paid for by insurance, unfortunately, but there are labs that can detect cancer far earlier when it's just in the microcirculation and when it's much easier to treat. In fact, if the Food and Drug Administration was really looking out for the folks, we'd all have it with our physicals, and we could detect cancer far earlier. But those labs are available today.

Ty: You talking about ONCOblot?

Valerie: ONCOblot and the RGCC.

Ty: These are labs that would be overseas then?

Valerie: I think they are overseas, but there are doctors here that, in the States, that will draw the blood and send it over for you. It's fairly easy.

Ty: You mentioned mammograms. What do you think about thermography?

Valerie: Thermography's great. Thermography can detect heat, which is produced by inflammation in the body. So you can use a mammogram to detect breast cancers probably eight years before …

Ty: Thermogram, you mean.

Valerie: Yeah, thermogram — eight years before a mammogram will pick it up. And the mammogram causes cancer. So every year a woman goes in to get her mammogram she increases her risk of breast cancer because of the radiation exposure, which a thermogram does not have.

Ty: So that sounds like a little bit better of a choice for a female that's supposed to be getting your mammograms, right.

Valerie: Yeah.

Ty: Go get your mammograms. Get your thermogram and you can detect it years earlier, and not have the detrimental effects of the ionizing radiation.

Valerie: Right. Exactly.

Ty: Talk about stress on the immune system and cancer.

Valerie: Yeah. Stress really diminishes the immune system because it increases your cortisol, which suppresses your immune system, which depletes your melatonin, your vitamin C, your niacins. So there's this big cascade actually where chronic, continuous stress will deplete your micronutrients.

Ty: And then that has a kind of cascading effect.

Valerie: Right, and raise your cortisol levels, really.

Ty: And once the cortisol raises, then the cascade happens. And then, I've seen the studies where they show that a minute of anger, a minute of stress actually depletes your immune system for a period of hours.

Valerie: Right. Right. And sugar. Eating sugar will shut down your immune system for four hours after you eat it. So when you eat a high-sugar breakfast, your immune system is shut down for four hours right in time for lunch. And so you do it again.

Ty: So when we're feeding our children the breakfast cereal that has all this added sugar, we just basically cripple their immune system until they eat lunch.

Valerie: Right. Right. It's so horrible, and we really need to get back to eating whole foods and really need to take it seriously shopping at the farmer's market for our families because what they're offering in the supermarkets is poison. Our children are really at risk, our grandchildren are really at risk now because the foods are all packaged and they have no nutrients. So we're overall micronutrient depleted. Our bodies have nothing to work with. That's really important too, to teach our kids the important of whole foods and to buy non-GMO foods to protect our bodies.

Ty: Non-GMOs key.

Valerie: Yeah, it sure is.

Ty: Because we learned about the GMO foods over the last two years, the way that they do cross cancer. I think you're right. Education is the key. That's one of the things that we're about here with *The Truth About Cancer*, is to educate the masses. And if we can educate the next generation about the truth of nutrition and all of these natural healing modalities we're going to be a lot better off.

Valerie: Yes.

Ty: Last question for you. Speaking of nutrition, one superfood that many folks don't know is a superfood is hemp.

Valerie: Oh, that's right.

Ty: It's a super food. It's like chlorella or spirulina. So talk about hemp. It's not only a superfood, but actually as a treatment for cancer.

Valerie: Right. That really opened my eyes when I started hearing stories of people that used cannabis oil and they didn't have cancer anymore. I met two people in one day — one was a nurse who had lymphoma, just randomly, two people I met one day. A nurse who had lymphoma started using cannabis oil. And she had — yeah, lymphoma and it was gone in four months. And then a few hours later I met another gentleman who had tongue cancer, had metastasized to the jaw and they wanted to remove half his jaw, some of his tongue. And he said, "No." He was a pretty young man, and he used the cannabis oil and it was gone in four months.

Ty: What is it about the cannabis oil that does the healing? Was it the high CBD oil or was it THC?

Valerie: They used high THC and high CBD oil.

Ty: Okay. So they had both.

Valerie: Yeah.

Ty: So that would then be available in the states that allow medical marijuana, right.

Valerie: Medical marijuana.

Ty: But not in the other states.

Valerie: Not in the other states.

Ty: Because unfortunately, when you have the high THC, the Delta-9-Tetrahydrocannabinol, that's the psychoactive component that they've made illegal in many states.

Valerie: Right. And I think that's changing as people learn more about cannabis and its medicinal properties. People are going to vote for it because they want the medicine for their families. It's a wonderful medicine.

Ty: It is changing. I see the tide turning when it comes to cannabis. I don't even like to call it marijuana because that sounds sinister.

Valerie: Yeah, it has a negative connotation.

Ty: Well, yeah, actually, the truth of the matter is that in the 1930s, the DEA coined the term 'marijuana' to make it sound sinister.

Valerie: Yeah. Yeah.

Ty: And in reality, what we have is a very high-nutrient, medicinal plant.

Valerie: Good for so many things: anti-inflammatory, autoimmune problems, cancer.

Ty: Epilepsy.

Valerie: Epilepsy. Seizures. Yes. Yeah, yeah.

Ty: That's awesome. So you're a big proponent of medicinal hemp.

Valerie: I am. I am. I am. For sleep.

Ty: I am too, and, you know, I didn't use to be. I didn't use to be. I believed the propaganda years and years ago that, "Oh, we need to stay… this is an evil weed." But I now believe that we should call it "heavenly hemp."

Valerie: Yeah, that's right. So I just want to let people know that are facing cancer, that are newly diagnosed, that they do have options and there are science-based labs that can help guide them in their treatment. They can get personalized treatment. They don't have to take the chemo and the radiation and when you really think about intuitively what feels right to you, poisoning your body goes against that. Intuitively, you know that that's not really the right way to go, that your body needs a…

Ty: You mean cancer is not a deficiency of chemotherapy?

Valerie: No. No, it's actually probably a nutrient deficiency, and different viruses, and toxic. We're toxic. We're toxic. So we just need to get rid of those toxins and support our immune system so that it can do its job.

Ty: And then the body heals itself when you give it the proper nutrients and when you detoxify. And that's coming from a lady that was a registered nurse in the oncology department for 17 years.

Valerie: Yes.

Ty: So you know what you're talking about.

Valerie: Yes.

Ty: That's awesome.

Valerie: Yeah, I do. Took me a while.

Ty: You know, I'm so glad that you stepped outside the box and that you're now on the side of health and healing, and your story's really encouraging. I saw you initially interviewed by Chris Warwick, and I said, "I've got to interview her," because your story is so compelling because you're someone that's been on the other side for a long time, and you've seen the way that the big three treatments are just devastating the people. And now you're doing the best you can to help people, to educate them about the real treatments for cancer. So I really appreciate you.

Valerie: Thanks so much, Ty. I'm so glad to be on this side. I really am.

Ty: I'm glad you're on the team. We got to go educate the world.

Valerie: That's right.

Ty: Yeah, well, thank you for your time today, Val. Really appreciate it.

Valerie: Thank you so much.

Ty: God bless you.

Valerie: All right. You too.

[end of transcript]

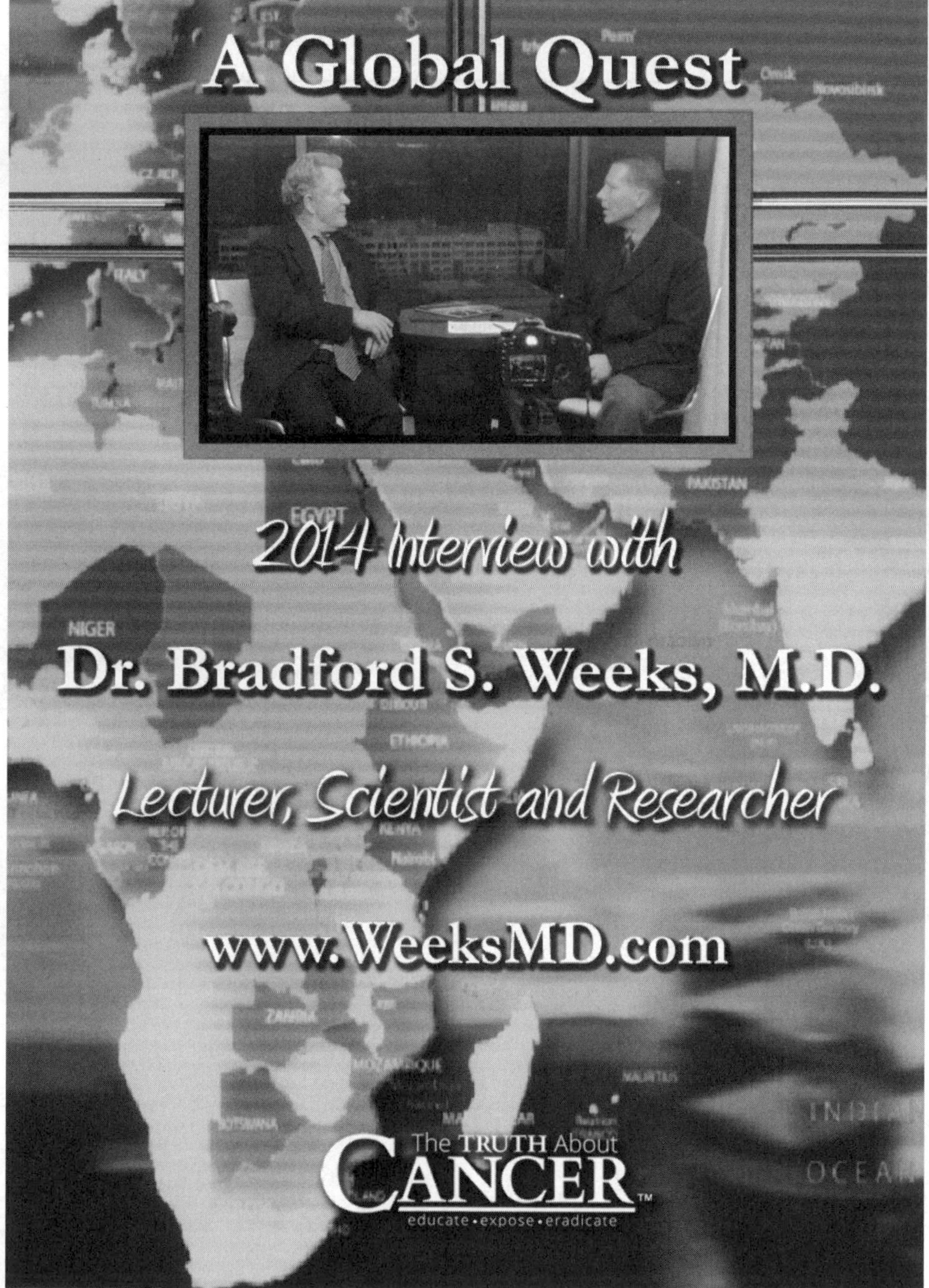
A Global Quest
2014 Interview with
Dr. Bradford S. Weeks, M.D.
Lecturer, Scientist and Researcher
www.WeeksMD.com
The TRUTH About CANCER
educate • expose • eradicate

THE TRUTH ABOUT CANCER

Ty: Okay. I'm here on a beautiful night in the "City of Angels" with Dr. Brad Weeks. Dr. Weeks, thank you for joining us.

Dr. Weeks: Ty, great to be here.

Ty: I look forward to getting some of the information out of your head about cancer treatments tonight.

Dr. Weeks: I am going to have to filter through my heart—heart warm thinking.

Ty: I will take it. I think that is a good process. So before we get into that, tell us a little about yourself, what you would want the viewers to know.

Dr. Weeks: I feel like a really fortunate person. I have been able to practice medicine for 25 years and it is a real honor to be able to help people who are suffering. A lot of people get up in the morning and they are not sure what their life has for them. My challenge has been to try to help people. Just a great honor. My wife, Laura, has been a fabulous supporter. I got four wonderful daughters so I feel like I am a pretty fortunate man.

Ty: You are. I have got four children. It is a blessing to have children and a great wife to support you.

Dr. Weeks: Especially you know when you are doing integrative holistic medicine we are always being, criticized is a light word. Attacked is maybe a more realistic word. We are innovators. We are ahead of the curve. We are doing things which I think are the, better than the standard of care. That is a tough situation for the family to be in because it is always a situation that people who are doing something different can be criticized. It is kind of an exciting time in medicine. I have been able to play a role which I am really excited about in helping bring innovative safe and effective treatment. I call them centsible. CENT centsible. It is cheap, effective and cost effective.

Ty: I like that word—"centsible."

Dr. Weeks: I am enjoying it.

Ty: So you talk about a standard of care. What do you mean by standard of care with cancer treatments?

Dr. Weeks: It is a really problematic reality. The standard of care is something which is not definable and yet it is used as an instrument for keeping doctors compliant with what could be called consensus. The real definition, what a reasonable doctor would do in a situation. But it is always something which the innovative doctors have to really exceed in order to stay helping patients. Conventional doctors are held to a conventional standard of care, but if we are doing something different we have to be much safer and much more effective in order to be able to offer that to patients. And what irritates me, Ty, is that it really should be between the patient and the doctor. If I can explain a concept to a patient where I clarify the risks and the benefits, even if it is for example a non-conventional cancer treatment, not a chemo, or not radiation, not surgery, I think in America still the patient should be allowed to choose that. The standard of care says not. There is a standard of care and the doctor must not vary his or her practice from that. I think the real issue is that the patient should be able to choose once they are fully and freely informed. Not happening today. It is a big challenge as you know.

Ty: Yes it is. So the standard of care in traditional well I say traditional, it's funny—the treatments that have been going for less than a 100 years are not really traditional. But in the typical treatments for cancer in the United States chemo, radiation and surgery.

Dr. Weeks: Right. And it is illogical because the, most cancer patients would say, I went for chemo and the doctor and the nurse told me any calorie is a good calorie. Eat this cake, eat this cookie, eat this donut, just keep the weight on. Totally oblivious to the very well-articulated, clearly demonstrated biochemical truths about, don't eat sugar, don't feed the cancer. I'm not a fan of the current standard of care for cancer. I can assure you that most oncologists, if they are honest with you, would say the same thing. They might say it is the best they have, but they are not happy with it. I don't think anybody is happy with 2.1 or 2.3 percent benefit over five years, which is what the research shows chemotherapy will give to an adult. My situation is that the standard of care is clearly something which needs to be improved upon with cancer. No one would disagree with that. The question is how can we let science and reason bring us forward into a new era of patient care?

Ty: What do you think about the quote I have heard many times from several doctors that most cancer patients today actually die from the treatments as opposed to the cancer itself?

Dr. Weeks: That has been—it is not a new idea. That has been clearly described in many publications. It is not surprising because these are toxic treatments. What I say to my clients when they go to see an oncologist is, ask the oncologist a couple of questions. One, ask the oncologist how they plan to take care of the patient while killing cancer. So we know it is a truism in surgery that the surgeon can really say, the surgery was successful, but the patient died. The surgeon can do a good job, and if the patient dies, it could be the anesthesiologist or something else. So it is not a surprise to hear a surgeon say—it is not a surprise to hear a surgeon say, the surgery was successful, but the patient died. And it is the same thing in cancer. I killed the cancer tumor but the patient dies a terrible, terrible death in the process. It is not okay. It is not the best we can do.

Ty: Because the tumor is a symptom of something that has gone wrong in the body, right?

Dr. Weeks: We talked about this a little earlier—Samuel Hahnemann, who is a medical doctor who actually was so frustrated with the standard of care in his day he gave up his medical practice. He gave up his MD. And he went in and informed a whole field of medicine called homeopathy, which is a whole other topic. It is a very fruitful study about healing. And one of his favorite quotes is that the symptom is a healing gesture. The body is no dummy. If the body is doing something it is probably a wise thing. It is maybe not a permanent solution. It is maybe a stop gap solution, but like a fever. Fortunately, if the child has a fever, guess what? The human being can live at a high temperature or a low temperature, but certain bacteria can't. The fever is a naturally, tremendously beneficial symptom which can help the child get healthy. Which is why after a fever our language says, I feel better. Nobody says, I had a fever and I am feeling like I felt before the fever. It has been a cleansing, detoxifying process. Of course, too much of a symptom can be, if not lethal, certainly terrible. Helen Keller is a classic example of too much of a fever. I am not advocating for excessive symptoms, but I am saying if the symptom happens the body should pay attention. Often it is the, if you will, the auto-pilot telling us dummies, hey, you are not doing something right. Cancer can be seen as a symptom, as a healing gesture.

What I have lectured on in the past is where I grew up in northern New Hampshire there was a town dump. And so we all knew we could take our trash over to Farmer Jones' back 40. And we put stuff there and we used to go there as kids and watch the bears and stuff. The fact of the matter, if God reached down with a big excavator and took all of the trash out of Farmer Jones' backyard and we couldn't use it anymore, we would go to Farmer Smith and we would pay him $40 a year to dump our trash there. Because we could take our trash to these back 40s, we could keep our front yards pretty clean. If you have a cancer in a breast I'm saying that is metaphorical, it is analogous to a cancer being like a dump. The body is saying something is wrong here. I am going to put everything, Farmer Jones' back 40, in the left breast, and there is a cancer. It is never the problem. It is always a symptom of other diseases or imbalances. If you just lop off the breast and say, Mrs. Jones, you are cancer free, you are ignoring the fact that unless you change your behavior the cancer will manifest somewhere else. If we can't go to

Farmer Jones' back 40 we are not going to put it on our front yards, we are going to go to Farmer Smith's back 40. It is a bit of a strange metaphor.

What I want to say is that when my clients show up with cancer, what I try to do is help them think through why they might have it, what the lesson might be. There is an expression, I think you know, that God gives nothing but gifts. So here is a cancer. I don't want to belittle the tragedy and the heartbreak and the terror that people experience, but given all of that, you are still in a position to say, is this telling me something? Is this a healing gesture? Is there a message here that I should pay attention to that I can actually become empowered and work through this in a healthy way?

Ty: It reminds me—I interviewed Dr. Francisco Contreras. He said that many people—many of his patients have told him that getting cancer was the greatest gift that ever happened because it gave them a perspective on life, it helped them to get really well. They looked at that as a healing gesture. Let me ask you this—the immune system is critical. Reducing inflammation is critical. Do they have any implication into the cancer equation—the immune system and inflammation how are they related to cancer?

Dr. Weeks: Well, it would be logical to argue that in an intact immune system there would be no room for cancer. And the immune system, which is kind of an indefinable entity, it is not like it is right over here or it is right over here. The immune system, it wraps around the GI tract. It is a nebulous, almost a vaporous process. It is hard to say in anatomy and physiology and dissection, here is the immune system. Having said that, if it is functioning well, its job is to enhance health and promote detoxification and so forth. Inflammation is one of the main instruments that the immune system uses to regulate health. One of the things we find in cancer, which is quite interesting, is that typically the guy that says, I haven't been sick a day in my life, I am thinking we have to worry about cancer here. Whereas a kid that gets a lot of fevers and has an immune system which is always up and running and not apathetic, that is a good sign. If you want to get a good prognosis for health, it is someone who has been able to have a challenge, regulate the immune system, have the big fever, burn through it and come out better.

Ty: Very similar to something Dr. Rashid Buttar told me. He said the people that I worry about are the people that never get sick because of the same exact reason.

Dr. Weeks: Yea. These are principles that go back. I mean I would like to say I invented them all, but they were long before any of us were alive. This is what people's grandmothers know. That is why in the old days when kids had the mumps, you go have mumps parties.

Ty: Mumps parties. Chicken pox parties. Yeah.

Dr. Weeks: Yea. Instead we are creating what is called anergy where we are giving all sorts of immune suppressing, sedating processes which thwart the immune system.

Ty: What are the most important foods in your opinion that have medicinal value that can help to prevent disease, cancer?

Dr. Weeks: Well, the first thing there is to be well-hydrated. Good quality water. I am against fluoride in water. I am against chlorine if possible. I am fortunate we have an artesian well. I like mineral water, spring water. I am not a big fan of the alkaline water process, but certainly the body has to be well-hydrated. What is important about that, Ty, you may not notice, but any addictive process, whether it is cocaine or heroin or coffee or cigarettes, is tougher to break if the person is dehydrated. So the first thing I do with someone who is, for example, an addict, is I rehydrate and I stabilize blood sugar. What is interesting about nicotine, for example, it clears the system quicker if you are dehydrated, so the patient is reaching for another cigarette. If you are well hydrated they are not quite sure when the nicotine left their system. It is the same thing. Cancer, all of the illnesses we pay attention to, are less problematic if the person is well hydrated. And water is a tremendous anti-inflammatory, of course. I am a fan of anti-inflammatory diets. I'm a fan of eating real food. Eating living food. It is astonishing to me that we even have this category called junk food. I like to tell my clients there is no such thing as junk food. There is food and there is junk and even though the junk can taste like food, it is not food. That is really not going to do what food is going to do.

Ty: It is kind of an oxymoron isn't it?

Dr. Weeks: It is. Indeed. The thing which I have paid a lot of attention to recently is eating seeds. I am going to use that term generally. Seeds will include nuts, will include beans. Anything which you can put in the grow that will grow—a pea would be a seed in that regard. Eggs, something like that. Caviar in particular. Fabulous. Seeds are tremendously valuable because the seed is such a wise little packet. It concentrates nutrients about 20 fold and 30 fold more than the rest of the fruit. It is this fabulous packet of concentrated nutrition. What we know is that it has got all sorts of genetic spare parts. If it is not going to be a seed that grows into a plant, that is available for you and I to repair our DNA and our RNA with. It also has tremendous stem cell precursors, especially in the husk of seeds. I encourage my clients to drink plenty of water. I like the urine to be light. I encourage them to eat seeds and nuts, raw, organic, non-X-rayed, non-radiated as much as possible and green leafy vegetables and so forth.

Ty: A living diet. A living food diet.

Dr. Weeks: Life comes from life. On the other, hand I had this gal today was saying to me, I eat a very strict diet, but sometimes I cheat. I said great. Good. Sometimes have a blast. The goal isn't we are taught in school it is not whether you win or lose it is how you play the game. And once you get cancer everybody forgets that. Now I'm thinking because as we are talking I should be careful with my terms. I now refer to these people I help as clients. And the reason is, for 20 years in the State of Washington, 21 years I had a very busy holistic practice. A lot of good cancer work and the State of Washington the medical board took my license. I consider it an illegal kangaroo court process, but it is the administrative process. So I am appealing at this point. I no longer practice medicine at this point. I'm hoping to get that back. But in the meanwhile as a consultant I can teach. Which is what we are doing with our time now we are helping people with information.

Ty: Got it. To me that tells me, they took your license, you were doing something right.

Dr. Weeks: For a lot of us it is kind of like a badge of honor. Like when Mahatma Gandhi was in prison in India, when he was fighting the British Empire in India, his lieutenant said to him, Mahatma, what are you doing in prison? We need you out here. And Gandhi said, under this regime, what are you doing not in prison. It is not the answer to have your license taken away. The answer is to empower patients so the patients will say to legislators, I insist on having freedom of choice in healthcare. In my case, patient complaints, it was fabricated by the State Medical Board because I am a thorn in their side. I make their doctors look relatively inept.

Ty: It reminds me of the story of Dr. Buttar, my good friend out of North Carolina. It cost him $10 million to fight the North Carolina medical board and eventually he beat them, but they tried to bankrupt him.

Dr. Weeks: And they are still after him.

Ty: They are. Yeah.

Dr. Weeks: I feel, Ty, that it is not my role as a medical doctor to fight for my license. It is the opportunity of clients to say we want Weeks to be caring for us. So that is why we stopped fighting in that regard and we are just going to put it in an appeal process at this point. For the record, Dr. Weeks still a doctor, no license because of the suspension, sees clients not patients.

Ty: Okay. You mentioned stem cells.

Dr. Weeks: Right. For the past seven years—I am one of four doctors now that is qualified to teach insulin potentiated chemotherapy IPT. And that is a fabulous way to do chemotherapy. So fabulous that I just think it is illogical for anyone who is going to get chemotherapy, if they want to do chemo, they should do IPT. A couple of quick reasons, and this might be included in other people discussing it. You have to know that when you give insulin it shifts the cancer cells to what is called the S phase or the synthesis phase or the active phase. And that is the only phase that chemotherapy can be effective. So you have really four phases that the cancer cell can be in. So you got a 25 percent chance if you give chemo that it is going to kill the cancer cell. If you give insulin beforehand, it pushes it to about 70 percent S phase. So now you got almost a three out of four chance to kill cancer cells. If you are going to give chemo, let's kill the cancer cells. Just giving a little insulin pushes the cells into a vulnerable phase.

The second thing I like about insulin potentiated chemotherapy is that when you give the insulin it makes the cell membranes not only more permeable to chemotherapy selectively compared to your other healthy cells, but it also inhibits the cancer cell from kicking out the toxic chemotherapy. As good as IPT is, I don't offer it anymore. The reason I don't is, it only kills tumors. Cancer tumors are not the real target. Cancer stem cells, which is usually about less than 3 percent of the tumor mass, would be the cancer stem cell, these are the ring leaders. These are the guys that are fomenting a riot and they have their lieutenants. For the most part a group riot is really composed of bystanders who watch and maybe go along. The tumor is not dangerous. The primary tumor rarely kills people unless it grows big enough to obstruct an airway or an artery or something. But it is the metastatic process that is dangerous. What we now know from people like Professor Max Wicha, Max Dean at Stanford, Wicha is in Michigan, the literature, if you search cancer stem cells and google it, if any of the patients will search cancer stem cells, they will see that the cancer stem cell is the real target. And one of my favorite quotes is Thomas Pynchon in *Gravity's Rainbow*. He says if you can get people to ask the wrong question, the answer doesn't matter. The wrong question being asked is, how can we shrink tumors, how can we kill tumors—all my good, wonderful colleagues are targeting the tumors. For the last six years, I have been the only one saying, you got to go after the cancer stem cells. If you shrink the tumor it is not correlated to longevity. If you attack the tumor effectively it will, as injured tissue, secrete an inflammatory cytokine to recruit uncommitted stem cells from the mezankine[ph] to migrate to the injured tissue, the cancer which was attacked by the chemo. Now here come these stem cells to the attacked tumor, injured tissue. And they say, here we come. By the way, what would you like us to become? And they become a tumor. That is why Max Wicha is on record, a distinguished professor of oncology. Max Wicha is on record for saying chemotherapy and radiation make your cancer worse.

You can't just stop a gazillion dollar industry in its tracks and have everyone say to their patients, sorry, no chemo today. Our gurus have told us not. Until they can start making money on an anti-inflammatory, which is what they are working on now, because the anti-inflammatory will stop the recruitment of the cancer of the non—of the stem cells which become cancer stem cells. Anyway, the thing I wanted to say there is that the real target is to stop cancer stem cells for three reasons—only they metastasize. Tumor cells don't metastasize. The cancer stem cell metastasizes. The cancer stem cells are resistant to chemo and radiation. So you can do what you want with chemo and radiation. You are not targeting the real villain, the real culprit. The third thing is that if you don't address the cancer stem cells your cancer is coming back because those are the ones that can recreate a cancer. But nobody is targeting them. So I say to my clients, if you are going to see your oncologist, ask him or her what are you going to do to help me be healthy while you kill my tumor, because that is all they can do. Current oncologists are only killing tumors and patients, but they are not killing cancer stem cells.

The second question is, what is your treatment going to do to my cancer stem cells. And Ty, then they have to watch the eyes of the oncologist. Because if they get kind of a blank stare, like what are you talking about, then they are not up to speed on literature, and you have to run away. And if they give this, oh damn, I'm busted, kind of sideways look, then it is a really unfortunate situation, because they know that their treatments aren't helping. They are just using the patient as a renewable resource, which is tragic. So cancer stem cells need to be addressed and currently the only way to do that is anti-inflammatories.

Ty: And the anti inflammatories help to kill the cancer stem cells?

Dr. Weeks: There is literature that says for example metformin selectively targets cancer stem cells. There are a lot of agents out there that selectively target cancer stem cells.

Ty: And metformin is that a drug?

Dr. Weeks: It is a blood sugar lowering drug. But there are arthritis drugs—aspirin. Too much aspirin will kill you, but you got to have some anti-inflammatories. We use a product called Soul which is ground up black cumin seed, black raspberry seed, and chardonnay grape seed. These are very powerful anti-inflammatory seeds, which have been well studied. Water. Tremendous benefit just by having good quality water to flush your system. Seeds have oil in them and oils help restore a membrane of cell's integrity. A lot of benefits to eating the seeds.

Ty: What does the Bible say? I have given you all of the fruit bearing seed in first chapter of Genesis.

Dr. Weeks: Exactly.

Ty: Interesting. Can you talk about a few natural cancer treatments, other than what you already listed? Any other natural cancer treatments that you are aware of that are effective?

Dr. Weeks: The first is really to ask the patient why he or she wants to live. And it is shocking, Ty. I think probably at least over 50 percent of my male clients, let me say, my former patients, 60 percent of the males, once the wife is out of the room, they say to me something like look, doc, with all due respect, I really don't want to live anymore. I certainly don't want to bankrupt my family. I have had a great life. Everything is good. I don't want to be a burden. I'm done. I'm only here because my wife wants me to be here. I respect that, because these are guys who know from friends and so forth that the next five years of conventional cancer treatment is going to be a debacle. They don't want to go through that. My first job is to try to get them inspired. If they could see a way through where we could focus on helping their body be healthy with a buy-in. What I have to tell you, most patients have given up by the time they have seen an oncologist. They don't believe they are going to do well. They don't think it is possible and they know they can't afford it and they are dreading it. If an oncologist doesn't put on a psychiatrist's hat and say, how are you feeling about this Mr. Jones, or what would you like to do Mrs. Jones, and not get those thoughts and ideas out on the table, then you are just wasting time.

The first treatment really is to have a relationship with a patient where they can really share their concerns. And then you can say, I'm not god, I can do my best. What are the criteria? You don't want pain or this and that? And you can formulate something. I have to tell you, it is shocking what oncologists get away with, when they simply lay out a plan, they don't really listen to no's and they say the patient has no choice. You know, it is even worse with parents with their kids with cancer.The first treatment is really to have a relationship and try to learn what the patient wants. Now in the current way that medicine is practiced in America, nobody has time for that kind of a discussion, but it is critically important.

The second thing is, I will ask my clients, why do they think they have cancer. A lot of them will say I don't know. I say well, why do you think you have cancer? They will say well, I don't know. And I say well why do you think you have cancer. And they know I am not going to stop until they tell me. And it could be that they feel like they have sinned. Or they could feel they could have some guilt or something. Then if one doesn't exorcise, so to speak, that, and help them understand that whatever they have screwed up in the past, their main commitment is what they can do today, and going forward. Again, the best chemo drugs in the world aren't going to be helpful. You have to have people understand that it is their life and help them feel empowered. You and I can appreciate the word enthusiasm means god within entheus. So if the patient can't be enthusiastic about each day, then that is a big immune drain as well. It is not about prolonging life and suffering. It is about quality of life. You want to prolong quality and quantity. But I, like, I would encourage my medical colleagues my oncologists to have those types of discussions with the patients. I think it is critically important. Then we deliver smart therapies. I call them centsible early on—C E N T so safe, effective and cost effective. That is diet, nutrition, exercise. My wife is a big proponent of yoga. Yoga has been, excellent studies on yoga. Excellent studies on walking.

This sounds a little simplistic, but I got to tell you, in my practice over the years, I can tell you it is abiding by the simple principles which really work. And the newest drug is never going to do it.

Ty: You mentioned safe and effective and so that would be abiding by the Hippocratic oath, which you took—first do no harm. You are keeping your patient safe. You are not harming them with a treatment.

Dr. Weeks: Yea.

Ty: That is what these natural treatments do.

Dr. Weeks: Unless the patient wants something. If they want something which I think would be not safe and not effective, it is still their choice. It is still their choice. I am not going to want to participate necessarily, but I'm not going to denigrate them for having a different idea. My rule is to educate, to try to inform to the best of my ability, to create a forum where they feel safe to get their questions answered. And then like a coach to kind of help them on their way.

Ty: Well, Dr. Weeks, I appreciate your obvious concern for your clients. I appreciate your passion. I appreciate you sharing your knowledge with us. I know that it is going to help a lot of people that have seen the show.

Dr. Weeks: Good for you, Ty. My pleasure.

Ty: God bless you.

Dr. Weeks: Thank you, sir.

[end of transcripts]

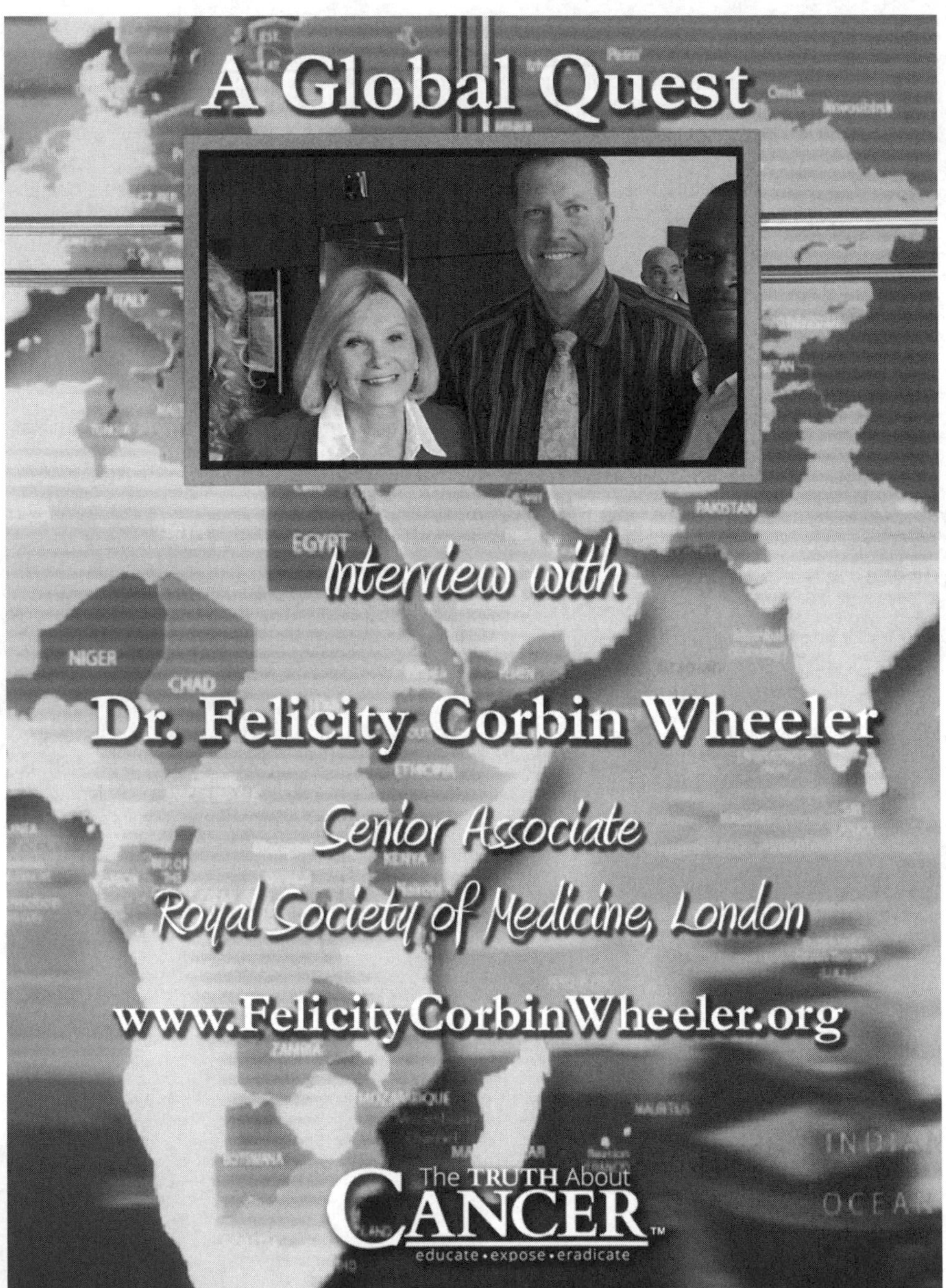
A Global Quest
Interview with
Dr. Felicity Corbin Wheeler
Senior Associate
Royal Society of Medicine, London
www.FelicityCorbinWheeler.org
The TRUTH About
CANCER
educate • expose • eradicate

Ty: I'm here in sunny London—it's sunny now—with Felicity Corbin Wheeler. Thank you for joining me today. You flew in all the way from Spain.

Dr. Wheeler: Thank you, Ty. I did indeed. Yes. I'm making television programs there called *Get Well Stay Well* which are actually teaching people how to eradicate, expose, and educate on cancer.

I'm a great proponent of that because I nearly died of pancreatic cancer in 2003, having already lost a daughter. And I had a son also with cancer when they were 14 and 16 so a terrible, terrible shock. I had been a British Red Cross nurse originally and then I worked in the Houses of Parliament so I have a medical and a slightly political background.

I just realized that there are so many myths. There is so much misinformation about cancer, so I love what you are doing. I love your *Quest for the Cure* and all the work that you're doing in America.

Ty: Thank you. Appreciate it. Tell us about your—you mentioned your son and your daughter both had cancer.

Dr. Wheeler: Well, we went back to live in Jersey, which is one of the Channel Islands and we thought an idyllic lifestyle to bring children up in. But we grow a lot of potatoes and tomatoes in Jersey. We had an old farmhouse and the chemicals, the pesticides, and all the other chemicals that they had used to grow more potatoes and more tomatoes were actually getting into our well water and we had absolutely no idea.

Firstly, my son had a carcinoid tumor in his appendix at 14 and I was horrified because I'd had my nursing background. I had worked for one of the top London cancer surgeons called Harvey White and was absolutely shattered that my son at 14 could produce this carcinoid tumor in the appendix. Luckily that was encapsulated. He had a full body scan and he was clear.

Then my daughter, six months later, is diagnosed with stage four B Hodgkin's disease and died in two years. So my whole life changed completely to researching better ways because I had my son to save and another child to save as well. So it completely changed my life.

I started researching. I started discovering all kinds of information that had been hidden. If my daughter had known about these cures, I'm sure that she would be here today. And the oncologist who was at the Royal Marsden Hospital—when I suggested going perhaps to America or looking at DART he said, "If you think lettuce leaves will kill your daughter, take her away and stop wasting my time."

My daughter of course, was horrified and said, "Mom, no. Don't say things like that or he won't look after me." She really believed the chemo and the radiation would cure her, but sadly it did not.

Anyway, I then got myself together. I went and trained in London. I trained in America. I've trained all over the place on natural cures. Quite unexpectedly, in 2003, I was getting a lot of indigestion and went and had a scan. I was by then yellow with jaundice and was told I had pancreatic cancer, a huge mass in the head of the pancreas where it's impossible to operate.

My husband, who was RAF brought me to London to the military hospital here. I had a wonderful professor there who stented the common bile duct to release the toxins in the liver which were actually killing me. I would have been dead in about six weeks. Terrible pain I was in, and terrible nausea. Anyway, there was nothing that they could do. He just stented it and said, "Well, that will relieve the worst of it. You know, hospice is the thing."

But my husband took me back to Church at Holy Trinity Brompton, that's my London church, and there—it was most amazing God incidence because I was prayed for by a woman called Emmy Wilson who is the Pastor, but also had been a gastroenterology nursing sister.

She said to me after she prayed for me, "Have you heard about B-17?" And my husband, who was RAF, said, "Oh, that's a bomber." She said, "No. Actually it's a vitamin as well."

Ty: RAF, Royal Air Force, and he thought of a B-17 plane. Okay. Funny.

Dr. Wheeler: Absolutely. Anyway we went back. I went and laid on the bed at the Royal Air Force Club and read my Bible, looked at Genesis 1:29 and 30 which tells us the right way we should eat.

Ty: What does it say in those verses?

Dr. Wheeler: It says, "Behold, I have given you every seed bearing plant on the face of the earth and every tree with fruit with seed in it. And this will be to you as food. And to every living thing I give green plant."

I'm laying there in agony being sick and feeling really dreadful, thinking, "I think this is probably right. We've got to detox." I then did lots of research. I got onto the Gerson Therapy. I got B-17 from Mexico from Dr. Francisco Contreras. And I got well.

Ty: From pancreatic cancer?

Dr. Wheeler: I did. It took me eight months for the actual tumor to be reduced to a scar. It is still there as a scar. Then it took me about two years to get my strength back and then I wrote the book *God's Healing Word*, which has got the whole story.

I just wanted to get the word out. I self-published, I didn't even wait to find a publisher. I thought I would rather spend my money on doing this for other people than wait for a publisher and try to do things commercially. So I got the book out there.

Then I was interviewed by Revelation TV who was a very brave channel run by Howard and Lesley Conder. They came out with the truth about things and they call it Revelation TV. They asked me to do some programs which I did and now I do a weekly program for an hour on natural health.

Ty: So you have your background as a nurse, you had the background in Parliament and are very well connected here in London. But that is kind of all the stepping stones for what you're doing today with your weekly health show.

Dr. Wheeler: Absolutely.

Ty: When you were diagnosed with pancreatic cancer, what was the prognosis from the doctor?

Dr. Wheeler: Six weeks to maybe six months.

Ty: Six weeks to six months to live.

Dr. Wheeler: But I know so many people who have had pancreatic cancer since and no one has survived. The only people who have survived are the doctors who are cited in Phillip Day's book, *Cancer: Why We're Still Dying to Know the Truth.*

There were two doctors there. One a doctor and one a dentist, in fact. And they got well with the B-17 and the colonics and the Gerson Therapy. I think, Ty, you have to put the whole thing together. You have to really detox the body, you have to restore the deficiency of living enzymes. You have to re-hydrate the body with the good juices and you have to address the stress in your life. And I'd had a lot of stress.

Ty: We'll hit a couple of things you just said. You said you have to re-hydrate with the juices. People don't realize that the purest water that you can get is actually vegetable juice.

Dr. Wheeler: Absolutely. It is the only thing to drink, really. I've just been in Mexico with Dr. Patrick Vickers.

Ty: Whom we will be interviewing in a few weeks.

Dr. Wheeler: Right. And also Dr. Francisco Contreras, he directed my treatment. We've been filming out there to really try and spread the word. You know, these guys are amazing because they give a lot of free information. If people can't afford to fly out to Mexico, they can actually follow these treatments.

This is what I do with my *Get Well Stay Well* days and weeks. I'm very lucky. I've been—I'm very blessed actually, because I've been elected a member of the Royal Society of Medicine. I'm absolutely amazed and delighted. So I'm holding a *Get Well Stay Well* day there and I invite these special doctors as guests to speak to a private group. It's just getting the word out there.

Ty: When you were diagnosed and you had this very bleak prognosis, six months at most—and you're right, with pancreatic cancer, nobody lives past a year if they are treated conventionally. So you are—this 12 years, 12 years now?

Dr. Wheeler: The year 2003.

Ty: So in addition to the vitamin B-12—did you take apricot pits or did you actually take the vitamin?

Dr. Wheeler: I actually got the laetrile sent over from Mexico.

Ty: Intravenous?

Dr. Wheeler: Intravenous.

Ty: Intravenous Laetrile.

Dr. Wheeler: And then I had great difficulty to find a doctor who was prepared to give it because my own doctor refused to. He said, "It's illegal. I can't do that." The second one also said, "My partners would throw me out if I did that."

Then my son—he's a lawyer in Jersey—had a lady who wind surfed with him on those beautiful beaches in Jersey. And she was a very free-thinking doctor, young, and she said, "I can do it for your mother. I believe it works."

So she did it. She has now come out of NHS, the National Health Service and she's actually doing natural medicine. She lives in France and Jersey and travels quite a bit.

The difficulty is, unless you are a doctor or a nurse yourself, to put up the IV and give it to yourself. This is how the doctors who did get well were able to do it, because they ministered to themselves.

Ty: They'd give themselves IVs? So in addition to the laetrile? Did you do any kind of a radical change of your diet or any other complementary treatments?

Dr. Wheeler: I think the greatest thing was doing the coffee enemas. Absolutely fantastic.

Ty: Which is what Dr. Nicholas Gonzalez recommends as well as his partner, Dr. Linda Isaacs who we interviewed last year. Especially for pancreatic cancer. Why is that?

Dr. Wheeler: It really works because we have to detox and the only way that the body can really detox radically is through the colon. The colon has years and years and years of backed up toxicity in it.

You see, Dr. Max Gerson cured his migraines to start with and then found that Dr. Albert Schweitzer came to him to cure the TB and cure the diabetes. Everything gets well when you detox. Detox is the beginning of getting well.

The thing is, when people go on the juices they release an awful lot of toxins in their body. And unless they wash those toxins out, they are going to really make themselves very ill.

Ty: Reabsorb them.

Dr. Wheeler: Reabsorb it through the gut, absolutely. I believe in the colonics, I also believe in the pancreatic enzymes that Dr. William Kelley talked about. You know, it's interesting because a lot of this came from UK as well.

There was a Professor John Beard who was an embryologist and was working up at a University in Edinburgh. He also got a degree from Freiburg University in Germany. He was promoting all this 100 years ago, Ty, but it's all been hidden and disparaged by Big Pharma who make all the money out of the chemo.

Ty: Sad, isn't it.

Dr. Wheeler: It's tragic. I've lost my daughter to it. Tragic.

Ty: I'm sorry for your loss.

Dr. Wheeler: So am I. And I'm sorry for your losses as well in your family. I think it's really great that you and I have changed our lives to really try and spread this word. I think this is what life is all about. We leave a legacy at the end. And it's what you do while you're here that counts.

Even if I go home tomorrow, I have actually produced a good legacy for my children, for the grandchildren. That's what we're here for.

Ty: Yes, it is. You talked about detoxification. You also mentioned stress. Do we need to detox the stress in our lives?

Dr. Wheeler: Absolutely, and how difficult is that?

Ty: So how do we do it?

Dr. Wheeler: I think God is really the only answer. I really do. So I went into ministry. I've studied an awful lot about meditation, detoxing the mind. You can do meditation with yoga. You can do meditation with the Lord, and I find that is the best way to do it.

Jesus said, "Go into your quiet place." It was the Jewish prayer shawl, the tallit. I actually prayed under my tallit when I was getting well. I'm a Christian, but I do believe in the Judaic heritage, the Old Testament. You know, that's where the Genesis 1:29-30 comes from. So we have to get back to our roots and then we heal.

Ty: We have to get back to our roots in two ways. Back to our roots or heritage, but also you mentioned roots. Talk about the roots of plants and how valuable they are from a nutritional perspective.

Dr. Wheeler: Absolutely vital and that's why I teach people in my courses you need to go back to the onions, the garlic, the carrot, the root vegetables which are really so much better than having fruit because fruit has got quite a bit of sugar in it. Although it's a much healthier sugar than the refined sugars.

But of course, Big Farma, with an F, is getting us all addicted to the wrong fats, sugars, and salts. They pay scientists a lot of money to get us addicted. They test all these things to see what is really hitting in the brain, the pleasure center in the brain.

These foods, these sugars do that. So I think there's this sort of mass genocide going on where the world population has been—a lot of people said it was a good idea to bring it down to 500,000.

You know, we have the Georgia Guidestones. We've heard a lot of these elite people saying on television how they want to reduce the world population. And what a way to do it? Getting people addicted to the wrong foods that kill them.

Ty: It's kind of a slow kill, isn't it.

Dr. Wheeler: It is. But devastating when you see people dying unnecessarily. So I do these courses either for a day or for a week where I try to teach people. I can give them the tools. I trained at Hippocrates Health Institute in America as well, and as Dr. Brian Clement says, "You can give people the tools, but they have to heal themselves." They have to do the colonics, they have to juice the juices, and they also have to address the stress in their lives.

Ty: We were just in Florida last week and I got two or three videos from ladies that were patients at Hippocrates, and they both knew who you were, as a matter of fact.

Dr. Wheeler: Oh, really?

Ty: Yes. And they had healed themselves through the treatments at Hippocrates.

Dr. Wheeler: That's great. I think there's a great worldwide network now of people who have healed. I think through the Internet we've now got a whole new way of transmitting the information, which is wonderful.

Ty: It is. What would your advice be to somebody that has recently been diagnosed with a cancer that the doctor says there is no hope for?

Dr. Wheeler: Well, the great thing is to keep calm and educate yourself. Because it's not the rush that the doctors push us into, "You've got to have chemo tomorrow" sort of thing.

It is really important to see your options, to see what the real statistics are from the people who are curing cancer like Dr. Francisco Contreras who is getting 56 percent better cure rates than orthodox medicine. You have to find out who these doctors are, what they are teaching. A lot of that you can do on the Internet. It's not expensive. You can actually research this stuff. Just do it.

The great thing is not to listen to well-intentioned friends who may be very misinformed. You also have to ask your oncologist, "Exactly what are the statistics for the particular kind of cancer I have?" In my case, of course, there was no chance of a cure anyway.

God was good in that way because I was pushed right into doing the right thing. And you also open doors and it's amazing how many people on my television shows write to me—I get hundreds of emails every week—and they say, "It was a God incidence. I just happened to be flicking channels. I went on and I saw you talking about the juices and the colonics."

It's like Chris Wilk said. He was just about to capitulate to the chemo when Jack LaLanne came on the TV.

Ty: I think you recently did an interview with Chris, didn't you?

Dr. Wheeler: I did, yes, in America.

Ty: Because we were in San Diego.

Dr. Wheeler: We were in San Diego together, yes. Yes, and we had dinner at the first inaugural Cure to Cancer conference. I was actually on your table.

Ty: I remember that. I was looking back at pictures a few weeks back and said, "That's right. We sat together."

Dr. Wheeler: I think it's amazing what Nathan Crane has done in setting up this conference. That's really going to open it up.

Ty: They've got a huge reach.

Dr. Wheeler: Yes, it's all wonderful. We want to get one in Europe as well if we can.

Ty: Concerning stress and the fear factor, in light of the fact that we know that cancer is made worse by stress and fear, what kind of sense or logic does it make to you for an oncologist to tell a cancer patient, "You have X number of months to live?" Are they God?

Dr. Wheeler: It's amazing how many patients obediently die exactly when they've been told to. My daughter was told that she would—if the bone marrow transplant didn't work, she'd be dead by Easter. And she obediently died on Maundy Thursday which is the Thursday before Passion Friday.

This is hugely important. It's what we speak out and say we have to be armed with the Armor of God in Ephesians 6 where we put on the Helmet of Salvation and the Breastplate of Righteousness. I think we really have to take control of our mind like a remote control with the TV. You switch the channels and you can do that. I think you have to immerse yourself in truth, which is what we're trying to help people with.

Ty: To me, it is almost a crime for an oncologist to do that to someone. We put our faith in these doctors, that what they say is true. So they instill the belief that you're going to die into somebody that's already sick, and you really lose hope at that point.

Dr. Wheeler: The white coats are very impressive, aren't they? And all the high tech stuff that people see when they go into the hospital. They think, "Oh, this must be right." But in fact, Dr. Lorraine Day, who I love, cured her own breast cancer many years ago as well. And she says, "Now, I'm going to take off my white coat and tell you the real truth." I think that is a very good DVD that she's made.

Ty: What did she use to cure her cancer?

Dr. Wheeler: She used DART and prayer and detoxing completely. She was a doctor, her husband was a doctor.

Ty: She's a medical doctor, right?

Dr. Wheeler: Yes. She was a Professor of Orthopedics at San Francisco [General] Hospital. When she was literally on the point of death—they thought she was going to die that night—I think her husband did the wheatgrass enema and colonic and re-hydrated her.

The wheatgrass is amazing. The wheatgrass has all the vitamins, all the minerals. It has B-17 in it as well. It's very healing inside the body and outside the body. I have people who have arthritis in hands. When you pack the hand with a flannel with the wheat grass in it, you'll find that the pain will come out of the hand, or any joint if you just sleep with the hand wrapped in wheat grass. I find people's skin problems completely clear up with the wheatgrass as well. You have to take it inside and apply it outside as well.

Ty: Is that something that you use with the patients that you work with now?

Dr. Wheeler: Absolutely. Yes. I was trained in barley grass at Hallelujah Acres and then with wheatgrass at Hippocrates Health Institute so I know both. Basically, you've got to get those good greens into your body because they've got the chlorophyll. They have all these healing enzymes. We have to get the raw, living enzymes into the body.

Ty: So God knew what he was talking about when he talked about the seeds and the herbs and the plants. He's given us everything we need in nature, right?

Dr. Wheeler: Absolutely. I think God always knows what He's talking about. We all try to do it our way, don't we, like Frank Sinatra, "I'll do it my way." And then we fall on our face and we realize we have to come back to the word.

Ty: Perfect example of that is when we try to manipulate genetically the food supply. In all of the cancers that it is causing and all the other health problems that these GMOs are causing, if we just ate food in its natural state, we wouldn't even have to deal with the issues.

Dr. Wheeler: And I'm really appalled that in the last Government, the Health Minister talked about promoting GM foods. I'm absolutely horrified. I'm hoping with the new change in Government that there may be a brighter and more intelligent perspective on that.

Ty: In the US, the GMOs are everywhere. They are in all the processed foods and we're even having debates about whether they should be labeled, which is absurd. Of course it should be labeled. But the same issues here in the UK?

Dr. Wheeler: Yes, absolutely. And people are lazy, they don't want to read labels. And anyway, I don't think you should buy anything with a label on it. I think you should just buy, as I do, I just go to the gypsy market which is down in Spain near me, it's on a Wednesday, it's on Saturday. And I can buy the organic fruit and vegetables from the farmers who I know and whose farms I visited. There are more and more people getting educated about these things.

Ty: That's interesting that you mentioned that. Somebody else recently—I can't remember who it was—said that real food does not have labels.

Dr. Wheeler: That's right. That's right. Just buy the good things. And I used to think we didn't need supplements. That's another thing. Because the ground has now become—the soil is so deficient in minerals that even when we have fruit and vegetables, they can be quite deficient. So I think now, sadly, we do need supplements as well. And you have to find a natural supplement, not a chemical one.

Ty: Right, not synthetic.

Dr. Wheeler: Not synthetic. No.

Ty: Name a couple of supplements that most people might be deficient in.

Dr. Wheeler: I think magnesium is the big one. Magnesium, selenium, zinc. I take CoQ10 as well. I think that is very good.

Basically, people have to watch out for themselves. I think you have to go to a naturopathic doctor who does a blood test and sees where you are on your own blood test and then can supplement what you need to supplement. It is quite individual. I think most people are devoid of magnesium and, of course, vitamin D, which is huge.

Ty: We've got a lot of vitamin D out here today.

Dr. Wheeler: We do, but most people in the Northern Europe, and also in Canada, of course, are living very deficient in vitamin D.

Ty: Well, that's actually a misnomer. We have a lot of ultra violet rays. Your body actually has to turn those rays into vitamin D with the cholesterol in your skin and it doesn't work very well if your body is full of toxins. It doesn't convert to vitamin D.

A lot of different issues. Just because you go out in the sun doesn't mean you're getting good vitamin D. That's why that's another thing to be checked, for the levels of vitamin D.

Dr. Wheeler: This is why I think it's really important to get a proper test. The Birmingham City Hospital do one, a postal one that you can do. Then I think it is important for people to take exercise and be out in the fresh air. Because you and I are probably sitting at our computers all day long or in the editing room making our films and we are not out in the sunshine. We may see it outside, but how many hours a day do you get out in the sun?

Ty: I have to make myself.

Dr. Wheeler: Exactly.

Ty: Which is one of the many reasons I love my wife, because she'll say, "Honey, let's go outside for an hour."

Dr. Wheeler: That's great.

Ty: So she grabs me and we go outside. Then during the summer we try to do that every day. You have to kind of pull yourself away from work and the computer to do it.

Dr. Wheeler: Yes, absolutely. It is vital. And also we have to walk on the grass or walk on the beach barefoot.

Ty: Earth.

Dr. Wheeler: Hug a tree.

Ty: Earthy.

Dr. Wheeler: Yeah, absolutely you've got—

Ty: Become a tree hugger. In a good way.

Dr. Wheeler: Absolutely. But the thing is to tell the truth.

Ty: Tell the truth. Well, you've been telling the truth. I've seen your work for the last few years and I appreciate what you're doing. Thank you for your television show each week and I'm looking forward to being a guest on your show. You're about to have me on this afternoon.

Dr. Wheeler: Absolutely. That's going to be wonderful, Ty. Looking forward to it.

Ty: It's going to be fun. Thank you for spending the time with us today. God bless you and we really appreciate you.

Dr. Wheeler: God bless.

[end of transcript]

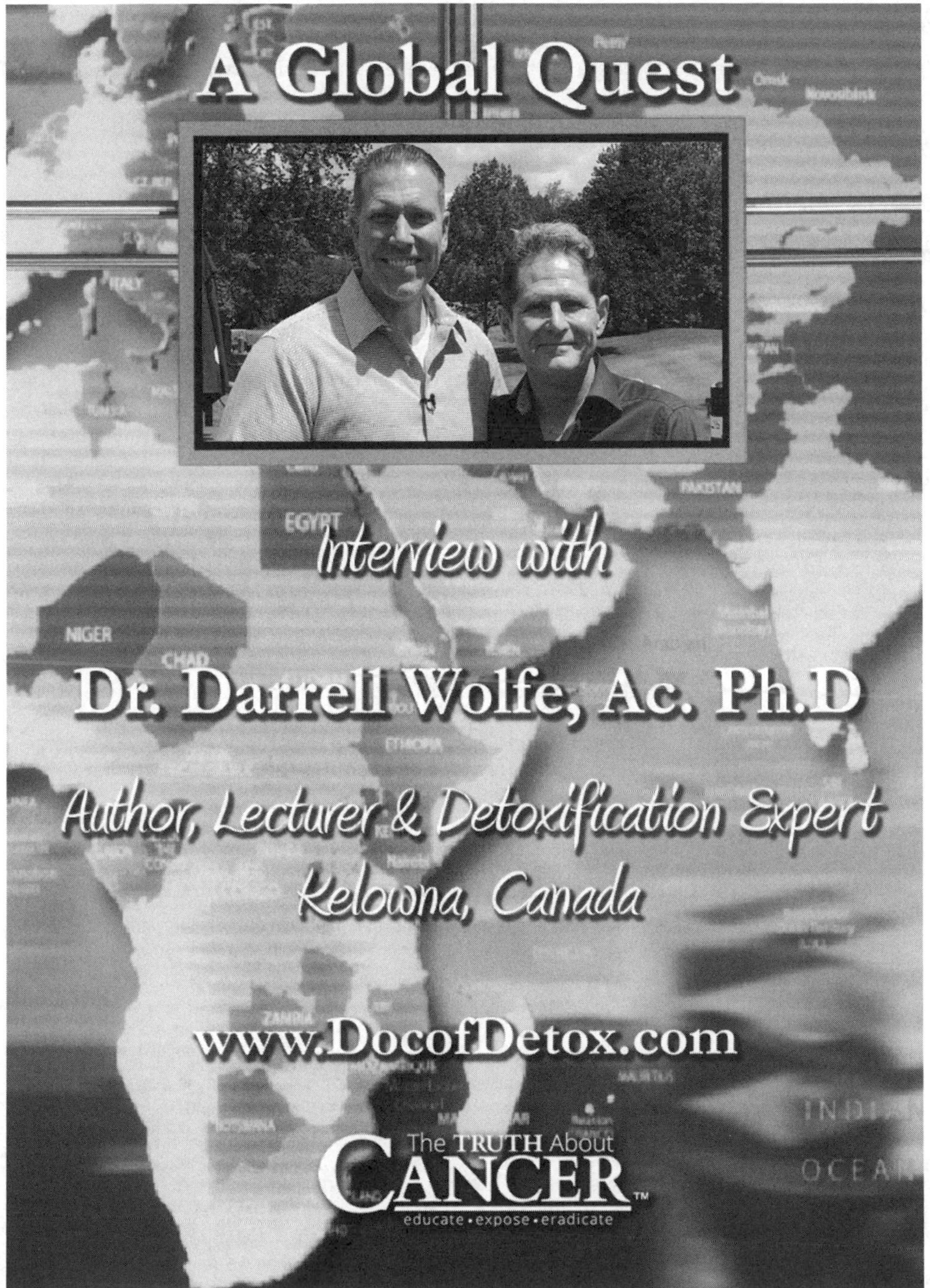
A Global Quest
Interview with
Dr. Darrell Wolfe, Ac. Ph.D
Author, Lecturer & Detoxification Expert
Kelowna, Canada
www.DocofDetox.com
The TRUTH About CANCER
educate • expose • eradicate

Ty: I'm here in Toronto, Canada. Just north of Toronto. We meet again, Dr. Darrell Wolfe.

Dr. Wolfe: How are you doing, Ty?

Ty: Doing great, buddy. Good to see you again. Let's see, last year for *The Quest for the Cure* we met in Las Vegas initially.

Dr. Wolfe: That's right.

Ty: Then we were in, was it in LA, or was it San Diego?

Dr. Wolfe: It was LA.

Ty: LA. And now we're up in Darrell's home turf in Canada. I'm really excited to have you be a part of this documentary as well. I think you're one of only maybe two or three doctors that are going to be in all three of the first documentaries that we've done with the *Truth About Cancer*. We're really excited to pick your brain on some other issues today that we haven't covered in the past. But initially, for those who are watching, in case they haven't seen the previous ones, share with us a little bit about your background and your education.

Dr. Wolfe: Well, my history on my education is that I have a doctorate in homeopathic acupuncture. Also, I ran the North American Institute for the Advancement of Colon Therapy for 12 years. Right now, my website is called *The Doc of Detox* and I have a clinic in Kelowna, British Columbia. I also run the International Training Institute of Health. What's that? The Training Institute of Health, it's where we do different programs where we teach lay people. They come in for what's called a Weekend Warrior. They come in Friday night, they leave on a Sunday, knowing everything they need to on how to protect themselves and how to master their own lives and become the cure.

Then, we also have people that fly into our clinic and we call it "Couples One-on-One," where couples actually come and they learn how to do therapy on each other and heal each other the way couples should, right? I also teach a professional training class in deep tissue, on how to remove scar tissue from the body. And also we teach people and professionals how to consult properly, which is called "Whole Life Consultant Certified."

Ty: So, "Doc of Detox," it's an appropriate name, too. To be honest with you, those who are watching, if you read my book on cancer, the first edition had nothing to do with detoxification. Darrell and I met shortly after that. And it's because of your book, *Spoiled Rotten*, that you wrote, that now, the entire chapter in my cancer book is based upon that pamphlet that you wrote on how to detoxify the whole body. So, I want to thank you for that because that was really—I didn't know anything about detoxification. It's really amazing to me how many people, even in natural medicine, don't know much about detoxification. I learned it through you. So thank you for that.

Dr. Wolfe: Well, thank you. But, you know, Ty, there it is right there. You just said it in a nutshell. Here you are, you are an author, researcher, and the most important step for the human body is daily gentle detoxification. Natural health practitioners still don't have it today. They don't understand it today. They still look at trying to do cleanse on somebody every few months. So, they still teach people to pile their crap up, create a manure pile, and then start to feel sick. And let's do a deep cleanse and then dump all those toxins out real fast, overload the body that is already overloaded.

It's like everything in life. If you exercise a little bit each day, you show that you love your family a little bit each day, and you show you love your body a little bit each day, then we wouldn't get into this mess, would we?

Ty: Daily gentle detox. There's a tea that you developed that we drink in our family.

Dr. Wolfe: It's called the Daily Cleansing Tea.

Ty: Daily Cleansing Tea, okay.

Dr. Wolfe: You know what? It's like this, your large intestine is the mother of all organs. It houses almost 60 percent of your immune system. And whenever you are in trouble, what's the first thing that sticks out?

Ty: Your belly.

Dr. Wolfe: Yes. If it sticks out, it is full of gas. If it sticks out and hangs down, that's your immune system falling down. That's your guts falling out. Meanwhile, you can walk down the street, you see three guys talking together in the corner and rubbing it and seeing which one gets the wish first.

Ty: Like little Buddhas.

Dr. Wolfe: Yes, it's an epidemic. But you know what? We have been educated into ignorants. Take a look at it and when people talk about, "I eat healthy." They don't even know what eating healthy is.

If you walk into a grocery store, 90 percent of the groceries in the grocery store are toxic and they'll cause cancer. Ninety percent.

You know what? If it's not from a farmer, it's not worth eating.

Ty: Real food doesn't have labels.

Dr. Wolfe: That's right. I heard somebody say that recently and it really resonated. Because most of the stuff that you're talking about, this 90 percent of the foods that cause cancer that are in the stores—I've heard that statistic from others and it's because of the fact that the foods that are in the middle aisles, they are all processed. They all contain cancer-causing agents, chemicals, additives, GMOs, whatever.

So you really want to shop around the outer edges of the store when shopping.

You know what it really comes down to?

Ty: What's that?

Dr. Wolfe: We are just so programmed. You know what? We are so dummied down. And I mean, we are all dummied down. I mean, you've got basically three percent of the population is in control of 97 percent of the money. The same families that have been controlling the planet for almost 200 years now, they've got it down to a fine art. They own the media and they download us, continually, download us all this stuff.

I mean, who else would play in to all this stuff and make themselves so toxic. And grow tumors, and bathe in chlorinated water, drink chlorinated water, eat processed foods, and just keep piling garbage into in, unless you have lobotomy.

Ty: It is programming, isn't it?

Dr. Wolfe: Is it ever. Everything is about programming. That's why the only way we are going to break this program is if you spend 15 minutes in the morning and 15minutes at night actually working on yourself and become self-centered. You have to become self-centered. And you have to know one thing, everybody lies. And all the corporations, they don't just lie, they will take your life. They do not care. You have to understand that there are very few families that own and control all these corporations.

Did you ever hear of the queen bee? There's only one queen bee in the hive and all the rest of them are workers and they will all be put to death to save the queen bee. Now, if you lived in a family and you've got four generations of this family to five generations in this family, and you were born and raised and you don't even know, you couldn't even count how much money you had, and you have the power to manipulate countries, you wouldn't know even better, would you?

So, these families, they manipulate us and they maneuver us and they get us to eat what they want and it's just a big game.

Ty: They get us to eat what they won't eat, right? When you talk about the big corporations, one of the big corporations that manufactures or that produces the GMO foods is Monsanto. They don't even serve their own GMO foods in their cafeteria but they get us to eat them. So, this brainwashing is taking place. Let's go back. You mentioned that for the last couple of hundred years, the country has been controlled by these families. Let's go back a hundred years to really—when we looked at the rates of cancer, maybe one in 80 people in 1900 had cancer. And now, the statistics are almost one in two people alive today will face cancer. Why this huge increase over the last century in cancer?

Dr. Wolfe: Well, because we have given our control away. We don't have our own garden. You don't have your own garden. You don't have own control. Today—for one thing, if I can say this, let's really take it where it was, okay? Why don't we go back to Nixon. He was the president that was going to end all cancers, the War on Cancer.

You know what? What they wanted to do is they wanted to galvanize us. How can we get everybody in fear, in panic, and get them motivated into our big thing which is cancer. The big money maker. If you can give somebody cancer then you are going to jack up your sales. And remember something, you know what? When it really comes push to shove, you would save your family before you save me.

Well, they'll save their family before they'll save all the other families. So now, Nixon is going to end the War on Cancer. He was either lied to or he was a big crook, "I'll never tell a lie." But what happened was, now we are going to end the War on Cancer so we're going to get everybody involved. We're going to get them to run for it. We're going to get them to jump for it. We're going to get them to pray for it. We're going to get them to beg for it.

So now you can't go anywhere without giving money. I can't buy groceries without somebody wanting money from me. And now they know they can't get it from other places. So now it's about the children. Or it's breast cancer because they're sexy. Meanwhile, we got lung cancer more.

So, why is cancer so big? Well, you are what you think about. My little girl, she got a pimple and she's said, "Daddy, is this a tumor?" That's programming. But it's not just that. At the same time they've got us panicking in fear, we're drinking out of plastic bottles, our foods are loaded with chemicals, GMOs. It doesn't end, does it?

Ty: You mentioned children. Why the increase in children's cancer over the last few decades. Any idea?

Dr. Wolfe: Well, any idea why children's cancer, is the way we feed them. We're always on the run. Microwave foods. Drive-thrus. Kids aren't getting their nourishment.

Also, what about the EMF? What about the Wi-Fi in the house?

Ty: What about infants that are born with cancer. Why might that be?

Dr. Wolfe: Well, because of the parents. Because the parents are so toxic. I mean, you create what you are. If we just learned how to gently cleanse every day. And if we are just drinking enough water. And if we're drinking structured hydrogen water every day. We're walking bags of water. We don't even think to detoxify.

The medical system will never talk about a few things, nutrition or detoxification, because the medical system is not into health.

Ty: So, Dr. Wolfe, what is the medical industry into then?

Dr. Wolfe: The medical industry? Well, let's take a look at it. Can we look at it like a pyramid thing? What we've got is—first, we've got the petroleum, pharmaceuticals, food conglomerates. They're all just one big company and that company is to control.

So, what are they in to? They are in to making money off of everybody else's pain. I already told you that if you were one of these families, you would believe that you were actually a God. That you're here. And it was your job to just rape and pillage. And that's how it is and that's what they do.

So, we've got the pharmaceutical industries, they created the medical industry back in 1910. The AMA would have folded it if it wasn't for Rockefeller coming and pouring a billion dollars. Then, they created what was the AMA in the medical industry. But you've got to understand something, the pharmaceutical created the medical industry so that they could have soldiers on the ground that could go out and sell their products and legitimize the poisoning.

So medical doctors—if pharmaceuticals are the pimps, what are the medical doctors? So now, a medical doctor, he becomes a doctor because he's intelligent, he's done a lot of schooling and he really wants to help people. But a lie is a lie no matter who tells it and no matter who's playing it out. So, it's not going to end there, is it?

It is only going to end with, maybe, practitioners, natural health practitioners and medical doctors that breakaway from the system that want—what do they want to do? They want to train people. Not treat them. Because I don't care how good a practitioner you are, whether you are a medical or whether you're a natural health practitioner. If you are in the business of treating, then guess what? Your patient is only going to be feeling good until the next treatment. It's going to be treatment, treatment, treatment until we actually train. That's why everything I do now is about training.

And why don't we want to treat them? Because natural health practitioners have the same medical model as the medical doctors do. And we also live in fear because we would like to be like them, making all that money.

So, we get caught up in that medical model when we're supposed to be natural health people. We're supposed to give back to the people. We're supposed to show people how they can get up in the morning and worship and love their bodies all day long so that their bodies are a light and a beacon. But we don't do that.

What we do is we try to sell them treatments and we try to sell them lots of great products but we don't teach them how to look after their bodies. We don't teach them to respect their bodies.

See, what happens is that pharma, the media, have stripped everybody of their dignity. People have lost control. They've given up. They feel helpless. They feel hopeless. And you know what? Who's going to save them, Ty?

Here we got the War on Cancer. They spent billions of dollars and your videos have done more than all these billions of dollars will ever do because you put hope back into these people's hearts. You put hope back into their minds. You've galvanized them. When somebody comes to me and they have cancer, when they leave my clinic they know that they are not going to die. For the first time, they are not full and reeking with fear.

You know what? Anybody out there, if you go to a health practitioner and you feel fear, then never go back there. You find a health practitioner that is going to empower you because we have the power to heal ourselves. And we have to give that back, Ty.

And as far as I'm concerned, if you're a practitioner and you're not training people or giving back their power, then you shouldn't be in business. And that's my thing right now. That's where I am at.

Ty: I appreciate your passion on that. I would have to agree. That's really our position as well, that we need to educate people. We need to give them the knowledge that they need so that they can implement whatever it might be that can heal their body. They need to be the ones that are empowered, not the practitioner but the person needs to have the knowledge because it's the body that heals.

And if we don't have that knowledge, then our bodies can't be the self-healing mechanisms that they are supposed to be. If we don't have the knowledge about how to detoxify, what to put in to our bodies, how to get rid of the bad stuff and so forth. And if we don't have that, we can't be self-healing machines.

Dr. Wolfe: You know what? People are going to go, "Oh my gosh. Why is he so dramatic or is he angry?" Well, I'm not. I'm awake. And people need to understand that you are being butchered and we're going to continually be butchered until we wake up and until we stand together.

Because the medical doctors aren't going to change because, guess what? They've got mortgages and they like the respect they're getting. And even when they know that their treatments aren't even working—take a look at oncologists. Seventy percent of oncologists won't even opt for their own therapy for themselves or their families. They'll opt for natural health. The proof is on the pudding.

We got to stop being scared. Are you tired of being scared? What scares you, Ty? What scares you? You know what? Ten years ago, I was scared of everything, the government, I was scared of cancer. I was scared of everything. They want us to be scared. Are you sick and tired of being scared? Get an elastic band, put it on your wrist and every time you think about cancer and it's going to take you down, give it a little click and go, "I'm everything. I was created by something very powerful. And the day that I take control and start learning to respect and put love back into my body and time back into it and respect it, then, nothing can take [me] down."

And we all need to know that everybody lies. But when it comes to corporations, they don't have blood, they don't have feelings and they will just strip you of everything you have. They'll strip your family of everything and they will lie right in front of you.

Ty: I think the thing for people to realize about these multinational conglomerates, these corporations, whether it's a big farmer or big agra, the big industries, is they are publicly traded. They only have one obligation that is to make money. That's their only job.

Dr. Wolfe: They're traitors.

Ty: That's their only job. The pharmaceuticals' company job is not to get us healthy. It is to make more money.

Dr. Wolfe: It's their bottom line.

Ty: It's the bottom line.

Dr. Wolfe: And their bottom line is fat and so is everybody else's bottom line now. So the reason why we can't lose the weight, the reason why we don't have energy is because we're in pain all the time.

We're in pain for two reasons, we're in pain mentally because we know that this is wrong. We're in pain physically because of all the garbage we bring in that rots inside of our intestines. And what happens is that that creates bad bacteria, fungus, and, parasites, and worms. And they all start brewing inside of us. All of those things we give off a toxin called endotoxin that gets dumped into your bloodstream. That's the only reason why you feel pain, because you are rotting inside. You are causing your own self-poisoning. Those toxins get it to your bloodstream and your body goes, "Oh my god! We got to save this guy."

So, your body creates what we call pain. Pain is your best friend. But what is the main thing that the medical system teaches you?

Ty: Suppress it.

Dr. Wolfe: Run. Run from pain. Suppress pain. And have you ever noticed something? Everybody that you ever noticed that runs from pain, they are all drug addicts.

And the other thing that I want to say is that if you are selling drugs on the street, you go to jail. But a doctor can sell drugs because he is being covered by pharmaceuticals that are so powerful that he can get away with—

So now, let's get back to it. We suppress our pain with the drugs. Pain causes more acidity and that causes more pain in your body. They know this and if we weren't so brainwashed, we ignore too, because why am I having more pain? Why am I getting older? Why are my joints stiff?

Because what happens is when you get the pain and if you don't shut the pain down by detoxifying gently every day, drinking proper water, eating whole plant-based organic foods—that's all you've got to do. And you've got to love yourself. Tell yourself 300 times a day, "I love myself. I approve of myself. I'm everything."

Detoxification is so big. Now, if you don't do that, you're in pain and if you don't shut that down by detoxifying, then your body creates scar tissue.

What's a tumor made out of, Ty?

Ty: Fibrin, scar tissue.

Dr. Wolfe: Oh my God. Isn't that something? Guess what? You have to feel pain to create fibrin, to create scar tissue. To create a massive scar tissue you have to be in pain for 20 years. What's the one thing, if we leave today, that we need to know?

If we don't take drugs and we're not in pain, then we must be living pretty good. If we can eat properly we're not going to have the pain that creates the inflammation that creates the fibrin that causes the stiff joints, that causes endometriosis. That causes the lumps in the breasts, all of those. And then, calcium.

So now what you do is you get scar tissue and then you get calcium coming from the bones to try to buffer down the acid. That's like the last stage before cancer. So even if you've got kidney stones, you've got gall bladder stones, then you know that you're already on your way to cancer.

Here's another one. How many people have foot fungus? A lady that I know, she's been a podiatrist for 30 years and she says that everybody that comes in with foot fungus, they all end up with cancer. Because to have fungus on the end of your toes, it grew in that manure pile into your large intestine. So to have it at the end of your toes and a sinus infection in your nose, means you're full of it. So, you're moldy.

Just like when a person doesn't detoxify and they get older, they smell like pepperoni. Do you know what that is? That's mold oozing out of their pores.

Ty: I'm chuckling but yes. I understand that there is a certain smell.

Dr. Wolfe: So these are just basic things that we need to be taught and that's why I say, "We need to train. We need to get on the ground and we need to train people." And you know what? Practitioners are scared to go out there and train people. Why? They actually believe we're going to run out of sick people.

Ty: I don't think we're in danger of that.

Dr. Wolfe: No, I don't think so either.

Ty: Talk about World War II, World War I, the World Wars. The infiltration of the World Wars by the pharmaceutical companies and any link that might have to the first chemotherapy drug?

Dr. Wolfe: Well, World War I was perpetuated by three pharmaceutical companies. Bayer, you know Bayer aspirin. And then there was Hoechst and then there was BASF. They created that war for one reason only, to collect hundreds of thousands of different patents on different things that were going to be marketed around the world. That was the only reason why they did it.

After that, the three of them came together and they call themselves, IG Farben. They knew that they had to be stronger because they didn't accomplish what they wanted to in the first place. So then they found a guy named Hitler, Adolf Hitler. And they empowered him and backed him. And they started the Second World War.

The Second World War was to go and to accomplish what they had begun in the first place but they didn't get to do it. But in the Second World War, Bayer, the same people that brought you Bayer aspirin are the same people that created mustard gas. And mustard gas was used in the Second World War. Mustard gas does many things, from causing you to spit-up blood, to causing different types of bone cancers. It basically destroys the body. It was one of the worst things that they ever used in war.

So, what happened was that these pharmaceutical companies, they actually built a plant. And I think the plant was as big as—it was in Auschwitz and the plant was 25 square kilometers.

Ty: Not to cut you off here, but we recently did an interview with Dr. Matthias Rath in Netherlands. And he showed us photographs of the plant that they built, the Auschwitz plant. I think it was 25 square miles or —it was five kilometers by five. Huge.

Dr. Wolfe: You know, they did that and then they studied and used people as their guinea pigs. They study all their pharmaceuticals. And then they went and took the mustard gas and made chemo by changing the sulphur atoms to nitrogen atoms. That was the first time, now we have chemo. And that's how chemo was created.

Ty: By a multinational drug conglomerate.

Dr. Wolfe: That's right.

Ty: Chemical conglomerate.

Dr. Wolfe: That's right. I don't mean to be like this and everybody is going to think it is really bad but whenever there's really horrific problems in the world, it is always because of the same people. They're the same troublemakers. The same people, but they just shift the blame to other places.

It will always be the same thing. It's not you and me.

Ty: What about natural cures for cancer? Are there any natural cures for cancer even though the word "cure" is passe and we're not supposed to say "cure." Are there treatments for cancer that might mitigate cancer that are natural?

Dr. Wolfe: Thousands. There are thousands of them. In comparison to what—well, for one thing, what the medical system has is very archaic. The only reason why people use the medical system, whether it be chemotherapy, radiation, or surgery—sometimes, surgery is needed—but it is because of fear or panic. So that's the only reason.

When it comes to natural cures, there's thousands of them, Ty. In my practice, I use curcumin and cayenne together with great success. I used another product which is atomic mineral spray. I use atomic mineral spray on the lymph nodes for almost every type of cancer. And I'll tell you, people who say they don't have cancer, within days, they've got scabbing on their lymph nodes. And that's the killing off of the cancer cells.

So there are thousands of cures out there. And what is a cure? A cure is something that takes something away. But remember something Ty, that's not really a good name is it? Because a cure is not permanent. People think it is permanent. The only thing that is permanent is you learning how to look after your body. You're not worried about cancer, but I'll tell you something, almost everybody watching this video right now is worried about cancer. They are on the couch, crapping themselves.

You know what? You are crapping yourself because you haven't been trained. You have been trained so you are confident. Am I confident? Like I said, I don't want to be scared anymore. If you don't want to be scared anymore then you need to train to how to look after yourself and not count on me.

You know what I say? I say to my patients this, "I'll give a money back guarantee that the work that I do, that is the first treatment that you come to me, you will learn more and you'll get more than everything else that you've done or you don't pay me."

Now, do I do that because I need the money or am I doing that because it's not difficult to outdo other practitioners because all you have to do is start empowering the people? And what great thing

You know what? This is the greatest thing that's ever been done on this planet, is your video series. And I'm not saying that to stroke you but this is a tidal wave. This has got me going. This has got me excited. This has put life back into me.

This will put courage back into practitioners so they can grow some. So that they can train people. So that people can become the masters of their own bodies. And guess what? That is the only cure. The only cure is you, not outside of you.

Ty: Well, thank you for the compliment. I really appreciate that. That's our role to create this tidal wave, as you put it, of education and knowledge for people to be able to be empowered. And as my co-host on a radio show, Robert Scott Bell says, "The power to heal is yours." And we want to give that power back to people.

Dr. Wolfe: Yes. And you know what? They don't even know that they don't even have it because they trust all these guys. All I have to say is, "Everybody at home, get off your lazy butt and stop being a scared chicken and take your life back and be what you are meant to be, great."

Ty: And I would say this interview has been great. Dr. Wolfe, I appreciate it.

Dr. Wolfe: Thank you, Ty.

[end of transcript]

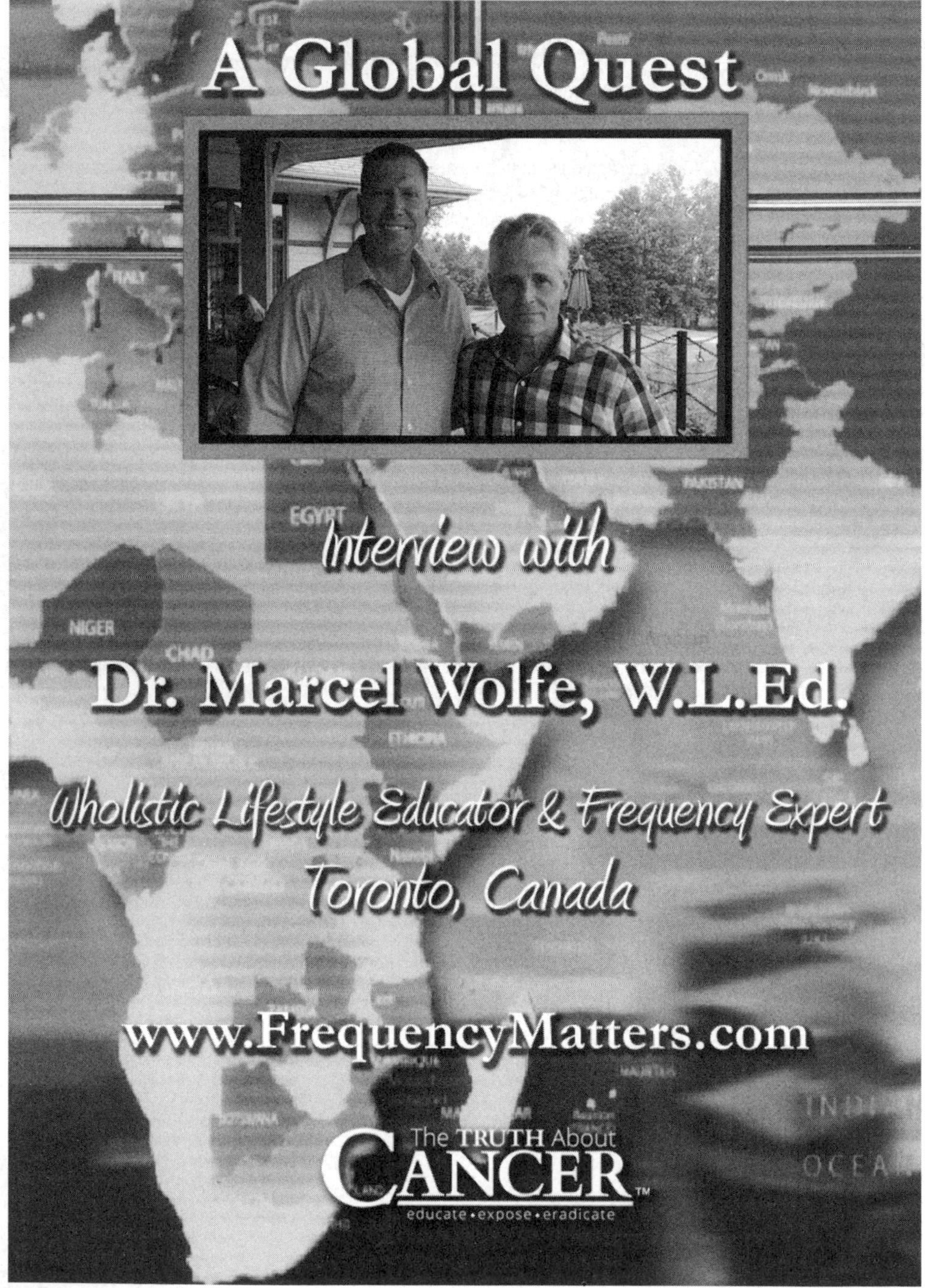
A Global Quest
EGYPT
Interview with
NIGER
CHAD
Dr. Marcel Wolfe, W.L.Ed.
Wholistic Lifestyle Educator & Frequency Expert
Toronto, Canada
www.FrequencyMatters.com
The TRUTH About
CANCER
educate • expose • eradicate

Ty: I'm here in Canada just north of Toronto with Marcel Wolfe. Marcel, thanks for being with us today.

Dr. Wolfe: It's good to see you.

Ty: We're going to talk about frequency, electricity. The interview should be electrifying. Thank you, Daryl, Dr. Wolf. So talk about frequency and cancer.

Dr. Wolfe: The connection is so strong and Albert von Szent-Györgyi, Nicola Tesla, Royal Raymond Rife, Dr. Samuel Milham, Dr. Robert Becker, they all understood this. How many more studies do we need to have, right? Can we not just take it that these gentlemen knew what they were talking about?

Albert von Szent-Györgyi said that cancer is due to a sub-molecular electronic disturbance. He's the one that understood vitamin C. He won the Nobel Prize for metabolism. He is considered the father of modern biochemistry. Maybe he knew what he was talking about.

Maybe Tesla, the inventor of electricity, who knew electricity—he brought to us two things, AC electricity and he tried to bring us DC but, of course, that wasn't good for the money people. And he also brought us ozone and PEMF, two forms of—

Ty: What is PEMF?

Dr. Wolfe: Pulsating electromagnetic energy fields. So not a static magnet. Everything in life pulses, we need a pulse. On the moon there is no PEMF, there is no pulse and that's why nothing lives there.

We have evolved, adapted to, and now are dependent upon energy that we weren't aware even existed. It wasn't until we sent somebody into space in 1962, Yuri Gagarin, who was only out there for an hour and 48 minutes, but because he was beyond the reach of these frequencies in our environment, in an hour and 48 minutes he had severe bone loss to the point of osteoporosis, decreased metabolism, loss of perception and depression which affected him for the rest of his life. He committed suicide at the age of 37.

When we expose ourselves to PEMF, you can actually flip those things, reverse them—increase bone density, increase perception, increase metabolism, and increase the sense of wellbeing.

Ty: Let me ask you this, Marcel. We hear about EMF being bad for us, electromagnetic frequencies, we're getting them from all directions. But what you're saying is that if you have PEMF, pulsed EMF, then it can be positive.

Dr. Wolfe: Exactly.

Ty: So how do we create PEMF?

Dr. Wolfe: Basically what we're trying to do is mimic. I say whether it's an air purifier, water purifier, or PEMF technologies, those technologies which best mimic nature are the ones you want to line up for.

There is a range of frequencies that are in our environment that are conducive to our health and that is what we are duplicating. The cell phone frequencies are billions of hertz per second. If you could imagine instead of being in nature—this is a sign wave, right? Even to look at it, it looks like the waves on the ocean and it's very calming.

If you can imagine putting your finger up and down, billions of cycles per second, even to look at it is annoying. If I turn on one of these meters it actually screeches. Our ears are not picking it up but the meter is and it's affecting our cells. We are primarily frequency.

Not only are we frequency, but even beyond that, we are actually light beings. Basically things that we've had faith in for over 5,000 years are now being proven by science. This is the most exciting time to be alive. We're this close to Star Trek health.

Ty: You mentioned frequency. One of the men that you mentioned previously was Royal Raymond Rife. He had a device that used specific frequencies that targeted cancer cells. The cells had a specific frequency. He was able to selectively target those through introducing this into the body.

Dr. Wolfe: Bacteria, viruses, parasites, pathogens, cancer are not good or evil. They are doing exactly what nature intended. They are getting rid of entities that are vibrating below the standard of nature. At 42 millihertz or less, that cell is cancerous. If it's at 70, it can't be cancerous. So, hmm. Does frequency sound like it might be an answer? Yes.

When the cells actually get the proper frequency, then we're talking about it has the ability to detox better, to uptake whatever it is that you're consuming. PEMF I'd have to say is one of the most powerful tools that I've seen in 35 years in holistic health.

Ty: What types of devices can generate PEMF?

Dr. Wolfe: We now have PEMF devices for cats and dogs. I'm working with a number of different companies. One company actually is the largest seller of PEMF for the equine industry—horses, race horses, jumpers. The beauty about nature is that there is no placebo effect.

Back in 2007 we had a world renowned horse trainer and breeder throw a PEMF human device on top of a horse's back. It had shipping fever, basically it was suffocating. And the vet heard the horse breathing, knowing the horse, and said, "I'm sorry, I'm 90 minutes away. By the time I get there the horse will be dead."

So she figured, "What have I got to lose?" This lady from Switzerland who came to visit her had this technology. She dragged it out, threw it on the horse's back, and within seconds the horse was breathing better. By the end of the day it was fine.

Another horse with a hip displacement—normally they shoot the horse—another horse confirmed. The vet came out, took the blood and confirmed, "Yes, it has Cushing's" which is a form of cancer for horses. And after about 14 sessions, gone. Hip displacement, fine. The thing about animals is that they don't go to Tim Horton's, they don't stay up late at night on the computer. They are doing more of what they should be doing.

I was just thinking about it earlier today. Anyone that says ozone cures, PEMF cures they are doing a huge disservice to themselves and other people. As we say—a good friend of mine, Dr. Howard Fisher who you had here—"a hammer is a great tool but it's not the only tool in the toolbox."

If you've got cancer, we're not just going to rely on ozone or PEMF or moringa. We're going to do everything we can so that that enemy says, "This isn't my place, I'm out of here. The frequencies are too high, too healthy. This is not my place." As a service to ourselves and to other people, yes we can be excited about PEMF. We can be excited about moringa or ozone or anything else. But in order to be fair, let's tell people, "Look. Do as much as you can that is practical for you."

That four ounces of organic, freshly squeezed wheatgrass juice and you've never had it before, when you take it you could have vomiting, diarrhea, nauseous feelings and figure, "Oh, this is bad for me." Well, no. It's actually good. It's just that when you clean house you make a mess. Do it at a level which is practical and that you can deal with. That all takes education, that all takes training.

What is the purpose of giving people wisdom? The purpose of wisdom is action. We want to empower people. As my brother says, "Enough of selling stuff. Let's train them." We're at a point in history right now. We just heard here in Canada—you got the same message as we did—we're looking at an increase of what, 40 percent in cancer because people are getting older?

It doesn't matter whether you are four or 84, a cat or a dog, it is all about quality of life. We don't know how long we're going to be here, but let's make the best of it. Let's stop denying. I want to see humans reach their potential.

The idea of still burning fossil fuel—what the hell? We had electric cars in New York and in the 1930s we had more electric cars on the road than what we have today. We had homeopathy, acupuncture, hands-on healing. We had more PEMF devices in medical schools than what we have today.

But what is happening now is a curious thing. Our government, in 2010, the Premier of our Province said, "If we continue, we're not going to be able to afford to help anyone." In 2010 we're using 42 cents out of every dollar raised in taxes for that present model, what I call, "Crisis Healthcare System."

They are good at a crisis, but in terms of anything else, forget it. They weren't educated. And as I say to people, "Look, before you ask your doctor about spirulina, cayenne, PEMF, first ask them how much did they study it? Have they ever had any experience in it? If the answer is no, then their opinion isn't worth anything."

We had those things in the 20s and 30s and people said, "Well, if this is so good, why are we just hearing about it now?" I know that people don't want to believe that there are actually people out there that are willing to sacrifice them just so they can make more money, but that is reality. That's the truth. So we need to figure that out, deal with it, and move on.

The thing I like about frequency is that I call it the truth serum for the future. We're going to pay more for this tomato over this one. Why? Because it has a higher frequency. It's got nothing to do with size, color, and taste. It is frequency.

Charlie Chaplin on his 70th birthday decided to get rid of those things which drew him down. And we're talking about frequency—people, food, situations. I tell people, "Don't wait till your 70th birthday, start doing it today." We need to actually empower this miracle, the human cell.

This is phenomenal. I have to show this to you. You've heard in different settings, in different religious communities, "Come into the light. Be part of the light." We're actually not just frequency beings, we're light beings.

This is actually a cross section of the DNA. Do you know anything about sacred geometry? When I looked at that, it just made me shiver. This is actually a cross section of the DNA. This is the DNA as we know it. It is actually the perfect antenna for picking up frequency.

But this shows us here that the DNA—as I call it, a thing of beauty and complexity, sacred geometry—this is a cross section of DNA revealing 4 billion photonic flashlights in one cross section of DNA.

What I would like to see is actually in schools, in churches, let's start with children and say, "Hey, look. We want you to understand that you are living in something, this human body, that is miraculous. It's amazing. You can be Super Girl, you can be Super Ty, you can be Super Daryl, you can be Super Howie. Here, we're going to show you how to do it. We don't know how long we're here but let's make the most of it. "

If they could actually see how incredible, miraculous the human cell is—I call it the most miraculous, most intriguing, most complex single entity that we'll encounter in this lifetime—if they could see how amazing this mobile home is, this temple, this bag of water shaped like a human being. If they could see how incredible it is, then maybe they would respect themselves more, and they wouldn't waste their time.

Ty: What's up with the fly swatter?

Dr. Wolfe: Basically I have two gifts here for you. I'm part of Tesla-mania. Tesla was, hands down, no question, the greatest mind in human history. If I could go back in history and spend some time with somebody, it would be him. He had the answers then. We just have to revisit his technology.

Can you imagine living in a world where we didn't use fossil fuel? We didn't use nuclear? What would it be like? We'd be living in paradise. If we had next to free energy, right? As Einstein said, "The most important thing is imagination."

If we had unlimited resources, where would we be by now? We're still burning fossil fuel. This is ridiculous, people. And people say, "Oh, you know, WiFi is all around. What are we going to do?" and they just put up the hands and say, "Oh, it's in God's hands." No. It's in your hands, okay?

Ignorance is no longer an excuse, not for you or the politicians. Because we can have current information [fingers snap] like that. And if you're a politician, it's your responsibility. If you're propagating ignorance we're going to find out about it now quicker than we ever have. We are calling you on it.

One example I love is Coca-Cola. They never wanted to be in the water business, but they were forced to. Why? Was it because we gave enough money to the government to educate people? By the way, the sugar causes cancer. The caramelization causes cancer. The carbonization causes cancer. There isn't one redeeming quality in this thing we call Coke, and guess what? We are now buying more water. And fewer people—you don't see many people around here with Coke cans anymore.

Why? Was that the government saying, "We need to step in and do the right thing," or was that Coca-Cola saying, "We've made enough money. We need to come forth and be honest about this." No. They were forced to because we increased the conscious awareness around what actually quenches thirst. It's water, the best water, frequency water. Not Coca-Cola.

Two months ago, Coca-Cola reported—I don't know if it was just Canada or North America—the worst financial record in their history. They can't sell their crap anymore, so they got into water and it is even ozonated. Let's bring things up to speed. Toronto still doesn't ozonate water.

Just for kicks, this is back probably about 12 years ago, I called up the water department in Toronto. I actually got the engineer in charge of Toronto water. And I was just playing around, I said, "When are we going to use ozone to purify water?" "Oh, we're doing studies." I said, "You know what? I have to be honest with you. We know everything that has ever been needed to know about ozone. Montreal is doing it, Vancouver is doing it."

Let's call these people and get them up to speed. They want to keep their jobs? Let's get them up to speed. I think politicians, if they screw up kick them out right away. Don't wait for for years. And I want to see the Canadian Prime Minister—pay him $20 million. I don't care. Get the best person. He's going to say, "I'm only being paid this much." We should actually put people in positions where they have no opportunity to do anything but the right thing. I'm getting off topic, but it's all connected.

Ty: Are you trying to keep the fly swatter a secret?

Dr. Wolfe: The fly swatter, sir, this represents—you have, actually, have better odds of you walking into a swamp and killing all the mosquitoes than our present medical system has at finding a cure for the hundred different forms of cancer that exist today.

You know that Ronald Raymond Rife—we just talked about him, an amazing person. And how did he end up? Pretty sad. We know that cancer has the ability to mutate. So does bacteria. Finally they've admitted, "We're fighting this bacterial war all wrong." It is because everything that is designed by nature has superior innate intelligence. If that bacteria needs to mutate or go under the fence or over the fence, it will.

When man designed something like anti-bacteria, antibiotic—"anti" means against, "biotic" means life. Why would you take something that is against life? It's going to wipe out all the good and bacteria and now leave you more vulnerable for something even more serious when we have things like ionic silver, oregano oil. And guess what? It's all frequency.

First, secondary chemistry and who said that? Oh, I don't know, Einstein? Albert von Szent-Györgyi? All these great individuals? It's time to get on. Let's make things happen. Every generation wants better for the children, but we're being told now that this generation of children are less likely to outlive their parents. Yet we're still being told life is better. Does that make sense to you?

Ty: All of the devices that we're using, all of the electromagnetic frequencies we're exposed to, you do worry about the next generation. But I see that you've got some devices over here that might help. Show us a few of the devices that you've got here and explain how they might help to mitigate some of this bad electricity, these bad frequencies that we are exposed to.

Dr. Wolfe: I say that it's time for us to become armed, not armed and dangerous, but armed and ready to find danger. Our environments are changing all the time. Even if you live in a house, you don't know if your neighbor is putting in WiFi or if he's got a cordless phone. With these meters we can actually find out and it's measurable.

According to North American standards, everything is okay until your cells start to cook by one degree. Well, things happen way before that. You don't want the cordless phone in your home. When I'm talking to people, they could be anywhere in North America, the first thing I'll say is, "Are you talking to me right now on a cordless phone?" "Yes." "You need to get rid of that yesterday."

And you've got cancer? You could be taking all these great things. You could have your PEMF mag. You would have been taking moringa and silver and all this good detoxification stuff, but if you are immersed in an EMF environment, you are undoing all the good.

Ty: Are there things that we can use to mitigate that?

Dr. Wolfe: Yes.

Ty: Because I'll guarantee you that not everybody that is watching is going to want to get rid of their cordless phone.

Dr. Wolfe: No.

Ty: Are there things that they can do?

Dr. Wolfe: We're not going back to living in caves or living in trees, but we need to use technology mindfully, not mindlessly. We're not going to die because of convenience. One of the reasons why I'm so passionate about this is because, as my brother said, "We've seen our relatives perish way before their time."

My father slept in an electric blanket in 1987. We told him not to. We said, "That form of energy so close in proximity to the human body is not conducive to your health." He said—and I quoted him, he's actually part of my presentation—"They wouldn't sell it if it wasn't safe." We can go down the list—mercury fillings, asbestos was called the miracle mineral, formaldehyde, no, not formaldehyde. What was the drug that we gave the children? Pregnant women in Canada? A huge settlement now.

Ty: Thalidomide.

Dr. Wolfe: Exactly. That was called the miracle drug. The government doesn't have a very good track record. Actually, I like one of the quotes from Einstein. He said "The greatest enemy of truth is to have faith in authority." It's like what? Why would you say that? It's because he knew. He tried to give people a heads up.

We have things that we can actually do. If I turn this on [vibrating sound]. Of course the frequencies way out here are not as bad as they are in the city. But if I just simply drape this—this actually has metal in it—it goes silent. I actually have put it in my home.

Ty: What is it made of?

Dr. Wolfe: This actually has metal in it. So basically, my sheer curtains at home are made of this material. I have a neighbor which is probably known internationally. It's called Baycrest. It has the closest cell tower. So here they are and they've got nice beautiful TV ads about how they are doing all this research to improve the quality of life. Meanwhile they've got a stinkin' cell tower on their institution and we call that our nasty neighbor. Measurably, it's doing everyone harm.

This is actually a cheaper meter. What I like about this is that it actually gives you an audible as well as a digital reading and you don't even have to take the course like I did for two years to become a building biologist. You can see that if this is in the yellow it's not so bad. If it's green it's better. If it is orange or red it is not so good.

Ty: So you've got your curtain there that can mitigate some of the electric fields coming in. Let's just assume that everybody is living in dirty electricity. Without the meters, what solutions do you have?

Dr. Wolfe: For a lot of people, they may not understand this. But I suggest that they just look into it. Even if they don't have the money for all of this, something as simple as dousing. Actually a pendulum can tell you, if it's a right spin, it's healthy. If it's a left spin it's negative. But the first thing that you want to do is you want to start with your bedroom.

Ty: Start doing what?

Dr. Wolfe: You want to make sure that that is the safest place in your home because you are spending eight hours a day.

Ty: I guess I'm not asking the question properly. I'm assuming we're all living in toxic, dirty electricity. So let's say that's a given. What do we do about it? What solutions do you have?

Dr. Wolfe: Here is one solution out of Germany. From what I understand, 400 of the staff of the Lufthansa Airlines are all wearing this.

Ty: What is it?

Dr. Wolfe: Basically it is putting out—and I can actually plug some of the technology I have into this so you can actually hear the different frequencies—it puts out eight different frequencies. So you can look up a frequency for sleep, for jet lag, for all the different situations in life.

Ty: It's putting out PEMF?

Dr. Wolfe: Yes, it's putting out pulsating electromagnetic energy fields. This other little device that we have here—

Ty: Does a device like this mitigate the effects of the other dirty electricity in the house?

Dr. Wolfe: A lot of people that sell these technologies—I probably have right now five different technologies on me. Because if this one helps me 15 percent and this one helps me 86 percent—we're living in extreme times and I have a saying that, "The extremes of today will be the norm of tomorrow."

If my grandparents knew that I'd pay $5 for a bottle of water at the airport they'd think I was loony. It's just the times require us to take further measures than what they had to. This one puts out eight different frequencies, PEMF.

Ty: Okay, hold on. Let's say somebody's talking on their cordless phone. Can they put that on in their house and then mitigate the negative effects of the cordless phone? That's my question.

Dr. Wolfe: As a building biologist, the first thing you want to do is remove the source of the problem. It's the same thing we do in holistic health, remove the source of the problem. We can actually use what I call holistic bandages but it gets back to your daily routine. Is that daily routine supporting the human cell, its functionality? If it is, then you're going to be a healthy person.

A lot of people sell these different devices, pendulums and the different things that they wear as blocking frequencies. If it actually blocked your cell phone frequencies you wouldn't be able to communicate. It is at best, making it less harmful. These things are now measurable.

We can use darkfield microscopy blood analysis, thermal imaging, infrared, electro interstitial scanner. We now have more of these scientific means of seeing an increase in terms of before and after.

What this will do and what this device does is that it enhances your own energy field which you've heard of, aura. It actually exists and we can actually see this using powerful film and camera. We can actually see it before and after. This is enhancing my own aura. This is actually putting out not only PEMF, scalar, and also color light therapy, all three.

This used to be a box that was $3,000 and now it's all into this. And soon we will actually have a cell battery in here so that you can charge this once every—it will go for two weeks. And you can put it in your car, you can put it in your computer.

It is actually going to send out healing frequencies while you're on your computer, while you are in your car, and you can also be able to wear this in your pocket, around your neck. It's going to enhance your energy field which acts—it's like the invisible buffer against all of this stuff that is happening to us.

Let's say you're in a room of 25 people and 24 people are speaking a language that you don't know what they are saying. But there is one person in that room that is speaking English. That is the one you are going to gravitate to and that one is the one that is going to enhance your overall energy. That's what the body is able to do.

Even right now we are surrounded. How many cell phone frequencies are we being hit by—TV, radio, WiFi, GPS, all of that. By enhancing your own body energy, you are increasing your opportunity to be shielded from these frequencies.

Ty: I guess it doesn't really block the bad frequencies. It just magnifies the good.

Dr. Wolfe: Yes. Your cells will resonate with 8 hertz, 5 hertz, and 7.83 hertz. But billions of hertz cycles per second? They are going to have an effect, they're disruptive. But if we can at least enhance our body's ability to protect ourselves that's the key here.

I highly recommend that people take the opportunity to investigate frequency and what role it plays in their lives and their environment. Something as simple as we were talking about earlier, linen. In the Bible it says, and also in the Torah, we're not supposed to wear linen and wool together. Well, okay, whatever I guess it's a rule. Let's try and abide by it. But there is a reason for everything.

Linen has a signature frequency of 5,000 and so does wool. The problem is one is positive and the other one is negative. What happens is that if you wear the two of them together—and this is important for cancer or for anybody that wants to optimize their health—is that it not only will put you into illness but also in pain.

Basically, like I was saying earlier, things that we've had blind faith in for over 5,000 years are now being proven and justified by using frequency, by using science showing measurable results before and after.

Chlorophyll has a frequency. A plant, an apple that we pick from the tree has its highest frequency and that is why this whole fresh and raw movement is so huge. Because the energy can be measured and it is higher than if we transport that fruit or vegetable from Mexico to Canada, nuke it, whatever. If you eat that food, you're going to be dead.

There was a device called a BT3. It had the ability to measure human frequencies, plant, soil, food, all of that. We have the ability. What I'm saying is that in making choices, whether it's about people or about food or about clothing to cover ourselves—the polyester, the synthetics have a frequency level of zero. It's actually going to detract from your energy.

If you've got cancer, you are going to want to put all of your options in your favor. You're going to want to eat the food with the highest frequency, drink the water with the highest frequency, and sleep in a bed that is not metal, that you don't have the cordless phone and the cell phone on your pillow, and all these crazy things. You need to become more mindful about what you're doing in your life to enhance your opportunity and your children's opportunity to have the best life possible.

Ty: Last question. Let's say that you're living in an urban area. There are cell phone towers everywhere. Some areas in the United States, I know we've got thousands of towers that are within 10 or 20 miles. What is the best way to protect yourself in an environment like that? Let's say maybe you turn your WiFi off at night. So what? In the big scheme of things, all these cell towers—what do you do to protect maybe your whole household?

Dr. Wolfe: There is a free app that is called Tower Locator. If you look at the cell towers in downtown Toronto which has some of the highest property values in Canada, right next to the CN Tower you're going to have to take some extreme measures.

We have black carbon paint. Literally you could paint all four walls, the ceiling and the floor, close the door and it's absolutely silent. You could paint over it any color that you want.

Ty: That stopped the electricity, the…

Dr. Wolfe: It stops the radio frequencies, which is the things that we're worried about in terms of the CN tower. We have children that are born with acute leukemia. "What the hell has that up with?" They haven't even had the opportunity to make good or bad choices.

We find out that the mother was sleeping next to a wall. On the other side of that wall was a fridge, a furnace, an air conditioner that threw off a huge AC electromagnetic energy field that mutated that new life form.

And how are we going to know this unless we have somebody like myself come in with a bunch of meters or at least buy one of these little meters, we're not going to know that. But there are things that we can do.

I've already helped friends of mine with million dollar condos. And she had to spend $12,000 but it was better than having to move in an area that she didn't know what was going to happen. There are things that we can do. But some people are so electro- hypersensitive they actually have to move out of the city.

Ty: Right. Marcel thanks for sharing with us today. It's been fascinating. I really appreciate it.

Dr. Wolfe: Thank you. I appreciate you, too.

[end of transcript]

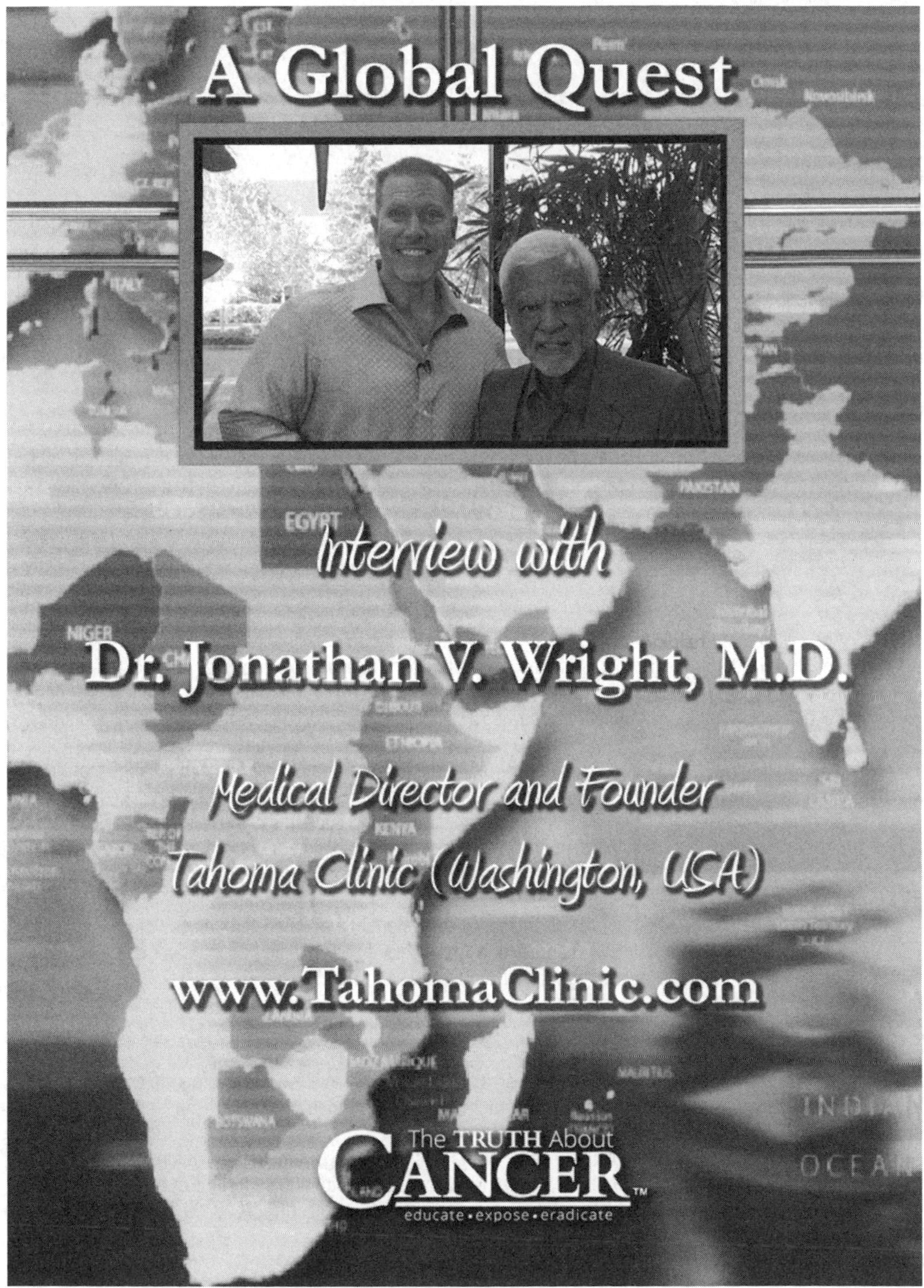
A Global Quest
Interview with
Dr. Jonathan V. Wright, M.D.
Medical Director and Founder
Tahoma Clinic (Washington, USA)
www.TahomaClinic.com
The TRUTH About
CANCER
educate • expose • eradicate

Ty: Well, I'm really excited to be here in Tacoma, Washington with Dr. Jonathan Wright. Thank you so much for joining us.

Dr. Wright: Thanks for coming out.

Ty: Beautiful clinic you have here. I love your office. We had several options to film here and we came in here and said, "this is the place to film."

Dr. Wright: You must like giraffes or something.

Ty: I like the eclectic nature of the office. It's great. I think it fits your personality. So I'm really interested to get your take on a lot of different subjects today. But first of all if you could, just for the people that are watching, could you go over your education? Where did you go to school and what got you to becoming a doctor?

Dr. Wright: All right. Where do I start? High school? Kindergarten?

Ty: Start wherever you feel like.

Dr. Wright: Well, let's see. Seems that the university happened to be Harvard and I happened to get into it when I was 16. So I managed to graduate when I was 20 and get an early start on medical school which was at the University of Michigan. And I was in the University of Michigan Medical School for four years. I should back up a little bit and say that one thing that was an important influence on the type of health care that I work with people on was that in college I did dual major. It was pre-med and it was cultural anthropology.

And cultural anthropology is a lot of different things having to do with different people around the world. The thing I got interested in is health all around the world with different peoples. I looked at what they were eating and what kind of things they were doing and how their health was. And that wasn't done deliberately to influence anything I'd learned in medicine. I was just interested in health all together.

It turned out that it was quite an influence. And the reason for that is that one of the things that's real clear from studying anthropology is that people who live close to the land and eat unprocessed unrefined foods—it doesn't matter what it is, it can be fishing coconuts if you're in the Pacific, it can be deer and elk if you're up in the mountains, and vegetables and stuff. It doesn't matter what it is. If it is unprocessed and unrefined we just do not see the higher rates of certain diseases that we see today.

The so called, as you know very well, diseases of western civilization. We don't see them. And so that taught me for later that a lot of times it doesn't matter what you're eating as long as it's totally natural, totally unrefined, and prepared right away. You might say it's eating local.

Ty: Sure. Farm to table.

Dr. Wright: Well, there you go. After good old University of Michigan, then a residency program as they're called,there was an internship residency after the medical school. And that was in family medicine.

And there, as well as in medical school, I was taught everything there was—that they taught medical students anyway—about human anatomy, physiology, chemistry and so forth. But when they got around to teaching therapies, they gave us a whole hour on nutritionals. A whole hour.

Ty: A whole hour.

Dr. Wright: In four years of medical school, they told us that there's vitamin A, and B1, and B2, and C, and D, and they're in alphabetical order and you can look them up. And then they told us some really basic facts. We got a whole hour of it.

On the other side of things, we got hours and hours and hours on how to use basically patented medicines. Which, as you know, are what usually go on the prescription pad as a molecule that can be patented with which means it's not found in nature. Because you can't patent it if it's found in nature. And that what's we get educated in. Well, I didn't know any better. Except for this little bit I had in Harvard in the cultural anthropology.

So when I was in the internship and residency program, that's most of what I did until a couple of three patients woke me up in the second year of the residency program. They came in and woke me up about what medicine should be about.

Ty: Dr. Wright, tell me about your "aha" moment that really opened your eyes. How did these patients help you to see the light?

Dr. Wright: Well, let me tell you about a couple of them. A lady comes in. I looked at her entire record. Same problem all time, intense leg cramps, just bad ones. And she had been tried on every patent medicine in the book that's supposed to stop leg cramps.

Plus they'd even used calcium because medical doctors were taught about calcium. And none of it had worked. And what had worked to control them but not get rid of them—in other words they weren't as bad—was quinine. It turns out if you take enough quinine to make your ears ring sometimes it will stop leg cramps.

So she was on all this quinine. I looked through her records. That's what she's been in for every time, everything had been tried. So when she came in and told me, "I'd like to get my leg cramps taken care of." I said, "everything has been tried. I don't know anything else to do for you. Besides that I'm a new graduate. I'm a rookie. So it's all in there. You've tried everything." She said, "no, no, no, no. I don't want you to try something for me. I want you to tell me if something is safe." Well, what's that?

So she pulls this book out and she says, "it says right here that vitamin E sometimes stops leg cramps." And I said, "okay. So did you try vitamin E?" "Oh no. The FDA tells us we can overdose on fat soluble vitamins and kill ourselves. But other places say it's safe. So I'm just here to ask you if it's safe for me to take vitamin E?" And remember this is in 1971 or 1972. So I told her that the one thing they told us about vitamin E in medical school is that you can't kill yourself with it.

You can kill yourself with vitamin D if you take way too much, vitamin A if you take too much. But you can't kill yourself with vitamin E. "Okay. That's all I needed to know." Basically, she was there to teach me something.

Any doctor will tell you that some of their patients are there to teach the doctor, not to be treated. Because I never saw her again. But she called up about six weeks later and says, "I just thought that I'd let you know that I took that vitamin E and the third week I quit having leg cramps. And I haven't had leg cramps since. And I flushed all those patent medications and quinine down the toilet."

And she said, "I think I'll just keep taking vitamin E." I thought, "Damn. There's a hole missing in my medical education here." Very fortunately I copied the titles of the books that she brought in. So I went down to the store and got one.

And the next time somebody came in—this is the second one, I won't bore you with a third one—she was having nausea from birth control pills. Now, early 70s, higher dose birth control pills. A fair minority of women got nausea from them. And she said, "this is the only kind of birth control I can use. IUD doesn't work for me and I can't trust some of the other means and so forth." So she wants to be on birth control pills but she doesn't like the nausea.

She says, "what can I do?" And I said, "I don't know. Excuse me a minute." And that's sometimes what the doctor is doing when they get up and say, "excuse me a minute." I went the next room and looked in that book that the lady brought in that I bought a copy of.

And it said right in that book that if you get nausea from estrogens, whether they're birth control pills or other estrogens, take some vitamin B6. It'll will go away. So I came on back and said, "well, you know I haven't actually worked with anybody on this. But I know vitamin B6 is safe in small doses. So here, take some vitamin B6 and see if your nausea goes away." Her nausea went away. I never saw her again either. And she didn't call me. She called my assistant and said, "my nausea is gone just thought I'd let you know."

So it's one of those times when somebody is there to teach you something as well as maybe to get better themselves. So I picked up that book and went to the University of Washington library. That book had a lot of nice footnotes to the medical studies. And I started—oh my gosh, look at all this stuff about vitamins and minerals and herbs that I never learned in medical school. And it's right there in the medical journal. How come I never learned it in medical school? And for anybody who wants to know, this was Adelle Davis' book.

Remember that name, Adelle Davis. It was one of her books. So at that time we had photocopies and we had to put a nickel in. So I spent a lot nickels up at the University of Washington library photocopying all this stuff. And that started a collection that I've continued. And also Dr. Alan Gaby, who you know of, he actually came out just after his internship and worked at the office that, at that time, was further south but here in this area. He worked there for about 18 months before he decided he wants to go back to where his family lives. Which you can't blame him for. But he picked up a lot of clinical stuff during that.

But I hardly ever saw Alan. When he wasn't at the practice, he was always up at the library. He's another library hound. So we had all this on-paper research and by the time we switched from on-paper to computerized which was the 90s, we'd accumulated about 60,000-70,000 articles. And they're all in this storage trailer in file cabinets and they are all titled and cross-referenced and so forth. When we finally learned how to run a computer—we were a little slow, both of us, on that—by then we collected another 20,000-30,000 articles. So we have close to 100,000 references from scientific journals that tell us about the diet, vitamins, minerals, botanicals, natural energies, and so forth and their influence on health.

So don't let anybody ever tell you that this isn't scientific. There's just tons of science. It's just that nobody pays attention to it because, I'm sorry folks, it isn't patentable. And if you can't patent it, you can't make big bucks. And I think we all know that the trend in, lets call it regular medicine, right now is for the newest patent medicines to be more expensive, more expensive, more expensive. What is it? $73,000 a year? $1,000 a pill for hepatitis treatment, that kind of stuff. You can charge that if you got a patent and you got a monopoly. And you cannot do that with unpatentable stuff. So that's why most medical doctors simply haven't even heard of it. It's not that they're, "I hate nature." It's just that they don't know the science is there.

Ty: And the science is there, in 100,000 articles.

Dr. Wright: Close to. We're not quite to 100,000. Either paper or electronic.

Ty: It really seems to me unfathomable that with that much scientific basis that they're not taught. But the medical schools may be co-opted. Who knows?

Dr. Wright: Of course. You've told everybody about the Flexner Report. I heard you on the radio doing that. And you know where that got started.

Ty: Sure. People hear this and they may say this sounds conspiratorial, right? You've heard the Fitzgerald Report, right?

Dr. Wright: I got a copy of some of the conclusions over here. Shall I read them to people?

Ty: Absolutely. The Fitzgerald Report. Tell the viewers what the Fitzgerald Report was.

Dr. Wright: I'll tell them. Or you can tell them and I'll just read it.

Ty: You go ahead and tell them.

Dr. Wright: The Fitzgerald Report was published in the *Congressional Record*, folks. Actually, it was an appendix to the *Congressional Record*. And Fitzgerald was an investigator for the Interstate Commerce Commission. I'm going to read this because I have to read you the citations because people will otherwise think it is conspiracy theory. In 1953 he was an investigator for the Interstate Commerce Commission. A senator whose grandson had been cured of cancer by natural means, and had a lot of trouble getting that cure done, asked him to investigate.

Now, here's just one quote everybody can read if they wish. All they have to do—folks if you want to see this, you put, "Fitzgerald Report 1953" into your search engine, up it comes. Fitzgerald says, "My investigation to date should convince this committee that a conspiracy does exist." This is testimony before Congress by a chief investigator for the Interstate Commerce Commission. "A conspiracy does exist to stop the free flow and use of drugs." Now, he calls it all drugs but most people even in conventional medicine call even vitamin drugs. If it's a treatment, it's a drug. And you do know that the FDA declared stool a drug some two years ago? And then they got so much ridicule from the academic centers that we're doing these fecal transplants that they undeclared stool a drug. But for a while, feces was a drug. How do you like that?

Anyway back to Fitzgerald. I know. It just seems weird. "To stop the free flow and use of drugs in interstate commerce which allegedly has solid therapeutic value. Public and private funds have been thrown around like confetti at a country fair to close up and destroy clinics." Notice he uses the word destroy. What he is talking about is the occasions when FDA went in with sledge hammers and broke up royal rife equipment in the office of Dr. Ruth Drown. Where they made someone throw all of his books that he had written on one aspect of energetic medicine. They were all burned at a bonfire in New Jersey. Book burning, sledge hammers. Now, Fitzgerald didn't say that. You can find that other part. I'll go back to Fitzgerald. But that's what he means by destroy. That's why he used the word destroy.

Okay, "to destroy clinics, hospitals, and scientific research laboratories which do not conform to the viewpoint of medical associations." Where this report comes from folks—and I'm sorry, I'm going to have to read it to you because my memory isn't that good. *Congressional Record*, Appendix, page A 5350. "A Report to the Senate Interstate Commerce Committee on the Need for Investigation of Cancer Research Organizations. Extension of remarks of Hon. William Langer of North Dakota in the Senate of the United States, Monday, August 5th, 1953." Not a conspiracy.

And what he says is, again, "public and private funds have been thrown around like confetti at a country fair to close up and destroy clinics, hospitals, and scientific research laboratories which do not conform to the viewpoint..."—it's got nothing to do with the law, it's got to do with the viewpoint—"...of medical associations." Benedict F. Fitzgerald, Junior Special Council, United States Committee on Interstate Foreign Commerce, 1953. And his report goes into a pages long report of suppression of natural treatments and it's in the *Congressional Record*.

And did anybody ever do anything about this? No. And part of what he says in that report is that the collusion, the actual conspiracy, is between Les Federales at FDA, the patent medicine companies, and the AMA. That's where the conspiracy that Fitzgerald identifies as is. And the fact that this printed in the *Congressional Record*, I think gets it sort of out of the, "this is nonsense" sort of thing. This guy is chief council—I'm sorry, Chief Special Investigator for the Interstate Commerce Commission.

Ty: Well, it certainly moves it from conspiracy theory to conspiracy fact.

Dr. Wright: There you go.

Ty: Doesn't it?

Dr. Wright: It sure does.

Ty: But the good thing is that since 1953 the FDA has never done anything like that, have they?

Dr. Wright: Sure they have.

Ty: Oh, they have?

Dr. Wright: Of course.

Ty: You want to share some of the stories that you have about that? Maybe personal stories?

Dr. Wright: Well, I do have this personal kind of story but I want to tell you about Dr. Ruth Drown first. You want to hear about her?

Ty: Yes.

Dr. Wright: There you go. We'll tell your faithful viewers about Dr. Ruth Drown. Dr. Ruth Drown was using equipment originated with Royal Rife. And Royal Rife was celebrated on page 1—do you know this? Perhaps some of your audience doesn't—of the Los Angeles times in 1932 or 33. A celebratory dinner for having cured cancer as attested to by 15 members of the faculty at the University of Southern California. Fifteen members.

They had sent him cancer patients. Some with not so bad cancer, some with really bad cancers. They were cured. So they had this celebration. "Cancer is now cured." How did Dr. Rife do it? Well, to try to condense it, he was an engineer. He'd invented this terrific optical microscope and he could see things almost to the point that an electron microscope can see today.

So he looked at cancers and he found that with each and every cancer there was an associated microorganism. He didn't say it was the same microorganism but it was and associated microorganism. He did something very smart. Taking from Einstein the cue that everything has its own vibratory frequency. Molecules do, people do. Everything has its vibratory frequency. He determined the vibratory frequency of those microorganisms and then he sent in a beam—which is why the machine was called a beam ray—he sent in a beam that had a dissonant frequency.

What's that? Have you ever tried to tune your radio and you tune it just right and it's nice and clear but you go a little bit off and it's, "meh meh meh" in addition to the talk. That's dissonance. You're almost on the right frequency but not quite.

So he sends in a dissonant frequency that's almost what these bacteria do. But they can't stand that because they're vibrating and are really close. So basically they rupture and die. All the bacteria do. He beamed them. And the cancers were cured. Now it's more complicated than that. He had to follow certain doses of rays and certain days and so forth. But anyway, the cancers were cured and it was celebrated on the Los Angeles Times..

He reports that he was visited by two people. One being Morris Fishbein at the AMA who was president at the time and another person. And I believe him because I've read that same report in a doctor's book from Alabama who's curing cancer with intravenous hydrochloric acid. I'm not kidding you. It was published for three years. I've got all of his reports. He was visited by two men from the AMA saying that he should sell them his treatments or he would never be published again. And he refused to sell and he was never published again.

I have the three years worth of reports. I can't get any more. There weren't anymore. Rife had the same visitation and so did other cancer-treating practitioners. Visitations from AMA telling us, "you sell us your stuff or we'll do you."

So that's why I believe Rife when he gave that because two other books reported the same thing. So he wouldn't sell. Rife wouldn't sell. So an employee turned up with kind of a shady background but I guess Rife didn't look into it good enough. And they got into some inter-company problems.

Rife, unfortunately, had an alcoholic family and he started drinking heavily. And that wasn't too good for Dr. Rife. So anyway, he wasn't doing his stuff anymore. His equipment was—actually in a lot of doctor's offices they bought Rife equipment.

Ruth Drown was one of those. She was a chiropractor. She was treating for cancer with Rife's equipment which again had been demonstrated and attested to by the newspaper in Southern California, the Los Angeles Times. I blank on the name. Attested that stuff cured cancer. Her equipment was bashed with sledge hammers by people from guess which federal agency?

Ty: FDA.

Dr. Wright: Yes. That's what I mean. Smashing with sledge hammers.

We'll fast forward to our clinic here. Now, it seems that—and this is 1982 now—it seems that 22 years before then, an FDA agent had shown up and gone, along with the member of the state board of pharmacy, to the part of our clinic where vitamins were on display.

And people could buy them from their health food store, they could buy them from us, they could buy them from wherever they got the best deal. But it was convenient to get it from us and a lot of people did. And they demanded that we give up all of our tryptophan to them. Give it to them. 110 bottles of it.

Ty: Tryptophan?

Dr. Wright: Tryptophan. Now why they did that was, as I say, 88, 89 was the world's first known GMO disaster. You've heard?

Ty: Yes.

Dr. Wright: Showa Denko Company in Japan had genetically modified a bacteria to make tryptophan. And guess what? It didn't make tryptophan. It made a tryptophan dimer which means two tryptophans stuck together. That's a GMO disaster because they put it in a bottle with capsules labeled "tryptophan" and it was sold in the United States. And that tryptophan stuck together. The body can't metabolize it and 38 people died. If that's not a GMO disaster, I don't know what is. But nobody wants to label it as a disaster caused by genetically modified organisms. That's what it was.

Ty: That was the first.

Dr. Wright: The very first. Showa Denko. So 38 people died. So FDA puts out this thing, "Thou shall not sell tryptophan." They didn't say exactly that but they said something like that. But everybody wondered, why didn't anybody in Canada die from tryptophan? How come Mexicans didn't die of tryptophan? How come people in Japan didn't die of tryptophan? Only in the United States were people dying of tryptophan. So they must not be dying of tryptophan. It must be something else. Because otherwise they'd die around the world.

It doesn't matter to the FDA, "Thou shall not use tryptophan." Now, we had some people who tryptophan helps so much that they were no longer trying to commit suicide from depression. We worked with them and the tryptophan would be a mood elevator. In fact, at that time somebody had done spinal taps on people with depression and found that people with depression were much lower in tryptophan metabolites than people who didn't have depression. They compared them.

So, logical good sense, it had been indicated by science that it was useful. After a couple of years and no more deaths, we took our bottles out of storage, 110 of them, and put them back on the shelves. But first we sent them to the Mayo Clinic. One bottle—it was all the same batch. Because the Mayo Clinic had discovered that it was the tryptophan dimer that was killing people. And so we wanted to make sure that we didn't have any tryptophan dimer in ours.

So we sent it to the Mayo Clinic. Report came back clean. Our batch happened to be all negative for tryptophan dimer. It was just tryptophan. So we put it back on the shelf. But we required a prescription because we wanted to keep track of everybody who had it. After we put them on the shelf, that's when the FDA guy came around with the lady from the State Board of Pharmacy and managed to get it all.

Funny thing about the timing, I was teaching at a medical convention in Chicago at the time. I wasn't there. And they bullied the manager of a—you can call it a vitamin store. In Washington State those are called dispensaries but I hate to use that term anymore because we don't sell pot at our dispensary. But that's what's used. They bullied that guy into giving them the 110 bottles of tryptophan.

So what are our patients supposed to do? Drive to Canada? So I called my attorney and said, "look they have no legal authority to do this." And my attorney says, "I'll look that up" and he did. And he says, they had no legal authority to do it. Recalls are voluntary.

And, by the way, it wasn't just me and my attorney who found that it was illegal. Dr. David Kessler, head of FDA at that time, testified before the Congress in 1993, the year after the event we're going to tell you about, that he needed more authority because voluntary recalls weren't good enough. And he needed to have the authority to have a mandatory recall. So he testified that he didn't have the authority two years ago to do what he did. And what did he do?

We put it back on the shelves. They came and stole it. We sue them. We want the tryptophan back. And my attorney says, "look, how much are 110 bottles of tryptophan worth?" About maybe $1,500. It was cheap at the time, it's really pricey now. Maybe $1,500. He says, "you really want to sue these people over $1,500?" I said, "it's not the $1,500, it's that patients are going to have to drive to Canada to get their remedies. And I'd like to get this stuff back for them here so they don't have to drive to Canada."

That was in August of 1991 that we filed the suit. And what we didn't know but found out later during all the proceedings is FDA spent the winter investigating our clinic. They sent an undercover agent to our clinic. And he tried to get one of our employees to ship something across state lines. And, of course, we knew better than to do that. So she says, "No. I can't ship thing across state lines."

So that didn't work, darn it. Another FDA agent went through the trash outside of our clinic. And how do we know that? Because on TV later they held up a bottle of injectable magnesium that was contaminated with fungus that they had gotten out of our trash. That's how I know they got it out of our trash. They said so on TV.

And I'm thinking, "excuse me, but that was why it was in the trash." We put it in trash for a reason. But that was another supposed evidence of our guilt. So they sent these people through our clinic. They investigated and investigated. And on May 6th, 1992 they raided our clinic with guns drawn.

Ty: No kidding.

Dr. Wright: No kidding. Yes. They told the King County sheriff that we were selling drugs. Because remember they called feces a drug and so vitamins are drugs. Anything you use for treatment is, according to them, a drug. We were selling drugs.

So the King County sheriff's office was expecting drug dealers and they raided with guns. One of them came in and stuck his gun within a few feet of the receptionist's face. And one thing though they didn't have is jack boots. You've heard of the jack boot? They all had regular shoes. And even though they had guns they wore regular shoes and kicked the doors in with their regular shoes. The doors were locked.

They had their raid shortly before 9am. And how do we know they kicked the doors in? Because somebody was sitting outside in a wheelchair waiting for his appointment. And he saw these guys come and kick the doors in. They came in with guns. And what did they do? They herded all the employees into a corner of the reception area and they proceeded to start seizing equipment, and medical records, and payroll records, and banking records, and everything.

And they told the King County police that it was because we were dealing drugs. So that day I was late for work. So I didn't get the gun pointed at me. Holly and I usually go to work together. And she and I parked the car and this really nice King County policeman came up and said, "Sir, I think you want to put all of your stuff in the trunk of your car." He had figured out by then what was going on. And I had my briefcase and stuff. And he said, "I think you want to put all your stuff in the trunk of your car." I looked at him and said, "really?" He says, "yes, really. And then follow me inside." Holly decided to drive the car home. It was a good thing she did. She said, "I'm not coming here today," and took the car home.

So I went inside with the briefcase and here's all the employees in the corner. And here's these people going through all of our records and taking—they actually drove up a semi truck and loaded it with equipment, and medical records, and financial records. That was by the end of the day. They didn't load it all while I was there. But by the end of the day they'd done that. And I asked them what they were doing here. So they presented a search warrant. If it hadn't been such a—"what are you doing?" They had the guns holstered, by the way, by then. They only pulled them when they ran in.

Ty: Well, that was nice of them.

Dr. Wright: That was nice of them, yes. Anyway, if it hadn't been such an, "oh, my God" moment, I would have laughed. Because that search warrant specified that they were there to seize our B complex vitamins, and our vitamin B12, and our folate, and other injectable substances which are all vitamins and minerals.

They were there to seize that. Can you imagine someone seizing B complex with guns? Which is why in the Seattle newspapers it became known as "The great B-Vitamin Bust." And that was the headlines in the different papers. And Holly probably showed you outside of her office all the agglomeration of the newspaper articles that are on. You can get a picture of those if you want some of them. It was called "The Great B-Vitamin Bust" because they were there to take our B vitamins.

But they also—funny thing, they took our whole financial records. And when they had a press conference about this afterwards—they didn't, we did—guess who was sitting in the audience? Two IRS agents. And what do they have to do with health care? IRS agents only supervise health care under Obamacare. They didn't supervise it back in 1992. They were really looking for every way to get us that they could. Because we had sued them.

Me, I would think that if somebody sued me, I'd defend myself in court. Not these guys. They came in and disrupted everything and they started to take—they didn't start to take—they took every one of our financial banking records. They took all of our patients records, every one. And we never got them back.

My attorney later on said, "would you give them back, please?" They said, "No. You can sue us again." And we didn't have the money at that point. So all the medical records, all the banking records, and various equipment, and B complex vitamins, and so forth. They basically said we all could go home. And our office manager said, "I don't think so. I think I'll stay here." She just wanted to keep an eye on them. So I called Holly and Holly says, "I think I know what to do."

She called up a talk radio show host that she knows who called the afternoon drive host and persuaded him to have me on the radio from 3-7pm that evening. Now, he was, what he called, a self-recovering attorney. And he read that warrant over the air. And he had asked me, "you got a bottle of that B complex?" I said, "Sure." And he opened it up and drank it while he was talking on the air and says, "okay FDA, come get me."

Ty: He was using the drugs.

Dr. Wright: He was using the drugs. So, actually, I wasn't down at the clinic the next few days except passing on the way going home. Because I was up in Seattle on the radio from four to seven, three nights in a row.

He urged all of his listeners to call the US Attorney who had not released the charging papers. Anyway, that's what they did. And they impaneled a grand jury. Eighteen months later, nothing. They impaneled a second grand jury. Another 18 months, nothing. No indictments. After the second grand jury failed to return any indictment, and the first one did to, they then announced to the newspapers. Not to me. They didn't call me and my attorney. They announced to the newspapers that they were closing the investigation. And both my attorney and me, we read about it in the newspaper.

Ty: Classy.

Dr. Wright: Look, our employees had to figure out why this happened. What are we doing to attract this? So our receptionist—the one who had the gun about that far, from here to the camera—she says, "you know, I was having to tell people at that time that to get an appointment here at Tahoma clinic especially with Dr. Wright, it's going to take three or four weeks. When that guy pulled out his gun at me, I gave him an appointment right away. It must be that he wanted an appointment."

But our clinic nutritionist had a different point of view. And she says, "Oh no. Have you ever read the symptoms of severe B vitamin deficiency?" And I said, "Tell me." And she says, "Oh look, it's right here. If you're severely B vitamin deficient you get mentally unstable. That must be why they came in with guns to seize our B vitamins. Because, you see, we haven't heard from them since. They must have used the B vitamins."

Ty: They must have used them. And you never got any of these papers back after this?

Dr. Wright: No. Never got the patients records back, never got the banking records back. We had to reconstruct, as best we could, all the banking records. And the patients records, we just had to ask people to tell us what they told us before.

But no, that never came back. And the whole thing was done for one purpose. All of that, we had to have a separate attorney for each employee because they were all called before the grand jury. And they can't have one attorney for two people. It's a conflict of interest, they said. And so up go the legal bills. Very fortunately, a colleague started a legal defense fund. And that legal defense fund not only collected, but spent on legal fees $500,000 over the years between 1992 and plus two grand juries. Five hundred thousand dollars.

And if we'd had to do that out of our personal—Holly and myself—if we'd had to do that, no way we could have done that. But thank you to anybody of you who are watching who donated to our legal defense fund back then. Thank you so much. Because we were able to re-equip from the equipment they'd stolen, and I do mean still stolen, because remember they didn't have legal authority to do this. It was not legal for them to do a mandatory recall at that time.

So they stole our stuff. Our tryptophan. And they came and raided our office. The whole thing was illegal. We were able to get enough equipment to get back and going. We were closed for a week and we opened up again. And we would not have been able to pay the employees or anything else if it hadn't been for that legal defense fund. Basically, again, "The Great B-Vtamin Bust"at Tahoma Clinic in May of 1992.

Ty: That's really unbelievable. It blows my mind that that's the country that we live in when it comes to health. When it comes to trying to give patients what they need as far as supplements to be healthy.

You have to deal with this kind of tyranny. You would think that this was a third world nation under some kind of a communist dictator.

Dr. Wright: They behave that way in this area. Health is not at all something that one can freely do for their own self. They can only do it under intense scrutiny. And most of the things that are useful can become unavailable at any time.

Ty: Dr. Wright, tell us about BEC5. What is it? And what does it do?

Dr. Wright: BEC5 is a compound derived originally from an Australian plant called devil's apple. And it's also found in eggplant and it's found in green pepper.

Ty: Eggplant.

Dr. Wright: Yes. It's one of the—any one of the things called solanaceae for those of you who are botanists. They all have some of this BEC5 in them. The technical term for them is solasodine glycosides. And all that glycoside means is that there's a sugar attached to something. It could be a string of sugars too.

It was discovered by a doctor William Cham. He likes to go by Bill. So we all call him Bill. He is a PhD. He is a brilliant guy. He was working at a university in Australia.

And someone came out to talk to him—even though his major field is lipid chemistry—they wanted to talk to him because they heard he was interested, about why their livestock, when they developed cancer in the eyeball—there's a certain kind of livestock that developed a lot of that—they go rub themselves up against the devil's apple plant with their eyes. Damn, their cancer would go away. And so they talked to Dr. Cham about that. And Dr. Cham was intrigued.

So, he went to research it and he isolated these things called salosodine glycosides. There are two or three of them but they're all lumped into the name BEC5. BEC5 is Bill Edward Cham-5. So here's what Dr. Cham found very quickly. What he found is that there was a membrane change in the membrane that surrounds a cancer cell. And if any cancer cell—and as you'll hear later on from Dr. Gaston, every cancer cell has this membrane change.

But normal cells that are not cancerous do not have that membrane change. And the key thing is that the solasodine glycosides, this sugar that sticks down, has a particular type of plant sugar that connects with the cancer cells' change membrane and it connects. And the cancer cell pulls that stuff inside the cancer cell where it doesn't mess with the DNA of the cancer cell. It goes to little baggies called lysosomes which are filled with enzymes and they are the storage depot for enzymes that the cell uses.

But this stuff, the BEC5, goes into the cancer cell. It goes to the lysosome somehow. It enters the lysosomes, and all the storage membranes are ruptured. And so this cell is flooded with digestive enzymes that digest itself to death.

Seriously. Now, if I have a skin cancer right here and I put it on there, it is not going to hurt the normal skin at all. That is the key thing. This is a beautifully targeted thing. If you heard about the latest thing in cancer treatment is targeting individualization and all that.

This has been around since 1980s by the way. Except not in these United States, of course. But there are legal jurisdictions for it. And that's where one has to get it. It's from a legal jurisdiction. So anyway I get this BEC5. It's a skin cream and I rub it all over there. And remember, it can't get into my normal cells. It can only get into cancer cells. And I put a Band Aid over it. I'll leave that for 12 hours, take the Band Aid off, renew the skin cream, put the Band Aid back on again. If I do that, usually within 12-14 weeks this process happens.

The cancer cells first start to turn a little red and they look a little granular. And then they start to turn red-grey and red-black and the whole thing collapses and implodes. And it leaves a little hole. But the cool thing is, you just keep putting skin cream on and the whole thing grows back in and you can hardly ever tell you had a cancer.

There's a whole book on this, folks. In fact, there are two books. One of them is called *The Eggplant Cancer Cure* because this stuff is found in eggplant. And the other one is a more recent book, *Inspired by Nature Proven by Science*. Both of them are by Bill Cham. So you can find these online. Bill Cham, *Inspired by Nature Proven by Science* and *The Eggplant Cancer Cure*.

Both of them come with pictures. For example, there's a picture in one of those books, I think it's *The Eggplant Cancer Cure*, of somebody who had this big cancer that encompassed part of the nose here and it went all around in a big circle like that. They started to putting on the BEC5 cream. At the worst stage, a person looked like they had a hole in the side of their face. Remember though, this cream cannot kill normal cells. And so when it got to the last cancer cell, it stops. It can't go any further. So here's this big hole. There's a picture of after it all healed—and this one took about 16-20 weeks because it was such a big cancer—you could not tell one side of the nose from the other unless you took a really close-up picture. And then it was just a little bit more grainy and the other side was a little more smooth. And that's the only way you could tell the person ever had cancer. And otherwise that person would have to have a humongous surgery and they'd have to have skin grafting. And this stuff can cure the cancer without all that.

What happened to it? Well, Dr. Cham was in Australia and by the time the Australasian Society for Dermatology [Research] complained to the Therapeutic Goods Administration, which is the same as FDA down there down under, they had documented that 70,000 people cured their own skin cancer with his stuff. And he was selling it over the counter. Can you imagine a cancer cure being sold over the counter and 70,000 people cured themselves?

Ty: We can't have that.

Dr. Wright: We cannot have that even if we're in Australia. So there's a complaint from the Australasian Society for Dermatology [Research] to the Therapeutic Goods Administration. "Put this stuff on prescription. Only doctors should treat."

So the Therapeutic Good Administration put it on prescription. There goes Dr. Cham's over the counter business. Guess what? Hardly any of the dermatologists prescribed this stuff. They couldn't get it anymore.

Ty: So they basically eliminated BEC5 by making it prescription only?

Dr. Wright: Almost. However, there are couple of three doctors who are still prescribing it. That's all. And Mrs. Cham, she got a phone call. "I can't afford to go to those doctors. My mother has a skin cancer. Would you please sell me just one tube?" "I can't do that it's not legal."

But the person called back and called back and just played on her charitable feelings or whatever, her empathy. And so she finally sold that person a tube of skin cream and was promptly arrested for selling it. It was entrapment in other words. She was taken to court for selling an illegal substance. I'm sorry. Illegally selling a substance. The substance was okay, if you're a doctor. But she can't sell it. She was taken to court. Now, how do I know? Because she told me along with Dr. Cham. This isn't hearsay. They told me they went to court. The judge, thank goodness, was sane and dismissed the case. He says, "you deliberately tried to entrap her. You deliberately did it. I'm going to dismiss this thing."

But what both—he's a PhD doctor, Dr. Cham, although not a medical doctor. His wife said that then the judge said, "and I want to see you two in my chambers." So they went into chambers with the judge. And the judge says, "I have seen this pattern before." This is what they told me. I was not there. But the Chams told me that the judge said, "I have seen this pattern before. They're not going to get off your case." He says, "I advise you to move out of Australia." The judge. In private of course.

They took his advice and moved to what was called in the past the French New Hebrides. It is now called Vanuatu. Which is a small island nation out in the Pacific Ocean. And guess what? It's legal to cure skin cancer in Vanuatu. And it's legal to sell this stuff in Vanuatu. So there's a website that people can look for. It's called Curaderm. It's under that tile, curaderm.net. And one can buy it legally because it's being bought from a legal jurisdiction for one's own use.

And I've had people come in and show me time after time, "I'm putting this on the cancer. I'm I doing it right?" And the only side effect I've ever seen is that the cream it's in contains some salicylate which is basically aspirin. Because that makes it penetrate better. And there are a few of us, including me, who are salicylate sensitive and so people get real red. And when I saw it getting real red on me, I just quit using it. You can't use it if you're salicylate sensitive. Nobody dies but you get all red and swollen up if you keep it.

So, people who are not salicylate sensitive can use it. And Dr. Cham is pretty clear in his books that it should be used on skin cancer. Dr. Gaston will tell you potential other uses because, remember, this membrane change happens on every cancer cell there is. But it's easiest to reach for yourself on a skin cancer.

Now, another little detail here and then I'll shut up because I do tend to go on for too long. And that is that there's a company in New Jersey, I believe. I'm not positive. But I think it's New jersey. They're still in business. They're called Lane Laboratories. Now, remember you can't patent this stuff. So they just made up their own batch. Dr. Cham had no patent. And they started selling it from New Jersey. Oh my God. And they were selling it and people were curing their own skin cancers.

And here comes FDA. And they go to court. And the final decision is Lane Laboratories shall pay, I think, it was two million. It might have been more. But I'll say a two million dollar fine for helping people to cure cancer by natural means because it wasn't approved by those Federales.

Ty. How dare they

Dr. Wright: How dare they cure skin cancer without approval? It reminds me very much, Ty, of King George III. You couldn't do a damn thing without his approval. And we have the same thing in health care now. Without approval, even if it's natural, and the only thing it hurts is the people with salicylate sensitivities, you cannot cure your skin cancer unless you go to a jurisdiction where it is legal. And it isn't legal in New Jersey. I sometimes wonder why our troops don't fight for freedom here at home.

Ty: That's a great question because we're lacking a lot of health care freedom here.

Dr. Wright: We're lacking a ton of it. So why send troops overseas to fight for freedom? We got plenty of freedom to fight for right here including taking care of our own health in the way that we would like.

Ty: I'm really struck by the similarities between the TGA and the FDA, the Australian version, right? They both have the same tactics. The FDA tried to entrap you, right? The TGA tried to entrap the Chams in Australia by planting someone with the phone call.

Dr. Wright: Excuse me. But I'm going to take three to four minutes to tell you about another entrapment.

State medical boards are this way too. You probably know that. Well, it seems that in 2007 we hired a physician who had been practicing in Texas. This is at Tahoma Clinic. We hired a physician who had been practicing in Texas. We insisted that he apply for a Washington state license. That's necessary. So he applied for a Washington state license in 2007, in the Fall of 2007. And the state medical board— which in this state is called the Washington State Medical Quality Assurance Commission. The state medical board, they have a website where you can look up any doctor and find out if they're licensed or not and so forth. And we looked him up once a month and his license was always listed as pending. We even took some screenshots. Pending.

So, he did not get his license granted. And we're back to King George III granting things. He did not get his license granted. Clear into 2009 it was still pending. So at that point he says, "look, I'm not waiting around any longer. I'm out of here." And he left the state. He gave us a couple of weeks notice. He was nice. But he gave us a couple of weeks notice and left.

Shortly after that I get a phone call. I'm being charged with aiding and abetting the unlicensed practice of medicine. And therefore endangering the public health. I'm being charged with that by the state medical board. One is not allowed to go to court. You have to go through administrative hearings with the Department of Health. Now, who are the people who are doing the hearings? They're all employees of the Department of Health.

So basically, your judge, jury, etc., are all employees of the people who are charging you. So we held these hearings. By the way, here goes another quarter million dollars because we had to hire attorneys. So we brought in an attorney from New York who was really, really good at this kind of stuff. As well as having our local attorney who was also really, really good. But this one from New York has more experience.

So he interviewed all these staff members at the State Board of Medicine. And he found out that four of them knew that this guy's license had been revoked in Texas on the very day his application came into the State Board of Medicine. They knew.

On the website of the State Board of Medical Quality Assurance Commission it says there that the "mission is to protect the public."

Ty: So why did they not?

Dr. Wright: So why didn't they call me? Can you say entrapment? They sat on it from 2007 to 2009. And I'm guilty of endangering the public. And all they had to do in 2007, "Dr. Wright that guy whose applied for a license, why he's had his license revoked in Texas." That's all they had to do.

And if they truly were there to protect the public interest or protect the public's health and safety, they would have done that. Because their mission is to protect the public health and safety except when they can nab somebody for it which is what they did. And they nabbed me for that and I had to hang my license from the ceiling on a string for three months. That's called the suspended license. That's what they did. Took the license, hung it on a string from the ceiling suspended. The license suspension and probation and all this stuff.

And if they'd just placed a phone call following on their true mission as stated on their website and called me up and said, "this man has had his license removed." Then we wouldn't have endangered the public health and safety. But they charged me with it. And as far as I'm concerned, they did it by letting it go for two years. But, you see, I haven't got a hearing where I can find them guilty. I haven't got a hearing method. So it's not just the FDA that does this.

Ty: It's nifty for them, isn't it?

Dr. Wright: Yes. The state board of medicine does this to alternative medicine doctors in nearly every state. Let's get back to what you want to talk about.

Ty: Alternative medicine doctors. That's an oxymoron isn't it?

Dr. Wright: It really is.

Ty: This isn't really alternative.

Dr. Wright: It's nature's medicine. And has been that way ever since there's been people. The wise grannies and some of the wise grandpas learned that this herb or that thing helped with this problem. And they passed it down, and passed it down, and passed it down.

But it's medicine that is derived from our planet. Now, the reason it's so important that it's derived from our planet is that our bodies are made up of the substance and energy of planet earth. Unless we're space aliens. And that's a different story. But if we're not space aliens—

Ty: Maybe the FDA is space aliens.

Dr. Wright: I don't know. One wonders sometimes. If we're regular people, substance and energy of planet earth. The molecules are all from planet earth and the energies are all from planet earth.

What's going to work best in your Chevy if it's broken? Chevy parts. If the body is broken do we put in original body parts which are original molecules and original energies? No. We take them and we twist them a little bit so we can patent them. And of course they don't fit quite right anymore if it's a molecule or we use an energy that isn't natural to the body. And we expect the body to heal with that? The best it can do is cover up symptoms.

So you get to buy it for the next 40 years while you're covering up your symptoms. Your blood pressure suppressor—instead of finding the cause of the blood pressure and getting it to go away. All those things. Patent medicines do not belong in human bodies. And I know I keep saying patent medicines and people aren't accustomed to that. They think of the 19th century. I'm sorry but all the giant pharmaceutical companies are holders of patents for molecule, after molecule, after molecule.

It's sort of like what belongs in the body. It's just sort of enough to do something but enough to cause a lot of damage too. So if we're going to be as healthy as we can in the bodies we now have, we have to use only the substance and energy that belongs in the body. And it makes no sense using patent medications. Patents are wonderful for certain things, protection of intellectual property rights and so forth. But patents have no place in health care.

I just said that and over there there's somebody from a big pharmaceutical company watching. They're going to be on my case. I just said patents have no place in health care.

And have you noticed that when a new drug comes out and they call it a blockbuster drug, they're not talking about, "it cures cancer." They're not talking about, "it's blockbuster for health." They're talking about how many bucks you can make. And that's what it always is. It seems that the number one goal of a lot of health care is to make money. And if we happen to do some good with it, that's fine. But our number one goal is to make money. And in health care—I mean go into banking if that's what you want. They do a good job of making money. And you're not messing up people's individual health nearly as bad.

Now, given the last banking crisis I don't know about them not messing up health at all. But that's another story. So anyway, I'll settle down.

Ty: No. That's great. Great information. I love that perspective because I think it's accurate. It's very accurate that we've got this business aspect to health care that's driving these decisions.

Last question Dr. Wright. Bioidentical hormones, do they cause cancer?

Dr. Wright: Let's see. Did your own hormones cause you cancer yet? No. Bioidentical hormones are no more dangerous and no more safe than a person's own hormones when they got hormones.

And we have to admit that young women do get breast cancer in their 30s, occasionally. It's not very often. So there is a little hazard. That's from her own hormones. I'm sorry, it's estrogen-related cancer, it's from her own hormones. But funny thing there's lots of research papers that say that's because she's not metabolizing her hormones properly.

There are certain estrogens that are pro-carcinogenic. There are certain estrogens that are anti-carcinogenic. And if we're doing bioidentical hormones responsibly we always, after the woman starts on her bioidentical hormones, within a month or two have her check completely how her estrogens and progesterone and so forth are metabolizing.

And we can tell her that her risk of cancer is quite low, thank you. Or her risk of cancer is high because she's not metabolizing properly. And even then there are no means of persuading a person's body to make more anti-carcinogens and less pro-carcinogens and to restore the balance so that bioidentical hormones when done that way are actually less risky than our own hormones were.

We can't ever say they're never risky. But we can say they are a lot less risky when they're done properly than the hormones we had when we were younger. And bioidentical hormones do so much good. Remember, bioidentical just means identical to the molecules found in our body. And that's important. No patents here.

For one, for men testosterone and for women estrogen dramatically reduces risk of Alzheimer's disease, dramatically. And it's known how it does it. I won't go into that. But the so-called mechanism of action, as they call it in medicine, is known how it does it. It reduces the risk of Alzheimer's dramatically.

Secondly, those bioidentical hormones for ladies, of course, they protect against osteoporosis. You're much less likely to get osteoporosis. They help you to mitigate your risk of heart disease. They're not the main thing that does that. And if you allow me, there's a super way of cutting your risk of heart attack. Just super. I'll tell you about that after. And it's well documented too. Anyway, estrogens somewhat cut you risk of heart attack.

But here's the important thing that estrogens do for ladies. And this information is not from me. It's from the Lung [Regeneration Laboratory]at Georgetown University, doctors Massaro. It's always Massaro and Massaro. So that's why I say doctors Massaro and they have these string of publications. And what they have proven is that a woman's lungs deteriorate at a much more rapid rate than men's lungs do after menopause.

So let's say we have a 50-year-old woman and a 50-year-old man and she just went through menopause. And a guys hormones glide down slowly. Her lung capacity deteriorates much more rapidly than a man's. And that's why if a woman has never smoked ever, her risk of COPD is still six to eight times the risk of a man who has never smoked.

We have six to eight ladies with COPD, non-smokers, compared to one non-smoking man with COPD. So if a woman wants to keep her lungs intact—and this is from on research institute, this isn't from me—she better at least think about estrogen. If she wants to be an athlete how is she going to do it without her lungs? If she wants to swim?

One other thing, estrogen helps a woman maintain her vocal quality and she never ends up sounding like granny, ever. And I've had a number of choir masters tell me how much better the women are singing since they got on their bioidentical hormones.

So that's for women. Now for men, testosterone again lowers the risk of Alzheimer's. That's very important. It does not raise the risk of heart attack if it's done properly. Now properly is you follow to make sure it's not too much. Because too much can make you make too many red blood cells. And if you have too many red blood cells things get kind of clogged up and your risk of heart attack is higher. But testosterone also has the osteoporosis benefit. But one of the big deals is muscle mass. Men can maintain their muscle mass with testosterone.

Bioidentical hormones are not just estrogen and testosterone. There's another one called oxytocin which is made by the pituitary. That's been found just last year by some very solid research to maintain muscle mass also. It won't re-grow new muscle, testosterone can help you do that. But it helps, it stimulates the muscle cell stem cells. And the muscle cell stem cells repair and regenerate the muscle.

So for women it's very important to use a smidgen of testosterone because estrogen does not do anything for muscle than we know about. So she needs a little bit so she doesn't turn into a little old lady. She doesn't need a great deal. But for women oxytocin will help them maintain their muscles too. And there are many other bioidentical hormones.

There's melatonin and there's aldosterone. There's lots of them. So I'll conclude on that by saying that if we copy the type of hormone precisely, bioidentical, we use the amounts that belong in the human body. Not greater not lesser. The amounts that belong in the human body. We check the metabolization of them to see how they are doing. If we do all of that we've got a very safe program that does something that you're staring to hear about. It's called extending the health span.

You met my wife today. Did she happen to tell you how old she is?

Ty: She didn't.

Dr. Wright: Would you care to guess?

Ty: I'm guessing 60.

Dr. Wright: She's 74. I'm sorry. She's 75. And just about everybody guesses her at least 15 to 20 years younger. Now, she's 75 and she's bouncing around this clinic like crazy. You saw her today. And that's what it will do for people. Nobody is going to live forever. But at least we can live healthy for a lot longer.

Heart attack and stroke. Real quick. As quick as I can. Remember if you give too much testosterone to some guys, they make more blood cells and that thickens the blood and it gets clogged. And you can get clogged and have a heart attack. Well, there's this terrific book out there, folks. It's called *The Origins of Atherosclerosis*, it's by a Dr. Kenneth Kensey and another doctor by the name of Young Cho. And what they show is that heart attack is not caused by cholesterol.

Let's be real clear here. It's caused by the thickness of the blood. It's a matter of physics not chemistry. It does not have anything to do with the chemistry. It's has everything to do with the physics of blood flow.

Now, you've seen pictures of the heart and here's the heart that's got all these blood vessels wrapped around it. Have you ever noticed that when they put on the cholesterol deposits it's not going everywhere on the arteries around the heart? It's only the branch points, isn't it? It's the branch points. And cholesterol accumulates here at the branch points. At the carotid arteries. And it accumulates as a branch point at the bottom of the artery. Here are the vessel legs, there's a branch point there.

Why does cholesterol accumulate at branch points? Can't be inflammation. Because if we have inflammation all over the body, which is currently what we blame a heart attack and cardiovascular disease on, we should have cholesterol up and down every artery because it should be equal inflammation.

Why should it inflame the branch point? There's no special nerve going in there to cause inflammation. What Dr. Kensey and Cho show in their book is that the thicker the blood when it comes to a branch point it creates turbidity, it abrades at that branch point. And the abrasion sets up the inflammation. It's the physical abrasion, like sandpaper. It's got that chemistry. It's the physical abrasion that sets up inflammation.

What happens to inflammation on my hands when I go garden? My body makes a callus. Lots of calluses. I don't garden anymore. No more calluses after a while. My arteries can't grow a callus even though it's inflamed and abraded. So what happens? The body pastes cholesterol all over it. And that's to cover the inflammation.

But the problem is if the blood remains too thick it's still going to create more inflammation where it will paste more cholesterol, more inflammation, more cholesterol.

Now, a couple of facts. If you are a woman between menarche and menopause and you don't smoke, you never take birth control pills, your risk of heart attack is zero. How's that happen? How come guys aren't immune doing that age? What are women doing? Loosing blood once a month.

So a woman's blood count—I'm going to use the hematocrit. That's the percent of red blood cells and total blood volume. And red blood cells are the major thing that goes into blood thickness.

A woman's hematocrit is normally 37-45. And a guy's hematocrit of the same age is normally 45-50. Look how much thicker that guy's blood is. So women up to menopause, unless they smoke or take birth control pills, they don't get heart attacks.

Men start having heart attacks in their 40s even before women start going through menopause and their risk goes up after that. But a woman, she still has that zero risk until menopause. If she does nothing to stop this problem, the viscosity, her blood thickness gets thicker and thicker and thicker. And by the time she is 61 to 62, women are having just as many heart attacks and strokes as men.

But Kensey and Cho point out one other thing and that is—and thank you for letting me get this out, Ty. Because for your audience, if they take heed, they're possibly going to do themselves a lot of good. I'm not going to sell them a thing. I'll get to that. I'll not try to sell them a thing. When a woman has menstrual bleeding every month her body has to replace that blood, otherwise she'd be bled out in a couple of years. She has to replace the blood.

So her body has to make a whole lot of new blood cells. New blood cells are more flexible. And they can fold over. And there are many areas in both male and female bodies where the capillaries are so small that the only blood cells that can get through are the ones that fold themselves in a half and they go through.

So women have always a population of juvenile blood cells and they fold these blood cells in half. They don't, they fold themselves in a half. And they get through there. And so a woman actually has better body perfusion.

The perfusion is the technical word for blood flow. All over the body she has better perfusion than guys do in the small areas where the small capillaries are. Us guys, unless we're out bleeding in a battle or something, we don't bleed. And so we don't make new blood cells very often.

So it's a combination of us guys having thicker blood and very many fewer new blood cells. And so we get many more heart attacks and strokes. Because this here will lead to the stroke and a heat attack too. We get many more than the ladies do.

So, over in Finland a number of years ago, 1990s, an experiment with 2,800 men was done. All they did was sign them up for observation, that's it. They didn't tell them to do anything. They just observed for nine years. And hold on to your hat here—the men who donated blood had 88 percent less heart attacks than the men who didn't donate blood, 88 percent.

And there it is in the medical journal. Why didn't we ever hear about it? Well you can't patent donating blood. I'm sorry. That was the best result I've seen. There was one done in the United States where they did the same thing, comparing men who donated blood and men who didn't donate blood. It was only a 55 percent reduction, Ty. Sorry. Only 55 percent instead of 88 percent.

Ty: Still not bad.

Dr. Wright: Still not bad. And all you got to do is go donate blood. What could be better? It doesn't matter whether you're a Republicat or a Dominican, I get them mixed up. It doesn't matter whether you're one of those or a Libertarian or a Socialist. This everyone can agree on. It does us some good and it does somebody else some good to donate blood.

So why, why, why hasn't this word gotten out? I talked to the head of Seattle blood—not the head, she was a high official in the Seattle blood banking community—she says, "we know that." I said, "why don't you tell people? You're always telling us help, help, help we need blood. It's Christmas and nobody is donating blood, not even Santa. Give us some blood. Why don't you just tell people that you will cut your risk of heart attack and stroke dramatically and you'll be flooded with people."

Remember this is Seattle, Ty? And I couldn't see what she was doing, but I could hear her voice and I imagined she was doing this. "We only want to have people donate blood for altruistic reasons," says she. That's a direct quote into my ear. Come on. Altruistic reasons? We want to donate blood to save somebody's life. Never mind altruistic reasons. But that's what she said.

And I just had a person come in to consult two days ago. And he told me that he's been to this blood bank and employees there have never heard of the fact that if you donate blood you cut down your blood viscosity and you reduce your risk of heart attack dramatically. They'd never heard of it.

So would you please get that word out, please? And you can make the terrific impact on heart attack in the United States here.

Ty: We will.

Dr. Wright: Just by spreading it. Thank you.

Ty: But you can't patent that like you can a statin drug.

Dr. Wright: You can't patent it. Now for people who the blood bank won't take because they just had a trip Mexico and you can't do that if you were just in Mexico. You just see a doctor who does this sort of thing and knows how to do IVs, and they get vacutainer bottle and put a needle in and they take out the unit of blood. You don't have to go to the blood bank. It's just nicer if you can donate it to somebody.

Ty: Fascinating. This information is really incredible. It blows your mind.

Dr. Wright: It does. And thank you so much for getting it out to folks.

Ty: Thank you for sharing today. I really appreciate it.

Dr. Wright: You're welcome. And thank you for coming.

[end of transcript]

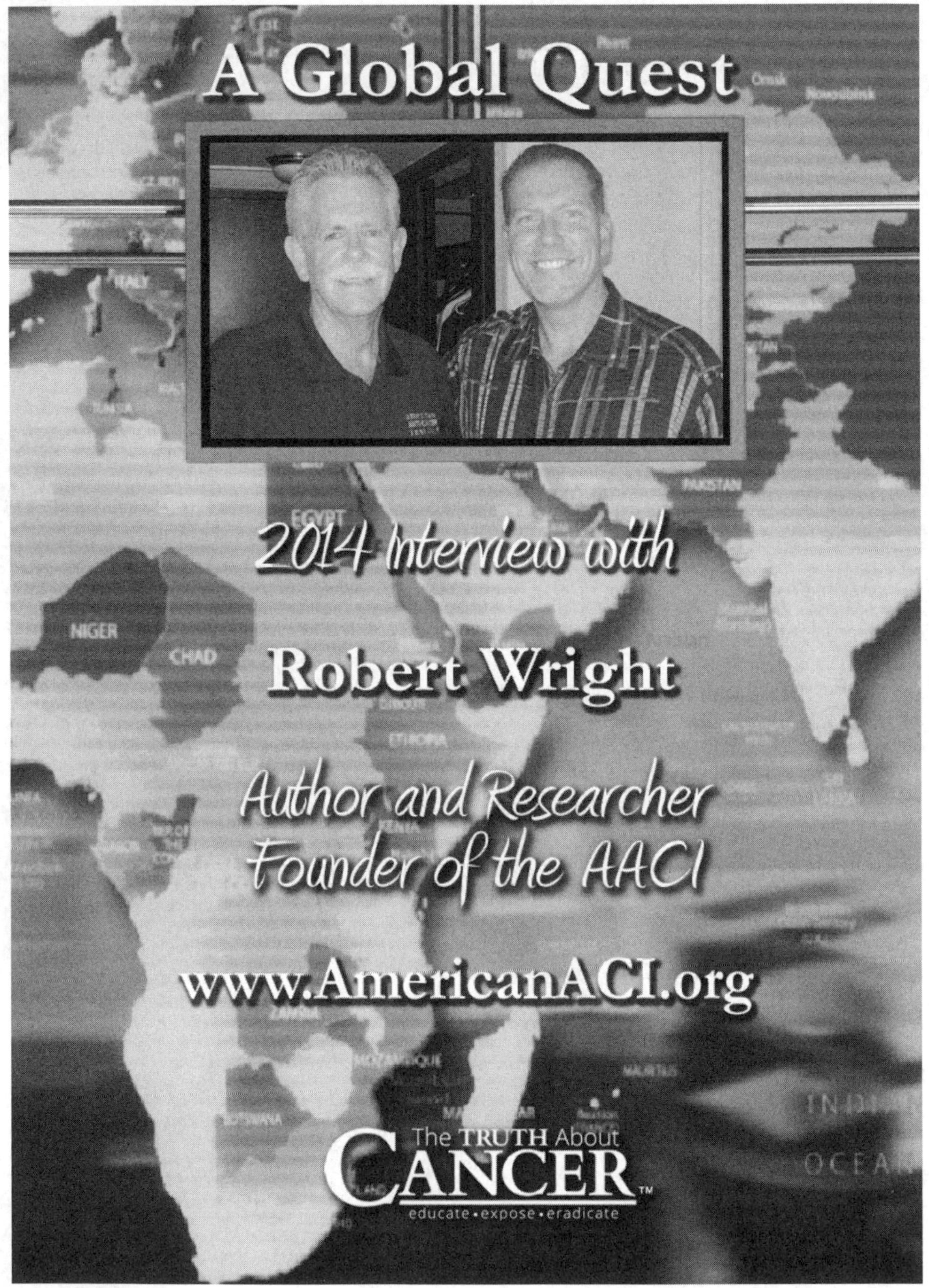
A Global Quest
2014 Interview with
Robert Wright
Author and Researcher
Founder of the AACI
www.AmericanACI.org
The TRUTH About
CANCER
educate • expose • eradicate

Bob: Cancer spreads by inflammation, why do you want to inflame it?

Interviewer: So you see sugar as being one of the big causes?

Bob: It's the cause of not just cancer. Think about this. If you drink a 12-ounce Pepsi Cola, it's got about 9 or 10 teaspoons of sugar in it.

That's enough to effectively shut down half of your immune system for four hours. It can't be good for you, can it? And that's one can, and our kids are drinking the Big Gulps today. It's no wonder they are sick.

Interviewer: That's a pretty big shame, isn't it?

Bob: It's a huge shame.

Interviewer: Do you think you could ever find yourself doing any advertising for Coke or Pepsi or any of those brands?

Bob: We will not compromise, even if it means we go out of business because we don't have the money. We don't do Google ads because we're not going to have them put any chemotherapy ads on our website. We will not compromise no matter what. No. I would never do ads for them, ever. I would do ads saying that, "This is death, folks, don't drink it." I would do those ads because I know what it is.

And the diet drinks with the aspartame, it's an excitotoxin. You want to put that in your brain? I'll tell you, you want brain cancer? Drink diet pop. I guarantee if you don't die of something else, you'll get brain cancer. That's a pretty bold statement, isn't it?

I mean, the proof is there. We're not paying any attention to it. Betty Martini, a doctor, sits on our Advisory Board. She goes all around the world teaching about aspartame, NutraSweet. It is poison. It turns to fumaric acid, which is the sting of the fire ant and formaldehyde in your body. After you die you are already embalmed, right?

We need to ask ourselves a question, if allopathic medicine really knows what they are doing. Do we think they know what they're doing? Do they have intent? It's a question that needs to be answered because do they believe, "When I give this patient chemo and radiation, that it actually can help them?"

Because we know the studies. Eighty plus percent of doctors, oncologists, would never undergo the chemotherapy they are prescribing. They must know what they are doing. And if they know what they're doing, then it becomes willful, does it not?

So, are they killing people? I'm asking the question now. Everybody listening needs to answer that question. We know that 97 percent of people who undergo chemotherapy are dead in five years. That study was placed in the 2004 edition of the *Clinical Oncology* journal.

It was the cancer doctors telling on themselves. Do I know this study to be true? It was a massive study done by epidemiologists who themselves were doctors. I interviewed the lead of that study just within the last six months and I said, "Is this still true today, this was published in 2004?" Dr. McDowell says, "It's absolutely as true today as it was when we published it back in 2004 and it may be getting worse."

So yes, in Australia and the United States where these studies were compiled, less than three percent of patients who undergo chemotherapy are alive in five years. Most of your listeners here won't know that or won't understand it because we live in an allopathic community within our country, within our world today. We don't believe that doctors would deceive us or lie to us. And when they tell us that chemo is our only chance, it's the first lie you hear.

And then you have the surgery. The second lie is, "We got it all." You can't get it all if you're focused on tumors. You simply can't. The cancer is probably already metastatic. Surgery spills it. Radiation, proven not to kill the stem cells, but to enhance them.

That's why we always hear, "Well, cancer came back." It didn't come back, folks, it just never left because chemo and radiation can't cure the cancer. It can't kill it all, and they grow it and expand it. It is a sad state of affairs we have today and the people need to know that, and they don't. Largely they don't, they are buffaloed into believing a lie.

That's why we do what we do and you guys do what you do. Because we need to educate the public about what works and what doesn't work. Chemo and radiation don't work except for maybe the four or five very rare cancers, testicular cancers and some others, that are what we call *in situ*. In other words, they don't move, they don't grow. They are just there and they are so slow growing that chemo can whack them.

In those cases—and that is only four or five percent of cancers—than chemo does have some effectivity. We all know people who have survived chemo so it must work, right? No. It is still a small percentage of the people.

We just have no concept of how many people have cancer and how many undergo the chemotherapy. You may know five people that survived out of the 1000 people that you know, not good stats.

We want to forward the truth so people can grab ahold of it and make a plan that will actually help them instead of hurt them. Most people really love testimonials because, in the final analysis, all that we are talking about,"What does it do in the human body?" Who cares what it does in the test tube or the petri dish. If it doesn't work in the human body, it makes no difference.

We really need to pay attention to that. The proof is in the pudding, it's not in the test tube. Until we get that, we're still going to have more and more drugs that perform well in the test tube or in the petri dish, but it's not the same thing.

The human body is a magnificent entity, machine, as it were. There is no one on earth that understands everything that goes on within the human body, all the interactions, all the pathways.

There are things yet, proteins and things, we've never discovered yet. What do they do? We don't know. But we know that these things are epigenetic. So let's boost that system. And we do.

Interviewer: Tell me about the role of epigenetics in cancer prevention and treatment.

Bob: Doctors would like you to believe that cancer is genetic. That we've got genetic abnormalities and cancer rises from a genetic predisposition or a break in your DNA or whatever it might be, but it is not true. It has actually been proven that it's not true. Doctors should, in fact, know this but they don't.

Let's say that your body and your genetics is the computer, that's the hardware. People can understand this. The epigenetics is the software. The software runs the hardware. We know that from computers. We don't seem to understand that with the human body.

What we need to do is not dwell upon the genetics, but the epigenetics. In other words, what works that computer? If the software is working, generally the hardware is working.

We need to be concerned about the things that are epigenetic in our body, that we put in our body. The right foods, the right liquids. We need to detox the body because your body is set up of pathways, enzymatic pathways, methylation pathways, detoxification pathways. If these are working, your body is working.

But in cancer, these aren't working and they are not working well. Doctors then want to back that up and say, "Well it's your genetics." No it's not. It comes from the epigenetics and, ultimately, it produces the cancer which then might break the genetics.

But no, it's the cancer first, the genetics second. It is twisted around as are so many things in the cancer industry today. The only way we can heal is chemo and radiation. It's another either misinterpretation or outright lie to the people.

There are so many misrepresentations and misconceptions in cancer today that the American people, by and large, believe a lie. We can't have that anymore because they don't heal and they know they don't heal. That is why they are out searching for natural methodologies to bring their bodies to healing.

That's why we have such a great crowd here at the Cancer Control Society today. That is why, if we ever get what we do covered by insurance, people will flee allopathic medicine as rapidly as they possibly can. Because in the final analysis, they just want to be healed.

They don't want to be poisoned, they don't want to be irradiated, they want to be healed. And when they understand that that is what we're doing and they can see it and we're more out there, they are going to flood to what we're doing.

It is helpful for everyone. Even those of us who think we know a little bit, we always learn. We always learn something because someone looks at it a different way or someone has got something new that we haven't heard about. That is always interesting.

We can't stop learning. We can't stop researching. As a matter of fact, the more I learn, the more I understand that I don't know. We need to realize that, as researchers and doctors and whatever we might be, that we can't stop this process. It needs to be ongoing.

Interviewer: So the *Truth about Cancer* has a been beneficial to even you.

Interviewer: Absolutely. And I bet, if you ask all of the people who participated, if they don't tell you the same thing, I would be surprised. Because some of those people—I know a lot of them, some of them haven't seen me. I haven't seen a few of them.

I picked up a few gems myself. I can't tell you right now because I'm always learning, I'm always going for something new. I'm always wondering, "What do you have? What is this supplement?"

We're seeing game changers every year now in this industry, whether it is a supplement, a therapy, a protocol, a treatment. We're seeing game changers and that is why we need to pay attention.

Was it about producing a natural protocol for someone and they don't follow it?

Interviewer: Yes. That was it.

Bob: Well, it's actually true. When you have cancer, you want to try and do everything right. It is not like being in the hospital and getting chemotherapy where they allow you to drink soda pop and eat ice cream cones because they think that sugar is not important and also the food you eat is not really important.

As a matter of fact, if you are suffering from cachexia, or if you are losing weight with your cancer, they give you anything they can to try and beef you up and put on weight. It really doesn't matter to them what is in it.

You look at these products that are given in the hospital, they are full of high fructose corn syrup and other types of sugars and canola oils and things which are really poison to the human body. They really don't care.

What we do is a little bit different. We think if you do something against a protocol that is designed for you—which should be relatively the same for most people with some nuances—that if you do anything against that you harm that protocol.

It is important for cancer patients to try and do everything right. You're battling a sickness here that you want to try and get rid of. If you are given a protocol that has all the right foods, the right supplements, the right water, the right liquids, the detoxification and the exercise, the five things that are very important for healing, then you need to make sure that you grab ahold of that and you follow it. Because if you fall off, things change. You don't want to go back to doing the things that got you here in the first place.

People will ask me, "Okay, Bob, I love your protocol. I'll get on and I'll do it, but tell me, how long do I have to do it for?" And I'll look at them in amazement and say, "You're missing the point."

"This is a lifestyle change. You want to do this for three months, for four months, for six months? Your cancer now is deemed to be in remission or gone, and then you want to go back to living the way you were living? Thinking—mistakenly—that you are cured now and you can do anything you want because you know if it comes back, you are able to go back and follow that protocol again and you'll be well again." It simply doesn't work that way. It doesn't.

This is a lifestyle change. People need to understand that they need to get on a protocol that largely they will follow for the rest of their life. It doesn't need to be necessarily as strict as it was in the beginning, but you need to change how you live.

You live for 60 years, you eat all the wrong things, drink all the wrong things, you put toxins in your body. And then when you have cancer, you think the doctor is going to give you the pill. "Just give me the pill and I'll be better and then I can go back to living how I was living." It doesn't work that way, never has, never will.

We need to get on a protocol that actually supports our body, supports the mechanisms in our body that detoxify our body, that brings us back into the homeostasis where we need to stay. It's very important that people follow the protocol and they stick with it.

I'm sure your doctor would tell you that, too, if you are undergoing chemotherapy. Actually doctors go overboard. If you are taking chemotherapy and you say, "Well, Doc, okay, but I want to take this supplement too, and I want to drink this ionized water." The doctor will say, "Oh, no. Don't do that, it hurts the chemo." It's not true. Actually, it will help the acidification of the body that chemo produces, it will help to ameliorate that.

We've known people who have gone through chemo and they've been on a natural plan at the same time. They never had a sick day, they never missed a day of work, they never lost their hair. We know these things support your body in whatever state that you're in.

Interviewer: If I was to take what Ty is doing down to the very simple thing. And it is just simply, he had the closest people in his life die from cancer. Like he and his dad—they weren't just father and son, they were pretty much best friends. And Ty just couldn't make sense of that. He couldn't make sense that his hero could die of something that was preventable, something that was treatable.

And until he created this, it never made sense. But now he can make sense of it. He has a way to be able to deal with that even though he still experiences pain, like he hasn't resolved. When you hear that story, what does that bring up for you? Hearing what Ty has experienced and the quest that he's on?

Bob: Well, Ty and I come from the same place. We're like brothers from a different mother you might say. We have struggled and suffered through stories that are similar. When I first saw his book come out, I got it and I read it cover to cover. Because my story started the same way when my mother died of cancer. She was diagnosed and within two weeks she was dead.

My dad was diagnosed subsequent to that and it took him 16 years to die. He was basically tortured by the medical community—24 drugs a day, the cancer moving from his removed kidney to his other good kidney. My dad suffered immeasurably over 16 years. My mom went fast.

The medical establishment could not help either one of my parents. You know, I was there when both my mom and dad took their last breath. I held my mom's head in my hands when she took her last breath. And I can tell you, that changes you. I watched my dad at 4:02 in the morning. I watched his chest heave for the last time, his last breath. These things change you.

Since I was already in an industry that was similar, I decided to find out what this cancer racket was all about. So Ty, you and I have taken similar pathways and I know you know that and I'm delighted that we've become great friends through this process.

But I see other people jumping on board and that is why I'm so happy and satisfied with the work that you guys are doing. Because we are getting more people involved, more experts, more people who have had similar circumstances, more people that are asking, "Why? Why me? Why my folks, my family?"

Now they are starting to get answers. Yes, some of them are simple. Some are more complex, but it drives them to search out more of this cancer industry. Where does cancer come from? Because doctors don't know. And how do you treat it? How do you live with it? What are the best things to do?

That's what people are finding out. This is the meat that they have been looking for for so long, and now they are getting it. I'm just delighted. I'm delighted to be a part of it. This is what we've needed for so long. And the methodology of getting it out to the people now, means that more and more people are becoming aware of, I want to say alternative, but we're mislabeled as alternative and it is really not true. We're natural and we're doing the things that really do work in the human body.

People are becoming aware. They are seeing all of these different faces from doctors to researchers telling similar stories. And it is impactful, and it is more and more. It is not tens and twenties now, it's hundreds, it's thousands of people telling similar stories. It carries a lot of weight.

Americans and people around the world are seeing this and they are saying, "There must be something to this." They are starting their own study and research and it is making a difference. So you guys stick with it.

Interviewer: It's incredible, man. Thank you. Thank you and I'm grateful for you sharing that story that I didn't know. Ty, obviously knows it. You guys connected on that.

I do want to ask you about that because I recently was talking to Ty about what that experience was like just in those final moments. When you go back into that moment, do you remember the feelings that you were feeling at that time?

Bob: You know, so many people have never seen anyone die, never seen anyone pass on. So it's a traumatic experience even if it is not a loved one. Ty talks about his parents and I get it because I went through the same thing.

You think this person that has raised you and has taught you is now leaving the face of the earth. You'll never talk to them again. You'll never see them again. It's a moment of realization, I guess you could say, of, "This is really it. This is the end. This person that I've known and grown with and loved will never be a part of my life again. What have I missed?"

That's part of what we all say,"What have I missed? What did I not ask?" It really hits home and all those emotions kind of rise up. They are cumulative and they rise up and you realize it. All of a sudden you realize it. "What has been left undone? What has been left unasked?"

Now my dad is gone, my mom is gone. It is really an emotional thing that can't really be explained unless you go through it. Different people have different types of situations. I was close with my mom, not as close with my dad, but still those memories come rushing back.

You have to depend on those now because that is what you have left. You've got photos and you have memories. That is what you fall back on then at that point, but it cumulates in that.

Interviewer: You talked about, "What did I not ask?"And I appreciate you going there because I think that is something that it is hard to process and it is hard to talk about because it's so painful. For you, did you experience regret?

Bob: I think that everyone, to a degree, will experience regret. Well, some people will not because they weren't close to their parents. I'm referring to people that you're close to whether it's your parents or, in Ty's case, your aunt, your uncle and people that you have been inherently close to throughout your life.

Are there regrets? I think there are because I'm left with—like I said, I never grew as close to this family member as maybe I could have. My dad and I weren't nearly as close as I was to my mom. Still, there were questions with my mom that I didn't ask. Things that I wanted to know about her and about her family.

"She's my mom. I'll always have time—right?—to ask more questions." But as I said, my mom went within two weeks or less of diagnosis and in hospice and out of it the last three or four days of that.

So you can't ask questions then. It's too late and then it starts to hit you. You can't ask any more questions about family, about her childhood, about where you came from. About questions you have even about your own childhood that you may have forgotten and about your family.

Those things rush up, maybe not all at once, some at that point. But even afterwards for a period of time. You'll stand over the grave site and you'll say, "Gee, I missed so much." Even if you were close with that family member, you'll understand that you still missed things.

So I tell people, "Ask the questions now. Draw close now. Do the things. Tell the people that you love that you love them, because you may not get another chance."

Interviewer: You only had two weeks to say goodbye to your mom.

Bob: Really not even that long.

Interviewer: It wasn't enough time, was it?

Bob: It really was not enough time because now you're concerned, "Is Mom really going to die? Is there something we can do to help her?" Of course that's been a long time ago. I did not have the expertise per se at that time to really help her.

Interviewer: Do you wish you did?

Bob: I do wish I did, but at the same time so many families are so mired in allopathic medicine that you can't draw them out sometimes no matter what you do. That is so painful for so many families.

I've heard the stories time and time again, "There was nothing I could say, there was nothing I could do. Bob, tell me, please, what do?" Because the rest of the family is pulling them to chemo and radiation. And I said, "Sometimes there is nothing you can do except pray for them. And tell them, 'I'll be there for you. If you need any help, if you have any questions.'"

Even if you have all of the information, that I think I have now ,and that others in this field have, sometimes you can only stand by and watch and tell them you'll be there for them, you'll pray for them, you'll hope for them, and if they have any questions or concerns, "I'm there for you." Well, it's really a hard thing. You're right, until you've experienced it, and many people have, you really need to be there.

As I said it will be a different experience for some than it is for others. Those that are really close to their folks or at least have a measure of closeness to their parents or their loved ones whoever they may be, they will struggle through similar experiences that I did and that Ty did. But it will be different for some.

I always tell them, "If you know someone only has two or three weeks left, they may survive it and we hope they do and we put together the protocols that hopefully they will survive, but at the same time if you haven't done it, get close at that time and ask the questions."

Interviewer: Right. Thanks man. Do you believe that Ty's movement, the Truth about Cancer, is saving lives?

Bob: There is no question. The Truth about Cancer—you wouldn't believe when the first and then the second series came out. We were bombarded. Of course, I was in five or six of those videos. But we were just bombarded with emails saying, "You asked us this, or you gave this point in the series. Tell me."

I want to expand upon that because in the series we do have little nuggets that are shown at times. And you don't necessarily get to expand and expound on things, but people grab ahold of those. And are they changed? You bet they are. And now they are questioning. They are questioning. "Huh. This makes sense to me now."

So is the Truth about Cancer changing lives? You bet it is. That's why I say, "Keep going. Keep going." I can see that. But what it does most of all is it gives people hope. And where there is hope, people will investigate and they will go about doing the things that help them to prosper. It is that hope. Don't ever forget that hope.

We can talk about therapies and protocols and treatments and supplements till we're blue in the face. But if you're not giving someone genuine hope, then they may not grab ahold of those things. They may not gravitate towards the things that really will help them. That's what you're doing.

We see that in people who are calling us after seeing this series. They have hope now. They are starting to do the things that will enable them to save their own lives in many occasions. It's hope.

Interviewer: That is beautiful.

Bob: It's true.

Interviewer: You can feel it. When you're on the phone and you can feel that they are being given that hope.

Bob: You know, I have people that talk to me all the time that are crying on the phone. We've talked for 20 or 30 minutes and they are crying. And I said, "Are you okay? What's wrong?" They said, "No. No. It's good. You've given me hope. I'm not getting hope anywhere else. You are giving me hope."

So that is what I say about this series. You are giving people hope and that makes all the difference in the world.

Interviewer: That's awesome, man. And I think there's nothing that Ty would want to give to people more than that because it's definitely something that he wasn't given.

Bob: That's what he does. That's what he does. You can see it, you can watch it. I can see it. I can see it in every interview he does. I watch all these interviews and I can see it.

He's compassionate, but he's interested. He's interested in what they are telling him. He's not sitting there looking over his, "What am I going to ask next?" He's sitting there looking them in the eyes and listening to them because he cares about them.

He wants to do the things that give them hope. But he's also drawing the hope out of them that, during that interview, is giving other people hope. You can distill it down any way you like, but distill it down to hope because hope changes things. It really does.

Interviewer: That's awesome. Because when his dad was diagnosed, the mother was there and she said, "As soon as I heard the word cancer, I couldn't hear anything else after that."

Bob: It's true.

Interviewer: Because after that, and definitely during that time—definitely without this information, that was it. It was like cancer and the word death were the same thing.

Bob: Synonymous, yes.

Interviewer: Yes. It was literally the same thing because she didn't stay to listen to the rest of it because if she knew, "Well what stage, what's happening—"

Bob: Yes. Cancer was basically termed the plague of the 20th century, but now it's the plague of the 21st century too, as we know. People don't think other people or themselves can survive the plague. The plague is known as the Black Death. People die when they get the plague.

You are right. Cancer is synonymous with death. When people do hear that, they shut down because they don't see hope. Many times they follow the doctor's orders. The doctor says, "You have six months to live. Get your affairs in order." They do what the doctor tells them to do and they die.

We give them hope. This series gives them hope. When you give someone hope then they have a chance to live and they do, many of them do. I would say most of them who pursue it do. Whereas, on the other end, most of them die.

Hope. They grab onto hope. You need to keep giving them hope and that's what we do and The Truth About Cancer. There's no other way that I can frame it. There is a lot of stuff in there that is great. But hope, that's where it is distilled down to and that changes lives and that saves lives and we need to know that.

Interviewer: Thanks Bob. I want to give you a hug for that, man.

Bob: I'm still attached here.

Interviewer: Thanks, Buddy.

Bob: You bet. Are we good now?

Interviewer: Yes.

[end of transcript]

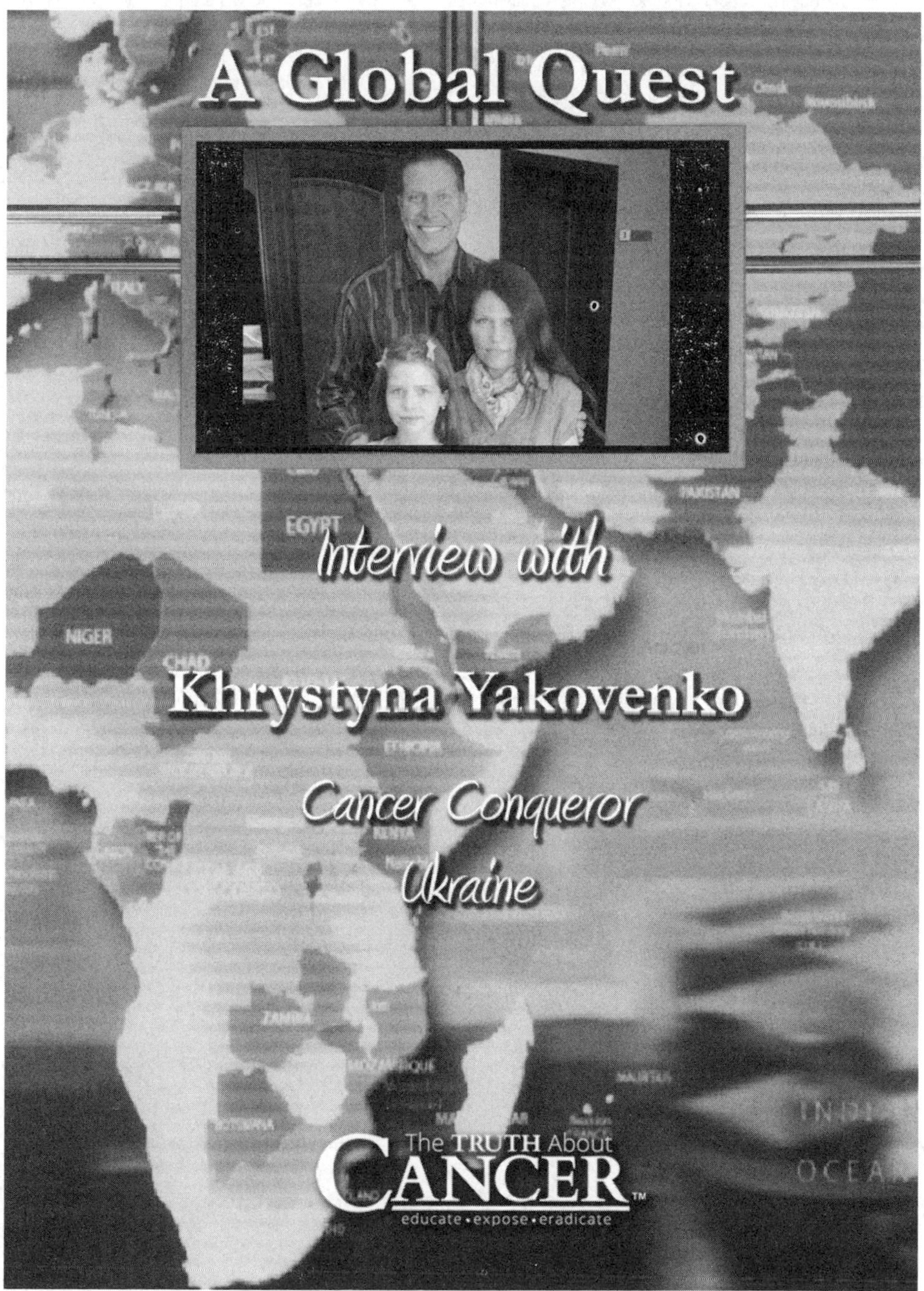
A Global Quest
Interview with
Khrystyna Yakovenko
Cancer Conqueror
Ukraine
The TRUTH About
CANCER
educate • expose • eradicate

Ty: I'm really happy to be here in Riga, Latvia, this morning. And I'm sitting across from a lady named Khrystyna. Thank you for joining us today. She is going to share with us her story of overcoming melanoma cancer. And so, Khrystyna, first of all, thank you for being here. And could you tell us a little bit about your background, your history?

Khrystyna via interpreter: It all started at the end of 2012.

Ty: You were diagnosed with cancer at the end of 2012?

Khrystyna via interpreter: I got my mole on the back injured accidentally. When I contacted my doctor, he diagnosed the melanoma in the fourth stage with metastasis in the liver.I had my surgery in December and they prescribed the first course of palliative chemotherapy.And starting from 2013, 25th of February I am the patient of International Virotherapy Center. And I am receiving virotherapy.

Ty: Okay, so you were diagnosed with malignant melanoma that had metastasized to the liver and you said that they prescribed palliative chemotherapy. What do you mean by palliative chemotherapy?

Khrystyna via interpreter: They prescribed the palliative chemotherapy, and at that time, I even didn't understand what is what. I completely trusted our Ukrainian doctors and I trusted the methods they are using and I trusted this palliative chemotherapy. I simply didn't realize the effect of this diagnosis completely entirely at that moment.

Ty: So, if I understand it correctly, by palliative chemotherapy, they did not offer you hope that it would cure your melanoma. Just that it would maybe give you a few more months to live, if I'm correct?

Khrystyna via interpreter: This palliative type of chemotherapy, of course, it is not thought to treat the melanoma. It is thought to maintain the life, at this latest period of a patient's life. It has to ease the pain, which actually, I didn't have at the time. And as melanoma is not sensitive to chemotherapy, so it's simply just to maintain the person's ability to spend these last periods.

Ty: So, they did not offer you much hope as far as curing your cancer with the chemotherapy. How many months or years did they approximate that you had left?

Khrystyna via interpreter: Maximum of half of the year, six months.

Ty: So, six months. Yesterday, I saw you with your daughter, I think. How old is she?

Khrystyna via interpreter: She's ten-and-a-half, and she's the younger daughter.

Ty: So, tell me about how it felt to you to have daughters that you may not be able to see.

Khrystyna via interpreter: ....

Ty: Take your time.

Khrystyna via interpreter: I think that my younger daughter was the one who prayed for me to God. Just one second.

Ty: Tell her it's okay.

Khrystyna via interpreter: It's a very hard topic to discuss. When I found out about my dad, it was not a secret from my family. My kids were aware about it, and my mom was also aware of it. My kids were realizing what cancer means, and we all together tried to find a way out of this situation. I was not feeling afraid. I was not falling into panic. Simply I understood that I had no right to leave it, I had to fight. In 2009, my father passed away and my mom and my kids, I was responsible for all the family. I was the one who was responsible.I had to make it, I had to make it over, and I said, "Please don't worry I'll make it anyway."

I think it is my daughter who actually prayed for me to God and when we first time came to the church, I received already the palliative chemotherapy. And after a month-and-a-half, I found out about Rigvir and I started to use Rigvir. When I first came to Virotherapy Center, the doctors didn't say, "Yes, we will do it." They said, "We will try because the stage was late." Sometimes on the initial stages people who have this very scary diagnosis they sometimes, by themselves, they lose hope. They stop to fight and they simply leave it. Sometimes there are people who even at late stages they continue to fight, they continue to find the way out of the situation. In these cases, the disease simply just is over.

Ty: I could tell yesterday at the other office, everyone was sitting around the table and your daughter was there with a little puppy dog and y'all were talking. I could tell she is really strong and an encouragement to you. You are fortunate to have a daughter like that and you also have another daughter as well.

Khrystyna via interpreter: Yes, I have an older daughter also. She is 16 now.

Ty: Once you began the Rigvir, the virotherapy here, and you began to improve, describe how the emotions in your family changed, especially with your daughters to see that you were getting better.

Khrystyna via interpreter: When I first found information about Rigvir, it was initiative that I realized that this will work on me. I simply, I knew for 100 percent that this is the way. And I trusted, entirely trusted, this method.

Ty: Good for you, because one of the very important parts about a successful cancer treatment is that you believe in it and you're ready to fight to save your life and that's exactly what you did. You determined that you were going to live, and you believe in the treatment, and that's a big part of the reason that you're healthy today, I believe.

Khrystyna via interpreter: I believe that this is the very important part of your treatment to entirely trust your doctors, and to be sure that it will work on you. In case you don't trust, simply, there is no use to starting then. So I trust it, and that's why I start it.

Ty: And so you not only trusted your doctors, but you trusted your doctors that were using a very, very successful treatment in Rigvir. So you had, as we call it in the United States, a double whammy. You had two for two.

Khrystyna via interpreter: After a month-and-a-half after I receive the palliative chemotherapy, I started, and I realize these effects of it. I realize that I have to find another way, and I was searching internet all through. I was searching, I was listening and watching the patients stories, the forums and I think that I found the whole information about melanoma and I realized what it is.

Ty: So, how did it feel once you realized that you had this successful Rigvir treatment for melanoma and that it was in Latvia, a country very close to home for you?

Khrystyna via interpreter: When I found out that information about Rigvir, at the very beginning I realized that this is the one that I need. And I started to find opportunities to receive it as soon as possible. And I'm really thankful for all the people working in the center, Virotherapy Center headed by Yurgos, the chairman. And they gave me so much support that I did not receive in my own country from our doctors. So I'm really thankful for this.

Ty: I've actually only met them, the people here, yesterday for the first time. And I agree with you. There are some incredible people here in this clinic that seem to have a lot of compassion for cancer patients and they give them hope. I think that your choice to come here was a very good choice.

Khrystyna via interpreter: They are really doing everything to help the patient regain his health. They provide all the help possible from their side and the rest is depending on patient, how he will fight. These specialists, they're not like ordinary doctors who for example, when it's the end of the day, they close their room, they leave their clinic, and they forget about everything. They are live all these experiences, all of these bad experiences with the patients through all of the way. They're walking through all of the way. They are trying to find an opportunity to make the medicine available. They don't simply say there is no way out of the situation. They still try to do everything to help the patient to find his way to fight the disease. And I know that I am not the only one with this late-stage cancer who really survived. There are many people, and many people now have a healthy and happy life. It is very important to start the treatment at the very right time, because most of the patients, they don't actually die from the disease, they die from the treatment, and due to the lost time.

***Ty**:* That's a real good point. Many patients do die from the conventional treatments like chemotherapy, but with Rigvir over the last three years you've not had any negative side effects like you would have had if you had been treating with chemotherapy. Correct?

***Khrystyna via interpreter**:* My treatment was already lasting for the third year, and I have not felt any side effects nor in the beginning, neither now. I feel completely normal. It's hard for people to believe that it is so simple and everything is so easy because it is comfortable. You don't feel discomfort. But simply, all the genius is simple. So it's even easier, you feel even better than just when you're having an ordinary slight flu. It's even lesser.

***Ty**:* So I guess this last questions is a bit rhetorical. I can tell by the smile on your face that you would definitely recommend this clinic to somebody else that might have been diagnosed with a late-stage cancer.

Khrystyna via interpreter: From my side, I also make some videos for other people and post it on the internet for other people to share my story for them to gain information on this therapy, and to also share my experience to encourage them. Because usually, patients tell their doctors that you can't understand me because you're not in my shoes. You don't have this diagnosis. For example, as for me to show it in figures, when I was diagnosed with cancer, I had 1,956 metastasis in liver. After the first chemotherapy, the one I discussed, I had 196. And only after six month of Rigvir therapy, there were left only 56. I am being contacted by many people via these videos and they asked me to share my story, to share how the treatment is going, and I think it's very important, because not everybody is ready to share their story. Because for someone it's hard, because it is really a very dramatic moment for every person. But I think it's important to share my experience, to give the support, to give my opinion, to share my experience so people can find these treatments earlier and they can save their own lives. And many people have, I think that many people have already, via my videos, they have saved their lives.

I believe and I know that Rigvir can treat cancer, it also stops the progression. It not only improves the quality of life, it really treats this disease. As I have searched through the internet for very long time, I watch the videos of every country. The medicine of any region. I didn't find the same medicine that could do the same for the health of the patient, and I can't understand those doctors who were still prescribing this conventional treatment for the patients because the melanoma is not sensitive. The radiotherapy, chemotherapy is simply a kind of treatment makes the disease progress, not to treat.

Ty: Well, thank you for being open to share your story today. Thank you for your strong willpower to live, and I look forward to being in touch with you in the future several years down the road and continued health for you, and looking forward to seeing pictures of you with your little girls growing up and getting married.

Khrystyna via interpreter: I still understand those doctors who don't prescribe this effective medicine, and I think that in this case is that the most important is where the person is. If the person is ready find, to look for the treatment, then he will find this therapy, and I hope that my video will give information about this. I hope my girls, when they grow up, they will be doctors, and they will be specialist in virotherapy. Will be helping people.

Ty: Well, thank you so much for sharing. This has been very inspiring and encouraging interview. And I know that the people who are watching this today are just going to be wanting to follow you, and they're going to be really looking into Rigvir therapy for cancer, because of your story. So thank you.

Khrystyna via interpreter: I hope so. Yes, I hope that it will motivate other people, because I could not think when I will be 40 that I will have this situation in my life. Because it's just an ordinary mole, and the disease is so serious.

Ty: Thank you.

[end of transcript]

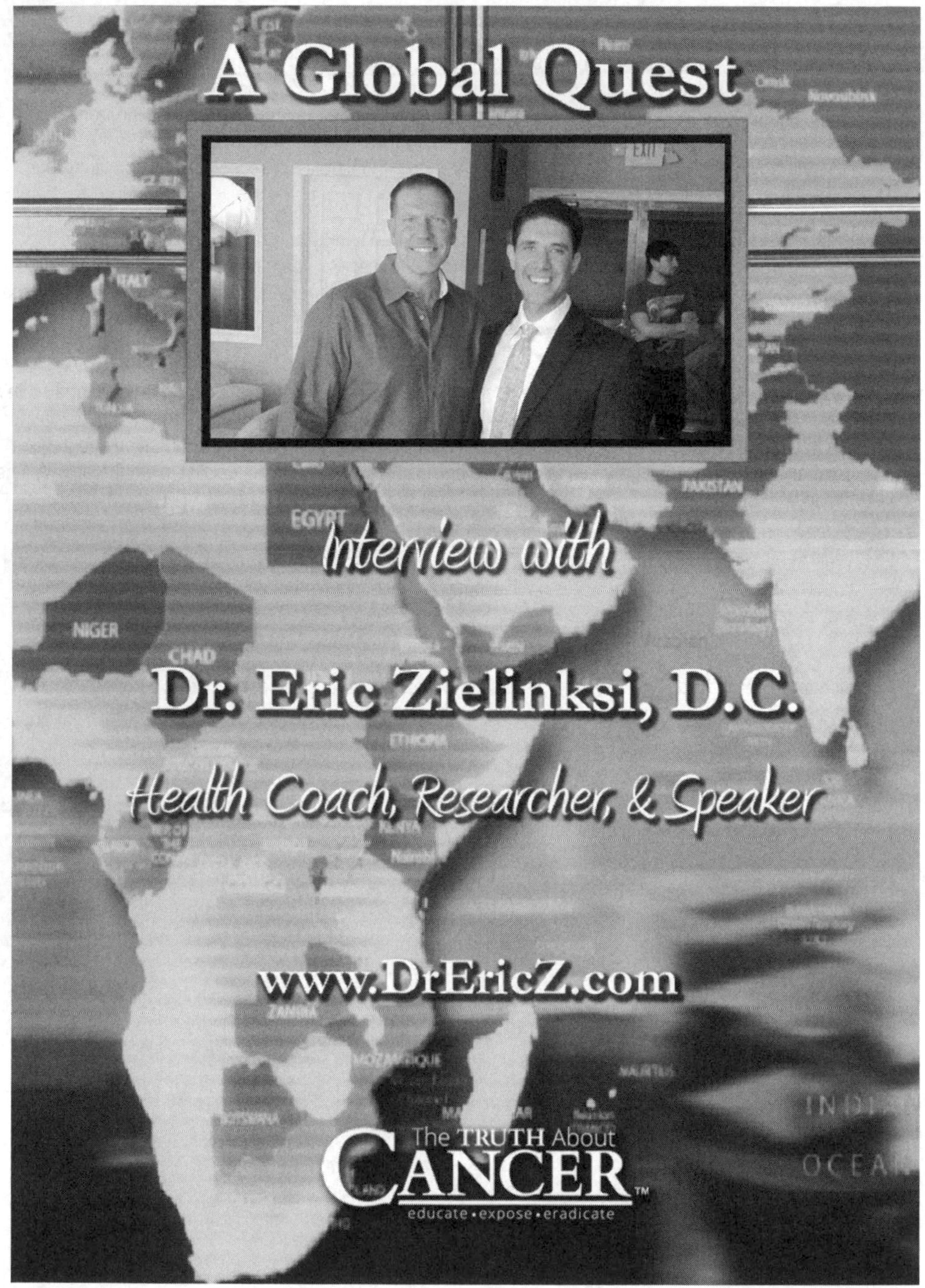
A Global Quest
Interview with
Dr. Eric Zielinksi, D.C.
Health Coach, Researcher, & Speaker
www.DrEricZ.com
The TRUTH About
CANCER
educate • expose • eradicate

Ty: I'm really honored to be here just outside of Atlanta, Ga., today with Dr. Eric Zielinski, Dr. Z.

Dr. Zielinski: Ty, I really appreciate it. What an honor.

Ty: Yeah, it's an honor for me to be able to talk to you today about essential oils. I'm really excited about this because this is a big piece of the overall health puzzle that we haven't discussed before so, Dr. Z, again, thanks for joining us.

And so I want to go back to the start with you. What got you interested in health and nutrition and eventually essential oils?

Dr. Zielinski: Well, how much time do we have because …

Ty: That's kind of an open-ended question.

Dr. Zielinski: It is. Oh my Lord. So, 12 years ago, I accepted Christ as my Savior and I had one of those dramatic, "I was blind, now I see, I was lost, now I'm found" experiences. And my mentor in Christ, his name is Enoch, and he's 71 years old today. He will run circles around you and me. He could still bench-press 250 lbs. and he's the healthiest person I know. He's not on any pharmaceuticals and just lives a very clean, healthy life.

And he told me, he looked me straight in the eye — I was a young man at the time — and he said, "Eric, you have to honor God. You have to honor your body as the temple of the Holy Spirit." And so what that did was really imparted to me a focus and a vision in my life. So when I started seeking out scripture and when I started seeking out just how to live and what it was to be a Christian, I also was seeking out natural health as well.

And so it's been a very great ride. I've been researching on my own for over a decade—actually, 12 years—natural health solutions and remedies. It wasn't until recently that I fell in love with essential oils. And that was because I'm a public health research writer and one of my clients asked me to write a series of public health reports.

And it was interesting because my wife has been using essential oils since we've been married, and she has her thing. She puts them here, there, and she just does her thing. She has her own little protocol. I just thought it was smelly stuff. I had never really given two thoughts about it. And here's the test though, developed athlete's foot a few years ago. I went to the gym, something happened, I got — what do you think? Tea tree or melaleuca. I got some knock-off brand at the health food store and nothing worked. And I'm like, "This stuff stinks. I mean …"

Ty: Doesn't work.

Dr. Zielinski: I threw it away. Yeah, I completely dismissed it until I started doing research and, being trained in how to sift through the literature, it blew my mind. I started doing research and I started seeing how oregano is more effective at antibiotic-resistant bacteria like MRSA and different sources of staph strains than current medications. I started doing research on cancer and you name it — and I was convinced. I went to my wife and I'm like, "What are you doing? And why are you enjoying these?" And she started explaining to me the difference between a therapeutic-grade oil and the knock-off brand at the store and, long story short, that's where it all began. Then I started looking into the different grades and brands.

Ty: So what are essential oils? Let's go back to the basics.

Dr. Zielinski: So an essential oil is a volatile organic compound. What I think people need to recognize when it comes to essential oil is that there is no nutrition in it. There is no vitamin or mineral. It's a chemical that essentially God gave to the plant to protect the plant from outside threats – whether it's bacteria, viruses, fungus, or even vectors like flies, bees, whatever that might attack the plant.

And so what it includes are organic compounds. Not organic as we think, meaning organic having a carbon chain included in it. Organic compounds like terpenes, alcohols, ketones, esters, and you-name-it is, basically chemicals.

Ty: From the plant.

Dr. Zielinski: From the plant. Natural chemicals from the plant. And with that, there are antioxidant properties, and we can talk a lot about that as time permits.

Ty: So basically, what the theory behind essential oils is then, is you take this natural protection for the plant and you are somehow able to move it over to yourself.

Dr. Zielinski: Basically.

Ty: With essential oils.

Dr. Zielinski: Well, you have to think of it. God inspired the writers of the Bible long ago when he said, "The leaves of the trees are for the healing of the nations." And that's exactly what this is.

Ty: That's essential oils.

Dr. Zielinski: Exactly.

Ty: So let's talk about some essential oils, specifically as they relate to cancer. Let's talk about some essential oils that might be good at treating cancer because I know that you've come across them in your research. And one of the things that I'm really glad about, with you specifically, is that you're such a researcher.

None of this stuff that you're saying is just conjecture. There is medical literature that is replete with what you talk about today so I really want to make note of that for the people that are watching. These are not Dr. Z's theories. This is steeped in medical literature.

Dr. Zielinski: Yes, and just because I understand my aromatherapist friends are going to be listening, and I'm going to get crucified if I don't say this statement: There is a fact that we have to be careful about invivo and invitro studies. We've got to recognize that even bleach will kill cells in a petri dish, but we're not going to drink bleach.

Ty: Right.

Dr. Zielinski: So to take the extrapolation that a certain essential oil is going to cure cancer when it was shown to kill, let's say, a bladder cancer cell line—be careful. However, it's important to recognize that the burden of proof is on the scientist at this point to show what's safe and what's not safe.

So when it comes to essential oils, it's really important to recognize one awesome thing too. There is no oil for one specific issue. What we have found, and this is pretty fascinating, is that, let's use the ayurvedic model—Indian folk medicine, for example. There is an abundance of lemons in India, so you'll find that Indians use lemon essential oil for virtually everything — detoxification, internally, externally, whether or not you're going to clean the counter or whether or not you want to clean your skin. They use lemon essential oils for everything from nausea to halitosis to diabetes, cancer.

Well, when you go to Australia, they're using melaleuca, tea tree and eucalyptus. When you go to Oregon and Washington, they're using peppermint for everything. So it's important to realize that these oils — a lot of them do the same thing. When I report on research it's limited because we've only done a limited amount of research, but, as far as I know, there is no essential oil that does not have a cancer effect.

Ty: Okay.

Dr. Zielinski: It's important because you're going to get helped one way or another. Most research has been done regarding frankincense. And just going back to the baby Jesus and the magi, it just rings so true to me. Why would these three wise men, we call them, travel halfway across the world to give the king of the Jews gold, frankincense and myrrh? Because it was — and still is, in my opinion — one of the most precious commodities on the planet.

And what frankincense does, it does multiple things. It produces what's called apoptosis, which I know you're very familiar with. It's a programmed cell death. So when you ingest frankincense, apply it topically over a tumor, or even inhale it via aromatherapy, what we have found was frankincense essential oil can trigger the cancer cell to die — basically commit suicide. ,It also gives your body what it needs to kill cancer as well, so it's a dual mechanism.

I just recently read a report of over 130 research articles regarding essential oils. And what the researchers came to understand was what essential oils do is prevent angiogenesis, which is the growth of veins and arteries. It stops metastatic growth. It prevents DNA repair, which is pretty key.

That's really key because there is one study that compared sandalwood and frankincense. It found that frankincense again triggered that apoptotic effect where the cancer cell died, but sandalwood killed cancer another way. Sandalwood went around the back end, in a sense, and flanked the cell by triggering the DNA to not have the ability to repair itself so that cancer just died that way too.

So there are multiple mechanisms. There are various other ways plus increasing reactive oxygen species and working at the cellular level to bring out oxidative stress.

Ty: So the essential oils – the different ones work with different mechanisms

Dr. Zielinski: Yes.

Ty: So you really would be wise then, I guess, to take multiple essential oils, especially if you're battling disease, because they're going to have different methods of action.

Dr. Zielinski: Okay. I have a 4-year-old son, and he loves everything to do with superheroes so I'm all about Avengers and everything.

There is a research study that actually uses the terminology "synergistic approach." So in a sense, it's like this. Iron Man, he can kick butt. Hulk, he's unstoppable. And same thing with Captain America. But when you get them together, they save the world.

And that's exactly what research has found was in the chemicals in the essential oils. They work together in a synergistic approach. Meaning this—you could take a ketone, you could take an ester out of an essential oil, and test that viability to kill certain cancer lines, but when you use the actual essential oil itself, it is a synergistic approach. But when you combine other oils too, it's like boom, Avengers Part 2. I can't wait to see that one, right?

Ty: It is like superheroes on steroids.

Dr. Zielinski: I love it. So that's where we're at right now. And it's unbelievable. And the thing is, we don't really know exactly how it works, but we're learning.

Ty: Well, one of the things interesting that you said was oregano oil. You mentioned oregano oil.

Dr. Zielinski: Yes.

Ty: I interviewed Dr. Josh Axe, and I think that was the primary oil that they used for his mother whohad cancer. So a lot of anti-cancer properties I know of in oregano oil. You also mentioned frankincense. Let's talk about one of the other gifts of the magi—myrrh.

Dr. Zielinski: Yes.

Ty: Can you talk about some properties of myrrh that might be good for a cancer patient?

Dr. Zielinski: Oh, myrrh is unbelievable when it comes to being able to affect people at increasing immunity, healing at diminishing side effects, yet I haven't reached any studies on myrrh specifically in cancer yet.

That doesn't mean it's not there, and it doesn't mean that it's not effective. What we have found was, again, is that myrrh is a very intuitive healing agent. And that's the other part. When it comes to aromatherapy and using oils internally and topically, these oils not only help with cancer, but the side effects. And that's so critical because, as you've traveled the world, Ty, you've talked to people that are cancer survivors and people struggling with cancer, it's really the side effects that get them. And often times, it's not the cancer that kills them. It's a common cold or a flu or you-name-it, right? It compromises the immune system.

Ty: From a devastated body.

Dr. Zielinski: And that's what the essential oils do when it comes to sleeplessness, nausea, especially with myrrh. The research on myrrh, when it comes to the side effects inadvertently related to cancer are pretty encouraging for folks.

Ty: Yeah. So talk about aromatherapy versus rubbing them on topically. That's the best way to use essential oils? You said they don't have nutrition per se, so would you ever take them through your mouth? Would you ever put drops on your tongue or swallow the oils, or do you rub them or burn them? What's the best way to use them?

Dr. Zielinski: Very good question. I want to dispel a myth. The myth is that essential oils are dangerous to consume orally. And it is a myth because research has been done. It's limited research, but there's one recent study that was done out of Iran, and it showed that just one drop of peppermint oil in the mouth—and also another study showed one drop of peppermint oil in a 16-ounce glass of water—has shown to increase athletic performance for college students. Which is pretty cool because it opens up the airways, it gives you energy, it lowers the blood pressure. So it is safe.

Enteric-coated peppermint has been shown to help with irritable bowel syndrome. So they're safe, but it has to be done in propriety. I've got to say, don't go on Pinterest and look at these morphine bombs and Valium bombs that say, "Hey, put 50 drops of oil on it and take a capsule." Use moderation. Use wisdom. Use common sense.

Ty: Right.

Dr. Zielinski: But there is every reason to show and believe that you could internally consume them and also apply topically. Apply topically — it's such a great way — and also aromatically. Now, aromatically, in my opinion, is the most effective way of benefiting from essential oils. And not to use a crude analogy, but it's the best one that I have come up with — the reason why cocaine addicts snort cocaine instead of injecting cocaine is it's the fastest way of getting a high.

If you just walk into this room and if you smell, let's say they have an air freshener, that's a volatile organic compound that reaches our nose. It gets into our nasal mucosa and there's millions of little nerve cells right here. Well, what happens is the compound immediately crosses the blood-brain barrier and starts to affect up to the hypothalamus and our brain. Then it gets into your lungs and once it gets into your lungs, it gets to the system relatively immediately.

Ty: Right.

Dr. Zielinski: So that is the most important way, in my opinion, to get the whole body affecting in a positive way. But we use all three approaches, in my opinion, under the guidance of a health care provider who is trained in this area and knows very well how to use them.

Ty: Right, right. I mean, I guess it's the same principle for somebody – you put chloroform over your mouth, it knocks you out immediately. That same immediate effect is the aroma therapy effect, only you're using good stuff instead of chloroform.

So what about the effects of essential oils on the immune system? Any noticeable effects on the immune system?

Dr. Zielinski: What doesn't it help? I mean, really, what doesn't it help? Everything. I mean, really, in my opinion. Oxidative stress is the number one cause of disease. It's been linked to everything from heart disease to cancer to you-name-it. And it's caused by the foods that we eat, the toxins that we consume, the air that we breathe, and the stress that we deal with in just being in American society, but also it's global.

Essential oils have been shown to help with every single aspect of oxidative stress. We're talking working at the cytokine level, working at cellular rejuvenation. And here's a cool thing. I love what these things do, especially frankincense. Regarding frankincense and cancer, it has what's known as cell selectivity. So when you're looking at cells in a petri dish or at the very few human studies that we have, what essential oils do is they target pathogens and they leave the healthy cells alone.

Ty: Selectively toxic.

Dr. Zielinski: Love it. If you're going to take out an enemy target, you're going to use a sniper instead of a nuclear bomb approach unless you want to take out a whole nation. And that's what chemotherapy, and that's what antibiotics do. They are basically a nuclear approach and they are killing people — mass destruction. But essential oils aren't like that.

"I'm telling you the wisdom of man," the Bible says, "is foolishness to God." And that's what we're experiencing right now. So when it comes to microbial infection, bacteria, virus, you name it, the essential oils kill that stuff. And the same thing with hand sanitizers and all these other things. You can use essential oils to replace all the toxins in your life so you don't have to be exposed.

Ty: Right. And the hand sanitizers, by the way, they kill all the good stuff on your skin, right? The antibacterials.

Dr. Zielinski: Yes. And 75 percent have an ingredient called triclosan, which has been a registered pesticide since 1969. I'm only 35 years old, but I'm telling you, I've seen a drastic change when I was a kid. When I was a kid, we used to just wash our hands with Dove soap and everything's smelly nowadays.

You go into a room, they got these wall flowers. That's poison. These volatile organic compounds and the smells from your lotions and your potions and your aerosols have all been shown to affect the brain at a cellular level. We're talking neuro-degeneration, Alzheimer's, ADD, autism, even cancer. It's killing us. Smell is vitally important.

Ty: Changing directions a little bit. And this is a sure theory because everybody's got a theory on this, but we've seen a huge increase in childhood cancer over the last couple of decades. Why?

Dr. Zielinski: I think because of the smells. I think because of the chemicals. I think because these kids don't know what it's like to not have all this aromatic toxin poison around them in addition to the GMOs, in addition to the non-organic food, the pesticides – it's everything. We live in such a toxic environment that I actually share with people to use essential oils and a natural solution approach for prevention. I eat really well, but when I walk outside the door, I'm being poisoned by all the smog. And how hard is it to even find good pure water nowadays? These poor kids are just being poisoned left and right, and it's a multi approach, it's a multifaceted approach. That makes sense and we could talk a lot about that so I want to be careful because that's a whole hour's segment right there.

Ty: No, that's good input. That's good input because I try to ask everyone who I'm interviewing that because I really want to try to get to the bottom of some of these reasons so that we can help. We can help stop this epidemic.

Dr. Zielinski: And we've got to get off our butts. We've got to get walking again, playing again. When I was a kid I used to play a lot, I used to eat a lot more fruits and vegetables and stuff. Now, kids are sitting down, they're watching TV. And I have to battle it because my kids are the odd kids. They've never been immunized, they've never had a shot, they don't know anything — they've never been to McDonald's. We go to McDonald's on a rest stop to go to Michigan when we drive home to see our family. That's what they think McDonald's is. I get them a fun toy or they play at the play area. They're like, "We're going to McDonald's to play?" They don't know what that is. It's poison. So that's the other thing. From the very beginning.

Ty: Right.

Dr. Zielinski: And also, I'll end with this because this is so vitally important because we've delivered three natural home births — my wife did. I was there for support, but I take a lot of credit because, hey, I was there, right? It all starts at the breast, and a lot of children right now aren't being breastfed. They're missing the vital nutrients in the colostrum and in the breast milk that they need. And so, in a sense, we're giving kids an automatic head-start to get autoimmunity because it's not helping their gut system.

Ty: Right, because they're missing that.

Dr. Zielinski: Oh, and they're also missing the vaginal flora that's helping the gut flora as well. So the C-sections—I mean, there's so much, Ty, again ...

Ty: But then we shoot them as soon as they get out to help them, right?

Dr. Zielinski: Oh, and you know the shots, compared to what it used to be, it's unbelievable. I was immunized, but the reality was, I only got like 15, 20 shots. Now it's like 50-plus. It's unbelievable. So that's all another topic though.

Ty: You throw that all together, they've got a stacked deck against them.

Dr. Zielinski: That's it. I think that's important and that's one of the reasons why I share with people, "Yeah, you can take an essential oil to fight cancer, but if you're going to go to McDonald's, you're wasting your time."

Ty: Right.

Dr. Zielinski: It's one step forward, three steps back. And the same thing, it's a multifaceted approach. It's all about balance.

Ty: Speaking about children with cancer, we've got a guest here today that I want to pull in on the interview. Allison, if you could come and sit down here next to Dr. Z? Allison Huish.

Dr. Zielinski: Yes, our dear friend.

Ty: Yes.

Dr. Zielinski: I love Allison. She's such a sweetheart. Hi.

Allison: Hi.

Ty: Thanks for joining us, Allison.

Allison: Thank you.

Ty: So while I was interviewing with Dr. Z here, he mentioned a couple of things that made me think of you. Number one, child with cancer. And number two, he'd spoke about frankincense oil being so potent against cancer. So could you share a little bit about your personal testimony of frankincense oil that Dr. Z was just speaking about?

Allison: Yeah. I have a love for frankincense oil. I think it is so powerful. All of the research that I had done shows what it can do. It is anti-tumoral. It helps boost the white blood cell count, so it definitely played a huge role in my tumor. It is by far the number one oil that I used to help get rid of my tumor. I did a lot internally, I did some topically. I have a great love for that oil.

Ty: And you were diagnosed with a brain stem tumor at the age of 13.

Allison: I was diagnosed at age 13. One thing that's interesting about my tumor, like I said, it was a pilocytic astrocytoma. That tumor is normally found in 6-, 7-year-old boys. It's not found in teenage girls. But it's a tumor that's starting to appear in much younger kids and especially more in males now.

Ty: And why do you think that is? Any theory?

Allison: Why I have my tumor?

Ty: Yeah, you said it was predominantly in males.

Allison: Predominantly in males. One thing that was interesting is, we have never been able to figure out what caused my tumor. We don't know. That is the great mystery. Years ago I did have one chiropractor who did some testing and he firmly believed that my tumor was caused by a DPT immunization. He thought that I had an immunization and maybe I fell down the stairs or off the tramp or something and so that immunization went to the localized spot and started to form a tumor.

Dr. Zielinski: We just don't know. We are walking experiments. And one reason why, Ty, I really appreciate what you're doing and I appreciate what we've done with the Essential Oil Revolution Summit. We're trying to create awareness because people just don't know.

Ty: Right, right. And that's the common mission, isn't it? To educate.

Dr. Zielinski: Yeah, you have to.

Ty: So to finish your story, Allison, you were 13, diagnosed with a brain tumor, used frankincense amongst other things, and then tell us the happy ending.

Allison: Yeah, so I was diagnosed when I was 13.

Dr. Zielinski: You're here.

Allison: I know. I'm here today, right?

Dr. Zielinski: Praise God.

Allison: I know, really. I do thank my Heavenly Father for many, many blessings.

Dr. Zielinski: Awesome.

Allison: So I was 13 years old when I was diagnosed. It took me about three years to get rid of it completely. But about three years into my process of using a lot of essential oils, frankincense oil, clove oil, good diet — my tumor started to shrink and about three years later, I was diagnosed to be completely tumor-free. So several years ago I did hit my five-year mark and ever since then have loved sharing my story in teaching other people about health and alternative medicine and finding natural solutions in your life.

Ty: And now you're the picture of health along with Dr. Z. If the two of you don't make people want to use essential oils, there's something wrong with them. Because you're obviously healthy, you're happy, and the concern that you have for other people is evident. And so, I just want to thank you for that. What's your message, Dr. Z, to end this interview, to the cancer patients who might be watching?

Dr. Zielinski: There's hope. We can't give up hope. I don't care what the diagnosis is. I don't care what the number is. Don't believe it. Believe that God's given you an unbelievable ability to heal yourself as Allison found out. She experienced firsthand because He is our healer. He not only is our healer, but He has given our body that ability to combat anything so don't give up hope. Try, seek, research, stay plugged into the things that you're involved with, and go forward.

Ty: Awesome. Well, thank you so much for spending the time to share your knowledge today.

Dr. Zielinski: Thank you so much.

Ty: And thank you too, Allison.

Allison: Thank you.

[end of transcript]

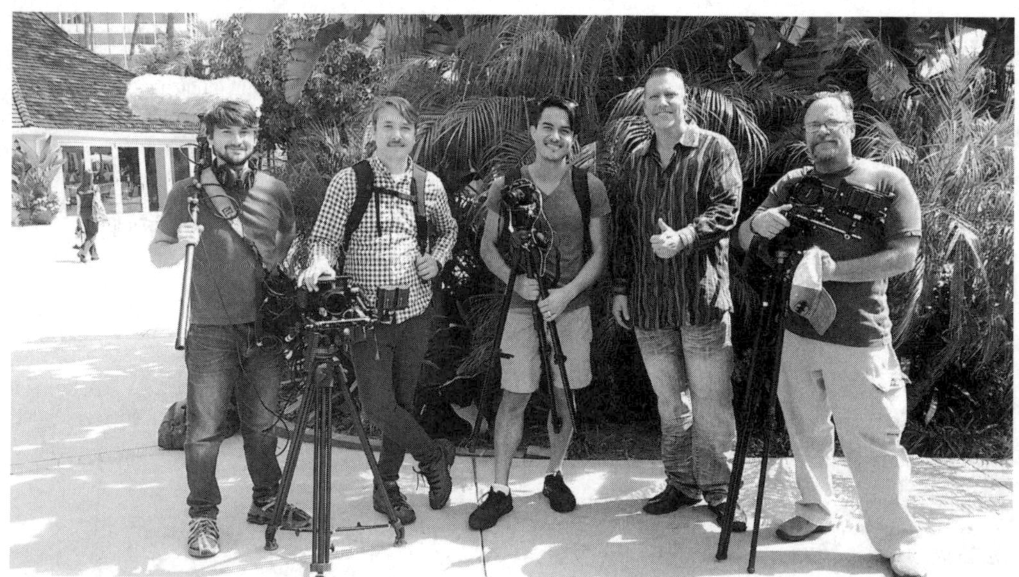

In San Diego (From Left to Right) Zachry Karisch, Travis Jones, Jonathan Otto, Ty Bollinger, Alan Ray

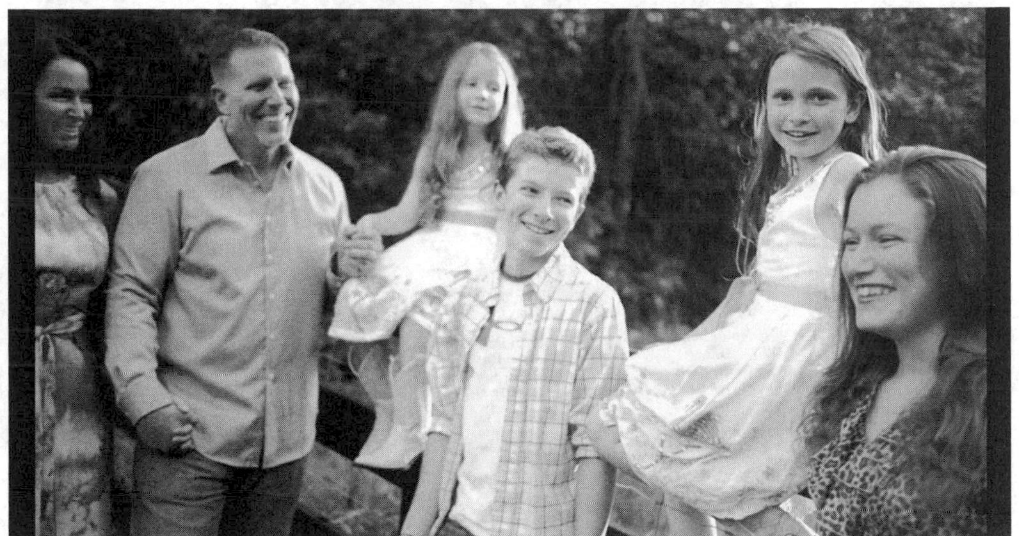

ABOVE – The Bollinger Family (From Left to Right) Charlene, Ty, Charity, Bryce, Tabitha, Brianna
BELOW – TTAC Founders - Jonathan Hunsaker & Ty Bollinger

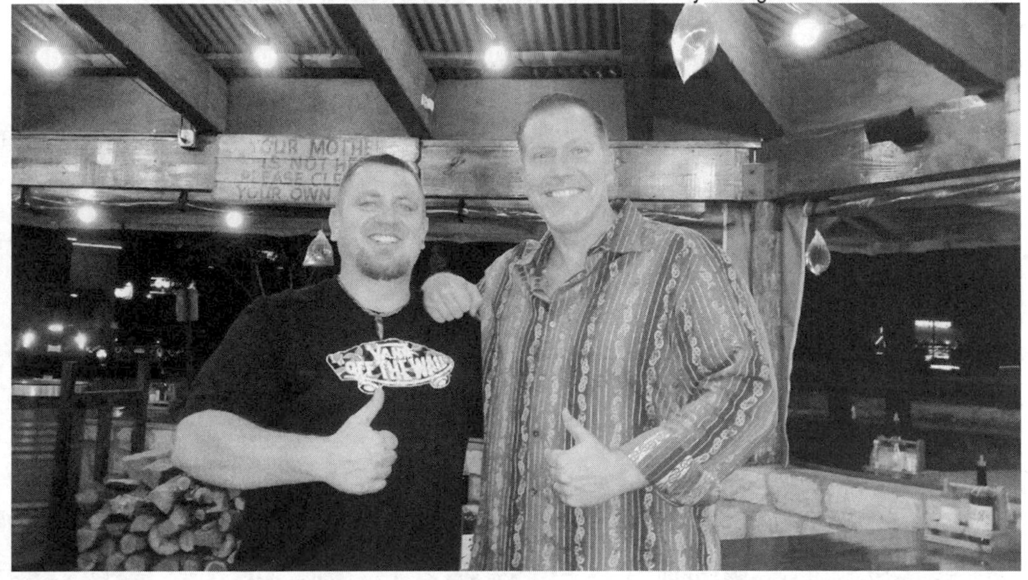

THE EXPERTS

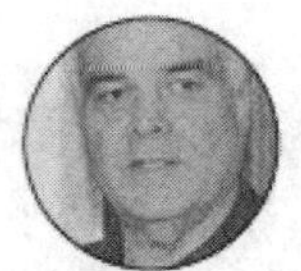

Dr. Matthias Rath, M.D.
Founder of Dr. Rath Research Institute (Netherlands)

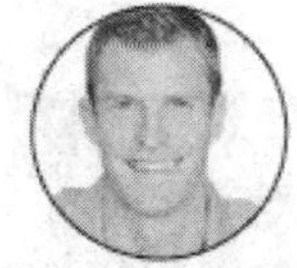

Dr. Josh Axe, D.N.M., D.C., C.N.S.
Nutrition Expert, Author & Founder of DrAxe.com

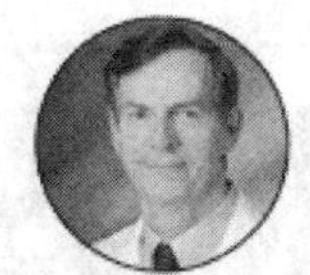

Dr. Russell Blaylock, M.D.
Neurosurgeon, Scientist & Editor of the Blaylock Wellness Report

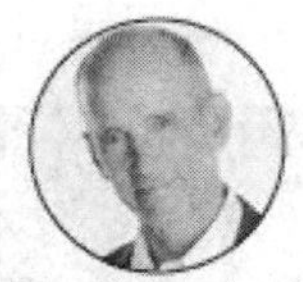

Dr. Joseph Mercola, D.O.
Founder of Mercola.com, New York Times Best-selling Author

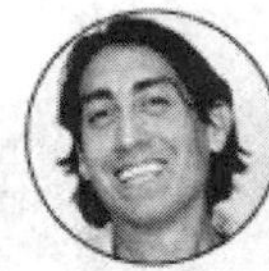

Sayer Ji
Author, Lecturer, National Healtl Federation Advisory Board

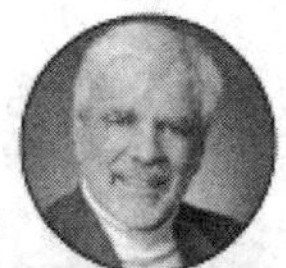

Dr. Jonathan V. Wright, M.D.
Medical Director and Founder - Tahoma Clinic (Washington, USA)

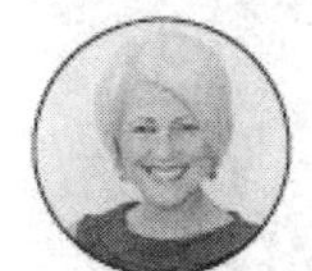

Dr. Véronique Desaulniers, D.C.
Breast Cancer Conqueror, Author, Physician & Lecturer

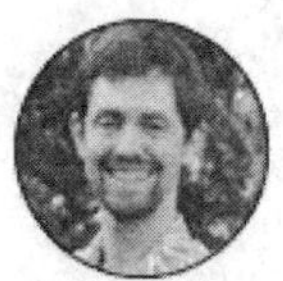

Ocean Robbins
CEO of Food Revolution Network, Author, Speaker & Facilitator

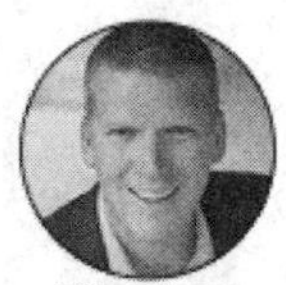

Mike Adams
aka "The Health Ranger" - Food Scientist, Author, and Lecturer

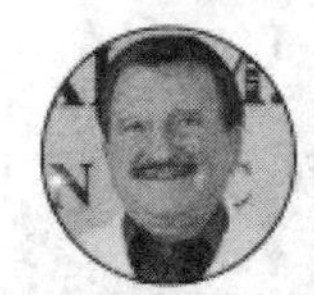

Dr. Stanislaw Burzynski, M.D., Ph.D
Scientist and Biochemist, Founde - Burzynski Clinic (Texas, USA)

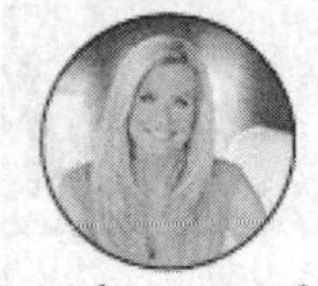

Dr. Leigh Erin Connealy, M.D.
Medical Director - Center for New Medicine (California, USA)

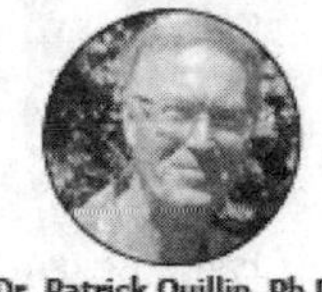

Dr. Patrick Quillin, Ph.D, R.D., C.N.S.
Author, Lecturer & Former VP of Nutrition - Cancer Treatment Centers of America

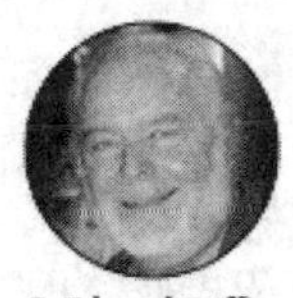

G. Edward Griffin
Author, Lecturer, and Filmmaker

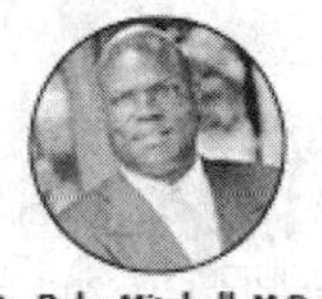

Dr. Roby Mitchell, M.D.
aka "Dr. Fitt" - Orthomolecular Medicine Physician

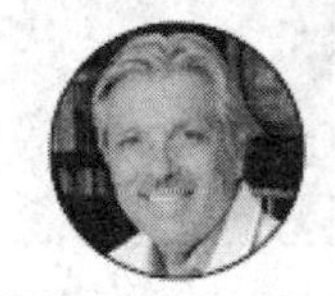

Dr. Francisco Contreras, M.D.
Oncologist and Surgeon

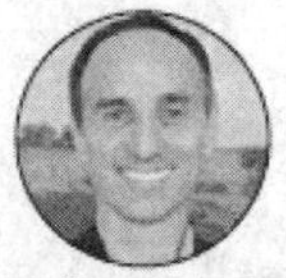

Jeffrey M. Smith
GMO Expert, Filmmaker, Researcher & Lecturer

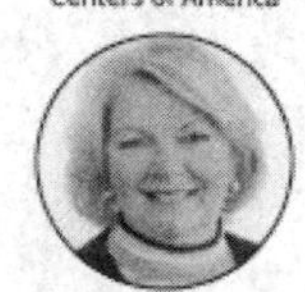

Dr. Sherri Tenpenny, D.O.
Author, Lecturer, Consultant & Vaccine Expert

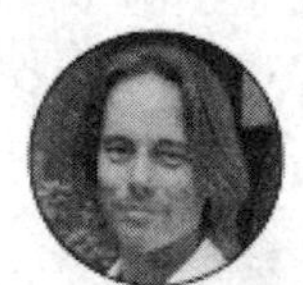

Dr. Edward F. Group III, D.C., N.D.
CEO - Global Healing Center, Speaker, Author & Educator

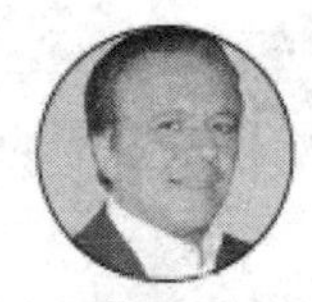

Dr. Tullio Simoncini, M.D., Ph.D
Oncologist, Pioneer in Sodium Bicarbonate Therapy

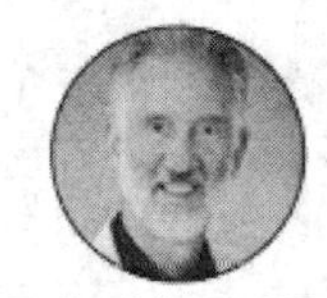

Dr. Ben Johnson, M.D., N.M.D., D.O.
Author, Lecturer, and Researche

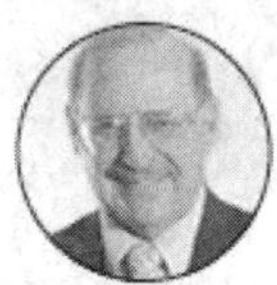

Dr. Joel Wallach, D.V.M., N.D.
Founder of Youngevity, Biomedical Researcher, Best-selling Author

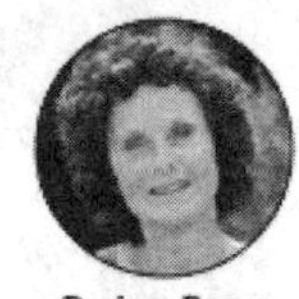

Desiree Rover
Medical Research Journalist, Author & Radio Host

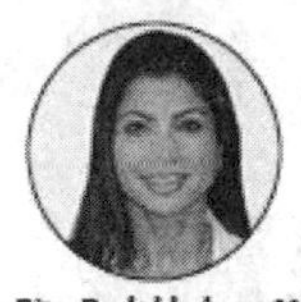

Dr. Bita Badakhshan, M.D.
Integrative Medicine Physician - Center for New Medicine (California, USA)

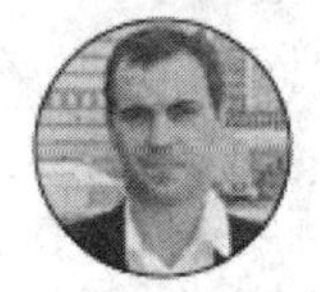

Dr. Boris Grinblat, M.D.
Naturopath & Medical Researcher

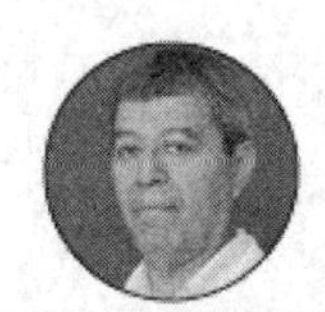

Dr. Elias Gutierrez, M.D.
Medical Director - Biomedical Center (Tijuana)

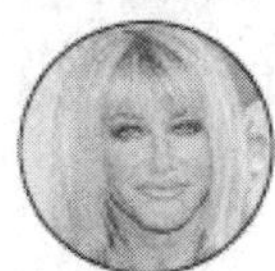

Suzanne Somers
Cancer Survivor, Author, and Actress

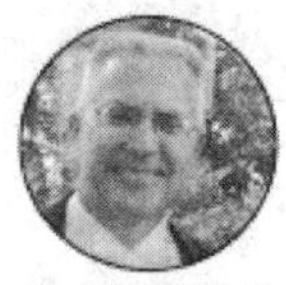

Jonathan Emord
Constitutional Attorney "The FDA Dragonslayer"

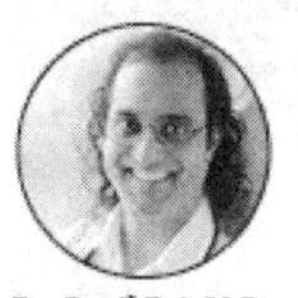

Dr. Sunil Pai, M.D.
Integrative Medicine Physician, Lecturer and Researcher

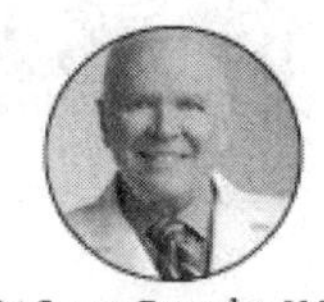

Dr. James Forsythe, M.D.
Oncologist and Homeopath

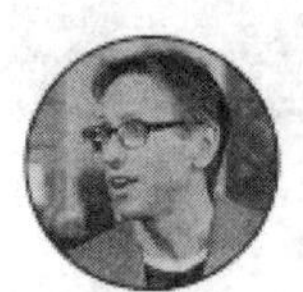

Dr. Robert Scott Bell
Author, Lecturer, and Syndicated Host of the "Robert Scott Bell Show"

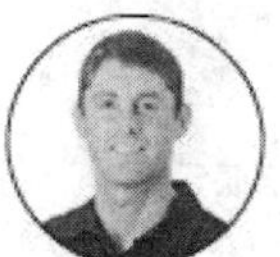
Dr. David Jockers
Author and Lecturer
Exodus Health Center

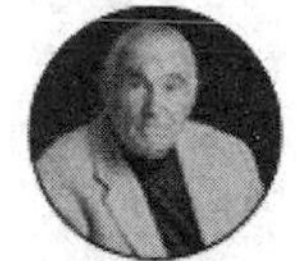
Burton Goldberg
aka "The Voice of Alternative Medicine"
Author and Lecturer

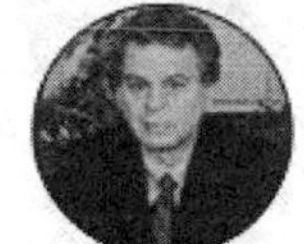
Dr. Nicholas Gonzalez, M.D.
Lecturer and Author

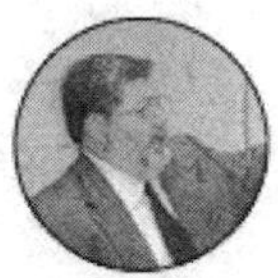
AJ Lanigan
Author, Lecturer, and Immunologist

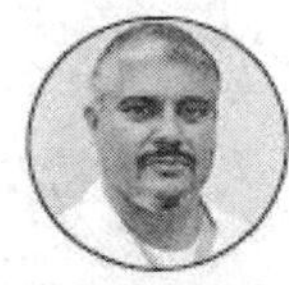
Dr. Rashid Buttar
Best-selling Author

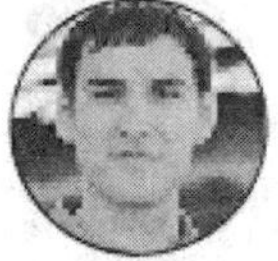
Chris Wark
Cancer Survivor, Author, and Lecturer

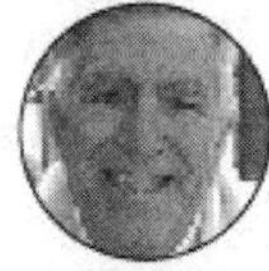
Bill Henderson
Cancer Coach, Lecturer, and Author

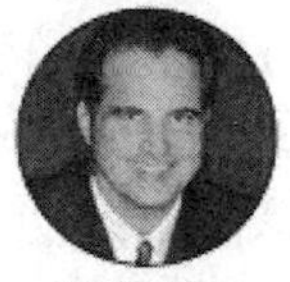
KC Craichy
Author and Nutritional Expert

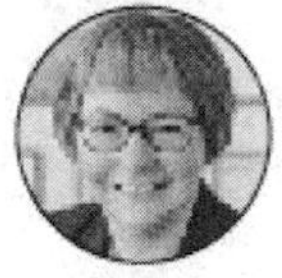
Dr. Linda Isaacs, M.D
Lecturer and Author

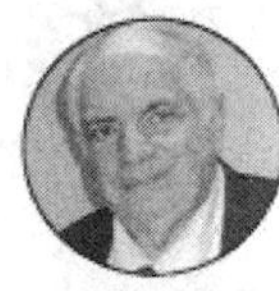
R. Webster Kehr
aka "The Cancer Tutor"

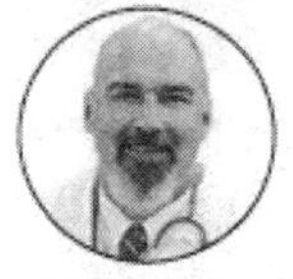
Dr. Keith Scott Mumby, M.D., PhD
Author and Lecturer

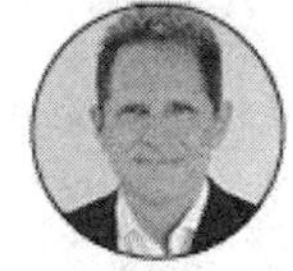
Dr. Darrell Wolfe, Ac. PhD
Author and Lecturer

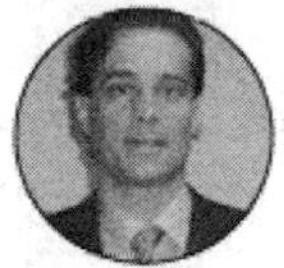
Jason Vale
Cancer Survivor

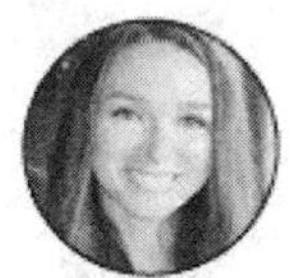
Charlene Bollinger
Researcher & Health Freedom Advocate, Co-Founder of www.CancerTruth.net

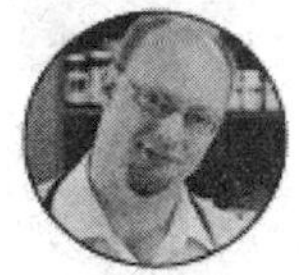
Dr. Daniel Nuzum, D.O., N.M.D.
Toxicologist, Professor, Scientist and Researcher

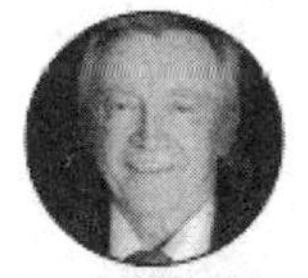
Dr. Murray "Buzz" Susser, M.D.
Integrative Physician and Lecturer

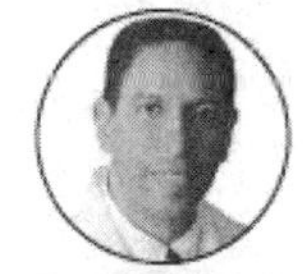
Dr. Tony Jimenez, M.D.
Scientist, Lecturer and Researcher

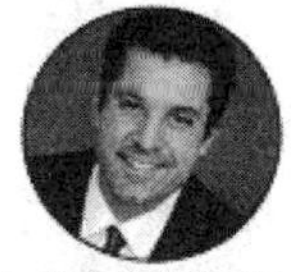
Dr. Irvin Sahni, M.D.
Lecturer and Scientist

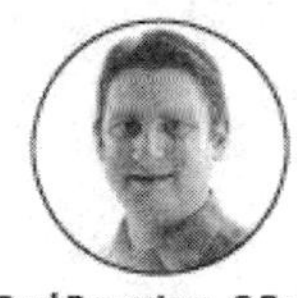
Paul Barattiero, C.Ped
Hydration Specialist

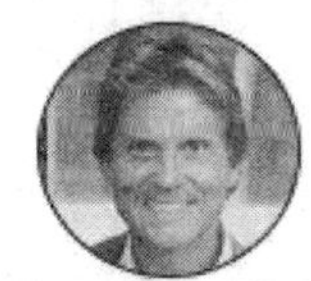
Dr. Robert Verkerk, Ph.D
Executive Director of Alliance for Natural Health-International

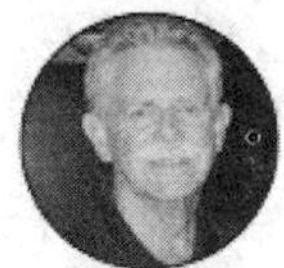
Bob Wright
Author and Researcher, Founder of the AACI (American Anti-Cancer Institute)

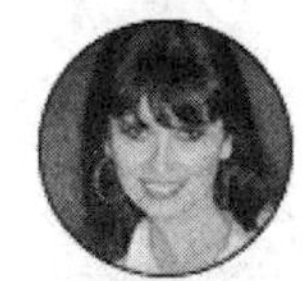
Dr. Galina Migalko, M.D., N.M.D
World-renowned Expert in Cancer Diagnosis; Integrative Physician

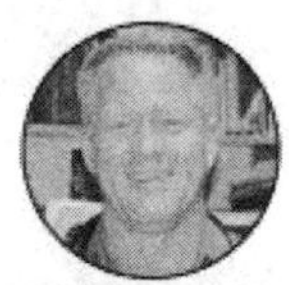
Dr. Bradford S. Weeks, M.D.
Lecturer, Scientist and Researcher

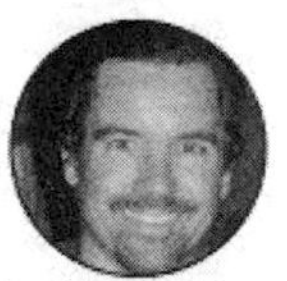
Dr. Patrick Vickers
Founder - Northern Baja Gerson Center

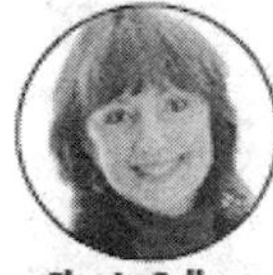
Cherie Calbom
"The Juice Lady"

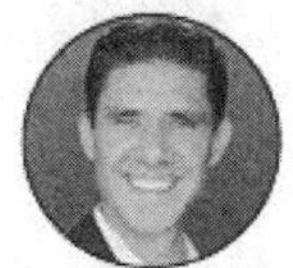
Dr. Eric Zielinksi, D.C.
Health Coach, Researcher, & Speaker

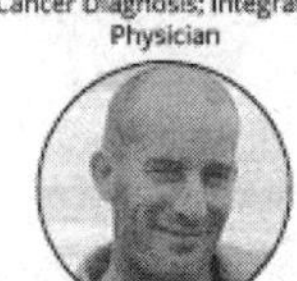
Dr. Gaston Cornu-Labat, M.D.
Author, Holistic Physician & Surgeon

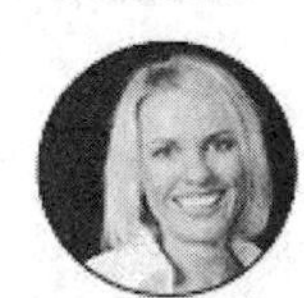
Dr. Gosia Kuszewski, N.D.
Functional Medicine Naturopath & Medical Herbalist

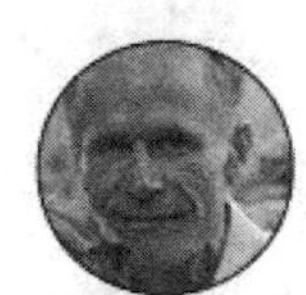
Dr. Henk Fransen, Ph.D
Natural Healer, Speaker & Author

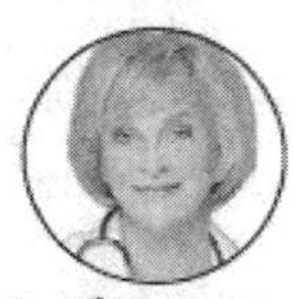
Dr. Hila Cass, M.D.
Integrative Medicine Physician, Author & Lecturer

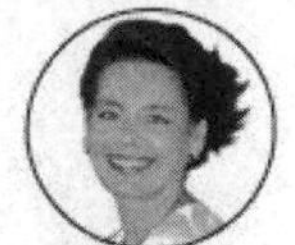

Dr. Irina Kossovskaia, M.D., Ph.D, N.M.D.
Physician, Scientist, Professor, Author & SCENAR expert

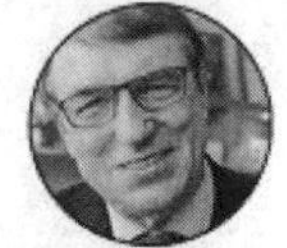

Dr. Ivars Kalvins, Ph.D
Scientist & Inventor, Director - Latvian Institute of Organic Synthesis

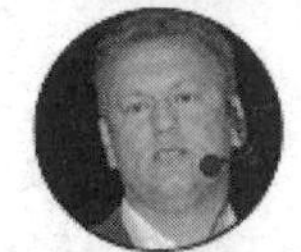

Dr. John Consemulder
Neuropsychologist, Author & Healer

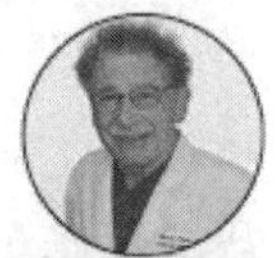

Dr. Jolly-Gabriel, Ph.D
Specialist in Hyperbaric Oxygen Therapy

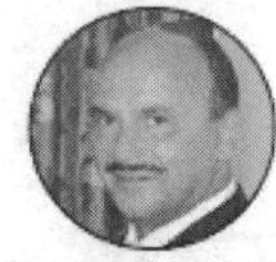

Dr. Leonard Coldwell, N.M.D., Ph.D
Syndicated Radio Host and Best-selling Author

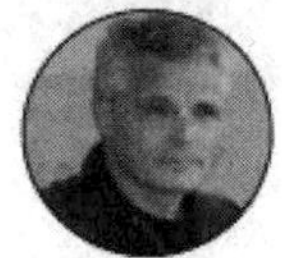

Dr. Marcel Wolfe, W.L.Ed.
Wholistic Lifestyle Educator, EMF & Frequency Expert

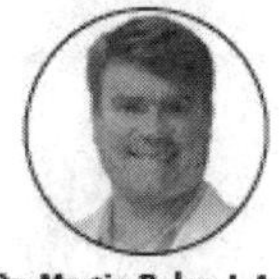

Dr. Martin Bales, L.Ac., D.A.O.M.
Certified Thermologist, Licensed Acupuncturist

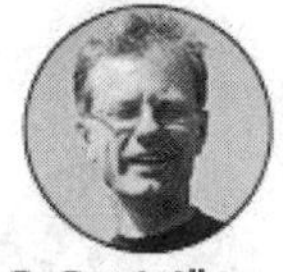

Dr. Peteris Alberts, M.D., Ph.D
Head of Research & Development - International Virotherapy Centre

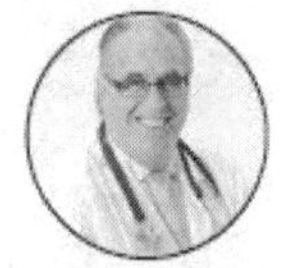

Dr. Steven Klayman, D.C.
Holistic Chiropractor

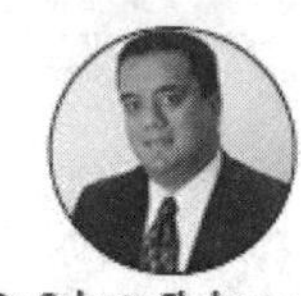

Dr. Subrata Chakravarty, Ph.D.
Chief Scientific Officer at Hope 4 Cancer Institute (Tijuana)

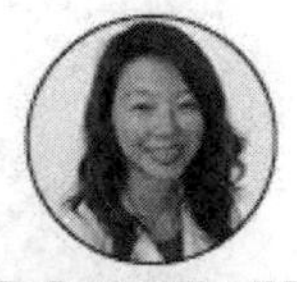

Dr. Suzanne Kim, M.D.
Integrative Medicine Physician - Center for New Medicine (California, USA)

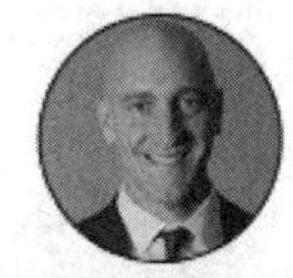

Dr. Terry Harmon, D.C.
Chiropractor, Member of the U.S. Wellness Advisory Council

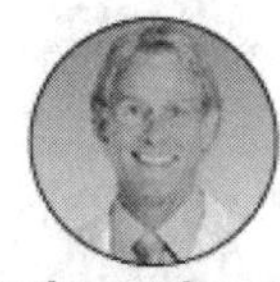

Dr. Thomas Lokensgard, D.D.S., N.M.D.
Holistic/Biological Dentist & Naturopath

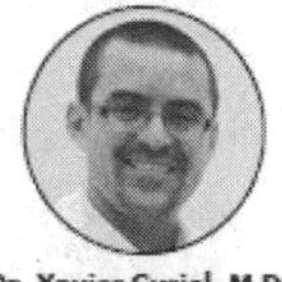

Dr. Xavier Curiel, M.D.
Integrative Medical Director at Hope 4 Cancer Institute (Tijuana)

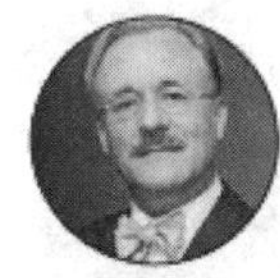

Dr. Robert Gorter, M.D., Ph.D
Director - Medical Center Cologne (Germany)

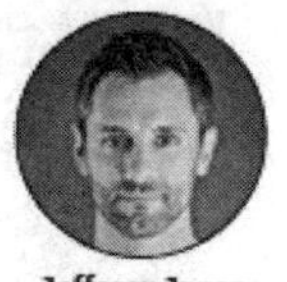

Jefferey Jaxen
Author, Researcher & Investigative Journalist

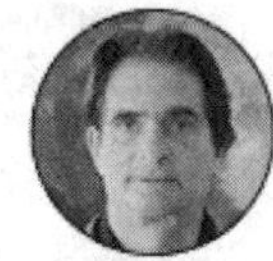

Jon Rappoport
Investigative Journalist (30+ years), Nominated for Pulitzer Prize

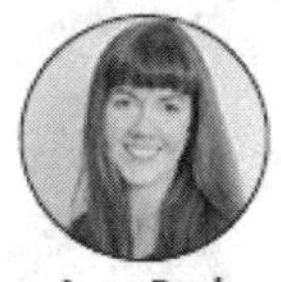

Laura Bond
Investigative Health Journalist & Author

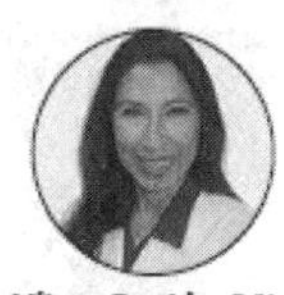

Liliana Partida, C.N.
Certified Nutritionist

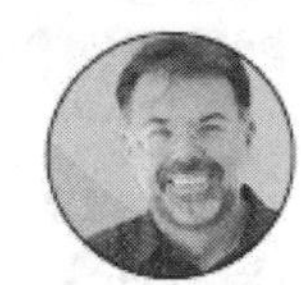

Marcus Freudenmann
Author, Documentary Film Director/Producer & International Lecture

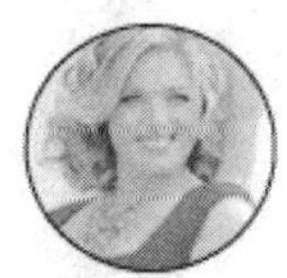

Tara Mann
Founder - Cancer Crackdown, Former Big Pharma Sales Rep

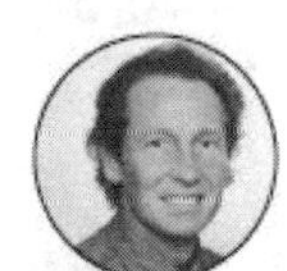

Dr. Igor Smirnov, Ph.D
Inventor, Scientist, Radiation Expert, Author & Speaker

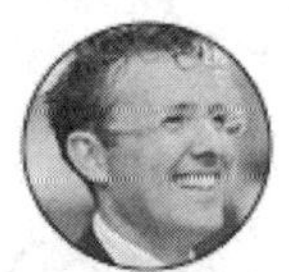

Ard Pisa
Author, Researcher & Speaker

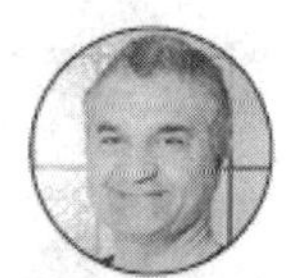

Dr. Raymond Hilu, M.D.
Founder and Medical Director - The Hilu Institute (Spain)

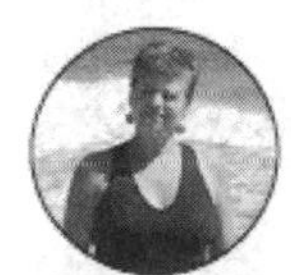

Valerie Warwick, R.N.
Cancer Conqueror, Oncology Nurse Specialist

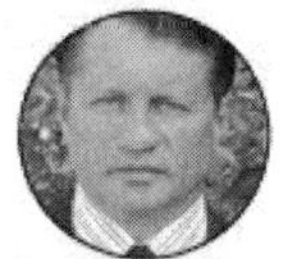

Dr. Howard Fisher, D.C.
Anti-aging Expert, Lecturer & Best-selling Author

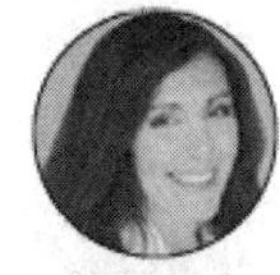

Dr. Manuela Malaguti-Boyle, Ph.D, N.D.

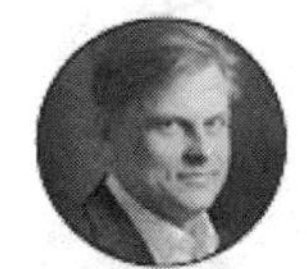

Dr. Kaspars Losans, M.D.
Oncologist, Medical Director - International Virotherapy Centre

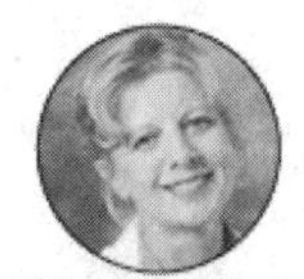

Dr. Aleksandra Niedzwiecki, Ph.D
Director of Research - Dr. Rath Research Institute (Netherlands)

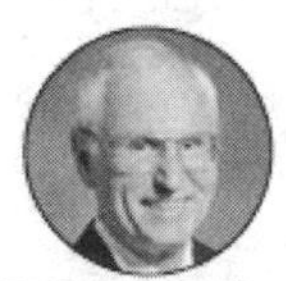

Dr. Garry F. Gordon, M.D., D.O.

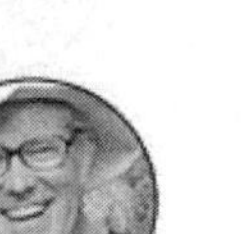

Joel Salatin
International Speaker, Farmer & Best-selling Author

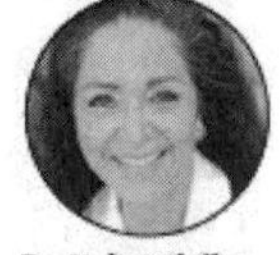

Dr. Nalini Chilkov, L.Ac., O.M.D.
Author, Clinician & Cellular Bilogist

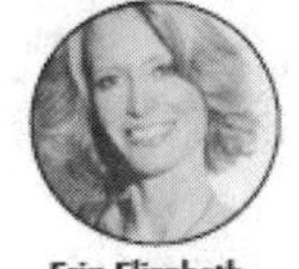

Erin Elizabeth
Author, Researcher & Public Speaker

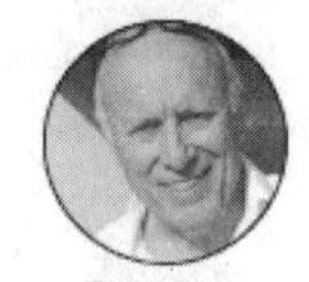

Peter Starr
Documentary Film Maker & Cancer Survivor

For more information about the experts who were interviewed in
THE TRUTH ABOUT CANCER: A GLOBAL QUEST
please visit the following website:
http://go2.thetruthaboutcancer.com/global-quest/experts-info-sheet/

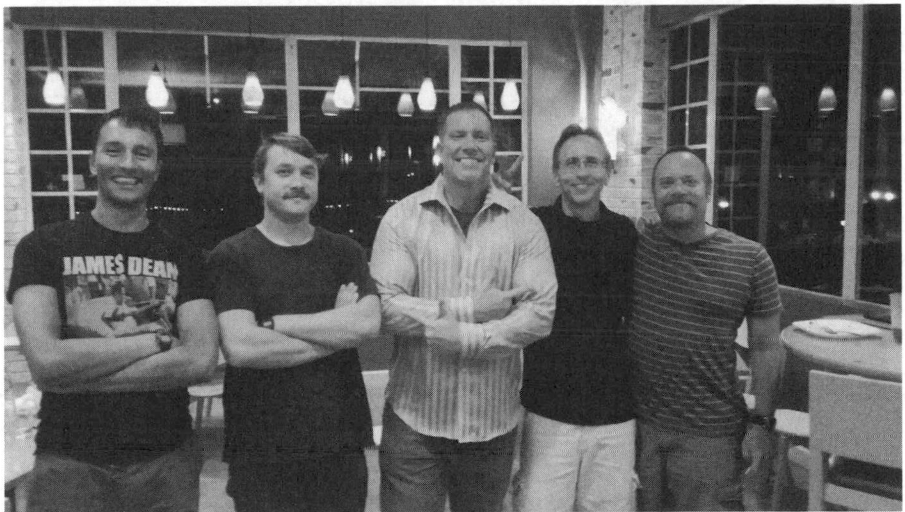

(ABOVE) With Edward Szall, Travis Jones, Robert Scott Bell, and Alan Ray in Naples, Florida

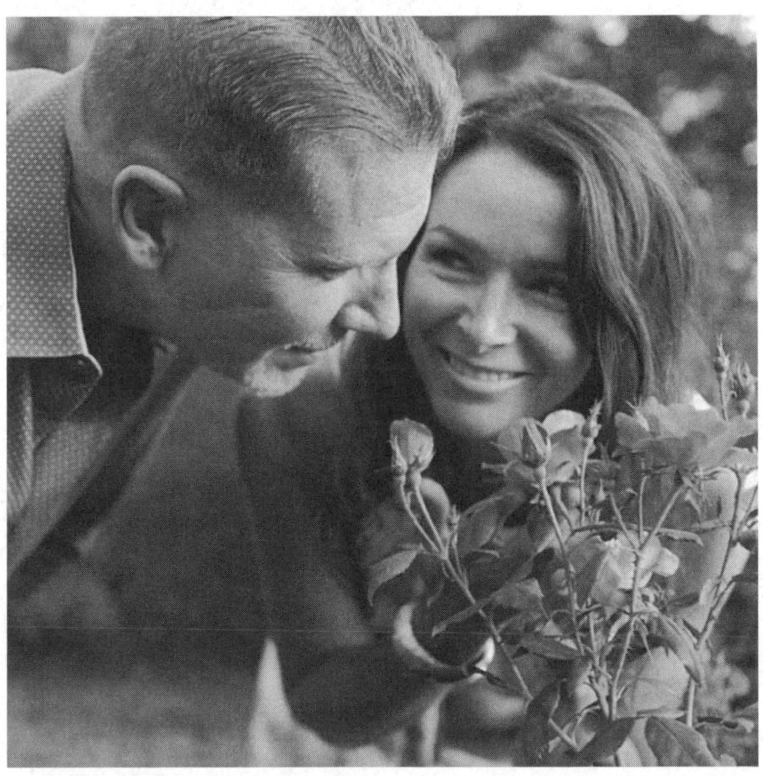

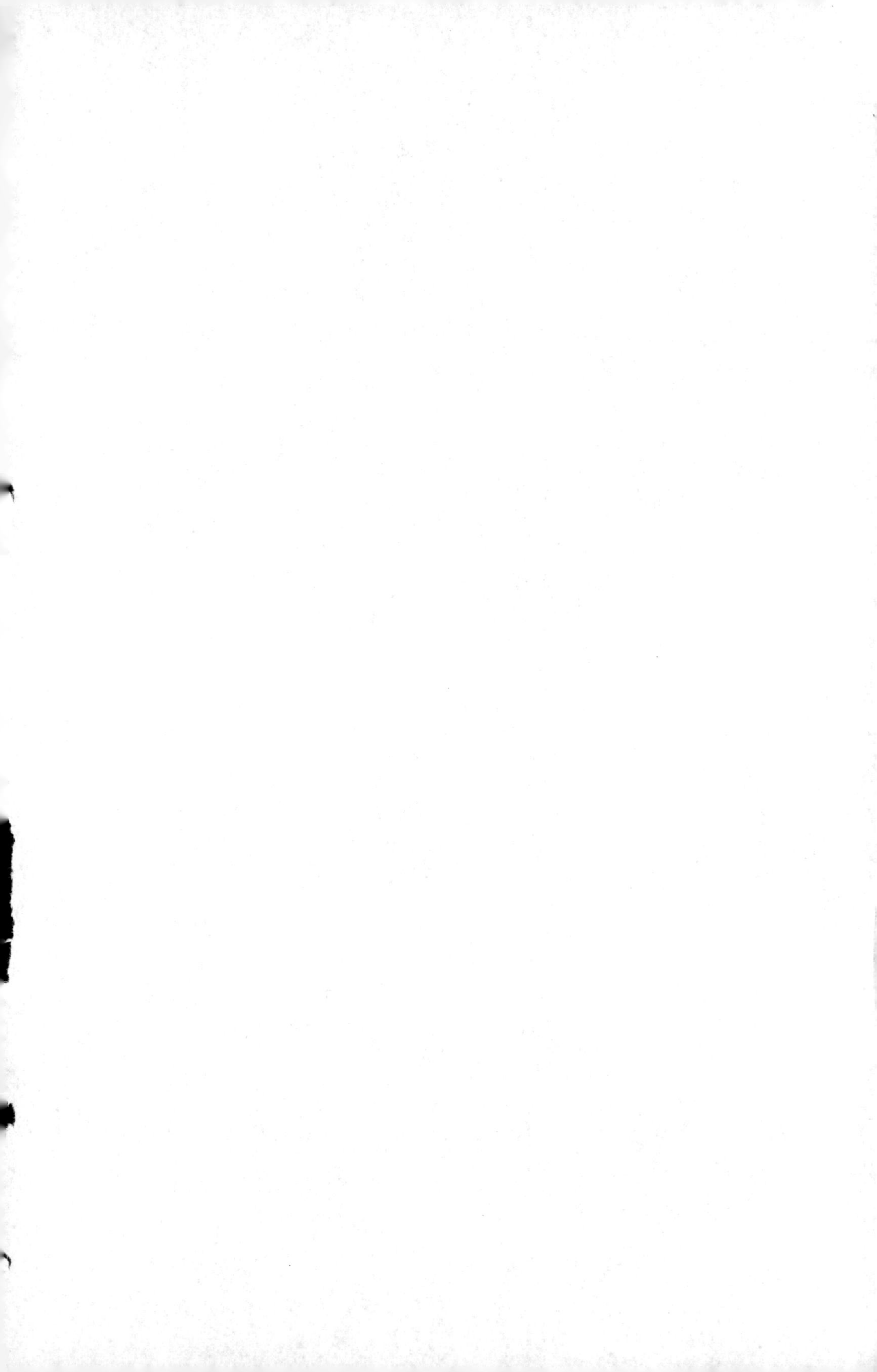